U0942218

Encyclopedia of Neuroscience

神经科学百科全书⑩

Intelligent Activities of the Brain

脑的智能活动

Editor-in-Chief

Larry R. Squire

Departments of Psychiatry, Neurosciences, and Psychology
University of California
San Diego and VA Medical Center
San Diego, CA
USA

科学出版社

北京

图字：01-2010-2764 号
Encyclopedia of Neuroscience
Larry R. Squire
ISBN: 978-0-08-044617-2

Authorized English language edition published by the Proprietor.
ISBN: 978-9-81-272714-5

Elsevier (Singapore) Pte Ltd.
3 Killiney Road
#08-01 Winsland House I
Singapore 239519
Tel: (65) 6349-0200
Fax: (65) 6733-1817

First Published 2010
2010 年初版

图书在版编目（CIP）数据

脑的智能活动 = Intelligent Activities of the Brain：英文 / (美)斯奎尔（Squire,L.R.）主编. — 北京：科学出版社，2010 （神经科学百科全书；10）

ISBN 978-7-03-028080-0

Ⅰ. ①脑… Ⅱ. ①斯… Ⅲ. ①脑神经－英文 Ⅳ.①R322.85

中国版本图书馆 CIP 数据核字（2010）第 117922 号

责任编辑：田慎鹏　贾明月/责任印制：钱玉芬/封面设计：耕者设计工作室

科学出版社 出版
北京东黄城根北街 16 号
邮政编码：100717
http://www.sciencep.com

北京佳信达欣艺术印刷有限公司 印刷
科学出版社发行　各地新华书店经销
*
2010年8月第　一　版　　开本：787×1092　1/16
2010年8月第一次印刷　　印张：42 3/4
印数：1—1 500　　字数：1 013 000

定价：158.00 元
（如有印装质量问题，我社负责调换）

导 读 一

自然界中没有什么比大脑更神奇、更令人迷惑不解的了。神经科学则是研究大脑工作原理和脑疾病机理的学科，也是一个新兴的交叉学科，涵盖神经生物学、神经生理学、心理学、认知科学、计算神经科学、神经解剖学、神经药理学、神经化学，以及神经内科、神经外科和精神科等临床学科。神经科学作为独立的学科 20 世纪 70 年代起始于美国，随后得到迅速发展，成为新世纪最具有挑战性和发展机遇的前沿科学，并促进了人工智能、脑-机接口、信息处理等相关学科的发展。

神经科学的重要性，不仅在于它是重要的基础学科，还在于它是与人类身心健康最密切相关的重要应用学科。随着人类健康的改善和寿命的延长，老龄化已成为众多国家发展面临的问题。我国 60 岁以上老人已达 1.3 亿，并正以每年 600 万的速度递增。老年痴呆、帕金森病等各种神经退行性疾病日益增加。我国老年人群中各种病因引起的痴呆病人已近 1000 万，并正逐年增加。脑中风已成为我国首位的死亡原因，也是单病种致死、致残率最高的疾病，是家庭和社会的巨大负担。社会和经济的高速发展、竞争和压力的增加，使精神和心理疾病日益增多，并成为威胁人民身心健康的严重问题。根据世界卫生组织统计，到 2020 年，精神和神经疾患带来的负担将占所有疾病经济总负担的 15%左右。吸毒成瘾成为影响社会安定和发展的严重问题，由静脉注射毒品引发的艾滋病也急剧增多。网络成瘾也成为危害青少年身心健康的严重问题。此外，各种感觉障碍（失明、聋哑）、智力发育障碍、癫痫、慢性痛、脊髓外伤等都是严重影响人类健康的神经疾病。由于神经系统的复杂性，目前我们对这些严重神经精神疾病的发病机理还缺乏深入的了解，并因此而缺乏有效的治疗手段。这些都是神经科学家面临的巨大挑战。

由于神经科学的前沿挑战性和重要社会意义，各个国家都对其给予了特别的重视。美国和欧洲在 20 世纪 90 年代推出“脑的十年”， 日本则提出“脑科学时代”，都对神经科学都给予了倾斜性的大力支持。神经科学的研究队伍也得到快速发展，美国神经科学年会的参会人数从 1971 年开始的几百人，到现在每年有 3 万多人参加。我国神经科学的研究队伍目前还比较小，今后应该会有很大的发展潜力和前景。

鉴于神经科学的复杂性、综合交叉性及其快速的发展，单一的神经科学专著已经难以在深度和广度上涵盖神经科学的全貌，也不能满足神经科学与相关交叉学科的相互了解和交融。出于这一需求，美国加州大学圣迭戈分校著名神经科学家 Larry R. Squire 教授协同其他四位神经科学家，组织编写了这套由 46 个各研究领域的学者作为副主编、2400 多名专家参与写作的《神经科学百科全书》。该书于 2008 年 10 月出版，并有电子版由 ScienceDirect 网上在线发行。全书包括约 1500 篇专论，每篇专论都是一篇针对某一主题的独立成章的综述，并附有重要参考文献。原书按照文章标题的 ABC 顺序分为 10 卷，共 1 万多页，是目前为止内容最全面、篇幅最大、最有影响力的神经科学百科全书。为便于读者查阅，原书中除了给出这些文章相关的主题检索（subject index）外，还将神经科学分为若干领域（subject classification），并在每个领域中列出了书中可能相关的文章目录。

本书在中国的出版实际上是进行了重新组织，全书的分卷不是按照原来文章标题的 ABC 顺序，而是按领域分类组织了 14 卷出版，每卷包括一到数个领域。领域分类以及该领域包含的文章内容基本上按照原书 subject classification 的范围，删节了一些可能被认为比较冷僻的内容。

出版社对该书的组织进行这样调整的好处是显而易见的。①原书内容太广，篇幅太多，按照 ABC 顺序排列的分册只能作为查询的工具，不宜做系统学习的材料。经重新组织按领域分卷出版，每一卷都可以作为相对独立的专著，使读者比较容易找到感兴趣的内容，有利于系统的学习。②缩减了篇幅，降低了出版和购买成本。③读者如果购买全套书籍，既可将其作为百科全书查询之用，还拥有了神经科学几乎每个领域的全套权威性专著；同时，读者也可以根据自己的兴趣和需要，选购其中的分册而不必购买全套书籍。

当然，这些按照领域分卷出版的专著和一般性专著还是不同的。一般的专著是对该领域进行全面的、系统的、分章节的渐进式论述，而本书各分卷的每篇文章则是对领域内的某一重要问题进行独立的论述。从这个意义上讲，本书的结构更像我们小时候读过的《十万个为什么》，每一分卷都是对某一学科存在的若干重要问题分别进行独立的深入浅出的阐述。应该指出的是，由于这是一套由众多学者参与写作的丛书，每篇文章的风格、对领域内问题把握的深度和准确性等可能存在不可避免的差异。

不可否认，本书的结构经过这样的调整后也存在一些缺点。例如，一篇文章可以和若干个主题相关，当决定每个领域中应该包括哪些文章，或者一些文章应该归属到哪些领域时难免会存在界定的困难，有些文章也会重复出现在不同的领域。不同背景的读者可能会有不同的判断，觉得有些关联不大的内容被放到了一起，而有些密切相关的内容却没有包括在同一分卷内。这些主题分类的困难和问题虽然在原书中就已经存在，但由于其在原书中只是作为检索参考用，不会引起明显的问题，而按照现在这样的领域分类分成专集出版时就难免存在不足。当然这些都是所谓鱼和熊掌不能兼得的问题，我们相信这套经过重新组织的《神经科学百科全书》仍不失为目前为止在中国出版的最具特色、篇幅最大、内容最广泛，也可能是最具影响的神经科学英文论著。

这套丛书可以作为在神经科学各领域及其交叉领域学习和工作的参考书。不同背景的读者还可能会在这套书中找到不同的用处。对于初入门者或交叉领域工作者，这套丛书可以作为你掌握神经科学重要基础知识、快速了解领域前沿问题的工具。对于在神经科学领域的年轻科研工作者，该书可能会帮助你找到领域内尚未解决的重要问题，并可能在科研思路上甚至具体方法上有所帮助。如果你已经在该领域有所建树，这套书还有一个作用：当你发现自己发表的工作被写进了这套百科全书时，一定会很高兴。但如果你觉得自己的工作很重要，却没有在这套书的相关文章里得到应有的反映，也不必耿耿于怀。一方面，每篇文章引用的参考文献很少，且多是引用综述性文献；另一方面，作者也可能对这个领域的把握不够准确。实际上我自己就有这样的体验，看到自己的一些工作在书中被讨论和引用时感到高兴，而看到书中有些文章在讨论相关问题时没有引用自己较早的原始发现，却引用了其他实验室后来的重复性工作时，不禁感到愤愤不平，甚至抱怨作者的无知。

虽然一般认为百科全书应该是权威性的著作，但对于科研工作者来说，权威往往会成为障碍。如果你对书里一些文章的观点有不同看法，找出他们不足的地方，或者发现你自己的实验结果和书中“权威”观点不一致，那么这也许是你拥有这套书的最大收获，因为它可以作为你工作的起点和创新的依据。科学就是要不断发展，神经科学也是进展最快的学科之一。若干年后你再读这套书，可能会发现不少内容已经过时，因而会感叹知识更新的快速或者取笑作者的短见，并可了解该领域发展的历史和变迁；另一方面，如果若干年后你发现书里很多内容仍然是权威性的，很多问题仍然没有得到解决，你可能会感叹科学发展的艰难；你也可能发现作者的一些预见已经被证实，不由得对该作者又增加了一分敬意。这些都是拥有这套百科全书所能得到的另外的乐趣吧。

最后要说明的是，这套书在中国的出版及其内容编排的调整等过程我都没有参与。出版社找我写个导读，由于杂事缠身，很长时间没能把这套书好好浏览一下。最后出版社告诉我，所有工作都已经完成，只等我写的导读出来后就可以出版时，才意识到竟然由于自己的拖拉而可能推迟了书的出版，在此深表歉意。

段树民

浙江大学医学院

2010 年 7 月

导 读 二

广大读者翘首以盼的第4版《神经科学百科全书》终于出版了。

该书是一套主要面向神经科学领域的学生和专业研究人员的大型理想参考书，由斯奎尔（Larry R. Squire）教授领衔主编，46位权威专家担任副主编。经过二十余年（该书第1版首发于1989年）的磨砺，该书已被打造成一本皇皇巨著，其主旨——成为神经科学所有领域信息的权威来源，已经逐渐为业内有识之士所认可。

原书共有13个大的主题，每个主题下有若干子主题。但由于全书篇幅太大，科学出版社此次从中选择了4个主题组成了14卷，每卷含某一主题中的一个或几个子主题。这4个主题分别是细胞间通信（Intercellular Communication；拆为4卷，即第①~④卷）、方法与技术（Methods and Techniques；拆为2卷，即第⑤~⑥卷）、神经系统的分子与细胞生物学（Molecular and Cell Biology of Nervous Systems；拆为3卷，即第⑦~⑨卷），和行为的神经基础（Neural Basis of Behavior；拆为5卷，即第⑩～⑭卷）。

为便于读者浏览、阅读和利用此套书，现将其特点和阅读注意点简介如下。

（一）主要特点

一是编辑阵容强大。原书由美国加利福尼亚大学圣迭戈和VA医学中心精神病学、神经科学和心理学系Larry R. Squire教授主编，索尔克（Salk Institute）生物科学研究所系统神经生物学系Thomas D. Albright教授、遗传学实验室Fred H. Gage教授，及美国斯克利普斯研究所分子和整合神经科学系Floyd E. Bloom等4位教授任资深编辑，所涉及的参与者数以千计。这些人都是本专业的专家和精英。

二是覆盖领域广泛。原书选取了近1500个条目，涵盖了神经科学的46个主要领域，分成10卷。可以说，凡是读者感兴趣的研究主题，基本上都能在该书中找到，或者通过线索得到相应的启发。

三是研究工作优异。书中所收入的每一篇文章，都是当今世界神经科学中优秀文章的代表。它反映了该领域中最重要的研究成果、最有力的研究工具、最光明的应用前景。它脉络清晰，取材丰富，分析透彻，解说详明；它插图精良，颇有创意，图文并茂，相得益彰。

四是读者层面兼容。该书所收录的内容注意基础性、应用性和前卫性，这就为不同层面的读者提供了普及和提高的广大空间和伸缩性。因此，本书既可用于教学，又可用于科研，是一套必备参考书。

五是参考文献丰富。每篇文章末尾都列有详尽的参考文献。各相关文章有众多的交叉参考文献，进一步阅读部分有成书前的最新信息。整个书系构成了纵横交织的文献网，可谓“文网恢恢”。

六是浏览检索便捷。原书编有两大索引，即主题索引和主题分类索引。各索引都列出了尽可能详细的下位条目，检索起来十分方便、省时。同时，该书全部内容在科学指引数据库在线发布，可在www.sciencedirect.com网站订阅。

（二）如何阅读

首先是高瞻远瞩，了解全貌。读者可充分利用主题索引，先粗略浏览原书所覆盖的主题，以便对其主要框架有一个大概的了解。再在自己感兴趣的主题下面，寻求对口的条目，这样从大到小的浏览方式，是一种从宏观到微观的、对了解全貌有极大帮助的阅读方式。

其次是管中窥豹，略见一斑。读者如果研究方向和目的都很明确，那么可以采取直接查找主题分类索引的方式，做到单刀直入，直奔目标。这样可以就某一点形成较深入的了解。此法适用于有一定教学和科研经验的读者。

再则是深入阅读，寻求新解。若采取上述两法仍不能得到理想的阅读效果。建议采取深入阅读之法。该法主要是偏重于书中所编列的进一步阅读部分（成书前新获取的信息），这有助于读者查阅更详尽的技术资料、综述文章及研究论文。

最后是交叉阅读，融会贯通。上述方法可以综合运用。读者还可以从本书索引进一步查找到其他的著作和网站，形成纵横交错，多头、多点查找路径，以便对某一主题形成全面的、深入的、前卫的了解，并尽可能地付诸实施。

上述看法，仅为一家之言和一孔之见，不一定适合所有人。但若能对大多数读者有所帮助，那我就如释重负了。

路长林
第二军医大学

导 读 三

探索脑的奥秘是自然界最诱人的科学问题之一。神经科学是研究动物和人类神经系统与脑的结构和功能的科学，是研究行为、心理活动乃至智能，以及神经系统疾病如何产生的科学，是 20 世纪下半叶到 21 世纪初生命科学中发展最快的领域之一。

神经科学由于其研究对象的复杂性，一开始就是高度跨学科的综合学科，它得到了神经生理学家、神经解剖学家、神经化学家和神经药理学家、心理学家、医学家乃至工程科学家们的重视和参与。1969 年北美神经科学学会（Society for Neuroscience，SFN）成立时，仅有会员几百人。其现已发展到拥有 4 万多名会员，出席年会的人数达 35 000 人以上，SFN 已成为世界生物医学学会中规模最大的学会。

伴随着分子生物学和计算机科学技术的飞速发展，神经科学 40 年来获得了突飞猛进的发展。从基因、分子神经科学到系统和行为神经科学，新概念、新技术、新规律的提出、应用与发现与日俱增，不断地增添和修正着人们对自身脑功能的认识。与此同时，爆发式地涌现出的新知识，使得同一个神经科学家不可能完全掌握所有神经科学的知识和方法。例如，化学导向的细胞和分子神经生物学家，往往不甚熟悉物理、数学导向的系统和计算神经科学方面的名词、概念和方法，反之亦然。然而，神经科学的蓬勃发展，又要求神经科学家不断更新自己的知识，尽可能地了解全局。这不仅是为了使自己跟上时代的发展，寻找新的突破点，更是为了将最新的知识和方法传播给学生。《神经科学百科全书》就是在这个背景下应运而生的。第一版《神经科学百科全书》（两卷本）于 1987 年出版，包括约 700 个词条；第二版《神经科学百科全书》（两卷本）于 1999 年出版，包括约 800 个词条；第三版《神经科学百科全书》是电子版的，于 2004 年出版。

现在由 Larry R. Squire 主编的第四版《神经科学百科全书》包括了 1500 个词条，由 Science Direct 在 2008 年在线出版，后又发行纸质版。Squire 和美国加利福尼亚州圣迭戈的四位资深神经科学家组成了主编小组，预先确定了 46 个神经科学的主要领域，共 13 个主题，然后邀请了 46 位在这些领域科研第一线的科学家组成副主编队伍，由他们进一步发动更大范围内的神经科学专家参加写作，集体合作完成了全部内容。书中的每一个词条都由科学家精心写作而成，类似一篇短小的综述和评论文章，读者可从阅读中获其精华。显然，它是 21 世纪初最权威、最详尽的关于神经科学知识的综合性信息来源。

《神经科学百科全书》内容浩瀚，篇幅巨大，显然不是一般个人所需和所能购置的。科学出版社在第四版《神经科学百科全书》的 13 个主题中，选择了 4 个最为通用的主题，做成了 14 个分卷，每卷含某一主题中的一个或几个研究领域，以便于我国广大神经科学工作者学习和使用。这 4 个主题分别是细胞间通信（分为 4 卷）、方法与技术（分为 2 卷）、神经系统的分子与细胞生物学（分为 3 卷），以及行为的神经基础（分为 5 卷）。这 14 个分卷的出版是一件有利于我国神经科学发展的大好事。它将为活跃在神经科学及与其有关领域的从事教学和科研的科学工作者、工程技术人员们提供一个相对完整的、有相当深度的知识库，使他们能方便地找到自己不熟悉的内容，扩大他们的视野；它也为学习和从事神经科学有关研究的研究生、本科生们提供一个自学和自选研究课题的有力工具。可以相信，科学出版社《神经科学百科全书》的问世，必将为我国神经科学及相关学科的发展提供一个有力的武器，并做出历史性的贡献。

寿天德

复旦大学生命科学学院

前　言

什么是百科全书？这一名词来自于两个希腊单词：*enkuklios*（意思是循环的）和 *paideia*（意思是教育）。在 16 世纪早期，拉丁手稿的抄写者们将这两个单词合而为一，其在英语中演化为一个单词，意思是具有广泛指导意义的工具书（*The American Heritage Dictionary*，2000，Boston：Houghton Mifflin, p.589）。从其来源可见，其希腊文原词中蕴含着以探索、综合的方式努力获取知识的含义。无论是拉丁文还是英文，该单词泛指涵盖广泛领域知识的工具书。

希腊文中强调的以创造性手段获取知识，在神经科学领域尤其适用。神经科学本身就是一个非常新的名词。Francis Schmitt 在本书第一版的前言中指出，本书的编写过程就是将不同领域的科学家们聚集在一起，冲击大脑研究中最顽固的难题。他推动建立了神经科学研究项目（Neuroscience Research Program，简称 NRP）。早期的 NRP 成员包括一些学术巨匠，如因关于光合作用的研究获得诺贝尔奖的 Melvin Calvin、诺贝尔奖获得者物理化学家 Manfred Eigen、生物化学家 Albert Lehninger，和当时正在努力破解基因编码的年轻分子生物学家 Marshall Nirenberg。

Schmitt 建立 NRP 的时候，神经科学作为一门综合学科还几乎不存在。微电极的发明使神经生理学家们得以记录单细胞的电活动，但是几乎不可能甄别其生物化学特性。一个重要的推进来自 20 世纪 60 年代中期涌现的 Falck-Hillarp 荧光显微镜技术，它能够选择性地观察儿茶酚胺和 5-羟色胺能神经元。这些胺类通路的研究又很快使得检测选择性损伤后效应的行为学家们和生化学家们开始合作研究，使得后者的工作不再局限于在整个脑组织匀浆的水平研究神经递质。20 世纪 70 年代关于神经递质受体的生化研究、它们位点的放射自显影研究，以及神经多肽的免疫组织化学研究，更是进一步促进了神经生理学家、神经解剖学家、神经化学家和神经药理学家们的对话。而过去两个世纪以来，分子生物学技术手段的应用更加丰富了这一交流。

神经科学的爆炸性发展也体现在神经科学学会（Society for Neuroscience, SFN）的历史上。SFN 于 1970 年（译者注：SFN 网站中所写的时间为 1969 年）由几百名研究人员在华盛顿特区创立，首任会长是 Vernon Mountcastle。而当我于 1980 年担任会长时，会员人数已经增长到 7000 人。我当时的一个主要任务是应对关于学会存在合理性的争论。有人认为"我们学会的科学家人数太多了。应当将其一分为二，如实验类的和理论类的"。与此相反，为了强调该领域的整体特点，我们推出了《神经科学杂志》（*Journal of Neuroscience*）。同时，我们认为学会的增长可能会最终进入平台期，精心的会议组织将可以避免会员个人"在会议的人潮中迷失"。现在看来，我当时关于平台期的预言偏离了实际。截至 2007 年 5 月，神经科学学会的会员人数已经超过了 38 000 名，其中超过 35 000 人参加每年的年会，这样的规模超过了其他任何生物医学类的学会。

很多人会认可神经科学是一门整合性最强的科学学科。基于此，如果从希腊语"学习的循环"的本意出发，编写关于它的百科全书相当必要，但又是非常有挑战性的。同之前的版本一样，这一版非常注意全书的知识结构，尤其重要的是，本书选择了最合适的副主编来组织每一个课题领域。每一位副主编都是长期活跃在该领域第一线的研究者。神经科学的所有重要领域都在本书中有所体现。其中分子和系统神经科学的权重都经过了仔细的衡量。

在这一快速发展的时期，人们可能会质疑，这样一版反映当前这一时刻的百科全书是否有意义。该书所提供的信息是否会在不久的将来过时？实际上，以前的几个版本已经证明，一本好的百科全书可以将不同的领域以浅显易懂的、有利于读者理解的语言整合起来。对于专业人士而言，它可以兼具启发和激励作用。对于初入此途的研究者而言，它将是进入神经系统研究领域的理想切入口。

Solomon H. Snyder

Distinguished Service Professor,

Johns Hopkins University

俞洪波 译

序

20 世纪中叶以来，关于神经系统的研究从以往生物与心理学研究的边缘地位跃升，成为神经科学这一交叉学科。这一新学科将生物化学、细胞生物学、解剖学、生理学、心理学、神经病学、精神病学等具有不同背景的科学家与临床医生们联系起来，研究令人激动的脑的秘密。他们专注于探索神经元的功能机制，澄清行为与认知的神经基础，了解神经系统疾病。1969 年神经科学学会的创建大大促进了该学科的发展，如今该学会已经拥有近 37 000 名会员。第一个针对神经科学的学术培训项目建立于医学院（1965 年加州大学圣迭戈分校建立神经科学系，1966 年哈佛大学建立神经生物学系）。第一个本科生培训项目于 1972 年建立于 Amherst 学院和 Oberlin 学院，后者培养了诺贝尔奖获得者 Roger Sperry 和三位神经科学学会会长。时至今日，全世界已经有超过 300 个神经科学系或相应的培养项目。

《神经科学百科全书》旨在将本学科丰富多元的内容条理化并仔细介绍，从而推动不同学术分支之间的沟通，提供权威的信息来源。该书面向较为广泛的读者群体，既包括初入神经科学研究的学生，也包括寻求特定专题知识的普通读者。无论是神经科学家，还是正在学习神经科学的本科生和研究生，或生命科学领域的教师、科普作家，都会从该参考书中获益。

《神经科学百科全书》的第一版，也是该学科的第一本详尽的参考书，于 1987 年在 George Adelman 卓有成效的领导下出版；该版本分为两卷，共 700 多个条目。本书的第二版由 George Adelman 和 Barry Smith 主编，包括超过 800 个条目，于 1999 年分两卷出版，同时配发了光盘版。2004 年的第三版仅以电子版本发行。

本次出版的版本包括近 1500 个条目，全书在 Science Direct 网站上发行，读者可以注册登录 www.sciencedirect.com 阅读。主编小组在神经科学中划分出 46 个主要领域，并邀请各个领域的专家担任副主编，由他们组织该领域的内容。每位副主编再邀请 30~40 位作者准备各个专题条目，这些专题将努力涵盖该领域的所有内容。许多专题作者都是该领域享有盛誉的领导者。这使得该书成为当今神经科学学科的汇编，其中囊括了最重要的研究、最有力的研究工具、最有潜力的应用。

许多条目本身就是一篇自成一体的独立综述。同时，在结论部分又有大量的交叉引用，它们可以将读者引入其他相关的条目。此书主体上以字母顺序组织所有条目。此外，详尽的主题分类又可以帮助读者找到相关的专题，以了解本学科的结构。

虽然没有一本神经科学的参考书能够囊括大脑研究每一个值得注意的想法和成果，主编们仍希望本书能够成为一本既翔实又具指导意义的、反映当代神经科学研究的汇编。神经科学还在不断发展向前，如果本书能够在征服神经系统疾病，和了解脑、思维及我们自身的征程中发挥作用，它就获得了成功。

本书的主编小组特此感谢 Elsevier 的编辑 Michael Bevan、Joanna De Souza 和 Richard Berryman，以及主编助理 Caroline Phipps、Afandi Mohamed 和 Nicky Carter，感谢他们将这一庞

大纷杂的工程组织得井井有条。感谢项目经理 Andrew Lowe 和 Laura Jackson，他们勤奋的工作推动着本书一步步向前，直至最终出版。

Larry R. Squire

俞洪波 译

SENIOR EDITORS

ASSOCIATE EDITORS

Charles D. Gilbert
The Rockefeller University
New York, NY
USA

Yukiko Goda
MRC Cell Biology Unit
University College London
London
UK

Lawrence S. B. Goldstein
Howard Hughes Medical Institute
UCSD School of Medicine
La Jolla, CA
USA

Antony W. Goodwin
Department of Anatomy and Cell Biology
University of Melbourne
Victoria
Australia

Tomas Hokfelt
Department of Neuroscience
Karolinska Institute
Stockholm
Sweden

Leslie Iversen
Department of Pharmacology
University of Oxford
Oxford
UK

Eugene M. Johnson
Department of Neurology
Washington University School of Medicine
St. Louis, MO
USA

Edward G. Jones
Center for Neuroscience
University of California
Davis, CA
USA

Jon H. Kaas
Department of Psychology
Vanderbilt University
Nashville, TN
USA

Helmut Kettenmann
Max-Delbrück Center for Molecular Medicine
Berlin
Germany

Christopher R. Kintner
Salk Institute for Biological Studies
La Jolla, CA
USA

Keith R. Kluender
Department of Psychology
University of Wisconsin
Madison, WI
USA

Richard J. Krauzlis
Salk Institute for Biological Studies
La Jolla, CA
USA

William B. Kristan
Division of Biological Sciences
University of California San Diego
La Jolla, CA
USA

Joseph E. LeDoux
Center for Neural Science
New York University
New York, NY
USA

Greg E. Lemke
Molecular Neurobiology Laboratory
Salk Institute for Biological Studies
San Diego, CA
USA

David A. Lewis
Departments of Psychiatry and Neuroscience
University of Pittsburgh
Pittsburgh, PA
USA

Pierre J. Magistretti
Center for Psychiatric Neuroscience
Prilly
Switzerland

Robert C. Malenka
Department of Psychiatry and Behavioral Sciences
Stanford University School of Medicine
Palo Alto, CA
USA

Peter R. Marler
Department of Neurobiology, Physiology and Behavior
University of California
Davis, CA
USA

Bruce S. McEwen
The Rockefeller University
New York, NY
USA

Earl K. Miller
The Picower Institute for Learning and Memory and Department of Brain and Cognitive Sciences
Massachusetts Institute of Technology
Cambridge, MA
USA

Paul E. Sawchenko
Salk Institute for Biological Studies
La Jolla, CA
USA

Wolfram Schultz
Department of Physiology, Development and Neuroscience
Cambridge University
Cambridge
UK

Terrence J. Sejnowski
Computational Neurobiology Lab
Salk Institute for Biological Studies
La Jolla, CA
USA

Gordon M. Shepherd
Department of Neurobiology
Yale University
New Haven, CT
USA

Clarke R. Slater
Institute of Neuroscience
Newcastle University
Newcastle upon Tyne
UK

Craig E. L. Stark
Department of Neurobiology and Behavior
University of California
Irvine, CA
USA

Robert Stickgold
Psychiatry Medical Department
Harvard Medical School
Boston, MA
USA

Peter L. Strick
Pittsburgh Veterans Affairs Medical Center and Department of Neurobiology
University of Pittsburgh
Pittsburgh, PA
USA

Edward M. Stricker
Department of Neuroscience
University of Pittsburgh
Pittsburgh, PA
USA

Thomas C. Südhof
Stanford University of Medicine
Palo Alto, CA
USA

Fred W. Turek
Center for Sleep and Circadian Biology
Northwestern University
Evanston, IL
USA

Stephen C. Woods
Department of Psychiatry
University of Cincinnati
Cincinnati, OH
USA

FOREWORD

What is an encyclopedia? The term is derived from two Greek words: *enkuklios*, which means cyclical, and *paideia*, which means education. In the early sixteenth century, copyists of Latin manuscripts combined the two words into a Latin designation which comes to us in English with the same spelling and with the meaning 'general course of instruction' (The American Heritage Dictionary, 2000, Boston: Houghton Mifflin, p. 589). The original Greek provides a dynamic connotation, an effort to approach knowledge in a probing, integrated fashion. In Latin and then English, the term has generally been applied to reference volumes addressing broad areas of knowledge.

The Greek emphasis on creative approaches to information is particularly apt for the neurosciences. The term 'neuroscience' is of remarkably young vintage. Francis Schmitt, in his foreword to the first edition of this encyclopedia, related his process of concatenating scientists from disparate fields into an invisible college whose workshops attacked the brain's most recalcitrant puzzles. He dubbed the organization the Neuroscience Research Program (NRP). The early NRP 'associates' included giants such as Melvin Calvin, whose Nobel Prize honored his work on photosynthesis; the Nobel laureate physical chemist Manfred Eigen; the biochemist Albert Lehninger; and Marshall Nirenberg, then a young molecular biologist in the throes of breaking the genetic code.

When Schmitt established the NRP, neuroscience as an integrated endeavor hardly existed. The invention of the microelectrode was permitting neurophysiologists to record from single cells, but characterizing them biochemically was impossible. A major step forward was the emergence in the mid-1960s of the Falck-Hillarp fluorescence microscopic techniques, which permitted selective visualization of catecholamine and serotonin neurons. Mapping the aminergic pathways soon led to collaborative efforts of behaviorists, who could examine the consequences of selective lesions, and biochemists, who no longer were relegated to monitoring neurotransmitters in homogenates of the whole brain. Advances in the 1970s in receptor biochemistry, their localization by autoradiography, and neuropeptide immunohistochemistry further enhanced discourse among neurophysiologists, neuroanatomists, neurochemists, and neuropharmacologists. In the past two decades, the tools of molecular biology have furthered the dialogue.

The explosion of the neurosciences can also be documented through the chronicles of the Society for Neuroscience (SFN). The SFN was founded in 1970 with Vernon Mountcastle as the first elected president, and its inaugural annual meeting in Washington, DC hosted a few hundred researchers. When I served as president in 1980, SFN numbered 7000 members. One of my key tasks was to combat attacks on the *raison d'être* of the society. Some argued, "We have too many scientists in this organization. Let's split into two societies, the 'Wets' and the 'Drys.'" Instead, to emphasize the integrated nature of the field, we launched the *Journal of Neuroscience*. Also, we argued that growth might plateau and that careful meeting organization would prevent individuals from getting 'lost in a crowd.' My prediction about a plateau was off the mark. As of this writing, May 2007, SFN numbers about 38 000 active members, with up to 35 000 people attending each annual meeting, dwarfing any other biomedical research society.

Most would agree that neuroscience is the most integrated scientific discipline. As such, the concept of an encyclopedia, in the original Greek sense of a circle of learning, is notably appropriate yet immensely challenging. The current edition, like earlier ones, succeeds by careful attention to organization and, most importantly, to the selection of the finest researchers as Associate Editors for individual topics. The Associate Editors are all seasoned veterans yet active researchers whose vision remains at the forefront of their field. All areas of importance are covered, from 'soup to nuts.' Emphasis is elegantly balanced between molecular and systems neuroscience.

In this era of rapid advances, one can question whether an encyclopedia, comprising a snapshot in time, serves a meaningful function. Might not all the information in such an enterprise be obsolete soon after publication? An effective encyclopedia, exemplified in these volumes, integrates disparate areas in a lucid, reader-friendly format. Such a publication can be provocative and invigorating to the most sophisticated professionals. At the same time, the entries are presented in such an inviting fashion that the encyclopedia serves for novices as the ideal entrée into the world of the nervous system.

Solomon H. Snyder
Distinguished Service Professor,
Johns Hopkins University

PREFACE

During the second half of the twentieth century, the study of the nervous system moved from a peripheral position within the biological and psychological sciences to become an interdisciplinary field called neuroscience. The new discipline brought biochemists, cell biologists, anatomists, physiologists, psychologists, neurologists, and psychiatrists – scientists and clinicians from diverse backgrounds, all drawn to the promise and excitement of studying the brain. They aimed to discover the mechanisms of neuronal function, elucidate the neural substrates of behavior and cognition, and learn about the diseases of the nervous system. The development of the discipline was catalyzed in 1969 by the formation of the Society for Neuroscience, which now has nearly 37 000 members. The first academic training programs for neuroscience were established in medical schools (the Department of Neurosciences at the University of California, San Diego in 1965 and the Department of Neurobiology at Harvard University in 1966). The first undergraduate training programs in neuroscience were established in 1972 at Amherst College and at Oberlin College, alma mater of Nobelist Roger Sperry and three Past-Presidents of the Society for Neuroscience. Today, there are more than 300 neuroscience departments and programs around the world.

The *Encyclopedia of Neuroscience* is intended to catalog and explicate the rich, diverse subject matter of the discipline and to facilitate communication among its subspecialties. It is meant to be an authoritative source of information for all areas of neuroscience. It will hopefully make neuroscience more accessible to a wide range of readers, from students making their first acquaintance with the field to general readers seeking information about specific topics. It should also serve as a useful reference for working neuroscientists and be useful as well to undergraduate and graduate students in neuroscience training programs, teachers in the life sciences, clinicians, and science writers.

The inaugural edition of this encyclopedia, which was the first comprehensive reference work for the field, was published in 1987 under the able leadership of George Adelman. It included some 700 entries and appeared in two volumes. The second edition, edited by George Adelman and Barry Smith, appeared in 1999 in two volumes and included more than 800 entries. A CD-ROM version of this edition was also published. A third edition, published only in electronic form, appeared in 2004.

The *Encyclopedia of Neuroscience* includes nearly 1500 entries. The full work will be published online at Science Direct, which can be accessed with subscription at www.sciencedirect.com. To assemble the entries, the Senior Editors identified 46 major areas of the discipline and then invited 46 Associate Editors, all experts in their field, to survey the content of neuroscience within each of these areas. Each Associate Editor then invited 30 to 40 authors to prepare articles on specific topics, with the objective of obtaining complete coverage for each area. Many of the authors are the recognized leaders in their field. The result is a compendium of expert articles representing the current world of neuroscience – the most important research, the most powerful tools, and the most promising applications.

Most of the entries are self-contained reviews that can be read as independent articles. Extensive cross-listing at the conclusion of each entry directs readers to articles on related topics. The principal organization of the *Encyclopedia* lies in the alphabetically arranged list of entries. In addition, the comprehensive subject classification will help readers find related topics and appreciate the structure of the discipline.

While no single reference work in neuroscience can claim to include every notable idea and fact about the brain, the Senior Editors hope that these volumes provide a summary of contemporary neuroscience that is both comprehensive and instructive. Neuroscience is still a developing field, but the *Encyclopedia* will have succeeded if it conveys the considerable promise that neuroscience offers for conquering the diseases that affect the nervous system and for understanding the brain, the mind, and ourselves.

The Senior Editors are grateful to the Developmental Editors at Elsevier, Michael Bevan, Joanna De Souza and Richard Berryman, and the Editorial Assistants, Caroline Phipps, Afandi Mohamed and Nicky Carter, for capably managing the formidable task of assembling and organizing the contents of the Encyclopedia. Andrew Lowe and Laura Jackson, the Project Managers, diligently brought the project through its several stages of production.

Larry R. Squire
Editor-in-Chief

目　　录

决策与神经经济学

执行功能与高级认知

半球特化

智能

振荡神经活性

决策与神经经济学

Animal Communication: Honesty and Deception

S L Vehrencamp, Cornell University, Ithaca, NY, USA

Definitions

Communication is defined as the transmission of information from a sender to a receiver via signals. True communication occurs when the information encoded in the signal enables the receiver to make decisions about behavioral responses and actions that subsequently benefit both the receiver and the sender. There are two ways in which this mutually beneficial exchange can break down in such a way that one party exploits the other: deception and eavesdropping.

Deception is the provision of inaccurate information by the sender such that the sender benefits from the interaction but the receiver pays the cost of a wrong decision. Types of deceit include 'exaggeration' or 'bluff' (using a signal whose rank among ordered alternatives is different from that for the corresponding condition values), 'lies' (use of the wrong signal among an unordered set of alternatives), and 'withholding information' (not giving a signal when appropriate). The evolution of such deceptive signaling is the focus of this discussion.

Eavesdropping typically occurs when a third-party receiver detects a signal directed at another receiver and uses the information to make decisions. The effect of eavesdropping on the sender could be positive or negative. For example, a countersinging interaction between two territorial male birds could provide information for eavesdropping females to make mate-choice decisions and for eavesdropping males to learn about the presence, relative dominance, or fighting ability of future rivals.

Both deception and eavesdropping can also take place in interspecific interactions. There are numerous examples of predatory species that mimic the mate attraction signal of their prey, but in such deceptive interactions between two different species, there is no selection pressure on the predator to be honest, and there is little the prey can do to avoid being exploited. The prey, as receiver, can try to improve its discrimination between true mates and impostors, but this process will simultaneously select for better mimicry by the predator. Similarly, predators can eavesdrop on the signals of their prey to locate their next meal. Prey can attempt to reduce the conspicuousness of these signals to predators while maximizing conspicuousness to conspecifics, but predators will counter with increased sensitivity. Such costs of signaling do affect signal design and receiver discrimination but are outside of this discussion of signal honesty. However, as shown below, some signals do appear to transmit honest information to heterospecifics for the benefit of both parties and provide a strong test of honest signaling models.

Honest signals, whether visual, vocal, olfactory, or tactile, are those in which some characteristic of the display (e.g., presence/absence, alternative forms, or a continuously varying parameter) is reliably associated with some attribute of the sender or its environment about which receivers want to know. Identifying this attribute specifies the kind of information transmitted by the signal. To fully demonstrate an honest signaling system, we would need to show that receivers not only attend to the signal and its variants but also benefit from knowing this information to make decisions. No signal is likely to be perfectly accurate. Senders make errors, but if errors lead to both positive and negative payoffs for the sender, we would not call it deception. Receivers will tolerate a certain level of sender error and deception as long as the signal is honest on average (see the section titled 'Do animals cheat?').

Context of Deception

When the sender and receiver in a signaling exchange both rank the payoffs of alternative receiver responses in the same order, selection will favor the accurate exchange of information within the limits of encoding, transmitting, and receiving error. However, sender and receiver often have conflicting interests because they rank the payoffs of alternative receiver responses differently. Under these conditions, animal senders will be tempted to provide misleading information so that the receiver performs the act that most benefits the sender. The strength of the selective pressure to deceive depends on the signaling context and the degree of conflict between the parties. Conflict of interest is greatest when two more or less equal competitors both desire the same nonsharable resource. Each would like the other to back down without a fight, and each would benefit from persuading the other that it is the better fighter by any means possible, including bluff. In the mate attraction context, both male and female benefit from mating with the correct species and therefore agree about the accurate transmission of species information. But females may want to mate only with a high-quality male, putting pressure on low-quality males to hide or exaggerate their quality. Similarly, an offspring in a brood of siblings may exaggerate its need for food to the parent in order to garner a larger share of the food for itself. Even in cooperative groups, where all members benefit from coordinated flock cohesion, two individuals may disagree about the direction the flock should move and lie to ensure that their directive is heeded.

A Brief History

In the early days of ethology, signals were shown to evolve through the ritualization of behaviors that are or were functionally appropriate to the contexts in which the signals are now given. Signals were believed to be honest indicators of underlying motivations because they were derived from physiologically or anatomically linked sources. With the rise of evolutionary game theory in the 1970s, this notion of signal honesty was questioned. Why should a sender give an honest signal? Similarly, if senders wear their emotions on their shirtsleeves, what prevents a clever receiver from using that information to exploit the sender? Richard Dawkins and John Krebs suggested that senders were best characterized as deceitful manipulators trying to mask their true intentions and trick receivers into actions benefiting senders. Receivers in turn were best viewed as mind readers trying to discount false signals, anticipate the true intent of the sender, and thus identify their own best countermove. This scenario leads to a never-ending arms race, with increasing deceit and concealment of true intentions by senders parried by increased discrimination and exploitation by receivers. Except when sender and receiver have common interests, the resulting signals would be largely deceitful and uninformative.

Amotz Zahavi challenged this pessimistic view of signal honesty. He asserted that receivers have the upper hand and ought not respond to signals unless they carry some guarantee of honesty. One guarantee is to require that the signal impose a cost such that deceitful senders cannot afford to produce an exaggerated signal or that they produce it only in an ineffective way. Signals characterized by such costs are called handicap signals. Although Zahavi's idea was viewed skeptically at first, subsequent game theory models demonstrated the evolutionary feasibility of handicap signaling, and the handicap principle is now widely accepted.

Since the mid-1980s, several dozen game theory models of biological communication have been developed, each depicting different signaling contexts and comprising different game structures and sets of assumptions. The common feature in all the models that found at least some conditions for stable signaling was the assumption of some type of cost imposed on dishonest senders. Without such costs, senders become dishonest, receivers ignore the signals, and no evolutionarily stable state with informative communication signals can be attained. These costs ranged from signal production costs to receiver retaliation costs, reputation costs, and various types of physical and physiological constraints. The realization that the type of cost affects both the form of a signal and the specific kind of information it can encode then led to the useful classification of signals based on the type of cost. Independent attempts to classify signals in this way have largely converged and provide a very powerful framework for understanding the evolution and diversity of animal communication signals.

Classifying Signals Based on the Type of Cost That Guarantees Honesty

Table 1 summarizes the simplest scheme for the relationship between the type of cost that maintains signal honesty, the form or design of the signal, and the kinds of information the signal can encode. Three signal categories have been distinguished here: handicap, index, and conventional signals.

Table 1 Signal classification based on the type of cost that maintains signal honesty

Signal class	*Cost*	*Signal design*	*Information*
Handicap	Signal production, time lost, risk of predation	Graded display, intensity correlated with sender quality	Fighting ability, stamina, condition, territory quality, need, motivation
Index	Physical or physiological constraints	Form linked to sender attributes	Body size, age, strength, pointing at intended receiver
Conventional	Retaliation by receivers	Antithetical discrete or graded display, arbitrary form	Motivation to escalate versus retreat, aggressive intentions, fighting ability, condition

Based on Maynard Smith J and Harper D (2003) *Animal Signals.* Oxford, UK: Oxford University Press; Vehrencamp SL (2000) Handicap, index, and conventional signal elements of bird song. In: Espmark Y, Amundsen T, and Rosenqvist G (eds.) *Animal Signals: Signalling and Signal Design in Animal Communication*, pp. 277–300. Trondheim: Tapir Publishers; Hurd PL and Enquist M (2005) A strategic taxonomy of biological communication. *Animal Behaviour* 70: 1155–1170.

Handicap Signals

The key concept of the handicap principle is that the cost imposed on the sender should be one that 'uses up' the particular sender attribute about which the receiver wants information. Receivers are selected to pay attention only to those types of signals that impose costs linked to the type of information receivers need. Thus the form of the signal is linked to its information content, typically a continuously varying signal parameter correlated with some sender attribute. Directional selection pressure from receivers favoring the most costly signal variants often results in extreme elaboration and exaggeration of the display character. Handicap signals are strategic signals, in the sense that all senders can produce all signal variants in principle, but senders of poor quality or condition tend not to produce the more intense variants because of the high signaling cost. **Figure 1** illustrates the classical handicap model, in which poor quality senders pay a higher cost for a given intensity of display. Their best option is to display at a lower intensity than a high-quality individual does, so signal intensity is reliably correlated with sender quality. Such signals are also called quality indicators and condition-dependent signals. Handicapping costs can be subdivided into production costs paid at the time of display and developmental costs paid earlier to grow the structures and organs needed for displaying. Several examples below show how such costs can be linked to useful information for receivers.

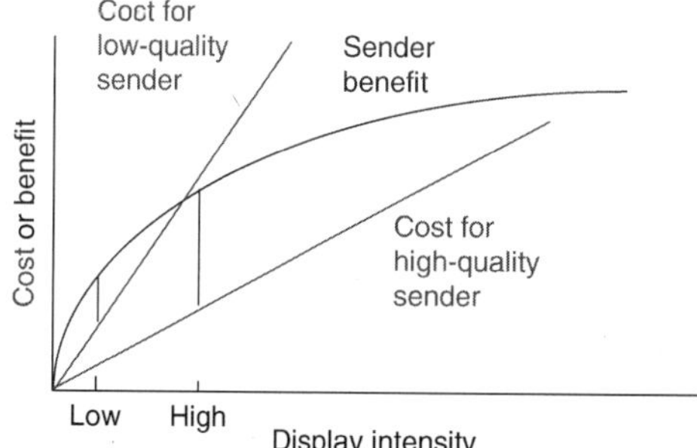

Figure 1 A graphical model for a handicap signal of sender quality. A key assumption is that displaying is costly, but high-quality senders pay a lower cost for a given display intensity than low-quality senders do. High- and low-quality senders receive the same benefit for a given display intensity. The optimal display level occurs at the point where the difference between benefit and cost is greatest. At equilibrium, high-quality senders display at a higher intensity than low-quality senders do, so display intensity is correlated with sender quality or condition. From Johnstone RA (1997) Evolution of animal signals. In: Krebs JR and Davies NB (eds.) *Behavioural Ecology: An Evolutionary Approach*, 4th edn., pp. 155–178. Oxford, UK: Blackwell Science.

Signals with energetically expensive production costs can inform receivers about the health, vigor, or foraging abilities of senders. For example, vocal and visual mate attraction signals must be repeated again and again. Female preference for males that not only produce high-quality displays but also repeat them at a high rate will increase the selection pressure on males to perform at the highest possible energetic level they can sustain. Unhealthy or poor-quality males cannot maintain such an expensive display rate, and this fact will be detectable to females. Choosy females will therefore benefit by selecting vigorous mates who are good genetic fathers or better parental providers or who possess food-rich territories (**Figures 2** and **3**). Repetitive countercalling contests between rival males can facilitate the assessment of relative condition, fighting ability, or motivation without their having to engage in a physical fight (**Figure 4(a)**). As a final example, energetic jumping displays are given by gazelles to approaching predators. Only individuals in good condition can afford to perform these actions well, and this provides honest information to the predators, which discourages them from chasing the more able displayers (**Figure 4(b)**).

Developmental costs are borne before the onset of display and can reveal either nutritional condition during development or more intrinsic aspects of genetic quality. The development of exaggerated display organs can also result in high maintenance costs for the bearer. A well-documented example is the elongated tail feathers of the barn swallow (*Hirundo rustica*) studied by Anders Møller. Females prefer males with longer tails, pairing much more quickly with males having artificially enlarged tails than with males with shortened tails. Long tails are a handicap for males; barn swallows are aerial foragers that capture flying insects on the wing. Artificial tail elongation increases the drag on the tail and reduces agility and foraging efficiency. Males with naturally long tails are stronger, healthier, and more parasite-resistant individuals who can not only grow long tails and cope with the foraging handicap but also pass on their parasite resistance to their genetic offspring. Females thus obtain better-quality offspring by selecting long-tailed males (**Figure 5**). Another good example of a handicap signal with a development cost is red coloration in birds and fish. Bearers of such color patches may also sustain the maintenance cost of increased conspicuousness to predators. Males in many songbird species possess repertoires of song types that they learn in the first months of life, and females have been shown to prefer larger repertoires and more complex songs. One promising explanation for this preference is the developmental stress

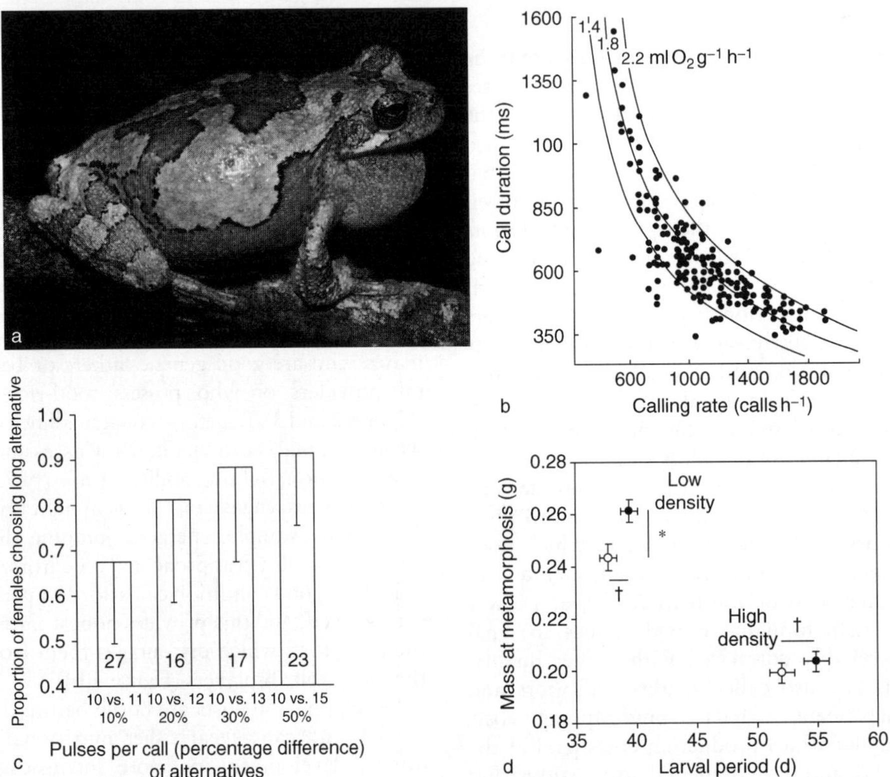

Figure 2 Call duration in the gray tree frog (*Hyla versicolor*) (a) is a costly handicap signal of male quality. (b) Calling is energetically expensive, with call duration and calling rate showing a trade-off in the field. An increase in both parameters is associated with an increase in oxygen consumption. Males increase their call duration when singing in dense choruses and when interacting vocally with other males. (c) Females strongly prefer males and experimental stimuli with longer call duration. (d) The offspring of females mated to long-calling males exhibit greater mass at metamorphosis than offspring of females mated to short-calling males, especially in contexts of low food density. In (c), error bars show the lower 95% confidence limits, and numbers in each bar indicate number of females in the sample. (d) The offspring of females mated to long-calling males (filled symbols) exhibit greater mass at metamorphosis than offspring of females mated to short-calling males (open circles), especially in contexts of low food density; error bars represent ±1 standard error, asterisk indicates significance at $P < 0.05$, and daggers indicate $P < 0.10$. (a) Photo courtesy of H Carl Gerhardt. (b) From Wells KD and Taigen TL (1986) The effect of social interactions on calling energetics in the gray treefrog (*Hyla* versicolor). *Behavioral Ecology and Sociobiology* 19: 9–18. (c) From Gerhardt C, Tanner SD, Corrigan CM, and Walton HC (2000) Female preference functions based on call duration in the gray tree frog (*Hyla versicolor*). *Behavioral Ecology* 11: 663–669. (d) From Welch AM (2003) Genetic benefits of a female mating preference in gray tree frogs are context-dependent. *Evolution* 57: 883–893.

hypothesis, which argues that young birds require good nutrition to develop the brain nuclei for song learning and production.

Two other types of handicap models involve signaling costs but provide different kinds of information. Models of sender need, developed with the context of begging in mind, require a signal whose intensity is correlated with increasing immediate costs (energetic or predation risk). The key features that stabilize the correlation between signal intensity and need are the greater benefit of food for a needier sender and the fact that the beggar sender and the donor receiver are genetic relatives. The other handicap model variant was developed in the context of aggressive signals, in which the performance of a signal makes the sender vulnerable to attack by the receiver. This has been called a vulnerability handicap or an interaction handicap because it represents a hybrid between the handicap model and the conventional signal model (see the section titled 'Conventional signals'). Signals in this category typically vary in their tactical impact such that a strong signal places the sender at greater risk of injury but is more effective in threatening the opponent.

Index Signals

Handicapping is not the only mechanism for generating honest signals. Recent models suggest that if coevolving senders and receivers can hit on a cost-free signal that reliably correlates with important sender

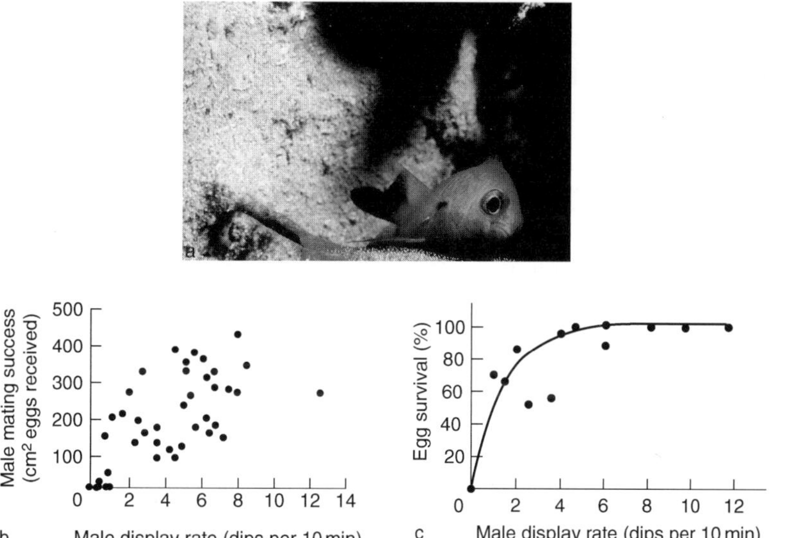

Figure 3 Example of display intensity as an indicator of male parental ability in the bicolor damselfish *Stegastes partitus* (a). This courting male is in the process of fertilizing recently laid eggs visible at the bottom. (b) Females prefer males that display at a high rate. Displaying is energetically costly and uses up calories, but males that are in good condition can afford high display rates and are more successful at guarding eggs (c). (a) Courtesy of Ken Clifton, with permission. (b, c) From Knapp RA and Kovach JT (1991) Courtship as an honest indicator of male parental quality in the bicolor damselfish, *Stegastes partitus*. *Behavioral Ecology* 2: 295–300.

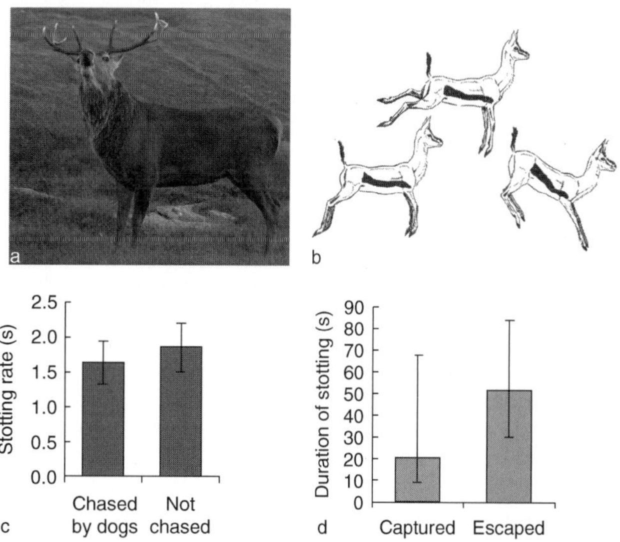

Figure 4 Examples of costly handicap signals in contexts other than mate attraction. (a) Male red deer (*Cervus elaphus*) engage in extended roaring contests with rivals. Roaring is an energetically expensive behavior that uses the actions and muscles employed during fighting. It is thought that only those males in good enough condition to fight can afford to roar at a winning level (Clutton-Brock TH and Albom SD (1979) The roaring of red deer and the evolution of honest advertisement. *Behaviour* 69: 145–170). (b) Stotting in Thomson's gazelles (*Gazella thomsoni*) involves leaping off the ground with all four legs held stiff and straight while running from predators (Walther FR (1969) Flight behaviour and avoidance of predators in Thomson's gazelle (*Gazella thomsoni* Guenther 1884). *Behaviour* 34: 184–221). They are far more likely to stot when chased by coursing wild dogs (78%) than when hunted by stalking cheetahs (9%). Wild dogs concentrated their chases on individuals that stotted at slower rates (c). Captured gazelles also stotted for shorter durations than gazelles that escaped (d). Gazelles were less likely to stot, and stotted at slower rates, during the dry season when food was lower and animals were in poorer condition. Stotting is therefore believed to be an honest signal to coursing predators of the prey's ability to escape capture. The error bars in (c) are ± 1 standard deviation and in (d) are interquartile ranges. (a) Photo courtesy of Alison Donald. (b) Reproduced from Walther FR (1969) Flight behaviour and avoidance of predators in Thomson's gazelle (*Gazella thomsoni* Guenther 1884). *Behaviour* 34: 184–221, with permission from Koninklijke Brill NV. (c, d) From FitzGibbon CD and Fanshawe JH (1988) Stotting in Thomson's gazelles: An honest signal of condition. *Behavioral Ecology and Sociobiology* 23: 69–74.

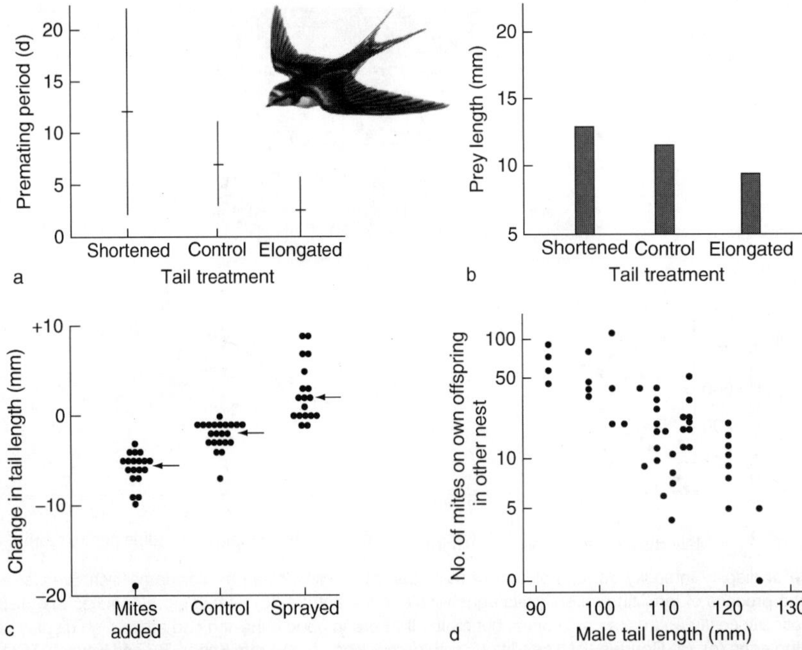

Figure 5 Tail length as a male quality indicator in the barn swallow (*Hirundo rustica*). (a) Females prefer (pair earlier with) males with experimentally lengthened tails. Error bars are ±1 standard deviation. (b) The cost of a lengthened tail in this aerial forager is increased drag, which reduces foraging efficiency and survivorship; males with naturally long tails suffer less of an aerodynamic cost than males with naturally short tails. (c) Long-tailed males possess fewer blood-sucking mites than do short-tailed males; removing the mites results in better tail growth. (d) Nestlings of males with longer tails and fewer parasites pass on their resistance to their offspring, even when they are raised in foster nests. (a) From Møller AP (1988) Female choice selects for male sexual tail ornaments in the monogamous swallow. *Nature* 332: 640–642. (b) from Møller AP, Lope F, and Lopez Caballero JM (1995) Foraging costs of a tail ornament. *Behavioral Ecology and Sociobiology* 37: 289–296. (c, d) from Møller AP (1990) Effects of hematophagous mite on the barn swallow *Hirundo rustica*: A test of the Hamilton and Zuk hypothesis. *Evolution* 44: 771–784, with permission from Blackwell publishing.

attributes, it will be favored over the costly signal. Some signals are constrained by physiology, anatomy, or physical principles to be honest indicators of certain types of sender attributes. Such signals are called unbluffable or index signals. Like handicaps, the form of the signal is strongly linked to the sender attribute of interest to the receiver. Unlike handicaps, they are not strategic signals, because some senders simply cannot produce some signal variants.

Examples of index signals include low-frequency vocal threats that are obligatorily linked with body size in many vertebrates, tailbeating displays in fish, and side-by-side head-high postures in ungulates. Similarly, push-pull and mouth-wrestling forms of ritualized fighting are reliable index signals of weight and strength. Signals that are linked with aging processes or health, such as silver backs in gorillas and song repertoire size in birds, indicate age, experience, and ability to survive (**Figure 6**). In song bird species with age-restricted (predispersal) song learning, song-type sharing between newly settled males and their neighbors is inversely correlated with dispersal distance and could serve as an index of fighting ability if good fighters are more likely to gain territories close to their tutors. Olfactory signals that are directly derived from reproductive hormones and by-products should also be classified as index signals. They directly reveal reproductive status in both males and females. Similarly, plant volatiles released by herbivores feeding on species-specific host plants are often used to attract conspecific mates. Although still controversial, alarm substances used by many schooling fish to disperse or cluster during predator attacks appear to be an antibacterial agent sequestered in the vacuoles of skin cells that is released on injury and would therefore qualify as an index signal.

Another cost-free constraint that leads to a type of index signal is an informational constraint. In this case, use of the signal is constrained by having access to some information. An example is stalked prey staring at a hidden predator, thereby signaling to the predator both its alerted state and the futility of continuing the hunt. The signal can be performed only by a sender who knows the location of the hidden predator.

Both index and handicap signals may have associated with them traits that make direct assessment of the relevant sender attributes easier or more accurate. Typically these are color patch markings or body

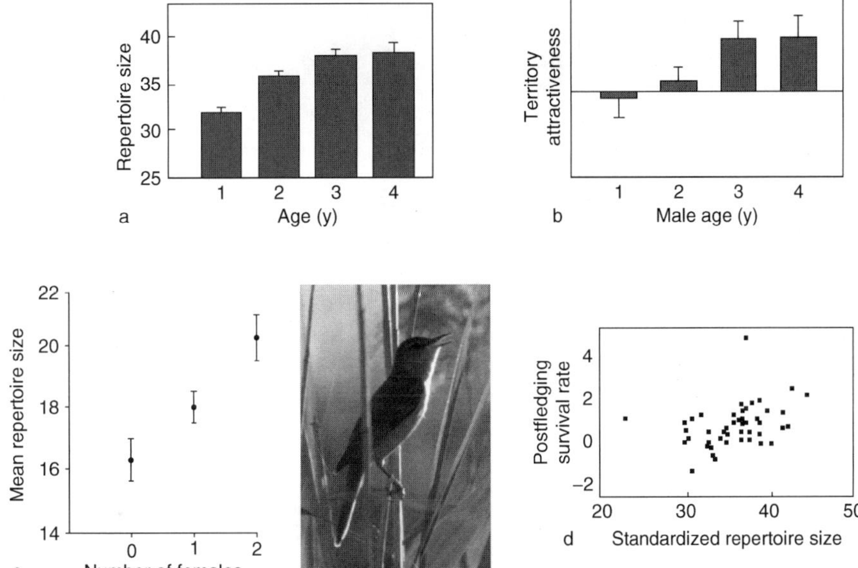

Figure 6 Repertoire size in an open-ended learner, the great reed warbler *Acrocephalus arundinaceus*, as an index of age. (a) Repertoire size increases with age for the first few years of life. (b) Older males possess better territories, as measured by occupancy and vegetation cover. (c) Males with larger repertoires (and better territories) attract more females in this polygynous species. Nine of ten females who sought extrapair fertilizations selected a neighboring male with a larger repertoire than their social mate. (d) The offspring of males with larger repertoires had higher survival, including return rate after migration, suggesting that larger-repertoire males pass on their inherently higher quality to their offspring. Error bars in (a), (b), and (c) are ±1 standard error. (a, b) From Hasselquist D (1994) Male attractiveness, mating tactics and realized fitness in the polygynous great reed warbler. PhD Thesis, Lund University, Sweden. (c) From Catchpole CK, Leisler B, and Dittami J (1986) Sexual differences in the responses of captive great reed warblers (*Acrocephalus arundinaceus*) to variation in song structure and size. *Ethology* 73: 69–77. (d) From Hasselquist D, Bensch S, and von Schantz T (1996) Correlation between male song repertoire, extra-pair paternity and offspring survival in the great reed warbler. *Nature* 381: 229–232. Photo courtesy of Bengt Hansson.

structures, called 'amplifiers,' that enhance visual perception of the physical attribute or movement display. Many fish have contrasting lines demarcating their body margins, which make assessment of body size easier. Similarly, a contrasting triangular marking on the abdomens of spiders makes assessment of nutritional condition, and thus fighting ability, easier. Contrasting stripes on the head in many birds, or outlining of the ears in many mammals, make it easier for a visual receiver to assess where a sender is looking.

Conventional Signals

Some communication signals are neither costly to produce nor obligatorily linked with physical properties of senders. The code by which these signals are associated with contexts is an arbitrary convention, and therefore these are called conventional signals. If there is no conflict of interest between sender and receiver, senders will not be tempted to cheat and conventional signals can be honest and stable without further guarantees. However, conventional signals are seen even during conflicts of interest, and in this case there must be a stabilizing cost that maintains honesty. The cost is receiver retaliation, which must come in the form of receiver skepticism or a retaliation rule in which receivers approach and check the sincerity of senders. In the most compelling model of conventional signaling with conflict of interest, both contenders must signal, and retaliate when both give a similarly strong signal, but retreat when the opponent gives a stronger one. Conventional signals are often discrete, with alternate antithetical signals for the strong versus weak message. This type of signal can convey information about aggressive motivation as well as fighting ability.

Prominent color patches in some birds and lizards are the classic example of this type of signal (**Figure 7**). The size or hue of the patch is correlated with the dominance rank of the individual, hence their designation as badges of status. Large badge size deters aggressive challenges by small-badged individuals. The cost of possessing a large badge is aggressive retaliation from other large-badged individuals. The evolution of such signals must be accompanied by frequent testing of the honesty of other individuals with a badge size similar to one's own and avoiding or ignoring individuals with larger or smaller badges.

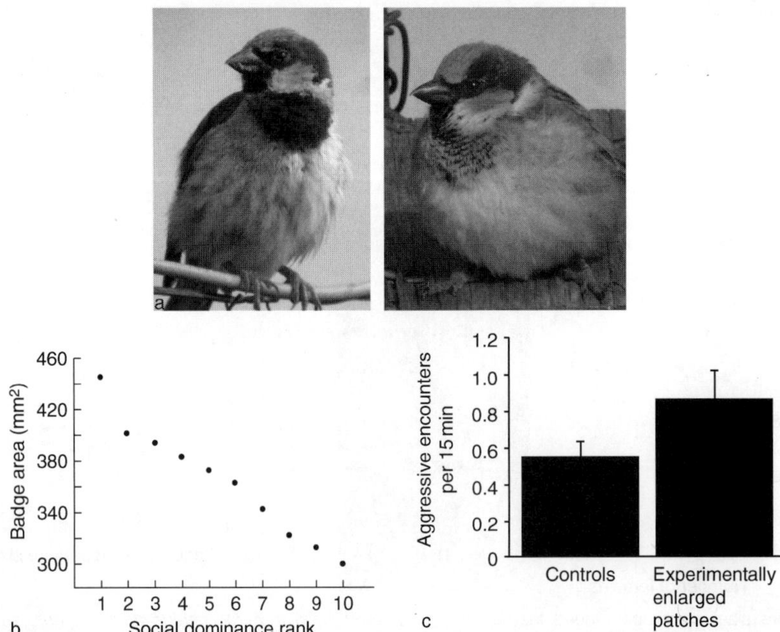

Figure 7 Badge of status in house sparrows, *Passer domesticus*. (a) The black bib on the chest of males varies greatly in size. (b) Size of the patch is strongly correlated with dominance rank. (c) Males with experimentally enlarged patches were involved in more aggressive encounters than were controls, and their attackers had larger than average patches. In Harris sparrows with a similar black chest patch, males with normally large bibs whose patch size was experimentally reduced had to fight very hard, but eventually won. Error bars in (c) are ±1 standard error. (a) Photo courtesy of Kevin McGowan. (b) From Møller AP (1987) Variation in badge size in male house sparrows. *Passer domesticus*: Evidence for status signalling. *Animal Behaviour* 35: 1637–1644. (c) From Møller AP (1987) Social control of deception among status signalling house sparrows *Passer domesticus*. *Behavioral Ecology and Sociobiology* 20: 307–311.

Such a rule makes it very dangerous and costly for a low-status individual to cheat by sporting a large badge. Certain vocal signals, such as song type matching and song type switching rate, are also believed to be conventional signals of aggressive intention.

Receiver skepticism is a type of receiver retaliation cost that can potentially stabilize honesty of conventional signals among group-living animals that recognize each other and interact repeatedly. Thus individuals who are observed to signal deceptively are remembered and tagged with a poor reputation or lack of trust, which may result in their failing to obtain certain benefits in the future. Reputation models with repeated interactions can even maintain honesty of cheap conventional signals when receivers have conflicting interests.

Do Animals Cheat?

Most signals are believed to be honest most of the time because conflicts of interest are minimal or appropriate costs are imposed on cheaters. But dishonest signaling does occur. Receivers will tolerate a certain amount of deception as long as they obtain a net gain by attending to signals (i.e., the probability that the signal is accurate times the payoff of making the right decision, plus the probability that the signal is inaccurate times the payoff of making the wrong decision, is positive). In theory, there are several contexts in which senders may be able to get away with some dishonesty. One context is a high level of perceptual error on the part of receivers, which favors less accurate mapping of sender quality on signal characteristics. A second context arises from a nonequilibrium outcome of dynamic coevolution between sender and receiver. A third model results when there are several classes of sender, each with its own costs and benefits of signaling, and receivers cannot distinguish between sender types; honest sender types must be sufficiently common relative to dishonest types to maintain the signaling system. A fourth situation occurs when receivers pay a very high cost for failing to respond to a signal, which leaves receivers vulnerable to deceit if senders figure out a way to benefit from the response. Documented examples of dishonesty fit several of these models.

Deceitful bluffing and exaggeration of body size or condition have been documented for competitive signals in several species. For example, mantis shrimp (*Neogonodactylus bredini*) defend their burrow from intruders with a claw-spreading threat display, which is effectively given even when the resident has recently molted and has a soft exoskeleton. In snapping shrimp (*Alpheus heterochaelis*), chela (claw) size is positively correlated with body size and ability to win fights, but individuals with chelae larger than expected for their body size give more open-chela displays than individuals with smaller-than-expected chelae. Males of the mealworm beetle (*Tenebrio molitor*) release a pheromone that attracts female mates, but males whose immune system has been experimentally challenged with a foreign material implant increase their pheromone production and are even more attractive to females than normal males are. These examples may fit the multiple-sender model above, in which receivers cannot accurately distinguish the intrinsic quality of senders and honest senders are more common than dishonest ones.

A good example of an outright lie has been described in birds foraging in flocks; one individual may give a false alarm call to scare competitors away from a rich food find. Initially it was believed that senders would not 'cry wolf' too often, because receivers would learn to ignore the signal and it would cease to be effective in true alarm contexts. However, several studies have shown that the incidence of alarm calls in the absence of a predator is quite high, 55–63%. Although a certain amount of alarm unreliability is caused by errors (e.g., by young individuals who haven't learned which heterospecifics are truly dangerous), senders have been shown to give false alarms in which they clearly benefit, and the likelihood of false alarming varies with the costs and benefits to senders. The reason such a high level of dishonesty can be sustained is clearly a result of the high cost of a miss to receivers (i.e., death) relative to the cost of falsely fleeing and losing a bite of food, supporting the fourth model above. False alarm calls are also given by some male birds and squirrels during the fertile period of female mates to interrupt extra-pair copulations with competitors.

The withholding of information is a much more difficult form of deceit to document than is the provision of false information. Not only must one demonstrate a reliable association between a specific context, a signal, and a specific response, but one must also show that there is some behavioral flexibility on the part of senders to either give or fail to give the signal in different circumstances in a way that benefits the sender. This last point has been termed the 'audience effect' of signaling. Food calls may be given by males in some species (falsely at times) to attract mates, but food calls are always withheld in the presence of rival males. Food calls may also be withheld in group-living species that expect group members to share rich food finds. In this case, there needs to be a significant cost of withholding information to sustain mostly honest notification of food. Such a cost has been described only in primates who fail to advertise a rich food find. If other group members catch an individual feeding on such a find without having called, the individual is aggressively punished. But receivers may have a difficult time detecting a lie in this case, supporting the first model above.

In conclusion, low levels of dishonesty may persist in many signaling systems, but signals must be reliable enough on average to justify receiver response. Otherwise, receivers will ignore signals, senders will no longer benefit from giving dishonest information, and the signals will disappear from the species' repertoire. A variety of costs and constraints maintain signal honesty, and signals must be costly in a way that explains why they provide reliable information.

See also: Communication Networks and Eavesdropping in Animals; Game Theory and the Economics of Animal Communication; Pheromones and other Chemical Communication in Animals; Sexual Selection and the Evolution of Animal Signals; Signal Transmission in Natural Environments; Signal Design Rules in Animal Communication; Visual Signaling in Animals; Vocal Communication in Birds.

Further Reading

Catchpole CK, Leisler B, and Dittami J (1986) Sexual differences in the responses of captive great reed warblers (*Acrocephalus arundinaceus*) to variation in song structure and size. *Ethology* 73: 69–77.

Clutton-Brock TH and Albon SD (1979) The roaring of red deer and the evolution of honest advertisement. *Behaviour* 69: 145–170.

Fitch WT and Hauser MD (2003) Unpacking "honesty": Vertebrate vocal production and the evolution of acoustic signals. In: Simmons AM, Fay RR, and Popper AN (eds.) *Acoustic Communication*, pp. 65–137. New York: Springer.

FitzGibbon CD and Fanshawe JH (1988) Stotting in Thomson's gazelles: An honest signal of condition. *Behavioral Ecology and Sociobiology* 23: 69–74.

Gerhardt C, Tanner SD, Corrigan CM, and Walton HC (2000) Female preference functions based on call duration in the gray tree frog (*Hyla versicolor*). *Behavioral Ecology* 11: 663–669.

Hasselquist D (1994) Male attractiveness, mating tactics and realized fitness in the polygynous great reed warbler. PhD Thesis, Lund University, Sweden.

Hasselquist D, Bensch S, and von Schantz T (1996) Correlation between male song repertoire, extra-pair paternity and offspring survival in the great reed warbler. *Nature* 381: 229–232.

Hasson O (1994) Cheating signals. *Journal of Theoretical Biology* 167: 223–238.

Hurd PL and Enquist M (2005) A strategic taxonomy of biological communication. *Animal Behaviour* 70: 1155–1170.

Johnstone RA (1997) Evolution of animal signals. In: Krebs JR and Davies NB (eds.) *Behavioural Ecology: An Evolutionary Approach*, 4th edn., pp. 155–178. Oxford, UK: Blackwell Science.

Knapp RA and Kovach JT (1991) Courtship as an honest indicator of male parental quality in the bicolor damselfish, *Stegastes partitus*. *Behavioral Ecology* 2: 295–300.

Maynard Smith J and Harper D (2003) *Animal Signals*. Oxford, UK: Oxford University Press.

Møller AP (1987) Social control of deception among status signalling house sparrows. *Passer domesticus*. *Behavioral Ecology and Sociobiology* 20: 307–311.

Møller AP (1987) Variation in badge size in male house sparrows. *Passer domesticus*: Evidence for status signalling. *Animal Behaviour* 35: 1637–1644.

Moller AP (1988) Female choice selects for male sexual tail ornaments in the monogamous swallow. *Nature* 332: 640–642.

Møller AP (1990) Effects of hematophagous mite on the barn swallow. *Hirundo rustica*: A test of the Hamilton and Zuk hypothesis. *Evolution* 44: 771–784.

Møller AP, Lope F, and Lopez Caballero JM (1995) Foraging costs of a tail ornament. *Behavioral Ecology and Sociobiology* 37: 289–296.

Vehrencamp SL (2000) Handicap, index, and conventional signal elements of bird song. In: Espmark Y, Amundsen T, and Rosenqvist G (eds.) *Animal Signals: Signalling and Signal Design in Animal Communication*, pp. 277–300. Trondheim: Tapir Publishers.

Walther FR (1969) Flight behaviour and avoidance of predators in Thomson's gazelle (*Gazella thomsoni* Guenther 1884). *Behaviour* 34: 184–221.

Welch AM (2003) Genetic benefits of a female mating preference in gray tree frogs are context-dependent. *Evolution* 57: 883–893.

Wells KD and Taigen TL (1986) The effect of social interactions on calling energetics in the gray treefrog (*Hyla versicolor*). *Behavioral Ecology and Sociobiology* 19: 9–18.

Decision-Making and Neuroeconomics

A Rustichini, University of Minnesota, Minneapolis, MN, USA

Decision Theory in Economics

Decision theory as developed in economics is an axiomatic analysis. The theory proceeds by first defining a set of choices that a subject (the decision maker, DM) faces. A choice is a finite set of options that are offered to the DM; a decision is the selection of one of these options. These are the observed data: it is in principle possible to collect them by explicitly asking a real DM to choose among the options, under the condition that the object selected is actually delivered to him. No speech acts (that is, statements like "I prefer this option to this other option") are necessary or allowed among the potential observations.

The method and the main results of the theory are best illustrated in a simple and concrete example of choice environment, choice under risk. In this environment the options are lotteries. A common lottery ticket provides an example: a winning number is drawn at random, and with such a ticket, a person is entitled to a payment if the winning number is the one he has, and he receives no payment otherwise. In general, a lottery is a contract specifying a set of outcomes (the payments made to the subject in our example) and a probability for each of these outcomes. The probability is typically specified in advance and precisely known to the subject.

For example, a lottery with two outcomes can be formally described with a pair $(x, p, y, 1-p)$, to be interpreted as this lottery gives the outcome x with probability p, and the outcome y with probability $1-p$. With this notation, a lottery with monetary payments (\$10, 1/2, \$0, 1/2) gives a 50/50 chance of a payment of 10 dollars and nothing otherwise. Lotteries do not need to award a monetary amount: the theory applies also to situations where x is an expensive jewel and y is a night in jail (if, for example, you are contemplating robbing a jewelry store and considering the risk of getting caught in the act). For simplicity of exposition we confine ourselves mostly to lotteries with monetary amounts in the rest of the article.

Revealed Preferences

The only feature that we can observe of our subject is the decisions he makes. We do not, of course, observe his preferences directly. However, we may interpret his choices as a 'revelation' he makes of his preferences: if when he is presented with a choice between lottery L_1 and L_2 he chooses L_1, we may say that he reveals he prefers L_1 to L_2. It is in this sense and in this sense only that we can say that the DM prefers something. The two descriptions of his behavior, one with the language of decisions and the other with that of preferences, are by the definition we adopt perfectly equivalent. Since the language of preferences seems more intuitive, it is the one used typically by decision theory, and is the one used here. But how do we describe the behavior or preferences of our subject?

Axioms

Even with simple lotteries with two monetary outcomes, by varying the amounts and the probabilities we can obtain an infinite set of possible lotteries, and by taking pairs of these lotteries we can obtain infinitely many choices. So to completely describe the behavior of a subject we should in principle list the infinite set of decisions he makes. The theory considers instead subjects whose decisions can be described by a short list of simple principles or axioms.

The first axiom requires that the preferences are complete: for every choice between the two lotteries L_1 and L_2, either L_1 is preferred to L_2 or L_2 is preferred to L_1. The occurrence of both possibilities is not excluded: in this case, the subject is indifferent to the two lotteries. When the subject prefers L_1 to L_2 but does not prefer L_2 to L_1, then we say that he strictly prefers L_1 to L_2. The second axiom requires the preferences to be transitive: if the DM prefers L_1 to L_2 and L_2 to L_3, then he prefers L_1 to L_3.

The next two axioms are also simple, but have more of a technical nature. Suppose we have two lotteries, $L_1=(x, p, y, 1-p)$ and $L_2=(z, q, w, 1-q)$. Take any probability r, a number between 0 and 1. Imagine the following contract. We will run a random device, with two outcomes, *Black* and *White*, the first with probability r. If *Black* is drawn, then you will play according to the lottery L_1; if *White* comes out, you will play according to the lottery L_2. This new contract is a lottery as well. If you do not care about how you get the amounts of money, then this is the lottery with four outcomes described as $(x, rp, y, r(1-p), z, (1-r)q, w, (1-r)(1-q))$. We write this new lottery as $rL_1+(1-r)L_2$. The two axioms that we mentioned are expressed using this new concept.

The next axiom, third in our list, requires that if you strictly prefer L_1 to L_2, then for some number r, you strictly prefer $rL_1+(1-r)L_2$ to L_2. This seems reasonable: when r is close to 1, the composite lottery is very close to L_1, so you should strictly prefer it to L_2 just like you strictly prefer L_1.

Finally, suppose that you strictly prefer L_1 to L_2. Then for any lottery L_3, you also strictly prefer $rL_1 + (1-r)L_3$ to $rL_2 + (1-r)L_3$. Again, this seems reasonable. When, in the description we gave above, *White* is drawn, then you get in both cases L_3; when *Black* is drawn, you get in the first case L_1 and in the second L_2. Overall, you should prefer the first lottery, $rL_1 + (1-r)L_3$.

Representation of Preferences

A fundamental result in decision theory (due to von Neumann and Morgenstern (vNM)) is that subjects having preferences that satisfy these four axioms behave as if they had a simple numerical representation of their preferences. A numerical representation of a preference is a function that associates to a lottery a single number, called the utility of the lottery, that we can write as $U(L)$. This function is called a representation of the preferences if whenever L_1 is preferred to L_2, then the utility of L_1 is larger than the utility of L_2, that is, $U(L_1) > U(L_2)$.

It should be clear that the existence of such a function restricts the preferences of the subject. For example, suppose that L_1 is preferred to L_2 and L_2 to L_3. If such a function exists, then $U(L_1) > U(L_2)$ and $U(L_2) > U(L_3)$. It follows that $U(L_1) > U(L_3)$, and since the utility is a representation of preferences, L_1 is preferred to L_3. That is, preferences with a utility representation must be transitive.

The vNM theorem also states that the preference order satisfies the four preceding axioms if and only if there exists a utility function with a very simple form that represents the preference. The form is simple because it is the expectation of the utility of each outcome, according to some function u of outcomes. For example, the expected utility of the lottery $L = (x, p, y, 1-p)$ is

$$U(L) = pu(x) + (1-p)u(y). \quad [1]$$

Cardinal and Ordinal Utilities

For neuroeconomics, and any research program that tries to determine how decisions are implemented, the utility function is probably the most interesting object. This function ties observed behavior with a simple one-dimensional quantity, the utility of the option, and predicts that the decision between two options is taken by selecting the option with the highest utility. If one is interested in determining the neural correspondents of the objects we have introduced, he must first know whether these objects are unique. For example, we may formulate the hypothesis that the decision is taken depending on some statistics of the firing rate of a group of neurons associated with each of the options. We may also consider that this firing rate is proportional to the utility we determine from observed choice behavior. Then we need to know whether this utility is uniquely determined. This introduces us to a fundamental distinction in decision theory, that between cardinal and ordinal representation.

An ordinal representation of a preference is any utility function such that $U(L_1) > U(L_2)$ if and only if L_1 is strictly preferred to L_2. There are clearly many such functions. For example, if M is any increasing function, then $M(U(L_1)) > M(U(L_2))$ if and only if L_1 is strictly preferred to L_2. So we say that an ordinal representation is unique only up to increasing (or monotonic) transformation, like the one we have used from U to $M(U)$.

Consider now the function u is eqn [1], and take two numbers $a > 0$ and b. Replace the u function in (1) with the new function v defined for any value z by $v(z) = au(z) + b$. If we replace the u in eqn [1], we obtain a new function on lotteries which also represents preferences and has the form of expected utility. Since these transformations leave the observed choices and preferences unchanged, the u in [1] is not unique. However, these are the only possible transformations we can apply. A second remarkable part of the vNM theorem is that if two functions u and v represent the preferences of a subject as expected utility (that is, as in [1]), then it must be that $v(z) = au(z) + b$ for some positive number a and some number b. In this case, the two functions are said to be linear transformations of each other, and representations like these are said to be cardinal representations. A different but equivalent way of saying this is that if we consider functions on a range of monetary prizes between a minimum of 0, say, and a maximum value M, and we agree to normalize the utility function u to $u(0) = 0$ and $u(M) = 1$, then there is a unique such function that, once substituted in eqn [1], represents the preferences of the DM.

However, the observed decision between two choices is determined by the function U, and this is unique only up to monotonic transformations. So even if we agree to normalize $U(0) = 0$ and $U(M) = 1$, still there are infinitely many such Us. Can we do better than this? We can, if we agree to extend the set of observed data to include errors and time in the decision process.

Stochastic Choice

The next step in our survey brings us closer to the models and results currently applied in neuroscience: the theory of stochastic choice.

To illustrate and motivate this new point of view, we begin with an interesting finding, discovered in the 1940s by an Iowa researcher, D Cartwright. He asked subjects to pick one of two alternatives. In keeping with our previous exposition, one may think of these alternatives as lotteries, although the original experiments were based on cognitive tasks, such as discriminating among geometric shapes or angles of different width. By changing the parameter appropriately, the experimenter could make the choice more or less difficult. For example, setting the width of two angles to be more similar would make choosing the wider angle a more difficult task. Also, by asking the subject to make the same choice repeatedly, at some time distance, he could test the frequency of the choice of one or the other of the alternatives in different decision problems. He could then construct what we can call the empirical random choice: the frequency of choice of each of the options from a given set of alternatives.

He had, however, also measured the response time for each choice (that is, the time that passed between the moment the choice was presented and the time the choice was made by the subject), and he then plotted the average response time for each decision problem against the minimum frequency of any of the two choices in that same problem. The key finding was that the longest response time was observed when the minimum frequency was approaching 50%. In other words, those problems in which the subject was more likely to select, over time, both options were also those in which he was taking more time to decide.

The result is robust and has been replicated since in many different environments. A related test is the measure of the response time measured as function of the distance between the two options, when a measure of distance is natural, for example, the distance between two numbers when the subject has to pick the largest. A robust finding is that the response time decreases with the distance (typically the log of the time is linear in the log of the distance). This is the 'symbolic distance' effect.

The finding of Cartwright suggests a model of decision in which two opposing forces push in the direction of each of the options. When the difference between these two forces is large, the decision is frequently in favor of the favored option, and the decision is taken quickly. When they are the same, the frequency of choice of the two options becomes closer, and the response time becomes longer.

For our purposes of outlining a theory of the decision process when the decision considers economic choices, it is important to note that for economic choices the same result holds. Suppose we determine the utility of a subject from the observed choices, that is, the quantity $U(L)$ for every lottery L. We can now measure the distance between the utility of any two lotteries in a choice and conjecture that the analog of the Cartwright results hold in this situation: the closer the two options in utility, the longer the time to decide, and the higher the minimum probability of choosing any of the two. This conjecture has been confirmed in several studies. There is one last hurdle: we have just seen that the U in [1] is not unique; in fact, even after normalization we have infinitely many such functions. So how can we measure in a meaningful way the distance in utility between two options?

Economic Theories of Stochastic Choice

The experimental evidence reviewed in the previous section suggests that when faced with a choice between two options many times, the subject may not always choose the same option in each instance. This is the opposite of what the utility theory we have reviewed so far predicts: in that theory, if the utility of one of the two is larger, it should always be chosen. Still, a large body of experimental and empirical evidence suggests that at best we can determine the frequency according to which one option is chosen, and that this frequency is not necessarily (in fact, is typically not) concentrated on one option. The key idea of the stochastic theory of choice is that the relative frequency of the choice of one option over the other gives a way to get a better measure of the utility of the two options.

The method of analysis is again axiomatic. Let $p(L_1, L_2)$ denote the frequency according to which lottery L_1 is chosen out of the set $\{L_1, L_2\}$, that we called the empirical random rule. Thus, it gives us evidence on whether L_1 is preferred to L_2: for example, this is plausible if that frequency is larger than 1/2. But it tells us more. If we compare the same frequency of choices out of two other lotteries $\{L_3, L_4\}$, and we observe that $p(L_1, L_2) > p(L_3, L_4)$, then we may say that the difference in utility between L_1 and L_2 is larger than the difference between L_3 and L_4. An appropriate set of axioms on the new evidence (the frequency of choice) guarantees that there is a utility function (that we denote V to distinguish it from the very different object U) such that

$$p(L_1, L_2) > p(L_3, L_4)$$

if and only if

$$V(L_1) - V(L_2) > V(L_3) - V(L_4) \qquad [2]$$

This function is a cardinal object: that is, if a different function W also satisfies [2], for the same p, then W is a linear monotonic transformation of V. That is, there are two numbers $a > 0$ and b such that $W = aV + b$. Another way of stating this delivers us the unique object that we were looking for: if we normalize V to $V(0) = 0$ and $V(M) = 1$, then this function is unique. This is the object we were looking for: a unique summary, entirely constructed from behavioral observations, of the value that the DM attaches to different options.

In the plan of determining the neural basis of decision, we have now two final steps. First, we have to produce a reasonable model of the decision process that produces a stochastic choice with the required coherence expressed formally by the axioms underlying the representation in eqn [2]. Second, we have to specify and test the neural basis implementing this process. Let us begin with the first.

The Random Walk Model of Decision

The random walk model is a model of the decision process, originally formulated by Ratcliff. The process was originally thought of as an explanation of memory retrieval. In this task, a subject is presented with an object and is asked to decide whether it is the same he saw some period earlier. The model describes the two objects (one in front of the subject, the other in his memory) as a vector of characteristics. The decision is taken by marking, for each characteristic, whether it is the same in the two objects (in this case mark a score of 1) or not (and then mark -1). When the sum of the evidence in favor and against the conclusion that the two objects are the same reaches a critical threshold, then the decision is taken.

The process provides the basis for a general model of decision. Let us consider for simplicity the case in which the DM has to choose between two alternatives. The essential elements of the model are a space of evidence, a stochastic process on this space, and two barriers. In the memory retrieval example, the space of evidence is the set of integers, where a number is the number of agreements minus the number of disagreements. The process on the space is a random walk: as the DM proceeds to consider the next characteristic in the list, he can add or subtract one unit to the current evaluation state, depending on whether he finds an agreement or a disagreement. Finally, the process stops and the decision is taken when a barrier (high or low) is reached. The decision process has been reduced to a random walk on a space and a stopping time described by two barriers. At the stopping time, the decision corresponding to the barrier is taken.

The Predictions of the Model

The model has several parameters: first, those describing the process, for example, the mean and the variance of the random walk. The other parameters are the barriers. The model yields two observed variables: the probability that one of the two decisions is taken, and the time needed to reach the decision. Of course, an important qualitative aspect of this model of the decision process is that choice is not deterministic: when the subject is presented with the same choice, he may sometimes choose one option, and sometimes the other. The connection between the theory of stochastic choice in economics and the random walk model is clear: the probability of choice of each option studied in the model of stochastic choice is the same object induced by the random walk model when the latter hits the barrier.

The model gives sharp predictions on the two variables. For example, if the drift in favor of one of the two options is stronger, then the probability that that option is chosen increases. Also, when the difference in drift between the two choice is small, then the time to take a decision increases. The model provides a good fit with the observed data on choice and on response time in a variety of situations. The question is: do we have any evidence that suggests a neural basis for this?

Decision Theory in Neuroscience

Intense research on the neural foundation of the random walk model of decision has been developed in the past years. To illustrate the method and the findings, we begin again with a classical experiment.

In the experiment, the subject (for example, a rhesus monkey) observes a random movement of dots. A fraction of the dots is moving to the left and a fraction to the right. The monkey has to decide whether a larger fraction of dots is moving to the right or to the left, being instructed to do this after intensive training. If it makes the right guess, it is compensated with a squirt of juice. Single neuron recordings of neurons show that the process of deciding on the direction is the outcome of the following process. Some neurons are associated with the movement to the left, and others to the right. The overall firing rate of the 'left' and 'right' neurons is of course roughly proportional to the number of dots moving in the two directions.

The decision is taken when the difference between the cumulative firing in favor of one of the two alternatives is larger than a critical threshold.

We suggest that the mental operation that is performed when the subject has to choose between two economically valuable options consists of two steps. First, the individual has to associate a utility to each of the two options. Second, he has to decide which of these two computed quantities is larger. This second step is a simple comparison of quantities. The first is completely new and is specific to economic analysis. Note two important features of this model: first, even if the DM assigns (somewhere in his brain) a strictly larger utility to one of the two options, he still does not choose for sure that option; he has only a larger probability of doing so. Second, the DM has a single utility or preference order over outcomes. The choice outcome is not deterministic, because the process from utility evaluation to choice is random.

What is the evidence supporting this view? Let us begin from the step involving comparison of quantities. There are experiments involving comparison of numbers, run with human subjects, that confirm the basic finding that the response time is decreasing with the distance between the two quantities that are being compared. For example, if subjects have to decide whether a number is larger or smaller than a reference number, then the response time is approximately decreasing exponentially with the distance between the two numbers. So there is experimental evidence that suggests that the operation of comparing quantities follows a process that is close to that described by the random walk model.

The last missing element is this: do we have evidence that there are areas of the brain where neurons fire in proportion to the utility of the two options?

The Computation of the Utility

Building on previous results, we examine the neural basis of the computation of the utility. In this experiment, a monkey is offered the choice between two quantities of different food or juices, for example, three units of apple or one unit of raisin.

By varying the quantities offered of juice of each type, the experimenter can reconstruct, from 'revealed preferences', the utility function of the monkey. This function can be taken to be, for the time being, an artificial construct of the theorist observing the behavior. The choices made by the subjects have the typical property of the random choice. For example, between any amount less than or equal to 2 units of apple-tea and 1 unit of raisin, the monkey always chose the apple juice. With 3 units of tea and 1 of apple, the frequency of choice was 50/50 between the two. With 4 units of tea, the monkey always went for the tea. This is the revealed preference evidence.

At the same time, experimenters can collect single neuron recordings from areas that are known to be active in evaluation of rewards (for example, area 13 of the orbito-frontal cortex). They could then plot the average firing rate over several trials (on the y-axis) against the estimated utility of the option that was eventually chosen on the x-axis. One then obtains a clear, monotonic relationship between the two quantities.

A Synthesis

We have now the necessary elements for an attempt to provide a synthesis of the two approaches, one based on economic theory and the other on neuroscience.

Consider a subject who has to choose between two lotteries. When a subject considers each of them, he can assign to it an estimate of the expected utility of each option. This estimate is likely to be noisy. When he has to choose between the two lotteries, he can simply compare the (possibly noisy) estimate of the two utilities, so the choice between the two lotteries is now determined by the comparison of these two values. At this stage, the choice is reduced to the task of comparing of two numerical values, just as the task that the random walk model analyzes.

In summary, this model views the decision process as the result of two components. The first reduces the complex information describing two economic options to a numerical value, the utility of each option; the second performs the comparison between these two quantities, and determines, possibly with an error, the larger of the two. The comparison in this second step is well described by a random walk model of decision.

Risky and Ambiguous Choice

In this final section we illustrate how this theory can provide a simple explanation of the choice behavior of subjects facing a special type of uncertainty: ambiguity. We begin with a precise definition of this idea. Our simple examples of lotteries were meant to illustrate the uncertainty that individuals face in real economic life: any choice is typically between options that promise not certain, but rather random, outcomes. In our examples, the probability over the outcomes was clearly defined: the description of a simple random device (for example, a toss of a coin) would not leave any doubt. But in common real choices, the outcomes do not come with clearly defined probabilities attached. For example, a car insurance is a contract stipulating payments depending on events (car accidents) for which we do not know the exact probability of their occurrence, although we can formulate a subjective estimate of it, or perhaps gather information from actuarial data. When the situation defining the probability of an option is not familiar, the ambiguity of the option may be particularly troubling. For example, an investor considering two different assests may look very different at those of a US company compared to those of a company in Malaysia: the confidence that he has on his forecasts may be fundamentally different in the two cases.

Ambiguity can be produced in experiments by reducing the information available to the subject on the likelihood of the outcomes. For example, he may be told that a lottery L will pay an amount x if a white ball is drawn from an urn containing 90 balls and y if a black one is drawn. He is not told, however, the proportion of black and white balls.

The barrier in the random walk model of choice that we have considered can be interpreted in the case of economic choices as expressing the level of satisfactory evidence which is considered necessary to make a decision. If this level is independent of the quality of the information, then the prediction on response time is clear: when the information is inferior, it would require a longer time to reach the same level of satisfactory evidence. We argue that the information-processing device (the brain) should also consider that inferior information gives a smaller incentive to wait and see. In the random walk model of decision, the trade-off between waiting and the accuracy of the information translates into different distances of the barrier from the initial point of the decision process: a barrier which is farther will require, all else being equal, more time and will allow more accurate evaluation. How should the barrier be set? This depends on the quality of information that the *DM* has. Consider, for example, the case in which the signal observed provides no information at all. Then clearly it is optimal to decide immediately, since observing the signal is not going to improve the quality of the decision. In this case the barrier is very close to the initial starting point of the process. Let us apply this to choices involving risky or ambiguous lotteries. For example, let us compare the situation in which a subject has to choose between a risky lottery and a certain amount to be paid for sure with a similar choice in which the lottery is ambiguous.

In these two types of choice, the quality of the information is different. When the quality is inferior (as in the case of ambiguous choices), the barrier should be closer to the initial point than in the risky choice because the evidence gathered is less useful. So a less informative signal has the effect of reducing the level of evidence considered necessary before the information processing stops and a decision is reached.

The main hypothesis we derive is that the choices made with a less informative signal (an ambiguous lottery compared to a risky one) may induce a shorter response time. Correspondingly, we should observe a weaker activation than those found during choices made with a more informative one. This is exactly what we find in several experimental analyses of choice.

See also: Decision-Making in Financial Markets; Delayed Reinforcement: Economics; Game Theory and the Economics of Animal Communication; Games in Monkeys: Neurophysiology and Motor Decision-Making; Neuroeconomics: History; Reward Decision-Making; Social Cognition.

Further Reading

Block HD and Marschak J (1960) Random orderings and stochastic theories of responses. In: Olkin J, Ghurye S, Hoeffding W, Madow W, and Mann H (eds.) *Contributions to Probability and Statistics*, Stanford: Stanford University Press.

Cartwright D and Festinger L (1943) A quantitative theory of decision. *Psychological Review* 50: 595–621.

Cartwright D (1941) The relation of the decision time to the categories of response. *American Journal of Psychology* 54: 174–196.

Davidson D and Marschak J (1959) Experimental tests of stochastic decision theory. In: West Churchman C (ed.) *Measurament Definitions and Theories*, New York: Wiley.

Debreu G (1958) Stochastic choice and cardinal utility. *Econometrica* 26(3): 440–444.

McFadden D and Richter M (1991) Revealed stochastic preferences. In: Chipman JS, McFadden D, and Richter MK (eds.) *Preferences, Uncertainty and Optimality.* Boulder: Westview Press.

Padoa-Schioppa C and Assad J (2006) Neurons in the orbitofrontal cortex encode economic value. *Nature* 441: 223.

Ratcliff R (1978) A theory of memory retrieval. *Psychological Review* 85: 59–108.

Schall JD (2001) Neural basis of deciding, choosing and acting. *Nature Reviews Neuroscience* 2: 33–42.

Shadlen MN and Newsome WT (1996) Motion perception: Seeing and deciding. *Proceedings of the National Academy of Sciences of the United States of America* 93: 628–633.

Shadlen MN and Newsome WT (2001) Neural basis of a perceptual decision in the parietal cortex (area LIP) of the rhesus monkey. *Journal of Neurophysiology* 86: 1916–1936.

Sigman M and Dehaene S (2005) Parsing a cognitive task: A characterization of mind's bottleneck. *PLoS Biology* 3(2): e37.

Tremblay L and Schultz W (1999) Relative reward preference in primate orbitofrontal cortex. *Nature* 398: 704–708.

Decision-Making and Vision

A K Churchland and M N Shadlen, University of Washington, Seattle, WA, USA

Introduction

Vision involves more than processing the light information received through the eyes. It involves interpreting information, classifying it, drawing inferences, and making decisions about its meaning in the context of goals, plans, and attitudes. The study of visual processing dovetails with the study of cognitive function. When we approach the study of vision from the 'processing' perspective, we tend to ask questions about the mathematical transformations of low-level features, such as contrast contours, to more complex entities, such as depth, motion energy, curvature, texture, objects, and faces. When we approach the topic from the cognitive perspective, we tend to ask questions about how information leads to a behavioral response, inference, or decision. Thus, a central question in the study of both vision and cognition is how the brain processes information to select among different behavioral alternatives. In this article we exploit knowledge about the neurobiology of vision to gain insight into the neurobiology of decision making.

A decision is a commitment to a particular choice or proposition at the expense of competing alternatives. It is usually based on evidence bearing on the likelihood of the alternatives and on the costs and benefits associated with the choices. This blanket formulation applies to complex decisions, like for whom to vote or what car to buy, and to simple ones, like whether to stop or go or whether a note is sharp or flat. The latter type of decision can be studied using the tools of neuroscience, especially those developed to study perception. We think understanding these simple decisions opens a window onto higher brain function in general.

Many decisions involve contingency and deliberation. By contingency, we mean that the process can occur without necessitating a particular outcome. Contingencies defy an 'if A then B' recipe. Instead we are inclined to use the language of probability to describe the outcome, or at least to predict it: if A then probably B, but maybe C or D. Of course, sometimes decisions are based on such overwhelming evidence that one outcome is guaranteed. We might view such decisions as diminutive examples, especially if they are part of a continuum. How we classify such easy decisions is not so important, but as objects of study, they are of limited utility to the neurobiologist. This is because the decision process is hard to separate from the cause and consequence – stimulus and response in the laboratory setting.

By deliberation, we mean that process is guided by more than one piece of information that is acquired from the environment or retrieved from memory over time. Again, not all decisions contain this element, but from a purely practical point of view, if the process of deciding is drawn out over time, it is easier to study. In short, decisions that do not necessitate immediate action can be peeled away from the evidence and outcome of the process. Decisions that incorporate deliberation also necessitate a stratagem for terminating the process. Thus many decisions are really double – they are a decision about the alternatives and a decision to commit based on the current state of knowledge.

The combination of these elements – contingency, deliberation, and a rule for termination – has led to the idea that many decisions are accomplished by a mechanism that accumulates evidence until some criterion level has been achieved. The neurobiology of decision making exploits this condition because it permits exposure of neural responses associated with the decision process and dissociated at least partially from the immediate representation of evidence or the outcome of the decision, typically a motor act. This separation of motor response from sensation – both temporally and logically (via contingency) – is a basic element of higher cognition.

The Basic Accumulator Model for Decisions

In the laboratory, stimuli can be configured so that the evidence for each alternative is present but sometimes weak. These kinds of stimuli are ideally suited to accumulation of evidence. We will describe work from a number of laboratories that have created stimuli of this kind to encourage animals to accumulate evidence over time. However, we are confident that this kind of decision making is not constrained to artificial laboratory situations. As we will detail at the end, a number of ecological situations are well suited to this kind of strategy also.

The premise behind the accumulator model for decision making is that evidence accumulates to better inform the decision. This is not always the case. Which decisions benefit from accumulation of evidence? A reasonable benchmark is the improvement in accuracy expected from an accrual of independent samples of evidence. The simplest example of when accumulation of evidence is beneficial is a process that adds a series of independent values in time. Suppose that a series of independent samples with mean μ and standard deviation σ arrive at rate kt. The accumulated signal at $t = T$ would have a mean μkT and standard deviation $\sigma\sqrt{kT}$. (Recall that the sum of two independent random numbers has mean and variance equal to the sum of the their means and variances, respectively.) Thus the signal-to-noise ratio should improve as $\sqrt{t}$.

If accumulation is truly benefiting the subject in a psychophysical experiment, we might expect the threshold stimulus intensity that is required to achieve some level of accuracy to fall by the square root of the stimulus duration. The graph in **Figure 1** shows results, which conform reasonably well to this prediction. Note that slope of threshold versus viewing duration is very close to -0.5. It is often the case that performance improves at a rate substantially less than what is predicted from the $\sqrt{t}$ relationship. That could be a sign that the samples of evidence (in time) are not independent, or that not all are used, either because there is some forgetfulness (e.g., a leak of an integrator) or that some samples are ignored (e.g., because the process has terminated before all the samples were counted). In other words, a departure from $\sqrt{t}$ does not rule out accumulation.

Formal models of the process just described are termed accumulator models. In these models, a decision variable reflects the evidence accumulated over time (**Figure 2(a)**). Models of this kind are also known

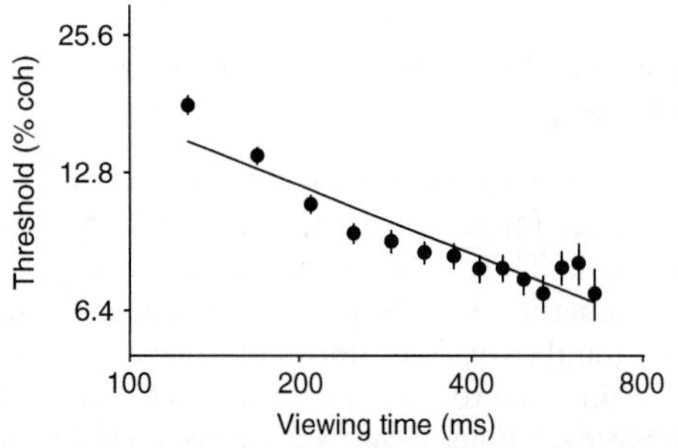

Figure 1 Accuracy improves as a function of viewing time in the motion discrimination task. Each point in the graph was obtained by measuring the monkey's accuracy as a function of motion strength for one viewing duration. From these data, we estimate a threshold: the motion strength required to reach 81% correct. The graph shows that when given extra viewing time, the monkey achieves this level of accuracy with weaker motion strength (coh, coherence). The best fitting line has a slope of –0.46 (95% confidence interval is –0.59 to –0.33). Adpted from Gold JI and Shadlen MN (2003) The influnce of behavioral context on the representation of a perceptual decision in developing oculomotor commands. *Journal of Neuroscience* 23(2): 632–651.

as sequential sampling models because new evidence is added at each moment in time. The rate of accumulation (k) might depend on a number of factors, including the salience of the sensory stimulus being evaluated to make the decision. When a sufficient amount of evidence has been accumulated, the decision variable reaches a threshold value, known as a bound, and the decision process is terminated. The bound provides a reliable way to determine when to cease accumulating evidence and commit to a course of action. When decisions are among two alternative courses of action, the process might be modeled by two accumulators, each accumulating evidence for one alternative (**Figure 2(b)**). And if the evidence for one alternative is evidence against the other, then the race can be conceived as a single process/accumulation terminating in an upper or lower bound, for the two alternatives, respectively (**Figure 2(c)**).

This last scenario is termed a diffusion or random walk to bound model. It has special status in the field of statistical decision making because, under appropriate assumption, it offers the most efficient algorithm for deciding between two alternatives. It also played a key role in Alan Turing's scheme to break the German enigma cipher during World War II. In all cases, a higher bound requires more evidence before the decision process is terminated, while a lower bound requires less evidence. As we will describe, bound height may be somewhat flexible and slowly change depending on the demands of the decisions being made. A variety of accumulator models have been proposed on theoretical grounds or to explain different data sets. Some restrict accumulation to positive quantities, some to positive or negative values drawn from normal distributions; some contain leak and some involve strong interactions between accumulators. Though the details of the models differ, they share a common theme, which is that they attempt to describe both the content of a decision and the time it takes to reach it with a single mechanism. Further, by using a bound to terminate the decision process, accumulator models collectively describe a process that is controlled by internal signals in the brain, rather than by external sensory cues. Here, we highlight differences between kinds of accumulator models only as needed.

We focus on a number of different kinds of decisions that appear to rely on the accumulation of evidence. We begin with perceptual decisions whereby individuals are required to make judgments based on visual stimuli. Next, we describe a simpler kind of decision to act or not. Last, we outline decisions that may be well-described by the accumulation of evidence, but require some key changes to the models described elsewhere in this article.

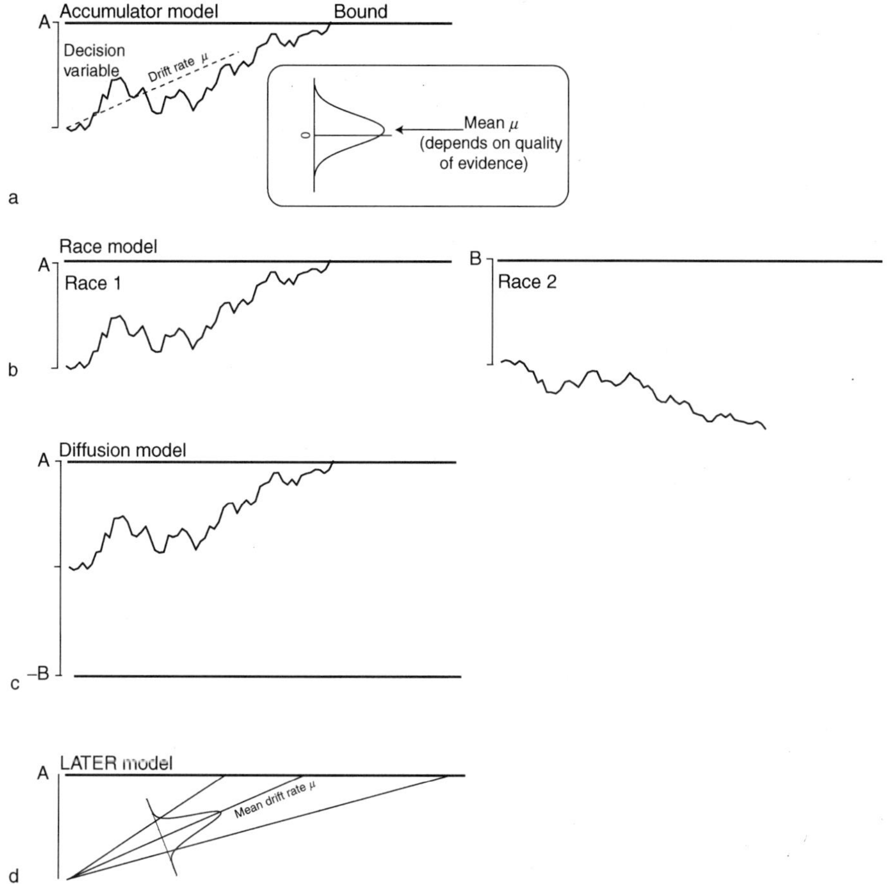

Figure 2 Accumulator models. (a) Basic accumulator model. Samples of momentary 'evidence' are accumulated into a decision variable. The process terminates when the decision variable reaches a bound. The momentary evidence is modeled as a probability distribution with mean μ and variance σ^2 (insert). The decision variable has the appearance of a random walk. The jagged trace shows one example. The average of many such traces would have a slope equal to μ and a variance equal to $n\sigma^2$, where n is the number of samples drawn in time. (b) Race model for decisions between two alternatives. Conventions are the same as in a except that there are two races, one for each possible outcome. Each decision variable is the accumulation of momentary evidence for one of the outcomes. (c) Diffusion model. In a two-choice decision, if the evidence for one choice is evidence against the other, then the two decision variables are identical except for a sign change. The accumulation can be drawn on a single graph with an upper and a lower bound. Horizontal line labeled 'A' reflects the bound for one choice; horizontal line labeled 'B' reflects the bound for the other choice. (d) The LATER (linear accumulation to threshold with ergodic rate) model for decisions to 'go' or not. The decision signal rises linearly from a starting point until the bound is reached. The rate of rise during this time varies from trial to trial and can rise slowly (thin, shallow line), at an intermediate rate (medium line), or quickly (thin, steep line). The variability in slope explains reaction time variability. The linear rise approximates the accumulation of a fixed value, which is drawn from a normal (Gaussian) distribution on each trial. The slopes are therefore normally distributed and so are the reciprocals of the reaction times.

Simple Perceptual Decisions

Behavioral Observations

Considerable behavioral evidence suggests that both humans and monkeys suffer more errors when they make decisions quickly. In a recent study by our group, humans performed a random-dot motion-discrimination task. Individuals viewed a dynamic random-dot kinematogram and decided the net direction of motion of the dots. Some of the dots moved together, in the same direction, while the remaining dots moved randomly. On each trial, the percentage of dots moving in the same direction, termed the coherence, was set to make the trial easy or more difficult. In our version of the task, individuals terminated the dot motion when they were ready with a decision by making an eye movement to one of two choice targets (**Figure 3(a)**). Accuracy (percentage of trials whereby the individual correctly reported the direction of motion) and speed (reaction time) were measured

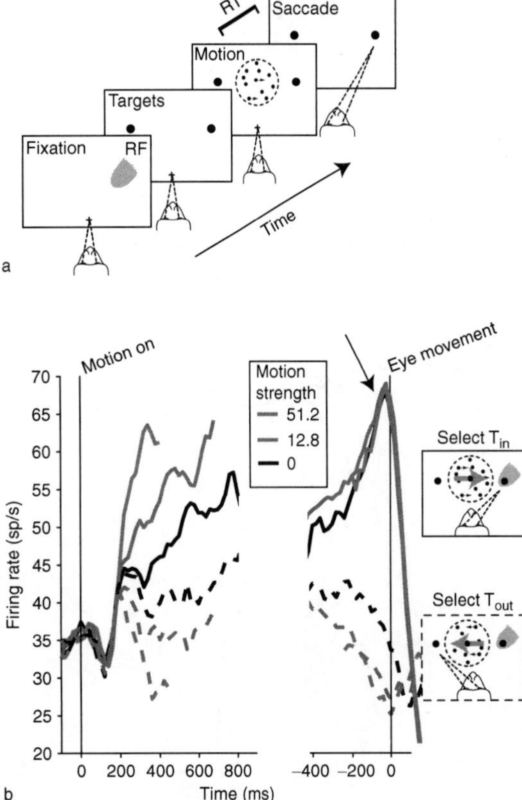

Figure 3 A neural correlate of a decision variable. (a) Reaction-time (RT) direction-discrimination task. A random-dot motion task is used to study decision making in humans and monkeys. The task begins with the appearance of a fixation point and two choice targets. After a random interval, a patch of moving dots appears. Some of the dots in the stimulus move coherently in the same direction while the remaining dots move randomly. When the individual is ready with a decision, he terminates the trial by making a saccade to one of two choice targets. When monkeys are performing the task, they are rewarded for correct responses with a drop of juice or water. (b) Average response from 54 lateral intraparietal area neurons on the direction-discrimination task. The firing rates (sp/s, spikes/second) of neurons in the lateral intraparietal area were measured while the monkey performed a RT version of the random-dot direction-discrimination task shown in (a). In each experiment, one of the choice targets was in the neuron's response field. Responses are grouped by motion strength (line color) and the choice the monkey made at the end of the trial in favor of the direction associated with the target in (T_{in}; solid) or out (T_{out}; dashed) of the neuron's response field. The responses are aligned to two events in the trial. On the left, responses are aligned to the onset of stimulus motion. Response averages in this portion of the graph are drawn to the median RT for each motion strength and exclude any activity within 100 ms of eye movement initiation. On the right, responses are aligned to initiation of the eye movement response. Response averages in this portion of the graph show the buildup and decline in activity at the end of the decision process. Only correct choices are included in these graphs for motion coherences >0%. Arrow indicates the approximate time at which responses to different coherences coalesce for T_{in} choices. From Roitman JD and Shadlen MN (2002) Response of neurons in the lateral intraparietal area during a combined visual discrimination reaction time task. *Journal of Neuroscience* 22: 9475–9489.

both when individuals were given no instructions about reaction time and when they were instructed to aim for a specified reaction time on the most difficult trials. Both individuals were able to comply with the instructions, and their reaction times changed accordingly. Changes in accuracy accompanied the changes in speed: when a fast reaction time was specified, both responded quickly, but both made more errors and hence had reduced accuracy.

An accumulator model described the individuals' behavior well, and also helped explain how both speed and accuracy changed with instruction. Because the model was required to account for both speed and accuracy with a single mechanism, it provided a stringent test of accumulator models. The model successfully described the behavior; further, changes in each of the model's three parameters were examined to see whether the model could produce the behavioral effects that were observed: rate of accumulation and bound height (both described previously) as well as residual time (an additional contributor to response latencies meant to encompass sensory and motor delays that are not part of the decision process). There was little change to drift rate and residual time when the speed–accuracy trade-off changed. Instead, changes in the speed–accuracy trade-off were best explained by changes in bound height. Specifically, when the individuals had fast reaction times and low accuracy, they had a low bound height, and when they had slow reaction times and high accuracy, they had a high bound height. Intuitively, this makes sense: increasing the bound height can be thought of as raising one's standards for how certain one has to be in order to make a decision. Raising one's standards improves performance, but it also takes more time. Similar findings have been obtained by BA Reddi and colleagues.

Notice that the rate of evidence accumulation – that is, the average drift rate of the decision variable – is governed by the intensity of stimulus motion. In contrast, the level of the bounds is controlled by the brain. J Palmer and co-workers showed that this level governs the trade-off between speed and accuracy. That may yield important insights into why performance may be different among individuals or even for the same individual under different circumstances. Unless decision time is measured, it is possible that the reason for poor performance is a low level for the bound. Put simply, the decision maker might ignore useful information because the brain has already come to the end of the decision process. This also accounts for improvements in performance that fall below the expected $\sqrt{t}$ improvement.

The brain might employ deeper principles to set the bound. For example, it has been suggested that the bound could be set to maximize the overall rate of harvesting reward. RY Cho and colleagues tested this using a variant of the choice-reaction-time (RT) motion task. Reaction time as a function of error rate for a number of different task difficulties (coherences) was measured and was observed to be very close to that of an optimal estimator for some individuals. The estimator took into account the overall reward rate, which depended on the individual's reaction time, error rate, and the intertrial interval. Although not all of the individuals tested appeared to have adopted an optimal strategy, the close match between the optimal estimator and the best 30% of individuals suggests that neural systems may invest in trying to find the speed–accuracy trade-off that maximizes reward.

Taken together, these behavioral studies provide evidence for accumulators by demonstrating that the time it takes to reach a decision is linked to the accuracy of that decision. The model is not without its drawbacks. For example, in its simplest form, it fails to account for the RT on error trials, and it tends to overestimate the degree of skew seen in the distribution of RTs measured experimentally. A variety of extensions have been proposed to remedy these failures. In our view, they should not allow us to lose sight of the essential computational principle. The appeal of the accumulator model is that it provides an explanation for both choice and decision time, using a single mechanism – hence their success in a wide variety of decision tasks, including brightness discrimination, letter discrimination, and lexical decisions.

Physiological Observations

The key features of the accumulator model have been observed in neural recordings obtained from awake monkeys while they performed the choice-RT direction-discrimination task. Monkeys perform this task almost identically to the way humans do. Just as in the Palmer experiments with humans, monkeys indicated their decisions about direction by making a saccadic eye movement to a 'choice target.' By recording from neurons that encode one of the choice targets – its salience, importance, or the fact that it will be a target of an upcoming eye movement – it is possible to observe a neural correlate of an evolving decision during the period in which it is formed. Recordings from several brain areas have shed light on the process, but only one area has been studied during the choice-RT version of the random-dot motion task.

Neurons in the lateral intraparietal (LIP) area are candidates for providing evidence for the neural basis of accumulator models. Area LIP receives input from sensory areas (middle temporal (MT) and medial superior (MST) areas) that are sensitive to the motion stimulus used in the task. Further, it projects to areas known to play a role in the generation of saccadic eye movements. The position of area LIP in a sensory-motor middle ground suggests it is suited to participate in decisions that use incoming sensory information to make choices about outgoing movements. LIP neurons are selective for the direction of a saccade, so they respond more vigorously on decisions when the choice target is in the neuron's response field relative to when the choice target is in the opposite hemifield. In other words, their firing rates indicate the outcome of the monkey's decision on the motion task. However, the dynamics of the LIP response in the period leading up to the saccade suggest that these neurons play a role in the formation of the decision.

There is a gradual change in firing rates of LIP neurons in the period between onset of random-dot motion and the end of the decision process signaled by an eye movement. These changes are depicted by the traces in **Figure 3(b)**. These traces are averages from many neurons over many trials. All of the solid traces correspond to trials that ended with an eye movement to the target in the neuron's response field (T_{in}). All of the dashed traces correspond to trials that ended with an eye movement to the opposite target (T_{out}). Not surprisingly, at the end of the decision, when the monkey is about to make an eye movement, the responses are clearly larger for T_{in} choices than for T_{out} choices (compare solid to dashed curves). In fact, the responses look like they reach the same firing rate, regardless of motion strength for all of the T_{in} choices (arrow). At the beginning of the trial, when the motion is first turned on, the responses are nearly identical for all choices and for all motion strengths.

What is happening in area LIP between the onset of random-dot motion and the eye movement response? In the first 100 ms after the dots appear there is a dip in the firing rate. This dip does not depend on the direction and strength of the motion, and it is the same regardless of the choice. It seems to signal the beginning of the decision process, but there is no sign yet of an accumulation of evidence for the T_{in} or T_{out} choice. The first sign that the neurons are affected by the direction of motion occurs ~200 ms after onset of the motion, when the solid and dashed curves begin to separate. From this point forward, the trajectories represent the accumulation of evidence for and against the T_{in} choice. When the motion is strong and toward T_{in} (solid orange), the evidence from the visual cortex is overwhelmingly positive: the accumulation has a large positive slope. When the motion is strong and toward T_{out} (dashed orange), the evidence is overwhelmingly negative: the accumulation has a large negative slope. When the motion is weak, the evidence is less definitive and the accumulation has a smaller positive (for T_{in} choices) or negative (for T_{out} choices) slope.

Consider the case when the motion is entirely ambiguous (0% coherence motion). From moment to moment, the direction-selective neurons in the visual cortex are providing evidence that is sometimes positive and sometimes negative, but whatever the sign, the evidence is weak. The accumulation of such evidence is a random walk that meanders away from its starting point in either the positive or the negative direction. The average of all such random walks would be a flat line with zero slope. But we have sorted the responses in accordance with the monkey's choices. According to the accumulator model, the trials that end in a T_{in} choice (**Figure 3 (b)**; solid dark blue) are those random walks that happen to wander to high firing rates – high enough to reach the bound (threshold) that terminates the decision process. The average of this half of the data should have a positive slope, and that is exactly what we see in **Figure 3(b)**. The other half of the trials ended in a T_{out} choice. According to the accumulator model, these are the random walks that never wandered far enough in the positive direction to cause a T_{in} choice. Instead, the decision terminated when the LIP neurons with the other target in their response field (our neurons' T_{out}) reached a high firing rate. Accordingly, this half of the data should appear to meander in a somewhat negative direction. That is exactly what we see in the dashed dark blue curve. The intermediate motion strengths (light blue) can be understood in much the same way.

The hallmarks of evidence accumulation and bound crossing just described are present in LIP neurons. First, as the monkey watches the motion stimulus, LIP neurons undergo ramplike changes in firing rate (**Figure 3(b)**, left panel). Importantly, responses to motion that is in the direction of the monkey's response field ramp up progressively at a buildup rate that is dependent on the quality of the evidence – the motion coherence. Around the time of the saccade, neural responses that have diverged, as a function of motion strength, coalesce to a common firing rate. About 70 ms after the responses come together, the saccade is executed (**Figure 3(b)**, right panel). This is a signature of the bound: when the firing rate of the LIP neurons reaches a critical value, the decision process ends with a decision in favor of the direction associated with the choice target in the neuron's response field. On the other hand, when the monkey chooses the opposite direction, the responses do not achieve a stereotyped level (**Figure 3(b)**, right panel, dashed curves). This observation suggests that these choices do not occur when the spike rate reaches a lower bound. Rather, the absence of a stereotyped termination value suggests that another process terminates the decision, presumably neurons with the chosen target in their response field. The observation thus supports a race between accumulators, like LIP neurons with each of the choice targets in their response fields, rather than the diffusion model in **Figure 2(c)**.

An accumulation to threshold model is able to reproduce the firing rate dynamics of LIP neurons well. Further studies have suggested that the momentary evidence that is accumulated in area LIP comes from a difference signal in area MT, that the accumulation represented in area LIP appears to be through a process resembling integration, and that LIP activity appears to be causally linked to the monkey's choice and response time.

Decision-related activity resembling the patterns in **Figure 3** have been observed in a number of brain areas for a variety of tasks. A gradual rise and decline in firing rates during decision making has been reported in the superior colliculus (SC), frontal eye field (FEF), and dorsolateral prefrontal cortex in studies using the random-dots task, although these studies did not measure reaction times. There is some evidence from human functional magnetic resonance imaging (fMRI) studies that a similar process underlies decision making in the human brain. In the SC, where neurons are associated with saccade-related and preparatory activity, responses of monkeys performing a two-choice position-identification task are related to reaction times and perhaps accuracy. And, in premotor cortex, responses appear to reflect different stages of the decision process when monkeys are engaged in a somatosensory discrimination task. Whether an accumulation to threshold model can explain the neural responses and behavior in all of these systems is not yet known.

Deciding to 'Go'

The behavioral and physiological observations thus far have been about perceptual decisions. However, accumulator models have been successful at describing even simpler decisions: whether to make a particular movement or not. These decisions arise when the evidence is overwhelming for one choice, or in which there is only one possible choice. In that case, the only real decision is whether to go or not. Such decisions take more time than one would expect based on simple sensory and motor latencies. Even a simple eye movement to a single target takes ~200 ms to initiate, and there is a lot of variability in this response time from trial to trial. RHS Carpenter has championed the idea that this variable latency furnishes contingency – the possibility of doing something else – thereby imbuing even a simple motor act with the seeds of higher brain function.

A simple accumulator model has been proposed to describe these kinds of decisions. In this model, known as LATER (linear accumulation to threshold with ergodic rate), a decision signal rises linearly from a starting point until it reaches a threshold. Because (1) these decisions take very little time and (2) the accumulation is mainly positive, the process can be described very simply as a ramp with variable slope (**Figure 2(d)**). It is very easy to see from the geometry in **Figure 2(d)** that the distribution of decision times will have its median where the mean accumulation ramp intersects the bound. The distribution of decision times will be skewed to the right. Indeed, if the distribution of ramp slopes is Gaussian, then the reciprocals of decision times will also obey a Gaussian distribution.

Because the LATER model primarily describes reaction times (i.e., how long it takes to reach the bound) rather than accuracy, it is well suited to decisions about when and whether to 'go.' The simple model has been exploited to study the role of prior probability (i.e., bias), urgency, and stimulus strength on the decision process. Bias might arise when there is some uncertainty about which action is about to be instructed. Urgency refers to a time pressure on initiation after an instruction to go. Stimulus strength might be something like the intensity of the instruction or the ease of its interpretation, much like the coherence of random-dot motion. These studies exploit the change in the median reaction time and the shape of the distribution to gain insight into the process. It seems that bias and urgency affect the height of the bound in **Figure 2(d)**, whereas stimulus intensity affects the rate or rise – what we would term the evidence accumulation.

This simple idea has been elaborated slightly to incorporate a race between two processes. As we have already noted, when there are two or more options, it may be sensible to conceive of two or more accumulators that reach a decision point, thus committing the organism to acting and selecting. In our view, the LATER type of accumulation makes sense when a single random number can effectively characterize the rate of accumulation. This will tend to be true when decision times are short and/or when the momentary evidence is the same at each moment in time. These conditions do not hold in the motion experiments reviewed earlier, but they do hold in some circumstances.

The countermanding task is a case in point. In countermanding, a second 'stop' signal instructs an individual to cancel a movement in the period between the onset of any eye movement target and movement initiation. When the stop signal is presented a long time before the individual is to make a saccade, the movement is easily withheld. However, when the stop signal occurs close to the time when the individual makes his saccade, the individual is sometimes unable to withhold the movement. The decision to go or cancel is well described by a race between a go and a stop signal.

There is physiological support of the kind of simple rise of a decision variable to a threshold, as postulated by LATER, to explain decisions to go. DP Hanes and JD Schall showed that movement neurons in the FEF exhibit a rapid rise in firing rate just before eye movement begins. These neurons, which are known to project to brain stem oculomotor structures, undergo a linear rise in firing rate after a target appears to instruct an eye movement. Hanes and Schall showed that the saccadic reaction times measured in monkeys could be explained by the rate of this rise in firing rate (**Figure 4**). Moreover, the firing rate reached a common value ~10–20 ms before the eye movement began, consistent with the presence of a threshold for initiation (**Figure 4**).

In countermanding, Hanes and Schall showed that these movement neurons also fail to achieve a critical level of discharge rate on trials in which the monkey successfully cancels a saccade. When the 'stop' signal comes too late and the saccade ensues, the FEF movement cells discharge as they do for saccades. This provides partial evidence for the type of race model hypothesized to underlie the decision process in countermanding. Indeed, a putative neural correlate of the other race – the stop signal – has been observed in the FEF and SC. However, the evidence for an accumulator-race model is still preliminary. It rests on the observation that fixation cells fire more and movement cells fire less when an eye movement is canceled. This is hardly surprising: by definition, the fixation cell responds when the animal does not make an eye movement. Thus, the argument that these cells participate in a race rests on subtle comparisons of firing rates in epochs predicted by the computational theory.

It seems secure that a rise in firing rate to a threshold level will account for the variable interval between

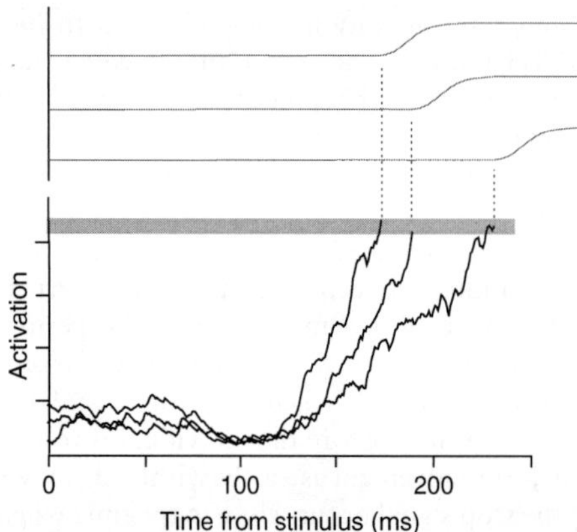

Figure 4 A neural correlate of a decision to go. Responses from a neuron in the FEF were recorded while a monkey made saccadic eye movements to a peripheral target. The three responses accompanied saccades to the same visual target in the response field of the neuron. Eye position traces (gray traces, top) show that the eye movements were nearly identical in amplitude, duration, and velocity but occurred at short, intermediate, and long latencies after the instruction to go. The firing rate began to increase at roughly the same latency from onset of the target (go signal), but the rate of increase was faster for the shorter latency saccades. Notice that the firing rate reaches a common value (horizontal gray bar) just preceding saccade initiation, consistent with the basic accumulator and LATER models in **Figures 2(a)** and **2(d)**. Adapted from Schall JD and Bichot NP (1998) Neural correlates of visual and motor decision processes. *Current Opinion in Neurobiology* 8: 211–217.

the onset of a visual target and movement initiation. It remains to be seen what role neurons in the FEF and other candidate structures play. Responses in the LIP, FEF, and SC can be altered by prior probability, reward expectation, uncertainty, and urgency, but it remains to be seen whether these responses interact with accumulation in the manner prescribed by LATER.

Limitations and Extensions of Accumulator Models

Certain kinds of tasks are less well suited to the simplest form of accumulator models. Some might necessitate modifications to the models in **Figure 2**, whereas others may simply require a different mechanism altogether. Simply put, accumulating evidence as it arrives in time is not always an optimal strategy for decision making. For example, when attempting to detect a relevant stimulus that occurs at an unpredictable time, accumulating evidence may be a poor strategy. If the brain were to accumulate evidence at the start of the trial, it might accumulate nothing but noise for the lengthy period of time while no stimulus is present. The accumulation of noise would cause a decision variable like the one depicted in **Figure 1** to drift away from the starting point (in a random walk) toward one of the bounds, before the relevant information is even present. Not surprisingly, visual detection tasks typically do not appear to be mediated by the kind of accumulation strategies discussed here. When attempting to detect a low-contrast visual stimulus, humans perform only slightly better when the stimulus is presented for a longer durations. Up to $\sim$80 ms, there is very clear improvement, as if stimulus intensity were accumulating in time (a phenomenon known as Bloch's law). But longer durations support only modest improvement in sensitivity. The improvement is explained by assuming that there is no accumulation of signal at all, but that longer viewing durations afford more independent opportunities to detect the stimulus. More opportunities decrease the probability that the stimulus will be missed.

Even without accumulation, it is possible to preserve the architecture of decision mechanism in **Figure 2** for detection tasks. A time-varying decision variable is compared to a threshold in a race against other competing interpretations. Suppose the accumulation of momentary evidence is not perfect, but 'leaks' away. This way, even if noise causes the decision variable to drift toward one of the bounds, it will return to a neutral position fairly quickly. In principle, such a leaky accumulator could obey a time constant appropriately matched to the time course of the signals it is trying to detect – in other words, those governed by physiological responses to the visual stimulus. This approach has been championed with great success in psychophysics and cognitive decision making.

There is some evidence for this type of decision mechanism in neurophysiology. EP Cook and JH Maunsell trained monkeys to detect the onset of coherent motion. The monkey stared at a fixation point while random dots appeared in a patch of a video display. At the beginning of each trial, the dot display was completely random, like the 0% coherence condition in the discrimination task described earlier. On half of the trials, the motion became coherent after a random time interval. The monkey released a lever to indicate that he detected the coherent motion. Cook and Maunsell recorded from direction-selective neurons in area MT and the ventral intraparietal (VIP) area while the monkey performed the detection tasks. Neurons in area MT are strongly selective for the direction of stimulus motion when it is presented in a part of the visual field known as a neuron's receptive field. Neurons in area VIP receive a strong input from MT neurons and many exhibit responses that are selective for the direction of motion as well. The patch of random dots was aligned to the neuron's response field and the motion was in the direction that would cause an increase in firing rate. Indeed, on trials in which the patch changed to coherent motion, the neurons increased their firing rates. The monkey detected the change when the instantaneous firing rate exceeded a criterion level. Importantly, the detection decision does not appear to be based on an accumulation of the MT response but rather on an instantaneous measure of firing rate. This makes sense because the brain cannot know when to begin accumulating evidence. (The actual estimate of instantaneous firing rate, whether performed by the brain or in data analysis, is achieved by smoothing the time series of spikes using a filter. The process can be described as leaky integration, but this should not be confused with accumulation.)

Accumulation of evidence in time may be misguided for other kinds of decisions as well. For example, some decisions involve comparing information across time. It would be detrimental to accumulate information in the time gap between two stimulus presentations. There is a need for some flexible control of integration in neural circuits. Indeed, as evidenced by R Romeo and colleagues in a two-interval vibrotactile comparison, neurons in the prefrontal cortex appear to encode both the vibration of the first stimulus, its memory in the time gap before a second comparison stimulus, and then the accumulation of evidence as the second stimulus is compared to the first. Clearly this requires an elaboration of the accumulation models depicted in **Figure 1**. On the other hand, storage (i.e., working memory) and accumulation are close cousins. Both rest on integration in the calculus sense, for both involve a stable value at a particular moment based on the history of inputs up until that moment. In this sense, working memory is just an accumulation of an impulse. In principle, a common mechanism might underlie both working memory and accumulation of evidence. Thus investigating not only the circuits involved in decisions, but also the cellular mechanisms of the neurons in those circuits, will be illuminating.

Real-World Decisions

The simple accumulator model will need to be elaborated to handle more complex decisions. There is some evidence that it can explain choice and decision times in decisions that are more complicated than a direction discrimination. However, a critical limitation is that samples of momentary evidence are accumulated in a single number, what we term a decision variable. But some decisions involve combining apples and oranges: perhaps evidence arrives from two different sensory modalities. One possible solution is that the brain does not accumulate raw evidence but rather evidence as it bears on a decision. For example, evidence from different sources may be more or less reliable. Studies of human perception and action suggest that the brain can combine such evidence by giving appropriate weights to the more and less reliable sources. The simple accumulators in **Figure 2** need to be elaborated to explain such observations.

Certainly much work is still needed to bridge the gap between simple decision making in the laboratory and complex decision making in the real world. However, it would be a mistake to think that the kinds of mechanisms that have successfully described decision making so far would be ill suited to decisions in a more natural context. Some interesting examples from ecology suggest that animals accumulate evidence for and against particular choices. In prey selection, for example, a predator may observe a number of potential prey before making a decision about which to choose. Wolves are known to do this, and it is a strategy which greatly assists their hunting: a wolf might survey a herd of moose, for example, for quite some time, taking into account each animal's age, size, physical health, and even dental health before launching an attack. Making a choice too quickly could be detrimental to a wolf because a young healthy moose can retaliate quite effectively, injuring or even killing a wolf. This kind of decision making raises the question of how accumulators might work on different timescales. The difference between a LIP neuron responding to dot motion for about 800 ms and a wolf surveying his prey for several hours or even days is considerable. Nevertheless, these ecological observations suggest that animals in the wild might accumulate evidence and fine-tune speed–accuracy trade-offs the same way that monkeys and human subjects do in a laboratory setting.

See also: Contextual Interactions in Visual Perception; Contextual Interactions in Visual Processing; Retina: An Overview; Vision for Action and Perception; Vision: Light and Dark Adaptation; Visual–Vestibular Interactions.

Further Reading

Carpenter R and Williams M (1995) Neural computation of log likelihood in control of saccadic eye movements. *Nature* 377: 59–62.

Colby CL, Duhamel JR, and Goldberg ME (1993) Ventral intraparietal area of the macaque: Anatomic location and visual response properties. *Journal of Neurophysiology* 69: 902–914.

Cook EP and Maunsell JH (2002) Dynamics of neuronal responses in macaque MT and VIP during motion detection. *Nature Neuroscience* 5: 985–994.

Ernst MO and Banks MS (2002) Humans integrate visual and haptic information in a statistically optimal fashion. *Nature* 415: 429–433.

Gold IJ and Shalden MN (2003) The influence of behavioral context on the representation of a perceptual decision in developing oculomotor commands. *Journal of Neuroscience* 23(2): 632–651.

Gold JI and Shalden MN The neural basis of decision making. *Annual Review Neuroscience* 30 (in press).

Good IJ (1979) Studies in the history of probability and statistics. XXXVII A.M. Turing's statistical work in World War II. *Biometrika* 66: 393–396.

Hanes DP and Schall JD (1996) Neural control of voluntary movement initiation. *Science* 274: 427–430.

Hanks TD, Ditterich J, and Shadlen MN (2006) Microstimulation of macaque area LIP affects decision-making in a motion discrimination task. *Nature Neuroscience* 9: 682–689.

Heekeren HR, Marrett S, Bandettini PA, et al. (2004) A general mechanism for perceptual decision-making in the human brain. *Nature* 431: 859–862.

Link SE (1992) *Wave Theory of Differnce and Similarity.* Hillsdade, NJ: Earlbaum Associates.

Link SW and Heath RA (1975) A sequential theory of psychological discrimination. *Psychometrika* 40: 77–105.

Machens CK, Romo R, and Brody CD (2005) Flexible control of mutual inhibition: A neural model of two-interval discrimination. *Science* 307: 1121–1124.

Palmer J, Huk AC, and Shadlen MN (2005) The effect of stimulus strength on the speed and accuracy of a perceptual decision. *Journal of Vision* 5: 376–404.

Platt ML and Glimcher PW (1999) Neural correlates of decision variables in parietal cortex. *Nature* 400: 233–238.

Ratcliff R and Rouder JN (1998) Modeling response times for two-choice decisions. *Psychological Science* 9: 347–356.

Reddi BA, Asrress KN, and Carpenter RH (2003) Accuracy, information, and response time in a saccadic decision task. *Journal of Neurophysiology* 90: 3538–3546.

Roitman JD and Shadlen MN (2002) Response of neurons in the lateral intraparietal area during a combined visual discrimination reaction time task. *Journal of Neuroscience* 22: 9475–9489.

Romo R, Hernandez A, and Zainos A (2004) Neuronal correlates of a perceptual decision in ventral premotor cortex. *Neuron* 41: 165–173.

Schall JD and Bichot NP (1998) Neurol correlates of visual and motor decision processes. *Current Opinion in Neurobiology* 8: 211–217.

Shadlen MN and Newsome WT (2001) Neural basis of a perceptual decision in the parietal cortex (area LIP) of the rhesus monkey. *Journal of Neurophysiology* 86: 1916–1936.

Sugrue LP, Corrado GS, and Newsome WT (2004) Matching behavior and the representation of value in the parietal cortex. *Science* 304: 1782–1787.

Watson AB (1986) Temporal sensitivity. In: Boff KR, Kaufman L, and Thomas JP (eds.) *Handbook of Perception and Human Performance*, pp. 6.1–6.43. New York: Wiley.

Decision-Making in Financial Markets

P Bossaerts, California Institute of Technology, Pasadena, CA, USA

Finance

Financial markets are a relatively recent phenomenon. They are markets where agents trade claims to future monetary payoffs, commonly referred to as securities or assets. Almost invariably, the payoffs are uncertain. That is, they entail financial risk. The first modern organized financial market was set up in Antwerp, in the lower countries (present-day Belgium), in 1460. At the time, the securities were claims on future payments by established buyers of goods and services, as well as sovereigns. Only much later (around the middle of the nineteenth century) was the type of asset – namely, equity – that most people would be familiar with in modern-day financial markets introduced. Equity, or common stock, is a claim on the residual earnings of firms, which means that the holder is entitled to the cash flow of the firm after the firm pays all debtors (which includes suppliers, employees, and banks). Much more recently, derivative securities were introduced (although many of them were already occasionally traded by the Dutch in the sixteenth century). These are claims on the payoffs on other securities. Options constitute the classical example of derivatives. Nowadays, a bewildering variety of securities are traded on and off organized exchanges.

Finance studies the behavior of agents when faced with financial risk, as well as the pricing of such risk in markets. Finance is both descriptive (why are prices the way they are?) and normative (how to compute optimal portfolios?). In many respects, finance is a subfield of economics, but there are a couple of features that really set it apart. The differences will be discussed shortly, because they may lead to fresh insights for neuroscience. Far more than economics, finance relies on probability theory. This is not surprising: early developments of probability theory derived from attempts to understand monetary games, as exemplified by Pascal's proposal for computing winning odds. That is, probability theory originated in many respects from efforts to formalize financial risk.

Many Facets of Risk

One dimension in which finance and economics differ substantially is that the former explicitly deals with the many facets of risk. Rather than summarizing the attractiveness of monetary gambles in terms of a single-dimensional index, ever since the work of Harry Markowitz, in the early 1950s, finance scholars have represented risk in terms of expected payoff, payoff variance, skewness, and even kurtosis. These constitute mathematical characterizations of payoff distributions. The expected payoff is just the mean payoff that one anticipates. The variance is the (square of the) typical ('standard') deviation from the mean. The skewness measures whether payoffs below the mean are more likely (negative skewness) or not (positive skewness). Kurtosis measures to what extent extreme payoffs (both above and below the mean) are more likely, compared to a benchmark payoff distribution – namely, the well-known bell-shaped gaussian distribution.

Analyzing Risky Payoffs

Let p_t denote the payoff on a monetary gamble in trial period t. Let x_t denote the anticipated, or expected, payoff. Mathematically:

$$x_t = \mathrm{E}[p_t]$$

where E denotes the expectations operator (whereby all possible outcomes are multiplied by their respective probabilities and summed). The payoff variance is defined as follows:

$$v_t = \mathrm{E}[(p_t - x_t)^2]$$

So, the payoff variance is the anticipated deviation from the expected payoff.

The skewness is defined as the expectation of the third-order power of the difference from the expected payoff:

$$\phi_t = \mathrm{E}[(p_t - x_t)^3]$$

The kurtosis is proportional to the fourth-order power:

$$\kappa_t \sim \mathrm{E}[(p_t - x_t)^4]$$

(The constant of proportionality is such that the kurtosis of a gaussian random variable equals 3, independent of its expected outcome and its variance.) Like variance, skewness and kurtosis are anticipated deviations from the expected payoff, but negative deviations are counted separately in computing skewness (because the third power of a negative number is negative, unlike the second and fourth powers), and the fourth power with which the kurtosis is computed effectively puts a heavy weight on outliers.

While there may be many other facets of risk, finance in general limits its attention to these four relationships. In the case of common stock, often only the first two (expected payoff and payoff variance) are considered (see **Figure 1**). It is known, however, that expected payoff and payoff variance provide an incomplete description of the risk of other securities, such as options. Humans are sensitive to skewness and kurtosis as well, and the most convincing way to confirm this is to consider the prices of options, which include huge premia for the skewness and the kurtosis of their payoffs.

Economists take a different approach. Ever since Bernoulli proposed logarithmic expected utility, economists have generally insisted on representing the attractiveness of risky gambles in terms of a single-dimensional index. There are very few exceptions. Even the celebrated Prospect Theory remains a representation of preferences in terms of a single-dimensional expected utility index. In Prospect Theory, the index is basically a multiplication of (subjective) probabilities of each of the possible payoffs with their respective utilities (nonlinear transformations of the payoffs). Of course, one can justify the finance approach in terms of a mathematical operation on expected utility – namely, a Taylor series expansion in terms of expectation, variance, skewness, and kurtosis. As such, an agent with logarithmic expected utility (i.e., Bernoulli's agent) prefers higher expected return, is averse to variance, prefers positive skewness (while averse to negative skewness), and is averse to kurtosis.

But the Taylor series approach is by no means necessary. Moreover, by not insisting that monetary gambles are ranked in terms of a single-dimensional index, one avoids properties that many would find counterintuitive. For instance, in expected utility theory and its variations (such as Prospect Theory), there is a tight relationship between the curvature of the utility function and risk aversion. In particular, the degree to which the utility function becomes less curved as wealth increases and, hence, the degree to which utility of an extra dollar decreases with wealth determine one's risk aversion. The faster the utility of an extra dollar decreases, the more risk averse one is. As such, fear of uncertainty is tied to decreasing utility for (certain!) extra monetary units, a rather counterintuitive property (see **Figure 2**).

After it was introduced in the 1950s, the finance 'mean-variance' approach proved extremely useful for determining optimal portfolios of securities. Indeed, it is rather complicated mathematically to

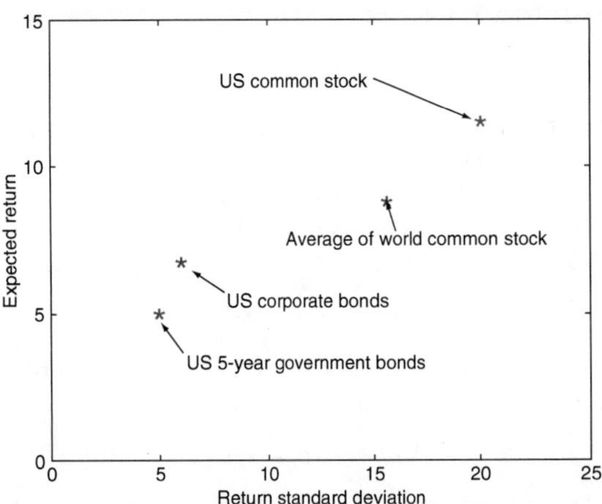

Figure 1 Trade-off between expected payoff and payoff standard deviation (square root of variance) from investing in several asset classes, based on historical data from 1926 to 2004. Payoffs are expressed in percentage returns (i.e., in percent per dollar invested). Returns are computed from investing at the end of the year and selling at the end of the subsequent year. Notice the trade-off: higher expected returns (e.g., on US common stock) imply higher risk (higher payoff variance). The degree to which one requires higher expected payoffs in order to be willing to accept higher risk measures one's risk aversion. Based on data from Center for Research in Security Prices of the University of Chicago.

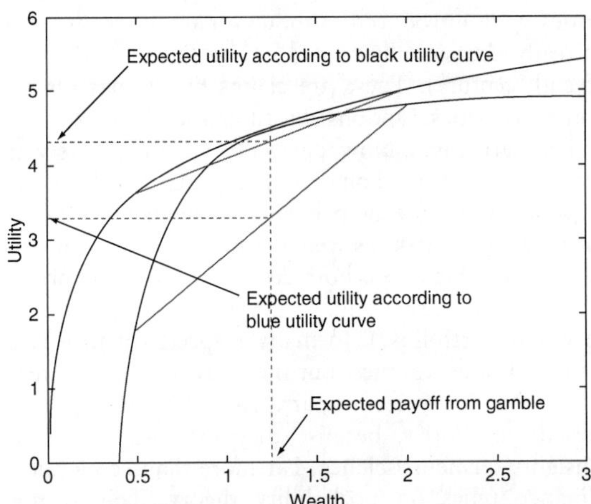

Figure 2 Effect of curvature of the utility function on risk aversion in the context of expected utility preferences. Shown are two utility functions. The black one is less curved than the blue one, in the sense that the degree to which additional utility of a dollar decreases with wealth is smaller for the former. This translates into lower risk aversion: the expected utility of a gamble that pays 0.5 or 2 with equal chance is higher for the black utility curve than for the blue one, implying that a person with the black utility function is willing to pay more for the gamble compared to someone with the blue utility curve. Using a simple geometric trick, the expected utility can readily be located by intersecting the vertical line through the expected payoff (vertical dotted red line) and the chord that connects the utility of the low payoff (0.5) with that of the high payoff (2) (solid red lines).

analyze the attractiveness of simultaneous risky gambles with correlated risks if one insists on, say, logarithmic expected utility, let alone Prospect Theory. In contrast, the properties of optimal portfolios in a simple mean-variance framework are very intuitive, and, after their discovery, led to profound insights in the 1960s about the pricing of risk in financial markets. In particular, it was realized that financial markets would not compensate investors for the entire risk as measured by a security's payoff variance, but only to the extent the payoff covaries (correlates) with the payoff on all other available securities. The covariation risk has become known as the 'beta' risk of a security. Laboratory experiments have demonstrated that the principle is correct. In such experiments, groups of human participants trade securities over anonymous, electronic markets. The securities are short-lived and their payoff patterns are deliberately kept simple and intuitive.

But there are other reasons why the finance approach is convenient. Among other things, it allows one to describe risk differences in very intuitive, statistical terms, and it facilitates learning. Both properties are relevant to neuroscience.

Describing Differences between Environmental and Financial Risks

It is likely that, through evolutionary pressures, the human brain is optimized to deal with environmental risks. This would inspire one to believe that the human brain is well adapted to financial risks as well. Yet financial risks and environmental risks differ substantially.

Two differences stand out. First, many environmental risks are adequately described by the gaussian distribution. This is not so for financial risks, which often display substantial excess kurtosis (extreme events happen far more often than predicted under the gaussian distribution). See **Figure 3**, for instance, which compares the risks of investing in Microsoft common stock and weather-related risks. Second, environmental risks often emerge in clusters, which means that the chance of their occurrence depends on whether they have just occurred. In contrast, the expected payoffs from investing in securities are rather independent over time, as witnessed by the ubiquitous warning in investment prospectuses that "past performance is no indication of future performance."

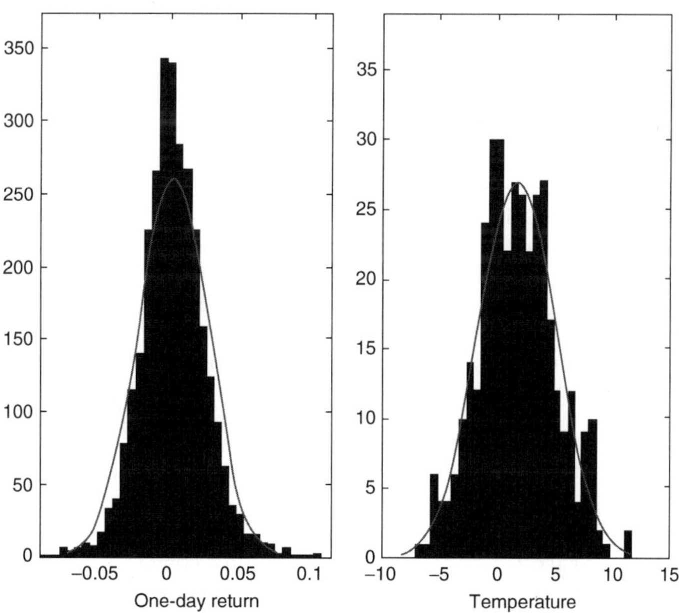

Figure 3 Histograms of daily returns (1-day payoffs per dollar invested) on Microsoft common stock (14 March 1986 till 31 December 1997; left panel) and of daily average temperature in Geneva, Switzerland in January (1995–2006). Red lines indicate best gaussian fit. The financial data (left panel) exhibit far more kurtosis than does the gaussian distribution, in the sense that extremely high and low returns are far more frequent. The histogram of the financial data is cut at a distance of about 4 standard deviations from the mean: seven data points are lost as a result; in particular, the maximum (17.97%) and the minimum (−30.12%) are not shown. The histogram of the temperature data (right panel) is not trimmed. The kurtosis of the financial data is estimated to be 15; the kurtosis of the temperature data is about 3, which is equal to the theoretical kurtosis of a gaussian random variable. Source: Center for Research in Security Prices of the University of Chicago (financial data) and the University of Dayton (Ohio) average daily temperature archive (temperature data).

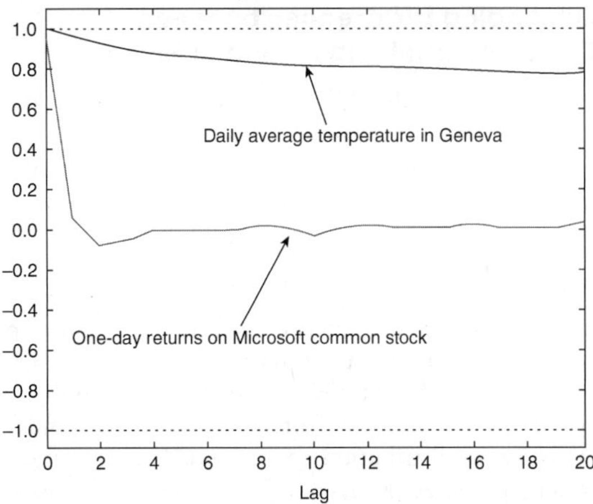

Figure 4 Time series correlation of daily returns on Microsoft common stock and of the average daily temperature in Geneva, Switzerland. Shown are the estimated correlations between the outcome of a series and its outcome *k* days in the past, where *k* is the lag indicated on the horizontal axis. A time series correlation close to zero indicates absence of predictability (past and future are uncorrelated); correlations close to 1 or −1 imply substantial predictability (the past is a very good indication of the future). Time series correlations of lag 0 are equal to 1, by definition (see **Figure 3** caption for data details).

Figure 4 illustrates the difference by comparing the time series correlation of payoffs on Microsoft common stock and that of the average daily temperature in Geneva, Switzerland.

One could claim that the differences between environmental and financial risks may explain why humans' attitudes toward financial risks are often 'irrational.' Before jumping to this conclusion, however, it is important to consider that, as we shall discuss soon, the brain seems to be using the very statistical language in terms of which the disparities between financial and environmental risks are most readily detected.

Learning in a Finance Framework

Learning is easy within the language of finance. This is because monetary gambles are described in terms of statistical moments of their payoffs (expectation, variance, skewness, kurtosis), and these moments can be estimated in an unbiased and efficient way using simple averages of past outcomes. This contrasts with learning in the context of single-dimensional utility indices. With the exception of classical expected utility indices, it is not obvious how updating should be done. Controversy remains even today, for instance, on how individuals with Prospect Theory preferences update their (biased) beliefs.

Predicting Changes in Prediction Risk

Financial payoffs are almost never equal to their predictions; actual and expected payoffs generally differ. That is, there is prediction risk. A second respect in which finance differs significantly from economics, and in fact from almost all other fields, is in its concern for tracking prediction risk. This is because financial prediction risk at times increases suddenly, generally after unusually large or small payoffs, and it decreases only gradually afterwards (see **Figure 5**). A simple statistical model known as generalized autoregressive conditional heteroskedasticity (GARCH) describes this process. As proposed by Robert Engle in the mid-1980s, in the GARCH model, risk increases after a large error in assessing prediction risk. If no further errors occur, prediction risk gradually decreases.

In computational neuroscience, one often distinguishes between estimation risk and (pure) risk. The former is the expectation of the size of the difference between estimates and true values of parameters that describe the distribution of outcomes; it reflects 'ignorance.' The latter is the expectation of the size of the difference between outcomes and the theoretical value of these parameters; 'output noise' is sometimes used as a synonym. When one is only concerned about prediction, this distinction may not be very relevant. All that matters is the prediction risk – that is, the expected size of the difference between outcomes and predictions. For other purposes, the distinction is crucial (e.g., when one is interested in testing whether the theoretical value of underlying parameters is different from zero). From a practical point of view, finance is about prediction, and, hence, the terms risk and prediction risk are used interchangeably. So, the payoff standard deviation plotted in **Figure 1** is really the prediction risk, measured as the historical standard deviation of the prediction error. (Likewise, the expected payoffs plotted in **Figure 1** are really predictions based on historical data.)

Prediction risk is of utmost importance in finance, among other factors, because the value of derivative securities such as options depends crucially on the risk in predicting the payoff of the underlying asset. Therefore, correct valuation of financial securities requires close monitoring of changes in prediction risk. This implies, in particular, tracking of prediction risk errors, to be used to update one's estimate of future prediction risk. The importance of this endeavor is further underscored by the recent introduction in many organized financial markets of securities with payoffs that depend on realized prediction risk (realized volatility).

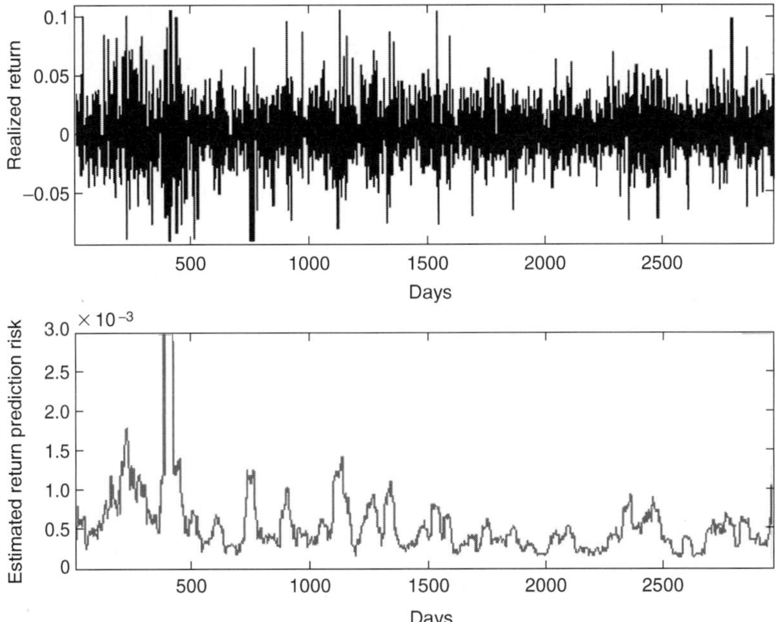

Figure 5 Historical daily returns on Microsoft common stock (top panel) and estimate of return prediction risk (bottom panel), over 2985 trading days (14 March 1986 till 31 December 1997). Return prediction risk is estimated as a 40-day moving average of the squared return. The sudden increases in prediction risk are visible despite the smoothness that the moving-average filter attempts to impose. Once prediction risk has increased, it decreases only gradually over time. These are the two main features of a generalized autoregressive conditional heteroskedasticity (GARCH) process. The GARCH model not only describes prediction risk in financial markets at the daily level (displayed here), but also at the minute or even subminute level.

Finance is one of the few fields in which prediction risk is considered to be stochastic. In many other fields, prediction risk is assumed to change deterministically. For instance, in the celebrated Kalman filter model, prediction risk changes according to a nonstochastic set of difference equations. The Kalman filter model applies to cases in which the underlying causes behind outcomes change slowly over time. The model is inadequate as a description of financial risk, however, wherein prediction risk often increases suddenly with past prediction risk errors, which means that prediction risk is stochastic. This is exactly what the GARCH model does capture.

Prediction Risk: Comparing The Kalman Filter and GARCH Models

Let p_t denote the payoff on a monetary gamble in trial period t and let x_t denote the predicted (expected) payoff. Let e_t denote the prediction error. That is,

$$e_t = p_t - x_t$$

Let υ_t denote the prediction risk, measured as the expectation of the square of the prediction error. In the Kalman filter model, υ_t changes over time deterministically, as follows:

$$\upsilon_{t+1} = a^2 \upsilon_t + q$$

for some scalars a and q. In the simplest GARCH model,

$$\upsilon_{t+1} = a^2 \upsilon_t + \kappa (e_t)^2$$

There are more complicated GARCH models, wherein the evolution of the prediction risk depends on lags of the prediction risk and of the squared prediction error beyond one period. But the essential difference with the Kalman filter model is that prediction risk changes stochastically because of the presence of a random term (the square of the prediction error e_t).

It may seem that the GARCH model is rather complicated. Yet, there is a relationship between the GARCH model and the Rescorla–Wagner reinforcement learning (RL) model from neuroscience. Specifically, a simple application to prediction risk of the Rescorla–Wagner rule produces a particular case of the GARCH model. This means that a simple RL model on prediction risk errors generates a GARCH model.

Reinforcement Learning Models for Risk Prediction as Special Cases of GARCH

The prediction risk error is defined as the difference between the realized prediction risk, measured as the squared prediction error $(e_t)^2$, and the anticipated prediction risk (υ_t):

$$\delta_t = (e_t)^2 - \upsilon_t$$

Applying the temporal difference (TD) model to update prediction risk, one obtains:

$$\begin{aligned}\upsilon_{t+1} &= \upsilon_t + \kappa\delta_t \\ &= \upsilon_t + \kappa[(e_t)^2 - \upsilon_t] \\ &= (1-\kappa)\upsilon_t + \kappa(e_t)^2\end{aligned}$$

which is a GARCH model with the restriction that the coefficient a^2 equals $(1-\kappa)$.

Neuroscience: The Finance Perspective

Evidence has accumulated recently that one of the primary roles of the dopaminergic system in the primate brain is to facilitate reward learning. Electrophysiology studies have confirmed that phasic firing of midbrain dopamine neurons correlates with errors in prediction (of cumulative anticipated rewards), and that these prediction errors affect future predictions through a simple but powerful Rescorla–Wagner rule. Functional magnetic resonance imaging (fMRI) scanning studies have found corresponding blood-oxygen-level-dependent (BOLD) signals in key subcortical dopaminoceptive areas such as ventral striatum and putamen. From a finance point of view, however, the Rescorla–Wagner rule is not fully satisfying as a model to predict rewards. This is because it does not take into account prediction risk.

Learning and Prediction Risk

Prediction risk is a key factor in determining how prediction errors should affect one's estimate of future payoffs. If the prediction risk is large, then a large prediction error is to be expected, and, hence, the prediction error should not have a large impact on future predictions. Conversely, if the prediction risk is small, then a large prediction error should cause one to substantially update one's prediction.

In terms of the Rescorla–Wagner rule of learning, this means that prediction errors should be scaled (normalized by) prediction risks in order to obtain a scale-free prediction error with which to update predictions. In general, the scaling is not simply a matter of dividing the prediction error by the (square root of the) prediction risk, but in certain cases it is. This suggests the hypothesis that the dopaminergic system encodes not just the prediction error, but also a scale-free version.

Accommodating Prediction Risk in the Rescorla–Wagner Learning Rule

When prediction risk is high, prediction errors should not change one's future predictions much because the prediction errors were expected to be sizeable anyway. Therefore, one should not update one's prediction with a constant κ, as in the traditional model. Using the notation introduced in previously, the traditional model reads as follows:

$$x_{t+1} = x_t + \kappa e_t$$

Instead, the update should be based on a scale-free prediction error η_t. In prediction of rewards in the model underlying the standard Kalman filter, the scaling takes on a very simple form:

$$\begin{aligned}x_{t+1} &= x_t + (\tilde{\kappa}/\upsilon_t^{1/2})e_t \\ &= x_t + \tilde{\kappa}(e_t/\upsilon_t^{1/2}) \\ &= x_t + \tilde{\kappa}\eta_t\end{aligned}$$

where, as before, υ_t denotes the prediction risk for trial period t $(\upsilon_t = \mathrm{E}[(e_t)^2])$. (Optimal prediction can be shown to imply that $\tilde{\kappa}$ should be proportional to the covariance between the outcomes and the scaled prediction error η_t.) Recent electrophysiological evidence from the nonhuman primate brain obtained in Wolfram Schultz' lab supports this hypothesis: at the time of reward delivery, the encoding of prediction errors in midbrain dopamine neurons appears to be scale-free (see **Figure 6**).

If dopaminergic neurons are able to attune firing to prediction risk, the brain must not only keep track of predictions, but also prediction risk. It seems that the brain does so, and the relevant signal may even be in the dopaminergic system itself. First, Schultz' lab has discovered that (other) midbrain dopamine neurons fire with delay during the anticipation period and throughout the period of reward delivery and that this delayed firing increases with prediction risk. This may provide the input signal with which raw prediction errors are scaled at the time of reward delivery. Second, fMRI analysis of certain subcortical dopaminoceptive regions of the human brain has also revealed a delayed signal that increases in prediction risk (see **Figure 7**).

One could go a step further. Because prediction risk generally changes over time, there is a need for the brain to encode prediction risk errors, with which to update prediction risk. To date, it is not known whether and where this is accomplished in the brain.

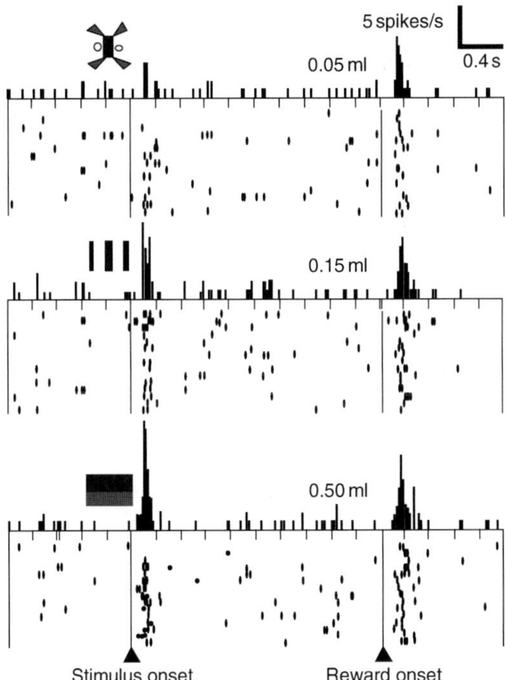

Figure 6 Spiking of primate midbrain dopamine neurons in three different types of trials involving a stochastic juice reward. In the first type, shown on top, the predicted reward (expected reward) and prediction risk (reward variance) are low. Predicted reward and prediction risk increase in the second trial type (middle) and again in the third trial type (bottom). The increase in predicted reward can be seen in the spiking of the neurons at stimulus onset, which is known to reflect prediction errors relative to baseline. The spiking at the time of reward is known to reflect prediction errors relative to expectation at stimulus onset. Only rewarded trials are shown, which is why the spiking at reward onset is always positive. Notice that the size of the spiking at reward onset does not reflect the differences of the sizes in prediction risk across trial types. In other words, the prediction error encoded in spiking at reward onset is scaled in a way that accommodates prediction risk. Reprinted from Tobler PN, Fiorillo CD, and Schultz W (2005) Adaptive coding of reward value by dopamine neurons. *Science* 307: 1642–1645, with permission from AAAS.

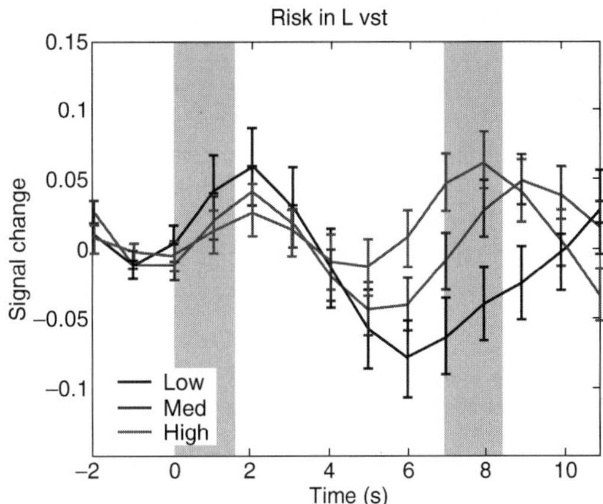

Figure 7 Functional magnetic resonance imaging evidence of activation of the subcortical dopamine system in the human brain modulated by prediction risk (measured as reward variance). Shown are time courses of the blood-oxygen-level-dependent signal in the left ventral striatum (L vst) in trials stratified by prediction risk. Left-hand gray area indicates period of stimulus onset (when reward prediction and prediction risk for the trial are conveyed); right-hand gray area indicates period of reward realization. Note that the prediction risk signal emerges with a delay: activation differentiation is maximal only after 7 s, which is approximately 2 s after peak activation in the canonical hemodynamic response. Reproduced from Preuschoff K, Bossaerts P, and Quartz S (2006) Neural differentiation of expected reward and risk in human subcortical structures. *Neuron* 51: 381–390, with permission from Elsevier.

There is some recent suggestive evidence that insula is crucial to encoding uncertainty-related phenomena, including prediction risk, but there is no account of prediction risk errors. Some of the evidence on activation of the midbrain locus coeruleus seems to suggest that norepinephrine may play the role for prediction risk errors that dopamine plays for prediction errors. Peter Dayan's group have recently started to distinguish between predicted and unpredicted uncertainty and have pointed to the role of norepinephrine in capturing the latter. Unpredicted uncertainty has an obvious relationship with prediction risk errors.

A Dual Role for Encoding Prediction Risk

The encoding of prediction risk not only facilitates learning: it can simultaneously play a crucial role in the determination of preferences. In finance, prediction risk is a crucial determinant of the desirability of a gamble. In **Figure 1**, the prediction risk of various securities is plotted on the horizontal axis (prediction risk is measured in terms of variance). As such, the encoding of prediction risk not only allows the brain to correctly update predictions, but at the same time, it also provides one of the parameters with which the brain can rank gambles. It is significant in this regard to note that the evidence for a prediction risk signal in the left ventral striatum of the human brain (see **Figure 7**) emerges even when there is no role for learning, and when individuals' behaviors (choice, reaction time) and brain activation (across trials) indeed do not show any evidence of updating. That is, the prediction risk signal plays a purely perceptual role.

The dual role of the encoding of prediction risk implies economy. The resulting efficiency is a powerful argument why the brain would not want to characterize the desirability of gambles in terms of a single-dimensional index, in contrast to economic theory. Of course, there is still the possibility that the brain does build a single-dimensional index on the basis of signals of expected payoff and payoff variance, but the point is that the raw inputs with which the index is computed come from a decomposition of the features of a random payoff in terms of statistical moments, as is done in finance. Moreover, the statistical inputs need not always be weighted in the same way, thus potentially explaining why attitudes toward risk appear to be unstable.

See also: Decision-Making and Neuroeconomics; Delayed Reinforcement: Neuroscience; Delayed Reinforcement: Economics; Games in Monkeys: Neurophysiology and Motor Decision-Making; Neuroeconomics: History; Reward Decision-Making.

Further Reading

Bossaerts P and Plott C (2004) Basic principles of asset pricing theory: Evidence from large-scale experimental financial markets. *Review of Finance* 8: 135–169.

Engle RF (1982) Autoregressive conditional heteroscedasticity with estimates of the variance of United Kingdom inflation. *Econometrica* 50: 987–1008.

Engle RF (2002) New frontiers for ARCH models. *Journal of Applied Econometrics* 17: 425–446.

Fiorillo CD, Tobler PN, and Schultz W (2003) Discrete coding of reward probability and uncertainty by dopamine neurons. *Science* 299: 1898–1902.

Huang CF and Litzenberger RC (1998) *Foundation of Financial Economics.* New York: Prentice Hall.

Markowitz H (1952) Portfolio selection. *Journal of Finance* 7: 77–91.

Preuschoff K, Bossaerts P, and Quartz S (2006) Neural differentiation of expected reward and risk in human subcortical structures. *Neuron* 51: 381–390.

Schultz W (1998) Predictive reward signal of dopamine neurons. *Journal of Neurophysiology* 80: 1–27.

Sharpe WF (1964) Capital asset prices: A theory of market equilibrium under conditions of risk. *Journal of Finance* 19: 425–442.

Tobler PN, Fiorillo CD, and Schultz W (2005) Adaptive coding of reward value by dopamine neurons. *Science* 307: 1642–1645.

Yu AJ and Dayan P (2002) Expected and unexpected uncertainty. Ach and NE in the neocortex. In: Becker S, Thrun S, and Obermayer K (eds.) *Advances in Neural Information Processing Systems,* 15, pp. 157–164. Cambridge, MA: MIT Press.

Relevant Website

http://nobelprize.org – R Engle's Nobel lecture, on GARCH models; H Markowitz' Nobel lecture, on portfolio theory; W Sharpe's Nobel lecture, on 'beta' pricing models.

Delayed Reinforcement: Economics

C Harris, University of Cambridge, Cambridge, UK

Introduction

In general, an economic subject faces many dimensions of choice. How much should she consume, and when should she consume it? What sort of career should she choose, and what sort of education and training should she undertake in order to prepare best for that career? What sort of spouse should she choose? Should she have children, and if so how many and when? How much should she work, and when should she retire? In which, among the bewildering array of assets on offer, should she place her savings?

This article focuses on just one of these dimensions: when should a subject consume? In other words, the focus is on the essence of intertemporal choice: time. The author does not consider the question of how much she should consume. The author does, however, allow for uncertainty. This is essential, for three reasons. First, in practice, most problems of intertemporal choice involve uncertainty. Second, even in the laboratory, there may be some uncertainty in a subject's mind as to whether she will actually receive the rewards being promised to her. Third, it is not possible to make sense of even the most basic concepts of the theory of intertemporal choice such as discount factors and discount rates unless the subject makes choices involving uncertainty.

Both economists and psychologists frequently analyze problems of intertemporal choice in terms of a subject's discount function. It is therefore important to begin by understanding what the use of a discount function does and does not entail. One thing that it does not entail is an assumption that the subject actually has a discount function. The point is that she behaves as if she had a discount function. The discount function itself is simply a convenient device that quantifies her choices. What the use of a discount function does entail is three assumptions about the nature of her choices: they must be complete, transitive, and substitutable. This is because a discount function is simply a particular kind of utility function: it assigns a utility to each date at which the subject could consume.

The three requirements of completeness, transitivity, and substitutability are controversial from both a theoretical and an empirical point of view. It is therefore somewhat surprising that psychologists are willing to work with discount functions. Nonetheless, there is one respect in which they are rather permissive: they are satisfied by essentially any discount function. Narrowing the range of possible shapes for the discount function therefore seems to be a higher priority than widening the enquiry to include behavior that is not consistent with having a discount function. Psychologists have taken an experimental approach to this problem, and they are inclined to interpret the data as suggesting that discount functions are hyperbolic. Following Samuelson, economists were inclined to assume for conceptual and mathematical convenience that discount functions were exponential. However, with the arrival of more powerful computers and more powerful analytical techniques, they have been increasingly willing to respond to the challenge to this paradigm contained in Strotz.

Much of the attraction of exponential discounting derives from the fact that it satisfies both dynamic consistency and stationarity. These requirements can be expressed as follows. Suppose that we are given two dates, $t > s > 0$. Then dynamic consistency means that, if the subject decides at date 0 that she would like to consume at date t, then she would not want to revise her decision at date s if given the opportunity to do so. Stationarity means that, if the subject decides at date 0 that she would like to consume at date t, then she would decide a date s to consume at date $s+t$.

Consider the following example. At 2 p.m., a subject is asked when she would like to eat supper. She chooses 7 p.m. Two hours later (i.e., at 4 p.m.) she is unexpectedly given the option of revising her choice. If she still chooses 7 p.m., then she is acting in a dynamically consistent manner. If, however, she chooses a different time (say 6 p.m.), then she is acting in a dynamically inconsistent manner. This change could be explained by the arrival of new information. For example, she may have learned at 3 p.m. that her 5 p.m. appointment had been cancelled. In this case, the dynamic inconsistency arises because she was asked to make an unconditional choice. Had she instead chosen a pair of times for supper, one to apply in the event that the appointment was on and the other to apply in the event that it was off, then she would have chosen the pair {7 p.m. if appointment, 6 p.m. if no appointment} and no revision in her choice would have been necessary. The dynamic consistency requirement embodied in an exponential discount function does not rule out changes that arise from the arrival of new information. It simply rules out changes that occur in the complete absence of any new information. As such, it is more reasonable than it might appear at first sight.

Now consider the same example, but from the point of view of stationarity. Stationarity requires that, when the subject is given the option of revising her choice at 4 p.m., she chooses 9 p.m.! The point is that, at 2 p.m., she wanted to have supper 5 h later. So, at 4 p.m., she should again want to have supper 5 h later. Stated in this way, the requirement of stationarity appears ridiculous: if the subject wanted to delay supper by 5 h at 2 p.m., then, at 4 p.m. when she is presumably hungrier, she should want (at the very minimum) to delay supper by less than 5 h. The problem does not lie with stationarity, however. It lies with an incompletely specified model. If hunger is an important factor in the subject's decision making, then it should be included in the model. Once it is included, the subject's choices become stationary again: for any given level of hunger, she will choose the same delay until supper. So stationarity too is more reasonable than it may appear at first sight.

Unfortunately, the exponential discounting model appears to be rejected by the experimental data. Dynamic consistency, stationarity, or both must therefore be wrong. From an experimental point of view, it would be hard to abandon stationarity: experiments are ultimately based on the idea that subjects will keep on doing the same thing if they are placed repeatedly in the same situation. It is therefore more sensible to abandon dynamic consistency, at least in its present form.

The experimental data also suggest that subjects are more patient with respect to any given delay, the further in the future that delay occurs. The present article proposes a method for deriving discount functions with this property and uses the method to derive a unified discount function that incorporates all three of the most popular discount functions (namely, exponential, hyperbolic, and generalized hyperbolic) as special cases.

Finally, if dynamic consistency is abandoned, then a subject's decision problem becomes an intrapersonal game. In this game, the interests of the future self are not necessarily aligned with those of the current self, and the current self has to try to anticipate the behavior of the future self. Anticipation is made easier by stationarity, which ensures that the outlook of the future self will be identical to that of the current self, but made harder by the fact that the future self may face circumstances different from those faced by the current self. Two extremes can be identified: a naive subject fails completely to anticipate the behavior of her future self (and fails to notice that she is failing to anticipate), and a sophisticated subject anticipates the behavior of her future self perfectly.

An Idealized Example

Consider the following idealized example of choice over delayed outcomes. Suppose that there is an infinite sequence of possible dates at which the subject can eat an apple: $t=0$ (today), $t=1$ (tomorrow), $t=2$ (the day after tomorrow), and so on. Denote the set of all possible dates by $\mathbb{T}=\{0, 1, 2, \ldots\}$; define a probability distribution p over $\mathbb{T}$ to be simple if the number of dates t for which $p(t)>0$ is finite; and denote by $\mathbb{P}$ the set of simple probability distributions (SPDs) over $\mathbb{T}$. The idea is then that:

1. The experimenter will offer the subject a choice of two SPDs.
2. The subject will choose between them.
3. The experimenter will use a suitable randomizing device to generate a date t according to the SPD chosen.
4. The subject will then wait until that date, at which point the experimenter will give her the apple and she will eat it straight away.

Faced with this problem, it can be argued that the perfect subject should proceed as follows. First, before she is actually asked to make any choice, she should formulate her preferences as between any pair of SPDs she could conceivably be offered. In other words, for any pair of SPDs p_1 and p_2, she must decide that (i) p_1 is at least as good as p_2; or (ii) p_2 is at least as good as p_1; or (iii) p_1 and p_2 are equally good. Second, her preferences should be consistent in the sense that, if she thinks that p_1 is at least as good as p_2 and that p_2 is at least as good as p_3, then she must also think that p_1 is at least as good as p_3. Third, if we start with three SPDs p_1, p_2 and p_3, and if we create two compound probability distributions $\tilde{p}_1$ (in which p_1 is chosen with probability γ and p_3 is chosen with probability $1-\gamma$) and $\tilde{p}_2$ (in which p_2 is chosen with probability γ and p_3 is chosen with probability $1-\gamma$), then the subject should again be consistent, this time in the sense that if she thinks that p_1 is at least as good as p_2 then she should also think that $\tilde{p}_1$ is at least as good as $\tilde{p}_2$. The logic behind this requirement is that, in moving from $\tilde{p}_2$ to $\tilde{p}_1$, we simply replace the intermediate outcome p_2 with the better intermediate outcome p_1. Substitutability, as defined later, incorporates a second requirement: provided that the probability distribution over final dates is the same, the subject should not care whether the probabilistic procedure used to arrive at this probability distribution takes place in two stages (as in a compound probability distribution) or in one (as in a simple probability distribution). This requirement is often called the reduction of compound lotteries.

More precisely, if we express the statement that the subject thinks that p_1 is at least as good as p_2 by writing p_1 B p_2, then it can be argued that the subject's preferences should satisfy the following three requirements:

Completeness: For all $p_1, p_2 \in \mathbb{P}$, we have either p_1 B p_2 or p_2 B p_1 or both.
Transitivity: For all p_1, p_2, $p_3 \in \mathbb{P}$, if p_1 B p_2 and p_2 B p_3, then p_1 B p_3.
Substitutability: For all p_1, p_2, $p_3 \in \mathbb{P}$ and all $0 < \gamma \leq 1$, if we put $\tilde{p}_1 = \gamma p_1 + (1-\gamma)p_3$ and $\tilde{p}_2 = \gamma p_2 + (1-\gamma)\, p_3$, then p_1 B p_2 if and only if $\tilde{p}_1$ B $\tilde{p}_2$.

These requirements can be challenged on both theoretical and empirical grounds. For example, why would the subject want to evaluate the vast number of hypothetical alternatives envisaged by the requirement of completeness? Why not simply wait until she is actually asked to make a choice, and only then evaluate the pair of dates that she is actually offered? Moreover, if she evaluates only a single pair of dates, then the consistency issue addressed by the requirement of transitivity – which in general involves three pairs of dates – never arises. Finally, the requirement of substitutability (for all its theoretical appeal) has not fared well when subjected to experimental testing. A full discussion of these challenges would, however, take us too far away from our main theme.

If the requirements of completeness, transitivity, substitutability, and a fourth technical requirement are all satisfied, then the following result holds:

Expected-Utility Theorem: There exists a utility function $u : \mathbb{T} \to \mathbb{P}$ that represents the subject's preferences in the sense that p_1 B p_2 if and only if

$$\sum_{t \in \mathbb{T}} p_1(t)\, u(t) \geq \sum_{t \in \mathbb{T}} p_2(t)\, u(t)$$

The fourth requirement says roughly that, if the subject strictly prefers p_1 to p_2, and if p_3 is a third simple probability distribution, then there is a small positive probability γ such that: (1) the subject strictly prefers the compound probability distribution $\widehat{p}_1$ (in which p_1 is chosen with probability $1-\gamma$ and p_3 is chosen with probability γ) to p_2; and (2) the subject strictly prefers p_1 to the compound probability distribution $\widehat{p}_2$ (in which p_2 is chosen with probability $1-\gamma$ and p_3 is chosen with probability γ). More precisely:

Archimedean axiom for all p_1, p_2, $p_3 \in \mathbb{P}$ such that p_1 B p_2 but not p_2 B p_1 (i.e., p_1 is strictly preferred to p_2), there exists $\gamma \in (0, 1)$ such that, if we put $\widehat{p}_1 = (1-\gamma)\, p_1 + \gamma\, p_3$ and $\widehat{p}_2 = (1-\gamma)\, p_2 + \gamma\, p_3$, then: (1) $\widehat{p}_1$ B p_2. but not p_2 B $\widehat{p}_1$ (i.e., $\widehat{p}_1$ is strictly preferred to p_2); and (2) p_1 B $\widehat{p}_2$ but not $\widehat{p}_2$ B p_1 (i.e., p_1 is strictly preferred to $\widehat{p}_2$).

We shall not discuss this requirement further.

In other words, there exists a utility function that characterizes the subject's choices in the sense that she chooses p_1 over p_2 if and only if the expected utility associated with p_1 exceeds the expected utility associated with p_2. (The expected utility of an SPD p is calculated by multiplying the probability $p(t)$ with which the date t is generated by the utility $u(t)$ associated with that date, and then adding up over all dates that occur with positive probability.) This result does not say that the subject has a utility function, only that she behaves as if she had one.

The utility function provided by the Expected-Utility Theorem is not unique: for all scalars $\alpha \in \mathbb{R}$ and $\beta > 0$, the utility function $\upsilon : \mathbb{T} \to \mathbb{R}$ defined by the formula $\upsilon(t) = \alpha + \beta\, u(t)$ does just as well. However, this is also the only sense in which u is not unique. More precisely, the following result holds:

Cardinal-Information Theorem: If there is a second utility function $\upsilon : \mathbb{T} \to \mathbb{R}$ that also represents the subject's preferences, then there exist scalars $\alpha \in \mathbb{R}$ and $\beta > 0$ such that $\upsilon(t) = \alpha + \beta\, u(t)$ for all $t \in \mathbb{T}$.

This result is essential for what follows. Indeed, important concepts in the analysis of intertemporal choice such as the discount factor and the discount rate are defined directly in terms of the utility function. Yet many different utility functions can be used to represent the subject's choices. We therefore need to make sure that any such concept is independent of which utility function is used to represent the subject's choices. In this way we can guarantee that it has a meaning directly in terms of what we observe, namely, the subject's behavior.

Consider the following analogy. We can measure temperature on the Celsius scale (corresponding to u) or on the Fahrenheit scale (corresponding to υ). Water freezes at 0° and boils at 100° on the Celsius scale, and it freezes at 32° and boils at 212° on the Fahrenheit scale. So statements like "the temperature is 0°" or "the temperature increased by 100°" do not make sense until one specifies whether the temperature scale is Celsius or Fahrenheit. However, statements like "when he heated the pan with a Bunsen burner the temperature rose by twice as much as when he heated it with a candle" make sense even if we do not know which temperature scale is being used. It is to statements like these that we must therefore confine ourselves. (The definitions of discount factor and discount rate given below both conform to this pattern.) Finally, in order to move between the Celsius scale and the Fahrenheit scale, we need to set $\alpha = 32$ and $\beta = \frac{9}{5}$.

Dynamic Consistency and Stationarity

Up to this point, we have assumed that, at date 0, the subject chooses a date at which to consume. She is then committed to that date. This is rather artificial: in an experimental setting, the experimenter can provide the external discipline that ensures that the subject really is committed to wait until the chosen date, but in everyday settings, a subject is likely to have opportunities to reconsider her choices.

Suppose by way of an example that $u(1) > u(2) > u(0) > u(3) > u(4) > \ldots$. In other words, while the subject knows that apples are good for her, given the choice of eating the apple today ($t = 0$) or tomorrow ($t = 1$), she would rather eat it tomorrow. Similarly, given the choice of eating the apple today ($t = 0$) or the day after tomorrow ($t = 2$), she would rather eat it the day after tomorrow. However, given the choice of eating the apple today ($t = 0$) or 3 days from now ($t = 3$), she would rather eat it today: even though she does not particularly like apples, she recognizes that she really must eat an apple from time to time.

Suppose further that the experimenter offers the subject a choice of eating the apple today ($t = 0$) or tomorrow ($t = 1$). Then the subject will certainly choose tomorrow. Suppose, however, that, when tomorrow actually arrives, the experimenter offers the subject a new choice: she can either have the apple right away (i.e., at $t = 1$, as originally planned), or she can have it on the following day (i.e., at $t = 2$). On the face of it, the subject is better off than she was before: she still has the option that she originally chose, but in addition she has the option of waiting another day. What will she do?

If we accept the logic of the preceding two sections, then the answer is that she should formulate a new utility function $\tilde{u}$ over the set $\tilde{\mathbb{T}} = \{1, 2, 3, \ldots\}$ of remaining dates. The question, then, is what relationship should this new utility function bear to the old utility function u? There does not seem to be a compelling answer to this question, but there are three possibilities.

Dynamic Consistency

One possible answer is that the subject will rank the dates $1, 2, 3, \ldots \in \tilde{\mathbb{T}}$ in exactly the same way that she ranked the dates $1, 2, 3, \ldots \in \mathbb{T}$. More explicitly, for all $t_1, t_2 \in \tilde{\mathbb{T}}$, $\tilde{u}(t_1) \geq \tilde{u}(t_2)$ if and only if $u(t_1) \geq u(t_2)$. In other words, the subject has preferences over absolute (or calendar) dates, and these preferences do not change with the passage of time. In the context of the example given above, that means that if (at date 0) the subject preferred to eat the apple at date 1, then (at date 1) the subject will still prefer to eat the apple at date 1.

Stationarity

Another possible answer is that the subject's preferences are really a kind of perspective on the future. The subject will therefore rank the dates $1, 2, 3, \ldots \in \tilde{\mathbb{T}}$ in exactly the same way that she ranked the dates $0, 1, 2, \ldots \in \mathbb{T}$. More explicitly, for all $t_1, t_2 \in \tilde{\mathbb{T}}$, $\tilde{u}(t_1) \geq \tilde{u}(t_2)$ if and only if $u(t_1 - 1) \geq u(t_2 - 1)$. In other words, the subject has preferences over relative dates, and these preferences do not change with the passage of time. In the context of the example given previously, that means that if (at date 0) the subject preferred to eat the apple 1 day later (i.e., at date 1), then (at date 1) the subject still prefers to eat the apple 1 day later (i.e., at date 2).

Exponential Discounting

Dynamic consistency ensures that a subject never wants to revise plans formulated at date 0, even if she is given the opportunity to do so. Stationarity means that a subject will approach a new planning problem in exactly the same way that she approached earlier planning problems. Can both of these advantages be incorporated within a single model? The answer is that they can, but only if the discount function takes a very particular form: it must be exponential.

In order to explain why, note that dynamic consistency implies that u and $\tilde{u}$ are simply two different representations for the same preferences over the dates in $\tilde{\mathbb{T}} = \{1, 2, 3, \ldots\}$. The Cardinal-Information Theorem therefore implies that we can find scalars $\alpha_{DC} \in \mathbb{R}$ and $\beta_{DC} > 0$ such that

$$\tilde{u}(t) = \alpha_{DC} + \beta_{DC}\, u(t) \qquad [1]$$

for all $t \in \tilde{\mathbb{T}}$. Similarly, stationarity implies that there are scalars $\alpha_S \in \mathbb{R}$ and $\beta_S > 0$ such that

$$\tilde{u}(t) = \alpha_S + \beta_S\, u(t-1) \qquad [2]$$

for all $t \in \tilde{\mathbb{T}}$. Inverting eqn [1] to express $u(t)$ in terms of $\tilde{u}(t)$, and then using eqn [2] to substitute for $\tilde{u}(t)$, we obtain

$$u(t) = \alpha_E + \beta_E\, u(t-1) \qquad [3]$$

for suitable scalars $\alpha_E \in \mathbb{R}$ and $\beta_E > 0$. (The scalars in question are $\alpha_E = \beta_{DC}^{-1}(\alpha_S - \alpha_{DC})$ and $\beta_E = \beta_{DC}^{-1}\beta_S$.)

Now, eqn [3] is a simple difference equation. If $\beta_E \neq 1$, then it has the unique solution

$$u(t) = \frac{\alpha_E}{1-\beta_E} + \beta_E^t\left(u(0) - \frac{\alpha_E}{1-\beta_E}\right) \qquad [4]$$

and, if $\beta_E = 1$, then it has the unique solution

$$u(t) = u(0) + t\,\alpha_E \qquad [5]$$

At first sight, these equations may appear to be rather complicated. Nothing could be further from the truth: they can be simplified dramatically by choosing a more convenient utility scale. More precisely, we can replace u with an equivalent utility function $v = \alpha + \beta\, u$ for suitably chosen α and β. If $\beta_E \neq 1$ and $u(0) = \frac{\alpha_E}{(1-\beta_E)} \neq 0$ then one uses $\alpha = -\frac{\alpha_E}{(1-\beta_E)}$ and $\beta = \left|u(0) - \frac{\alpha_E}{(1-\beta_E)}\right|^{-1}$; if

$\beta_E \neq 1$ and $u(0) - \frac{\alpha_E}{(1-\beta_E)} = 0$ then one uses $\alpha = -\frac{\alpha_E}{(1-\beta_E)}$ and $\beta = 1$; if $\beta_E = 1$ and $\alpha_E \neq 0$ then one uses $\alpha = -u(0)$ and $\beta = |\alpha_E|^{-1}$; and if $\beta_E = 1$ and $\alpha_E = 0$ then one uses $\alpha = -u(0)$ and $\beta = 1$. In this way, we find that there are essentially only five possible choices for the subject's utility function:

1. $\upsilon(t) = \beta_E^t$ for some $\beta_E \neq 1$;
2. $\upsilon(t) = -\beta_E^t$ for some $\beta_E \neq 1$;
3. $\upsilon(t) = 0$;
4. $\upsilon(t) = t$; and
5. $\upsilon(t) = -t$.

These cases occur, respectively, if (1) $\beta_E \neq 1$ and $u(0) - \frac{\alpha_E}{(1-\beta_E)} > 0$; (2) $\beta_E \neq 1$ and $u(0) - \frac{\alpha_E}{(1-\beta_E)} < 0$; (3) either $\beta_E \neq 1$ and $u(0) - \frac{\alpha_E}{(1-\beta_E)} = 0$, or $\beta_E = 1$ and $\alpha_E = 0$; (4) $\beta_E = 1$ and $\alpha_E > 0$; and (5) $\beta_E = 1$ and $\alpha_E < 0$. Cases 1, 2, and 3 could be summarized by saying that, viewed from the perspective of date 0, the utility of eating the apple at date *t* is the product of two factors: (1) an instantaneous utility (i.e., a utility that is obtained at the actual moment of consumption) that takes one of the three values 1, −1, and 0; and (2) a discount factor $\beta_E \neq 1$ raised to the power of *t*. There is nothing in the theory that we have sketched that requires that $\beta_E < 1$, so β_E can take any value in $(0,1) \cup (1, \infty)$. Cases 4 and 5 are limiting cases of cases 1 and 2, obtained when β_E tends to 1. This is easier to see when preferences are represented by the utility function *u*. Indeed, rewriting eqn [4] in the form $u(t) = \frac{(1-\beta_E^t)}{(1-\beta_E)} \alpha_E + \beta_E^t u(0)$, we find that $u(t) \to t\ \alpha_E + u(0)$ as $\beta_E \to 1$. In other words, we obtain eqn [5]. There are other ways of taking limits. For example, if we let $\beta_E \to 1$ in case 1, then $\widehat{u}(t) \to 1$. This is, of course, case 3, the case in which the subject is indifferent among all dates. Similarly, if we let $\beta_E \to 1$ in case 2, then $\widehat{u}(t) \to -1$. This is again case 3.

The Discount Factor

Intuitively speaking, the discount factor at date *t* tells us what fraction of the utility gain from an increase in consumption at date *t* the subject would still obtain if that increase in consumption were deferred until date $t+1$. This is a measure of the subject's patience at date *t*: the bigger the fraction of the utility gain that she still gets, the more patient she can be said to be.

Now, in our model, there are only two possible levels of consumption at date *t*: either the subject eats one apple or she eats no apples. However, to say that she eats no apples is ambiguous: it leaves open the question of when she does eat the apple. The best way to resolve this ambiguity is to introduce a new possibility into our model, namely, that the subject never eats the apple. This possibility can be captured by adding the new date ∞ (i.e., infinity) to the existing list of dates $\mathbb{T} = \{0, 1, 2, \ldots\}$. Choosing $t \in \mathbb{T}$ then means choosing to eat the apple at date *t*, and choosing $t = \infty$ means choosing never to eat the apple. It is also helpful to impose the requirement that $u(t)$ converges to $u(\infty)$ as *t* gets large. This ensures that deferring the consumption of the apple indefinitely and never consuming it yield essentially the same utility. Having to introduce the date ∞ into the model is the one small price that we have to pay for eliminating the level of consumption from the model.

We can now make precise the definition of the discount factor outlined previously. Indeed, the utility gain from eating the apple at date $t+1$ instead of never eating it is $u(t+1) - u(\infty)$, the utility gain from eating the apple at date *t* instead of never eating it is $u(t) - u(\infty)$, and the discount factor at date *t* is

$$\delta(t, 1) = \frac{u(t+1) - u(\infty)}{u(t) - u(\infty)}$$

For example, if $u(t) = \beta_E^t$ for some $\beta_E < 1$, then $u(\infty) = 0$ and $\delta(t, 1) = \beta_E$ for all *t*. Notice that $\delta(t, 1)$ is unchanged if we replace *u* by the equivalent utility function $\upsilon = \alpha + \beta u$. The discount factor is therefore a genuine behavioral measure.

The Discount Rate

In order to derive some alternatives to the exponential-discounting model, it will be helpful to treat *t* as a continuous variable. In the theory that we have sketched, a single indivisible good is consumed once. It is therefore relatively easy to adapt the theory to the continuous-time case. We can then ask what fraction of the utility gain from an increase in consumption at date *t* the subject would still obtain if that increase in consumption were deferred until date $t+\tau$. More precisely, we can introduce a generalization of the discount factor, namely,

$$\delta(t, \tau) = \frac{u(t+\tau) - u(\infty)}{u(t) - u(\infty)}$$

This is again a measure of the subject's patience at date *t*. Like $\delta(t, 1)$, $\delta(t, \tau)$ is unchanged if we replace *u* by the equivalent utility function $\upsilon = \alpha + \beta u$. It too is therefore a genuine behavioral measure.

Now, we would ideally like to make τ as small as possible, to ensure that we measure the subject's patience at date *t* as precisely as possible. However, $\delta(t, \tau) \to 1$ as $\tau \to 0$. We therefore look instead at the discount rate

$$\rho(t) = \lim_{\tau \to 0} \frac{1 - \delta(t, \tau)}{\tau}$$

This tells us how quickly $\delta(t, \tau)$ falls below 1 as the delay τ grows from 0. It is therefore a measure of the subject's impatience at date t. Elementary calculus shows that

$$\rho(t) = \frac{-u'(t)}{u(t) - u(\infty)} \quad [6]$$

For example, if $u(t) = \beta_E^t$ for some $\beta_E < 1$, then $\rho(t) = -\ln(\beta_E) > 0$.

In some respects, the terminology of discount factor and discount rate is unfortunate: it might have been better to use the terms patience factor and impatience rate instead.

Beyond Exponential Discounting

According to the exponential-discounting model, the subject's discount rate ρ is constant. However, if there is one thing on which the experimentalists all agree, it is that ρ decreases with time: a given delay is regarded as less serious, the further in the future it occurs.

One way of modeling this stylized fact is to make $\rho(t)$ a weighted average of a short-run discount rate λ and a long-run discount rate μ in which the weight placed on μ increases with time. For example, we could put

$$\rho(t) = \frac{1}{1+\nu t}\lambda + \frac{\nu t}{1+\nu t}\mu \quad [7]$$

Here v is a strictly positive parameter which measures the speed with which the discount rate moves from its short-run value λ to its long-run value μ, and the weight placed on μ increases from 0 when $t = 0$ to 1 when $t = \infty$.

If we substitute this formula for $\rho(t)$ in eqn [6], then we obtain a simple differential equation for the utility function u, $(1 + vt)\,u'(t) + (\lambda + \mu vt)\ (u(t) - u(\infty)) = 0$. It is easy to verify that this equation has the general solution

$$u(t) = C\ \exp(-\mu t)(t + \nu t)^{-\frac{(\lambda-\mu)}{\nu}} + u(\infty) \quad [8]$$

where C is an arbitrary constant. This solution is consistent with our requirement that $u(t) \to u(\infty)$ provided that either $\mu > 0$ and $\lambda \in \mathbb{R}$, or $\mu = 0$ and $\lambda > 0$. Assuming this to be the case, we can choose the utility scale in such a way that $u(\infty) = 0$. There are then three basic possibilities: $C = 1$, $C = -1$, and $C = 0$. Focusing on the case $C = 1$, we obtain

$$u(t) = \exp(-\mu t)\ (t + \nu t)^{-\frac{(\lambda-\mu)}{\nu}} \quad [9]$$

This is an attractively simple functional form with both exponential and hyperbolic features: $u(t)$ is the product of the exponential discount factor $\exp(-\mu t)$ and the hyperbolic discount factor $(1 + \nu t)^{-\frac{\lambda-\mu}{\nu}}$. Moreover, the parameters λ, μ, and v are all readily interpretable.

Equation [9] is sufficiently general to encompass both exponential and hyperbolic discounting. Indeed, if we set $\mu = 0$, then we obtain

$$u(t) = (1 + \nu t)^{-\frac{\lambda}{\mu}} \quad [10]$$

This is the generalized hyperbola of Harvey and Loewenstein and Prelec. And, if we specialize further by putting $\lambda = v$, then we obtain

$$u(t) = (1 + \nu t)^{-1} \quad [11]$$

This is the original hyperbola of Herrnstein. Third, if we put $\lambda = \mu$, then we obtain

$$u(t) = \exp(-\mu t) \quad [12]$$

This is the exponential used by Samuelson.

Equation [9] also offers a flexible functional form for statistical testing. For example, while it is widely thought that the discount rate $\rho(t)$ is decreasing in t, it would be desirable to be able to know the statistical significance of this finding. Because eqn [9] is valid for both $\lambda - \mu > 0$ and $\lambda - \mu < 0$, it can be used as the basis of a one-tailed test of whether $\lambda - \mu > 0$ (as expected) or not. Similarly, while it is widely thought that discount functions are not exponential, it would be desirable to know the statistical significance of this finding. Equation [9] can be used as the basis of a two-tailed test of whether $\lambda - \mu = 0$ or not (as expected). Third, it is sometimes claimed that discount rates are close to 0 for large t. Because eqn [9] is valid for all $\mu \geq 0$ (provided at least that $\lambda > 0$), it can be used as the basis of a test of whether the restriction $\mu = 0$ is rejected by the data or not.

Equation [9] does, however, have one fault. Except in the special case where $\lambda = \mu$ (i.e., the case of exponential discounting), it is difficult to incorporate into theoretical models in a mathematically tractable way. This difficulty can be overcome. Notice that there are essentially four elements in the construction of eqn [9]: (1) the short-run discount rate λ, (2) the long-run discount rate μ, (3) the pattern of adjustment $t \to \frac{t}{1+t}$, and (iv) the speed of adjustment v. The trick is to change the (seemingly simple) pattern of adjustment

$$t \to \frac{t}{1+t}$$

into the (seemingly complex) pattern of adjustment

$$t \to \frac{\theta(1 - \exp(-t))}{\exp(-t) + \theta(1 - \exp(-t))}$$

where θ is a nonnegative parameter. (Notice that θ is not the rate of adjustment.) Making this change leads to the (thankfully simple!) discount function

$$u(t) = \exp(-\mu t)\ (\exp(-\nu t) + (1 - \exp(-\nu t))\theta) \quad [13]$$

introduced by Harris and Laibson. This discount function is the product of two factors: the exponential discount function $\exp(-\mu t)$ and the supplementary discount function $\exp(-vt)+(1-\exp(-vt))\,\theta$. The supplementary discount function attaches weight 1 to date 0 and weight θ to date ∞, and the difference between these two weights decays exponentially at rate v. If $\theta<1$, there is therefore a transparent sense in which the present is overweighted relative to the future.

The idea behind eqn [13] is to divide time into two phases. During both of these phases, discounting takes place at rate μ. However, at the point of transition between them, an additional discount factor θ is applied. Finally, the transition between them takes place at rate v. The perceptive reader may wonder why we do not assume that discounting takes place at different rates in the two phases. For example, why not assume that discounting takes place at rate $\widehat{\lambda}$ during the first phase, that discounting takes place at rate $\widehat{\mu}$ during the second phase, that an additional discount factor $\widehat{\theta}$ is applied at the transition between the two phases, and that the transition between the two phases takes place at rate $\widehat{v}$? The answer is that this leads to no increase in generality: under these assumptions the discount function still takes the form given in eqn [13] with $\theta=\frac{\beta\widehat{v}}{(\widehat{v}+\widehat{\lambda}-\widehat{\mu})}$, $\mu=\widehat{\mu}$, and $v=\widehat{v}+\widehat{\lambda}-\widehat{\mu}$. In other words, one of the parameters $\widehat{\theta}$, $\widehat{\lambda}$, $\widehat{\mu}$ and $\widehat{v}$ is redundant. This construction is a compromise between the homogeneity of exponential discounting (which involves only a single phase) and the complete inhomogeneity of discount functions like that given in eqn [9] (which involve a continuum of phases).

Intrapersonal Games

If exponential discounting is rejected by the data, then dynamic consistency, stationarity, or both must be wrong. The author concludes this article by exploring the theoretical implications of abandoning dynamic consistency, but retaining stationarity, doing this in the context of an example.

Suppose that $u(1)>u(2)>u(0)>u(3)>u(4)>\cdots>u(\infty)$. This is the same as the example in the section titled 'Dynamic consistency and stationarity,' except that the new date ∞ has been added. Suppose, however, that the subject is now free to choose any date she wishes.

One possible approach to this problem is to assume that the subject is naive. At date 0, the subject's preferences are represented by the utility function $u_0=u$. More explicitly, we have $u_0(1)>u_0(2)>u_0(0)>u_0(3)>u_0(4)>\cdots>u_0(\infty)$. She will therefore plan to consume at her most preferred date, namely, $t=1$. However, at date 1, stationarity implies that her preferences over future dates can be represented by the utility function u_1 given by the formula $u_1(t)=u_0(t-1)$. More explicitly, we have $u_1(2)>u_1(3)>u_1(1)>u_1(4)>u_1(5)>\ldots>u_1(\infty)$. She will therefore plan to consume at her most preferred date, which is now $t=2$. And so on, indefinitely.

This reads like a textbook example of procrastination: every day the subject plans to eat the apple the following day, with the result that she never eats it. The weakness of the analysis is that the subject never learns from her repeated failure to eat the apple that her plan to eat the apple the following day is unrealistic.

A second possible approach is to assume that the subject is sophisticated. From the very outset, she recognizes that she cannot bind her future self to take the actions that she deems desirable today. So, instead, she tries to anticipate the choice c_t that she will make at date t in case she has not already consumed the apple. In this case, there are three stable patterns of behavior. They are summarized in **Table 1**. Each column of this table contains the choices made at a particular date. The first three rows contain the choices made in the three possible behaviors of the sophisticated subject. The fourth row contains the choices made by a naive subject, for the purposes of comparison. A value of 1 denotes that the subject decides to eat the apple, and a value of 0 denotes that she decides not to eat it.

If the behavior of the sophisticated subject follows the first pattern, then she ends up consuming the apple straight away. This is in marked contrast to the naive subject, who never consumes it. This pattern of behavior is supported by the following logic.

At date 0, the subject recognizes that if she does not eat the apple immediately, then (because she will not

Table 1

Date	*0*	*1*	*2*	*3*	*4*	*5*	*6*	*7*	*8*	*9*	*10*	...
Behavior 1 of sophisticated subject	1	0	0	1	0	0	1	0	0	1	0	...
Behavior 2 of sophisticated subject	0	1	0	0	1	0	0	1	0	0	1	...
Behavior 3 of sophisticated subject	0	0	1	0	0	1	0	0	1	0	0	...
Behavior of naive subject	0	0	0	0	0	0	0	0	0	0	0	

eat it at dates 1 or 2) she will end up eating it at date 3. Since $u(0) > u(3)$ (and therefore $u_0(0) > u_0(3)$), she decides to eat the apple straight away. Similarly, at date 1, she recognizes that if she does not eat the apple immediately, then (because she will not eat it at date 2) she will end up eating it at date 3. Since $u(2) > u(0)$ (and therefore $u_1(3) > u_1(1)$, by stationarity), she decides not to eat the apple. Similarly, at date 2, she recognizes that if she does not eat the apple immediately, then she will eat it at date 3. Since $u(1) > u(0)$ (and therefore $u_2(3) > u_2(2)$, by stationarity), she decides not to eat the apple. And so on.

Notice that the naive subject ends up with the lowest possible utility, namely, $u(\infty)$, and that (under behavior 1) the sophisticated subject ends up with the better utility $u(0)$. Sophistication, therefore, does pay in this example. However, the sophisticated subject does better still under behavior 3 (which results in a utility of $u(2)$) and best of all under behavior 2 (which results in a utility of $u(1)$).

Five other points are worth noting. First, we do not obtain a unique prediction for the behavior of a sophisticated subject. This is typical of all but the simplest games. But we do still get clear predictions. For example, a naive subject will never eat the apple, whereas a sophisticated subject will eat it within the first three periods. Second, although the model is stationary, none of the three predictions for the behavior of the sophisticated subject is stationary. While it may not be reasonable to rule out behaviors that are nonstationary, it is reasonable to look for behaviors that are. One way of obtaining stationary behavior is to allow the subject to randomize. Third, randomization can be given an attractive interpretation in this model. It need not mean that the subject deliberately randomizes between eating and not eating the apple (e.g., by tossing a coin). It could mean instead that she is unsure whether she will eat the apple tomorrow or not: all she knows is that she will eat it with some probability. Fourth, the game-theoretic approach we have adopted in the analysis of the sophisticated subject effectively reinstates dynamic consistency in a more subtle form. Previously, a subject was deemed to be dynamically consistent if the future self would always find it to be in her own interests to go along with any plan formulated by the current self. Now the current self recognizes that the interests of the future self may not coincide with her own and chooses the best plan that the future self will be willing to go along with. Finally, the behavior of a naive subject is absurdly naive: even pigeons can do better than that. Similarly, the behavior of the sophisticated subject is absurdly sophisticated: even the most intelligent human being would struggle to foresee as much as she does. The truth probably lies somewhere in between.

See also: Decision-Making in Financial Markets; Decision-Making and Neuroeconomics; Delayed Reinforcement: Neuroscience; Game Theory and the Economics of Animal Communication; Games in Monkeys: Neurophysiology and Motor Decision-Making; Neuroeconomics: History; Prediction Errors in Neural Processing: Imaging in Humans; Reward Decision-Making; Social Cognition.

Further Reading

Frederick S, Loewenstein G, and O'Donoghue T (2002) Time discounting and time preference: A critical review. *Journal of Economic Literature* 40: 351–401.

Harvey CM (1986) Value functions for infinite-period planning. *Management Science* 32: 1123–1139.

Herrnstein RJ (1981) Self-control as response strength. In: Bradshaw CM, Szabadi E, and Lowe CF (eds.) *Quantification of Steady-State Operant Behavior*, pp. 3–20. Amsterdam: Elsevier/North-Holland.

Koopmans TC (1960) Stationary ordinal utility and impatience. *Econometrica* 28: 287–309.

Koopmans TC, Diamond PA, and Williamson RE (1964) Stationary utility and time perspective. *Econometrica* 32: 82–100.

Kreps D (1990) *A Course in Microeconomic Theory*. New York: Harvester Wheatsheaf.

Laibson D (1997) Golden eggs and hyperbolic discounting. *Quarterly Journal of Economics* 112: 443–477.

Loewenstein G and Prelec D (1992) Anomalies in intertemporal choice: Evidence and an interpretation. *Quarterly Journal of Economics* 107: 573–597.

Mazur JE (1987) An adjustment procedure for studying delayed reinforcement. In: Commons ML, Mazur JE, Nevins JA, and Rachlin H (eds.) *Quantitative Analysis of Behavior: The Effect of Delay and of Intervening Events on Reinforcement Value*, vol. 5, pp. 55–73. Hillsdale NJ: Erlbaum.

O'Donoghue T and Rabin M (1999) Doing it now or later. *American Economic Review* 89: 103–124.

Rachlin H and Green L (1972) Commitment, choice and self-control. *Journal of the Experimental Analysis of Behavior* 17: 15–22.

Samuelson PA (1937) A note on measurement of utility. *Review of Economic Studies* 4: 155–161.

Starmer C (2000) Developments in non-expected utility theory: The hunt for a descriptive theory of choice under risk. *Journal of Economic Literature* 38: 332–382.

Strotz RH (1956) Myopia and inconsistency in dynamic utility maximization. *Review of Economic Studies* 23: 165–180.

Delayed Reinforcement: Neuroscience

C M Bradshaw, S Body, and E Szabadi, University of Nottingham, Nottingham, UK

Theoretical Bases

A basic principle of human and animal behavior is that organisms tend to carry out voluntary actions which lead to rewarding outcomes. Couched in such simple terms, this principle conveys little information, because the terms 'voluntary action' and 'rewarding outcome' are defined with reference to one another, leading to a proposition that is essentially circular. The problem is not resolved merely by replacing the everyday notions of voluntary action and reward by technical terms such as 'operant behavior' and 'reinforcement.' What is needed is first a formal statement of the reinforcing relation which allows the key terms to be defined rigorously, and second a means of anchoring the statement to some underlying biological mechanism. The burden of fulfilling the first requirement has been shouldered variously by psychologists, behavioral ecologists, and economists, while the task of addressing the second requirement has been taken on by behavioral neuroscientists. While considerable advances have been made with each of these endeavors, a complete understanding of reward-motivated behavior awaits a successful integration of the two approaches. This article argues that one area where such an integration is nearly within reach is the analysis of the effects of delayed reinforcement.

It is generally agreed that the efficacy or 'value' of a reinforcer is an inverse function of its delay. Specifying the mathematical form of this function is an important step in the direction of defining the reinforcement process. Choice schedules have played a crucial part in establishing the nature of this function. Faced with a choice between two reinforcers of different sizes, animals will, other things being equal, prefer the larger one. Similarly, faced with a choice between two reinforcers associated with different delays, animals will, other things being equal, prefer the one that can be obtained sooner. In real life, of course, other things are seldom equal, and choice between rewarding outcomes inevitably involves consideration of the relative merits of the two rewards along more than one dimension. For example, in the situation that has been most extensively studied in the operant behavior laboratory, the study participant must choose between a smaller reinforcer that may be obtained after a brief delay and a larger reinforcer whose delivery is considerably postponed; in such an 'intertemporal choice' situation, the participant's choice behavior necessarily reflects the influences of both size and delay of reinforcement.

In a pioneering experiment by George Ainslie, pigeons repeatedly chose between a smaller reward, A, delivered after a delay d_A, and a larger reward, B, delivered after a longer delay, d_B. With d_A set at zero, the birds showed a strong preference for A. However, when both delays were progressively increased by the same amount, D, preference for A weakened, and eventually reversed, so that at high values of D the birds actually preferred B to A. Ainslie's demonstration of preference reversal delivered, in the eyes of many psychologists, the coup de grâce to models of choice based on classical microeconomic theory, in which the value of a commodity is presumed to decline exponentially as a function of delay. Exponential delay discounting is epitomized by eqn [1]

$$V = qe^{-kd} \qquad [1]$$

where V is the hypothetical value of a reward, q is its size or quantity, d is delay, and k is an exponential decay parameter. In keeping with economic notions of 'rational choice,' exponential delay discounting functions decline in parallel (provided that k is held constant), with the result that if A is preferred to B when their respective delays are d_A and d_B, A will still be preferred to B when their delays are $d_A + D$ and $d_B + D$. However, as pointed out by Ainslie, preference reversal is entirely compatible with hyperbolic delay discounting, as shown in **Figure 1**.

An elegantly simple statement of hyperbolic delay discounting, championed by James Mazur, is given in eqn [2]

$$V = \frac{q}{1 + Kd} \qquad [2]$$

where K is a parameter expressing the rate of (hyperbolic) delay discounting.

In fact, exponential discounting (eqn [1]) can be made to accommodate preference reversal, provided that k is allowed to vary inversely with q, in other words, if the rate of discounting is allowed to be higher for small reinforcers than for large ones. Such may indeed be the case when humans make choices between hypothetical monetary reinforcers. However, there is good evidence that this so-called 'magnitude effect' does not apply when animals make choices between food reinforcers, suggesting that eqn [2] is to be preferred to eqn [1].

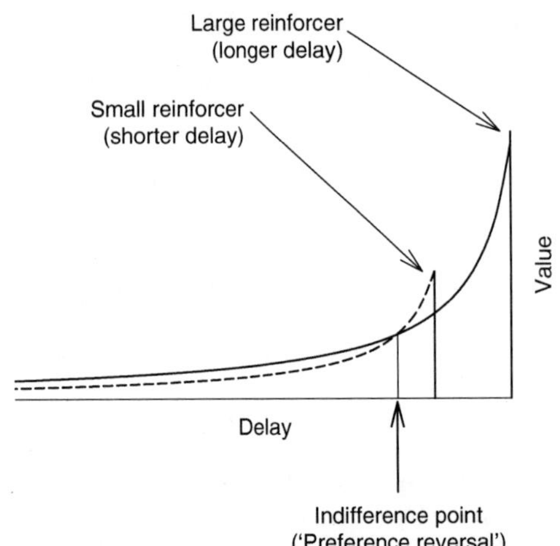

Figure 1 Ainslie's theoretical account of preference reversal, based on the principle of hyperbolic delay discounting. The vertical lines represent the instantaneous values of a large (continuous line) and a small (broken line) reinforcer. The curves show the decline in value that results from imposition of a delay between the response and the delivery of the reinforcer. At the indifference point ('preference reversal'), the values of the two reinforcers are equal. If the organism makes its choice when the delay to the small reinforcer is relatively short (i.e., at a delay value to the right of the indifference point), the smaller reinforcer is preferred. If the delays to both reinforcers are increased, so that the organism is required to make its choice at some time point to the left of the indifference point, the larger reinforcer will be preferred. Note that the intersecting value curves are a consequence of hyperbolic discounting (exponential discounting gives rise to curves that decline in a parallel fashion: see text).

Recent work in our laboratory suggests that eqn [2] somewhat oversimplifies the discounting function. The problem arises from the fact that eqn [2] implies that, if d is held constant, V is directly proportional to q, the physical size of the reinforcer. There are, however, good reasons to doubt this supposition. For instance, when rats make choices between reinforcers consisting of different numbers of food pellets, preference for the larger reinforcer is stronger when the two reinforcers consist of one and two pellets than when they consist of three and six pellets. This suggests a nonlinear relation between V and q. According to one model, the 'multiplicative hyperbolic model' (MHM), the relation is hyperbolic, as defined by eqn [3]

$$V = \frac{q}{q+Q}\frac{1}{1+Kd} \qquad [3]$$

where Q is a parameter which modulates the effect of reinforcer size upon value. It should be emphasized at this point that the role of Q is not merely to explain away embarrassing departures from the straightforward predictions of eqn [2]. As will be seen later in this article, neurobiological interventions can alter animals' choices between reinforcers by altering their sensitivity to delay and/or their sensitivity to size. Q provides a vehicle for formalizing and quantifying the effects of interventions on sensitivity to reinforcer size.

According to MHM, eqn [3] may be expanded in order to accommodate the effects of other variables on reinforcer value. For example, probability of reinforcement, p, can be accommodated thus:

$$V = \frac{q}{q+Q}\frac{1}{1+Kd}\frac{1}{1+H\theta} \qquad [4]$$

where θ is the odds against the occurrence of the reinforcer ($[1/p]-1$) and H is a an odds-discounting parameter. Equation [4] allows risky choice, a matter of great interest to students of foraging behavior, to be considered within the framework of MHM.

It will not have escaped the reader's notice that V is not a directly measurable quantity. As an intervening variable, it is useful only to the extent that it can be linked to some explicit feature of behavior. Two ways of dealing with V can be found in the literature. The first approach is to link it to notions of 'response strength' and to infer changes in V from changes in the rate or vigor of responding. The second approach is to write equations which allow V to be canceled out; this is the indifference or null equation approach. The fundamental assumption underlying the derivation of indifference equations is that when the animal displays indifference between two reinforcers, A and B, their values are equal: $V_A = V_B$. This equality may be expanded using the definition of V specified by eqn [4], and then reduced to simple relations among the quantitative features of the two reinforcers. For example, in an experiment in which an animal makes choices between a small reinforcer, A, delivered after a short delay and a larger reinforcer, B, delivered after a longer delay, the delay to B that results in indifference between A and B ($d_{B(50)}$) is a linear function of the delay to A (d_A):

$$d_{B(50)} = \frac{1}{K}\left[\frac{q_B(Q+q_B) - q_A/(Q+q_A)}{q_A/(Q+q_A)}\right] + d_A\left[\frac{1+Q/q_A}{1+Q/q_B}\right] \qquad [5]$$

Equation [5] is one member of a family of null equations that may be derived to describe indifference between two reinforcers; it is particularly suited to experiments in which the sizes of the two reinforcers are held constant and delays are systematically varied (see **Figure 2** for an example). Other equations can be derived to describe situations in which size, rather than

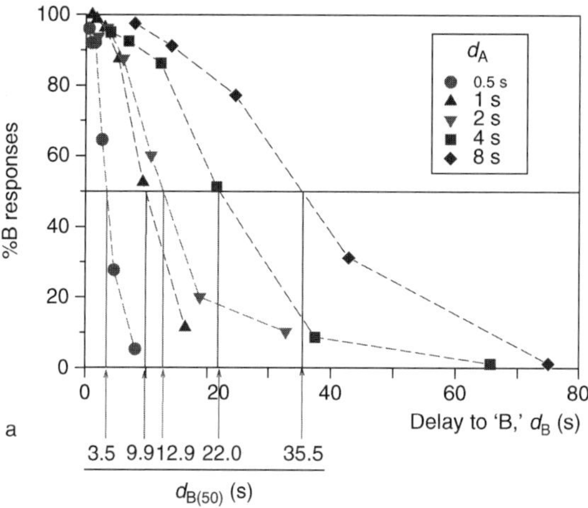

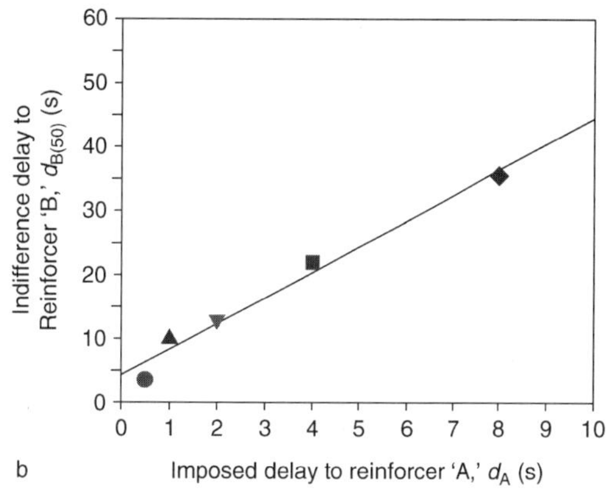

Figure 2 Derivation of a linear indifference function: example of data obtained from one rat. (a) Preference functions: percent responding on lever B (%B) is plotted against the delay to the larger of two reinforcers (d_B). Each plot shows the data obtained from one phase of the experiment, in which the delay to the smaller reinforcer (d_A) was fixed at the value shown in inset panel. The horizontal line signifies indifference (%B = 50), and the vertical lines indicate the indifference delays ($d_{B(50)}$) obtained in each phase (values shown under the abscissa). (b) Linear indifference function ($d_{B(50)}$ vs d_A) derived using the indifference delays shown in (a). The fitted line is the linear function specified by eqn [5]. Unpublished data from Kheramin S, Body S, Bradshaw CM, Szabadi E, Deakin JFW, and Anderson IM.

delay, is systematically manipulated, or in which reinforcer probability is the variable of interest.

As well as specifying the form of the indifference relation (in the case of eqn [5], a linear relation), null equations also offer a means of characterizing the effects of interventions on the discounting parameters. A more ambitious goal, which, unfortunately, is often thwarted by the intrinsic variability of the behavioral data, is to derive quantitative estimates of the discounting parameters pertaining to individual animals. For example, the slope of the linear function specified by eqn [5] is determined entirely by the sizes of the two reinforcers and the size-discounting parameter Q. The delay-discounting parameter K may be obtained using the formula $K = (\text{slope} - 1)/\text{intercept}$.

Indifference equations highlight a feature of choice behavior which has important implications for neurobiological analyses of reinforcement processes: choice usually entails a compromise. In the situation characterized by eqn [5], the compromise is one between size and delay. Indifference implies that a balance has been struck between the competing attractions of the larger size of reinforcer B and the shorter delay associated with reinforcer A. This balance can be upset, and hence the indifference point displaced, by altering the animal's sensitivity to either size or delay of reinforcement, or both. This is illustrated in **Figure 3**, which shows the effects of hypothetical interventions on the linear indifference function defined by eqn [5]. The left-hand graph shows the effect of an intervention that alters sensitivity to delay (via an increase in K), the middle graph shows the effect of an intervention that alters sensitivity to size (via a reduction of Q), and the right-hand graph shows the effect of an intervention that alters sensitivity to both of these features of reinforcers (via increases in both K and Q).

If the foregoing analysis is correct, it follows that the reluctance of an individual animal to select the larger and more delayed of two reinforcers does not necessarily indicate that it is especially sensitive to delay of reinforcement; it is equally possible that it differs from its peers only in its sensitivity to the relative sizes of the two reinforcers. Therefore, interpretation of induced shifts of preference favoring smaller, less delayed reinforcers in terms of 'accelerated delay discounting' or 'delay aversion' should be made with due caution. Moreover, the time-honored anthropomorphisms 'impulsive' and 'self-controlled' choice have little to recommend them. While they have served a useful purpose in highlighting the distinction between different uses of the term 'impulsiveness' in clinical and lay discourse, in particular the distinction between impulsive choice (selection of smaller earlier reinforcers) and impulsive action (acting rapidly in situations where delay is advantageous), they can be seriously misleading if they are identified with hypothetical behavioral processes. As we have seen, models such as MHM imply that altered sensitivity to delay of reinforcement is neither a necessary nor a sufficient condition for a shift in preference in favor of smaller earlier reinforcers.

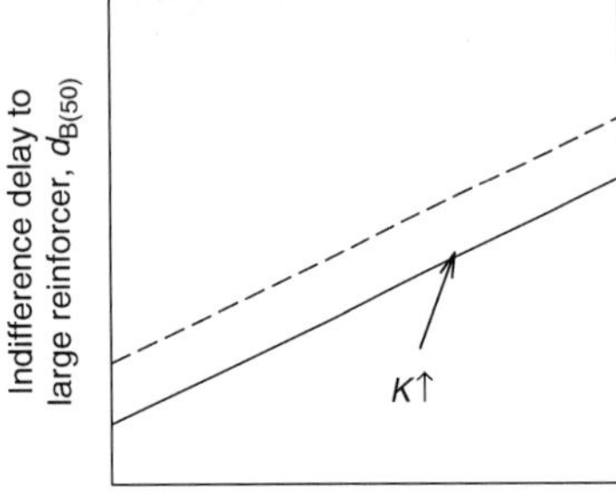

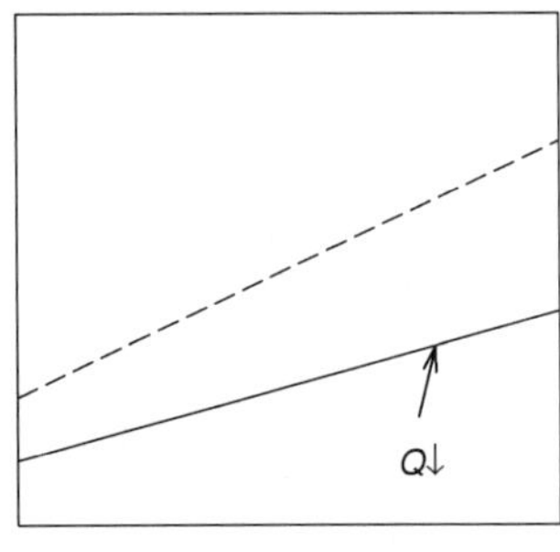

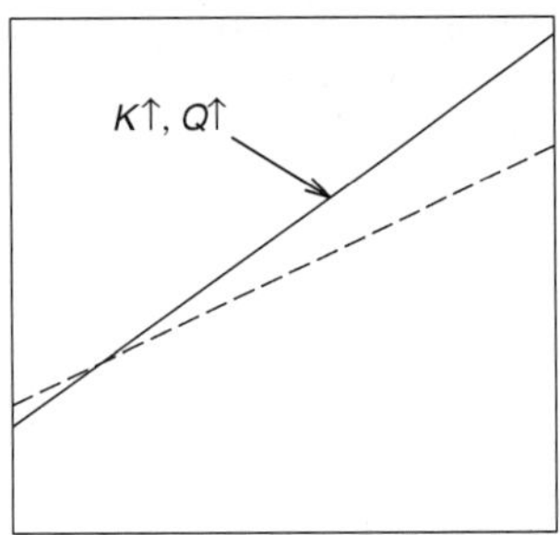

Figure 3 Effects of three hypothetical interventions on the linear indifference function defined by MHM (eqn [5]). Ordinates: indifference delay to the larger of two reinforcers, $d_{B(50)}$; abscissas: delay to the smaller reinforcer, d_A. In each graph, the broken line represents the 'baseline' function and the continuous line represents the function derived in the presence of an intervention that alters the delay-discounting parameter, K (left-hand graph), the size-discounting parameter, Q (middle graph), or both parameters (right-hand graph). Note that preference for the smaller, earlier reinforcer (A) can be promoted by either an increase in K or a reduction of Q, but the slope of the function is altered only in the latter case. If K and Q are both increased, the baseline and altered functions may intersect, resulting in stronger preference for A at low values of d_A, and weaker preference for A at high values of d_A, in the presence of the hypothetical intervention.

Methodology

Numerous methods have been devised to investigate intertemporal choice behavior. A full description of these methods is beyond the scope of this article, and the interested reader is referred to the articles listed in the 'Further reading' section. Some of the most commonly used approaches are outlined in this section.

Free-Operant Concurrent Schedules

In these schedules, the study participant has continuous access to two operanda that are associated with different outcomes. One type of concurrent schedule that lends itself well to studies of delayed or probabilistic reinforcement is the concurrent-chains schedule, in which equal initial-link schedules (e.g., a pair of concurrent variable-interval schedules) provide access to mutually exclusive terminal-link schedules (e.g., response-independent reinforcer delivery following different delays). Relative response rate in the initial links provides the measure of preference, and equality of response rates is taken to indicate equality of the reinforcing values of the terminal links. Of course, precise indifference may not be obtained in any one pair of schedules; however, the indifference point may be estimated from a series of concurrent schedules by application of the 'generalized matching law.'

The 'time-left' procedure is a concurrent chain schedule which yields continuous, graded measure of preference. Equal initial-link schedules provide access, at unpredictable times after the start of a trial, to two mutually exclusive terminal links which deliver reinforcement either after a fixed delay or, after a variable delay, at the end of the trial. Early in the trial, the fixed delay is shorter than the variable delay, whereas toward the end of the trial, the variable delay is shorter. Preference for the variable delay accordingly increases from approximately zero at the start of the trial, to near 100% at the end of the trial. The locus of the indifference point (50% choice of the variable delay) depends on the length of the fixed delay and the sizes of the reinforcers offered in the two terminal links. It has been shown that the indifference delay is a linear function of the length of the fixed delay, in accord with eqn [5].

Discrete-Trials Concurrent Schedules

These schedules comprise a series of trials in each of which the participant chooses between two mutually exclusive alternatives. Preference is measured as proportional choice of one alternative across a number of trials. Discrete-trials concurrent schedules tend to engender exclusive preference; this is the expected outcome of repeated exposure to choice between mutually exclusive alternatives, A and B, since alternative A will always be chosen whenever $V_A > V_B$, and vice versa (see earlier). However, indifference points may be determined by systematic manipulation of a relevant independent variable (e.g., delay to one reinforcer), and estimation of the value of that variable corresponding to 50% choice of each alternative.

Conventional T-maze tasks are a type of discrete-trials concurrent schedule; they can be adapted to the study of intertemporal choice by delaying reinforcer delivery in one of the goal boxes by some specified time. Most studies employing T-maze tasks have used proportional choice of the delayed reinforcer as a simple measure of preference, a measure which can only yield an indifference point if preference is tested using a range of delays.

J. L. Evenden and C. N. Ryan introduced a protocol for examining the effect of delay in a discrete-trials lever-pressing task. In each free-choice trial, lever A delivers a small reinforcer immediately, whereas lever B delivers a larger reinforcer after a delay, d_B; d_B is progressively increased in successive blocks of trials. The value of d_B at which preference switches from B to A may be taken as the indifference delay, $d_{B(50)}$. In our laboratory, the method has been extended, using a range of delays to the smaller reinforcer (d_A), to enable linear indifference functions to be obtained between $d_{B(50)}$ and d_A, as prescribed by MHM.

An important technical development in the estimation of indifference points was Mazur's introduction of the adjusting delay schedule. In this schedule, the participant undergoes a series of trials in which the sizes of the two reinforcers and the delay to the smaller reinforcer are fixed, while the delay to the larger reinforcer is allowed to vary in accordance with the participant's choices. When the participant shows a preference for the larger reinforcer, the delay to that reinforcer is increased; when preference shifts to the smaller reinforcer, the delay to the larger reinforcer is reduced. Extended training on this schedule results in the establishment of a quasi-stable delay to the larger reinforcer, which is taken as the indifference delay.

J. B. Richards and colleagues have devised a variant of Mazur's method, the adjusting-amount schedule, in which rats make repeated choices between a delayed liquid reinforcer of fixed volume and an immediate reinforcer, the volume of which is adjusted in accordance with the animals' choices. The volume of the variable reinforcer at which indifference is achieved is often taken as an index of the 'value' of the fixed-volume delayed reinforcer. However, it should be noted that the logic of this method is based on the assumption that value is linearly related to reinforcer size, in accordance with eqn [2], an assumption that is contradicted by models such as MHM, which assume that value is constrained by an asymptotic function such as that defined by eqn [3]. An important practical advantage of the adjusting-amount schedule is the rapid (within-session) attainment of stable indifference that has been reported in many studies.

Effects of Neurobiological Interventions on Choice of Delayed Reinforcers

The 5-Hydroxytryptaminergic Pathways

Twenty years ago, Phillipe Soubrié proposed that the ascending 5-hydroxytryptaminergic (5-HTergic, or serotonergic) pathways may play an important role in enabling organisms to tolerate delay of reinforcement, and that dysfunction of these pathways might therefore promote selection of small immediate reinforcers in preference to larger delayed reinforcers. Several studies have since investigated the effects of lesions of the 5-HT pathways, and acute treatment with drugs whose mode of action is believed to involve these pathways, on choice between small immediate and large delayed rewards. Unfortunately, these experiments have produced varied, and sometimes conflicting, results. The results of experiments investigating the effects of central 5-HT depletion are summarized in **Table 1**.

Several early experiments employed intraraphe injections of the selective neurotoxin 5,7-dihydroxytryptamine (5,7-DHT) to destroy the ascending 5-HTergic pathways. These studies generally indicated that loss of central 5-HT was associated with a shift of preference toward smaller, less delayed reinforcers.

Table 1 Effects of central 5-HT depletion on intertemporal choice behavior

5-HT depletion method	*Behavioral method*	*Number of preference functions/ indifference points*	*Effect on preference for smaller, earlier reinforcer*	*Reference*
Intra-raphe 5,7-DHT	Adjusting delay	1	↑	Wogar et al. (1993)
Intra-raphe 5,7-DHT	Time-left procedure	1	↑	Al-Ruwaitea et al. (1999)
Intra-raphe 5,7-DHT	Adjusting delay	5	↑	Mobini et al. (2000a)
Intra-raphe 5,7-DHT	Discrete-trials choice	1	↑	Mobini et al. (2000b)
i.c.v.5,7-DHT	Discrete-trials choice	1	0	Winstanley et al. (2003)
i.c.v.5,7-DHT	Discrete-trials choice	1	0	Winstanley et al. (2004)
i.c.v. 5,7-DHT	Discrete-trials choice	1	0	Denk et al. (2005)
*p*CPA	T-maze choice	NA	↑	Bizot et al. (1999)
i.c.v. 5,7-DHT	Discrete-trials choice	1	0	Winstanley et al. (2005)

5,7-DHT, 5,7-dihydroxytryptamine; i.c.v., Intracerebroventricular injection; *p*cpa, *p*-chlorophenylalanine.

More recent experiments, generally employing intracerebroventricular injections of the same neurotoxin, have not replicated this result. The reason for this discrepancy is unclear; obvious candidates are different techniques for inducing 5-HT depletion and different behavioral paradigms used to measure choice behavior. A weakness of most of these studies is the use of a single preference function or indifference point, which, as discussed previously, can cloud the interpretation of any changes observed. However, this is unlikely to be the sole reason for the discrepant results, because the only study to have used a multiple-indifference-point approach found that 5-HT-depleted rats showed a parallel displacement of the linear indifference function defined by eqn [5], consistent with a selective increase of the delay-discounting parameter K (see **Figure 3**, left-hand graph). This pattern of effect implies that the shift of preference favoring smaller earlier reinforcers should occur at all values of delay, and therefore the outcome of the experiments should not have been affected by the use of different delays in different experiments. The possible role of the 5-HTergic pathways in risky choice is a largely unexplored area. Two recent studies found no evidence that 5-HT depletion promotes selection of large low-probability rewards (a putative model of gambling); however, this is clearly a topic that requires further research.

There have been some attempts to explore the effects of drugs that interact with 5-HTergic mechanisms on intertemporal choice. Earlier studies, which mainly used T-maze-based choice paradigms, reported that 5-HT uptake-inhibiting drugs generally promoted choice of the larger, more delayed of two reinforcers, in keeping with Soubrié's proposal that endogenous 5-HT contributes a restraining influence on the selection of small immediate gains. More recent experiments, using discrete-trials operant procedures, have indicated that 5-HT_{1A} receptor stimulation tends to promote the selection of smaller earlier reinforcers, possibly via an interaction between 5-HTergic and dopaminergic mechanisms in the ventral striatum. Unfortunately, all these studies have examined the effects of drugs on a single preference function. Confirmation that the reported effects reflect changes in the rate of delay discounting must await the results of parametric studies that allow clear separation of delay discounting from sensitivity to reinforcer size.

The Dopaminergic Pathways

The possibility that the central dopaminergic pathways may contribute to the control of behavior by delayed reinforcement has attracted considerable interest because of the putative involvement of dopaminergic dysfunction in attention-deficit/hyperactivity disorder (ADHD), a condition in which 'impulsiveness' is a prominent feature. Unfortunately, a clear picture of dopamine's role in intertemporal choice has yet to emerge.

Selective dopamine depletion from the nucleus accumbens and local injection of dopamine receptor antagonists into this region have generally been found to have little effect on preference for the smaller and earlier of two reinforcers. This is in contrast to the effect of excitotoxic lesions of this structure, which have been found to promote the selection of small immediate reinforcers (see later). In one study, injection of the selective catecholamine-depleting neurotoxin 6-hydroxydopamine into the orbital prefrontal cortex (OPFC) had a complex effect on intertemporal choice, promoting the selection of the larger, more delayed reinforcer to an increasing degree as the delay to the smaller reinforcer was progressively increased (see **Figure 3**, right-hand graph). This finding can be interpreted on the basis of MHM (eqn [5]) in terms of a dual effect on delay discounting (K was increased) and sensitivity to relative reinforcer size (Q was increased).

A number of studies have investigated the effects of systemic treatment with psychostimulant drugs, which facilitate dopaminergic function. Earlier studies yielded disconcertingly disparate results; however, it now seems that these apparently inconsistent findings may be reconcilable. As shown in **Table 2**, there are reports that the catecholamine-releasing agent amphetamine can promote the selection of either the smaller immediate reinforcer or the larger delayed reinforcer in intertemporal choice schedules. A methodological factor whose importance has come to light in more recent experiments is the presence or absence of a cue during the delay interval. There are theoretical and empirical reasons for believing that an intradelay cue functions as a conditioned reinforcer whose reinforcing efficacy is inversely related to the duration for which it is presented. Consistent with this notion, it has been found that rats generally tolerate much longer delays to reinforcement when a cue is presented during the delay than when no cue is provided. Since amphetamine and related drugs are believed to enhance the effect of conditioned reinforcers, it might be expected that these compounds would promote the selection of the more delayed of two reinforcers when the delay is signaled by an explicit cue, and this indeed turns out to be the case. In the absence of such a cue, the predominant effect of amphetamine is to promote selection of the smaller earlier reinforcer. Unfortunately there are no published studies that have

Table 2 Effects of amphetamine and related drugs on intertemporal choice behavior

Drug	*Behavioral method*	*Number of preference functions/ indifference points*	*Effect on preference for smaller, earlier reinforcer*	*Reference*
d-Amphetamine 0.5 mg kg^{-1}	Discrete-trials choice	NA	↑	Charrier and Thiébot (1996)
d-Amphetamine 0.1 mg kg^{-1}	Discrete-trials choice	1	↑	Evendon and Ryan (1996)
Methamphetamine 0.5, 1, 2 mg kg^{-1}	Adjusting amount	1	↓	Richards et al. (1999)
d-Amphetamine 0.5, 1 mg kg^{-1}	Adjusting amount	1	↓	Wade et al. (2000)
d-Amphetamine 0.3, 1, 1.6 mg kg^{-1}	Discrete-trials choice	1	↑↓[a]	Cardinal et al. (2000)
d-Amphetamine 0.3, 1, 1.5, 2.3 mg kg^{-1}	Discrete-trials choice	1	↑	Winstanley et al. (2003)
d-Amphetamine 0.4, 0.6, 0.8 mg kg^{-1}	Discrete-trials choice	1	↑↓[b]	Isles et al. (2003)
Methamphetamine 0.3, 1, 1.7, 3 mg kg^{-1}	Concurrent-chains schedule	1	↓	Pitts and Febbo (2004)

[a]↑ when intradelay cue was not used; ↓ when intradelay cue was used.
[b]Dose-dependent effect: lower doses promoted choice of the larger reinforcer, higher dose promoted choice of the smaller reinforcer.

incorporated a range of indifference points, and therefore it remains unknown whether the effects of amphetamine on intertemporal choice reflect a selective influence on delay discounting.

The Nucleus Accumbens Core

Excitotoxic bilateral destruction of the nucleus accumbens core (NAC) has been found to displace preference functions in favor of smaller immediate reinforcers. However, it has yet to be established, on the basis of parametric studies, whether this is due to facilitation of delay discounting.

The Prefrontal Cortex

Excitotoxic lesions of the ventral–medial and dorsal–medial (anterior cingulate) prefrontal cortex have been found to have no effect on intertemporal choice behavior. However, destruction of the OPFC produced a complex pattern of effect (**Figure 4**); preference was minimally affected when short delays to the smaller reinforcer (d_A) were employed, whereas the lesion promoted preference for the larger reinforcer to an increasing degree as d_A was progressively increased. Analysis of the linear indifference functions using MHM (eqn [5]) indicated that the OPFC-lesioned subjects had a higher rate of delay discounting (K was increased) and a greater sensitivity to relative reinforcer size (Q was increased) compared to sham-lesioned control subjects.

Future Directions

There is, as yet, no unanimous agreement on the most appropriate model of delay discounting; however, there is a good level of agreement about the range of phenomena that a successful model should accommodate – preference reversal and indifference functions are prominent among these phenomena. More controversial is the issue of how the influences of different features of reinforcers, for example, delay and magnitude, may be disentangled. The model advocated in this article (MHM) is an attempt to address this problem; while we make no claim that MHM is unique in this respect, we are convinced that formal models, of which MHM is one example, can provide a framework for quantifying the effects of various features of reinforcers, which may be of considerable help in the quest to identify the neurobiological substrate of choice behavior.

Emerging evidence for the involvement of the NAC and OPFC in intertemporal choice, discussed earlier, is of particular interest in the light of recent neurophysiological evidence that these structures are active during prereinforcer delays. It has been suggested that neural activity in these areas may help the organism to bridge the gap between an operant response and a rewarding outcome, and may therefore play an important role in 'anticipation' of rewarding events. An important question that should be addressed in future research is whether the putative involvement of these structures in intertemporal choice reflects their

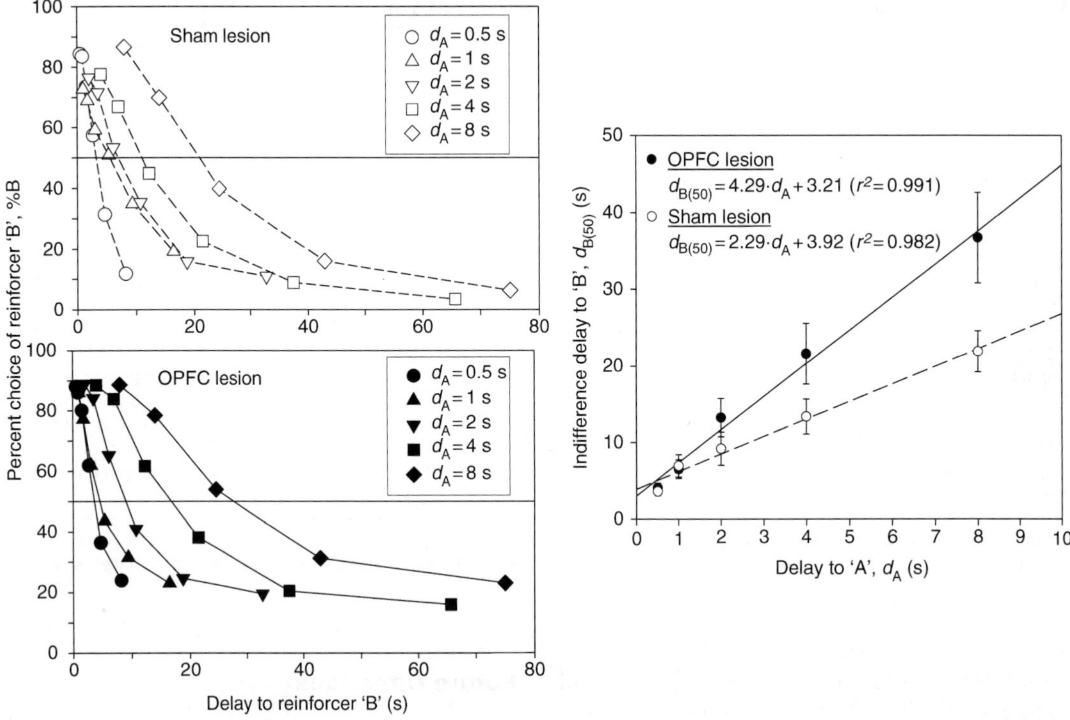

Figure 4 The effect of excitotoxin-induced lesions of the OPFC on intertemporal choice. (Left-hand graphs) Preference functions: percent responding on lever B (%B) is plotted against the delay to the larger of two reinforcers (d_B). Each plot shows the data obtained from one phase of the experiment, in which the delay to the smaller reinforcer (d_A) was fixed at the value shown in the inset panel. The horizontal line signifies indifference (%B = 50). (Right-hand graph) Linear indifference functions derived for the control group of sham-lesioned rats (open circles) and the OPFC-lesioned rats (filled circles). Ordinate: indifference delay to the larger reinforcer ($d_{B(50)}$); abscissa: imposed delay to the smaller reinforcer (d_A). Points are group mean data (± SEM); lines are best-fit linear functions. Data from Kheramin S, Body S, Mobini S, et al. (2002) *Psycyhopharmacology* 165: 9–17.

participation in integrated cortico-striato-thalamo-cortical circuits.

See also: Amphetamines; Delayed Reinforcement: Economics; Psychopharmacology of Reward and Appetite in Rats; Reinforcement Models; Reward and Learning; Reward Decision-Making; Reward Neurophysiology and Primate Cerebral Cortex; Reward Neurophysiology and Orbitofrontal Cortex.

Further Reading

Al-Ruwaitea ASA, Chiang T-J, Al-Zahrani SSA, Ho M-Y, Bradshaw CM, and Szabadi E (1999) Effect of central 5-hydroxytryptamine depletion on tolerance of delay of reinforcement: Evidence from performance in a discrete-trials 'time-left' procedure. *Psychopharmacology* 141: 22–29.

Bizot J-C, Le Bihan C, Puech AJ, Hamon M, and Thiébot MH (1999) Serotonin and tolerance to delay of reward in rats. *Psychopharmacology* 146: 400–412.

Cardinal RN, Robbins TW, and Everitt BJ (2000) The effects of d-amphetamine, chlordiazepoxide, alpha- flupenthixol and behavioural manipulations on choice of signalled and unsignalled delayed reinforcement in rats. *Psychopharmacology* 152: 362–375.

Cardinal RN, Robbins TW, and Everitt BJ (2004) Choosing delayed rewards: Perspectives from learning theory, neurochemistry, and neuroanatomy. In: Vuchinich RE and Heather N (eds.) *Choice Behavioural Economics and Addiction*, pp. 181–213. Oxford: Elsevier.

Charrier D and Thiébot MH (1996) Effect of phychotrophic drugs on rat responding in an operant paradigm involving choice between delayed reinforcers. *Pharmacology, Biochemistry, and Behavior* 54: 149–157.

Denk F, Walton ME, Jennings KA, Sharp T, Rushworth MFS, and Bannerman DM (2005) Differential involvement of serotonin and dopamine systems in cost–benefit decisions about delay or effort. *Psychopharmacology* 179: 587–596.

Evenden JL and Ryan CN (1996) The pharmacology of impulsive behaviour in rats: The effects of drugs on response choice with varying delays of reinforcements. *Psychopharmacology* 128: 161–170.

Ho M-Y, Mobini S, Chiang T-J, et al. (1999) Theory and method in the quantitative analysis of 'impulsive choice' behaviour: Implications for psychopharmacology. *Psychopharmacology* 146: 362–372.

Isles AR, Humby T, and Wilkinson LS (2003) Measuring impulsivity in mice using a novel operant delayed reinforcement task:

Effects of behavioural manipulations and d-amphetamine. *Psychopharmacology* 170: 376–382.

Kacelnik A (2003) The evolution of patience. In: Loewenstein G, Read D, and Baumeister R (eds.) *Time and Decision: Economic and Psychological Perspectives on Intertemporal Choice*, pp. 115–138. New York: Russel Sage.

Kheramin S, Body S, Mobini S, et al. (2002) Effects of quinolinic acid-induced lesions of the orbital prefrontal cortex on inter-temporal choice: A quantitative analysis. *Psychopharmacology* 165: 9–17.

Mazur JE (1997) Choice, delay, probability, and conditioned reinforcement. *Animal Learning & Behavior* 25: 131–147.

Mazur JE (2001) Hyperbolic value addition and general models of animal choice. *Psychological Review* 108: 96–112.

Mazur JE (2006) Mathematical models and the experimental analysis of behavior. *Journal of the Experimental Analysis of Behavior* 85: 285–291.

Mobini S, Chiang T-J, Al-Ruwaitea ASA, Ho M-Y, Bradshaw CM, and Szabadi E (2000a) Effect of central 5-hydroxytryptamine depletion on inter-temporal choice: A quantitative analysis. *Psychopharmacology* 149: 313–318.

Mobini S, Chiang T-J, Ho M-Y, Bradshaw CM, and Szabadi E (2000b) Effects of central 5-hydroxytryptamine depletion on sensitivity to delayed and probabilistic reinforcement. *Psychopharmacology* 152: 390–397.

Pitts RC and Febbo SM (2004) Quantitative analyses of methamphetamine's effects on self-control choices: Implications for elucidating behavioral mechanisms of drug action. *Behavioural Processes* 66: 213–233.

Richards JB, Sabol KE, and de Wit H (1999) Effects of methamphetamine on the adjusting amount procedure, a model of impulsive behavior in rats. *Psychopharmacology* 146: 432–439.

Sagvolden T, Johansen EB, Aase H, et al. (2005) A dynamic developmental theory of attention-deficit/hyperactivity disorder (ADHD) predominantly hyperactive/ impulsive and combined subtypes. *Behavioral and Brain Sciences* 28: 397–468.

Schultz W (2004) Neural coding of basic reward terms of animal learning theory, game theory, microeconomics and behavioural ecology. *Current Opinion in Neurobiology* 14: 139–147.

Soubrié P (1986) Reconciling the role of central serotonin neurons in human and animal behavior. *Behavioral and Brain Sciences* 9: 319–364.

Sozou PD (1998) On hyperbolic discounting and uncertain hazard rates. *Proceedings of the Royal Society, London, Series B* 265: 2015–2020.

Wade TR, deWit H, and Richards JB (2000) Effects of dopaminergic drugs on delayed reward as a measure of impulsive behavior in rats. *Psychopharmacology* 150: 90–101.

Winstanley CA, Dalley JW, Theobald DEH, and Robbins TW (2003) Global 5-HT depletion attenuates the ability of amphetamine to decrease impulsive choice in rats. *Psychopharmacology* 170: 320–331.

Winstanley CA, Theobald DEH, Cardinal RN, et al. (2004) Contrasting roles for basolateral amygdala and orbitofrontal cortex in impulsive choice. *Journal of Neuroscience* 24: 4718–4722.

Winstanley CA, Baunez C, Theobald DEH, et al. (2005) Lesions to the subthalamic nucleus decrease impulsive choice but impair autoshaping in rats: The importance of the basal ganglia in Pavlovian conditioning and impulse control. *European Journal of Neuroscience* 21: 3107–3116.

Wogar MA, Bradshaw CM, and Szabadi E (1993) Effect of lesions of the ascending 5-hydroxytryptaminergic pathways on choice between delayed reinforcers. *Psychopharmacology* 111: 239–243.

Game Theory and the Economics of Animal Communication

R A Johnstone, University of Cambridge, Cambridge, UK

Introduction

One may contrast signals with cues – traits that influence the behavior of others but have not been favored by selection for this reason. The rustling of a mouse running through long grass may, for instance, draw the attention of a predatory owl; the sound here serves as a cue to the location of the mouse, but it does not represent a signal (nor is this an instance of communication), because it is not adapted for this purpose. Selection has not favored mice who attract the notice of predators in this way; if anything, quieter individuals who minimize the noise they make are more likely to survive. By contrast, a display trait such as the song of a nightingale, the roar of a red deer, or the train of a peacock has been favored by selection precisely because of the responses it evokes, and thus it constitutes a true signal.

Selection of Signals – Efficacy versus Strategy

The first requirement for an effective signal, in any context, is that it should be readily detectable and identifiable by the appropriate recipient. Yet communication may often take place over long distances or in a noisy environment, so by the time they reach the receiver, signals are attenuated, degraded, and overlaid by irrelevant stimuli. Selection will therefore tend to favor conspicuous and distinctive signals that are easier to detect and identify, even in the presence of noise. At the same time, such displays may be energetically costly or time consuming to produce and may draw the unwanted attention of 'eavesdroppers' such as predators and parasites. The displays we see in nature should be those that strike the best balance between the opposing selective pressures for greater efficacy and lower cost.

Many studies have looked at the design of animal signals from this perspective, focusing on the features that enhance signal efficacy. There is evidence, for instance, that the details of visual and vocal signal design are often adapted to the particular physical environment in which communication occurs, and to the sensory capacities and 'psychology' of receivers, so as to facilitate efficient detection. But the emphasis in this article is on a different aspect of signal design. It is not enough that a display should be readily detectable. If it is to be favored by natural selection, it must also, once detected, tend to elicit responses that are beneficial for the signaler. This 'strategic' perspective on signal evolution emphasizes those properties of a display that render it effective in eliciting a beneficial response rather than those that facilitate detection.

To understand the strategic aspect of signal design, we must consider selection from the perspective of both the signaler and the receiver. Selection favors signalers that elicit favorable responses from receivers; it also favors receivers that respond appropriately to signalers. Game theory, with its emphasis on strategic interaction, is thus a powerful tool for modeling this aspect of signal evolution.

Conflicts of Interest and the Problem of Honesty

In some 'cooperative' contexts, the recipient of a signal also gains by responding in a manner that is beneficial for the signaler. Under these circumstances, the evolutionary interests of the two parties are aligned. Consider, for example, the 'dance language' of honeybees, by means of which a worker returning to the hive can convey to her sisters the location of a food source. The worker benefits by recruiting others to the food, just as they stand to gain by responding to the information she provides. Selection on both parties thus favors efficient communication.

In most cases, however, there is an evolutionary conflict of interest between signaler and receiver because the latter suffers by responding in a manner beneficial to the former. Bolas spiders, for instance, attract male insect prey by means of a pheromonal lure that mimics the sex pheromones of females of the prey species. Responding to such a chemical 'lure,' while it may benefit the spider, is clearly detrimental to the prey.

The conflict in the above case is extreme, but even in situations where there is a degree of common interest between signaler and receiver, there will usually be an element of conflict too. For instance, both males and females share a common interest in finding and identifying potential mates of their own species. However, males are typically under stronger selection to acquire many mates, and females to acquire better mates. This gives rise to a conflict of interest. Females stand to gain by accurately assessing the mating benefits (material or genetic) that a potential partner has to offer, in order to reject suitors of low value. Conversely, males stand to gain by misleading females as to their own value, in order to gain additional matings. In a similar way, conflict arises between parents and offspring, even though both have a genetic stake in each other's survival. Offspring are selected to demand more food than parents are selected to provide. As a result, parents stand to gain by accurately assessing offspring need, but offspring stand to gain by misleading parents as to their own condition in order to extract additional resources from them.

The first theoretical game models of animal communication suggested that because of the underlying conflict of interest between signaler and receiver, informative or honest signaling cannot persist. Consider, for instance, a population in which signalers reliably advertise their aggressive intentions by means of a threat display. Maynard Smith, using game theory to model conflict behavior, argued that threat displays that provided receivers with accurate information about an animal's intentions would not be evolutionarily stable. If a display provides honest information about an opponent's propensity to fight, receivers should attend to it and should be more likely to back down when they confront an opponent who signals strongly. Consequently, it seems that a 'deceitful' mutant that always announced a high level of aggression would prosper because its opponents would more often retreat. The spread of such mutants would, however, devalue the signal. Ultimately, it would no longer pay to attend to the display, because it would no longer provide reliable information.

The same argument seems to apply to any signaling system in which there is a conflict of interest between signaler and receiver. Any correlation between the production or intensity of a display and the underlying state of the signaler can be disrupted by the spread of a 'deceitful' mutant that gains by adopting a misrepresentative signal. Consequently, the models seemed to suggest that communication should be viewed, not as a cooperative exchange of information, but as the focus of an arms race between signalers as 'manipulators' and receivers as 'mind-readers,' the former standing to gain by effective exploitation, the latter by effective extraction of information. Honesty, from this perspective, merely represented a temporary phase of the arms race in which receivers have 'drawn ahead' of signalers.

Constraints and Costs – The Handicap Principle

Despite the potential benefits that signalers stand to gain by misleading receivers, the majority of signals seem to convey at least some reliable information. In other words, stable honesty is the usual outcome of the arms race between signaler and receiver. How can such honesty persist in the face of the evolutionary conflict between the two?

Honesty may endure if it is physically impossible for a signaler to produce a misleading signal. In some cases there is a material link between the signal and some underlying aspect of the signaler's state, such that the former is constrained to provide information about the latter. For instance, many animals display bright coloration attributable (in part at least) to carotenoid pigments. Since most cannot synthesize carotenoids themselves but must acquire them as part of their diet, the intensity of carotenoid coloration is inescapably linked to (past) foraging success. An individual that fails to acquire sufficient carotenoids through foraging simply cannot manufacture the pigments needed for vivid color. Studies of the house finch (*Carpodacus mexicanus*), for instance, a species in which males display patches of carotenoid pigment on the crown, breast, and rump, have shown that females prefer redder males and that vivid coloration reflects nutritional state at the time of molt. Since molting precedes mate choice by some time, redder males may not necessarily be in better condition when they are actually chosen as partners, but plumage coloration was correlated with nest attentiveness and overwinter survival, suggesting that brighter males do make, on average, better fathers.

While a few signals may be 'unfakable' because of such physical constraints, most are not. An individual's choice of one threat display or another, for instance, is not physically constrained by its fighting ability or motivation, nor is the length of a bird's tail inescapably tied to its value as a mate. To account for widespread honesty, therefore, an explanation is required that is applicable to situations in which the relationship between the signal and the underlying state of the signaler is open to behavioral or evolutionary change.

Amotz Zahavi was the first biologist to propose such a general explanation for honesty. He suggested that a signal could provide reliable or 'honest' information about the quality of the signaler if it were costly to produce. Consider, for instance, a population in which males reliably advertise their value as mates by means of some sexual display. The correlation between signal and mate value would seem vulnerable to disruption by the spread of a deceitful mutant that adopts the display typical of the most desirable males, regardless of its own quality. Suppose, however, that the signal is costly to produce but that superior males can more easily bear these costs than can inferior males. Under these circumstances, it might pay an inferior male to refrain from signaling, even though it would be physically able to do so, because the costs involved would outweigh the benefits to be gained. At the same time, for superior males who can more easily bear the costs of display, production of the signal would yield a net benefit. Under these circumstances, honesty can persist.

While Zahavi initially focused chiefly on sexual displays, he has subsequently argued that the handicap principle is applicable to many and perhaps all forms of communication. Costly signals could serve to advertise fighting ability, for instance, and thereby to deter rivals, or could deter predators by advertising ability to escape or fend off attack. Costly contributions to group activities could, in a similar way, advertise social status, provided that only dominant, high-quality individuals can afford to invest time and energy in such pursuits. In short, receivers in most contexts can obtain reliable information about signaler quality by attending to displays that are costly to produce.

A Simple Model

Zahavi's handicap principle suggests a possible solution to the problem of honesty. At first, however, it was widely dismissed as unworkable. In part, this rejection of the idea was due to Zahavi's verbal formulation, which was open to different interpretations, leaving some doubt as to precisely what was meant. Acceptance had to wait until the development of formal models, in many cases based on game theoretical techniques. Indeed, the problem of honesty has been, and remains, the chief focus of game theoretical models of animal communication, and such models have played a key role in establishing the plausibility of honest, costly advertisement (it must also be noted that economic game theory had reached similar conclusions rather earlier).

To illustrate this approach, this article presents a very simple (perhaps the simplest possible) game theoretical model of honest signaling. Suppose that one individual, the signaler, is informed of the value of an uncertain parameter q (possibly representing some aspect of the external environment, but more likely some aspect of its own type or state). The signaler than chooses an action s, referred to as a signal. Another individual, the receiver, who is unaware of the value of the parameter q, observes the signal s and decides, on this basis, to adopt some response r. In our simple case, q, s, and r all take values of either 0 or 1. Each player then receives a payoff that may depend on q, s, and r.

The problem of honesty arises when receivers gain by responding differently to signalers of different type, but at least some signalers stands to gain by eliciting a response that is, from the perspective of the receiver, inappropriate for their type. Suppose, for instance, that the receiver obtains a payoff of 1 if its response matches the signaler's type (i.e., if $r=q=0$ or $r=q=1$), but a payoff of 0 otherwise (if $r\neq q$). All signalers, by contrast, obtain a payoff equal to r and therefore prefer a response of 1 to a response of 0. How is a separating equilibrium, at which signalers of different types adopt different signals, possible under these conditions? Any such equilibrium appears vulnerable to invasion by a rare class of mutant signaler that, regardless of its true type, adopts the signal typical of individuals of type $q=1$, thereby eliciting the favorable response $r=1$.

Suppose, however, that the signal adopted by individuals of type 1 is costly to produce. The handicap principle suggest that this can serve to maintain honesty. For simplicity, let us restrict our attention to the potential separating equilibrium at which individuals of type $q=1$ adopt the signal $s=1$ (eliciting the response $r=1$), while individuals of type $q=0$ adopt the signal $s=0$ (eliciting the response $r=0$). Now suppose that production of the signal $s=1$ entails an additive cost of magnitude c_i (≥ 0) for signalers of type i, whereas the signal $s=0$ is cost-free. Provided that $c_0 > 1 > c_1$, the separating equilibrium is stable against invasion by the cheating mutant suggested above because the cost of adopting signal $s=1$ outweighs the benefits to be gained thereby for individuals of type 0 but not for those of type 1. Cheating in this case may be possible, in the sense that a mutant individual can arise that adopts signal $s=1$ when of type $q=0$, but it proves unprofitable.

In the above case, signalers differ in the cost they pay to produce the 'favored' signal $s=1$, but all stand to gain the same benefits by eliciting the 'favorable' response $r=1$. Suppose, by contrast, that all signalers pay the same cost, of magnitude 1, to produce the favored signal, but that the benefit they stand to gain by eliciting the favorable response $r=1$, denoted b_i for signalers of type i, differs according to their type. Provided that $b_1 > 0 > b_0$, the separating equilibrium is once again stable against invasion by the cheating mutant because the signal $s=1$ is unprofitable for individuals of type $q=0$. In this case, however, honesty is maintained not by the differential cost of the signal but by differential benefit. The former case is often described as a signal of quality, the latter as a signal of need.

In reality, of course, signalers may vary both in the cost of signaling and in the benefits they stand to gain, and some more-realistic models have incorporated both factors (though surprisingly many analyses continue to focus exclusively on one or the other).

Evidence for Honesty

Even the very simple model presented above suffices to demonstrate that signal cost can, in principle at least, serve to maintain honesty. But is there any evidence that the handicap principle plays such a role in nature? This article offers two illustrative examples of the kind of studies that have been undertaken to confirm its importance.

Perhaps the best evidence for honest, costly advertisement of quality comes from work by Mappes and colleagues on sexual display in the wolf spider *Hygrolycosa rubrofasciata*. Males of this ground-dwelling species attract mates by drumming on dry leaves on the substrate with their abdomen. Experiments have shown that drumming entails energetic costs – males kept under standardized conditions lose weight faster and experience greater mortality when induced to drum more often by exposure to females. At the same time, those males who were observed to drum more frequently and vigorously under natural conditions suffer less when subsequently induced to drum in the lab, indicating that the costs of the display are indeed lower for those males that signal more strongly, as the handicap principle predicts.

Turning to advertisement of need, some of the best evidence for honest, costly signaling comes from work by Kilner on the begging displays of captive canary (*Serinus canaria*) nestlings. When an adult canary returns to the nest with food, the offspring stretch and posture, gape and call as the adult empties its crop and distributes the regurgitated food among the brood. Chicks that attain positions closer to the parent are likely to receive more food, but when offspring proximity to the parent was experimentally controlled and hunger manipulated, parents were observed to preferentially feed hungrier chicks, suggesting that they respond to cues indicative of offspring need. What form might these cues take? The mouths of canary nestlings exhibit a rapid change in color intensity, the 'flush,' following the onset of begging, and subsequent experiments revealed that this change in color accurately reflects a nestling's state of need and that parents preferentially feed chicks with artificially reddened mouths. Gape color thus appears to provide parents with an honest signal of chick hunger (although parents may also respond to chick posturing and calling as well). Finally, when pairs of canary siblings were induced to beg for markedly different durations, greater begging was found to retard growth, both immediately and in the long term. This growth cost is likely to entail a reduction in fitness, because daily mass gain was strongly correlated with survival of chicks to independence. It thus appears that chick begging in this species constitutes a costly, as well as an honest, signal of hunger.

Occasional Deceit

The handicap principle seems to offer a simple and widely applicable solution to the problem of honesty. But if receivers can obtain reliable information about signaler quality or condition merely by attending to costly displays, how can one account for instances of deceit?

Selection will favor receivers who respond to a signal if, on average, they obtain a net benefit by doing so. But a benefit 'on average' is compatible with occasional exploitation. Suppose, for instance, that a rare class of signaler finds display cheaper than other individuals do, for the same level of quality, or stands to gain more by eliciting a favorable response, for the same level of condition. Such individuals do best to produce a 'misleading' signal, typical (in most cases) of signalers of higher quality or in greater need than themselves. This will lead receivers to respond more favorably to them than to other signalers. We might expect receivers to adjust their behavior to take account of the presence of these deceptive individuals – the risk of encountering one will favor lower responsiveness to intense displays. Nevertheless, provided that the frequency of such individuals is low enough, and the cost of responding to them inappropriately is not too great, they need not disrupt the signaling system altogether. Evidence of occasional deceit can thus support the handicap principle if it can be established that deceitful signalers do differ from others in the net benefit they stand to gain from display (and if there are constraints on the frequency of deceit).

A good example is the use of deceptive begging signals by avian brood parasites such as cuckoos. As discussed above, there is evidence that chick begging constitutes (in at least some cases) an honest signal of hunger. Models of begging predict that chicks who are less closely related to their nestmates and to the adults raising them should beg more intensely because they have less to lose by depriving their competitors of food and/or forcing the adults to work harder. A brood parasite chick is an extreme instance of this: Since it is entirely unrelated to the other chicks in the nest or to its host parents, it has no genetic interest in their survival. Accordingly, Kilner and colleagues have shown that chicks of the common cuckoo exploit the signaling system of reed warbler hosts by begging at a greater rate than do host chicks. Intriguingly, parents appear to respond to both the vocal and the visual signals of their offspring. Cuckoo chicks, which eject all host young from the nest, display a reduced gape area compared with a host brood yet apparently compensate by more rapid calling.

Exploitation of host parents by specialized brood parasites may appear an extreme and unusual instance of deceit. However, more subtle forms of intraspecific deception may be widespread. A nice illustration is the occurrence of bluffing in the marine stomatopod crustacean *Gonodactylus bredini*, studied by Adams and

Caldwell. Males of this species defend cavities in coral rubble and ward off intruders with a meral spread threat display. Following molt, an individual's soft condition means that it is unable to fight effectively, yet newly molted owners threaten more often than those that are capable of fighting, thus reducing the chances that intruders will attack and discover their opponents' vulnerability. That this deceit does not destabilize the signaling system entirely presumably reflects the relativey low probability of encountering a newly molted opponent.

Cost-Free Honesty?

The evidence discussed earlier shows that signal cost can indeed, as the handicap principle suggests, favor quality-dependent or condition-dependent expression of display traits. Cost, in other words, is sufficient to maintain honesty. But is it necessary? The more-enthusiastic proponents of the handicap principle have argued that honest signals must be costly, otherwise what is to prevent cheating? But more-recent analyses suggest that cost-free honesty is possible. Two rather different mechanisms have been proposed that might maintain signal reliability even in the absence of cost.

The first mechanism was suggested in the context of signaling of need by offspring to their parents. As pointed out above, offspring are selected to demand more resources than parents are selected to supply. Consequently, an honest signal of need is potentially subject to devaluation by deceitful mutants that misrepresent their need, thereby attaining additional resources. However, since offspring have a genetic stake in the well-being of their parents, selection will not favor unlimited selfishness on the part of young. Offspring stand to gain by simulating a level of need that is slightly greater than their true need, but not so great that they might elicit excessive investment that would be overly costly to the parent. Selection, in other words, will act against offspring that are too deceptive.

As a result of selection against excessive deception, a cost-free signaling equilibrium is possible at which offspring divide into two or more discrete categories, according to their need, in each of which all individuals adopt the same begging behavior (sometimes referred to as a 'pooling' equilibrium). In the simplest case, for instance, those whose need falls below some threshold refrain from begging while the remainder beg. Under these circumstances, the parent cannot distinguish among nonbegging young and must attribute to them all the same 'average nonbegging' level of need; similarly, the parent cannot distinguish among begging young and must attribute to them all the same 'average begging' level of need (greater than the average for nonbegging young). A nonbegging offspring may thus stand to gain by exaggerating its need slightly, but it cannot do so – by choosing to beg, it will cause the parent to greatly overestimate its level of need, to an extent that can prove disadvantageous, even if begging entails no direct costs.

Formal game-theoretical models have confirmed that a cost-free equilibrium of the above kind is possible in principle. Whether actual chick begging represents a cost-free or a costly signal remains, however, controversial. As described earlier, there is evidence that begging entails fitness costs in at least some cases. But in other instances, the costs are less obvious – most attempts to measure the energetic cost of begging, for instance, suggest that this is very small. Similarly, while experiments have shown that playback of begging calls can increase the risk of nestling predation, this result holds true only for offspring in open nests and perhaps overlooks the fact that parents may normally be able to warn their offspring to remain silent when predators are nearby, so reducing the effective cost of begging. Despite the paucity of evidence for substantial costs, however, offspring typically do not exhibit 'pooling' but instead show continuous variation in begging intensity, which better fits the predictions of costly signaling models. Perhaps, in reality, begging may involve both costly and cost-free components – it is certainly a composite signal, often combining posturing, calling, and gaping.

In any case, 'pooling' models of cost-free begging are based on the fact that signalers (offspring) have a genetic stake in the well-being of receivers (their parents). Because this is not the case in many other signaling systems, such models are of restricted applicability. A second mechanism for the maintenance of cost-free honesty, however, is of much broader scope. Looking back at the very simple model we introduced earlier, we showed that in the case of a signal of quality, stable honesty is possible provided that $c_1 > 1 > c_2$, that is, provided that the cost of signaling exceeds the benefit to be gained for individuals of class 1, but not for individuals of class 2. This condition allows for the possibility that $c_2 = 0$, that is, that the signal is entirely cost-free for individuals of class 2. Because it is only these individuals that employ the signal at equilibrium, the outcome is then one in which no cost is paid. What maintains honesty (in the face of a conflict of interest between signaler and receiver) is the fact that low-quality individuals 'would' incur a cost 'if they were to adopt' the display behavior typical of a high-quality signaler. This does not mean, however, that such display behavior must entail a cost for the high-quality individuals that actually employ it.

The above argument suggests that cost-free honesty is possible in any context, provided that cost is incurred only by those signalers that misrepresent their state. It is difficult to envisage a physical mechanism that could give rise to such conditional costs. When costs are socially imposed, however, it does seem plausible that receivers might punish only those signalers that are subsequently discovered to have employed misrepresentative or deceptive signals. For example, rhesus monkeys living on the island of Cayo Santiago, Puerto Rico, often (though not always) produce distinctive vocalizations when they discover or eat food, particularly high-quality food such as coconut. Following the discovery of food by one individual, other group members were in some cases observed to detect and approach the food source and its original discoverer. Some discoverers were then attacked and injured, whereas others were allowed to keep the food they had collected. It appears that individuals who call when they discover food are more likely to be approached by other group members, and as a result suffer from increased feeding competition. However, discoverers who call incur less aggression when subsequently detected than do those discoverers who remain silent. In this case, then, the threat of aggression directed at 'deceptive' individuals who refrain from calling may serve to maintain honest advertisement of food discoveries.

Further Questions

This brief review makes clear, the important role that game-theoretical models have played, and continue to play, in the study of animal communication. Because most forms of communication involve an evolutionary conflict of interest between signaler and receiver, they are potentially vulnerable to disruption by 'dishonest' signalers. Game-theoretical models have served to verify the logic of Zahavi's handicap principle and to confirm that signal cost may indeed support honest signaling in the face of a conflict of interest, a suggestion for which there is now some empirical support. At the same time, such models have also suggested that honesty need not always entail signal cost. This last issue remains the subject of much controversy, and the study of putative cases of cost-free honesty continues to attract much interest. There are also many further questions that fall within the scope of game theory, but which have not been touched on here. Three topics that are of particular interest, for instance, are the evolution and use of multiple signals, the dynamics of extended communicatory interchanges, and the evolution of signaling within a communication network in which multiple receivers may eavesdrop on a signal (and multiple signalers may compete for the attention of a receiver). Given the many questions that remain to be answered, it seems likely that game theory still has much to contribute to the study of animal communication.

See also: Animal Communication: Honesty and Deception; Communication Networks and Eavesdropping in Animals; Electrical Perception and Communication; Endocrinology of Animal Communication: Behavioral; Kinship Signals in Animals; Pheromones and other Chemical Communication in Animals; Referentiality and Concepts in Animal Cognition; Seismic and Vibrational Signals in Animals; Sexual Selection and the Evolution of Animal Signals; Signal Design Rules in Animal Communication; Visual Signaling in Animals.

Further Reading

Adams ES and Caldwell RL (1990) Deceptive communication in asymmetric fights of the stomatopod crustacean *Gonodactylus bredini*. *Animal Behavior* 39: 706–716.

Bergstrom CT and Lachmann M (1998) Signalling among relatives. III. Talk is cheap. *Proceedings of the National Academy of Sciences of the United States of America* 95: 5100–5105.

Grafen A (1990) Biological signals as handicaps. *Journal of Theoretical Biology* 144: 517–546.

Hauser MD and Marler P (1993) Food-associated calls in rhesus macacques (*Macaca mulatta*). II. Costs and benefits of call production and suppression. *Behavioral Ecology* 4: 206–212.

Hill GE, Inouye CY, and Montgomerie R (2002) Dietary carotenoids predict plumage colouration in wild house finches. *Proceedings of the Royal Society of London, Series B* 269: 1119–1124.

Johnstone RA and Grafen A (1993) Dishonesty and the handicap principle. *Animal Behaviour* 46: 759–764.

Kilner RM (2001) A growth cost of begging in captive canary chicks. *Proceedings of the National Academy of Sciences of the United States of America* 98: 11394–11398.

Kilner RM, Noble DG, and Davies NB (1999) Signals of need in parent-offspring communication and their exploitation by the common cuckoo. *Nature* 397: 667–672.

Lachmann M, Szamado S, and Bergstrom CT (2001) Cost and conflict in animal signals and human language. *Proceedings of the National Academy of Sciences of the United States of America* 98: 13189–13194.

Mappes J, Alatalo RV, Kotiaho J, and Parri S (1996) Viability costs of condition-dependent sexual male display in a drumming wolf spider. *Proceedings of the Royal Society of London, Series B* 263: 785–789.

Maynard Smith J (1974) The theory of games and the evolution of animal conflicts. *Journal of Theoretical Biology* 57: 239–242.

Maynard Smith J (1991) Honest signalling: The Philip Sidney game. *Animal Behaviour* 47: 1115–1120.

Maynard Smith J and Harper D (2003) *Animal signals*. Oxford, UK: Oxford University Press.

Searcy WA and Nowicki S (2005) *The Evolution of Animal Communication*. Princeton, NJ: Princeton University Press.

Zahavi A (1975) Mate selection: A selection for a handicap. *Journal of Theoretical Biology* 53: 205–214.

Games in Monkeys: Neurophysiology and Motor Decision-Making

D Lee, Yale University School of Medicine, New Haven, CT, USA

Stages of Decision Making

Decision making can be defined as choosing a particular option from multiple alternatives, and it is often carried out in order to maximize certain desirable quantity, such as reward or utility. Animals rely heavily on the sensory stimuli they receive from their environment to choose appropriate behavioral responses (**Figure 1**). A precise pattern of sensory stimuli impinging on the animal's nervous system is determined by the positions and orientations of the animal's sensory organs as well as the current state of the animal's environment. These sensory inputs are inevitably corrupted to a variable degree by the noise in the animal's nervous system. Based on this noisy representation, individual objects in the environment are recognized and additional properties of these objects that the animals have learned from their previous experience can be retrieved from their memory storage. This is the process of perceptual decision making. Based on the outcome of perceptual decision making, the animal chooses what to do, and this is referred to as cognitive decision making. For example, should the animal eat the apple it just discovered from a tree, or save it for a rainy day? Even when all the objects in the animal's environment are correctly identified, the animal's behavioral response may change depending on the animal's metabolic needs, and the animal's cognitive limitations may prevent the animal from selecting a behavioral response that produces the most desirable outcome. Finally, the number of various movement trajectories that can be chosen to accomplish a particular behavioral objective is often infinitely large, and the selection of a particular motor trajectory can be referred to as motor decision making. For example, a light switch can be turned on by the right or left hand or even by one's head if both hands are occupied or injured. This article focuses on the neural mechanisms of cognitive and motor decision making in monkeys with a particular emphasis on cognitive decision making in the context of social interaction.

Utility Maximization and Reinforcement Learning

Standard economic analysis of choice behavior, such as the expected utility theory, begins with the assumption that decision makers assign a numerical score to each available option according to the subjective desirability of its outcome, commonly referred to as utility function. It is also assumed that decision makers make their choices so as to maximize the expected value of utility function. Numerous studies of human choice behavior have shown that these assumptions are often violated. Many of these violations are accounted for by alternative theoretical proposals, such as the prospective theory of Kahneman and Tversky and the regret theory of Bell, Loomes, and Sugden. Nevertheless, the expected utility theory still remains as a core theory in microeconomics, and accounts for a wide range of choice behavior in both humans and animals.

To understand the neural basis of decision making within the framework of the expected utility theory, it is important to distinguish two different types of utility which Kahneman referred to as decision utility and experienced utility. Decision utility corresponds to the amount of subjective pleasure expected by the decision maker during the process of decision making. In contrast, experienced utility is the amount of actual pleasure or satisfaction derived from chosen actions or from the consumption of chosen objects. If the decision maker makes correct predictions regarding the outcomes of chosen actions during the time of decision making, experienced utility would be equal to decision utility. In reality, however, the decision maker's knowledge of his or her environment is seldom complete, and there is often a discrepancy between these two types of utilities. It is, therefore, possible that decision utility and experienced utility might be represented and processed in separate brain areas. The results from previous neuroimaging studies in human subjects, however, show that decision utility and experienced utility influence the level of metabolic activity in similar brain areas, including the dorsolateral prefrontal cortex, the orbitofrontal cortex, the anterior and posterior cingulate cortex, the posterior parietal cortex, and the basal ganglia. Activity of individual neurons in many of these brain areas has been examined in nonhuman primates, and the results are largely consistent with the findings from the human neuroimaging studies. Thus, signals related to decision and experienced utilities are encoded in a broadly distributed network of cortical and subcortical areas.

If the animal's environment is stationary, the probability that a given action would produce a particular outcome would be fixed, and, therefore, optimal decision-making strategies can be hardwired in the form of stimulus–response mapping. In reality, the environment is almost always dynamic, and the actual outcomes frequently differ from the outcomes

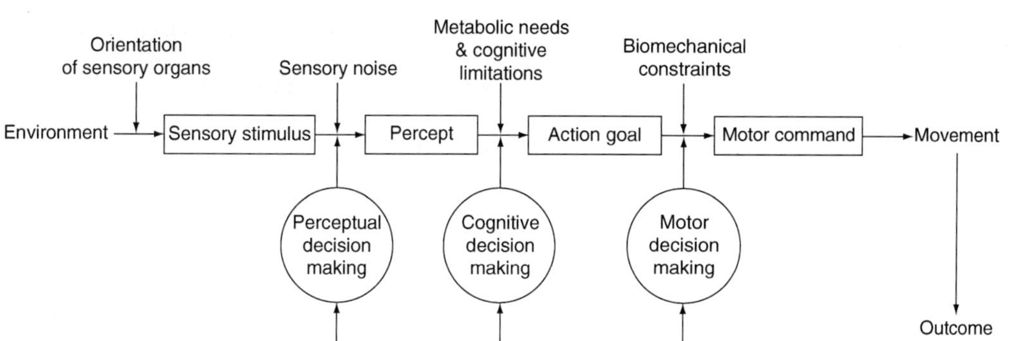

Figure 1 Different stages of decision making.

anticipated during the process of decision making, so decision utilities may deviate from the experienced utilities. To make choices optimally, therefore, decision makers need to adjust decision utilities according to their experience. In reinforcement learning theory, decision utilities are referred to as value functions and the difference between decision and experienced utilities is referred to as reward prediction error. The work of Schultz and his colleagues showed that reward prediction error is encoded by the activity of dopamine neurons in the primate ventral tegmental area and substantia nigra pars compacta. These dopamine neurons project densely to the striatum, and neuroimaging studies in human subjects found that the activity in the striatum also reflects reward prediction error. Therefore, dopamine neurons and their target neurons in the striatum might play a key role in updating and encoding the value functions during dynamic decision making.

Game Theory and Adaptive Social Decision Making

To make choices optimally, decision makers must be able to predict the outcomes of their actions correctly. For animals in a social context, the outcomes of their choices often depend on the behaviors of other animals, so they must be able to predict the choices of other animals. The mathematical problem of finding an optimal decision-making strategy in a socially interactive setting is addressed by the game theory introduced by von Neumann and Morgenstern.

In game theory, a game is characterized by a set of players, a set of available actions for each player, and a payoff function that assigns utility to each player according to the choices of all players. As in the expected utility theory, game theory assumes that players in a game seek to maximize their utility functions individually, and then provides normative predictions as to the choices that rational players should make. One such prediction is provided by Nash equilibrium, which is defined as a set of strategies for all players from which no players can deviate individually to increase their payoffs. Although game theory provides such solutions to many different types of games, many studies in behavioral economics have found that people often display systematic deviations from such theoretical predictions.

Matching Pennies Game

Barraclough and his colleagues investigated whether the choice behavior of monkeys during a simple zero-sum game, known as matching pennies (**Figure 2(a)**), follows the prediction of Nash equilibrium. In each trial, a monkey and a computer opponent each chose either the left-hand or the right-hand target, and the monkey was rewarded only when it chose the same target as the computer. The computer was programmed to simulate a utility-maximizing player capable of analyzing and exploiting the animal's behavior. In the matching pennies game illustrated in **Figure 2(a)**, choosing one of the options exclusively is not a part of the Nash equilibrium. For example, if the monkey and the computer always choose the left-hand and right-hand target, respectively, their payoffs would be both zero. This is not a Nash equilibrium, since the monkey can increase its payoff by increasing the probability of choosing the right-hand target. The Nash equilibrium for this matching pennies game is for each player to choose the two targets with equal probabilities. Barraclough and his colleagues found that the overall probability that the animal would choose each of the two targets was quite close to this equilibrium prediction. However, there was still a bias for the animal to choose the same target chosen by the computer opponent in the previous trial, which was exploited by the computer to reduce the probability of reward for the animal.

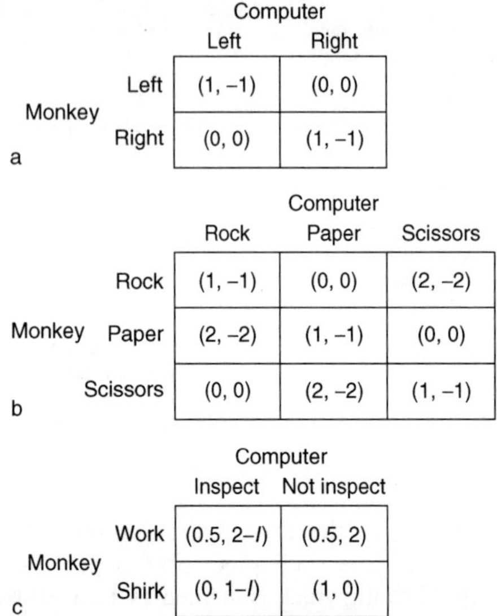

a

		Computer Left	Computer Right
Monkey	Left	(1, −1)	(0, 0)
	Right	(0, 0)	(1, −1)

b

		Computer Rock	Computer Paper	Computer Scissors
Monkey	Rock	(1, −2)*		

Figure 2 Payoff matrix for matching pennies game (a), rock–paper–scissors game (b), and inspection game (c). Each game is played by a monkey and a computer opponent. For each payoff matrix, rows correspond to the alternative choices for the monkey, and columns correspond to the choices of the computer opponent. Two numbers inside the parentheses correspond to the payoffs or utilities for the monkey and the computer opponent, respectively. In the matching pennies game, the optimal strategy, known as Nash equilibrium, is for each player to choose the left-hand and right-hand targets randomly with equal probabilities. The equilibrium strategy in the rock–paper–scissors game is to choose each option with a 1/3 probability. In the inspection game, *I* indicates the cost of inspection (0 *I* 1), and the optimal strategy is for the computer opponent to inspect with the probability of 0.5 and for the monkey to shirk with the probability of *I*.

The fact that monkeys displayed small but systematic biases in their choice behavior during the matching pennies game might reflect a specific learning algorithm used by the animal to approximate the optimal decision-making strategy. Therefore, the choice behavior of monkeys during the matching pennies game was analyzed further with a reinforcement learning model. Such a model formalizes Thorndike's law of effect and generalizes the so-called win–stay–lose–switch strategy. In this model, the probability of choosing each target is determined by the logistic function of the difference between the value functions for the two targets. In addition, value functions are adjusted according to the outcome of the animal's choice in each trial, and the effect of the animal's choice in a given trial decays exponentially during the following trials. Accordingly, the value function of a target increases gradually if its choice is rewarded frequently. The animal's choice behavior during the matching pennies game was indeed consistent with the predictions from this simple reinforcement learning model.

During the matching pennies game, neurons in the dorsolateral prefrontal cortex display several different types of signals that might reflect the process of reinforcement learning. First, many neurons modulate their activity according to the animal's choice in the previous trial. In many decision-making problems, the outcome of a particular choice is often revealed after some delay. In such cases, it is necessary to maintain information about the action taken by the animal until its outcome is revealed, so that its value function can be adjusted appropriately. In reinforcement learning, such memory of a previous action is referred to as eligibility trace. Therefore, activity in the dorsolateral prefrontal cortex related to the animal's choice in the previous trial might provide the neural substrate of eligibility trace. Second, activity of neurons in the dorsolateral prefrontal cortex often reflects whether the animal was rewarded in the previous trial or not. This suggests that the dorsolateral prefrontal cortex may be involved in adjusting the value functions for the recently chosen actions, since the outcome of a given choice determines how its value function would be updated in reinforcement learning. Finally, some neurons in the dorsolateral prefrontal cortex displayed modulations in their activity according to the combination of the animal's choice in the previous trial and its outcome (**Figure 3**). Such signals can provide information about the choice of the computer opponent, and therefore can also contribute to the process of updating value functions, since during the matching pennies game, the choice of the opponent determines the animal's choice that would be rewarded.

Rock–Paper–Scissors Game: Reinforcement Learning versus Belief Learning

Although the choice behavior of monkeys during the matching pennies game was relatively well described by a simple reinforcement learning model, the simplicity of this game makes it difficult to test whether the animal might rely on an alternative learning algorithm. For example, in belief learning, the decision makers update their beliefs about the choices of other players, and choose the best action that maximizes the expected payoffs based on such beliefs. For the matching pennies game, reinforcement learning and belief learning models cannot be distinguished. To understand this, imagine that the animal selects the left-hand and right-hand target in two successive trials while the computer selects the right-hand targets in both trials. The animal would then be rewarded only in the second trial. In a reinforcement learning model, the value function for the left-hand target would decrease after the first trial and the value

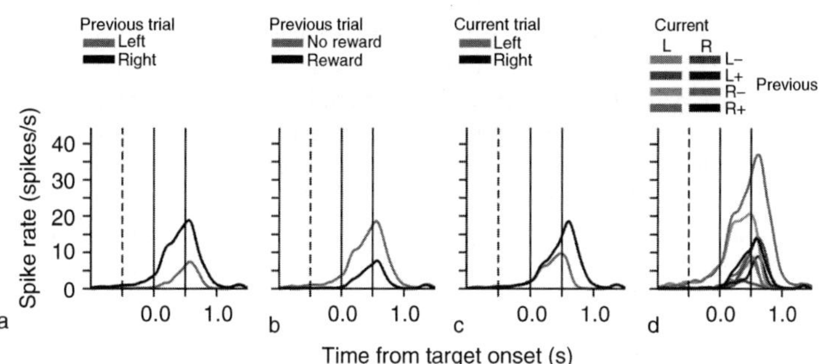

Figure 3 Temporal changes in the spike rate of a single neuron in the dorsolateral prefrontal cortex of a monkey during a matching pennies game. The activity of this neuron was modulated by the animal's choice in the previous trial (a), its outcome (b), and the animal's choice in the current trial (c). In addition, this neuron increased its activity significantly when the animal chose the right-hand target after the same choice was not rewarded in the previous trial (d). Adapted from Barraclough DJ, Conroy ML, and Lee D (2004) Prefrontal cortex and decision making in a mixed-strategy game. *Nature Neuroscience* 7: 404–410.

function for the right-hand target would increase after the second trial. Accordingly, after two such trials, the animal would be more likely to choose the right-hand target. In a belief learning model, the animal would strengthen its belief that the computer opponent would choose the right-hand target, and therefore the value function for the right target would increase after each trial. As in reinforcement learning, this would also increase the probability that the animal would choose the right-hand target. These two scenarios would become indistinguishable if the value functions are related to the probability of choosing each action through a logistic function that determines the animal's choice as a function of the difference between the two value functions.

The difference between reinforcement learning and belief learning can be revealed if a player has to choose from more than two alternatives. In such cases, belief learning might be a more efficient way to improve the strategy of a decision maker compared to reinforcement learning. This can be illustrated using the example of a rock–paper–scissors game (**Figure 2(b)**). In reinforcement learning, if a player chooses rock and is defeated by the opponent who chooses paper, the value function for rock and the probability of choosing it would decrease, but the value functions for paper and scissors would not be affected. In belief learning, the player would strengthen his or her belief that the opponent would choose paper again, so the value function for scissors and the probability of choosing scissors would increase more than for paper. It should be noted that if the opponent plays according to the Nash equilibrium strategy, the average payoff to the other player would be fixed regardless of his or her strategy and regardless of the learning algorithm used to update the strategy. However, if the opponent has a bias toward a particular choice, then belief learning may lead more efficiently to the strategy that can exploit such a bias.

The experienced-weighted attraction (EWA) model proposed by Camerer and Ho incorporates the features of both reinforcement learning and belief learning model according to a weight parameter that specifies the relative contribution of each learning algorithm. They found that the EWA model was more consistent with the results obtained from experimental games in human subjects compared to either reinforcement learning or belief learning models. Consistent with these findings, the choice behavior of monkeys during a computerized version of a rock–paper–scissors was also better accounted for by a model that incorporated the features of both reinforcement learning and belief learning.

Inspection Game

When multiple decision makers interact in a dynamic environment, their payoff matrix and therefore the optimal decision-making strategies might change unpredictably. Dorris and Glimcher investigated the abilities of monkeys to adapt to such unpredictable changes in the payoff matrix during an inspection game. Similar to matching pennies game, each of the two players in this game has two alternatives. For the monkey, these two targets correspond to work and shirk, respectively (**Figure 2(c)**). If the animal chooses the 'work' target, it receives a fixed amount of reward. Otherwise, it receives a larger or smaller amount of reward, depending on whether the computer decides to inspect or not. The Nash equilibrium for the computer is to inspect with the probability of 0.5, whereas the optimal strategy for the monkey is to shirk with the probability equal to the inspection cost (I). Although the probability that the animal would choose each of the two targets roughly followed the predictions of the Nash equilibrium, there was still a systematic discrepancy between the theoretical prediction and the animal's choice behavior. Specifically, the animal chose to shirk more often than the equilibrium prediction when the inspection cost for the computer opponent was small. It should be noted that during this inspection game, the animal was always rewarded by the same amount of reward for choosing to work, and therefore did not receive any information as to whether the computer opponent chose to inspect or not. Therefore, choosing to shirk might have additional advantage in that it provides some information about the behavior of the opponent, and this may explain why the animal chose to shirk more frequently than the Nash equilibrium solution, especially after an unpredictable change in the payoff matrix.

The lateral intraparietal area (LIP) is a region in the primate posterior parietal cortex closely connected with other oculomotor centers, such as the superior colliculus and the frontal eye field. Neurons in the LIP often modulate their activity according to the direction of eye movement during its preparation and execution, and might be actively involved in the process of decision making. For example, activity of LIP neurons is systematically related to the probability and magnitude of reward expected from certain eye movements. The possibility that the activity of LIP neurons reflects the subjective value of the expected outcome from an eye movement toward its receptive field was tested using the inspection game paradigm. Although the decision to shirk leads to a variable outcome depending on the choice of the opponent, the expected utilities for shirking and working must be equal at the Nash equilibrium. This prediction was tested by requiring an animal to indicate its choice to shirk by making an eye movement toward a visual target in the receptive field of an LIP neuron. Although the probability of making such eye movements varied according to the inspection cost and the corresponding Nash equilibrium, the activity of LIP neurons remained relatively constant. In addition, LIP activity was significantly correlated with the trial-by-trial variation in the utility of choosing the target in the neuron's receptive field. These results are consistent with the hypothesis that LIP neurons encode subjective utilities of eye movements.

Utility and Cost Functions in Motor Control

In combination with appropriately chosen utility functions, the principle of utility maximization can account for a wide range of choice behaviors in both humans and animals. Similarly, changes in the choice behavior during social interactions and other behavioral changes in a dynamic environment can be modeled with reinforcement learning algorithms. In order to produce the physical movement in the animal's body, however, the brain has to translate its chosen behavioral goal into a specific pattern of muscle activations.

Due to a large degree of redundancy in the motor system, there are practically an infinite number of muscle activation patterns that can accomplish more or less the same desired final configuration of the animal's body. For example, when a person or a monkey reaches for an object, either of the two hands can be used, and often a variety of grasp postures can be chosen. When monkeys are allowed to choose freely their hands to acquire a food item, they often display hand preferences. However, such hand preference is not complete, and the animals tend to switch their hands in successive trials. This indicates that utilities for reaching and grasping movements incorporate the relationship between successive movements. Similar to the cortical circuitry involved in the selection of a behavioral goal, the neural system responsible for motor decision making is also distributed. For example, neurons encoding information about the movement target and the hand chosen to acquire it are found in multiple cortical areas, including the dorsal premotor cortex, the dorsolateral prefrontal cortex, and the supplementary motor area.

Even the trajectories of simple movements, such as reaching or saccadic eye movement, have a large degree of freedom. Nevertheless, the trajectories of such movements tend to be highly stereotyped and typically bell shaped. This led to the assumption that specific movement trajectories are chosen as a result of optimization. For example, it has been proposed that the motor system chooses a particular trajectory to minimize the rate of change in acceleration (jerk) or torque. The function to be minimized during optimization, such as the total jerk, is referred to as the cost or loss function, and therefore can be considered as negative utility function. In general, the cost function computed from the error at the end of the movement does not make specific predictions about the movement trajectory, unless the effect of neural noise is considered. Trains of action potentials recorded from the neurons throughout the motor system, including the motor neurons in the spinal cord, display highly irregular patterns, and the amount of such neuronal noise tends to increase with the average activity. This is referred to as signal-dependent noise. The variability at the end point of a given movement, such as reaching, would increase if the hand is suddenly accelerated, requiring rapid muscle contraction and higher activity of motor neurons. In fact, the optimal trajectory that minimizes the variability in the end point in the presence of signal-dependent noise resembles those with minimum jerk. Motor errors are encoded by climbing fibers in the cerebellum, and such signals can be used to reduce the positional error by modifying the corresponding movement trajectory.

See also: Cognition: Basal Ganglia Role; Decision-Making and Vision; Dopamine Neurons: Reward and Uncertainty; Game Theory and the Economics of Animal Communication; Learning, Action, Inference and Neuromodulation; Posterior Parietal Cortex and Arm Movement; Reward Decision-Making; Reward Neurophysiology and Primate Cerebral Cortex; Reward Neurophysiology and Orbitofrontal Cortex; Social Brain: Evolution.

Further Reading

Barraclough DJ, Conroy ML, and Lee D (2004) Prefrontal cortex and decision making in a mixed-strategy game. *Nature Neuroscience* 7: 404–410.

Camerer CF (2003) *Behavioral Game Theory.* Princeton: Princeton University Press.

Camerer CF and Ho T-H (1999) Experience-weighted attraction learning in normal form games. *Econometrica* 67: 827–874.

Dorris MC and Glimcher PW (2004) Activity in posterior parietal cortex is correlated with the relative subjective desirability of action. *Neuron* 44: 365–378.

Harris CM and Wolpert DM (1998) Signal-dependent noise determines motor planning. *Nature* 394: 780–784.

Körding KP and Wolpert DM (2004) The loss function of sensorimotor learning. *Proceedings of the National Academy of Sciences of the United States of America* 101: 9839–9842.

Lee D (2006) Neural basis of quasi-rational decision making. *Current Opinion in Neurobiology* 16: 191–198.

Lee D, McGreevy BP, and Barraclough DJ (2005) Learning and decision making in monkeys during a rock-paper-scissors game. *Cognitive Brain Research* 25: 416–430.

Lee D and Schieber MH (2006) Serial correlation in lateralized choices of hand and target. *Experimental Brain Research* 174: 499–509.

Montague PR, King-Casas B, and Cohen JD (2006) Imaging valuation models in human choice. *Annual Review of Neuroscience* 29: 417–448.

Platt ML and Glimcher PW (1999) Neural correlates of decision variables in parietal cortex. *Nature* 400: 233–238.

Schultz W (2006) Behavioral theories and the neurophysiology of reward. *Annual Review of Psychology* 57: 87–115.

Sutton RS and Barto AG (1998) *Reinforcement Learning: An Introduction.* Cambridge, MA: MIT Press.

von Neumann J and Morgenstern O (1944) *Theory of Games and Economic Behavior.* Princeton: Princeton University Press.

Wolpert DM and Ghahramani Z (2000) Computational principles of movement neuroscience. *Nature Neuroscience Supplement* 3: 1212–1217.

Relevant Website

http://www.bme.jhu.edu – Reza Shadmehr Home Page, The Whitaker Biomedical Engineering Institute at Johns Hopkins.

Neuroeconomics: History

P W Glimcher, New York University, New York, NY, USA

Overview

Within the neurobiological community this rapprochement had its origins in the early 1990s. At that time, significant progress was being made toward understanding the neurobiological basis of simple sensory–motor decision making in nonhuman primates. The catalyst for that progress was Newsome and colleagues' work on the relationship between activity in the middle temporal area of visual cortex (area MT) and perceptual decisions. The goal of this work was to relate the activity of single neurons in area MT to the perceptual decisions of monkeys. They accomplished this using a formal mathematical model that defined an optimal perceptual decision-making process, a normative psychophysical theory, which was rooted in the theory of signal detection that had dominated behavioral studies of perception for several decades. As other research groups began to extend this work, studying more complicated and less perceptual forms of decision making, it became clear that the normative models of psychophysics that define optimal performance in perception could not be extended to situations in which choices relied on complex functions of nonsensory variables: a point made decades earlier, but often overlooked, by the mathematical psychologists Duncan Luce and Patrick Suppes.

At the same time, cognitive psychologists employing functional magnetic resonance imaging (fMRI) also became interested in understanding the neural basis of decision making. In the late 1980s and early 1990s, a number of early studies were conducted that also demonstrated the need for a unified theory of choice in the neurobiological setting.

This gap between theory and experiment led a number of physiologists and psychologists to begin to explore alternative models for understanding what constitutes efficient decision making. What quickly became clear was that the academic discipline of economics, although far behind neuroscience experimentally, possessed an extremely well-developed corpus of elegant normative models that could serve the same role for neuroscientific studies of decision making that signal detection theory had served for neuroscientific studies of perception.

At the same time that this gradual realignment was taking place in theoretical neuroscientific circles, economics was also experiencing the beginnings of an important sea change. Until the early 1970s, economics had developed as a theoretical and analytic discipline that lacked an experimental tradition. The goal of economics, since the neoclassical revolution of the first half of the twentieth century, had been to relate external-world variables to the choices made by individuals, or groups of individuals, using purely theoretical approaches. Within neoclassical economics, only preexisting data about choices in real-world situations served as acceptable dependent variables for tests of theories, and unsurprisingly many dominant theories were only weakly tested by these existing data sets. In the 1960s, a number of empirical demonstrations raised serious challenges to this approach, suggesting that the existing corpus of normative theory was not as predictive of choice as had been hoped. Partly in response to these challenges and in response to others, in the 1970s a number of economic scholars began to develop a homegrown experimental methodology to empirically explore how theories could explain behavior in laboratory, or artificial, markets and games, and how the trading behavior of human subjects was influenced by changes in the rules governing the operations of those markets.

Together, these two groups of scholars laid the foundations for what was essentially a new economic approach, one in which hypotheses could be posed and addressed experimentally. Like those that had come before them, however, they also believed strongly that the goal of economics was to predict and explain choice. As a result, they argued that while studies of hidden psychological or neurobiological processes might be of interest to scholars studying the algorithms by which choice was accomplished, these biological studies would add little in the way of predictive power to models of choice itself, the object of economic study.

The rise of fMRI in the 1990s, however, changed that assumption for some economists. During that period, brain scanners became relatively cheap to use and widely distributed in the academic community. The popular press also showed a tremendous interest in brain scanning, and a constant flood of articles describing 'how the brain worked' appeared in the general press. The result was an interest, particularly among younger economists, in the possibility that measurements of neural state could be used to test or refine economic models.

The two communities, neuroscience and economics, thus came toward a union from two very different directions. Neurobiologists largely turned toward economics as a source of normative theory while economists turned toward neurobiology for new measurements that could be used to test or constrain existing theory. Both of these approaches were, and remain, controversial in many circles. Neurobiologists opposed to the use of economic theory argued that the complex normative models of economics would be of little value for understanding the behavior of real humans and real animals. In a similar vein, many economists argued that algorithmic-level studies of decision making were unlikely to improve the predictive power of normative models in any meaningful way.

Critical First Steps

Despite the vocal criticism of mainstream elements in both communities, these social and technological trends led to a convergence of interest among a group of economists, neuroscientists, and cognitive psychologists in the late 1990s. This community of scholars, who began to call themselves neuroeconomists around 2002 or 2003, aggregated around a small set of meetings and papers during this period. Although the first explicitly neuroeconomic papers preceded the first interdisciplinary workshops by several years, these meetings were probably the critical step that allowed these social and natural scientists to develop a common language.

Probably the first of these interdisciplinary interactions was held in 1997 at Carnegie-Mellon University, organized by the economists Colin Camerer and George Loewenstein. After a hiatus of several years this was followed by two meetings in 2001, one held by the Gruter Foundation for Law at their annual meeting in Squaw Valley. At that meeting the Gruter Foundation chose to focus its workshop on the intersection of neuroscience and economics and invited several speakers active at the interface of these converging disciplines. The second meeting was focused more directly on what would later become neuroeconomics and was held at Princeton University. The meeting was organized by the neuroscientist Jonathan Cohen and the economist Christina Paxson. This meeting is often seen as the inception point for the present-day Society for Neuroeconomics. At that meeting, economists and neuroscientists met to explicitly discuss the growing convergence of these fields and to debate the value of such a convergence. There was, however, no consensus among the scholars present at that meeting that such a convergence would be desirable. In fact, when asked specifically at the end of the meeting what he thought of such a convergence, the internationally acclaimed economist Ariel Rubenstien (then at Princeton) concluded, essentially, that there was nothing in neuroscience that would change how he thought about economics.

Nonetheless, the Princeton meeting generated significant momentum and 2 years later (2003) a small invitation-only meeting that included nearly all of the active researchers in the emerging area was held on Martha's Vineyard and organized by Greg Berns of Emory University. This 3-day meeting marked a clear turning point in which a group of economists, psychologists, and neurobiologists began to identify themselves as neuroeconomists and began to explicitly shape the convergence between the fields. This led, the subsequent year, to an open registration meeting at Kiawah Island, South Carolina that was attended by 83 people in which the Nobel Laureate in economics Vernon Smith delivered the keynote address. At that meeting a decision was made to incorporate the existing group as an academic society that would sponsor an annual meeting that would serve as a focal point for neuroeconomics internationally. At that meeting Paul Glimcher was elected President of the Society for Neuroeconomics which held its first formal meeting the following year (2005) at Kiawah Island with a group of 114 people.

At the same time a group of European scholars undertook the establishment of a similar meeting in 2002. The first meeting of the European conference on neuroeconomics (ConNEcs) was held at the Westfalian Wilhelms University of Muenster in northern Germany. This was followed by a second meeting in 2004, establishing neuroeconomics as an international discipline.

Landmark Papers

Against this backdrop of meetings, a series of critical papers and books were emerging that shaped the interactions between these scholars and also served to communicate the goals of the emerging neuroeconomic community to the larger neurobiological and economic communities. Probably the first neurobiological paper to explicitly rest on a normative economic theory was Peter Shizgal and Kent Conover's 1996 review in *Current Directions in Psychological Science* entitled: 'On the neural computation of utility.' This was followed the next year by a related paper published in *Current Opinion in Neurobiology* entitled 'Neural basis of utility estimation' authored by Shizgal. The reason that these papers can be viewed as the first neuroeconomic papers is that they attempt to describe the neurobiological substrate for a behavioral choice using a normative theory rooted in neoclassical economics. In these papers, Shizgal analyzed the results of studies of intracranial self-stimulation in rats using a type of utility theory related loosely to the standard expected utility theories of Savage and VonNeuman and Morgenstern. The papers argue that the choices an animal makes about whether or not to work for direct electrical activation of the medial forebrain bundle can be construed as an effort to maximize the animal's instant-to-instant utility. In their analysis, changes in the desirability of brain stimulation reward, for example, as a function of stimulation frequency, can be formally interpreted as changes in the utility of the electrical stimulation. Unlike standard theories of utility, however, Shizgal proposed that the expected utility of an action is perceived by the animal as the expected utility of that action divided by the sum of the expected utilities of all available actions. This particular formulation had its origin in the work of the psychologist Richard Herrnstein who proposed that many choices reflect this 'normalization' with regard to the value of other alternatives, a phenomenon he referred to as the matching law (1997).

This equation was introduced to self-stimulation studies about 5 years earlier by Shizgal's mentor C Randy Gallistel. In the early 1990s, Gallistel used Herrnstein's work to inspire quantitative choice-based experiments intended to cardinally scale the desirability of any given set of self-stimulation parameters. Shizgal's extension of this work is critical for the history of neuroeconomics because he retained Gallistel's goal of quantitatively measuring, or more precisely cardinally scaling, the desirability of a neurobiological manipulation while focusing on the idea that such a scale implies an underlying utility theory. What Shizgal's work did not do, however, was to fully incorporate the standard economic model, but rather a more normative version of Herrnstein's approach.

In 1999, this work was followed by a paper published by Michael Platt and Paul Glimcher (another student of Gallistel's) in *Nature* that argued quite explicitly for a normative utility-based analysis of choice behavior in monkeys. As they put it in that paper: "Neurobiologists have begun to focus increasingly on the study of sensory–motor processing, but many of the models used to describe these processes remain rooted in the classic reflex. ... Here we describe a formal economic–mathematical approach for the physiological study of the sensory–motor process, or decision-making." The paper goes on to argue for an approach to the study of decision making rooted in standard expected utility theory. At an experimental level, the paper demonstrates that the activity of single neurons in the posterior parietal cortex is a lawful function of both the probability and magnitude of expected rewards. This was significant because standard expected utility theory predicates choice on lawful functions of these same two variables. The paper, however, makes a misstep in its final examination of choice behavior. The authors examine a matching-law type behavior, which they interpret in terms of normative expected utility theory. This is problematic because there is no normative standard for the analysis of the classical matching-law. The result is a mixing of normative and nonnormative approaches that characterized many of the early neuroeconomic papers from neurobiologists.

At the same time that this paper appeared in print, the economists Colin Camerer, George Lowenstein, and Drazen Prelec began circulating in economic circles a manuscript by the name of 'Grey matters.' In this manuscript the authors also argued for a neuroeconomic approach, but this time from an economic perspective. Over the course of the preceding decade behavioral economists, a group of scholars interested in deviations of actual choice behavior from normative theory, had argued that the choices of humans often did not reflect optimal calculations that perfectly maximized utility. Instead, these behavioral economists had noted that, particularly under conditions in which choosers experience strong emotions, decisions typically deviate systematically from the predictions of standard normative models. What these three scholars argued was that these systematic deviations may reflect neurobiological constraints on decision making and that future neurobiological studies might serve to reveal and define these constraints that cause deviations of behavior from normative theory. What was striking about this argument, in economic circles, was that it proposed an algorithmic analysis of the physical mechanism of choice, a possibility that has been explicitly taboo in economic circles. Prior to the 1990s it was a completely ubiquitous view in economic circles that models of behavior, like utility theory, were 'as if' models: the model was to be interpreted as if utility was represented internally by the chooser. But critically it was irrelevant whether this was actually the case because the models sought to link options to choices not to make assertions about the mechanisms by which that process was accomplished. Camerer and colleagues argued against this view suggesting that deviations from normative theory should be embraced as clues to the underlying neurobiological basis of choice. In a real sense then, the economists turned to neurobiology for exactly the opposite reason that the neurobiologists had turned to economics. They embraced neuroscience as a principled complement to the axiomatic reasoning that characterized the core features of standard economic practice.

In sum then, some members of the neurobiological community had turned toward economics in an effort to embrace a normative theory that they were just beginning to understand, but a normative theory that had only limited predictive power. Members of the economic community had turned toward neuroscience in an effort to find an alternative to normative theory that could account for the choices of real individuals. Of course, these conflicting goals were well aligned; both groups were becoming poised to meet in the intersection of their disciplines.

At this point there was a rush by several research groups to perform an explicitly economic experiment that would mate these two disciplines in human choosers. Two groups succeeded in this quest in 2001. The first of these papers appeared in the journal *Neuron* and reflected a collaboration between the fMRI pioneer Hans Breiter, Shizgal, and the Princeton psychologist/economist Daniel Kahneman (who would win the Nobel prize for his contribution to behavioral economics the following year). That paper was loosely based on prospect theory, a nonnormative form of expected utility theory that guided much research in judgment and decision-making laboratories throughout the world. In that paper Breiter and colleagues manipulated the perceived desirability of a particular lottery outcome (in this case, winning zero dollars in a 'wheel of fortune' game) by changing the values of the two other possible lottery outcomes it was competed with. When winning zero dollars is the worst of three possible outcomes, Kahneman and Tversky's prospect theory predicts, as do several related theories, that subjects should view it negatively, but when it is the best of the three outcomes then subjects should view it more positively. The scanning experiment revealed that brain activation in the ventral striatum matched these predicted subjective valuations.

The other paper published that year reflected a collaboration between the economist Kevin McCabe, his colleague Vernon Smith (who would share the Nobel prize with Kahneman the following year for his contributions to experimental economics), and a team that included economists, a psychologist, and a biomedical engineer. Their paper, which appeared in the pages of the *Proceedings of the National Academy of Sciences* in the United States, examined behavior and neural activation while subjects engaged in a strategic game. This also represented the first use of game theory, an economic tool for the study of social decision making, in a neurobiological experiment. In that paper, subjects played a trust game either against an anonymous human opponent or against a computer. In their game, two players interact regarding an investment. The game begins when the first player is given 45 monetary units and given a choice between keeping that money or investing it with an unseen partner, the trustee. Any money given to the trustee is then multiplied by nine, and the partner must decide whether or not to share 180 units of this windfall to the original investor. What is interesting about the game is that standard normative theory (which assumes a self-interested chooser) assumes that the trustee wishes to maximize her gain. This predicts that in a consequence-free laboratory environment the trustee should refuse to share the windfall. Her partner, the investor, is presumed to know this about her opponent and thus is expected, in the first round, to keep all of the money for herself. What is striking about the game, however, is that humans do not behave in accord with these normative predictions when playing against another, even anonymous, human. Some players, however, do approximate this approach when facing a computer opponent. What McCabe and colleagues therefore did was to scan subjects while they played against both humans and computers and to take the difference between activation in the two states. These neurobiological data revealed that in some subjects the medial prefrontal cortex is differentially active under these two conditions, becoming more active when subjects play this cooperative strategy that deviates from the normative prediction. From these data the authors hypothesized that this nonnormative pattern of cooperation has its origin in circuits of the prefrontal cortex.

The following year, many of these emerging trends were reviewed in an important special Society for Neuroscience conference issue of the journal *Neuron*, edited by Jonathan Cohen and Kenneth Blum, entitled 'Reward and decision.' As these editors wrote in the introduction to that issue: "Within neuroscience, for example, we are awash with data that in many cases lack a coherent theoretical understanding (a quick trip to the poster floor of the Society for Neurosciences meeting can be convincing on this point). Conversely, in economics, it has become abundantly evident that the pristine assumptions of the 'standard economic model' – that individuals operate as optimal decision-makers in maximizing utility – are in direct violation of even the most basic facts about human behavior." In that issue, although all of the articles are written by neurobiologists, particular attention is drawn to normative theories of decision. Of particular interest are articles by Montague and Berns, Schultz, Dayan and Balleine, Gold and Shadlen, and Glimcher, which all point toward the interaction of normative models and neurobiology. In particular, the issue draws attention to the ongoing debate about the role of the neurotransmitter dopamine in reward processing and draws upon previous work that had identified normative or near-normative models of learning that posit a role for dopamine. What followed was a literal flood of decision-making studies in the neuroscientific literature, many of which relied on normative economic theory.

At the end of this initial period a set of summary reviews began to emerge that served as manifestos for the emerging neuroeconomic discipline. In 2003, Glimcher published a book, directed primarily at neuroscientists, that reviewed the history of neuroscience and argued that this history was striking in its lack of normative models for higher cognitive function. Glimcher proposed explicitly in that book that economics could serve as the source for this much needed normative theory for cognitive neuroscience. Shortly thereafter, the Camerer, Loewenstein, and Prelec paper was published (2005), which also served as a manifesto for neuroeconomics, but this time from the economic side. More recently, an invited review detailing many of these advances appeared in the journal *Science*, marking the advancing visibility of neuroeconomics in the scientific community at large.

The next major step in neuroeconomics was probably the incorporation of game theoretic normative models into a broader neurobiological spectrum. In 2004, two key papers appeared that employed normative game theory for the study of single neurons in awake-behaving primates. A paper by Daeyeol Lee and colleagues studied animals trained to play a very simple classic game called matching pennies. In that game the monkeys had to choose between one of two responses, A and B. The monkeys' computer opponent made a similar choice. If they both chose the same response, the monkey earned a drop of juice, and if they made opposite choices, the monkey earned nothing. Lee varied across long blocks of trials the game theoretic sophistication of the monkey's computer opponent while recording from single neurons in the frontal cortex. What he and his colleagues found was that the behavior of the monkeys was responsive to the sophistication of the opponent and that neurons of the frontal cortex encoded properties related to both the monkeys' strategies and the recent history of the game.

In a similar vein, Dorris and Glimcher trained monkeys to play a slightly more complex game called work or shirk. Game theory, in this case Nash equilibrium theory (REF), predicts both a particular outcome for any set of payoffs in that game and that at behavioral equilibrium the monkeys should mix their responses, sometimes working and sometimes shirking. Regardless of the ratio of shirking to working, the normative theory (somewhat counterintuitively) predicts that the subjective value of working and shirking should be nearly identical at this equilibrium. They found that the behavior of the monkeys was fairly well predicted by the normative theory, and neurons in the posterior parietal cortex seemed to fire at a rate that was also predicted for elements encoding expected utility. Together, these two papers probably represented the first use of normative game theory for single-unit studies.

Within the economic community a role similar to that of the *Neuron* special issue was played by a special issue on Neuroeconomics presented by the journal *Games and Economic Behavior* and edited by the economist Aldo Rustichini, which appeared shortly after this in 2005. Within the economic community this issue was hugely influential and served to define neuroeconomics to a large degree. That issue included articles by several economists and neuroscientists, including scholars ranging from Gallistel to Smith.

Another major advance was presented in 2005 by Michael Kosfeld and his colleagues in Ernst Fehr's research group at the University of Zurich. This paper was important because it was the first demonstration of a neuropharmacological manipulation that alters behavior in a manner that can be interpreted with regard to normative theory. Subjects were asked to play a trust game much like the one examined by McCabe and colleagues. Fehr's critical manipulation was to increase brain levels of the neurotransmitter oxytocin (by an intranasal application of the compound) before some of the players made their decision. What Kosfeld and colleagues found was that trustees in the game (those players who had received money from the investors) returned more to the investors (in contravention of normative theory) if they had received oxytocin than if they had been treated with a control substance. What was most interesting about this study from a neuroeconomic point of view was the demonstration that administration of this endogenously produced hormone altered the choice behavior of subjects in a way that went against an existing and well-described normative economic theory.

Summary

The future of neuroeconomics, however, remains unclear. There is still significant opposition to neurobiological approaches within much of mainstream economics, and, in fairness, neuroeconomics has yet to revolutionize either economic theory or the culture of neuroscience. The next decade should prove a critical period for this discipline. During this second decade neuroeconomics, if it is to succeed, will have to make major contributions to both of its parent disciplines.

In 1998 the evolutionary biologist EO Wilson wrote that "The full understanding of utility will come from biology and psychology by reduction to the elements of human behavior followed by a bottom-up synthesis, not from the social sciences by top-down inference and guesswork based on intuitive knowledge. It is in biology and psychology that economists and social scientists will find the premises needed to fashion more predictive models, just as it was in physics and chemistry that researchers found the premises that upgraded biology." It remains to be seen whether neuroeconomic studies will provide major insights in either neuroscience, economics, or both over the next few years. Only time will determine whether this emerging discipline actually can revolutionize its parent disciplines.

See also: Decision-Making in Financial Markets; Decision-Making and Neuroeconomics; Delayed Reinforcement: Economics; Game Theory and the Economics of Animal Communication; Games in Monkeys: Neurophysiology and Motor Decision-Making; Prediction Errors in Neural Processing: Imaging in Humans; Reward Decision-Making; Social Cognition.

Further Reading

Barraclough DJ, Conroy ML, and Lee D (2004) Prefrontal cortex and decision making in a mixed-strategy game. *Nature Neuroscience* 7: 404–410.

Bechara A, Damasio H, Tranel D, and Damasio AR (1997) Deciding advantageously before knowing the advantageous strategy. *Science* 275: 1293–1295.

Breiter HC, Aharon I, Kahneman D, Dale A, and Shizgal P (2001) Functional imaging of neural responses to expectancy and experience of monetary gains and losses. *Neuron* 30: 619–639.

Camerer C, Loewenstein G, and Prelec D (2005) Neuroeconomics: How neuroscience can inform economics. *Journal of Economic Literature* 43: 9–64.

Dayan P and Balleine BW (2002) Reward, motivation, and reinforcement learning. *Neuron* 36: 285–298.

Dorris MC and Glimcher PW (2004) Activity in posterior parietal cortex is correlated with the relative subjective desirability of action. *Neuron* 44: 365–378.

Ellsberg D (1961) Risk, ambiguity, and the Savage axioms. *Quarterly Journal of Economics* 75: 643–669.

Gallistel CR (1994) Foraging for brain stimulation: Toward a neurobiology of computation. *Cognition* 50: 151–170.

Gallistel CR (2005) Deconstructing the law of effect. *Games and Economic Behavior* 52: 410–423.

Glimcher P (2002) Decisions, decisions, decisions: Choosing a biological science of choice. *Neuron* 36: 323–332.

Glimcher P (2003) *Decisions Uncertainty and the Brain: The Science of Neuroeconomics.* Cambridge, MA: MIT Press.

Glimcher PW and Rustichini A (2004) Neuroeconomics: The consilience of brain and decision. *Science* 306: 447–452.

Gold JI and Shadlen MN (2002) Banburismus and the brain: Decoding the relationship between sensory stimuli, decisions, and reward. *Neuron* 36: 299–308.

Herrnstein RJ, Rachlin H, and Laibson DI (1997) *The Matching Law: Papers in Psychology and Economics.* New York/ Cambridge, MA: Russell Sage Foundation/Harvard University Press.

Houser D, Bechara A, Keane M, McCabe K, and Smith V (2005) Identifying individual differences: An algorithm with application to Phineas Gage. *Games and Economic Behavior* 52: 373–385.

Kahneman D and Tversky A (1979) Prospect theory: An analysis of decision under risk. *Econometrica* 47: 263–291.

Kosfeld M, Heinrichs M, Zak PJ, Fischbacher U, and Fehr E (2005) Oxytocin increases trust in humans. *Nature* 435: 673–676.

Luce RD and Suppes P (1965) Preference, utility, and subjective probability. In: Luce RD, Bush RR, and Galanter E (eds.) *Handbook of Mathematical Psychology.* New York: Wiley.

McCabe K, Houser D, Ryan L, Smith V, and Trouard T (2001) A functional imaging study of cooperation in two-person reciprocal exchange. *Proceedings of the National Academy of Sciences of the United States of America* 98: 11832–11835.

Montague PR and Berns GS (2002) Neural economics and the biological substrates of valuation. *Neuron* 36: 265–284.

Newsome WT, Britten KH, and Movshon JA (1989) Neuronal correlates of a perceptual decision. *Nature* 341: 52–54.

Platt ML and Glimcher PW (1999) Neural correlates of decision variables in parietal cortex. *Nature* 400: 233–238.

Plott CR and Smith VL (1978) An experimental examination of two exchange institutions. *Review of Economic Studies* 45: 133–153.

Rilling JK, Sanfey AG, Aronson JA, Nystrom LE, and Cohen JD (2004) Opposing BOLD responses to reciprocated and unreciprocated altruism in putative reward pathways. *Neuroreport* 15: 2539–2543.

Sanfey AG, Rilling JK, Aronson JA, Nystrom LE, and Cohen JD (2003) The neural basis of economic decision-making in the Ultimatum Game. *Science* 300: 1755–1758.

Savage LJ (1954) *The Foundations of Statistics.* New York: Wiley.

Schultz W (2002) Getting formal with dopamine and reward. *Neuron* 36: 241–263.

Shizgal P (1997) Neural basis of utility estimation. *Current Opinion in Neurobiology* 7: 198–208.

Shizgal P and Conover K (1996) On the neural computation of utility. *Current Directions in Psychological Science* 5: 37–43.

Smith VL (1991) *Papers in Experimental Economics.* Cambridge: Cambridge University Press.

VonNeumann J and Morgenstern O (1944) *Theory of Games and Economic Behavior.* Princeton: Princeton University Press.

Wilson EO (1998) *Consilience: The Unity of Knowledge.* New York: Knopf (distributed by Random House).

Neuroethological Perspective

K K Watson and M L Platt, Duke University, Durham, NC, USA

Introduction

The unifying goal of ethology, as well as of newer fields of behavioral ecology and sociobiology, is to provide an evolutionary explanation for behavior. This approach proposes that both natural and sexual selection favor those behaviors that maximize the reproductive success of individuals within the context of their physical and social environments. Ethologically, rewards can be considered proximate goals that, when acquired, tend to enhance survival and mating success. Similarly, avoiding punishment is a proximate goal that ultimately serves to augment the long-term likelihood of survival and reproduction. These definitions thus extend the traditional psychological and neurobiological notions of reward and punishment, which are typically defined by the quality of eliciting approach and avoidance, respectively. As detailed herein, the assumption of evolutionary adaptation within ethology, behavioral ecology, and sociobiology has promoted the development of mathematical models that formally define rewards and punishments within specific behavioral contexts. Such models suggest that full understanding of the neurobiology of reward and decision making will require consideration of naturally occurring behaviors in the specific ecological and social contexts in which they are normally expressed.

The Economics of Natural Behavior

In one of the first direct applications of economic modeling to animal foraging behavior, MacArthur and Pianka proposed in 1966 a model that defined criteria for the consumption or rejection of prey by a foraging animal. Using feeding efficiency as a proxy measure for evolutionary fitness, the benefits of consuming a particular prey type were modeled as the ratio of the energetic benefit afforded to the animal relative to the time costs of seeking and handling that prey type:

$$R = E/(T_h + T_s)$$

R is the net benefit gained by the predator for consuming a particular prey type, E is the amount of energy gained, T_h is the handling time, and T_s is the search time. The model is solved to maximize R, which determines the diet offering the greatest net energetic return and thus maximizing evolutionary success.

One prediction of this model is that the greater the abundance of higher quality foods, the less an animal's diet will consist of lower quality foods (the 'independence of inclusion from encounter' rule). In the 1970s, Goss-Custard found evidence in support of this prediction in his studies of redshank, small wading birds found in estuarine habitats in Great Britain. Redshanks feed on crustaceans and worms; crustaceans offer higher energetic returns relative to worms, which offer lower energetic returns. As predicted, the birds did not indiscriminately consume every worm or crustacean encountered; instead, they exclusively ate crustaceans when their density was high, but included worms in the diet when crustacean density declined. This result makes intuitive sense because the cost of eating worms includes 'missed opportunities' to search for and eat more nutritionally profitable crustaceans. When crustaceans are rare, however, it is more profitable to focus on small but abundant worms rather than wasting time searching for higher value foods.

The general prediction of the prey model – that inclusion of a particular food in the diet is independent of its encounter rate – has since been replicated in a variety of species, including birds, insects, fish, mammals, and even humans. However, as is often the case in economics, MacArthur and Pianka's simple model does not perfectly describe behavior in the real world. In Goss-Custard's study, as well as subsequent studies of different species using different methods, the animals did not display the steplike preference shift predicted by the prey model. Instead, foragers exhibited 'partial preferences' for different types of prey (e.g., preferring one type 75% of the time) when prey density changed. Such partial preferences might reflect the implementation of sampling behavior, which allows the animal to acquire improved information about the statistics of the local environment. Alternatively, partial preference could reflect sensory or memory-related cognitive limitations.

Early models, including MacArthur and Pianka's, described behavioral optimization in a generic sense, without regard to the specific physiological or cognitive constraints of a particular animal. Prediction of a precise outcome in an individual species, on the other hand, requires consideration of the specific set of physiological and environmental constraints relevant to that animal. For example, moose foraging for terrestrial and aquatic plants must satisfy both energetic needs and sodium requirements within the limitations imposed by gut capacity. Terrestrial plants are richer in energy than aquatic plants are, and take up less room in the gut. However, aquatic plants contain more sodium than terrestrial plants do, and, because aquatic plants are buried under ice during the winter, moose must consume enough of them during the summer to satisfy their sodium requirements for the rest of the year. Belovsky developed a model of diet choice in moose, satisfying these constraints using linear programming. According to this model, if moose forage in a manner that maximizes energetic return while simultaneously satisfying sodium needs and rumen constraints, the model predicts a diet of 18% aquatic plants, in precise agreement with actual field observation data (**Figure 1**).

Early field studies using optimal foraging models, such as Goss-Custard's redshank study and Belovsky's moose study, demonstrated the strengths of the economic approach: formulation of models allows for clear and precise predictions that can be tested empirically, and provides a quantitative tool around which to organize explanations of behavior. Importantly for this discussion, such models make clear that defining rewards and punishments requires careful consideration of the behavioral and physiological capacities of a given species and the specific physical and social environments in which the species normally acts.

Neurobiology of Reward and Decision Making

Ultimately, the nervous systems of humans and other animals have evolved to promote behaviors that enhance fitness, such as acquiring food and shelter, attracting mates, avoiding predators, and prevailing over competitors. To achieve these goals, animal brains have become exquisitely specialized to attend to important features of the environment, extract their predictive value for success or failure, and then use this information to compute the evolutionarily optimal course of action. Traditionally, these brain mechanisms have been studied with regard to their roles in acquiring rewards and avoiding punishments.

As noted, rewards are traditionally defined as stimuli that elicit approach behavior, while punishments can be defined as stimuli that elicit avoidance. Recent studies have revealed elementary properties of the neural systems that process rewards and punishments as traditionally defined. Specifically, the circuit connecting midbrain dopamine neurons to the ventral striatum and prefrontal cortex appears to be crucial for processing information about rewards. For example, animals will work to receive current delivered via electrodes implanted in the dopaminergic ventral tegmental area (VTA) or medial forebrain bundle, which connects the VTA to the ventral striatum. In fact,

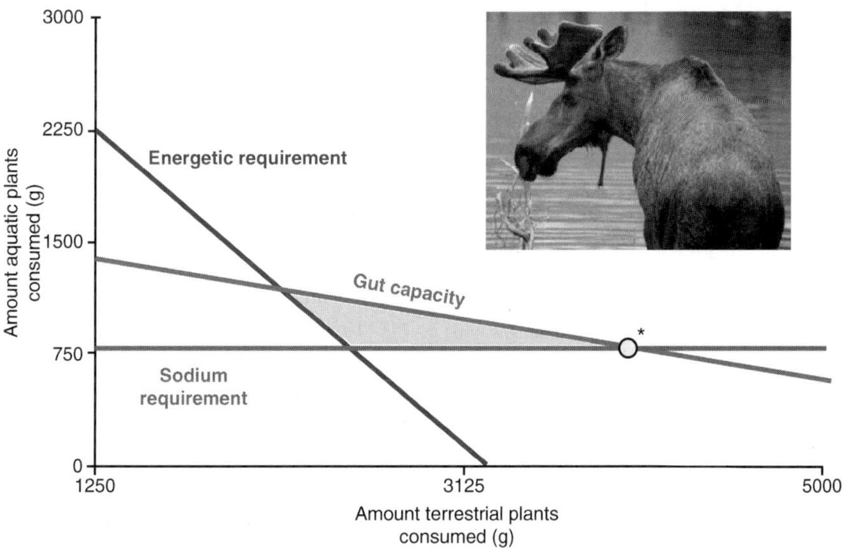

Figure 1 Optimal diet choice in moose (*Alces alces*). The daily ratio of aquatic plants to terrestrial plants consumed by moose must satisfy three constraints: the diet must meet energetic (blue line) and sodium requirements (red line), subject to digestive limitations (green line). Those ratios that meet these constraints are contained in the yellow shaded area. The vertex marked with an asterisk indicates the aquatic-to-terrestrial plant ratio that maximizes energetic intake while also satisfying all constraints. Adapted from Stephens PW and Krebs JR (1987) *Foraging Theory*, p. 120. Princeton, NJ: Princeton University Press. Photo courtesy of the National Park Service.

animals will preferentially work for such intracranial self-stimulation (ICSS), to the exclusion of acquiring food or mating opportunities, which are normally reinforcing.

Electrophysiological recordings from dopaminergic neurons show that these cells respond to primary rewards, such as food and water, as well as to conditioned stimuli that predict such rewards (**Figure 2**). Moreover, dopamine neuron responses scale with both reward magnitude and reward probability. Dopamine neurons do not, however, merely signal rewards and the stimuli that predict them. Current evidence suggests that phasic bursts by dopamine neurons may correspond to the reward prediction error term initially proposed in purely behavioral models of learning. According to this view, such phasic dopamine responses provide a mechanism for updating predicted valuation functions, which can be used both to learn about stimuli in the environment and to select profitable courses of action.

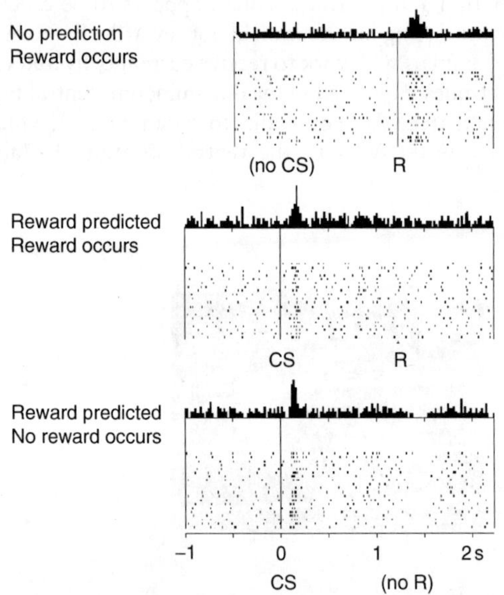

Figure 2 Reward-related responses by a single dopamine neuron recorded in a macaque monkey. (Top) When the animal is still learning the task, the fruit juice reward is unexpected, and the neuron responds at the time of reward delivery (R). (Center) After the monkey learns the relationship between a conditioned stimulus (such as a light or tone) and a reward, the neuron responds to the conditioned stimulus that predicts reward delivery (CS), but not to the reward itself. (Bottom) If the reward is omitted after the predictive stimulus, dopamine neuron activity is suppressed during the time of expected reward delivery. Each raster indicates the time of neuron spiking, and each row corresponds to a single trial for that neuron. The histograms summate the spikes over all the trials. Adapted from Schultz W, Dayan P, and Montague PR (1997) A neural substrate of prediction and reward. *Science* 275: 1593–1599.

These valuation functions can be thought of as the neural implementation of the optimization functions assumed to guide behavior in economic models of behavior developed in behavioral ecology and ethology.

Signals from the dopaminergic midbrain neurons influence processing within cortical decision-making areas, primarily in prefrontal and parietal cortex, that assign value to sensory stimuli and eventually transform that information into motor output. Platt and Glimcher probed the impact of expected value on sensorimotor processing in the lateral intraparietal area (LIP), a region of the brain previously linked to visual attention and motor preparation. In that study, monkeys were cued to shift gaze from a central light to one of two peripheral lights to receive a fruit juice reward. In separate blocks of trials, the authors varied the expected value of orienting to each light, either by varying reward size or by varying the probability of each cue onset. Platt and Glimcher found that LIP neurons signaled expected target value, the product of reward size, and saccade likelihood, prior to cue onset (**Figure 3**). In a second experiment, monkeys were permitted to choose freely between the two targets, and both neuronal activity in LIP and the probability of target choice were correlated with expected target value.

Sugrue, Corrado, and Newsome extended these observations by probing the dynamics of decision-related activity in LIP using a virtual foraging task. In this experiment, the rewards associated with each of two targets fluctuated over time. Under these conditions, monkeys tended to match the rate of choosing each target to its relative rate of reinforcement. Moreover, the responses of individual LIP neurons to a particular target corresponded to the relative rate of reward gained from choosing it on recent trials, with the greatest weight placed on the most recent trials. Together, these and other studies suggest that simple behavioral decisions may be computed by scaling neuronal responses associated with a particular stimulus or movement by its value, thus modifying the likelihood of reaching the threshold for eliciting a specific motor action.

Uncertainty and Decision Making

Early ethological models of behavior assumed that animals maintained complete knowledge of the environment and that reward contingencies were deterministic. In practice, however, uncertainty about environmental contingencies places strong constraints on behavior. The impact of uncertainty on choice has long been acknowledged in economics, which defines the spread of an outcome's known probability as risk. In the eighteenth century, Daniel Bernoulli proposed

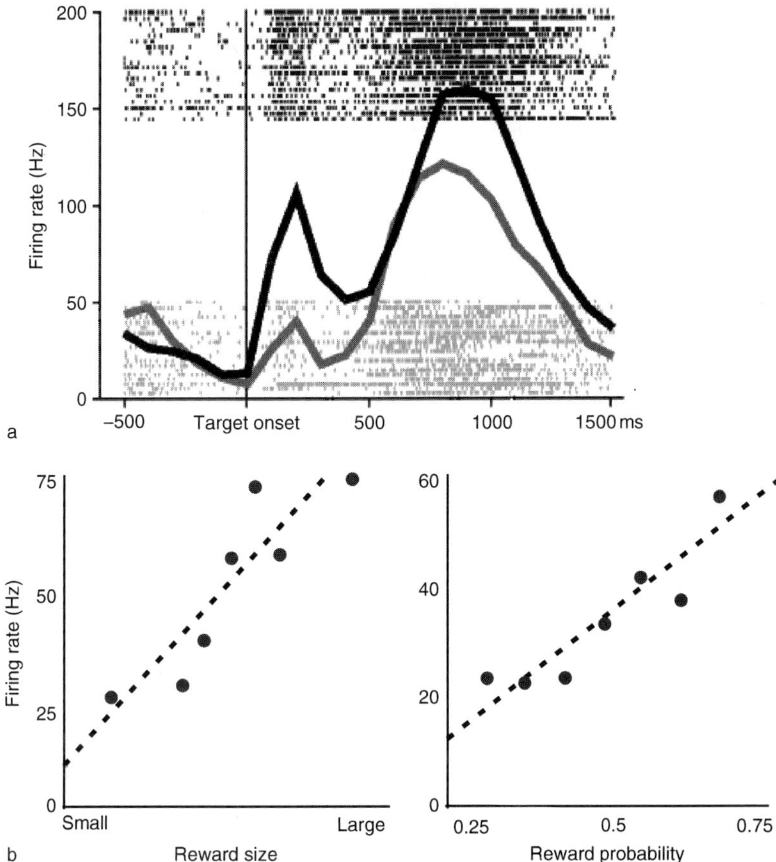

Figure 3 Lateral intraparietal area neurons encode expected target value. (a) Neuronal firing is greater during trials when the expected reward is large (black line) than when the expected reward is small (gray line). Black and gray rasters indicate the time of individual spikes for large- and small-reward trials, respectively; each line of rasters corresponds to a single trial. Curves represent the summation of activity over all the trials. (b) Firing rate of a single lateral intraparietal area neuron increases linearly with reward size (left) and reward probability (right). Adapted from Platt ML and Glimcher PW (1999) Neural correlates of decision variables in parietal cortex. *Nature* 400(6741): 233–238.

that the expected values of monetary transactions, particularly risky financial ventures, differ from their corresponding subjective utilities (as determined by the economic agent). This idea, which would eventually revolutionize the field of economics, challenged the traditional notion that people value outcomes strictly according to their financial returns.

Initial economic models applied to animal behavior explicitly ignored variance in reward outcomes. For example, Charnov's marginal value theorem, devised to predict when a foraging animal should leave a particular food patch, was based purely on the average distribution of resources. Although this model described behavior in simple contexts fairly well, it failed to account for behavioral sensitivity to variability within patches even when the average value of each patch was identical.

In a seminal ethological study probing the impact of risk on decision making, Caraco observed the behavior of yellow-eyed juncos, a species of small bird. These birds were given the option of choosing a tray with a fixed number of millet seeds or a tray with a probabilistically varying number of seeds, with the same mean as the fixed option. Preferences depended on the ambient temperature. At 19 °C, juncos preferred the fixed option, but at 1 °C, they preferred the variable option. The proposed explanation for this switch from risk aversion to risk seeking is that, at the higher temperature, the rate of gain from the fixed option was sufficient to maintain the bird on a positive energy budget. At the lower temperature, however, energy expenditures were elevated, so the fixed option was no longer adequate to meet the animal's energy needs. When cold, the bird's best chance for survival was to gamble on the risky option, since it might yield a higher rate of return, compared to the fixed option.

The relationship between energy budget and risk taking has been found to be generally true across a variety of animal species, including insects, fish, birds, and mammals. Moreover, this principle also describes human decisions in experiments using money as a reward. The convergence of behavioral results from animals and humans endorses the notion that studying risk-sensitive decision making in animals can illuminate the mechanisms underlying risk sensitivity in humans. These observations strongly suggest that sensitivity to risk is an evolutionarily ancient neural adaptation supporting adaptive decision making.

Neuroimaging studies in humans have revealed that preference for a risky option is associated with increases in neuronal activity in the ventral striatum and posterior parietal cortex. Moreover, choosing a risky option activates the dorsal striatum, precuneus, and premotor cortex. A recent electrophysiological study in monkeys probed how such risk-related activity might be translated into action. Monkeys were given a choice between juice rewards of fixed or variable sizes, with the same mean reward rate. Under these conditions, monkeys showed a strong preference for the risky option. Simultaneous recordings from single neurons in the posterior cingulate cortex, a region of the brain associated with spatial attention, visual orienting, and reward processing, revealed responses that were correlated with subjective preferences for the risky option. The foregoing discussion makes plain that the discrepancy between observable outcomes and subjective preferences in decision making under risk offers a powerful paradigm for investigating the neural mechanisms underlying adaptive decision making.

Social Rewards in Primates

In most neurobiological studies of decision making in nonhuman animals, food or water is delivered following performance of a particular action. Such direct and immediate reinforcers are typically referred to as primary rewards, and, as reviewed earlier, are associated with activation of midbrain dopamine neurons, as well as neurons in the ventral striatum and orbitofrontal cortex. In humans, a varied assortment of hedonically positive experiences can evoke activity in these regions, including eating chocolate, hearing pleasant music, or even reading a funny cartoon.

Although outcomes such as food consumption or the opportunity to mate clearly motivate behavior, abstract goals such as information gathering or social interaction can also motivate approach or orienting behavior in the absence of hedonic experience. For humans and other primates, in particular, many decisions are motivated by competitive and cooperative interactions with others in a social group. The adaptive significance of navigating a complex social environment explains why social stimuli and interactions, such as an attractive smiling face, a cooperative transaction, or the opportunity to punish a traitor, evoke activity in neural circuits that overlap with those activated by primary rewards. Physical features of the face, for example, provide information about genetic quality and thus can be useful in determining whether to pursue mating. In addition to attractiveness, people apparently also use information apparent in faces to assess the expected value of cooperation. Together, these observations implicate the operation of a neural system dedicated to linking social stimuli, such as faces, to the valuation functions guiding behavioral decision making.

Nonhuman primates also use social information to evaluate their behavioral options. For example, field studies of primate social behavior have revealed that monkeys preferentially invest in relationships with dominant individuals. Moreover, male primates often use visual cues to predict female mating receptivity. These observations suggest that primates maintain valuation functions for specific social and reproductive stimuli that guide behavior. Deaner, Khera, and Platt explored this hypothesis quantitatively in the laboratory using a pay-per-view task in which male rhesus macaques were given a choice between two targets. Orienting to one target yielded fruit juice but orienting to the other yielded fruit juice and the picture of a familiar monkey. By systematically changing the juice payoffs for each target and the pools of images revealed, the authors estimated the value of different types of social and reproductive stimuli in a liquid currency.

Their work revealed that male monkeys forego larger juice rewards to view female sexual signals or the faces of high-ranking males, but need overpayment to view the faces of low-ranking males (**Figure 4**). In contrast to the valuation functions governing target choice, the patterns of gaze associated with each class of image hint at the affective complexity associated with social stimuli. Specifically, monkeys looked at female sexual signals for longer times than they looked at either high-ranking or low-ranking male faces, perhaps reflecting differences in the hedonic qualities of these stimuli (**Figure 4**). Presumably, male monkeys value the opportunity to view the faces of high-ranking males not because they are hedonically pleasing, but rather because they are potentially threatening and thus highly relevant for guiding behavior. Thus, social stimuli and behaviors that are strongly motivating are not necessarily hedonically

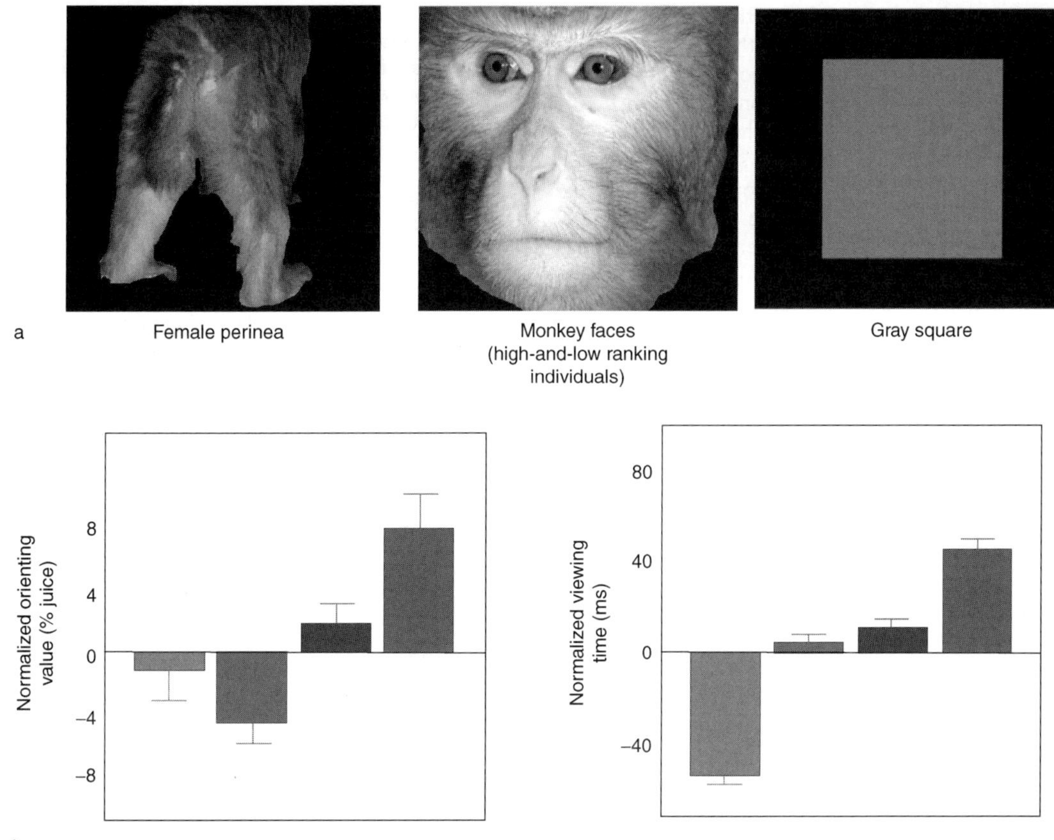

Figure 4 Monkeys value social and reproductive information. (a) Example images shown to monkeys during a 'pay-per-view' task used to assess valuation of socially relevant visual images. (b) Mean normalized orienting values (left) and looking times (right) for various image classes. Orienting values are significantly higher for both the perinea (red bar) and high-status faces (blue bar), in contrast to either the low-status faces (green) or gray square (gray). Although the monkeys choose to orient more frequently to the high-status faces than the low-status faces, the lengths of time they gaze at either of these image classes are both shorter than the time they spend viewing the perinea. Adapted from Deaner RO, Khera AV, and Platt ML (2005) Monkeys pay per view: Adaptive valuation of social images by rhesus macaques. *Current Biology* 15: 543–548.

pleasing, and it is likely that they engage distinct neural circuitry – a hypothesis yet to be tested empirically.

Social Games

One of the results of the dialogue between biology and economics was the development of evolutionary game theory. As a conceptual framework, game theory can be used to describe the ways in which behavior is influenced by the behavior of other animals when they compete for limited resources, such as mates and food, in order to survive and reproduce. A classical game describes the interaction of two or more agents with conflicting interests, both trying to maximize some gain. Each game makes precise the number of agents involved, the actions available to those agents, and the payoff that will result from all possible interactions. In economics, the participants in the game identify the costs and benefits available to each player, and are generally expected to adopt a 'rational' behavioral strategy. Typically, these behavioral strategies comprise a probabilistic distribution of responses for all players, often called the Nash equilibrium, invulnerable to penetration by other behavioral strategies. In biological applications of game theory, the economic assumptions of self-interest and rationality are replaced by the evolutionary assumptions of Darwinian fitness and population stability.

Lee and colleagues explored frequency-dependent decision making in monkeys while recording from neurons in the dorsolateral prefrontal cortex (DLPFC). Monkeys played an analog of matching pennies against a computer opponent. In this game, the animal is rewarded for choosing the target not chosen by the computer. By manipulating the algorithm governing the computer's choices, the experimenters were able to simulate social opponents implementing various strategies. When confronted with an opponent that tracked both the history of choices and the rewards received, monkeys' choice frequencies approached the optimal random solution. Neurons in the DLPFC were sensitive to the history of choices, rewards, and current movement plans. These signals could in theory be used to update the values of each alternative action, a computation necessary for the animal to choose optimally. Obviously, the ability to make such strategic changes in behavior would be highly favored in the natural social environment. However, the neural mechanisms underlying strategic interaction with other individuals, rather than a computer opponent, have just begun to be explored in humans using neuroimaging techniques, and have yet to be probed in animals.

Conclusion

Although still in the early stages, the union of ethology, economics, and neuroscience – the emerging field of neuroeconomics – offers a potentially powerful way to study the neural mechanisms underlying decision making and behavioral allocation. Just as in other animals, natural selection has shaped human behavior and its neural substrate. Thus, the behavior we display today may more strongly reflect the operation of a nervous system which evolved over eons to optimize hunting and gathering behavior in small groups, rather than being economically rational. These considerations predict that neuroethological studies will be crucial for understanding the neurobiology of reward and decision making in humans and other animals.

See also: Computational Neuroethology; Decision-Making in Financial Markets; Decision-Making and Neuroeconomics; Delayed Reinforcement: Economics; Game Theory and the Economics of Animal Communication; Games in Monkeys: Neurophysiology and Motor Decision-Making; Neuroeconomics: History; Reward and Learning; Reward Systems: Human; Reward Decision-Making; Social Interaction; Social Cognition.

Further Reading

Barraclough DJ, Conroy ML, and Lee D (2004) Prefrontal cortex and decision making in a mixed-strategy game. *Nature Neuroscience* 7(4): 404–410.

Deaner RO, Khera AV, and Platt ML (2005) Monkeys pay per view: Adaptive valuation of social images by rhesus macaques. *Current Biology* 15: 543–548.

Glimcher PW (2003) *Decisions, Uncertainty, and the Brain: The Science of Neuroeconomics*. Cambridge, MA: MIT Press.

Goss-Custard JD (1977) Responses of Redshank, *Tringa totanus*, to the absolute and relative densities of two prey species. *Journal of Animal Ecology* 46(3): 867–874.

Kacelnik A and Bateson M (1997) Risk-sensitivity: Crossroads for theories of decision-making. *Trends in Cognitive Science* 1(8): 304–309.

MacArthur RH and Pianka ER (1966) On optimal use of a patchy environment. *American Naturalist* 100(916): 603–609.

McCoy AN and Platt ML (2005) Risk-sensitive neurons in macaque posterior cingulate cortex. *Nature Neuroscience* 8(9): 1220–1227.

Platt ML and Glimcher PW (1999) Neural correlates of decision variables in parietal cortex. *Nature* 400(6741): 233–238.

Sanfey AG, Loewenstein G, McClure SM, et al. (2006) Neuroeconomics: Cross-currents in research on decision-making. *Trends in Cognitive Science* 10(3): 108–116.

Schultz WW (2002) Getting formal with dopamine and reward. *Neuron* 36(2): 241–263.

Schultz W, Dayanz P, and Montague PR (1997) A neural substrate of prediction and reward. *Science* 275: 1593–1599.

Smith JM (1982) *Evolution and the Theory of Games*. Cambridge, MA: Cambridge University Press.

Stephens PW and Krebs JR (1987) *Foraging Theory, p.120*. Princeton, NJ: Princeton University Press.

Reasoning and Problem Solving: Models

A K Barbey and L W Barsalou, Emory University, Atlanta, GA, USA

Introduction

Neuroscience research has increasingly provided evidence that informs theories of reasoning. We begin by defining classic forms of reasoning; and summarizing psychological contemporary theories. We then review empirical evidence from neuroscience that bears on these theories. Finally, we summarize current challenges and identify promising areas for future research.

Definition and Types of Reasoning

Reasoning is a hallmark of human thought, supporting the process of discovery that leads from what is known or hypothesized, to what is unknown or implicit in one's thinking. Reasoning can take the form of deductive inference, whereby the evidence guarantees the truth of the conclusion. Alternatively, when reasoning depends on conditions of uncertainty, it takes the form of inductive inference, whereby the evidence provides only limited support for the truth of the conclusion. The deductive inference that a storm has emerged is supported by evidence that it is raining, whereas observing lightning clouds provides only limited support for the inductive inference that it will rain. Many forms of reasoning typically depend on conditions of uncertainty, including problem solving, causal reasoning, and analogical inference.

Problem solving refers broadly to the inferential steps that lead from a given state of affairs to a desired goal state. For example, deciding who to vote for in a presidential election, diagnosing a patient on the basis of observed symptoms, or preparing for a mountain climbing expedition all depend on problem solving. Problem solving often requires the process of planning, namely, formulating a method for attaining a desired goal state. Planning a mountain climbing expedition, for example, requires scheduling the season of the expedition by predicting the consequences of taking the trip during different seasons. This is accomplished by modeling the situation and observing the consequences of possible actions (e.g., the occurrence of snow in winter introduces new challenges).

Prediction and explanation further depend on causal reasoning (i.e., the ability to infer causal relations). For example, knowledge that cold winter weather can cause an accumulation of snow in the mountains, which in turn can cause an avalanche, supports the prediction that an avalanche is possible during winter.

Finally, new predictions and explanations can be generated by analogical reasoning, whereby relations from one domain are mapped onto another domain. For example, students can conceptualize particle motion in an atom through an analogy to the solar system.

Theoretical Perspectives on Reasoning in the Psychological Literature

The psychological literature contains various theories that address the cognitive architecture and symbolic representations that underlie reasoning. After reviewing these theories, we turn to neuroscience evidence that bears on them.

Cognitive Architecture

One major distinction can be drawn between theories that view the mind as containing specialized reasoning modules, versus theories that view the mind as containing general-purpose reasoning systems. According to the modular view, the mind consists of specialized modules that are unavailable to conscious awareness and deliberate control (cognitively impenetrable), and that are only able to process specific types of information (information encapsulation). Advocates of this view have proposed a diversity of modules that underlie reasoning, including modules for semantic inference, communicative pragmatics, social exchange, intuitive numbers, spatial relations, naive physics, and biomechanical motion. If cognitive architecture emerges from an underlying neural architecture, then strong modular views predict that the neural systems for reasoning should be relatively localized, implementing modules that are cognitively impenetrable and informationally encapsulated.

Alternatively, dual-process theorists propose that reasoning is based on two general-purpose systems: an associative system and a rule-based system. The associative system uses basic cognitive operations such as association, similarity, and memory retrieval to produce primitive judgments quickly and unconsciously. The rule-based system reflects more evolutionarily advanced mechanisms that implement reasoning procedures deliberately and consciously. For example, inductive reasoning largely depends on the retrieval and evaluation of world knowledge, whereas deductive reasoning depends on rule-based, formal procedures.

The dual-process theory further motivates the cognitive demand hypothesis: when people have little time and limited processing resources, incentives, and/or external aids available for making a judgment, they only use the associative system when reasoning. Conversely, when people have more time and greater processing resources, incentives, and/or external aids available, they also use the rule-based system. The dual-process model predicts that reasoning recruits different neural systems, depending on cognitive demand. When tasks are easy, the associative system is sufficient for correct reasoning and primarily recruits left inferior frontal gyrus, especially Broca's area, in addition to the temporal lobes and posterior parietal association cortex. As tasks become more difficult, the rule-based system becomes required for correct reasoning and recruits the prefrontal cortex, especially the ventrolateral subregion, which has been implicated in rule maintenance.

A second theory that provides a general-purpose account of reasoning is grounded in a somewhat different pair of systems: the linguistic system and the conceptual system. According to this view, the brain's language system initially produces relatively superficial information about a reasoning problem, such as word associates, syntactic structures, etc. As linguistic forms become generated, their meanings become increasingly represented in the conceptual system. A key assumption of this approach is that superficial processing based on linguistic representations may often be sufficient for adequate reasoning performance. When it is not sufficient, conceptual representations must be generated to produce more sophisticated reasoning. Thus, consistent with the dual-process model, this view predicts that differences in the cognitive demands of a reasoning task (i.e., superficial vs. deep processing) will differentially engage neural systems.

In general, both dual coding frameworks predict that reasoning will recruit neural systems that support two forms of coding. One important set of systems underlies language processing, including the left frontotemporal language system. A second set of important systems underlies conceptual processing, mental simulation, and imagery, including bilateral sensorimotor areas.

Representation in Reasoning

A second major distinction can be drawn between theories of reasoning that are based on amodal versus modality-specific representations. According to standard theories, the modality-specific states that are active while perceiving an entity are redescribed into amodal representations that bear no correspondence to the neural systems producing them. For example, the concept 'chair' is represented by redescribing the modality-specific states that underlie the perception of a chair into amodal representations (e.g., feature lists, semantic nets), processed by classic symbolic mechanisms (e.g., predication, argument binding). Thus, amodal theories predict that conceptual processing will recruit brain regions outside sensorimotor areas that underlie language and rules, including left prefrontal and superior temporal regions implicated in formal, rule-based operations.

In contrast, embodied theories of knowledge propose that knowledge and meaning are grounded in modality-specific representations. Increasing empirical evidence from both the cognitive and the neuroscience literatures suggests that modality-specific representations underlie higher level cognition. According to this framework, concepts are represented by simulating the modality-specific states that were initially activated during perception, action, and interoception. Embodied theories propose that simulations are organized at a higher level by simulators that integrate information across a category's instances. Over time, for example, visual information about how cakes look becomes integrated in a 'cake' simulator, along with gustatory information about how cakes taste, somatosensory information about how they feel, motor programs for interacting with them, emotional responses to experiencing them, and so forth. The result is a distributed system throughout the brain's modality-specific areas that establishes conceptual content for the general category of 'cake.' Thus, embodied theories predict that conceptual processing will recruit a broadly distributed system of modality-specific brain regions.

Embodied theories further motivate the task specificity hypothesis. According to this hypothesis, the neural areas underlying a particular type of reasoning, such as deduction, may show little in common, as the specific materials and tasks vary. Because different materials and tasks produce different patterns of modality-specific activation, the same general form of reasoning does not show a single, stable pattern, and no common areas may emerge. In contrast to the 'cognitive demand hypothesis,' this view predicts that significant differences in the task and/or materials – even those that do not affect cognitive demand – are likely to dominate neural activation more than the type of reasoning performed.

Mental Models versus Mental Logic

A third major distinction can be drawn between theories of reasoning that are based on visuospatial models versus theories that are based on logical operations. Mental-model theory proposes that deductive and inductive reasoning depend on spatially organized mental models. According to this view, an argument is evaluated by generating alternative models of its premises, where each model represents possible circumstances that render the premises true. If all the models constructed from the premises are consistent with the truth of the conclusion, then the argument is judged to be deductive or valid. If, however, only a limited number of models render the conclusion true, then the argument is judged to be inductive or probabilistic.

Given the proposed role of mental models in both deductive and inductive reasoning, this theory predicts that these forms of reasoning will recruit common neural systems. Specifically, mental-model theorists have predicted that deductive and inductive reasoning will both primarily recruit right-hemisphere regions. Furthermore, to the extent that mental models represent situations spatially, this view predicts that parietal and occipital regions implicated in visuospatial processing will be engaged.

In contrast, mental logic theory offers an account of deductive reasoning that is based on the application of formal deductive rules according to formal syntactic operations. Thus, rule theorists have predicted that reasoning is likely to recruit left prefrontal and superior temporal regions implicated in formal, rule-based operations.

Empirical Evidence on Reasoning from the Neuroscience Literature

We next present empirical evidence from neuroscience that bears on the psychological theories just reviewed. We begin with research on deductive reasoning, and also address research that compares deductive and inductive reasoning. We then review research on problem solving, causal reasoning, and analogical reasoning.

Deductive Reasoning

The brain systems that implement deductive reasoning depend on whether the reasoning problem consists of familiar versus unfamiliar semantic content. When reasoning about familiar semantic content (e.g., All dogs are pets / All poodles are dogs / Therefore, all poodles are pets), a left frontotemporal system is engaged, including left inferior frontal cortex (BA 47), left middle/superior temporal cortex (BA 21/22), and left temporal pole (BA 21/38). Previous research has implicated this system, not only in deductive reasoning, but also in memory and language tasks that employ familiar semantic content. In general, linguistic processing appears central to all these tasks.

In contrast, reasoning about unfamiliar semantic content (e.g., All P are B / All C are P / Therefore all C are B) activates a bilateral frontoparietal system, including bilateral dorsal (BA 6) and inferior (BA 44) frontal lobes, bilateral superior and inferior parietal lobes (BA 7), and bilateral occipital lobes (BA 19). This pattern of activation is also found during the processing of spatial information, and is similar to the neural activity observed while people make transitive inferences about geometrical shapes.

Thus, deductive reasoning recruits left and right prefrontal cortex asymmetrically as a function of familiarity. Across both familiar and unfamiliar deduction problems, left prefrontal cortex is generally active, suggesting that this region is necessary for deductive inference. Conversely, right prefrontal cortex is engaged only when a problem involves unfamiliar semantic content or a conclusion that conflicts with prior beliefs (e.g., No harmful substances are natural / All poisons are natural / Therefore, no poisons are harmful). Whereas language may often dominate familiar reasoning, language and spatial/visual processing may often be central for unfamiliar reasoning.

The brain systems that implement deductive reasoning also depend on whether a reasoning problem produces correct versus incorrect conclusions. Research on this issue has used inhibitory belief problems, namely, problems whereby individuals must inhibit a highly accessible belief that could interfere with correct reasoning (e.g., No addictive things are inexpensive / Some cigarettes are expensive / Therefore, some cigarettes are not addictive). Drawing a correct conclusion on these problems requires that individuals (1) detect the conflict between their prior beliefs and the logical inference, (2) inhibit the prepotent response associated with their belief bias, and (3) engage the appropriate reasoning mechanisms. In contrast, drawing an incorrect conclusion on these problems results from failing to detect the conflict between beliefs and logical inference, and/or failing to inhibit the prepotent response associated with a belief bias.

When people draw correct conclusions on inhibitory belief problems, right inferior prefrontal cortex becomes active. When they draw incorrect conclusions, ventromedial prefrontal cortex is active instead. Activation in right inferior prefrontal cortex when drawing correct conclusions appears to reflect the detection and/or resolution of the conflict between belief and logic. Conversely, activation in ventromedial prefrontal cortex when drawing incorrect conclusions appears to reflect the role of nonlogical mechanisms, perhaps associated with greater affective processing.

In summary, the neural systems that underlie deduction vary considerably, depending on task factors and cognitive demand. Consistent with the task specificity hypothesis, the areas that support deduction vary with the familiarity of the materials, and with whether belief violations occur and are detected. Consistent with the cognitive demand hypothesis, more neural areas are recruited for difficult unfamiliar problems than for easier familiar ones. Consistent with the modularity view, left prefrontal cortex generally appears active across most deduction paradigms, suggesting that it is essential for deductive inference.

Deductive versus Inductive Reasoning

Many experiments have asked individuals to perform both deduction and induction in the same experiment, so that the neural circuits underlying these two types of reasoning could be distinguished. One neuroimaging experiment used a categorical syllogism task consisting of three conditions – deduction, induction, and baseline – to assess this issue. In the deduction condition, individuals received a valid or invalid categorical syllogism (e.g., None of the bakers play chess / Some of the chess players listen to opera / Therefore, some of the opera listeners are not bakers). The task was to indicate whether the conclusion was valid (i.e., whether the conclusion was guaranteed by the truth of the premises). In the inductive reasoning condition, individuals only received invalid categorical syllogisms (e.g., Some of the computer programmers play the piano / No one who plays the piano watches soccer matches / Therefore, some computer programmers watch soccer matches). The task was to indicate whether the conclusion was probable or improbable. The deduction and induction conditions were each compared to a baseline condition, in which a categorical syllogism with anomalous semantic content was presented (e.g., All the engineers own a computer / None of the engineers has been to school / Therefore, all the people who own computers are married). Importantly, the categorical syllogisms were fully counterbalanced across individuals so that the same materials occurred in every condition.

Deductive reasoning (deduction minus baseline) produced activation in the left dorsolateral frontal cortex (BA 6), broadly consistent with the left frontal activation observed by other researchers for familiar semantic content. When deduction was compared directly to induction, however, a different pattern emerged, namely, activation in bilateral posterior regions, with a right-hemisphere prevalence, including associative visual cortex (e.g., cuneus, precuneus, middle and superior occipital gyri), as well as right superior parietal lobe (BA 7) and thalamus. These areas have been reported for visuospatial tasks that require form discrimination and imaginative operations. These areas have also been reported for deductive reasoning tasks that employ visuospatial materials. Such activations suggest that people use visuospatial representations, such as Venn diagrams or Euler circles, to support deductive reasoning on categorical syllogisms. In addition, activation was also found in right anterior cingulate (BA 24/32), implicating attention and executive control in deductive reasoning. Inductive reasoning (induction minus deduction) revealed activation in left dorsolateral frontal (BA 8 and 10) and right insular cortices. These regions are known to be involved in probabilistic reasoning tasks that require the estimation of relative frequencies and other quantities (e.g., How fast do race horses gallop?).

A subsequent neuroimaging study extended the methods and design of the study just described to a deduction task that employed conditional statements instead of categorical syllogisms (e.g., If he is an electrician, then he spent two years in night school / He is an electrician and owns a computer / Therefore, he spent two years in high school). In contrast to the categorical syllogisms used in the previous study, visuospatial processing did not seem relevant to these conditional syllogisms. Thus, these researchers predicted that the new task and materials would not recruit brain regions that perform visuospatial processing. Consistent with this prediction, deductive reasoning (deduction minus induction) revealed a major focus of activation in right inferior frontal cortex (BA 44), in right anterior cingulate (BA 24), and in right middle temporal cortex (BA 21). These researchers concluded that this frontotemporal system constitutes a logic-specific network in the right hemisphere that is comparable to the language-specific network in the left hemisphere. Specifically, these researchers argued that this right-hemisphere system implements a calculus of mental transformations that underlie formal deduction.

In a further comparison, inductive reasoning (induction minus deduction) revealed large intense activations in the left inferior frontal (BA 47) and left insular cortices, in addition to left posterior cingulate (BA 31), parahippocampal (BA 36), left medial temporal (BA 35), and superior and medial prefrontal cortex (BA 9). These areas are broadly consistent with the left frontal (BA 8 and 10) and insular areas found in the previous study, known to be involved in the recall and evaluation of familiar world knowledge. Consistent with standard theories of inductive reasoning, the recall and evaluation of familiar world knowledge appear to play central roles during induction.

Another neuroimaging study developed a category learning task to assess the component processes of inductive reasoning. Of primary interest were the neural systems that support rule application versus rule inference during category learning. Stimuli consisting of novel animals were presented to individuals, who were asked to judge whether all the animals in a set were from the same category. In the rule application condition, a rule was provided that specified the criteria for category membership. In the rule inference condition, individuals had to infer the rule with no instruction. Each condition was further divided into an easy and difficult condition based on the computational demands of the task. These researchers found that rule inference (rule inference minus rule application) preferentially recruited bilateral hippocampus, an area in which activation is modulated by stimulus novelty. In contrast, rule application (rule application minus rule inference) revealed activation in the presupplementary motor area (BA 8). This area is implicated in the anticipation of motor activity and likely reflects an anticipatory response to category exemplars, a response that is absent when the categorization rule is unknown.

In addition to the episodic encoding of novel stimuli, inductive reasoning requires the generation and testing of hypotheses. For example, inferring the basis for category membership requires generating and testing possible rules, such as "has spots on the abdomen" or "has only two appendages" for a category of fictional animals. To assess the neural systems that underlie hypothesis selection, these researchers evaluated the task by difficulty interaction: {hard rule induction minus hard rule application} minus {easy rule induction minus easy rule application}. This comparison assessed the effects of increased difficulty due to subtle variations in the stimulus features of animals that satisfied or violated the category membership rule. The result was an activation in right lateral orbital prefrontal cortex (BA 47 and BA 11), an area implicated in complex reasoning tasks such as analogical and metaphorical transfer. Across different types of reasoning, difficult problems often activate this area.

In summary, current findings from neuroimaging studies of deduction and induction again suggest that the neural bases of reasoning are highly sensitive to the particular tasks and materials employed. For example, deductive reasoning from conditional statements engages a right frontotemporal system, thought to support the application of formal deduction rules, whereas deductive reasoning from categorical syllogisms activates a parieto-occipital system that supports visuospatial processing. Furthermore, the latter result differs from the findings of other researchers, who have found that a left frontotemporal system supports deductive inference in a categorical syllogism task. The observed differences on the same fundamental reasoning process – deduction – probably reflect methodological differences between the tasks and materials used across studies. Furthermore, the fact that different materials are often used on deduction and induction tasks suggests that different activations for these two forms of reasoning may often be driven by differences in materials rather than by differences in reasoning.

Consistent with the task specificity hypothesis, the neural processes that underlie a given type of reasoning (e.g., deduction) may depend more on the tasks and materials used than on the type of reasoning *per se*. Although left prefrontal cortex is often active on deduction tasks (as described in the previous section), it was not active for some of the studies discussed in this section. Perhaps the one consistent finding so far is that reasoning about familiar materials tends to utilize left-hemisphere language and knowledge networks. Conversely, reasoning about less familiar problems tends to utilize bilateral systems that include right-hemisphere mechanisms. This pattern is consistent with theories that postulate two different reasoning systems, one that processes language, and one that processes spatial/visual information.

Problem Solving and Planning

Depending on whether a problem-solving task is well structured or ill structured, different brain systems are engaged. On well-structured problems, such as the Tower of Hanoi, the starting state, the goal state, and possible transformations are specified completely. For example, the starting state consists of three pegs mounted on a platform and three disks of varying sizes stacked in descending order on the first peg. The goal state is to stack the disks in descending order on the third peg. The possible transformations are restricted to moving disks such that (1) only one can be moved at a time, (2) any disk that is not removed must remain on a peg, and (3) a larger disk cannot be placed on a smaller disk. In such tasks, well-structured planning typically recruits left prefrontal cortex, including frontopolar, dorsolateral, and ventrolateral regions.

In contrast, an ill-structured planning problem is specified incompletely. In the Multiple Errands Task, for example, individuals are taken to an unfamiliar neighborhood and asked to complete errands, such as buying a loaf of bread, according to the following rules: you are to spend as little money as possible (within reason) and take as little time as possible (without rushing excessively). You are not to use anything not bought on the street (other than a watch) to assist you. You may perform task steps in any order. In such tasks, ill-structured planning typically activates right dorsolateral prefrontal cortex

(DLPFC), in contrast to the left prefrontal regions that support well-structured planning.

The neural systems underlying planning are further differentiated into subsystems for plan formation versus plan execution. One finding is that DLPFC supports sequential operations during plan formation, whereas medial ventral prefrontal cortex (MVPFC) plays a motivational role in plan execution. More specifically, DLPFC appears to support the generation of hypotheses and the construction of plan steps, whereas the MVPFC appears to support the affective processing required for plan execution (e.g., initiative and determination).

Lesion studies complement the neuroimaging studies just reviewed. One representative study evaluated problem solving in patients with frontal lobe lesions (FLLs) on the Water Jug problem. Patients had to construct unique action sequences that transferred specific quantities of water between jugs of different sizes (e.g., Jar A = 8 units of water, Jar B = 5 units of water, Jar C = 3 units of water). Specifically, individuals had to construct an action sequence that achieved a goal state given by the experimenter (e.g., Jars A and B must contain 4 units of water, and Jar C must contain 0 units). The researchers found that patients with FLLs struggled to make counterintuitive moves that were required to solve the task but that appeared to deviate from the desired goal state. Furthermore, left and bilateral FLL patients were more impaired than right FLL patients were, suggesting that poor performance in the Water Jug task was primarily linked to left DLPFC damage.

In summary, these findings demonstrate that problem solving and planning generally depend on prefrontal systems. Because DLPFC appears important for most problem-solving tasks, modular views receive support. Differences in task conditions modulate the active areas of the prefrontal cortex, however, providing support for the task specificity hypothesis. For example, well-structured versus ill-structured problems rely on left versus right prefrontal regions, respectively. This pattern is also consistent with theories that assume two different systems, such as dual-process and dual-code theories, support reasoning. Finally, distributed theories receive support, given that multiple systems typically underlie problem solving. For example, problem solving requires both planning and execution, and also both reasoning and motivation, with different neural systems supporting each component process.

Causal Reasoning

Several studies have evaluated the neural systems that support the perception of mechanical causation in the classic Michotte launching event. In a launching event, a ball travels horizontally across a computer screen and collides with a ball located in the center. The collision results in the second ball 'launching' away from the first, horizontally, across the screen, thereby eliciting the perception that the first ball caused the second to move. One study compared the neural response produced by the launching event to the response elicited by a control event in which the first ball passed below the second ball without a collision (noncausal condition). Of primary interest were the neural systems engaged when individuals judged either (1) the presence or absence of causation versus (2) the direction of the ball's motion. A reliable increase in medial frontal activation occurred for judgments of causality relative to judgments of ball movement. Moreover, this increase occurred during both the causal and noncausal conditions, suggesting that the signal increase was specifically associated with the process of making a causal judgment, not with the perception of actual causality.

Another study evaluated whether causal perception and causal inference rely on common or distinct hemispheric regions. Two callosotomy (split-brain) patients and a group of neurologically intact patients were tested. Of primary interest was neural activity in the left versus right hemispheres during (1) the perception of causal events (i.e., the Michotte launching event) and (2) causal inference tasks when the relation between a candidate cause and an observed effect had to be inferred (rather than perceived directly). Perception of causality and causal inference depended on different hemispheres of the divided brain. Whereas causal perception engaged the right hemisphere, causal inference engaged the left-hemisphere.

Another study assessed the brain systems for processing evidence that was either consistent or inconsistent with an individual's existing causal beliefs. Individuals received evidence on the effectiveness of drugs designed to relieve depressive symptoms. Two factors were manipulated: the plausibility of the theory that explained the drug's action, and the consistency between theory and data. When individuals reasoned with evidence that was consistent with existing causal beliefs, a network of brain regions widely associated with learning and memory was engaged, including the caudate and the parahippocampal gyrus. In contrast, when they reasoned with inconsistent evidence, a different pattern of activation occurred that is widely associated with error detection and conflict resolution, including the anterior cingulate cortex (BA 24/32), posterior cingulate, and precuneus (BA 7). The researchers concluded that people's beliefs and expectations act as a filter during evidence evaluation. When evidence is consistent with existing causal beliefs, the neural systems underlying those beliefs implement causal reasoning. When evidence is inconsistent with existing beliefs, a different neural system detects this inconsistency and triggers the construction of a novel causal explanation.

The observed findings demonstrate that causal reasoning is supported by a broadly distributed neural system that is highly sensitive to the causal reasoning task (i.e., causal perception versus causal inference) and the consistency of causal evidence with existing beliefs. These findings provide support for theories of reasoning that are (1) based on distributed rather than localized representations (e.g., dual-process, dual-code, embodied theories), (2) incorporate the role of existing knowledge rather than operating on the basis of purely logical representations (e.g., dual-process, dual-code, embodied, mental-model theories), and (3) advocate the task specificity hypothesis (e.g., dual-process, dual-code, embodied theories).

Analogical Reasoning

Several studies have found that analogical reasoning engages frontopolar cortex. Furthermore, different components of analogical reasoning appear to differentially engage frontopolar versus dorsolateral prefrontal areas. Whereas dorsolateral areas are recruited for processing externally generated information (e.g., the monitoring and manipulation of presented facts), frontopolar areas are recruited additionally for the evaluation and manipulation of internally generated information.

One study assessed the neural systems that support analogical reasoning in the Raven's Progressive Matrices task. Study participants received a 3×3 matrix of figures with the bottom right figure missing, and had to infer the missing figure by selecting one of four possible alternatives. Participants received three types of problems that differed in their degree of relational complexity (0-relational, 1-relational, 2-relational). The 0-relational problems involved no relation of change and thus required no relational processing. The 1-relational problems involved one relation of change in either the horizontal or vertical dimension, and thus required relational reasoning. Finally, the 2-relational problems involved two relations of change, in both the horizontal and vertical directions, and thus required even more relational reasoning.

A region-of-interest analysis was performed to assess the role of prefrontal cortex in processing multiple relations simultaneously (i.e., relational integration). This analysis produced two main findings. First, activation occurred in frontopolar prefrontal cortex (BA 10), reflecting the internal generation of relations required to form complex analogies. Interestingly, this activation only occurred for 2-relational problems, not for 1-relational problems, suggesting that frontopolar cortex is important for processing complex relational structures. Second, activations also occurred in right DLPFC (BA 46), which reflected greater manipulation of externally presented information in more complex problems. Other studies using the Raven's Progressive Matrices task have found similar results, and have also reported bilateral posterior parietal activations (BA 7).

In another study, individuals received a source picture of colored geometric shapes, followed by a target picture of colored geometric shapes. Pictures that did not share similar geometric shapes but that did share the same system of abstract visuospatial relations were also presented. Individuals judged whether each source-target pairing was analogous (analogy condition) or identical (literal condition). Analogical reasoning (analogy minus literal) recruited the dorsomedial frontal cortex (BA 8) and left-hemisphere regions, including frontopolar (BA 10), inferior frontal (BA 44, BA 45, BA 46, and BA 47), and middle frontal (BA 6) cortices, and also inferior parietal cortex (BA 40). These findings suggest that analogical reasoning is mediated by a predominantly left-hemisphere frontoparietal system.

Another study systematically evaluated the component processes of analogical reasoning. Specifically, this study assessed the neural systems that underlie (1) the storage of abstract relations in working memory and (2) the process of integrating abstract relations to form analogies. These researchers also found that analogical reasoning activated a left frontoparietal system, with some regions of this circuit mediating working memory processes and others mediating abstract relational integration. In particular, left frontopolar regions (BA 9/10) were again central to the processing of relations that underlie analogical reasoning.

In summary, the observed findings for analogical reasoning are consistent with theories that advocate distributed rather than localized representations (e.g., dual-process, dual-code, embodied theories). As we saw, distributed frontal and posterior systems appear to play a wide variety of roles as representations are retrieved, stored, and integrated. Findings on analogical reasoning further support the cognitive demand and task specificity hypotheses (e.g., dual-process, dual-code, embodied theories). Different kinds of information recruited different prefrontal areas (e.g., external vs. internal information), and the harder the reasoning, the more areas recruited (e.g., 1-relation vs. 2-relation problems). The general importance of frontopolar cortex for generating relations internally suggests that this area is especially important for processing complex analogies.

Summary, Conclusions, and Future Directions

The findings discussed in this article support the following conclusions about the neural bases of reasoning. First, deductive reasoning does not appear to recruit a unitary neural system but instead engages different brain regions based on the particular reasoning task and materials employed. Second, inductive inferences drawn from familiar categorical syllogisms and conditional statements engage a left-hemisphere language and knowledge network implemented in frontal and temporal regions. Third, problem solving generally recruits prefrontal regions, including bilateral DLPFC and MVPFC. Fourth, causal reasoning does not engage a single neural system but instead recruits different systems based on the causal reasoning task and the consistency of causal evidence with background beliefs. Finally, analogical inference selectively recruits frontal and parietal regions, with frontopolar cortex becoming increasingly important as task complexity increases.

The neuroscience evidence reviewed helps evaluate current psychological theories. First, reasoning typically recruits broadly distributed neural systems, providing evidence inconsistent with the relatively localized predictions of modularity theory. Possible exceptions include the importance of certain frontal regions for problem solving (left DLPFC) and analogical reasoning (frontopolar cortex). Second, the results demonstrate that reasoning does not solely recruit left-hemisphere regions for language and rule-based operations. Instead, reasoning often engages bilateral and posterior regions beyond those implicated by amodal and mental logic theories of reasoning. Third, the predominantly right-hemisphere system predicted by the mental-models theory across both deduction and induction is inconsistent with many patterns of left-hemisphere and bilateral activation observed across studies. Fourth, dual-process, dual-code, and embodied theories are generally consistent with the reviewed findings. These theories receive support because they predict the presence of (1) broadly distributed neural systems and (2) multiple reasoning systems (e.g., associative vs. rule, language vs. knowledge). These theories also receive support from the many studies that exhibit effects of task specificity and cognitive demand. As task conditions change, so do the neural systems that represent and process the relevant information.

In general, reasoning tends to recruit broadly distributed and diverse neural systems. The difficulty of establishing specific neural systems for a given type of reasoning (e.g., deduction) strikes us as one major challenge for future research. Does a particular type of reasoning consistently activate a specific neural circuit across wide variation in tasks and materials? If so, what is this circuit? Another major challenge is that the multifaceted nature of the neurobiological evidence and cognitive theories results in a many-to-many mapping: neural regions often serve multiple cognitive functions that can be mapped onto multiple cognitive theories. Sorting out the functional roles of particular brain areas and their roles in psychological theories of reasoning should be another major goal in this research area.

Many other challenges also await future research in this area. For example, do the results from the laboratory tasks reviewed here generalize to everyday reasoning tasks? Rather than occurring in a vacuum, everyday reasoning often occurs in social situations and is associated with emotional affect. What are the neural bases of reasoning under these conditions? How do social and emotional processes modulate reasoning? Future research should also address the important distinction between reasoning to a conclusion versus recognizing a conclusion. Because many real-world situations require that people generate valid conclusions (not just recognize them), future neuroscience research should assess the neural bases of this process. Future research should also continue to address the role of task difficulty in reasoning. Does task difficulty result in the recruitment of more brain regions, or are the same regions activated more intensely? Future research should also address the effect of learning on the neural systems that underlie reasoning. Do novices and experts engage similar neural systems during reasoning?

Finally, researchers should develop psychological theories that motivate fine-grained neurobiological predictions, and should design experiments that distinguish between theories, rather than simply attempting to confirm one. Although much progress has been made in framing the issues and establishing preliminary evidence, neuroscience research on reasoning is still in its infancy. We anticipate major advances in coming years.

Acknowledgments

This work was supported by National Science Foundation Grants DGE-0536941 and DGE-0231900 to A K Barbey, and by National Science Foundation Grant BCS-0212134 and Defense Advanced Research Programs Agency Contract FA8650-05-C-7256 to L W Barsalou.

See also: Decision-Making and Vision; Executive Function and Higher-Order Cognition: Assessment in Animals; Games in Monkeys: Neurophysiology and Motor Decision-Making; Memory Representation; Prefrontal Cortex: Structure and Anatomy; Prefrontal Cortex; Referentiality and Concepts in Animal Cognition; Reward Decision-Making.

Further Reading

Barbey AK and Sloman SA (in press) Base-rate respect: From ecological rationality to dual processes. *Behavioral and Brain Sciences*.

Barsalou LW (1999) Perceptual symbol systems. *Behavioral and Brain Sciences* 22: 577–660.

Braine MDS (1990) The 'natural logic' approach to reasoning. In: Overton WF (ed.) *Reasoning, Necessity, and Logic: Developmental Perspectives*, pp. 135–158. Mahwah, NJ: Erlbaum Press.

Christoff K and Gabrieli JDE (2000) The frontopolar cortex and human cognition: Evidence for a rostrocaudal hierarchical organization within the human prefrontal cortex. *Psychobiology* 28: 168–186.

Christoff K, Prabhakaran V, Dorfman J, et al. (2001) Rostrolateral prefrontal cortex involvement in relational integration during reasoning. *NeuroImage* 14: 1136–1149.

Colvin MK, Dunbar K, and Grafman J (2001) The effects of frontal lobe lesions on goal achievement in the water jug task. *Journal of Cognitive Neuroscience* 13: 1129–1147.

Flombaum JI, Santos LR, and Hauser MD (2002) Neuroecology and psychological modularity. *Trends in Cognitive Sciences* 6: 106–108.

Fonlupt P (2003) Perception and judgment of physical causality involve different brain structures. *Cognitive Brain Research* 17: 248–254.

Fugelsang J and Dunbar K (2004) A cognitive neuroscience framework for understanding causal reasoning and the law. *Philosophical Transactions of the Royal Society of London. Series B* 359: 1749–1754.

Goel V (2002) Planning: Neural and psychological. In: Nadel L (ed.) *Encyclopedia of Cognitive Science*, vol. 3, pp. 697–703. New York: Macmillan.

Goel V (2005) Cognitive neuroscience of deductive reasoning. In: Holyoak K and Morrison R (eds.) *Cambridge Handbook of Thinking and Reasoning*, pp. 475–492. Cambridge University Press: New York.

Goel V, Buchel C, Frith C, et al. (2000) Dissociation of mechanisms underlying syllogistic reasoning. *NeuroImage* 12: 504–514.

Goel V and Dolan RJ (2003) Explaining modulation of reasoning by belief. *Cognition* 87: B11–B22.

Green AE, Fugelsang JA, Kraemer DJM, et al. (2006) Frontopolar cortex mediates abstract integration in analogy. *Brain Research* 1096: 125–137.

Holyoak KJ (2005) Analogy. In: Holyoak KJ and Morrison RG (eds.) *Cambridge Handbook of Thinking and Reasoning*, pp. 117–142. Cambridge, UK: Cambridge University Press.

Johnson-Laird PN (1983) *Mental Models: Towards a Cognitive Science of Language, Inference, and Consciousness*. Cambridge, UK: Cambridge University Press.

Novick LR and Bassok M (2005) Problem solving. In: Holyoak KJ and Morrison RG (eds.) *Cambridge Handbook of Thinking and Reasoning*, pp. 321–349. New York: Cambridge University Press.

Osherson D, Perani D, Cappa S, et al. (1998) Distinct brain loci in deductive versus probabilistic reasoning. *Neuropsychologia* 36: 369–376.

Over DE (2003) From massive modularity to meta-representation: The evolution of higher cognition. In: Over DE (ed.) *Evolution and the Psychology of Thinking: The Debate*, pp. 121–144. New York: Psychology Press.

Paivio A (1986) *Mental Representations*. New York: Oxford University Press.

Parsons LM and Osherson DN (2001) New evidence for distinct right and left brain systems for deductive versus probabilistic reasoning. *Cerebral Cortex* 11: 954–965.

Roger ME, Fugelsang JA, Dunbar KN, et al. (2005) Dissociating processes supporting causal perception and causal inference in the brain. *Neuropsychology* 19: 591–602.

Wharton CM, Grafman J, Flitman SS, et al. (2000) Toward neuroanatomical models of analogy: A positron emission tomography study of analogical mapping. *Cognitive Psychology* 40: 173–197.

Whitaker H, Savary F, Markovits H, et al. (1991) Inference deficits after brain damage. Paper presented at the International Neuropsychological Meeting, San Antonio, 1991.

Reward Decision-Making

P Shizgal, Concordia University, Montreal, QC, Canada

Introduction

A Northwestern crow (*Corvus caurinus*) swoops down to a beach from its perch atop a nearby cliff. Gliding a few feet above the intertidal zone, it scans attentively before alighting. The crow's beak probes the sand repeatedly and emerges holding a small whelk. After a brief pause, the bird drops the whelk and searches for another, eventually finding a larger one that meets its fancy. The crow then flies along the beach to a rocky area, ascends almost vertically, drops the mollusk, and dives to inspect the result. The spire has broken off, and the crow easily extracts the body, which it swallows in a single gulp. Returning to the water's edge, the crow again searches the sand, rejecting small whelks and eventually flying off with a large one. This time, the shell remains intact after the first drop and several subsequent ones. Rather than abandoning the obstinate prey, the crow persists until the shell has broken and then harvests its reward.

At multiple steps in this vignette, the crow is faced with consequential choices. Rather than setting off to search for new prey on its own, the bird may have the option of scrounging food from another crow that has procured a prey item too large to consume quickly, such as a fish. While gliding over the intertidal zone, the crow selects a propitious landing spot among multiple candidates. It seems particularly choosy in accepting or rejecting whelks it has dug out of the sand and very persistent in continuing to drop a whelk that has not yet broken open.

Experiments have revealed the adaptive quality of such choices. For example, the smaller whelks do not offer a net average energy gain; they have a low probability of breaking when dropped, and their energy content fails to offset the high cost of multiple ascents to the drop point. In contrast, the larger whelks are profitable because they break more readily and contain more food energy. The probability of breaking a whelk shell seems independent of the number of times it has already been dropped; if so, abandoning a whelk that has failed to open is inefficient, because after having paid the cost of procuring another, the crow, on average, would be no closer to mealtime.

The foraging behavior of the Northwestern crow highlights several variables critical to decisions about reward seeking: reward magnitude (as indexed by the size of the whelk), procurement and handling costs, and risk (a function of the probability that the whelk shell will survive a drop) all contribute to the choices made by the crow. Experimental paradigms have been developed to manipulate such variables under simplified, highly controlled, laboratory conditions. These paradigms have been used in conjunction with neurobiological methods, such as electrophysiological recording, neurochemical measurements, pharmacological treatments, brain stimulation, and lesions, to study the neural circuitry involved in adaptive decision making.

Many experiments that apply neurobiological methods to study decision making under laboratory conditions have been carried out using rodents working at operant tasks to obtain rewards. Responses, such as pressing a lever, serve as simplified analogs to procurement behaviors seen in the wild. Rewards such as food pellets are harvested after the operant requirement has been satisfied. Cost is manipulated by varying the amount of work (e.g., the number of lever presses) required to deliver a reward, the effort required to execute each response, or the time that must be invested. The work or time requirement for earning each reward may be either fixed or variable. Additional dimensions of reward that are commonly manipulated include amount (e.g., size of a food pellet or volume of liquid), intensity (e.g., concentration of sucrose), delay (time between meeting the work or time requirement and delivery of the reward), and kind (e.g., food vs. water).

Intensity, Rate, and Cost

Brain Stimulation Reward

An experimental model that has seen particularly heavy use in studies of the neural basis of decision making in laboratory rodents entails delivery of electrical stimulation via chronically implanted electrodes. Rats will work vigorously and insatiably for such stimulation when the electrode is appropriately positioned within the brain. The behavior performed to trigger the stimulation is called self-stimulation, and the effect that draws the rat back to the lever is called brain stimulation reward (BSR). Electrical stimulation of the medial forebrain bundle can compete with, summate with, or substitute for goal objects such as sucrose solutions, water, or food pellets. It has been proposed that a neural signal arising from the stimulation mimics those that encode the intensity of a natural reward.

Computing the Payoff from BSR

Gallistel and co-workers have carried out experiments employing rewarding brain stimulation to model the decision-making processes of foragers. They reasoned that to allocate its behavior adaptively, a successful forager must multiplicatively combine information about the intensity of the reward and the rate at which it is encountered. Imagine a bird foraging for berries that vary in sugar concentration and abundance. One bush offers sweet, ripe berries at a low density; while foraging there, the bird will encounter intense rewards at a relatively low rate. Another bush offers a higher density of less ripe berries. Under such circumstances, the product of intensity and rate should provide a reasonable estimate of the energy return from each bush. In the brain-stimulation experiments, reward intensity was controlled by varying the number of pulses in each stimulation train (and thereby the induced impulse flow in the stimulated neurons), and reward rate was controlled by varying the average delay to rearming of the lever after a reward had been harvested. The experimenters measured the preferences of the rats for stimulation trains that varied in intensity and rate. The rats behaved as if they had computed the payoff from the trains of stimulation pulses by multiplying the intensity and rate of reward.

Conover and Shizgal trained rats on a task that provides control over the opportunity cost of rewarding brain stimulation. In order to earn a reward, the rats had to be holding down a lever at the time that an unpredictable, unsignaled interval timed out; cost was controlled by varying the average duration of the interval. The longer the rat held down the lever, the less it could engage in alternate activities such as grooming, exploring, or resting. Thus, cost in this paradigm is roughly analogous to the average time required for the crow to harvest a whelk; during this time, the bird must forgo the benefits of alternate activities, such as nest building. The behavior of the self-stimulating rats is well described by a model that equates the payoff from the stimulation to the ratio of reward intensity and cost. This result is consistent with the finding of Gallistel's group in that opportunity cost is the inverse of the reward rate that a subject in the Gallistel experiments would achieve if it spent all of its time working at a particular lever.

The Role of Dopamine in BSR

In models of operant performance, such as the matching law, behavioral allocation is tied to the net payoffs from the competing options; the multiple components of payoff (such as the intensity and cost of reward) act in concert in determining choice (e.g., by scalar combination, as illustrated above). This makes functional sense, but it poses a challenge for experiments on the neurobiological underpinnings of decision making: if a given manipulation shifts the allocation of behavior to reward seeking, through which component(s) of payoff did the manipulation act? This problem is illustrated by the controversy over the role of dopaminergic neurotransmission in the evaluation, selection, and procurement of rewards.

The first experiments linking dopaminergic neurons to reward were carried out on self-stimulating rats, and it has been shown repeatedly that manipulation of dopaminergic neurotransmission profoundly alters the effectiveness of BSR. Reward effectiveness can be estimated from the strength of the stimulation required to sustain a given level of performance; if low-stimulation currents or frequencies suffice, then the reward produced per unit of stimulation must be high, and thus the stimulation is deemed very effective at inducing reward. The effectiveness of BSR is increased by drugs that boost dopaminergic signaling, such as those that block the dopamine transporter, and decreased by drugs that attenuate dopaminergic signaling, such as those that block postsynaptic receptors.

Either explicitly or implicitly, most of the reports detailing the modulation of BSR following perturbations in dopaminergic neurotransmission attribute the observed change in performance to alteration of the intensity of the induced reward signal. However, an alternative account is suggested by work conducted by John Salamone's group on the effects of dopamine-specific lesions on performance for natural rewards. They show that there is little change in performance when work requirements are low and a substantial change when requirements are large. The nature of the reward costs determines the effect of the dopaminergic modulation. Performance on tasks requiring intense physical effort, such as scaling a barrier or repeatedly pressing a lever at a high rate, is very sensitive to decreases in dopaminergic neurotransmission, whereas performance appears to be little affected on low-intensity tasks that entail few responses or merely waiting for a reward. Such results could be due to dopaminergic influence on the proclivity of the subject to invest effort in the pursuit of reward. Conversely, changes in reward effectiveness could have differential effects on performance for low- and high-cost rewards due to the nonlinear relationship between performance and reward strength. The degree to which changes in reward intensity and proclivity to pay high effort costs contribute to the effects of dopaminergic manipulations on performance for either rewarding brain stimulation or natural rewards has yet to be worked out definitively.

Different Roles for Phasic and Tonic Signaling by Dopaminergic Neurons?

Should dopaminergic neurotransmission prove to influence reward intensity, questions remain concerning the underlying mechanism. Two intertwined issues must be resolved: (1) Do dopaminergic neurons lie in series with the neural signals representing reward intensity, or do they modulate transmission in the reward-signaling pathway? (2) What are the relative roles of the phasic and tonic components of dopaminergic signaling? The neural signal that gives rise to BSR is short-lived: it builds up quickly, particularly when the stimulation is strong, and it decays quickly as well. One mode of dopaminergic signaling consists of brief bursts of action potentials lasting a few hundred milliseconds. Could this phasic activity underlie the phasic signal that gives rise to BSR? This seems unlikely. The phasic release of dopamine can be monitored *in vivo* by electrochemical means. In rats trained to self-administer brief trains of pulses via electrodes positioned near the cell bodies of midbrain dopamine neurons, phasic dopamine release in the ventral or dorsal striatum was rarely seen during self-stimulation; in the few cases in which it was observed at the start of a test session, the phasic dopamine signal declined quickly and was no longer detectable after a minute or so; in contrast, the rats continued to work vigorously for the stimulation. These results are difficult indeed to reconcile with the notion that the reward signal is encoded in the phasic release of striatal dopamine.

A second mode of dopaminergic signaling entails the steady release of the neurotransmitter over longer timescales. The existing data on the influence of dopaminergic manipulations on BSR are consistent with the notion that such sustained release gates transmission of the reward signal. In this view, the dopamine neurons do not compose part of the direct pathway that translates the neural activity induced by the electrode into the rewarding effect. Instead, these neurons regulate the strength of the reward signal by modulating transmission of the phasic signal induced by the electrode. In turn, dopamine tone is increased by the rewarding stimulation. Due to positive feedback between the rewarding effect and dopamine tone, performance is remarkably persistent when stimulation strength is high.

A distinction between a phasic reward signal and the phasic firing of dopaminergic neurons has also emerged from extensive research on dopaminergic responses to conditioned stimuli and natural goal objects. Schultz's group has shown that the firing of dopaminergic neurons resembles the reward-prediction error in reinforcement-learning models. The reward is a drop of juice, and the simian subjects are thirsty during testing. Delivery of the reward is preceded by an initially neutral stimulus. The initial presentation of the juice reward elicits a vigorous burst of firing from the dopamine neurons. However, as learning proceeds and the onset of the conditioned stimulus comes to predict the drop of juice that follows, these neurons no longer respond to delivery of the reward; if the now-expected reward is omitted, firing is suppressed below its baseline rate. Thus, the phasic activity of the dopamine neurons appears to encode the difference between the reward the monkey was expecting and the reward it receives. In this view, a nondopaminergic 'primary' reward signal is relayed to the dopamine cells and compared with a reward prediction to generate an error signal, which is encoded in the phasic firing of the dopamine neurons. This error signal serves to train the neural network that generates the reward prediction and to adjust action patterns to maximize the harvest of rewards. Perhaps the neural signal that gives rise to BSR corresponds to the primary reward signal in this model. The identity of the neurons that produce this signal has yet to be established, but there is accumulating evidence implicating the extended-amygdala network.

Risk

The introductory vignette illustrates a form of risk sensitivity in foraging behavior. Every time the crow makes the arduous ascent to the drop point, it runs a risk that its efforts will be for naught. Prey selection appears to take this risk into account, in the form of a preference for larger whelks that are more likely to break when dropped.

In laboratory rats, there is evidence that circuitry in a particular brain region plays a role in determining risk sensitivity. Lesions of the core region of the nucleus accumbens, a dopaminergic terminal field, shifted choices toward small certain rewards and away from larger probabilistic ones. The lesioned rats behaved disadvantageously, choosing rewards with lower expected values (e.g., 1 food pellet delivered with $p=1$) in preference to those with higher expected values (e.g., 4 food pellets delivered with $p=0.32$ or 0.7). Thus, the circuitry disrupted by the lesion, which is modulated by dopaminergic input, appears to contribute to the rats' ability to assign adaptive weights to low-probability rewards. In this light, is it interesting to note case studies in which pharmacological treatments that increase dopamine tone appear to boost the incidence of pathological gambling. These findings have been interpreted to suggest that sustained activity of dopaminergic neurons influences risk appetite in humans. Patients with lesions of the ventromedial region of the prefrontal cortex, another dopaminergic terminal field, show increased risk tolerance.

Delay

The effectiveness of rewards depends not only on their probability but also on their imminence. Imagine a cheetah lurking in the tall grass. Scanning the savanna, it spies two similar gazelles trotting towards its hiding place from different locations. Clearly, the gazelle that will first enter the cheetah's striking range is the better prospect. Thus, the values of the two gazelles can be said to be discounted according to their projected arrival times, and the value of the nearer one is less diminished due to the smaller delay. However, if the more distant gazelle is larger than the nearer one, the cheetah is faced with a dilemma: pursue the smaller, sooner reward or wait for the larger, later one? If there is a constant probability over time that either gazelle will change direction or will be pursued by another cheetah before it comes into range, then the present value of each gazelle should decline exponentially as a function of its predicted time of arrival. The cheetah will forgo the small gazelle and wait for the larger one if the size difference outweighs the difference in the temporal discounts, regardless of whether the expected arrival is imminent or far off.

Experiments carried out on many different animals paint a more complex and intriguing picture of the discounting problem. The discount function deviates from a simple exponential and is approximated by a rectangular hyperbola. This widespread finding implies that imminent rewards are attributed even greater relative weight than a simple exponential discounting model predicts. Moreover, the preference of a decision maker who discounts hyperbolically can reverse as a function of its temporal vantage point. A cheetah behaving in this way would fix its sights on the larger, later reward if both predicted arrival times are relatively far off in the future; as the gazelles approached, its preference would shift to the smaller, sooner reward. The latter behavior is said to be 'impulsive.' The steeper the discount curve, the more dramatic the preference reversal, and the more short-sighted the behavior of the cheetah will appear. Thus, it is not surprising that neural mechanisms involved in temporal discounting have been implicated in impulse-control disorders, which are believed to entail excessive discounting of negative long-term consequences in the pursuit of modest short-term gains.

Cardinal and colleagues have shown that lesions of the core region of the nucleus accumbens not only steepen probability discounting but also steepen temporal discounting, shifting the preference of laboratory rats toward smaller, sooner rewards. In the inferotemporal cortex, another dopaminergic terminal field implicated in decision making, dopamine release increases during performance of a temporal discounting task but release of serotonin does not; in contrast, serotonin release is boosted in the medial prefrontal cortex during the discounting task whereas dopamine release is decreased. It has been argued that there is a division of labor between cortical territories, with the temporal and reward-magnitude dimensions of the task processed preferentially in the medial prefrontal cortex and the orbitofrontal cortex, respectively; neurochemically distinct diffuse projection systems originating in the brain stem appear to differentially modulate the operation of the distributed cortical circuitry.

Kind

Animals must procure diverse resources in order to ensure survival and successful reproduction. These resources are sorted into differentially fungible categories (kinds) by physical, chemical, physiological, and ecological realities. An excess of stored food cannot offset a deficit in hydration or compensate for a lack of nest-building materials. In contrast, pathways of metabolism provide for partial convertibility of nutrients; although all macronutrients can be used as sources of cellular energy, carbohydrates provide a superior means of meeting short-term needs whereas fats provide a superior input to long-term stores. Thus, animals face what economists call a substitution problem. Their task is not merely to procure the most valuable single resource from a set of possible options but rather to assemble, at the lowest cost and risk, the basket of goods that best meets a diverse set of needs. Due to the variable degree to which items can be substituted for each other to meet particular needs, the contribution of each item to the value of the basket cannot be computed merely by adding the individual values. The computational task is rendered even more challenging by the fact that a given goal object may contain resources of many different kinds. For example, a prey item typically contains macronutrients from all three classes, water, minerals, and vitamins.

How does the nervous system go about solving the substitution problem? It has been suggested that functional subdivision of brain reward circuitry may contribute to this important task. Perhaps dedicated circuitry processes the reward value of resources of a given kind. Combining the outputs of such specialized circuits on the basis of the substitutability of the rewards they evaluate could then help distribute the choices of the decision maker so as to achieve an appropriate basket of goods. Evidence for functional specialization of brain reward circuitry is provided by studies of the effects of energy balance on BSR. When the tip of the stimulating electrode lies in a particular region of the lateral hypothalamus, dorsolateral to the fornix, depletion of the long-term energy stores boosts the rewarding effect; leptin, a hormone produced by adipocytes in proportion to their fat content, attenuates the rewarding effect of stimulation delivered to this region. In contrast, when nearby portions of the medial forebrain bundle are stimulated, the rewarding effects are unaltered by depletion of the fat stores and either unchanged or increased by administration of leptin. Such evidence suggests that physiological feedback signals differentially modulate the rewarding effects produced by stimulation of different brain sites.

The Origin of Reward Signals

The neural signals representing the intensity, amount, and kind of rewards interact with signals representing general information about rate, cost, risk, and delay. In addition to the evaluation of rewards, many fundamental psychological processes, such as interval timing and memory, are essential to such computations. Thus, it is not surprising that a wide array of brain structures has been implicated in reward-related decision making, including multiple territories in the prefrontal cortex, the striatum and ventral pallidum, the amygdaloid complex and extended amygdala, the hippocampal formation, the medial forebrain bundle, and the midbrain nuclei that give rise to ascending dopaminergic, noradrenergic, serotonergic, and cholinergic projections. Using the gustatory system as an example, the following section addresses the origin of reward signals and their processing prior to combination with other information required for decision making.

Taste plays a crucial and obvious role in determining the rewarding properties of food items, and a considerable body of research has been devoted to the origin of gustatory reward signals. A bifurcation of information flow is implicit in any sensory pathway that gives rise to reward signals. One function of sensation is to determine the identity and quality of a stimulus; another is to indicate what that stimulus is worth at the present moment. In contrast to the circuitry dedicated to determining what the stimulus is, the circuitry charged with computing stimulus value functions in an inherently subjective manner. No taste stimulus is inherently good: a food that seems irresistible when we are hungry may become disgusting after we have overindulged. Thus, the computation of gustatory reward by the evaluative channel implies a weighting of sensory information by internal signals reflecting the current physiological state, a process that Cabanac has labeled 'alliesthesia.' Further modulation of stimulus value occurs as a result of learning, short-term exposure, and modulation by hormonal, circadian, and photoperiodic factors.

In rodents, there is a bifurcation in the gustatory projection. Gustatory information from the nucleus of the solitary tract is relayed to the parabrachial region, which, in turn, projects in parallel to the gustatory thalamus and to basal forebrain targets in the lateral hypothalamus and extended amygdala. Norgren and Grill proposed that the informational function is subserved by the thalamocortical branch, whereas the evaluative function depends on the basal-forebrain branch. Consistent with this view is the finding that sucrose, a rewarding gustatory stimulus, fails to increase dopamine release in the nucleus accumbens following interruption of the basal-forebrain projection but continues to do so following interruption of the thalamocortical branch.

The parabrachial relay for corticopetal gustatory information appears to be absent in the primate, and there is abundant evidence for the processing of gustatory rewards by cortical circuitry. At early stages of processing in the primate gustatory system, up to and including the primary gustatory cortex, food deprivation does not appear to modulate the responses of taste-sensitive neurons. However, such modulation is seen in the secondary gustatory cortex, within the orbitofrontal region as well as in the lateral hypothalamus. Rolls has proposed that neurons in the latter regions are involved in evaluative processing, whereas the early stages of the pathway and the primary gustatory cortex are involved in informational processing. Within the orbitofrontal cortex, his group has demonstrated separate representations of multiple sensory characteristics of foods, such as sweetness, viscosity, and graininess, as well as neurons tuned to combinations of several different sensory qualities. Also represented there are rewards processed in different sensory modalities, such as somesthesis. The elaborate representations within the orbitofrontal cortex seem well suited to tackle the substitution problem by means of a weighted combination of signals representing the values of different goal objects and their components.

Conclusion

Animals searching for sustenance, shelter, or mates, must solve multidimensional decision problems on an ongoing basis, trading off the benefits and costs of rewards against those of territorial defense and predator avoidance. Neuroscientific research into the mechanisms underlying such decisions is at an early stage. Nonetheless, components of the computational processes underlying reward-related decisions have been brought under experimental control and linked to neurochemically and anatomically characterized circuitry in the brain.

See also: Connectivity of Primate Reward Centers; Dopamine; Dopamine in Perspective; Goal-Directed Behavior Theories; Neuroethological Perspective; Neuropsychology of Primate Reward Processes; Prefrontal Contributions to Reward Encoding; Representation of Reward; Reward Systems: Human; Reward Neurophysiology and Primate Cerebral Cortex; Reward Neurophysiology and Orbitofrontal Cortex; Reward Processing: Human Imaging; Transcription and Reward Systems.

Further Reading

Cabanac M (1971) Physiological role of pleasure. *Science* 173: 1103–1107.

Cardinal RN and Howes NJ (2005) Effects of lesions of the nucleus accumbens core on choice between small certain rewards and large uncertain rewards in rats. *BMC Neuroscience* 6(1): 37.

Cardinal RN, Winstanley CA, Robbins TW, et al. (2004) Limbic corticostriatal systems and delayed reinforcement. *Annals of the New York Academy of Science* 1021: 33–50.

Conover KL and Shizgal P (2005) Employing labor supply theory to measure the reward value of electrical brain stimulation. *Games and Economic Behavior* 52(2): 283–304.

Gallistel CR (1994) Foraging for brain stimulation: Toward a neurobiology of computation. *Cognition* 50(1–3): 151–170.

Hajnal A and Norgren R (2005) Taste pathways that mediate accumbens dopamine release by sapid sucrose. *Physiology & Behavior* 84(3): 363–369.

Hernandez G, Hamdani S, Rajabi H, et al. (2006) Prolonged rewarding stimulation of the rat medial forebrain bundle: Neurochemical and behavioral consequences. *Behavioral Neuroscience* 120(4): 888–904.

Rolls ET (2005) Taste, olfactory, and food texture processing in the brain, and the control of food intake. *Physiology & Behavior* 85(1): 45–56.

Schultz W (2002) Getting formal with dopamine and reward. *Neuron* 36(2): 241–263.

Shizgal P, Fulton S, and Woodside B (2001) Brain reward circuitry and the regulation of energy balance. *International Journal of Obesity* 25(supplement 5): S17–S21.

Waraczynski MA (2006) The central extended amygdala network as a proposed circuit underlying reward valuation. *Neuroscience & Biobehavioral Reviews* 30(4): 472–496.

Wightman RM and Robinson DL (2002) Transient changes in mesolimbic dopamine and their association with 'reward.' *Journal of Neurochemistry* 82(4): 721–735.

Winstanley CA, Theobald DE, Dalley JW, et al. (2006) Double dissociation between serotonergic and dopaminergic modulation of medial prefrontal and orbitofrontal cortex during a test of impulsive choice. *Cerebral Cortex* 16(1): 106–114.

Wise RA (1996) Addictive drugs and brain stimulation reward. *Annual Review of Neuroscience* 19: 319–340.

Zach R (1979) Shell dropping: Decision-making and optimal foraging in Northwestern crows. *Behavior* 68: 106–117.

Social Cognition

J L Marchant and C D Frith, University College London, London, UK

Introduction

In everyday life we constantly interact with the people around us, whether it is to cooperate, compete, or simply to go about our day-to-day business. For such interactions to be successful we must be able to understand and predict the actions of these other people. We typically understand actions in terms of minds: beliefs, desires, and intentions. This is termed having an 'intentional stance' or having a 'theory of mind,' while our ability to 'read' mental states has been called 'mentalizing.' A range of functional imaging studies have attempted to identify the neural correlates of mentalizing when participants make 'off-line' inferences about the mental states of interacting characters in stories, cartoons, and animations. A number of brain regions have been consistently activated by these tasks, including the medial prefrontal cortex (MPFC), temporal poles, and temporoparietal junction.

Yet, like most psychological and neuroimaging studies, these studies were investigations of people in isolation. Even imaging studies of social cognition do not typically involve true interactions. Brain activity is measured in various social contexts or when an individual thinks about her own mental states or those of another person. In all of these paradigms the flow of information is one way. The participant simply responds to a facial expression or to a social scenario. In a true interaction the information flows both ways. We do not simply read the signals of others. We send back signals for them to read. We do not simply respond passively to other persons, we respond actively in order to change them: to make them trust us or fear us. For such interactions, it is not sufficient to represent our own mental state or the mental state of the other. We need also to represent the other's representation of our mental state. In a successful interaction our mental states are effectively shared. Perhaps the simplest example of such an interaction is joint attention, in which each participant knows that there is mutual attention to the same object. However, it is only recently that studies have started to investigate how brain systems are engaged when we directly interact with another person in order to perform 'on-line' mentalizing.

The most basic form of social interaction is joint action in which two people cooperate in order to achieve some common goal. In order to successfully achieve their shared goal, participants must understand how they and their partner view each other's roles within the partnership. This process involves at least four levels of mentalizing: (1) our belief about our partner's role, (2) our belief about how our partner views his role, (3) our belief about how our partner believes we view our role, and finally (4) our belief about how our partner believes we view him. If we are able to represent all levels of this mentalizing structure, we should be able to understand the intentions of our partner and predict his actions.

This section summarizes findings from recent studies in which two participants socially interact in a variety of tasks. We start by noting some important behavioral studies and then discuss neuroimaging findings that suggest an important role for the medial frontal cortex, including the anterior cingulate cortex (ACC), in on-line social interaction. Next, we highlight the new breed of 'hyperscanning' studies that go beyond analysis of a single brain to look at systems of interacting brains.

What Can Behavioral Studies Tell Us?

A variety of experiments have been used to explore cooperative behavior between humans and nonhuman animals. Tasks have included attainment of a reward that is not accessible to the individual, successful completion of a joint action task, and exchange of information in a communicative partnership. Such cooperation is highly prevalent in human society. Children as young as 18–24 months old are able to interact with an adult human in a cooperative activity, unlike their chimpanzee counterparts.

Even though language plays a vital role in most cooperative endeavors, it is not necessary for successful cooperation. As long as we can monitor the actions of others we can identify their goals and intentions and modify our own behavior accordingly. Indeed, the mere presence of another person performing a task with us can modify our own response. Sebanz and colleagues used a spatial compatibility task wherein participants made one of two spatially distinct actions in response to a color cue and in the presence of an irrelevant spatial cue. When participants worked alone and assigned one hand to each of two response alternatives, reaction times were slowed when there was an incompatibility between the desired response and the irrelevant spatial cue. This effect disappeared when the participant responded to only one of the two alternatives. However, the incompatibility effect returned when a second participant was assigned to respond to the other alternative. This result suggests that we automatically represent the actions of the person sharing the task with us even though this impairs our own performance.

In the task used by Sebanz and colleagues the performance of one participant had no direct effect on the performance of the other. Reed and colleagues used a simple task in which a crank handle was used to align a cursor with a target. In the joint action condition both participants effectively held the same handle, but had no communication except via the force the other was applying. Participants perceived the contribution of the other as a hindrance, but, in practice, when they worked together, their performance became more efficient than when they worked alone. The force profiles of the participants' actions dramatically changed in the joint response as they developed strategies to work together. Most often one participant contributed more to acceleration and the other to deceleration of the movement of the crank, thereby achieving more efficient and faster movement.

Although cooperative behavior between nonrelated participants are uncommon in the animal kingdom, Mendres and DeWaal have shown that pairs of capuchin monkeys can work together to pull a tray forward in order to receive a reward. The monkeys made more communicational glances to their partner in the joint action task than when they acted alone, in an attempt to motivate their partner. Joint action performance became poorer when the partners were unable to see each other, and the authors suggest this was because the capuchins required visual contact to coordinate the timings of their responses.

The more complex tasks typical of human cooperative interactions are greatly helped by direct communication. Communication is not only a way to express our intentions to others, it also enables the exchange of information relevant to the task in hand. This bilateral process requires both participants to input their own information, monitor their partner, and update their action. Communicators must constantly evaluate and amend their actions to take account of the reactions of listeners, and listeners must inform communicators of any changes in their current understanding to make sure that both have common knowledge. Common knowledge acts to set a mutual base, where all participants are aware of the information and know that all the other participants are also informed. Much of this common knowledge emerges as a by-product of the interaction.

Communication does not rely solely on the monitoring of speech, but also on many other communicative signals, such as facial expressions, posture, and body movements, and what is happening in each participant's workspace and in the surrounding environment. When any part of this information is blocked, communication becomes less effective and less efficient. Understanding is further worsened if communication becomes a noninteractive process, as with written instructions. For example, Clark and Krych studied a task in which one participant gave directions while the other participant followed these directions in order to build a structure. Task efficiency was greatly reduced when a barrier obscured the view of each other's workspace. Furthermore, noninteractive communication using prerecorded directions produced the greatest number of errors.

Cooperative behavior is usually mutually beneficial to both participants, but often it requires at least one participant to invest their trust in the other with some degree of risk. To prevent betrayal of trust and loss of investment we must wisely choose our partners and invest the minimal amount to reap maximal reward. We must continually monitor our partner for trustworthiness and at the same time give out signals indicating that we are worthy of trust (reputation management). Trust and reciprocity have been studied in economic games such as the Prisoners' Dilemma. An optimal strategy in such games is 'tit-for-tat,' in which trust is repaid by trust and betrayal is repaid by betrayal. Players in economic games have a strong sense of the 'fairness' of interactions. Given the opportunity, they will punish those who make unfair offers, even at some cost to themselves (altruistic punishment). The occurrence of altruistic punishment increases group cooperation.

Neural Activity Associated with Social Interactions

To date the majority of imaging studies of on-line social interactions have involved various kinds of trust and reciprocity games in which the brain activity of each participant is recorded while each interacts with partners outside the scanner.

Some of these experiments have manipulated participants' 'intentional stance' by making them believe that they are interacting with a human or computer partner. In these studies, which have used both competitive and cooperative games, greater activity is seen in the MPFC and adjacent ACC when participants believe they are interacting with a human rather than a computer. This activity is located in the anterior rostral region of the MPFC (using the terminology of Amodio and Frith), where most of the MPFC activity associated with off-line mentalizing tasks has also been observed. A recent study in monkeys has shown that lesions in the ACC cause a loss of interest in social stimuli.

Brain regions concerned with emotion are strongly implicated in these trust and reciprocity games. For example, the ventral striatum and other regions concerned with reward are activated after episodes of mutual cooperation. Unfair offers, on the other hand, decrease activity in reward areas while activating the anterior insula. Insula activity also occurs in response to negative emotions such as disgust and pain. Given these effects, is not surprising that the faces of game partners who persistently cooperate or defect rapidly come to elicit positive and negative emotions, respectively. These effects are largely eliminated if the other player is believed to be a computer or a person who is not a free agent, but merely follows instructions.

When persistent defectors are seen to be punished, activity also increases in brain regions associated with reward. This involvement of reward systems suggests a mechanism whereby cooperation and altruistic punishment can be maintained during social interactions.

Two Brains, Two Scanners

Investigating the brain activations of one player only gives half the story, because another person (and their brain) is involved in a dyadic social interaction. To address this problem a new type of neuroimaging has been developed by Read Montague and his colleagues. This system, known as 'hyperscanning,' allows the simultaneous brain scanning of two socially interacting people by using an Internet link to temporally align two functional magnetic resonance imaging (fMRI) scanners and their presentation systems. Timing and presentation information, such as scanner onset or type and onset of stimuli and rewards, can be transmitted between different scanning laboratories. The Internet connection allows participants to interact with other participants in fMRI scanners located around the world and opens the opportunity to investigate the correlation between the activities of socially interacting participants.

The two hyperscanning studies published so far have both involved trust and reciprocity games. Participants played against the same human partner and were free to make their own choices to allow models of trust and reputation to be built. One participant, the investor, was given money and then decided how much money to share with the other participant, the trustee. Any shared money was tripled and then the trustee decided how much money to repay the investor.

As in previous studies, brain areas associated with reward (dorsal striatum) were activated when trust was reciprocated. However, in the course of the game this signal increasingly anticipated the time at which the investor knew that her trust had been reciprocated. The authors suggest this anticipatory signal is analogous to reward prediction in simple conditioning experiments. As trust builds during the course of the game, the investor becomes increasingly confident that her benevolent behavior will be rewarded by benevolent reciprocity.

However, the importance of the hyperscanning paradigm lies in the possibility of direct investigation of interactions between brains. For example, a cross-brain correlation analysis indicates whether activity in a region in one brain can predict activity in a region of the other brain. In the trust and reciprocity game a strong correlation was found between the investor's middle cingulate cortex and the trustee's ACC. These different locations in cingulate cortex could be related to representations of the 'self' (middle cingulate cortex active during submission of the participants' own responses) or the 'other' (ACC active during the revelation of their partners' responses). These representations were independent of the role of each participant or the type of reciprocity produced. The authors concluded that the cingulate cortex has a spatial map of response agency along the anteroposterior axis. Given this account of the representations in cingulate cortex, the cross-brain analysis indicates that the linked brain regions represent the same thing. Thus, the investor's representation of himself/herself (participant A) is linked to the trustee's representation of the other (participant A). This could be evidence, at the neural level, of the alignment between representations that is necessary for successful social interactions.

Conclusions

Investigations of the neural basis of interacting minds have only just begun. The possibilities are very exciting. As we have seen, there are many behavioral paradigms, in addition to economic games, that have yet to be adapted for brain imaging experiments. Hyperscanning is a particularly important development since interacting minds depend upon interacting brains. When we analyze activity in interacting brains, we need to treat the two (or more) brains as a single system, which has emergent properties that cannot be seen in the single brain. fMRI is perhaps not the ideal modality for such analysis, since we can only look at rather slow hemodynamic changes. Electroencephalography and magnetoencephalography, with their high temporal resolution and direct reflection of neural activity, will provide powerful ways for looking at links between brains during social interactions. Analytic techniques already developed for looking at functional connectivity within brains, such as structural equation modeling and casual modeling, can be applied without modification to analysis of connectivity between brains.

See also: Cognition: An Overview of Neuroimaging Techniques; Decision-Making and Neuroeconomics; Emotion: Neuroimaging; Neuroeconomics: History; Neuroimaging; Reward Decision-Making; Reward Processing: Human Imaging; Social Brain: Evolution; Social Emotion: Neuroimaging; Social Interaction; Social Interaction Effects on Reward and Cognitive Abilities in Monkeys.

Further Reading

Amodio DM and Frith CD (2006) Meeting of minds: The medial frontal cortex and social cognition. *Nature Reviews Neuroscience* 7: 268–277.

Axelrod R (1984) *The Evolution of Cooperation.* New York: Basic Books.

Barr DJ (2004) Establishing conventional communication systems: Is common knowledge necessary? *Cognitive Science* 28: 937–962.

Clark HH and Krych MA (2004) Speaking while monitoring addressees for understanding. *Journal of Memory and Language* 50: 62–81.

Fehr E and Gachter S (2000) Altruistic punishment in humans. *Nature* 415: 137–140.

Frith CD and Frith U (2006) How we predict what other people are going to do. *Brain Research* 1079: 36–46.

King-Casas B, Tomlin D, Anen C, et al. (2005) Getting to know you: Reputation and trust in a two-person economic exchange. *Science* 308: 78–83.

Mendres KA and DeWaal FBM (2006) Capuchins do cooperate: The advantage of an intuitive task. *Animal Behaviour* 60: 523–529.

Reed K, Peshkin M, Hartmann MJ, et al. (2006) Haptically linked dyads – are two motor-control systems better than one? *Psychological Science* 17: 365–366.

Rudebeck PH, Buckley MJ, Walton ME, et al. (2006) A role for the macaque anterior cingulate gyrus in social valuation. *Science* 313: 1310–1312.

Rilling JK, Sanfey AG, Aronson JA, et al. (2004) Opposing BOLD responses to reciprocated and unreciprocated altruism in putative reward pathways. *NeuroReport* 15: 2539–2543.

Sanfey AG, Rilling JK, Aronson JA, et al. (2003) The neural basis of economic decision-making in the Ultimatum Game. *Science* 300: 1755–1758.

Saxe R (2006) Uniquely human and social cognition. *Current Opinion in Neurobiology* 16: 235–239.

Sebanz N, Bekkering H, and Knoblich G (2006) Joint action: Bodies and minds moving together. *Trends in Cognitive Sciences* 10: 70–76.

Tomlin D, Kayali MA, King-Casas B, et al. (2006) Agent-specific responses in the cingulate cortex during economic exchanges. *Science* 312: 1047–1050.

Warneken F, Chen F, and Tomasello M (2006) Cooperative activities in young children and chimpanzees. *Child Development* 77: 640–663.

Wu JZ and Axelrod R (1995) How to cope with noise in the Iterated Prisoners' Dilemma. *Journal of Conflict Resolution* 39: 183–189.

Social Interaction

J K Rilling, Emory University, Atlanta, GA, USA
A G Sanfey, University of Arizona, Tucson, AZ, USA

Decision Making and Social Interactions

The study of decision making has as its goal the understanding of our fundamental ability to process multiple alternatives and choose an optimal course of action. A good decision is one that chooses the best available course of action in the face of characteristic uncertainty about the consequences. Although some decisions are straightforward, many are more difficult, either because the stakes are high (e.g., the choice of a mate or deciding between potentially life-saving medical treatments) or because there are difficult trade-offs to make between competing options (e.g., the respective benefits and side effects of a drug). To complicate matters, often our decisions are, in addition, dependent on the possible responses of others, for example when we are deciding whether to ask someone on a date or when entering a business negotiation.

Traditional economic models of decision making, such as the Utility family of theories, propose several aspects of a decision that must be integrated in order to choose the best option. Broadly speaking, these are the subjective values of the potential outcomes that may occur and the likelihood of these outcomes actually occurring. These factors are then weighed to produce a utility for each option, with the alternative with the highest utility chosen. In social decisions, this computation is complicated by the fact that we must also attempt to infer the values and probabilities of our partner or opponent in attempting to reach the optimal decision.

Given that humans live in highly complex social environments, many of our most important decisions are made in the context of these social interactions. This article focuses on research investigating social decision making in two-person interactions, although social decision making often involves considerably more than this. Nevertheless, even in the course of dyadic social interactions, humans are regularly confronted with a wide range of decisions that have far-reaching consequences for the welfare of both the people involved and others. Should I affiliate with or trust this person? Should I compete with or be deferential toward this person? How should I respond to a breach of trust by this person? What is the socially appropriate thing to do in this situation?

An additional reason to focus on the neural basis of decisions in the context of social interactions stems from evolutionary considerations. Primate social behavior is more complex than that of most other mammals because primates form alliances and coalitions that compete with one another. On average, primates also have larger brains for their body size than other mammals. Moreover, relative neocortex size is positively correlated with social group size, a presumed proxy for social complexity, across anthropoid primates. These facts suggest that large primate brains may have evolved in response to social complexity in order to support greater social intelligence that would, in turn, allow an individual primate to successfully negotiate these complexities. If humans represent an extension of this primate trend, then a reasonable claim is that the human brain was designed in some measure to deal with complex social interactions and that our brain's decision-making circuitry probably evolved in part to support these types of decisions.

Finally, a number of psychiatric disorders involve deficits in social decision making. For example, depressed patients often withdraw from social interactions, choosing instead to be alone. Psychopathic individuals often manipulate and objectify others, making it difficult for them to establish stable, long-term bonds. Mania is often accompanied by impulsive and frequently damaging decisions about sexual behavior, shopping, travel, and driving. In addition, several axis II personality disorders involve poor choices within interpersonal relationships. Endeavoring to understand the neural bases of these disorders therefore rests in part on an understanding of the neural bases of social decision making.

Tasks

In a similar fashion to the framework provided by Utility Theory for studying individual decisions, Game Theory offers well-specified models for the investigation of social exchange. However, much of the decision behavior actually observed in these tasks deviates, often quite substantially, from the predictions of the standard game theoretic model, suggesting that psychological and neuroscientific approaches may help our understanding of these decisions and judgments. Recent research has combined these tasks with neuroimaging in an effort to gain a more detailed picture of social decision making. This research probes the neural basis of decision making in the context of social interactions and combines behavioral paradigms from behavioral economics with a variety of methods from neuroscience.

A class of decisions has been investigated by experimental economics tasks, which, although beguilingly simple, require complex reasoning about the motivations and strategies employed by other players and thus offer a useful window into more complex forms of decision making – decisions that may better approximate many of the choices we make in real life.

One specific focus of these games is reciprocal exchange, exemplified by trust games and closely related Prisoner's Dilemma (PD) games. In the Trust Game (TG), a player (the Investor) must decide how much of an endowment to invest with a partner (the Trustee) in the game. Once transferred, this money is multiplied by some factor (usually tripled or quadrupled), and then the Trustee has the opportunity to return some or all of the amount to the Investor but, significantly, need not return any money if he or she decides against it. If the Trustee honors trust and returns money to the Investor, both players end up with a higher monetary payoff than was originally obtained. However, if the Trustee abuses trust and keeps the entire amount, the Investor ends up with a loss. Because the Investor and Trustee interact only once during the game, Game Theory predicts that a rational and selfish Trustee will never honor the trust given by the Investor. The Investor, realizing this, should never place trust in the first place and so will invest zero in the transaction. Despite these grim theoretical predictions, in most studies of the TG a majority of investors do send some amount of their money to the Trustee.

The well-studied PD game is similar to the trust game, except that both players simultaneously choose whether to trust one another without knowledge of their partner's choice (**Figure 1**). In the PD game, two players choose to either cooperate with one another or not (i.e., defection) and receive a payoff that depends on the interaction of their two choices. The largest payoff occurs when the player defects and the partner cooperates (DC = \$3). The second largest payoff is for mutual cooperation (CC = \$2), followed by mutual defection (DD = \$1), and finally player cooperation combined with partner defection (CD = \$0). Each outcome corresponds to a different outcome of a social interaction and typically elicits a different set of social emotions. Again, game theoretic predictions are that players will immediately default to mutual defection, but in most iterations of the game, players exhibit much more trust than expected, with mutual cooperation a common finding, at least in early rounds of the game. Mutual cooperation is often associated with friendship, love, trust, or obligation; mutual defection is often associated with feelings of rejection and hatred. Cooperation by one person and defection by the other typically results in the cooperator's feeling anger or indignation and in the defector's feeling anxiety, guilt, or elation from successfully exploiting his or her partner to advantage.

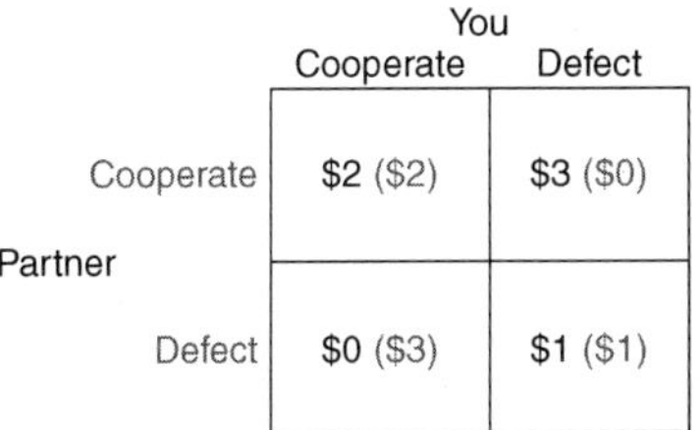

Figure 1 Payoff matrix used in PD game. The scanned player's choices are the column labels and nonscanned partner's choices are the row labels. Payoff to the scanned player is in black; payoff to the nonscanned partner is in red.

These games are good models for the reciprocal exchange of favors. Given that favors are rarely exchanged simultaneously in real life, the TG at first seems a better model for real-life behavior than the PD; however, the PD choices in round n can also be viewed as a response to the partner's choice in round $n - 1$. Both PD and TG can be played as either single-shot or iterated interactions. In the single-shot versions, cooperative moves by the trustee in the TG, or by either partner in the PD, are unambiguously altruistic insofar as individuals are sacrificing personal gain so that their partner can receive more. In the iterated versions of the games, in which several consecutive rounds are played with the same partner, cooperative choices are not necessarily selfless because consistent cooperation with a reciprocating partner generally yields the player higher cumulative earnings over the long term than does a noncooperative strategy that often settles into the equilibrium outcome of mutual selfishness. Whereas economists have emphasized the importance of these interactions being anonymous in order to eliminate reputation effects that could bias choices, others argue that humans are evolutionarily unprepared for such non-naturalistic social interactions and that subjects should meet and know the identity of their playing partners. Both anonymous and nonanonymous versions of these games have been studied with neuroimaging.

Bargaining games are another common focus of experimental economics, with the family of Dictator and Ultimatum games often used to examine responses to equality and inequality. In the Dictator Game (DG), one player (the Proposer) decides how much of an endowment to award to the second player (the Responder). Allocations in this game measure pure altruism, in that the Proposer sacrifices personal gain to share the endowment with his or her partner. The Ultimatum Game (UG) is a variant which examines more strategic thinking in the context of two-player bargaining. In the UG, the Proposer and Repsonder are also asked to divide a sum of money, with the Proposer specifying how this sum should be divided between the two. However, in this case the Responder has the option of accepting or rejecting the offer. If the offer is accepted, the sum is divided as proposed. However, if it is rejected, neither player receives anything. In either event, the game is over; that is, there are no subsequent rounds in which to reach agreement. The decision to reject an unfair offer is considered a form of altruistic punishment because the Responder chooses to receive no money rather than the amount offered by the Proposer, presumably to punish the Proposer for making a miserly offer. If people are motivated purely by self-interest, the Responder should accept any offer and, knowing this, the Proposer should offer the smallest nonzero amount. However, again Game Theory predictions are at odds with observed behavior, and in most industrialized cultures, low offers of less than 20% of the total amount are rejected about half the time. There are some interesting differences in more traditional cultures, but in general the probability of rejection increases substantially as offers decrease from 50% to 0%. Thus, people's choices in the UG do not conform to a model in which decisions are driven by immediate self-interest.

Methods

The neural correlates of decision making in these games have been investigated using a variety of methods. One approach uses functional neuroimaging, namely functional magnetic resonance imaging (fMRI) or positron emission tomography (PET), to image changes in blood flow while subjects are playing interactive games in the MRI or PET scanner. Subjects can view computer-projected visual stimuli from inside the scanner, either via goggles that display the visual stimuli or via a mirror that allows the subject to view a projection screen outside the scanner. Because verbal responses can create motion artifacts, subjects generally indicate choices by pressing specific buttons on a response box. With these imaging methods, it is possible to examine regional blood flow during the decision-making epochs of the task and to link these to specific choices.

Imaging studies of social interactions have emerged relatively recently within cognitive neuroscience. Many early fMRI studies presented subjects with stimuli of other human faces, given the obvious importance of faces in human social interactions. Typically, these stimuli were static, two-dimensional pictures of faces that subjects were instructed to either passively view or judge on some attribute (gender, age, etc.). Using similar types of stimuli, other studies examined face-processing deficits in patients with damage to specific brain regions such as the amygdala or the fusiform gyrus. Still others have attempted to probe social cognition by asking subjects to read stories or view cartoons and then make judgments about these hypothetical scenarios. For example, the neural correlates of both mentalizing and moral reasoning have been probed with this methodology. These studies have yielded valuable insights with respect to the neural underpinnings of human social cognition. However, for each, we can raise questions about the ecological validity of the stimuli. Does the pattern of brain activation in response to static two-dimensional face stimuli accurately reflect the brain's response to the dynamic embodied faces that we encounter in everyday life? Is the pattern of brain activation in response to reasoning about hypothetical fictitious scenarios the same as when grappling with significant real-life social problems? Is mentalizing about the actions of another person the same as making a consequential decision based on these actions?

One approach to improving the ecological validity of experiments in social cognitive neuroscience is to image brain function as subjects actually interact with other people in real social interactions. Recent innovative studies have imaged human subjects while playing both TG and bargaining games with partners communicating from outside the scanner. Potentially even more exciting, hyperscanning technology has been developed that makes it possible to image brain function in two or more interacting partners simultaneously, by using network connections between two separate scanners. Hyperscanning has obvious advantages in terms of data-collection efficiency (i.e., collecting twice as much data in the same amount of time), but will also open new vistas in social cognitive neuroscience. For example, it will allow the imaging of coordinated patterns of brain activity in people who are effectively working together toward a common goal. It could also be used to evaluate simulation theories of empathy, according to which we understand others by reproducing their neural states. Further applications for this method will undoubtedly emerge in the future.

Another approach to investigating the neural correlates of social decision making involves manipulating specific neurotransmitter systems and examining the effect on game-playing behavior. For example, dietary tryptophan depletion can be used to decrease brain serotonin levels, and central oxytocin (OT) levels can be elevated by intranasal self-administration of OT. Still another approach involves the use of transcranial magnetic stimulation (TMS) to temporarily activate or deactivate a brain region and then examine the effect on a decision-making task. Finally, patients with circumscribed brain damage to particular regions can be tested in these games to see if the damaged brain area has an impact on social decision making.

Findings

Although the methods and tasks outlined here seem to offer exciting prospects for research on social decision making in years to come, the very recent development of this field has meant that the definitive findings revealed thus far are understandably limited. However, studies have outlined a number of tantalizing findings with respect to both brain regions and neurotransmitter systems that appear to be involved in decision making in the context of social interactions.

The Caudate Nucleus

There is good reason to suspect that mesencephalic dopamine projections to the caudate nucleus are involved in decision making in the context of reciprocal exchange (**Figure 2(a)**). Single-cell recording studies in monkeys demonstrated that midbrain dopamine neurons track reward prediction errors. Unexpected rewards increase the firing rate of midbrain dopamine cells, whereas the omission of expected rewards decreases their firing rate. These reward prediction error signals are hypothesized to play a critical role in learning stimulus–response associations, thereby shaping decision making. Midbrain dopamine cells project to both the ventral and dorsal striatum, including the caudate nucleus, and the activation in the human caudate nucleus is modulated as a function of trial-and-error learning with feedback, suggesting that the caudate nucleus may allow an organism to learn contingencies between its own responses and either rewarding or punishing outcomes. Several neuroimaging studies have demonstrated that the human caudate tracks a social partner's decision to reciprocate or not reciprocate cooperation in the TG or PD. This caudate response is also related to future game decisions. Specifically, reciprocated cooperation activates the caudate nucleus and unreciprocated cooperation deactivates this area, in line with the reward prediction error already described (**Figure 3**). In addition, caudate activation is associated with increased cooperation in subsequent rounds. These findings suggest that the caudate registers social prediction errors that guide decisions about reciprocity. Interestingly, these prediction error signals from partner feedback

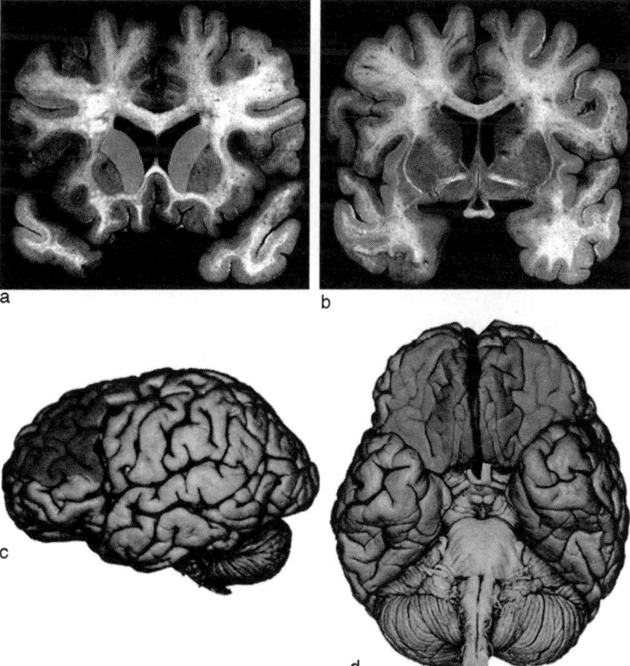

Figure 2 Brain regions involved in decision making in the context of social interactions: (a) caudate nucleus; (b) anterior insula; (c) dorsolateral prefrontal cortex; (d) ventromedial prefrontal cortex. (c, d) From Davidson RJ, Putnam KM, and Larson CL (2000) Dysfunction in the neural circuitry of emotion regulation–possible prelude to violence. *Science* 289(5479): 591–594.

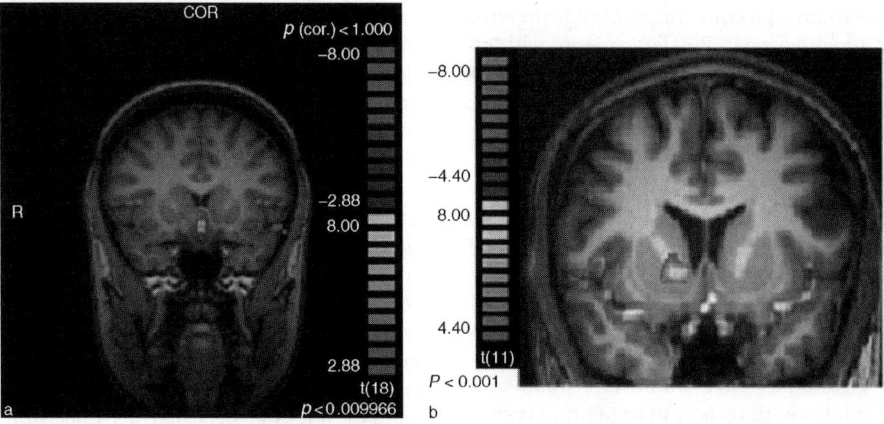

Figure 3 Ventral caudate activation for the contrast between partner reciprocation and nonreciprocation: (a) in an iterated PD game; (b) in an iterated Trust game. (a) From Rilling JK, Sanfey AG, Aronson JA, Nystrom LE, and Cohen JD (2004) Opposing BOLD responses to reciprocated and unreciprocted altruism in putative reward pathways. *NeuroReport* 15: 2539–2543. (b) From Delgado MR, Frank RH, and Phelps EA (2005) Perceptions of moral character modulate the neural systems of reward during the trust game. *Nature Neuroscience* 8: 1611–1618.

can be blunted or even absent when people instead base their decisions on the prior moral reputations of social partners. That is, moral reputations lead to a discounting of feedback information from social partners, demonstrating both top-down and bottom-up influences on the neural basis of social cooperation. Finally, activation in caudate nucleus is also related to satisfaction with punishing nonreciprocators for their norm violations, even when this punishment involves a financial loss to the subject.

Anterior Insula

Activation within the anterior insula has been observed in response to a variety of negative social interactions, from social exclusion in a virtual ball-tossing task to unreciprocated cooperation in an iterated PD game to receiving an unfair offer in the UG to watching a loved one receive a painful stimulus (**Figure 2(b)**). The anterior insula is also responsive to physically painful stimuli, and its activity is correlated with skin conductance responses. These results, and others, suggest that the anterior insula is involved in mapping physiological states of the body, including pain, touch, and visceral sensations of autonomic arousal. The right anterior insula, in particular, is thought to be a site of interoceptive awareness that gives rise to subjective feeling states that may play a role in decision making. Finally, recent fMRI data implicate the right anterior insula in aversive conditioning. In the UG, unfair offers that are subsequently rejected have a stronger average anterior insula response than unfair offers that are subsequently accepted (**Figure 4**), and activation in the anterior insula is related to the degree of unfairness of the offer. In the iterated PD game, individuals with a stronger anterior insula response to unreciprocated cooperation have a higher frequency of defection, suggesting that the anterior insula marks the social interaction as aversive and discourages trusting the nonreciprocating partner in the future. Thus, activation within the anterior insula may be involved in marking negative social interactions as aversive and biasing subsequent social decision making.

Although both the anterior insula and the caudate nucleus are involved in social decision making, both are also involved in nonsocial decision making such avoiding physically noxious stimuli and adaptive foraging, respectively. These neural systems probably initially evolved to support these more fundamental aspects of behavior. When social skills became more crucial with the evolution of primates, these systems may have been exapted for new functions, such as detecting harmful social stimuli and learning when, and to whom, altruism should be dispensed. However, in the process of adapting these old systems to novel demands, they may well have been modified and social pressures may have left their imprint. Indeed, this is the manner in which the evolutionary process typically unfolds. For example, some land mammals such as otters have evolved to fill aquatic niches. But rather than evolving completely novel structures to propel them through water, they modified their feet, the primary function of which is locomotion on land, to make them better suited to also travel through water. The end result is limbs designed for terrestrial locomotion combined with webbed feet designed for aquatic locomotion. That is, the otter limb is adapted to both forms of locomotion. Analogously, human brain systems may be designed for a combination of social and nonsocial functions.

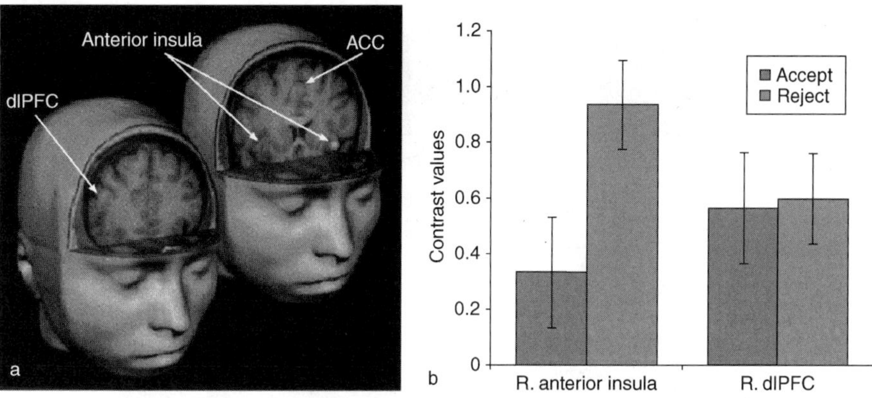

Figure 4 Brain responses to unfair offers: (a) activated brain regions in response to receiving an unfair (vs. fair) offer in the UG; (b) ratio of anterior insula to dorsolateral prefrontal cortex activation in response to unfair offers as a function of whether the offer was accepted or rejected. ACC, anterior cingulate cortex; dlPFC, dorsolateral prefrontal cortex; R., right. Reproduced from Sanfey AG, Loewenstein G, McClure SM, and Cohen JD (2006) Neuroeconomics: Cross-currents in research on decision-making. *Trends in Cognitive Science* 10: 108–116.

Dorsolateral Prefrontal Cortex

The dorsolateral prefrontal cortex (dlPFC) has long been recognized as critically involved in cognitive control, including cognitive control over emotions (**Figure 2(c)**). Recent studies suggest its specific involvement in overriding prepotent emotional biases, such as when delaying gratification or making utilitarian decisions in the context of moral dilemmas. The dlPFC is also activated by unfair offers in the UG, which subjects are more likely to accept when dlPFC activation exceeds anterior insula activation (**Figure 4(b)**). This has led to the hypothesis that UG decisions, and difficult social decisions more generally, often involve competition between emotional processing and higher-level controlled or deliberative processing that bias decision making in opposite ways. Emotional processes are driven by the subcortical, limbic, and paralimbic structures, whereas the deliberative processes rely on the anterior and dorsolateral regions of prefrontal cortex, as well as areas of posterior parietal cortex. Further evidence in support of the a role for the dlPFC in social decision making is provided by studies showing that application of repetitive transcranial magnetic stimulation (rTMS) to the dlPFC influences decision making in the UG. Finally, dlPFC activation is also associated with the choice to defect in the PD game, suggesting that most people may in fact have a prepotent emotional bias to cooperate in the game.

Ventromedial Prefrontal Cortex

Studies of patients who have suffered damage to the ventromedial prefrontal cortex indicate that this brain region is critical for appropriate social decision making. Previously well-adapted individuals who sustain damage to this region become unable to observe social conventions and unable to decide advantageously on matters pertaining to their own lives. Because these patients have generally well-preserved intellectual abilities and knowledge of appropriate social behavior, it has been hypothesized that their deficit lies in an inability to use emotions and feelings to guide social decision making. The result is that they often opt for behaviors that, although yielding immediate rewards, often have larger future negative consequences associated with them. This leads to the obvious but so far untested hypothesis that these patients should be less likely to endure the short-term cost associated with reciprocating altruism and should consequently have trouble sustaining long-term, mutually beneficial social relationships. This hypothesis could be formally evaluated by testing patients in an iterated PD game.

The Oxytocin System

In rodents, the neuropeptides oxytocin (OT) and vasopressin (AVP) facilitate social affiliation, making them attractive candidates for the neural modulation of human social relationships. Accordingly, in a TG, intranasal OT infusion was shown to increase initial monetary transfers by Investors. Recent research suggested that neuropeptides cross the blood–brain barrier after intranasal administration, bypassing the bloodstream, implying that these effects are due to OT's action in the brain. Intranasal OT administration has recently been combined with fMRI to assess the impact of OT on the neural response to fearful/threatening faces and scenes. Compared with

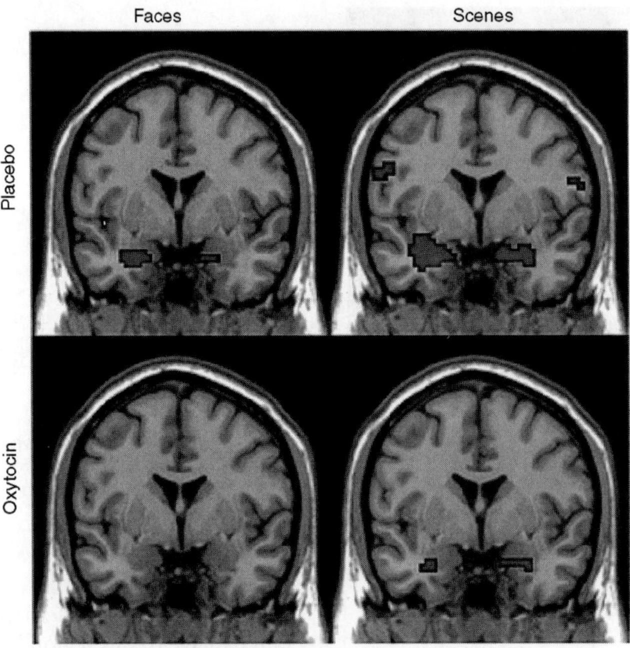

Figure 5 Intranasal oxytocin administration decreases amygdala response to threatening faces and scenes. Reproduced from Kirsch P, Esslinger C, Chen Q, et al. (2005) Oxytocin modulates neural circuitry for social cognition and fear in humans. *Journal of Neuroscience* 25: 11489–11493.

a placebo, OT decreased the activation in the amygdala for both types of fearful stimuli (**Figure 5**). These results are consistent with evidence that OT reduces stress and anxiety and are also consistent with the abundance of OT receptors in the rodent amygdala, although OT receptors have not yet been found in the human amygdala. This study suggests one potential mechanism by which OT could increase trust – by reducing anxiety about potential nonreciprocation. Another possibility suggested by animal experiments is that OT release in the nucleus accumbens renders social interactions more rewarding.

The Serotonin System

Serotonin plays a significant role in modulating prosocial behavior. Peripheral and central indices of serotonin function show negative associations with violent and aggressive behavior, but positive associations with socially affiliative behavior (such as grooming and approach) in primate models. Pharmacological interventions that increase serotonergic activity also facilitate affiliative behavior. These results suggest the possibility that serotonin levels could influence decision making in the context of social interactions. Indeed, depleting subjects of tryptophan, the amino acid precursor of serotonin, is associated with reduced rates of cooperation in the PD game. Given that serotonin is known to modulate dopamine reward pathways, these effects could be mediated by serotonin withdrawal's attenuating the rewarding and reinforcing effects of cooperation.

Conclusion

In summary, the neuroeconomics approach to social decision making has already yielded some interesting findings and hypotheses, and the combination of neuroscientific, economic, and psychological methods and tasks seems sure to uncover much more about the social brain in the coming years.

See also: Decision-Making and Neuroeconomics; Delayed Reinforcement: Economics; Game Theory and the Economics of Animal Communication; Games in Monkeys: Neurophysiology and Motor Decision-Making; Neuroeconomics: History; Neuroendocrinology of Social/Affiliative Behavior; Reward Decision-Making; Social Brain: Evolution; Social Cognition; Social Stress in Adult Primates.

Further Reading

Bechara A, Damasio H, and Damasio AR (2000) Emotion, decision making and the orbitofrontal cortex. *Cerebral Cortex* 10: 295–307.

Craig AD (2003) Interoception: The sense of the physiological condition of the body. *Current Opinion in Neurobiology* 13: 500–505.

Critchley H, Elliot R, Mathias C, and Dolan R (2000) Neural activity relating to the generation and representation of galvanic skin conductance responses: A functional magnetic resonance imaging study. *Journal of Neuroscience* 20: 3033–3040.

Davidson RJ, Putnam KM, and Larson CL (2000) Dysfunction in the neural circuitry of emotion regulation – possible prelude to violence. *Science* 289(5479): 591–594.

de Quervain DJ, Fischbacher U, Treyer V, et al. (2004) The neural basis of altruistic punishment. *Science* 305: 1254–1258.

Delgado MR, Frank RH, and Phelps EA (2005) Perceptions of moral character modulate the neural systems of reward during the trust game. *Nature Neuroscience* 8: 1611–1618.

Henrich J, McElreath R, Barr A, et al. (2006) Costly punishment across human societies. *Science* 312: 1767–1770.

King-Casas B, Tomlin D, Anen C, Camerer CF, Quartz SR, and Montague PR (2005) Getting to know you: Reputation and trust in a two-person economic exchange. *Science* 308: 78–83.

Kirsch P, Esslinger C, Chen Q, et al. (2005) Oxytocin modulates neural circuitry for social cognition and fear in humans. *Journal of Neuroscience* 25: 11489–11493.

Kosfeld M, Heinrichs M, Zak PJ, Fischbacher U, and Fehr E (2005) Oxytocin increases trust in humans. *Nature* 435: 673–676.

Knoch D, Pascual-Leone A, Meyer K, Treyer V, and Fehr E (2006) Diminishing reciprocal fairness by disrupting the right prefrontal cortex. *Science* 314: 829–832.

Lim MM and Young LJ (2006) Neuropeptidergic regulation of affiliative behavior and social bonding in animals. *Hormones and Behavior* 50: 506–517.

Miller E and Cohen J (2001) An integrative theory of prefrontal cortex function. *Annual Review of Neuroscience* 24: 167–202.

Montague PR, Berns GS, Cohen JD, et al. (2002) Hyperscanning: Simultaneous fMRI during linked social interactions. *Neuroimage* 16: 1159–1164.

Montague PR, Dayan P, and Sejnowski TJ (1996) A framework for mesencephalic dopamine systems based on predictive Hebbian learning. *Journal of Neuroscience* 16: 1936–1947.

Rilling JK, Sanfey AG, Aronson JA, Nystrom LE, and Cohen JD (2004) Opposing BOLD responses to reciprocated and unreciprocted altruism in putative reward pathways. *NeuroReport* 15: 2539–2543.

Sanfey AG, Loewenstein G, McClure SM, and Cohen JD (2006) Neuroeconomics: Cross-currents in research on decision-making. *Trends in Cognitive Science* 10: 108–116.

Sanfey AG, Rilling JK, Aronson JA, Nystrom LE, and Cohen JD (2003) The neural basis of economic decision-making in the Ultimatum Game. *Science* 300: 1755–1758.

Schultz W (1997) Dopamine neurons and their role in reward mechanisms. *Current Opinion in Neurobiology* 7: 191–197.

Singer T, Seymour B, O'Doherty J, Kaube H, Dolan RJ, and Frith CD (2004) Empathy for pain involves the affective but not sensory components of pain [see comment]. *Science* 303: 1157–1162.

van't Wout M, Kahn RS, Sanfey AG, and Aleman A (2005) Repetitive transcranial magnetic stimulation over the right dorsolateral prefrontal cortex affects strategic decision-making. *NeuroReport* 16: 1849–1852.

Wood RM, Billing JK, Sanfey AG, Bhagwagar Z and Rogers RD (2006) Effects of tryptophan depletion on the performance of iterated Prisoner's Dilemma game in healthy adults. *Neuropsychophamacology* 31(5): 1075–1084.

执行功能与高级认知

Agnosia

D Tranel and N L Denburg, University of Iowa Hospitals and Clinics, Iowa City, IA, USA

'Agnosia,' a neurological term of Greek origin (a + Greek *gnosis*), signifies a lack of knowledge and is virtually synonymous with an impairment of recognition. In the traditional literature, two types of agnosia were commonly described. 'Associative' agnosia referred to as failure of recognition that results from defective activation of information pertinent to a given stimulus. 'Apperceptive' agnosia referred to a disturbance of the 'integration' of otherwise normally perceived components of a stimulus.

Teuber in 1968 gave a narrower definition, in which agnosia was synonymous with having "normal percepts stripped of their meaning." In this sense, agnosia is conceptualized as a disorder of memory, and only associative agnosia qualifies for this stricter definition. In practical terms, however, it has been useful to retain the concept of apperceptive agnosia and to maintain a distinction between apperceptive and associative agnosia. In both conditions, recognition is disturbed. In the apperceptive variety, the problem can be traced, at least in part, to faulty perception, usually in reference to aspects of higher-order perceptual capacities (it is not appropriate to use the term agnosia for conditions in which perceptual problems are severe and obviously preclude the patient's apprehension of meaningful information). In associative agnosia, perception is largely intact, and the recognition defect is strictly or primarily a disorder of memory.

The difficulties of trying to separate apperceptive and associative forms of agnosia underscore the fact that the processes of perception and memory are not discrete. Rather, those processes operate on a physiological and psychological continuum, and demarcation of a clear separation point at which perceptual processes end and memory processes begin is simply not possible. Many patients with recognition defects will have elements of both conditions, that is, high-level perceptual problems and disturbances in memory. Some, however, can be classified unequivocally into one type or the other. For these reasons, the following operational definitions are appropriate. Associative agnosia is a modality-specific impairment of the ability to recognize previously known stimuli (or new stimuli for which learning would normally have occurred) that occurs in the absence of disturbances of perception, intellect, or language, and is the result of acquired cerebral damage. The designation appreciative agnosia applies when the patient meets the preceding definition in all respects except that perception is altered.

The term 'agnosia' should be restricted to situations in which recognition impairments are confined to one sensory modality, for example, vision, or audition, or touch. When recognition defects extend across two or more modalities, the appropriate designation is 'amnesia'. As noted, the term agnosia should not be used for patients in whom recognition defects develop in connection with major disturbances of basic perception. Nor should the term be applied to patients with major impairments of intellect. Finally, the term agnosia-should be reserved for conditions that develop suddenly, following the onset of acquired cerebral dysfunction.

One other important distinction is between 'recognition' and 'naming.' The two capacities are often confused. It is true that recognition of an entity, under normal circumstances, is frequently indicated by naming (e.g., that is a 'groundhog' or that is 'Joe Montana'). Studies of brain-injured subjects, however, have shown clearly that recognition and naming are dissociable capacities, and the two terms should not be used interchangeably. Damage in the left inferotemporal region, for example, can render a patient incapable of naming a wide variety of stimuli, while leaving unaffected the patient's ability to recognize those stimuli. For the two preceding examples, for instance, the patient may produce the descriptions of 'that's a roly-poly animal that digs holes under barns and hibernates in the winter,' and 'that's the guy from Notre Dame who was a famous quarterback and won lots of football championships.' Both descriptions indicate unequivocal recognition of the specific entities, even if their names are never produced. In short, it is important to maintain a distinction between recognition, which can be indicated by any number of responses signifying that the patient understands the meaning of a particular stimulus, and naming, which may not, and need not, accompany accurate recognition. The patient with agnosia fails to experience familiarity with the stimulus, and is thus unable to evoke its meaning, use, or relevant relationships in both verbal and nonverbal terms.

In principle, agnosia can occur in any sensory modality, relative to any type of entity or event. In practice, however, some types of agnosia are far more frequent. 'Visual agnosia,' especially agnosia for faces ('prosopagnosia'), is the most commonly encountered form of recognition disturbance affecting a primary sensory modality. Visual agnosia is a disorder of recognition confined to the visual realm, in which a patient cannot arrive at the meaning of some or all categories of previously known nonverbal visual stimuli, despite normal or near-normal visual perception and intact alertness, attention, intelligence, and language. Most patients manifest a comparable defect in the anterograde compartment; that is, they cannot recognize new nonverbal, visual stimuli that would normally have been learned after adequate exposure.

The condition of 'auditory agnosia' is rarer, followed by the even less frequent 'tactile agnosia.' A frequently encountered condition which also conforms to the designation of agnosia is a disturbance in the 'recognition of illness,' or what has been termed 'anosognosia'.

It is important to distinguish anosognosia from several closely related conditions. One is 'anosodiaphoria', a term that refers to the condition in which a patient acknowledges, but fails to appreciate the significance of, acquired impairments in physical or psychological function. Although anosodiaphoria is not a true form of agnosia, in practice there is a certain degree of overlap between anosodiaphoria and anosognosia. In fact, it is common to observe that blatant forms of anosognosia, for example, denial of hemiplegia, tend to evolve over time, as the patient recovers, into various degrees of anosodiaphoria. Another condition refers to a disorder of body schema. Body schema disturbances are conditions in which patients become unable to localize various parts of their bodies. The most common manifestations are 'autotopagnosia,' 'finger agnosia,' and 'right–left disorientation' (the latter two being essentially partial forms of the first). Autotopagnosia refers to a condition in which the patient loses the ability to identify parts of the body, either to verbal command or by imitation. In its most severe form, the disorder affects virtually all body parts; however, this is quite rare, and it is far more common to observe partial forms of the condition, including deficits in finger localization (finger agnosia) and right–left discrimination.

Accurate detection and diagnosis of agnosia are important on several accounts. Both visual and auditory agnosia are strongly associated with the presence of bilateral cerebral disease, and the presence of one of these conditions can be a useful clue regarding the localization of brain dysfunction. This can be especially helpful in the early stages of acquired cerebral dysfunction, when even modern neuroimaging procedures may fail to detect a lesion. Such conditions furnish additional diagnostic clues because they are typically associated with cerebrovascular disease affecting the territories of the posterior or middle cerebral arteries. Furthermore, unilateral disease involving the dominant parietal lobe has recently been implicated in both tactile agnosia and apraxia. To avoid misdiagnosis, it is important to note that the complaints or behaviors of patients with agnosia can seem so bizarre as to raise questions about their veracity. There was, indeed, a time when it was doubted whether such conditions existed at all. That agnosic conditions do occur is no longer a contentious issue; nonetheless, clinicians may be skeptical of a patient who suddenly claims an inability to recognize familiar faces, despite normal vision, or of a patient who suddenly behaves as though all auditory information had lost its meaning. A particularly unusual case of agnosia was recently reported in which a child with sleep-induced electrophysiological abnormalities involving the occipito-temporal regions and episodic seizure disorder demonstrated stable defects in visual–spatial abilities, as well as visual agnosia.

Despite their relative rarity, agnosias have also proved to be important 'experiments of nature,' and they have assisted with the investigation of the neural bases of human perception, learning, and memory. Careful study of agnosic patients over the past couple of decades, facilitated by the advent of modern structural (computed tomography, magnetic resonance) and functional (positron emission tomography, functional magnetic resonance) neuroimaging techniques, and by the development of sophisticated experimental neuropsychological procedures, has yielded important new insights into the manner in which the human brain acquires, maintains, and retrieves various types of knowledge.

See also: Amnesia: Declarative and Nondeclarative Memory; Prosopagnosia; Recognition Memory; Shape Representation in Inferotemporal Cortex.

Further Reading

Bauer RM and Demery JA (2003) Agnosia. In: Heilman KM and Valenstein E (eds.) *Clinical Neuropsychology,* 4th edn., pp. 236–295. New York: Oxford University Press.

Caselli RJ (1991) Rediscovering tactile agnosia. *Mayo Clinicical Proceedings* 66: 129–142.

Crutch SJ, Warren JD, Harding L, and Warrington EK (2005) Computation of tactile object properties requires the integrity of praxic skills. *Neuorpsychologia* 43: 1792–1800.

Damasio AR and Damasio H (1994) Cortical systems for retrieval of concrete knowledge: The convergence zone framework. In: Koch C and Davis JL (eds.) *Large-Scale Neuronal Theories of the Brain*, pp. 61–74. Cambridge, MA: MIT Press.

Damasio AR, Damasio H, Tranel D, and Brandt JP (1990) Neural regionalization of knowledge access: Preliminary evidence. *Symposia on Quantitative Biology* 55: 1039–1047.

Damasio AR, Tranel D, and Damasio H (1990) Face agnosia and the neural substrates of memory. *Annual Review of Neuroscience* 13: 89–109.

Damasio H, Grabowski TJ, Tranel D, Hichwa RD, and Damasio AR (1996) A neural basis for lexical retrieval. *Nature* 380: 499–505.

Denburg NL and Tranel D (2003) Acalculia and disturbances of the body schema. In: Heilman KM and Valenstein E (eds.) *Clinical Neuropsychology,*, 4th edn., pp. 161–184. New York: Oxford University Press.

Eriksson K, Kylliainen A, Hirvonen K, Nieminen P, and Koivikko M (2003) Visual agnosia in a child with non-lesional occipito-temporal CSWS. *Brain & Development* 25: 262–267.

Teuber H-L (1968) Perception. In: Weiskrantz L (ed.) *Analysis of Behavioral Change*, pp. 274–328. New York: Harper & Row.

Tranel D and Damasio AR (1985) Knowledge without awareness: An autonomic index of facial recognition by prosopagnosics. *Science* 228: 1453–1454.

Tranel D and Damasio AR (1996) The agnosias and apraxias. In: Bradley WG, Daroff RB, Fenichel GM, and Marsden CD (eds.) *Neurology in Clinical Practice*, 2nd edn., pp. 119–129. Stoneham, MA: Butterworth Publishers.

Vignolo LA (1982) Auditory agnosia. *Philosophical Transactions of the Royal Society of London* 298: 49–57.

Warrington EK and McCarthy RA (1987) Categories of knowledge: Further fractionation and an attempted integration. *Brain* 110: 1273–1296.

Alexia

D Tranel and N L Denburg, University of Iowa Hospitals and Clinics, Iowa City, IA, USA

Alexia is a neurological term of Greek origin (a + Greek *lex(is)*) that designates a partial or complete inability to read. There are a number of different subtypes of alexia, but all have in common the feature that the affected patient cannot read normally, so that reading is slow or impossible, and comprehension of read material is impaired. In the American literature, alexia is used nearly exclusively to designate acquired defects in reading, that is, reading impairments that occur as the result of a neurological condition in an individual who was previously literate. The British literature tends to use the term dyslexia to refer to this condition. Dyslexia in the American literature is typically applied to persons who have a developmental form of reading disorder – specifically, the not uncommon condition of being unable to learn to read normally, which becomes manifest during childhood and typically affects the acquisition of both reading and writing skills.

Stroke is the most common cause of acquired alexia, especially when the condition appears as an isolated or relatively isolated symptom. Other forms of neurological disease, including cerebral tumors, inflammatory processes, and head injury, can also cause alexia, and there are some cases of degenerative disease (e.g., Alzheimer's) in which a reading disturbance is a prominent early feature of the patient's cognitive dysfunction. Acquired alexia occurs in two main forms. One, termed alexia with agraphia, involves a reading impairment that is accompanied by writing defects; this form is common in patients with various aphasia syndromes. The other, termed alexia without agraphia (or 'pure alexia'), involves an isolated defect in reading that is not accompanied by impaired writing. Pure alexia is associated with lesions that disconnect both visual association cortices from the dominant, language-related temporoparietal cortices. Pure alexia can be caused by a single lesion strategically placed in the region behind, beneath, and under the occipital horn of the left lateral ventricle, by damaging pathways en route from the callosum and pathways en route from the left visual association cortex (**Figure 1**). Another setting is the combination of a lesion in the corpus callosum, which disconnects right-to-left visual information transfer, and a lesion in the left occipital lobe, which disconnects left visual association cortex from left language cortex (**Figure 2**). Such lesions are likely to produce a right hemianopia; this sign is a frequent, although not invariable, accompaniment of pure alexia. Another neuropsychological correlate of pure alexia is color anomia, that is, the inability to name colors.

The 'purity' of alexia without agraphia stems from the fact that patients with these lesions do not develop disturbances in writing or in other aspects of speech and linguistic functioning. This separates this type of alexia from the types of reading defects that are common in aphasic patients. (It is rather striking to observe patients who can write a sentence easily and then be unable to read what they have just written.) In this sense, pure alexia can be construed as a disturbance of visual pattern recognition. Patients with pure alexia are unable to read most words and sentences, and in severe cases cannot read even single letters. The problem is not one of visual acuity: the fact that the patients can see the sentences, words, and letters they cannot read can be readily demonstrated by having the patients copy those stimuli, a task that will be executed normally. Thus, most patients with pure alexia have normal visual acuity (although a quadrantanopia or hemianopia may be present), and most have normal recognition of nonverbal visual stimuli such as objects and faces.

In terms of treatment for pure alexia, there are two schools of thought. The first is to attempt to increase the speed and accuracy of letter-by-letter reading. The second, higher-level approach involves an abandoning of letter-by-letter reading for the adoption of whole word recognition, a more efficient approach.

As noted, the nonacquired, developmental varieties of reading disorder are subsumed under the term of developmental dyslexia. These reading impairments, almost invariably accompanied by writing weaknesses (especially spelling defects), constitute a learning disability which in fact is the most common form of learning disability in the general population. Some developmental dyslexias may be related to a disturbance of the cellular organization of language cortices, possibly originating *in utero*. A few older postmortem studies have suggested that abnormalities of cortical organization in the brains of dyslexic patients may have contributed to the reading disability. There is a strong association between developmental dyslexia and left-handedness. The older literature indicated that dyslexia was far more common in boys than girls, but recent and better-controlled studies have not supported this notion; the ratio may even be fairly close to 1:1.

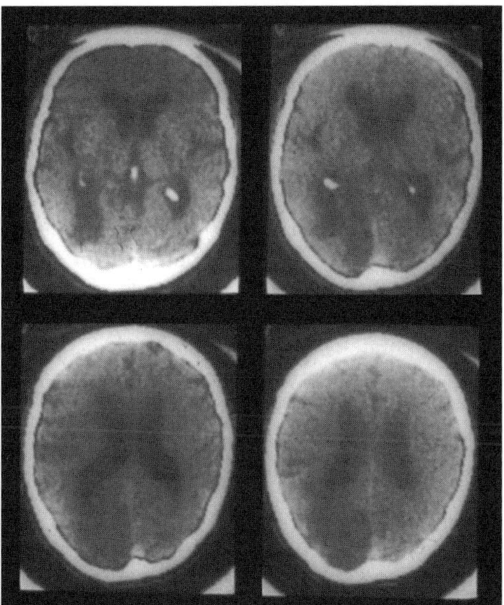

Figure 1 Illustration of the neuroanatomic findings of a patient with pure alexia, arising from a single lesion.

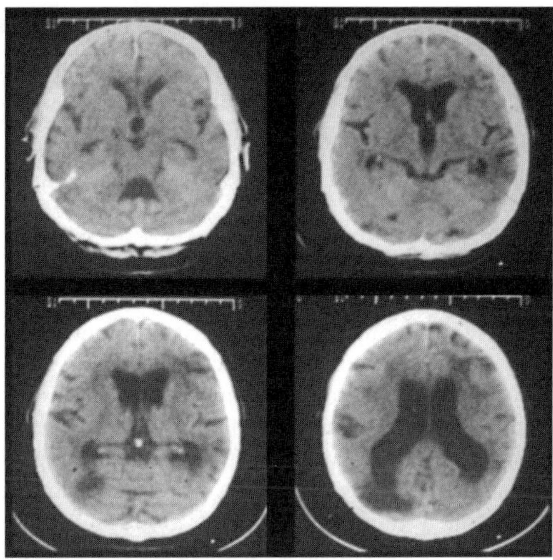

Figure 2 Illustration of the neuroanatomic findings of a patient with pure alexia, arising from a multiple lesion.

See also: Aging of the Brain and Alzheimer's Disease; Agraphia; Cerebrovascular Disease; Dementia; Dyslexia: Neurodevelopmental Basis; Reading; Stroke; Stroke: Neonate vs. Adult.

Further Reading

Benson DF, Brown J, and Tomlinson EB (1971) Varieties of alexia. *Neurology* 21: 951–957.

Coltheart M, Patterson K, and Marshall JC (1980) *Deep Dyslexia.* London: Routledge and Kegan Paul.

Geschwind N (1965) Disconnection syndromes in animals and man. *Brain* 88: 237–294, 585-644.

Greenblatt SH (1973) Alexia without agraphia or hemianopia: Anatomical analysis of an autopsied case. *Brain* 96: 307–316.

Petersen SE, Fox PT, Snyder AZ, and Raichle ME (1990) Activation of extrastriate and frontal cortical areas by visual words and word-like stimuli. *Science* 249: 1041–1044.

Tranel D (1994) Assessment of higher-order visual function. *Current Opinion in Ophthalmology* 5: 29–37.

Tranel D (1996) Disorders of color processing (perception, imagery, recognition, and naming). In: Feinberg T and Farah MJ (eds.) *Behavioral Neurology and Neuropsychology*, pp. 257–266. New York: McGraw-Hill.

Amnesia: Declarative and Nondeclarative Memory

L R Squire, P J Bayley, and C N Smith, University of California at San Diego, San Diego, CA, USA

Introduction

Amnesia refers to difficulty in learning new information or in remembering the past. It is important to distinguish the amnesia that occurs following brain injury or disease (neurological amnesia) from the rarer functional (or psychogenic) amnesia that can occur as the result of an emotional trauma. Neurological amnesia has a variety of origins, including prolonged alcoholism, a temporary loss of blood supply or oxygen to the brain, and diseases such as herpes simplex encephalitis. All these conditions preferentially damage the medial temporal lobe or diencephalon. Neurological amnesia causes severe difficulty in learning new facts and events (anterograde amnesia). Amnesic patients also typically have some difficulty remembering facts and events that were acquired before the onset of amnesia (retrograde amnesia). Functional amnesia shows a different pattern of anterograde and retrograde memory impairment. Functional amnesia is characterized by a profound retrograde amnesia that is transient in some cases, and little or no anterograde amnesia is exhibited.

Functional Amnesia

Functional amnesia, also known as dissociative amnesia, is a dissociative psychiatric disorder that involves alterations in consciousness and identity. Although no particular brain structure or brain system is implicated in functional amnesia, the cause of the disorder must be due to abnormal brain function of some kind. Its presentation varies considerably from individual to individual, but in most cases, functional amnesia is preceded by physical or emotional trauma and occurs in association with some prior psychiatric history. Often, the patient is admitted to the hospital in a confused or frightened state. Memory for the past is lost, especially autobiographical memory and even personal identity. Semantic or factual information about the world is often preserved, though factual information about the patient's life may be unavailable. Despite profound impairment in the ability to recall information about the past, the ability to learn new information is usually intact. The disorder often clears, and the lost memories return. Occasionally, the disorder lasts longer, and sizable pieces of the past remain unavailable.

Etiology of Neurological Amnesia

Neurological amnesia results from a number of conditions, including Alzheimer's disease or other dementing illnesses, temporal lobe surgery, chronic alcohol abuse, encephalitis, head injury, anoxia, ischemia, infarction, and the rupture and repair of an anterior communicating artery aneurism. The common factor in all these conditions is that they disrupt normal function in one of two areas of the brain – the medial aspects of the temporal lobe and the diencephalic midline. Global amnesia results from bilateral damage, whereas material-specific amnesia results from unilateral damage. Typically, left-sided damage affects memory for verbal material, and right-sided damage affects memory for nonverbal material (e.g., the recall of faces and spatial layouts).

Anatomy

Well-studied cases of human amnesia and animal models of amnesia provide information about the neural connections and structures that are damaged in neurological amnesia. Damage limited to the hippocampus itself is sufficient to cause amnesia. For example, in one carefully studied case of amnesia (patient R.B.), the only significant damage was a bilateral lesion confined to the CA1 field of the hippocampus. The severity of memory impairment is exacerbated by additional damage outside the hippocampus. Thus, severe amnesia results when damage extends beyond the hippocampus to include adjacent structures in the medial temporal lobe, including the parahippocampal cortex, entorhinal cortex, and perirhinal cortex. Another well-studied case (H.M.) had surgery in 1953 to treat severe epilepsy. Most of the hippocampus and much of the surrounding medial temporal lobe cortices were removed bilaterally (the entorhinal cortex and most of the perirhinal cortex). Although the surgery was successful in reducing the frequency of H.M.'s seizures, it resulted in a severe and persistent amnesia.

Functional magnetic resonance imaging (fMRI) of healthy individuals who are engaged in learning and remembering reveals neural activity in the same structures that, when damaged, cause amnesia. It is also possible through structural imaging (MRI) to detect and quantify the neuropathology in amnesic patients. Many patients with restricted hippocampal damage have an average reduction in hippocampal volume of about 40%. Two such patients whose brains were available for detailed, postmortem neurohistological analysis (patients L.M. and W.H.) proved to have lost virtually all the neurons in the cornu ammonis (CA) fields of the hippocampus. These observations suggest that a reduction in hippocampal volume of approximately 40%, as estimated from MRI scans, likely indicates the near complete loss of hippocampal neurons. The amnesic condition is associated with neuronal death and tissue collapse, but the tissue does not disappear altogether because fibers and glial cells remain.

As questions about amnesia and the function of medial temporal lobe structures have become more sophisticated, it has become vital to obtain detailed, quantitative information about the damage in the patients being studied. In addition, single-case studies are not nearly so useful as group studies involving well-characterized patients. In the case of patients with restricted hippocampal damage, one can calculate the volume of the hippocampus itself as a proportion of total intracranial volume. One can also calculate the volumes of the adjacent medial temporal lobe structures (the perirhinal, entorhinal, and parahippocampal cortices), again in proportion to intracranial volume. Last, when there is extensive damage to the medial temporal lobe, it is important to calculate the volumes of lateral temporal cortex and other regions that might be affected. It is important to characterize patients in this way in order to address the kinds of questions now being pursued in memory research.

To understand the anatomy of human amnesia, and ultimately the anatomy of normal memory, animal models of human amnesia have been established in the monkey and in the rodent. In the monkey, following lesions of the bilateral medial temporal lobe or diencephalon, memory impairment is exhibited on the same kinds of tasks of new learning ability that human amnesic patients fail. Cumulative work with animal models suggests that the full medial temporal lobe memory system consists of the hippocampus and adjacent, anatomically related structures, including the entorhinal cortex, parahippocampal cortex, and perirhinal cortex (see **Figure 1**). When these adjacent structures are damaged, the severity of amnesia is greater than when only the hippocampus itself is damaged.

The important structures in the diencephalon are the mediodorsal thalamic nucleus, the anterior thalamic nucleus, the internal medullary lamina, the mammillary nuclei, and the mammillo-thalamic tract. Because diencephalic amnesia resembles medial temporal lobe amnesia in the pattern of sparing and loss, these two regions likely form an anatomically linked, functional system.

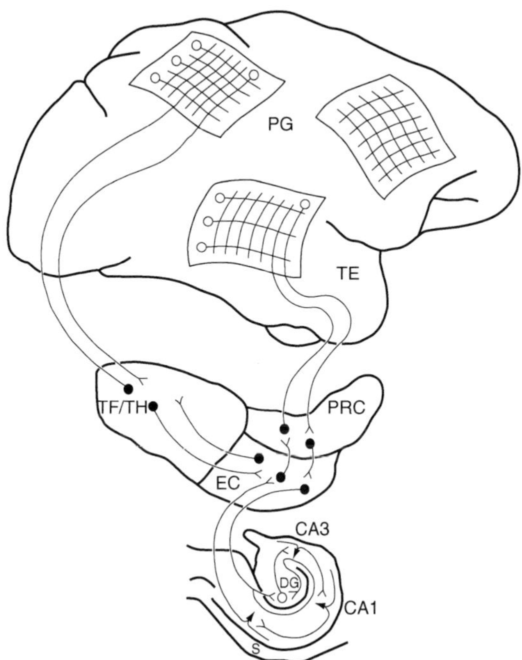

Figure 1 Schematic drawing of primate neocortex together with the structures and connections in the medial temporal region important for establishing long-term memory. The networks in the cortex show putative representations concerning visual object quality (in area TE) and object location (in area PG). If this disparate neural activity is to cohere into a stable long-term memory, convergent activity must occur along projections from these regions to the medial temporal lobe. Projections from neocortex arrive initially at the parahippocampal gyrus (TF/TH) and perirhinal cortex (PRC) and then at entorhinal cortex (EC), the gateway to the hippocampus. Further processing of information occurs in the several stages of the hippocampus, first in the dentate gyrus (DG) and then in the CA3 and CA1 regions. The fully processed input eventually exits this circuit via the subiculum (S) and the EC, where widespread efferent projections return to neocortex. The hippocampus and adjacent structures are thought to support the stabilization of representations in distributed regions of neocortex (e.g., TE and PG) and to support the strengthening of connections between these regions. Subsequently, memory for a whole event (for example, a memory that depends on representations in both TE and PG) can be revivified even when a partial cue is presented. Damage to the medial temporal lobe system causes anterograde and retrograde amnesia. The severity of the deficit increases as damage involves more components of the system. Once sufficient time has passed, the distributed representations in neocortex can operate independent of the medial temporal lobe. (This diagram is a simplification and does not show diencephalic structures involved in memory function.)

The Nature of Amnesia

It is important to appreciate that amnesic patients are not impaired at all kinds of memory. The major distinction is between declarative and nondeclarative memory. Only declarative memory is affected in amnesia. Declarative memory refers to the capacity to remember the facts and events of everyday life. It is the kind of memory that is meant when the term 'memory' is used in ordinary language. A declarative memory can be brought to mind as a conscious recollection. Declarative memory provides a way to model the external world, and in this sense it is either true or false. The stored representations are flexible and can guide successful performance under a wide range of test conditions. Finally, declarative memory is especially suited for rapid learning and for forming and maintaining associations between arbitrarily different kinds of material (e.g., learning to associate two different words).

Anterograde Amnesia

Amnesia is characterized especially by profound difficulty in new learning. This impairment is referred to as anterograde amnesia. Amnesia can occur as part of a more global dementing disorder that includes other cognitive deficits, including impairments in language, attention, visuospatial abilities, and general intellectual capacity. However, amnesia can also occur in the absence of other cognitive deficits and without any change in personality or social skills. In this more circumscribed form of amnesia, patients have intact intellectual functions and intact perceptual functions, even on difficult tests that require the ability to discriminate between similar images containing overlapping features. Patients also have intact immediate memory (as measured, for example, by the ability to repeat a short string of digits). Their intact immediate memory explains why amnesic patients can carry on a conversation and appear quite normal to the casual observer. Indeed, if the amount of material to be remembered is not too large (e.g., a three-digit number), then patients can remember the material for minutes, or as long as they can hold it in mind by rehearsal. One would say in this case that the patients have carried the contents of immediate memory forward by engaging in explicit rehearsal. This rehearsal-based activity is referred to as working memory. The difficulty for amnesic patients arises when an amount of information must be recalled that exceeds immediate memory capacity (typically, when a list of eight or more items must be remembered) or when information must be recalled after a distraction-filled interval or after a long delay. In these situations, patients will remember fewer items than will their healthy counterparts.

Amnesic patients are impaired on tasks of new learning, regardless of whether memory is tested by free recall, recognition (e.g., presenting an item and asking whether it was previously encountered), or cued recall (e.g., asking for recall of an item when a hint is provided). In addition, the memory impairment involves not just difficulty in learning about specific episodes and events that occurred in a certain time and place (episodic memory), but also difficulty in learning factual information (semantic memory). Finally, the memory deficit is present regardless of the sensory modality in which information is presented (visual, auditory, olfactory, and so on).

Retrograde Amnesia

In addition to impaired new learning, amnesia also impairs memories that were acquired before the onset of amnesia. This type of memory loss is referred to as retrograde amnesia. Retrograde amnesia is usually temporally graded. That is, information acquired in the distant past (remote memory) is spared relative to more recent memory. The extent of retrograde amnesia can be relatively short and encompass only 1–2 years, or it can be more extensive and cover a much longer time. For example, an amnesic patient can have retrograde amnesia covering the previous one or two decades. In contrast, memories for the facts and events of childhood and adolescence can be intact. The severity and extent of retrograde amnesia is determined by the locus and extent of damage. Patients with restricted hippocampal damage have a limited retrograde amnesia covering a few years prior to the onset of amnesia. Patients with large medial temporal lobe damage have extensive retrograde amnesia covering decades.

The sparing of remote memory relative to more recent memory illustrates that the brain regions damaged in amnesia are not the permanent repositories of long-term memory. Instead, memories undergo a process of reorganization and consolidation after learning, during which time the neocortex becomes more important. During the process of consolidation, memories are vulnerable if there is damage to the medial temporal lobe or diencephalon. After sufficient time has passed, storage and retrieval of memory no longer require the participation of these brain structures. Memory is at that point supported by neocortex. The areas of neocortex important for long-term memory are thought to be the same regions that were initially involved in the processing and analysis of what was to be learned. Thus, the neocortex is always important, but the structures of the medial temporal lobe and diencephalon are also important during initial learning and during consolidation.

Spatial Memory

Discussions of amnesia have focused especially on the status of spatial memory because of the discovery of 'place cells' in the rodent hippocampus and the possible importance of the hippocampus in forming spatial maps. In human amnesia, spatial memory is impaired along with other forms of declarative memory. Patients have difficulty acquiring new spatial knowledge, and they are impaired in remembering recently acquired spatial knowledge. However, as is the case with other forms of declarative memory, remote spatial knowledge is intact. One well-studied patient with large medial temporal lobe lesions and severe amnesia (E.P.) was able to mentally navigate his childhood neighborhood, use alternate and novel routes to describe how to travel from one place to another, and point correctly to locations in the neighborhood while imagining himself oriented at some other location. These findings show that the medial temporal lobe is not needed for the long-term storage of spatial knowledge and does not maintain a spatial layout of learned environments that is necessary for successful navigation. Accordingly, the available data support the view that the hippocampus and related medial temporal lobe structures are involved in learning new facts and events, both spatial and nonspatial. Further, these structures are not repositories of long-term memory, either spatial or nonspatial.

Nondeclarative Memory

It is a striking feature of amnesia that many kinds of learning and memory are spared. Memory is not a unitary faculty of the mind but is composed of many parts that depend on different brain systems. Amnesia impairs only declarative memory and spares nondeclarative memory. Nondeclarative memory refers to a heterogeneous collection of abilities, all of which afford the capacity to acquire knowledge nonconsciously. Nondeclarative memory includes motor skills, perceptual and cognitive skills, priming, adaptation-level effects, simple classical conditioning, and habits, as well as phylogenetically early forms of experience-dependent behavior such as habituation and sensitization. In these cases, memory is expressed through performance rather than recollection, and performance does not require reflection on the past or even the knowledge that memory is being influenced by past events. For example, in the case of motor skills, one can learn how to ride a bicycle but be unable to describe what has been learned, at least not in the same sense that one might recall riding a bicycle on a particular day with a friend. Perceptual skills include such things as reading mirror-reversed print and searching a display quickly to find a hidden letter. In formal experiments, amnesic patients acquire perceptual skills at the same rate as individuals with intact memory, even though the patients may not remember performing the task.

Priming refers to an improved ability to identify a word or other item as a result of its prior presentation. For example, suppose that a line drawing of a dog, hammer, and airplane are presented in succession, with the instruction to name each item as quickly as possible. Typically, about 800 ms are needed to produce each name aloud. If in a later test these same pictures are presented intermixed with new drawings, the new drawings will still require about 800 ms to name, but now the dog, hammer, and airplane are named about 100 ms more quickly. The improved naming time occurs independent of whether one remembers having seen the items earlier. Furthermore, amnesic patients exhibit this effect at full strength, despite having a poor memory of seeing the items earlier. Priming effects of this kind can persist across intervals as long as several weeks. In formal experiments, severely amnesic patients had intact priming for recently presented words, even when the patients performed at guessing levels (50% correct) on tests that asked them to recognize which words were presented previously and which were not. This result shows that priming is fully independent of declarative memory.

Adaptation-level effects refer to changes in judgments about stimuli (e.g., their heaviness or size) that are caused by recent experience. For example, experience with light-weighted objects subsequently causes other objects to be judged heavier than they would be if the light-weighted objects had not been presented. Amnesic patients show this effect to the same degree as healthy individuals, though they have difficulty remembering what they have done.

Classical conditioning refers to the development of an association between a previously neutral stimulus and an unconditioned stimulus. One of the best-studied examples of classical conditioning in humans is eyeblink conditioning. In a typical conditioning procedure, a tone repeatedly precedes a mild air puff directed to the eye. After a number of pairings, the tone comes to elicit an eyeblink in anticipation of the air puff. Amnesic patients acquire the tone-air puff association at the same rate as healthy individuals do. In both groups, awareness of the temporal contingency between the tone and the air puff is unrelated to successful conditioning. Simple classical conditioning, where the tone overlaps with the air puff and terminates with it, is dependent on the cerebellum.

Habit learning refers to the gradual acquisition of associations between stimuli and responses, such as learning to make one choice rather than another. Habit learning depends on the neostriatum (basal ganglia). Many tasks can be acquired either declaratively, through memorization, or nondeclaratively, as a habit. For example, healthy individuals will solve many trial and error learning tasks quickly by simply engaging declarative memory and memorizing which responses are correct. In this circumstance, amnesic patients are disadvantaged. However, tasks can also be constructed that defeat memorization strategies, for example, by making the outcomes on each trial probabilistic. In such a case, amnesic patients and healthy individuals learn at the same

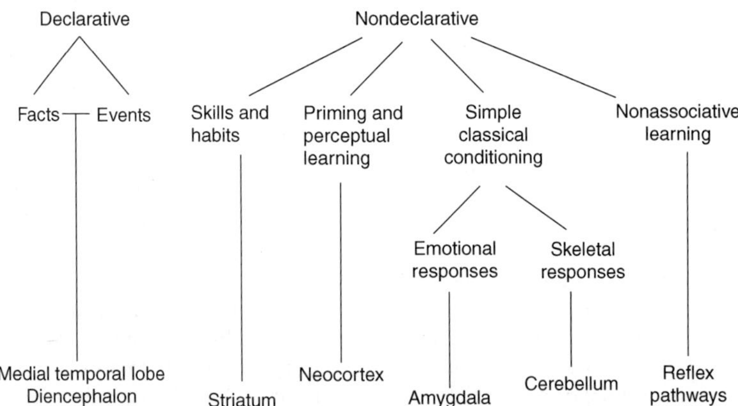

Figure 2 Classification of mammalian long-term memory systems. The taxonomy lists the brain structures thought to be especially important for each form of declarative and nondeclarative memory. In addition to the central role of the amygdala in emotional learning, it is able to modulate the strength of both declarative and nondeclarative learning.

gradual rate. It is also true that severely amnesic patients who have no capacity for declarative memory can gradually acquire trial-and-error tasks, even when the task can be learned declaratively by healthy individuals. In this case they succeed by engaging habit memory.

This situation is nicely illustrated by the eight-pair concurrent discrimination task, which requires individuals to learn the correct object for each of eight object pairs. Healthy individuals learn all eight pairs in a single test session. Severely amnesic patients acquire this same task over many weeks, even though at the start of each session they cannot describe the task, the instructions, or the objects. It is known that this task is acquired at a normal (slow) rate by monkeys with medial temporal lobe lesions and that monkeys with lesions of the neostriatum (basal ganglia) are impaired. Thus, humans appear to have a robust capacity for habit learning that operates outside awareness and independent of the medial temporal lobe structures that are damaged in amnesia.

These examples illustrate that nondeclarative memory is distinct from declarative memory. It is spared in amnesia, and it operates outside awareness. Nondeclarative forms of memory depend variously on the neostriatum, the amygdala, the cerebellum, and on processes intrinsic to neocortex (**Figure 2**).

Summary

The study of amnesia has illuminated the nature of memory disorders and has also led to a better understanding of the neurological foundations of memory. Experimental studies in patients, neuroimaging studies of healthy volunteers, and related studies in experimental animals continue to reveal insights about what memory is and how it is organized in the brain. As more is learned about the neuroscience of memory, about how memory works, more opportunities will arise for achieving better diagnosis, treatment, and prevention of diseases and disorders that affect memory.

See also: Animal Models of Amnesia; Episodic Memory; Functional Amnesia; Hippocampus: Computational Models; Memory Disorders; Recognition Memory; Semantic Memory.

Further Reading

Bayley PJ, Frascino JC, and Squire LR (2005) Robust habit learning in the absence of awareness and independent of the medial temporal lobe. *Nature* 436: 550–553.

Bayley PJ, Gold JJ, Hopkins RO, et al. (2005) The neuroanatomy of remote memory. *Neuron* 46: 799–810.

Eichenbaum H and Cohen NJ (2001) *From Conditioning to Conscious Recollection: Memory Systems of the Brain.* New York: Oxford University Press.

Gordon B (1995) *Memory: Remembering and Forgetting in Everyday Life.* New York: Mastermedia.

Milner B, Squire LR, and Kandel ER (1998) Cognitive neuroscience and the study of memory. *Neuron* 20(3): 445–468.

Schacter DL (1996) *Searching for Memory: The Brain, the Mind, the Past.* New York: BasicBooks.

Squire LR and Kandel ER (2000) *Memory: From Mind to Molecules.* New York: W. H. Freeman.

Squire LR and Schacter DL (eds.) (2002) *The Neuropsychology of Memory,* 3rd edn. New York: Guilford Press.

Squire LR, Stark CE, and Clark RE (2004) The medial temporal lobe. *Annual Review of Neuroscience* 27: 279–306.

Teng E and Squire LR (1999) Memory for places learned long ago is intact after hippocampal damage. *Nature* 400: 675–677.
Wais PE, Wixted JT, Hopkins RO, and Squire LR (2006) The hippocampus supports both the recollection and the familiarity components of recognition memory. *Neuron* 49: 459–468.

Relevant Websites

http://www.alzforum.org – Alzheimer's Research Forum.
http://whoville.ucsd.edu – Home page of Larry R. Squire.
http://www.nia.nih.gov – National Institute on Aging, Alzheimer's Disease Centers.

Animal Models of Amnesia

M Moss, Boston University School of Medicine, Boston, MA, USA

Early Contributions to the Study of Memory: The Pioneers

Perhaps the first major contribution to the formal literature on human memory came from the French psychologist Theodule Ribot in his treatise on the *Diseases of Memory* that produced his 'law' which states that older memories are better remembered than more recent memories. But it is also difficult to introduce this subject without mention of the seminal contribution by William James in his *Principles of Psychology*. James made the case that the processing of memory had a neural substrate and that memory could be fractionated into primary (short-term) and secondary (long-term) memory, concepts we still struggle with today. He also introduced what we now consider the two major systems of memory processing: declarative memory and habit (procedural memory). Nor can any introduction to the subject of memory ignore the contribution of Hermann Ebbinghaus, who made the first major attempt at the quantification and measurement of memory, which culminated in his work *On Memory*. Sergei Korsakoff described a disorder of memory associated with the effects of alcohol and that now bears his name, and Vladimir Bekhterev was the first to point to the possible relationship of memory impairment with damage to the temporal lobe.

While these individuals were laying the foundation for the study of human memory, others began to apply this body of work to animal models. Most notable among these were EL Thorndike, a student of James, and Ivan Pavlov, with his work on classical conditioning. It was also at this time that Shepard Franz began using formal training paradigms in his work on the effects of brain lesions in animals. His student, Karl Lashley, extended this work to a level that many now consider to have constituted the seminal phase of the utility and value of animal models in neuropsychology.

Amnesia: The Paradox and Animal Models

Perhaps the most informative and seminal case study in the field of amnesia and one that initiated major activity using animal models of amnesia was that of patient H.M. In 1953, H.M. underwent surgery for treatment of intractable seizures. The procedure entailed bilateral resection of the medial temporal lobes, including the anterior two-thirds of the hippocampus, the amygdala, and hippocampal gyrus (**Figure 1**). Although the surgery was successful in ameliorating the frequency and intensity of his seizures, H.M. was left with a devastating impairment in his anterograde short-term memory and to a limited extent his retrograde memory, extending to at least several months preceding the procedure.

Following the surgery, H.M. was able to remember events over very brief intervals. However, it was the fate of this immediate memory that was imperiled. After a period as short as 30 s, or with brief distraction, recall of immediate events was, in virtually all cases, permanently erased. Despite this striking condition, it soon became evident through formal experimentation that H.M. retained some learning capacity. H.M. was able to perform certain motor skill and perceptual learning tasks and could retain much of this learning for as long as a year. It was this case that cemented the theoretical notions that the ability to remember is subserved by at least two memory systems. It was Cohen and Squire who dubbed the impaired and spared memory in H.M. (and other amnesiac patients) as declarative and procedural systems, respectively. Accordingly, declarative memory has been ascribed to medial temporal lobe structures and their anatomic connections to polymodal association areas of the cerebral mantle, whereas procedural memory has been ascribed to nonmedial temporal regions, with the neostriatum and cerebellum as the leading proposed neural substrates.

To date, although studies in animals have explored the neural basis of nondeclarative memory, most have focused primarily on localizing and fractionating the anatomic and functional neuronal substrate of declarative memory. Hence, the thrust of research has focused on the hippocampal formation and the adjacent parahippocampal cortices (including the entorhinal, perirhinal, and parahippocampal cortices; see **Figure 2**).

Rodent Models of Memory Function

In light of the anatomic and connectional similarities of the medial temporal lobe across species, both rodents and nonhuman primates (as well as canines and felines) have been utilized to assess various aspects of memory function. To a great extent, behavioral paradigms that are equivalent in design have been adapted to each of these species. One such behavioral task is delayed nonmatching to sample.

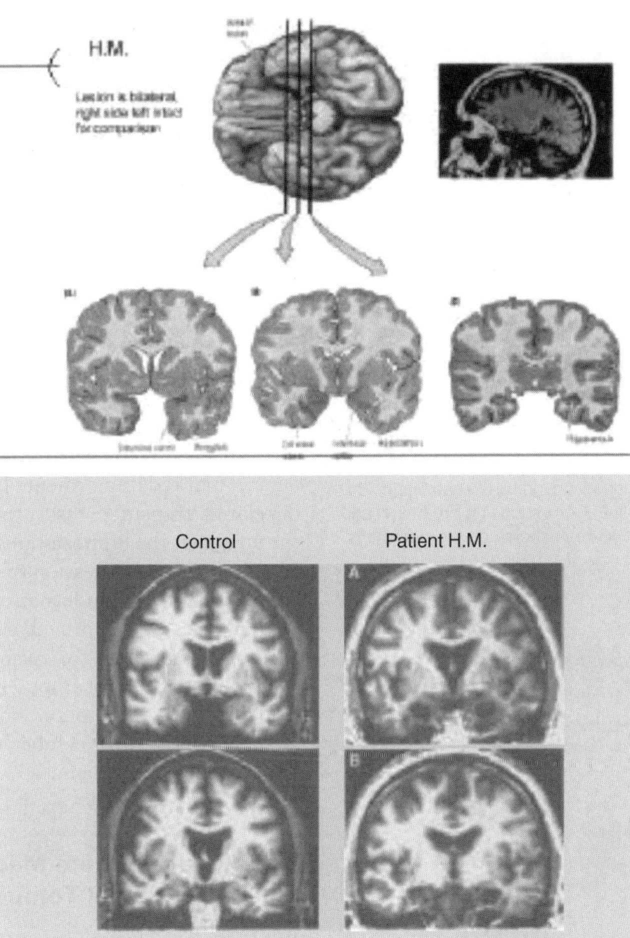

Figure 1 (Above) Representation of area of resection of medial temporal lobe areas in patient H.M. (Below) (A) Magnetic resonance image of coronal section of H.M.'s brain at rostral level showing resection of the amygdala (right) relative to normal control. (B) More-caudal level of H.M.'s brain showing removal of hippocampal formation (right) relative to normal control brain.

In this task, animals must respond to a sample stimulus and then, after a delay, must choose between a novel stimulus and the previously presented familiar one (**Figure 3**). Rats with damage to the hippocampus can learn the delayed nonmatching to sample task as efficiently as controls with delays of a few seconds but evidence a marked impairment when delays are extended to longer than a minute. These findings support the view that the hippocampus is essential in the ability to form associations between given stimuli and the context in which the stimuli appear.

Perhaps the most widely used method of assessing memory in rodents relies on the use of the Morris Water Maze. In the typical paradigm, the rat (or mouse) is placed into a pool of opaque water that contains an escape platform hidden a few millimeters below the water's surface. Visual cues, such as colored shapes, are placed around the pool in plain sight of the animal. When released, the rat swims around the pool in search of an exit. Several variables can be measured, including the time spent in each quadrant of the pool, the time taken to reach the platform (latency), and the total distance traveled. Rats with damage to the hippocampus are markedly impaired in this task. In contrast, rats with the same lesion can perform successfully on the task when the platform is visible above the water's surface. The data have accumulated to show that removal of the hippocampus in rats results in a marked impairment in tasks requiring spatial navigation and in those that specifically require the animal to remember recent locations it has visited. This effect appears more robust with

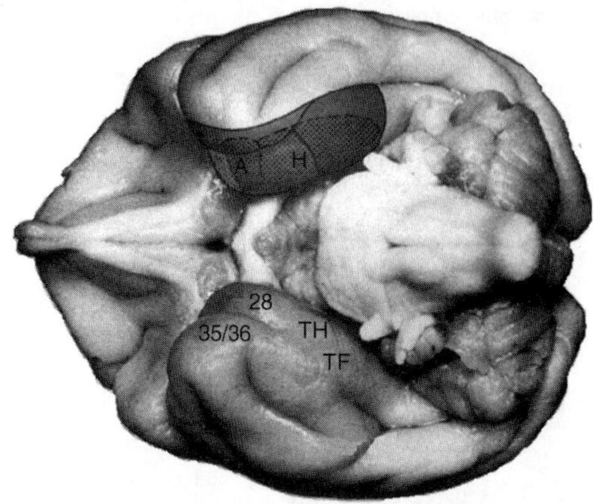

Figure 2 Ventral view of the rhesus monkey brain. Left hemisphere (top of photograph) depicts entorhinal cortex (purple), perirhinal cortex (blue), and parahippocampal cortices (green). Positions of subcortically positioned amygdala (A) and hippocampus (H) are depicted by dotted line. Corresponding Brodmann and Von Bonin and Bailey nomenclature is shown on the right hemisphere (bottom of photograph).

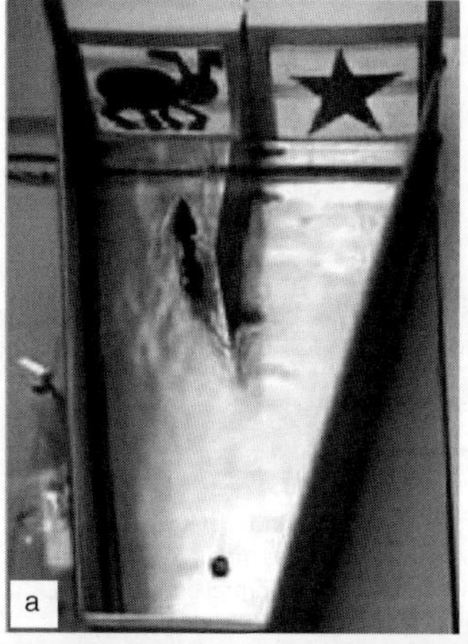

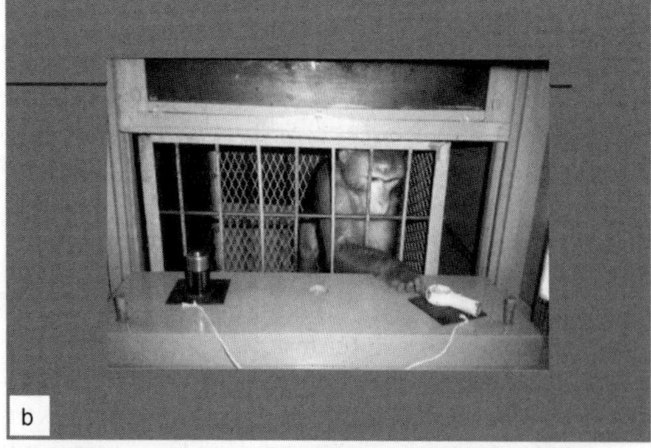

Figure 3 Photograph showing rhesus monkey in the Wisconsin General Testing Apparatus. The monkey is displacing the 'novel' object to obtain a reward (raisin) during the recognition portion of a trial on the delayed nonmatching to sample task.

damage to the hippocampus itself rather than to the surrounding rhinal cortices.

Taking advantage of rodents' exquisitely sensitive olfactory system, Eichenbaum and colleagues have used a novel paired associate odor task to demonstrate that the hippocampus is essential for memory function. In this task, rats first were rewarded for identifying an odor (A) that was paired with another given odor. Several such pairs were readily learned by normal rats as well as those with damage to the hippocampus. This basic stimulus–response learning task could easily be seen as supported by the nondeclarative memory system. On another phase of the task, rats had to infer an association between two odors that were not directly paired but that shared a common associate odor. Whereas control rats learned this task readily, those with hippocampal lesions evidenced marked impairment. Together with the results of related 'transitive' tasks, the data strongly support the view that the hippocampus is key to mediating the connection and expression of memory in a relational context. Eichenbaum has also shown that the hippocampus is essential in mediating sequential events, a working component for episodic memory. Rats with lesions of the hippocampus retain their capacity to recognize individual odors but are severely impaired in their ability to remember the sequential order of odors presented to them.

Nonhuman Primate Models of Memory Function: Medial Temporal Lobe

While evidence from human cases strongly implicated the hippocampal formation in subserving normal memory function, it was unclear whether specific components of this structure had selective roles in memory function. Indeed, the hippocampus represents the endpoint of the transition from a six-layer cortex of the adjacent parahippocampal gyrus to a three-layer cortex in the hippocampus itself. Two of these regions, the perirhinal and parahippocampal cortices, are the recipients of input from secondary sensory association areas, including visual, somatosensory, and auditory regions, that, in turn, project to the entorhinal cortex, which is the major cortical afferent to the hippocampus. The perirhinal, entorhinal, and parahippocampal regions were damaged in patient H.M. (**Figure 1**), and these regions had also been removed in the surgical approach to the hippocampal formation in the early stages of nonhuman primate studies. As a result, it was difficult to distinguish between deficits traditionally attributed to damage to the hippocampus proper and those that arose from damage to the rhinal and adjacent cortices.

Several studies over the past 10 years have been aimed at fractionating the specific contributions of the hippocampus and rhinal cortices. Findings regarding the effect of damage to the hippocampus in nonhuman primates have been equivocal, particularly regarding the most commonly used task in assessing memory, delayed nonmatching to sample (DNMS). Results from studies of the effects on DNMS performance of damage to the hippocampus of nonhuman primates range from virtually no effect to marked impairment, particularly when delays greater than 30 s are used. However, when certain experimental design variables are taken into account, the contribution of the hippocampus to this task is better revealed.

One striking methodological difference in these studies of memory in nonhuman primates is the point in the experimental paradigm at which the tasks are initially learned. In studies in which monkeys with hippocampal lesions were both trained on the DNMS task and tested on the delay conditions following surgery, a marked impairment obtained. In contrast, in monkeys that were trained on the DNMS task preoperatively and tested postoperatively for retention of performance, little or no impairment was found. This difference in procedure may play an important role in the results because it very likely affects how and where the initial memory is mediated.

Another task used to assess memory, and one that has been widely used with human participants, is the delayed recognition span test (DRST). The DRST is a short-term memory test that requires the participant to identify, trial by trial, the new stimulus within an increasing array of serially presented stimuli. The task is administered using different classes of stimulus material in order to help characterize recognition memory deficits across several stimulus domains. For the spatial condition, identical discs are used as stimuli. A disc is placed over one of 18 wells, which is baited. A screen is raised, and the monkey is allowed to displace the disc to obtain the reward. The screen is then lowered, and a second disc is placed on the board over a baited well while the first disc is returned to its original position over the now unbaited well. After 10 s, the screen is raised, and the monkey is required to displace the new disc in order to obtain the reward. Each successive correct response is followed by the addition of a new disc until the monkey makes an error (i.e., chooses one of the previously chosen discs). With the occurrence of the first error, the trial is terminated, and the number of discs on the test tray minus 1 (i.e., the number of correct responses) constitutes the recognition span score for that trial. The object condition is administered in a similar fashion. Within each trial, the position of the previously correct stimuli is changed in a pseudorandom fashion so that the animal has to identify the new stimulus on the basis of visual cues without the use of spatial cues. Ten trials are administered each day for 10 days (see **Figure 4**).

Monkeys with bilateral damage restricted to the hippocampal formation made with ibotenic acid injection guided by magnetic resonance imaging are, like patients with Alzheimer's disease, markedly impaired in both the spatial and the object conditions of the DRST. They achieve lower spans than controls, whether the spans are unique or have been presented repeatedly over several sessions.

With regard to the rhinal cortices, Murray and others have performed extensive experiments using neurotoxic lesion methods to produce selective lesions to the perirhinal cortex in the monkey. Damage to this region produces impairment in stimulus recognition and in the maintenance of stimulus–stimulus associations for individual objects that, taken together, suggests that the perirhinal cortices are important for the accurate representation of visual stimuli and have profound effects on both perceptual and memory functions.

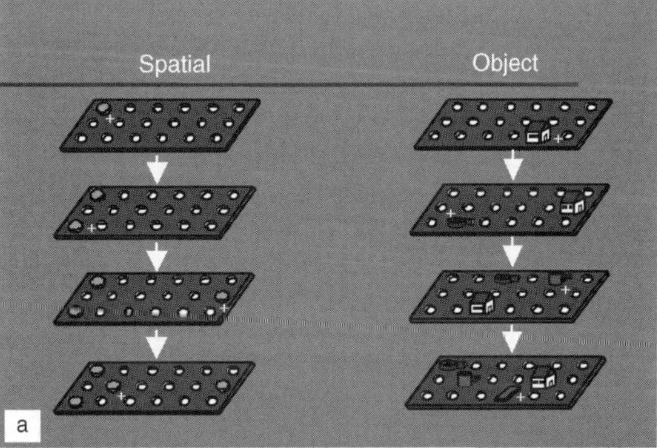

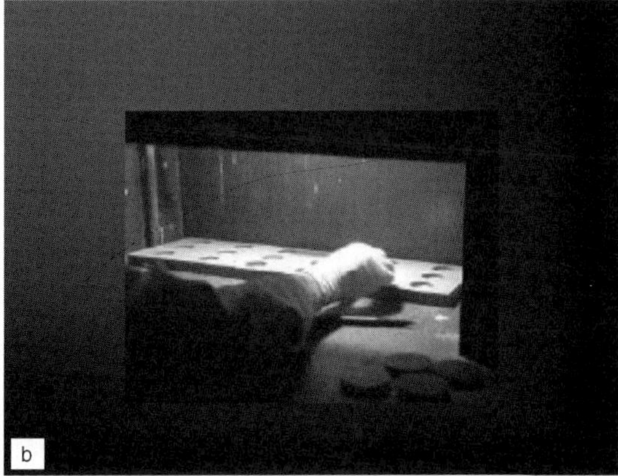

Figure 4 Schematic of the delayed recognition span test (DRST). Left: spatial condition; right: object condition.

Nonhuman Primate Models of Memory Function: Prefrontal Cortices

In the 1930s, researchers began to realize that the frontal lobe was involved in short-term memory processes. Jacobsen, taking the lead from findings of Brown and Schafer, advanced the notion that the frontal lobes may have a role in cognitive function. Jacobsen found that monkeys with damage to the prefrontal cortex were markedly impaired on a delayed response task. The findings were received as the first convincing evidence that the frontal lobes played a role in short-term memory function. Over the past 70 years, evidence for a role of the prefrontal cortices in memory function has been limited. It has become evident form the work of Goldman-Rakic that a small region of the prefrontal cortex plays a key role in working memory and that this area may be modality specific to spatial organization. It has been unclear whether damage to a specific region of the prefrontal cortex (e.g., dorsolateral region (area 9, area 46), ventrolateral region, or ventromedial region) has a specific role in memory or is related more to alteration of response control or some other aspect of so-called executive function.

More-recent evidence has shown that combined damage to areas 9 and 46 of the dorsolateral prefrontal cortex in the monkey results in an impairment on postoperative acquisition and delay conditions of the DNMS task. This deficit is quite severe, as monkeys with dorsolateral prefrontal cortex lesions take more trials to learn the task than do those with lesions of the hippocampus by a factor of almost 2 and perform as badly as monkeys of advanced age.

As is the case with findings from the DNMS task in nonhuman primates following lesions to the hippocampus, the findings following damage to the dorsolateral prefrontal cortex are not consistent. While it may be the case that combined, but not separate, lesions of dorsal prefrontal cortex that include both areas 9 and 46 are necessary to produce a measurable impairment on this task, it is equally plausible that preoperative versus postoperative acquisition of the task may represent the critical difference in findings.

Medical Temporal and Prefrontal Interactions?

While the exact temporal and anatomical sequence of memory processing remains to be elucidated, it is plausible that brain regions associated with visual recognition memory function (such as the hippocampal complex) and other medial temporal lobe structures, along with various parts of the prefrontal cortex, are differentially active in the course of acquisition and retention of qualitatively different cognitive tasks. Further, it is possible that declarative memory function may represent a functionally linked sequential network of mnemonic processing involving both medial temporal and prefrontal areas. According to this notion, one might speculate that during the initial acquisition of the nonmatching principle, both the hippocampus and the dorsal prefrontal cortex are active in processing and storing rules of the nonmatching paradigm. Hence, one would predict that damage to either structure alone would produce impairment in a postoperative acquisition paradigm, and both this report and previous work are consistent with this notion. Accordingly, one might predict that damage sustained by either structure alone following initial acquisition of tasks which employ the nonmatching rule would result in unimpaired or mildly impaired performance on the tasks, and indeed published reports of studies of such a postoperative retention paradigm are consistent with this. Moreover, one would predict that only combined damage to both the medial temporal lobe and the prefrontal cortex would produce significant impairment in such a postoperative retention paradigm, but this has yet to be tested. While these questions have yet to be tested directly, the notion of a complex interaction between prefrontal and medial temporal lobe systems in the acquisition and retention of recognition memory tasks can be tested empirically by making lesions of both the dorsal prefrontal cortex and medial temporal lobe concurrently in a postoperative retention paradigm.

Conclusion

While much progress has been made, greater effort must be made to bring tasks of memory function in animals into parallel with those in humans. It is also here that the great value of animal models can be brought to bear. One can more easily parcellate the anatomic and functional components of memory in animal models with carefully constructed experimental designs and then turn to mapping these onto studies of human memory.

See also: Aging and Memory in Animals; Amnesia: Declarative and Nondeclarative Memory; Episodic Memory: Assessment in Animals; Executive Function and Higher-Order Cognition: Assessment in Animals; Functional Amnesia; Spatial Memory: Assessment in Animals.

Further Reading

Beason-Held LL, Rosene DL, Killiany RJ, and Moss MB (1999) Hippocampal formation lesions produce memory impairment in the rhesus monkey. *Hippocampus* 9(5): 562–574.

Clark RE, West AN, Zola SM, and Squire LR (2001) Rats with lesions of the hippocampus are impaired on the delayed nonmatching-to-sample task. *Hippocampus* 11: 176–186.

Cohen NJ and Squire LR (1980) Preserved learning and retention of pattern analyzing skills in amnesics: Dissociation of knowing how and knowing that. *Science* 210: 207–210.

Eichenbaum H (2004) Hippocampus: Cognitive processes and neural representations that underlie declarative memory. *Neuron* 44: 109–120.

Eichenbaum H, Otto T, and Cohen NJ (1994) Two functional components of the hippocampal memory system. *Behavioral and Brain Sciences* 17: 449–472.

Goldman PS and Rosvold HE (1970) Localization of function within the dorsolateral prefrontal cortex of the rhesus monkey. *Experimental Neurology* 27: 291–304.

Mahut H, Zola-Morgan S, and Moss MB (1982) Hippocampal resections impair associative learning and recognition memory in the monkey. *Journal of Neuroscience* 2: 1214–1229.

Mishkin M (1978) Memory in monkeys severely impaired by combined but not separate removal of the amygdala and hippocampus. *Nature* 273: 297–298.

Murray EA (1990) Representational memory in nonhuman primates. In: Kesner RP and Olton DS (eds.) *Neurobiology of Comparative Cognition*, pp. 127–155. Hillsdale, NJ: Erlbaum.

Squire LR (1992) Memory and the hippocampus: A synthesis from findings with rats, monkeys, and humans. *Psychological Review* 99: 195–231.

Zola-Morgan S and Squire LR (1986) Memory impairment in monkeys following lesions limited to the hippocampus. *Behavioral Neuroscience* 100(2): 155–160.

Attention and Eye Movements

E Kowler, Rutgers University, Piscataway, NJ, USA

Eye movements are inextricably linked to visual attention because both are the principal tools available for selecting interesting portions of visual scenes for enhanced perceptual and cognitive processing. Selection is crucial for animals that rely on foveal images for making decisions about the visual environment or for guiding action. As a result, most of what is known about eye movements and attention derives from studies of human and nonhuman primates.

Eye movements are often taken to mark the path of attention through a scene, where attention refers to the internal (or covert) distribution of processing resources. Eye movements and attention are assumed to serve useful purposes connected to the visual task, an assumption that has fueled decades of efforts to use eye movements to study how people search, read, study pictures of scenes, or carry out all manner of visually guided actions involving reaching, pointing, manipulating objects, walking, or driving. All these tasks require serial processing of different parts of a scene, and all routinely call upon eye movements.

For eye movements to be useful, they must be able to bring the line of sight to relevant locations quickly and accurately, and to keep it there, with no deliberate effort or laborious decision stages beyond those already incorporated into the task itself. In order to meet these requirements – speed, accuracy, and low cognitive load – eye movements must be sensitive to both the physical structure of the visual array and to the momentary needs of the task. To see why this is the case, consider the two extreme possibilities. On the one hand, if eye movements were completely under the control of the stimulus, with gaze attracted to the most vivid or salient portions in a scene, cognitive load would be minimal, but the eye would continually be dragged off to useless and irrelevant locations. It would be impossible to choose targets according to the needs of the task. (Nevertheless, there are many models based on just this assumption.) On the other hand, too much emphasis on volition, choice, or effort to control gaze would create undue cognitive demands and interfere with the ongoing flow of the task. The effort devoted to eye movement control would be a continual distraction from the job of recognizing objects and making task-related decisions and plans. Over the past decades, oculomotor scientists have struggled to find ways of integrating these two extreme modes of eye movement control. The focus of these attempts, in behavioral, psychophysical and neurophysiological studies, has been the attempt to find and understand the relationship between the control of eye movements and the mechanisms of visual attention.

What Is Attention?

Before considering the relationship between eye movements and attention, it is useful to briefly summarize some aspects of attention as they apply more generally to perception.

In his classical treatment of attention, William James acknowledged that, although everyone knows what attention is ("experience is what I agree to attend to", p. 402) the question of what attention does is difficult to answer. Attention is credited with being able to enhance certain experiences at the expense of others, but at the same time it must do so without distorting the nature of these experiences. Attention, James said, might make it possible to notice a faint sound or light, but paying attention to faint sounds or lights does not make them suddenly appear unusually loud or bright.

Modern researchers grappling with James's paradox have devised a number of clever experimental paradigms to explore the effects of attention on perception in many different contexts. Attention can be summoned to locations or to objects by various sorts of cues or signals, or it can be drawn away by imposition of a competing task. Studies using these techniques have led to broad agreement about several characteristics of attention:

1. Attention can lower detection thresholds and increased perceived contrast, producing improvements resembling those produced by modest increases in the contrast of the stimulus itself. These effects may correlate with attention-induced changes in cell firing patterns (e.g., increased contrast gain) at neural levels as early as V1 or the lateral geniculate nucleus (LGN).

2. Improvements in perceptual thresholds can be produced by paying attention either to a selected location (the 'attentional spotlight'), to a selected feature, or to a selected object. In the case of feature-based attention, the attentional benefits can spread across broad regions of space; in the case of object-based attention, the benefits of attention can extend to the different features (color, size, orientation) making up the attended object.

3. Attention to an object serves to overcome potential perceptual interference from visual objects

nearby. The importance of attention in the presence of competing stimuli has contributed to the view that attention should be viewed as an internal processing resource that can be distributed among features, objects or regions, as needed, to accomplish task goals. The importance of competition for limited resources has also been reflected at the neural level (areas V4 or the middle temporal area (MT), for example) with observations showing that, in the presence of multiple stimuli falling in a cell's receptive field, attention determines the relative contribution of each to the response of the cell.

4. Attention may also control access to limited capacity visual short-term or visual working memory, including the visual memory that preserves information from one fixation to the next.

All four of these characteristics – demonstrated in experiments that took pains to eliminate a role for eye movements, often by restricting stimulus presentations to very brief intervals of time – have influenced thinking and research about the role of attention in oculomotor control and the role played by eye movements and attention in visual processing.

Attention and Gaze Stabilization

One of the most important functions of eye movements is to maintain stable gaze. Even modest rotations of the head, if not compensated by counterrotations of the eye in the orbit, can create sufficient motion of the retinal image to impair visual resolution, carry important visual details away from the fovea, and create the illusion that the environment itself is moving. The oculomotor system is equipped with sophisticated systems that use both visual and vestibular signals to compensate for head movements and maintain stable gaze. These traditional full-field gaze stabilization reflexes, however, are not ideally suited to environments containing multiple objects at various distances and locations, viewed by observers who continually pick up and handle some of these objects, and who continually shift their own position in myriad ways. These situations require the maintenance of a stable gaze on only one thing at a time, and this means overriding the global visual or vestibular gaze stabilization reflexes, or at least restricting the portion of the scene on which they are allowed to operate.

In the early twentieth century, physicist and philosopher Ernst Mach described the situation well. The problem, said Mach, is that the retinal motion generated by head movements and body movements as we move through the environment may "exert a peculiar motor stimulus upon the eye, and draw our attention and our gaze after them" (p. 146). But this attraction can be overridden:

> No special apparatus is necessary for observing the foregoing phenomena. They are to be met with on all hands. I walk forward by a simple act of the will. My legs swing to and fro without my having to attend to them particularly. My eyes fixed steadfastly upon my goal without suffering themselves to be drawn aside by the motion of the retinal images consequent upon progression. All this is brought about by a single act of the will. . . . The same process must also be set up if the eyes are to resist for any length of time the stimulus of a mass of moving objects. (Mach, 1906/1959: 146)

Mach's impression that we can override flows of motion on the retina and maintain stable gaze on chosen targets has been confirmed and extended many times in the modern oculomotor laboratory. It is possible, for example, to maintain gaze on even very small stationary targets superimposed on large and vivid moving backgrounds. It is also possible to smoothly track a target moving across a stationary background (although this has proven to be the more difficult task) and to track a target moving in the presence of a nearby moving nontarget. In the case of the target and nontarget, it may require about 100 ms or so for complete selectivity to be achieved. Observations such as these have been made in many studies since 1930, with different kinds of backgrounds and with fixation targets of different sizes and retinal locations, each time showing that it is possible to maintain fixation on selected targets and override the effects of the more plentiful motion signals originating from the background (**Figure 1**).

The ability to select the target for smooth eye movements has also been demonstrated with superimposed transparent sheets of dots, each moving at a different velocity (**Figure 1(b)**). With such patterns, attending to a discrete location would not be sufficient to select one sheet as the target because dots are superimposed everywhere. Thus, effective selection with transparent motions requires attending to a selected object or surface rather than to a discrete location within the pattern. Interestingly, the selection of one of the transparent surfaces does not disrupt the perceptual impression of transparency, nor does it disrupt perceptual interactions between the superimposed fields. For example, if one of the fields is moving and the other is stationary, the stationary field seems to be moving opposite in direction to the other, ignored moving field. The percept of induced motion shows that the selection of the target for the eye movements leaves intact basic operations of sensory and perceptual motion processing. This raises the possibility that the selective mechanism that determines the target for

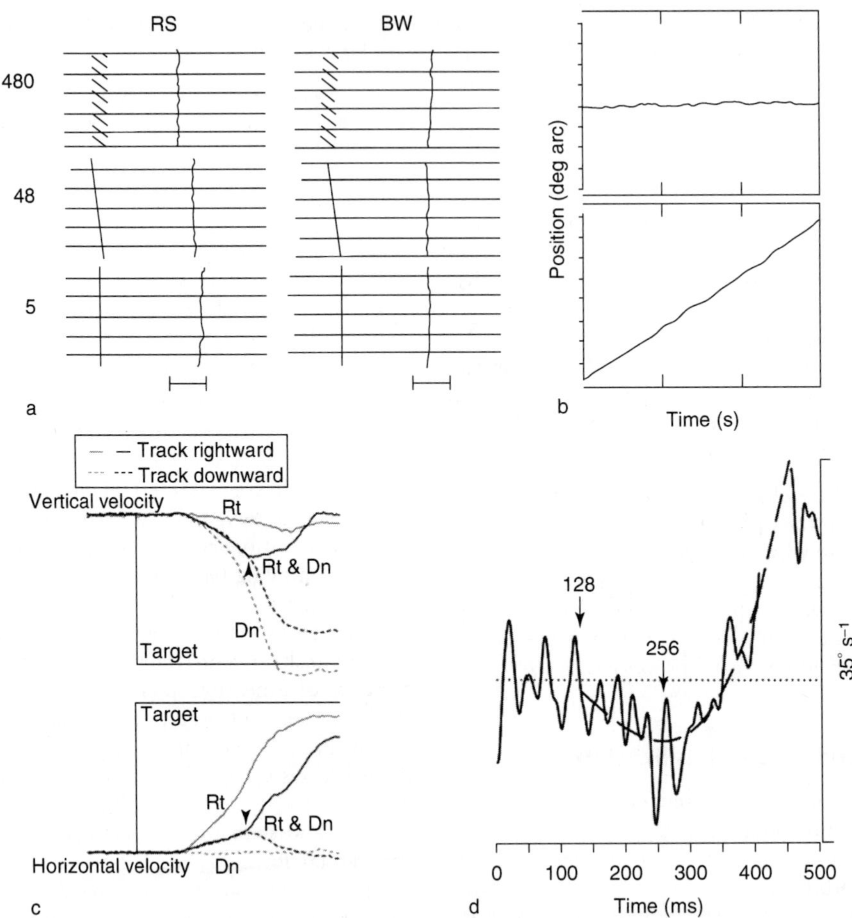

Figure 1 Smooth eye movements and attention: (a) examples of horizontal smooth eye movements maintaining a stable line of sight on a stationary fixation target superimposed on a background moving grating; (b) example of the independence of smooth eye movements from background motion with stationary and moving dots; (c) average eye velocity in response to a single target moving either downward (top) or rightward (bottom) or to a pair of targets, one moving rightward and the other downward; (d) horizontal eye velocity in the presence of two visual arrays of noise elements moving in opposite directions, one located above and the other below the line of sight. In (a), the data are from two observers, RS and BW. The left trace in each panel shows the stimulus motion (5, 48, or 480 min arc s^{-1}); the right trace shows horizontal eye movements. Horizontal lines are 1 s time markers, with time beginning at the bottom. The horizontal bar below the panels for each observer represents a 1° eye rotation. In (b), each trace shows horizontal smooth eye movements with two full-field superimposed arrays of random dots, one array stationary and the other moving at 1.2° s^{-1}. In the upper panel, the observer was told to fixate the stationary array and, in the lower panel, to pursue the moving array. There was virtually no effect of the unattended field on performance. In (c) average eye velocity is in response to a single target moving either downward (top) or rightward (bottom) (thin eye traces, labeled Rt or Dn) or to a pair of targets, one moving rightward and the other downward (bold traces labeled Rt and Dn). Traces labeled Target shows the stimulus which traveled over 20° for 400 ms. After 150 ms, one of the target motions of the pair disappeared, leaving only a single stimulus moving downward (top) or rightward (bottom). Eye velocity when both target motions were present was the average of the two target velocities until about 80 ms after one of the motions was removed (marked by the arrows) when the traces diverged. In (d), the eye trace shows the change in pursuit direction when first one, and then the other, moving field is selected as the pursuit target. (a) Reproduced from Murphy BJ, Kowler E, and Steinman RM (1975) Slow oculomotor control in the presence of moving backgrounds. *Vision Research* 15: 1263–1268, with permission from Elsevier. (b) Reproduced from Kowler E, Van der Steen J, Tamminga EP, and Collewijn H (1984) Voluntary selection of the target for smooth eye movements in the presence of superimposed, full-field stationary and moving stimuli. *Vision Research* 24: 1789–1798, with permission from Elsevier. (c) From Lisberger SG and Ferrera VP (1997) Vector averaging for smooth pursuit eye movements initiated by two moving targets in monkeys. *Journal of Neuroscience* 17: 7490–7502. (d) From Liston D and Krauzlis RJ (2003) Shared response preparation for pursuit and saccadic eye movements. *Journal of Neuroscience* 23: 11304–11314.

smooth eye movements may use its own dedicated attentional filter whose operation has minimal consequences for perception.

The Role of Attention in Perception versus the Role of Attention in Smooth Eye Movements

One way to find out whether smooth eye movements and perception share a common attentional mechanism is to expand the eye movement experiment to include a concurrent perceptual task. In one representative situation, an observer is presented with two sets of moving targets and asked to smoothly track one set and ignore the other (**Figure 2**). In this situation, perceptual judgments made about the tracked target are more accurate than those made about the untracked background (even after taking into account any differences in retinal position and retinal velocity), implying that a single filter and a single attentional decision determine the strength of signals reaching both perceptual and oculomotor systems. But there are important differences between eye movements and perception. Whereas the smooth tracking eye movements are nearly perfect, with virtually no effect of the unselected background motion, perceptual judgments about the unselected background are above chance, showing that some perceptual registration of the background remains. Thus, there is an asymmetry between the effects of attention on perception and eye movements. Analogous results have been obtained from neurons in the extrastriate cortical areas MT and medial superior temporal region (MST), the presumed sources of the motion signals that guide smooth eye movements and serve perception. Neurons in these areas respond more vigorously to attended and tracked motion than to unattended untracked motion, but the differences in firing patterns are small and do not explain the high degree of selectivity that can be demonstrated in smooth pursuit eye movements (although they are in general agreement with the magnitude of selectivity observed

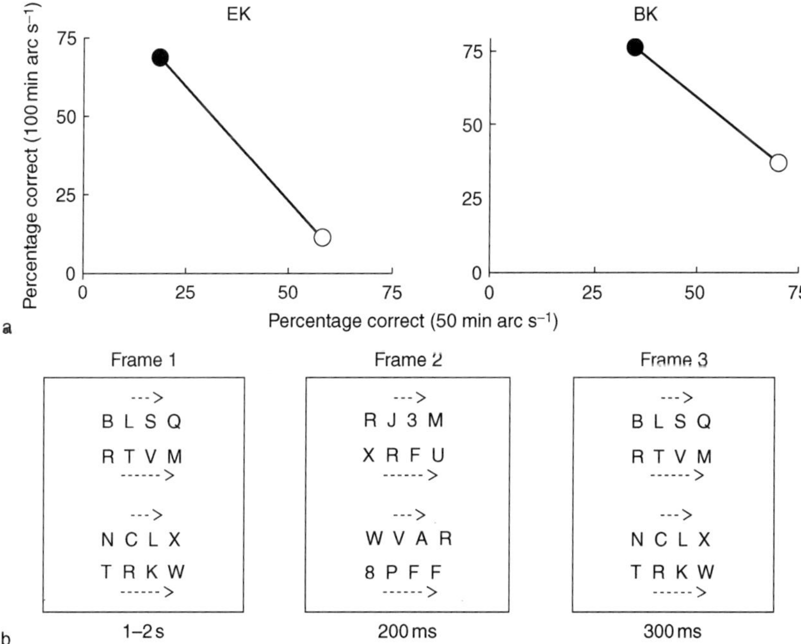

Figure 2 Smooth eye movements with a concurrent perceptual task: (a) perceptual performance for two observers; (b) representative sequence of display frames for a trial. The three display frames in (b) show four rows of letters moving rightward with the top and third rows moving at half the velocity of the second and bottom rows. Letters remained within the confines of the frame so that as portions reached an invisible boundary on the right they re-appeared immediately on the left side of the display. Vertical eye position remained in the gap between rows 2 and 3 while subjects attended and tracked either the faster or slower pair of rows. Frames 1 and 3 are masks. Frame 2 is the critical display, containing two numerals that had to be identified at the end of the trial. Tracking gains were >0.8. The perceptual performance shown in (a) for two observers depended on instructions. When observers attended and tracked the slower pair of rows (open symbols), identification accuracy was better for the slower rows than the faster rows. When they attended and tracked the faster pair of rows (closed symbols), identification improved for the faster pair at the expense of the slower pairs. Separate analyses showed that these results were not due to differences in retinal speed of tracked and untracked rows and were due solely to attention. Reproduced from Khurana B and Kowler E (1987) Shared attentional control of smooth eye movements and perception. *Vision Research* 27: 1603–1618, with permission from Elsevier.

at the perceptual level). The observed differences between the effects of attention on eye movements and perception, and the small effects observed in the motion areas MT and MST during the selective tracking tasks, imply that a given distribution of attention across target and background has different consequences for perception and for eye movements. This rules out early selection models, in which attention operates primarily at an early sensory level of visual processing shared by perception and eye movements.

The ability to eliminate almost all influence of the unselected motion signals from the eye movements suggests the involvement of a winner-take-all (WTA) network operating on the set of attentionally weighted motion signals emerging from areas MT and MST. WTA networks are often used in models of attention or perception and are effective ways to remove weak, and potentially interfering, signals. Although such a network operating downstream from sensory motion areas could account for the perfect or near-perfect selectivity observed for eye-tracking performance, an unconstrained WTA network places a strict limit on the options. It would not, for example, allow people to divide attention between a target and background and to track at a velocity intermediate between the two. An alternative to the WTA network is an executive controller that determines the relative weights assigned to different sets of sensory motion signals. A single executive controller could be used by both perceptual and oculomotor systems with different effects on each. For example, assigning maximum weight to a target could completely attenuate the representation of nontargets in neural areas devoted to smooth tracking and only partially attenuate the nontarget representation in perceptual areas. Different assignments of weight would produce different performance outcomes. Given that the neural circuitry that controls smooth eye movements includes several high-level cortical areas (frontal eye field (FEF), supplementary eye field (SEF), and lateral intraparietal area (LIP)) that also play roles in perceptual attention, there is considerable opportunity for executive intervention in the attentional weighting of motion signals from target and background.

Summary: Attention and Gaze Stabilization

Selective attention plays a crucial role in the control of smooth eye movements by ensuring that stable gaze can be maintained on either stationary or moving targets, regardless of the signals present in the background. Attention ensures that eye movements are controlled only by signals originating from the selected object. Performance of concurrent oculomotor and perceptual tasks have shown that a single attentional decision affects both – it is not possible to maintain gaze on one object while fully attending another. Unselected objects nevertheless remain perceptible and continue to generate neural signals in areas sensitive to motion. This outcome rules out early selection models of attentional control and raises still unanswered questions of how a common attentional decision can have different consequences for smooth eye movements and for perception.

Attention and Saccadic Shifts of Gaze

Saccadic eye movements are used to inspect the visual environment, with saccadic shifts of gaze occurring anywhere from once every several seconds to several times a second. Visual processing occurs during the pauses between saccades. Unlike smooth eye movements, which cannot be generated without some sort of representation of smooth motion, saccadic eye movements can be made at will to look at arbitrary locations.

Saccades are typically directed to useful or informative locations and are often taken to disclose the path of attention during performance of natural tasks. Attention, however, need not be locked to the fovea even as the eye jumps from place to place. Attention to locations remote from the line of sight is valuable for broad surveys of the scene and is indispensable for ensuring that saccades land on the selected object, regardless of the visual structure of the immediate surround.

Eye Position as an Overt Marker of the Locus of Attention

Figure 3 shows examples of saccadic patterns made during various visual tasks: reading, counting, geometry problem-solving, and visual scene recall. **Figure 4** shows eye movements during visual search. **Figure 5** replicates and extends the well-known experiment described by Yarbus in his 1967 book *Eye Movements and Vision*, in which people were asked to inspect the same painting in order to answer different questions. The scan patterns differed depending on the question, showing that the physical features of the pictures do not by themselves determine the landing locations of the eye but that there is considerable influence of purpose and intent. **Figure 6** looks at this issue from another angle, showing scan patterns obtained when looking at two versions of the same photograph, where in one version the image has been filtered and the fine detail removed. Although the task is the same in each, the scatter of the fixated locations is different.

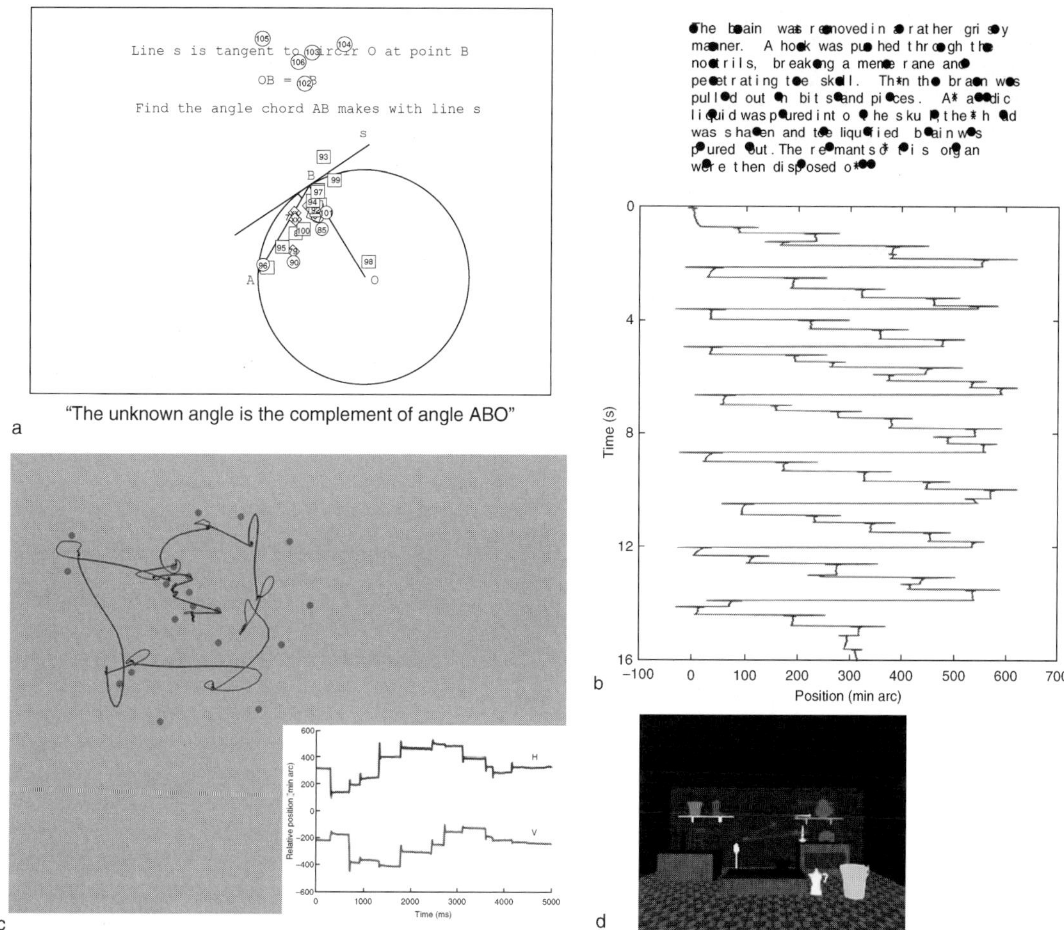

Figure 3 Examples of eye movements during various visual and cognitive tasks: (a) fixation positions of one observer during one stage of solving a problem in geometry; (b) eye movements during reading; (c) eye movements while counting an array of dots; (d) eye movements during a visual recall task. In (a), the problem is presented above the diagram and the excerpt from the protocol is below it. Important features of the diagram were refixated at regular intervals. Analyses of the timing and locations of fixations showed frequent revisits, consistent with a working memory capacity of five visual features of the problem. In (b), the same pattern of eye movements is shown as individual fixation locations superimposed on the text (top) and as a trace of eye positions over time (bottom). Eye position is on the abscissa, and time moves from top to bottom. These eye movements are typical of reading in that saccades were about seven characters long and intersaccadic pauses were about 275 ms. More than 40 readings of this same text showed little change in the pattern of eye movements and a high level of consistency in the distribution of landing locations. In (c), eye movements are shown both superimposed on the dot array and also as horizontal and vertical traces over time. In (d), subjects had to report the contents of the picture after periods of scanning ranging up to 4 s. Analyses showed that memory for the content of the pictures was preserved across successive viewings separated by several minutes and several intervening viewed scenes. (a) Reproduced from Epelboim J and Suppes P (2001) Eye movements during problem solving in geometry. *Vision Research* 41: 1561–1574, with permission from Elsevier. (b) Reproduced from Schnitzer BS and Kowler E (2006) Eye movements during multiple readings of the same text. *Vision Research* 46: 1611–1632, with permission from Elsevier. (d) Reproduced from Melcher D and Kowler E (2001) Visual scene memory and the guidance of saccadic eye movements. Vision Research, 41: 3597–3611, with permission from Elsevier.

Similar efforts to document sequences of fixations in different tasks have been made in more complex and dynamic situations, in which observers move about the environment, handling various objects for some specific purpose. The sequences of fixation positions of the two eyes are required when observers perform three different tasks: tapping a set of rods in prescribed order, grooming a fellow primate, and assembling a doll.

Data such as these have always been intriguing. They prove that ordinary visual experience, which seems smooth, continuous, and flowing, is really made up of sequences of brief, still frames and snapshots, whose detailed contents escape awareness. We do not notice

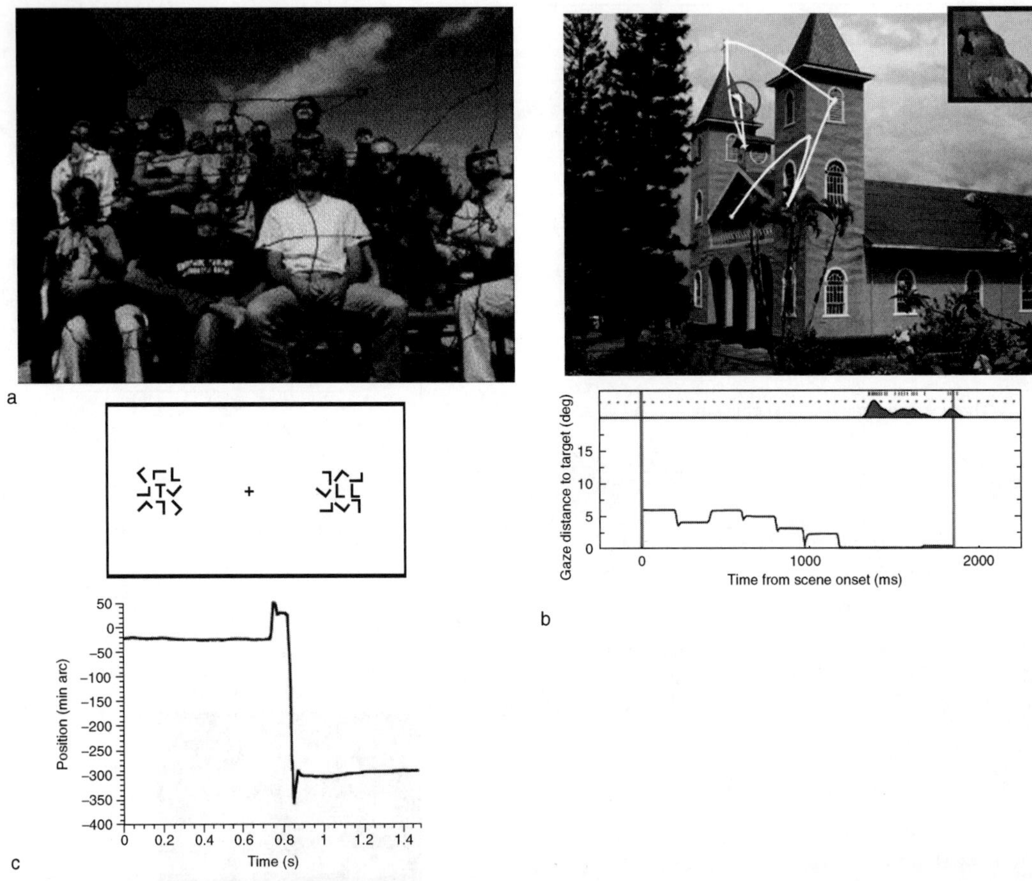

Figure 4 Eye movements during visual searche: (a) search for small gray crosses superimposed on the scene; (b) search in monkey for a small embedded target (reproduced in inset); (c) search for a target letter T embedded in one of two clusters of L's. In (a), analyses showed little or no bias to avoid returning to previously fixated location. In (b), eye traces show the distance to the target over time. Spike density functions show little response until just before the animal fixates the hidden target. Selection of the target as a saccadic goal was shown to be a necessary condition for the firing bursts. In (c), the probability that one of the clusters contained the T (0.8/0.2) was disclosed by a brightness cue. The eye traces show that often subjects looked first at the cluster with the lower probability, particularly when the cluster was closer to the line of sight, and then quickly with an unusually short latency interval (<100 ms) made a second saccade to the high probability cluster containing the target letter. (a) Reproduced from Hooge ITHC, Over EAB, van Wezel RJA, and Frens MA (2005) Inhibition of return is not a foraging facilitator in saccadic search and free viewing. *Vision Research* 45: 1901–1908, with permission from Elsevier. (b) Reproduced from Sheinberg DL and Logothetis NK (2001) Noticing familiar objects in real world scenes: The role of temporal cortical neurons in natural vision. *Journal of Neuroscience* 21: 1340–1350, with permission from the Society for Neuroscience (c) Reproduced from Araujo C, Kowler E, and Pavel M (2001) Eye movements during visual search: The costs of choosing the optimal path. *Vision Research* 41: 3613–3625, with permission from Elsevier.

each individual glance because we remember only what is most essential – the cumulative number of dots counted or the meaning of a word or phrase – or we use what we see to guide an immediate action. Observing sequences of eye movements reveals the sequential nature of vision and provides a view of underlying goals and strategies that would be hard to recover through other means.

Decisions, Attention, and Saliency Maps

Understanding the rules that govern saccadic planning in everyday life tasks is an enormous undertaking that must be based on models of the task, combined with knowledge of the relevant visual, cognitive, and motor capacities that limit performance and affect the strategies adopted. Although we still lack comprehensive and general models, progress has been made toward the goal. One of the influential constructs developed to account for the eye movements made during scanning of a scene is the salience map. As originally proposed by Koch and Ullman, the salience map is derived from the output of banks of visual filters, modeled after those present in early levels of the

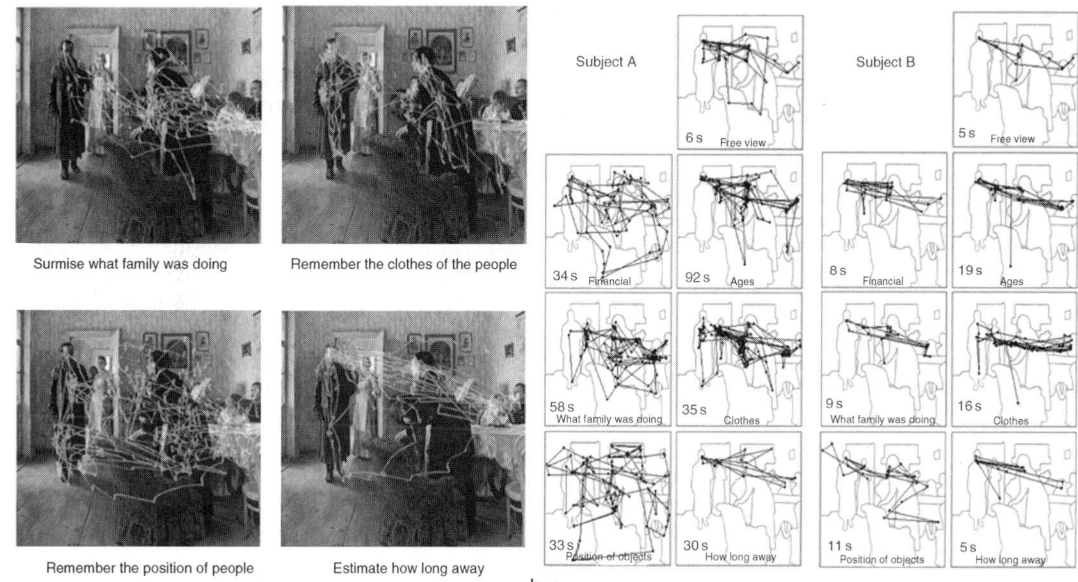

Figure 5 Effect of task motivation on eye movements: (a) people looking at Repin's painting *The Unexpected Visitor* altered the choice of fixation positions depending on the question they had to answer; (b) a replication of Yarbus's experiment, in which subject A shows the same sensitivity to task as Yarbus demonstrated but subject B tends to look in the same places regardless of the task. (a) Adapted from Yarbus A (1967) *Eye Movements and Vision.* New York: Plenum. (b) Figure provided by J Pelz and reproduced with permission. For discussion see Lipps M and Pelz JB (2004) Yarbus revisited: Task-dependent oculomotor behavior [abstract]. *Journal of Vision* 4: 115a, with permission from ARVO.

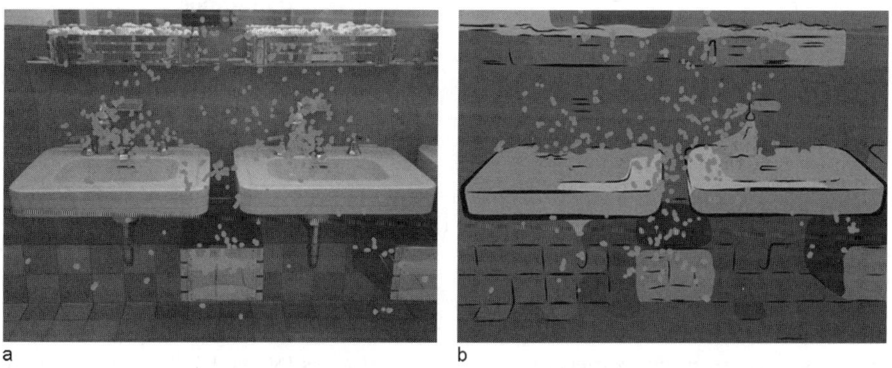

Figure 6 Fixations made by 10 viewers while looking at two variants of the same photograph: (a) original photo; (b) version in which computer graphics techniques were used to create a drawing-like version of the scene and remove detail throughout the image. Subjects were instructed to remember the picture for a subsequent recognition task. In (a), fixations are tightly clustered in a few key areas. In (b), fixations are more uniformly distributed. Figures provided by A Santella; original photo courtesy of Philip Green spun. For discussion see DeCarlo D and Santella A (2002) Stylization and abstraction of photographs. *ACM Transactions on Graphics* 21: 769–776; Santella A and DeCarlo D (2004) Visual interest and NPR: An evaluation and manifesto. In: *Proceedings of the Third International Symposium on Nonphotorealistic Animation and Rendering*, pp. 71–78. Annecy, France, 7–9 June. New York: ACM Press.

visual system (V1). These filters respond on the basis of local feature contrast (luminance, color, or orientation contrast) present in the scene. Models for the generation of salience maps integrate all three types of feature contrasts, taking the effects of retinal eccentricity into account. Saliency maps have been used to predict where people direct saccades and how they distribute visual attention (i.e., processing capacity) across a scene even when eye movements are not made.

In order to use a global salience map to predict a sequence of fixations, two additional assumptions have to be made. The first is that a WTA network (similar to that already discussed in the context of smooth eye movements) establishes the ordering of the fixations, with the region with the highest salience level designated as the next one to be fixated. The second assumption is that the salience map is subjected to inhibition of return; that is, once a location is examined its strength in the salience map will abruptly diminish, thus allowing the line of sight to proceed to new places and avoiding the need to store a list of already-scanned locations. Armed with a salience map and these two supporting assumptions, it has been possible to generate precise predictions about where people look during unconstrained free-viewing. The predictions have proven to be reasonably accurate, at least when computed salience is compared to the global aggregate of fixated locations over some period of inspection. Nevertheless, the approach has not been without controversy.

The main criticism of the salience map approach is the obvious one, recognized and discussed even by proponents of the approach. Strict control of eye movements or attention based solely on physical salience becomes counterproductive as soon as people are faced with real-world tasks (**Figures 4–6**). In real-world tasks, people look at the objects and details that are important, regardless of the physical salience levels. Gaze and attention may be drawn to novel or unexpected objects or to highly familiar objects, depending on the situation. None of these characteristics is represented by physical salience. Physical salience also does not capture the long-term changes in gaze preferences that develop as the contents of the scene are learned, nor does it capture effects of motivation. Do you look at something because it attracts your interest, because it contains some new information you need to perform a task, or because you need to confirm a detail that you already know is present? All of these so-called top-down variables that influence gaze and attention can be viewed as displacing the concept of a saliency map or, alternatively, as imposing an additional set of weights on the physical salience levels.

Neurophysiological studies using a variety of active saccadic tasks involving visual search or visual discriminations have addressed a portion of the problem of incorporating top-down variables by showing that neurons in areas related to saccadic planning (LIP, FEF, and superior colliculus (SC)) may be able to encode the top-down salience level at a given location. The evidence for this assertion is that neurons in these areas show enhanced activity when objects in their receptive fields contain information relevant to the guidance of an upcoming saccade, even when the location of enhanced activity does not correspond to the location of the saccadic target. Visual areas (the V4 or inferotemporal visual area (IT), for example), also show sensitivity to top-down salience. In these areas, neurons tuned to specific features show effects of attention, as well as patterns of presaccadic enhancement. Thus, there has been considerable progress in identifying brain areas that modulate responses to objects depending on their immediate behavioral significance, and these areas may constitute the core of a network that directs attention and saccades to objects or locations relevant to a task.

Incorporating top-down factors and physical salience levels into a single map may be a physiologically plausible means of deriving a single message to guide saccades and attention. Alternatively, there may be multiple maps that compete for control. Studies of eye movements during visual search have provided some support for the notion of competing maps. In these studies, saccades are drawn to physically salient locations that are not likely to contain the search target, followed quickly by corrective saccades to more appropriate, but less salient, places (**Figure 4(c)**). These rapid saccadic sequences could represent the results of the competition between different maps for momentary control of the neural centers that produce saccades. Although such competition seems inefficient, the amount of time lost by an occasional errant saccade may be small enough that an investment of time and resources in more prudent saccadic planning may not be warranted.

Saccades and Attention

Saliency – either stimulus-driven or top-down – is said to predict the distribution of both attention (internal processing resources) and saccades over time and space. Is there any important or necessary distinction between the distribution of attention and saccades? According to premotor theories of attention, saccadic eye movements and shifts of attention are essentially the same process, originating in the same neural areas, with an attention shift occurring only when the saccade is suppressed or inhibited. The premotor theory is supported by finding several neural areas (SC and FEF) whose activity can evoke or is correlated with both attention shifts and saccades. Nevertheless, it is troubling for premotor theories that attention can be distributed in parallel across the visual field or aligned symmetrically about the line of sight; spatial patterns do not readily map on to trajectories of saccades.

If we view attention not as a subthreshold saccade but rather as an internal processing resource that influences both perception and motor control, we can then ask how attention and saccades interact. Attention plays an important role in saccadic guidance in that, although it is possible to shift attention independently of the saccade, it does not appear possible to plan and carry out an accurate saccade without shifting some attention to the saccadic goal.

Dual-task studies, similar to those described earlier for smooth eye movements, have examined the distribution of visual attention prior to saccades, using various psychophysical tasks as indicators of local attentional strength. These dual-task studies require observers to do two things at once (in as brief a time as possible), namely, prepare to look at a specified object and identify a perceptual target presented while the preparation of the saccade is in progress. The perceptual target appears either at the saccadic goal or elsewhere. These experiments can succeed only if care is taken that the two tasks are done in the same brief interval of time because otherwise observers can decide to delay saccades in order to improve perceptual performance.

Dual-task experiments have shown that perceptual performance is better at the saccadic goal than elsewhere (see illustrative study in **Figure** 7), showing that saccades and attention do not functional independently. Yet, as was the case with smooth eye movements, perceptual performance at nongoal locations remained well above chance even when efforts were made to produce the saccades as quickly and accurately as possible (i.e., with the same latency and accuracy as observed with no concurrent perceptual task). Moreover, it only required a modest sacrifice in saccadic performance (10–20% latency increases) to achieve pronounced improvement in perceptual performance at nongoal locations.

Similar connections between attention and saccades are found during the execution of sequences of saccades (**Figure** 8(**a**)). Best perceptual performance is found at the saccadic goal, with elevations in perceptual thresholds at other locations, the amount of elevation depending on when and where the perceptual target appears. The pattern of activity observed during saccadic sequences suggests that the reduction in the attentional levels at nongoal locations is important for providing sufficient attentional contrast to guide an accurate saccade and prevent the line of sight from landing at salient, but incorrect, locations during scanning tasks. Thus, the main role of top-down attention in saccadic guidance may be to suppress the attraction of physically salient, but irrelevant, locations.

When the scan path to be followed is marked by a feature difference, rather than being followed from memory, the distribution of attention changes significantly. Attention spreads to locations along the feature-cued path, including targets of subsequent, as well as previous saccades (feature-based attention) (**Figure** 8 (**b**)). An interesting question raised by these results is how the saccades remain accurate when so many locations are attended at once. As was the case with smooth eye movements, there are two main alternatives. The first is a WTA network that directs the eye to the location where attentional strength is greatest. The second alternative requires the intervention of a central executive controller that imposes its own attentional weights. The controller could, for example, focus all active effortful attention on the upcoming target. The perceptual enhancement observed elsewhere along the featured-cued path could result from a passive process that facilitates the spread of attention across space to the selected features.

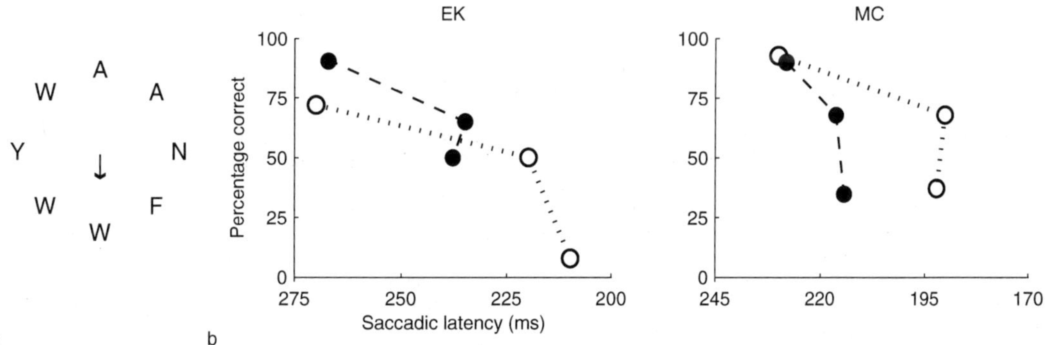

Figure 7 Saccades and attention: (a) the task display; (b) attentional-operating characteristics for two subjects showing the trade-off of saccadic and perceptual performance under two different conditions: saccade to a randomly chosen location (filled circles) and saccade to the same location on each trial (open circles). Shown in (a), the display contained eight randomly chosen letters. The task was to make a saccade (downward, in this case) while simultaneously identifying the letter in the right-hand position. Display timing was adjusted so that the critical letters appeared only during the saccadic preparation interval. In (b), The three data points in each function show performance under three instructions: (1) minimize saccadic latency (lowermost symbols), (2) sacrifice latency for improved perceptual accuracy (uppermost symbols), and (3) perform at a level intermediate between these two extremes. Achieving best perceptual identification accuracy required a sacrifice in saccadic latency (analysis of saccadic precision showed analogous results). Perceptual identification reached near-perfect levels with latency increases of only 10–20%. Reproduced from Kowler E, Anderson E, Dosher B, and Blaser E (1995) The role of attention in the programming of saccades. *Vision Research* 35: 1897–1916, with permission from Elsevier.

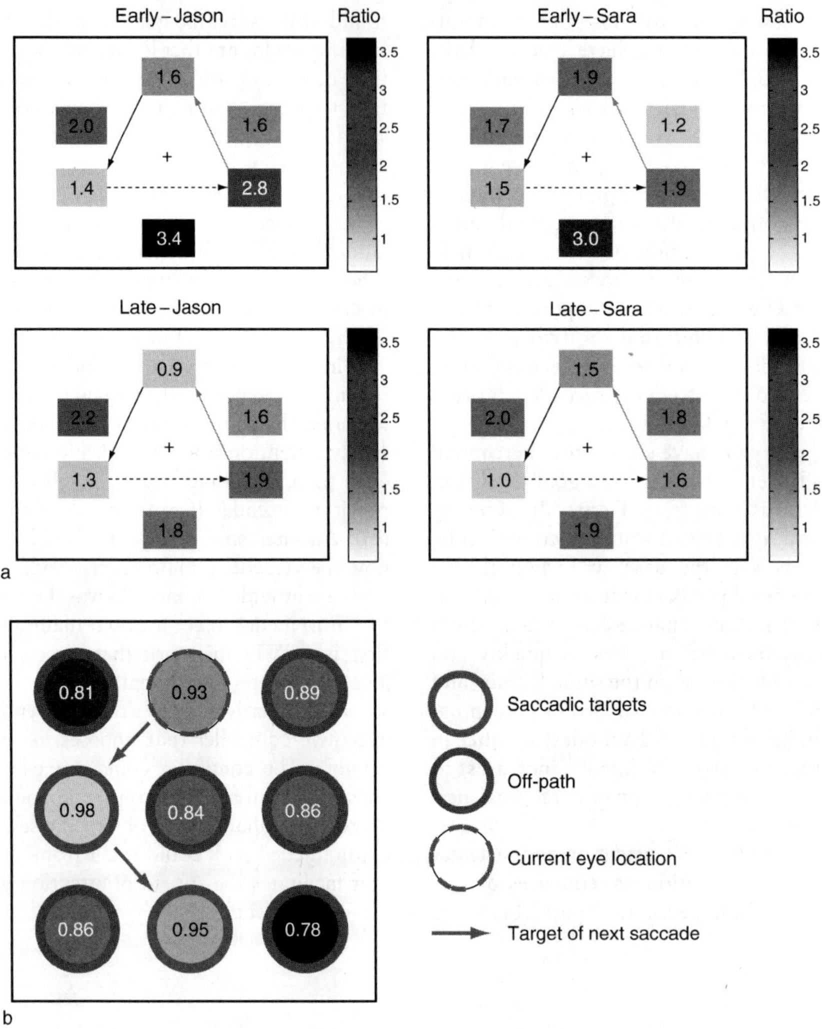

Figure 8 Attention during performance of sequences of saccades: (a) repetitive sequences of saccades; (b) nonrepetitive sequences of saccades. In (a), two subjects made saccades to rectangular boxes following a triangular pattern (shown by arrows) in which saccades were made to every other box. During a randomly selected fixation pause, an oriented Gabor patch was shown in one of the boxes either during the early (top row) or later (bottom row) portion of the pause. Current fixation position is in the top box. The colors of the boxes and the numbers in the boxes show the ratios of contrast threshold for correct orientation identification relative to thresholds during steady maintained fixation. Thresholds were significantly elevated at all locations except the currently fixated position (top of each graph) and target of the next saccade (lower left box in each graph). In (b), arrows represent a segment of a saccadic path. Current eye position is the top circle (dotted outline). Shading and numbers in the circles show percentage of correct orientation identification (two alternative forced-choice) for a Gabor patch shown briefly in one of the circles during a randomly selected intersaccadic pause. Perceptual performance is best for locations on the saccadic path, including the targets of the next two saccades. Performance for on-path locations is better than for off-path locations, including off-path locations of equal or smaller retinal eccentricity. (a) Reproduced from Gersch TM, Kowler E, and Dosher B (2004) Dynamic allocation of visual attention during the execution of sequences of saccades. *Vision Research* 44: 1469–1483, with permission from Elsevier (b) From Gersch TM (2007) *Attentional Filter Used during Scanning Influent Both Perception and Memory.* Doctoral thesis, Rutgers University.

Summary: Attention and Saccades

The picture of saccades and attention that emerges from these psychophysical and behavioral studies, which is in agreement with neurophysiological work, is that saccades and attention normally operate in a connected fashion, with saccades landing at the object that is the main focus of attention. Nevertheless, attending to the goal of saccades still allows significant perceptual processing at different locations, perhaps with the aid of other mechanisms that passively distribute attention to relevant locations in parallel across the visual array.

Overall Summary and Conclusion

The connection between eye movements and attention described in this article gives some support for the prevalent assumption that eye movements can provide reliable indicators of the main focus of attention in active visual tasks, such as reading, search, or object manipulation. Attention plays a crucial role in oculomotor control by enhancing signals from selected targets relative to those in the background, thus ensuring that eye movements are planned and programmed on the basis of selected visual signals, regardless of the visual configuration of objects nearby. Following the classical treatment of William James, it is useful to distinguish between the distribution of attention and the effects of attention. Attending to a given target can completely eliminate the influence of visual backgrounds on eye movements (smooth or saccadic) while continuing to allow perceptual processing, albeit at reduced levels. This asymmetry between perception and eye movements has the desirable consequence of allowing eye movements to be accurate without disrupting global perceptual analysis across the visual field.

See also: Attentional Functions in Learning and Memory; Contextual Interactions in Visual Perception; Perception and Eye Movements; Saccades and Visual Search; Saccadic Eye Movements; Sensorimotor Integration: Attention and the Premotor Theory; Vision for Action and Perception; Visual Attention.

Further Reading

Araujo C, Kowler E, and Pavel M (2001) Eye movements during visual search: The costs of choosing the optimal path. *Vision Research* 41: 3613–3625.

Corbetta M, Akbudak E, Conturo TE, et al. (1998) A common network of functioning areas for attention and eye movements. *Neuron* 21: 761–773.

DeCarlo D and Santella A (2002) Stylization and abstraction of photographs. *ACM Transactions on Graphics* 21: 769–776.

Deubel H and Schneider WX (1996) Saccade target selection and object recognition: Evidence for a common attentional mechanism. *Vision Research* 36: 1827–1837.

Epelboim J and Suppes P (2001) Eye movements during problem solving in geometry. *Vision Research* 41: 1561–1574.

Gardner JL and Lisberger SG (2001) Linked target selection for saccadic and smooth pursuit eye movements. *Journal of Neuroscience* 21: 2075–2084.

Gersch TM (2007) *The Attentional Filter Used during Scanning Influences Both Perception and Memory.* Doctoral Thesis, Rutgers University.

Gersch T, Kowler E, and Dosher B (2004) Dynamic allocation of attention during sequences of saccades. *Vision Research* 44: 1469–1483.

Hayhoe M and Ballard D (2005) Eye movements in natural behavior. *Trends in Cognitive Science* 9: 188–194.

Hooge ITHC, Over EAB, van Wezel RJA, and Frens MA (2005) Inhibition of return is not a foraging facilitator in saccadic search and free viewing. *Vision Research* 45: 1901–1908.

James W (1890/1950) *Principles of Psychology*, Vol. 1, p. 402. New York: Dover.

Khurana B and Kowler E (1987) Shared attentional control of smooth eye movements and perception. *Vision Research* 27: 1603–1618.

Koch C and Ullman S (1985) Shifts in selective visual attention: Towards the underlying neural circuitry. *Human Neurobiology* 4: 219–227.

Kowler E (1990) The role of visual and cognitive processes in the control of eye movement. In: Kowler E (ed.) *Eye Movements and Their Role in Visual and Cognitive Processes*, pp. 1–70. Amsterdam: Elsevier.

Kowler E, Anderson E, Dosher B, and Blaser E (1995) The role of attention in the programming of saccades. *Vision Research* 35: 1897–1916.

Kowler E, Van der Steen J, Tamminga EP, and Collewijn H (1984) Voluntary selection of the target for smooth eye movements in the presence of superimposed, full-field stationary and moving stimuli. *Vision Research* 24: 1789–1798.

Lipps M and Pelz JB (2004) Yarbus revisited: Task-dependent oculomotor behavior [abstract]. *Journal of Vision* 4: 115a.

Lisberger SG and Ferrera VP (1997) Vector averaging for smooth pursuit eye movements initiated by two moving targets in monkeys. *Journal of Neuroscience* 17: 7490–7502.

Liston D and Krauzlis RJ (2003) Shared response preparation for pursuit and saccadic eye movements. *Journal of Neuroscience* 23: 11305–11314.

Mach E (1906/1950) *Principles of Psychology, Vol. 1, The Analysis of Sensations.* New York: Dover.

Melcher D and Kowler E (2001) Visual scene memory and the guidance of saccadic eye movements. *Vision Reearch* 41: 3597–3611.

Murphy BJ, Kowler E, and Steinman RM (1975) Slow oculomotor control in the presence of moving backgrounds. *Vision Research* 15: 1263–1268.

Santella A and DeCarlo D (2004) Visual interest and NPR: An evaluation and manifesto. In: *Proceedings of the Third International Symposium on Nonphotorealistic Animation and Rendering*, pp. 71–78. Annecy, France, 7–9. June New York: ACM Press.

Schnitzer BS and Kowler E (2006) Eye movements during multiple readings of the same text. *Vision Research* 46: 1611–1632.

Sheinberg DL and Logothetis NK (2001) Noticing familiar objects in real world scenes: The role of temporal cortical neurons in natural vision. *Journal of Neuroscience* 21: 1340–1350.

Sperling G and Dosher BA (1986) Strategy and optimization in human information processing. In: Boff KR, Kaufman L, and Thomas JP (eds.) *Handbook of Perception and Human Performance Vol.1: Sensory Processes and Perception.* New York: Wiley.

Steinman RM, Menezes W, and Herst AN (2005) Handling real forms in real life. In: Jenkin MRM and Harris LR (eds.) *Seeing Spatial Form*, pp. 187–212. New York: Oxford University Press.

Yarbus A (1967) *Eye Movements and Vision.* New York: Plenum Press.

Relevant Website

http://www.philip.greenspun.com – Philip Greenspun.

Attention: Models

P H E Tiesinga, University of North Carolina at Chapel Hill, Chapel Hill, NC, USA
T J Sejnowski, Salk Institute and University of California at San Diego, La Jolla, CA, USA

Introduction

Our sensory environment is represented in the cortex as the electrical activity of billions of neurons. The neural activity in the visual pathway reflects not only the current visual environment but also the goals and expectations of the organism as well. Suppose that one is at the airport picking up a friend who is wearing a red coat. In general, red objects will activate specific neurons in the visual cortex, but, because they are now relevant to the current goal, their responses will be enhanced and preferentially processed. Selective attention is a general strategy for selecting the currently relevant information out of the overwhelming amount of information that enters the brain via the senses. This article reviews models for selective attention in the visual system at the level of single neurons and the local circuit they are embedded in.

Parametric Models for Stimulus Response Properties of Early Visual Neurons

The response of a visual neuron depends both on the stimulus that is driving it (bottom-up) and attention (top-down). The purely sensory responses of cortical neurons were originally characterized in anesthetized cats and primates and with simple stimuli such as oriented bars and gratings. In the primary visual cortex (V1), many neurons respond best to a stimulus of a specific orientation placed at a specific location in the visual field. The receptive fields (RF) of middle temporal (MT), V2, and V4 cortical areas downstream to V1 are much larger than those of V1 neurons and involve more complex combinations of features.

When an oriented bar is placed at the center of the RF of a V1 simple cell, the mean firing rate varies approximately as a bell-shaped curve with the stimulus orientation (**Figure 1(a)**) that can be approximated mathematically as

$$R(\theta) = R_0 + A \exp\left(\frac{(\theta - \theta_{\mathrm{pref}})^2}{2\sigma^2}\right) \qquad [1]$$

where R is the firing rate in response to a stimulus of orientation θ, θ_{pref} is the neuron's preferred orientation, σ is the tuning width (related to the half width at half height), R_0 is the neuron's firing rate in the absence of the stimulus, and A represents the strength of firing rate modulation. Studies using anesthetized cats and macaques as well as alert macaques to investigate the orientation selectivity of V1 neurons have revealed spontaneous activity R_0 ranging from zero to about 20 Hz and A varying from a few hertz to 100 Hz. The tuning width σ could be as low as 10° with a median value of 30° across all layers in V1 in alert macaque monkeys.

Luminance contrast is the absolute difference in luminance values across the stimulus expressed relative to the background. It is a measure of stimulus strength, and it takes values between zero and 100%. The firing rate increases monotonically with stimulus contrast (**Figure 1(b)**). Mathematically, this relationship is summarized in terms of the contrast response function (CRF), a commonly used expression for which is

$$R(c) = R_0 + R_m \frac{c^n}{c_0^n + c^n} \qquad [2]$$

where c is the contrast, R_m is the maximum firing rate, c_0 is the contrast for which the firing rate above baseline is half R_m, and n is the power of the nonlinearity. Typical values for cat and primate V1 are $c_0 \approx 10\%$, $n \approx 2$. The CRF has three regimes. For low contrast ($c \ll c_0$), the firing rate increases supralinearly as a power of the contrast c. The largest rate of change in firing rate is at medium contrast, around c_0, and the firing rate saturates at high contrasts ($c \gg c_0$).

Orientation tuning is approximately contrast invariant. For a range of contrast values, the orientation-tuning curve has approximately the same shape but a different maximum firing rate (the parameter A). Mathematically, this implies that the rate above baseline can be written as a product of the orientation-tuning curve and the contrast response curve (**Figure 1(c)**):

$$R(\theta, c) = R_0 + R_m \frac{c^n}{c_0^n + c^n} \exp\left(\frac{(\theta - \theta_{\mathrm{pref}})^2}{2\sigma^2}\right) \qquad [3]$$

This functional form reflects a normalization model. A given stimulus activates not only the neuron that is recorded but also a pool of other neurons. The recorded neuron receives input proportional to the orientation-tuned output of a filter L and the

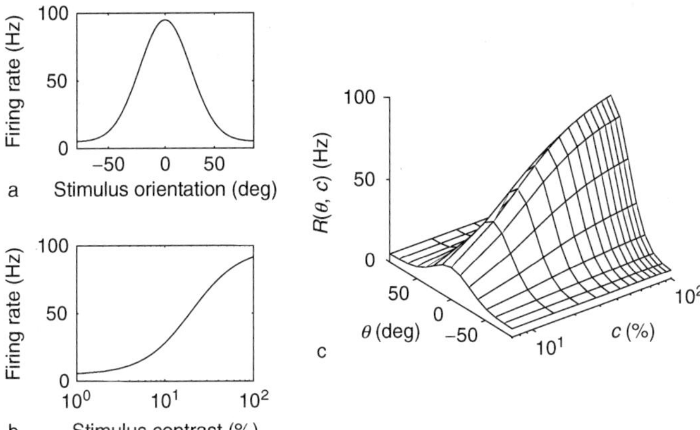

Figure 1 (a) Orientation-tuning curve. (b) Contrast response function. (c) The firing rate, according to eqn [3], as a function of orientation θ and contrast c.

contrast c. The combined activity of neurons in the pool is independent of stimulus orientation, but it increases with contrast as c^n. This activity divisively normalizes the response of the recorded neuron. The normalization model can account for a large number of experimentally measured responses. Model studies and *in vitro* experiments show that a number of biophysical mechanisms yield divisive normalization. An alternative means of achieving normalization involves the short-term plasticity of the synapses onto the neuron.

Parametric Models for Attentional Modulation of Early Visual Responses

The modulation by selective attention of neural responses has been studied in awake nonhuman primates. The strongest modulation of individual neurons was recorded in the MT, V4, and inferotemporal cortical areas, which all are downstream of V1. In one experimental paradigm, two equivalent arrays of stimuli are presented, typically on opposite sides of the vertical meridian. The monkey is rewarded for detecting a subtle change in the stimulus at a cued location. It is not rewarded for reporting a change in a stimulus at the noncued location. Since this is a difficult task, the monkey needs to pay attention to the cued location in order to observe and respond to the stimulus change. The neuron that is recorded has its receptive field at one of the two locations. Hence, the response of that neuron to the same stimulus with attention can be compared with when attention is directed at the location outside the neuron's RF.

Attention modulates the firing rate. For spatial attention, the firing rate typically increases when the neuron's receptive field overlaps with the area where attention is directed. The neuron receives feed-forward synaptic inputs and transforms them into a firing rate. Attention could act in several ways: it could make the feed-forward input stronger, or it could change the gain of the input-to-output transformation. The former is referred to as contrast gain and the latter as response gain. In **Figure 2(a)**, illustrating contrast gain, the CRF with attention (left curve) is plotted together with the curve for attention directed away from the RF (right curve). Attention shifted the curve to the left, which implies that a neuron responds to a stimulus as if it had a contrast higher than its actual (veridical) contrast. Contrast gain has three distinguishing properties. First, with attention the neuron will respond to low-contrast values that it did not respond to without attention. Second, the largest change in firing rate will occur for moderate firing rates corresponding to contrasts around c_0. Third, the saturation firing rate remains the same, but it is reached for a lower value of the contrast than without attention.

Response gain is illustrated in **Figure 2(b)**. The CRF with attention is obtained by multiplying the CRF without attention by a gain factor larger than unity. Response gain can be distinguished from contrast gain. First, if the neuron does not respond to a low-contrast stimulus without attention, neither will it do so with attention. Second, the largest change in firing rate will occur at the highest value of the contrast where the neuron fires at its highest rate. Third, the saturation rate will be higher for attention compared with no attention.

Experiments in a spatial attention paradigm in cortical areas MT and V4 of macaque show that attentional modulation of the CRF is best described as contrast gain. This matches the results of psychophysical experiments: Human observers report that the perceived contrast of a stimulus is higher if it is in the focus of attention. Other experiments on the

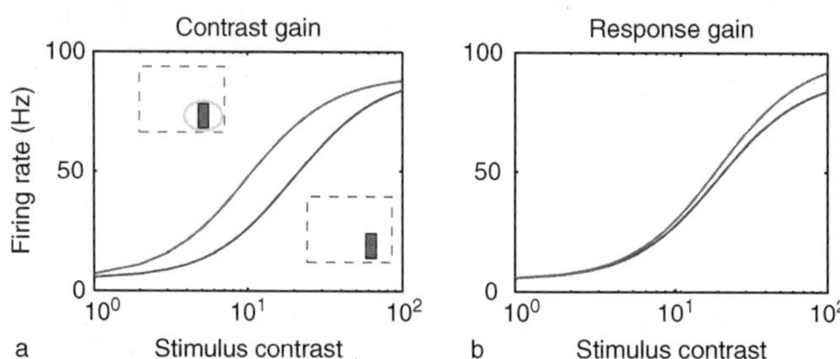

Figure 2 Attentional modulation of the contrast response function when attention is directed away from (blue) or directed toward (green) the receptive field of the recorded neurons. Illustration of (a) contrast gain and (b) response gain.

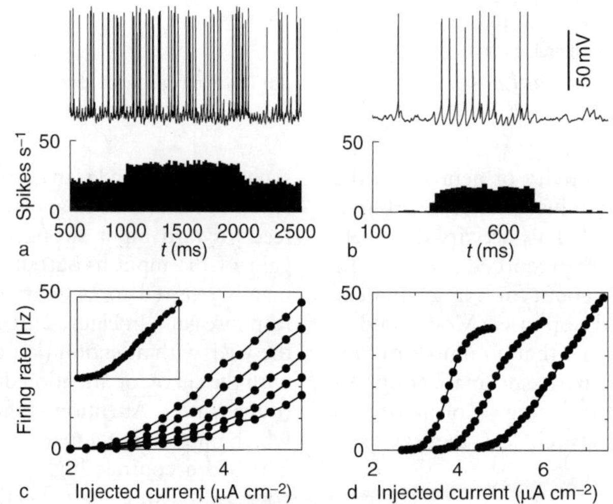

Figure 3 Response gain and contrast gain can be mediated by modulation of inhibitory synaptic inputs. (a, b): (top) Example voltage trace and (bottom) spike time histogram based on 500 trials. (a) The model neuron was driven by synchronous inhibitory and asynchronous excitatory inputs. During the interval between 1000 and 2000 ms, the jitter of the inhibitory volleys was decreased from 4 to 2 ms. During the period of increased inhibitory synchrony (low jitter), the firing rate was increased from 22 to 35 Hz. (b) The model neuron was driven by synchronous inhibition and a constant depolarizing current. During the interval between 300 and 700 ms, the jitter of the inhibitory volleys was decreased from 8 to 2 ms. The inhibitory inputs act as a gate. During periods of low inhibitory synchrony (high jitter), the neuron does not spike, whereas during periods of high inhibitory synchrony, it does spike. (c) and (d) The firing rate vs. current curves. Response gain: in (c) the synchronous inhibitory volleys consisted on average of ten presynaptic spikes, the jitter was, from top to bottom: 1, 2, 3, 4, and 5 ms. Inset: the five curves were made to overlap by scaling the firing rate and by small shifts in the current. Contrast gain: in (d) the synchronous inhibitory volleys consisted on average of 50 presynaptic spikes, and jitter was, from left to right, 1, 3, and 5 ms. Reproduced from Tiesinga PH, Fellous JM, Salinas E, Jose JV, and Sejnowski TJ (2004) Inhibitory synchrony as a mechanism for attentional gain modulation. *Journal of Physiology-Paris* 98: 296–314, with permission from Elsevier.

modulation of orientation tuning curves were best described as a response gain with attention. Overall, there is evidence in support of response gain, as well as contrast gain, depending on the specific details of the behavioral task by which attentional modulation was studied. In experiments designed to study feature-based attention in area MT, effects consistent with response gain were found. The neuron's response was multiplied by a gain factor that monotonically increases with the difference between the attended feature (direction, color, or shape) and the feature value preferred by the neuron. A similar effect of feature-based attention was obtained in fMRI experiments with human participants. The response of MT to a moving random dot pattern was increased when it was task-relevant. In macaque visual cortex, attention led in some, but not all, cases to an increase in baseline rate (R_0).

Thus, the response to a stimulus of contrast c and orientation can be described by eqn [3]. In this expression, attention 'a' enters via the baseline rate $R_0(a)$ and the contrast threshold $c_0(a)$. The effects of attention are consistent with either response gain or contrast gain depending on which stimulus parameter is varied. This form makes a prediction that has recently been confirmed experimentally: the response to a stimulus of nonoptimal orientation should saturate at the same contrast as a stimulus with optimal orientation.

Biophysical Models for Attentional Response Modulation

A biophysical model must account for the inputs a neuron receives from three sources: feed-forward input that represents stimulus aspects (bottom-up), modulatory feedback input (top down), and recurrent connections within the same cortical area (but potentially different layers). The recurrent activity depends both on bottom-up and top-down inputs. Furthermore, the bottom-up input includes the influence of top-down projections on the earlier cortical area. Response mechanisms can be studied theoretically and *in vitro* at the single-neuron level under the assumption that the three sources of synaptic inputs can be split up in two sets of independent inputs, one of which depends only on the stimulus identity and contrast, the other only on the locus of attention. The rate of stimulus-related synaptic inputs depends, as a bell-shaped tuning curve, on the stimulus orientation, with excitatory inputs dominating inhibitory inputs. The attention-related inputs consist of approximately equally strong excitatory and inhibitory inputs. Thus the main contribution of attention consists of modulating fluctuating inputs. Two mechanisms have been proposed that are based on the idea that attention modulates the amount of fluctuation. First, in gain modulation by balanced synaptic inputs, attention causes a proportional change in rates of excitatory and inhibitory inputs such that the variance of the membrane potential changes but its mean remains the same. Second, in gain modulation by correlation, there is a change in correlation between inputs such as the synchrony of inhibitory inputs or the delay between excitatory and inhibitory inputs. Both of these proposed mechanisms are supported by *in vitro* experiments. The basic paradigm is as follows: in the experiments, feed-forward inputs are presented by a constant depolarizing input current I injected at the soma, whereas the modulatory inputs are injected at the soma using dynamic clamp. The firing rate versus current curve (f–I) is then constructed by calculating the firing rate for a set of different values of I in the presence of the modulatory inputs. Chance and co-workers have shown that an increase in the level of balanced synaptic inputs yields a decrease in the gain of the f–I curve. Tiesinga et al. have shown that an increase in inhibitory synchrony also leads to an increase in gain of the f–I or a shift in the f–I along the current ordinate (**Figure 3**).

The single-neuron studies show how the response could be modulated, but they do not provide a mechanism at the local circuit level by which the necessary changes in the modulatory inputs come about. Furthermore, in the model as well as *in vitro*, the inputs were somatic, but the modulatory and feed-forward inputs may impinge at different locations on the neuron's extensive dendritic tree, which could introduce more complex dynamical interactions.

Discussion

This article has focused on the effects of attention on the response of a single neuron to a simple stimulus. Current experimental investigations are extending these results in two ways. First, in higher cortical areas, the receptive fields are so large that they accommodate multiple stimuli. Attentional modulation is much stronger when there are multiple stimuli in a receptive field. Phenomenological models are presently being developed to quantitatively account for these data. Second, even when attention does not change the firing rate, it may change the correlation between neurons. Experiments in V4 show that attention increases the coherence in the γ-frequency range between neurons and the local field potential. This suggests an important role for the synchrony in networks mediating the effects of attention. Future theoretical research is directed at exploring the synchrony hypothesis at the level of the cortical circuit.

See also: Attention and Eye Movements; Attentional Networks; Attentional Functions in Learning and Memory; Neglect Syndrome and the Spatial Attention Network; Sensorimotor Integration: Attention and the Premotor Theory; Visual Attention; Visual Motion Models.

Further Reading

Albrecht DG, Geisler WS, Frazor RA, and Crane AM (2002) Visual cortex neurons of monkeys and cats: Temporal dynamics of the contrast response function. *Journal of Neurophysiology* 88: 888–913.

Bichot NP, Rossi AF, and Desimone R (2005) Parallel and serial neural mechanisms for visual search in macaque area V4. *Science* 308: 529–534.

Chance FS, Abbott LF, and Reyes AD (2002) Gain modulation from background synaptic input. *Neuron* 35: 773–782.

Ferster D and Miller KD (2000) Neural mechanisms of orientation selectivity in the visual cortex. *Annual Review of Neuroscience* 23: 441–471.

Fries P, Reynolds JH, Rorie AE, and Desimone R (2001) Modulation of oscillatory neuronal synchronization by selective visual attention. *Science* 291: 1560–1563.

Maunsell JH and Treue S (2006) Feature-based attention in visual cortex. *Trends in Neurosciences* 29: 317–322.
Reynolds JH and Chelazzi L (2004) Attentional modulation of visual processing. *Annual Review of Neuroscience* 27: 611–647.
Salinas E and Sejnowski TJ (2001) Correlated neuronal activity and the flow of neural information. *Nature Reviews Neuroscience* 2: 539–550.
Tiesinga PH, Fellous JM, Salinas E, Jose JV, and Sejnowski TJ (2004) Inhibitory synchrony as a mechanism for attentional gain modulation. *Journal of Physiology* 98: 296–314.
Williford T and Maunsell JH (2006) Effects of spatial attention on contrast response functions in macaque area V4. *Journal of Neurophysiology* 96: 40–54.

Attentional Functions in Learning and Memory

M Sarter and C Lustig, University of Michigan, Ann Arbor, MI, USA

Attention and Memory: Conceptual Issues

Attention describes a set of cognitive processes which act to optimize stimulus detection, discrimination, and processing. Attention operates in part by top-down tuning of sensory systems to facilitate the detection of selected stimulus characteristics, such as location and modality, by switching the cortical processing from associational to input modes, and by allocating attentional resources to these operations. Different forms of attention have been categorized, such as sustained, selective, and divided attention. Sustained attention describes the subject's state of readiness to detect rarely and unpredictably occurring changes in the stimulus situation over extended periods of time. Selective attention brings targeted information into the focus of consciousness, while suppressing the detection and processing of nontarget signals. Divided attention emphasizes the allocation and the management of limited attentional resources in situations that require attention to multiple stimuli or tasks.

The assumption that attended stimuli are encoded more effectively into memory than less-attended ones is straightforward and supported by substantial evidence. However, theoretical frameworks that more fully describe the relationships between attention and learning and memory (L&M) have remained unexpectedly rare. Furthermore, empirical analyses of interactions between attention and L&M focused on selected aspects of attention and a rather small number of experimental paradigms. For example, increased demands on the division of attention impair stimulus encoding, but generally do not impede the retrieval of previously learned information. Conversely, high demands on memory operations impair attentional capacities, particularly the ability to filter nontarget stimuli from being processed. A second major paradigm used in research on the interactions between attention and L&M concerns the impaired learning of extradimensional shifts, as such shifts require the processing of a previously unattended stimulus dimension (e.g., shape, when one had been attending to color).

Attentional processes and capacities represent a cluster of variables contributing to the efficacy of L&M. At the extreme, it is difficult to envision meaningful acquisition of declarative information in the absence of attention. Furthermore, levels of attentional performance vary considerably, and this variation affects the rate of learning and thus the efficacy of memory. Therefore, it is not unexpected that brain mechanisms mediating attentional functions and capacities are also part of the neuronal circuitry mediating L&M.

Functional neuroimaging studies provide strong evidence for the interplay between attention, learning, and memory. Meta-analytic and experimental studies reveal large overlaps between prefrontal and parietal regions activated in attention and memory tasks that are not shared with other (e.g., language processing) domains. Dividing attention at learning leads to reduced activity in prefrontal brain regions associated with subsequent memory, and has long been known to reduce memory performance. Conversely, recent evidence suggests that higher levels of tonic or baseline activity in regions involved in stimulus perception (e.g., parahippocampal regions for perception of scenes) are associated with higher levels of attention to those stimuli, and with better subsequent memory than those preceded by lower tonic activity. Memory also serves to guide attention: memory-guided visual search activates similar brain regions as does cue-guided visual search, and may even provide greater performance benefits than a visual cue.

In summary, attention, learning, and memory are highly integrated, dynamically interactive processes. This interactivity is reflected both in heavy overlap between the brain systems involved in attention and those involved in L&M, and in the mutual influences of attention on memory processing. The following sections describe the neurobiological mechanisms of attention–memory interactions in more detail.

Neuronal Macrosystems Mediating Attentional Functions and Capacities: Major Research Themes

Both lesion studies and functional neuroimaging provide evidence for a distributed cortical network of prefrontal and posterior parietal regions involved in attention. The specific regions involved vary according to the nature of the attentional task. Demands on sustained attention, irrespective of the modality of targets, activate frontal and parietal regions primarily in the right hemisphere. Selective attention and demands for nontarget filtering recruit cingulate and other prefrontal regions, again primarily in the right hemisphere. Bilateral frontoparietal regions typically are activated by tasks requiring the division of attention between multiple targets.

Ongoing research, particularly experiments employing functional magnetic resonance imaging (fMRI), continues to refine the attribution of aspects of attentional performance to specific cortical networks. Results from this research confirm the conceptualization of anterior and posterior attention systems. Posner and Peterson proposed that the anterior attention system, consisting mainly of cingulate and other prefrontal regions, mediates target detection or the processes involved in the subject's consciousness of a signal's presence through producing a response documenting its detection. The posterior attention system involves the posterior parietal cortex and collicular and thalamic regions and controls management of the visual-attentional space.

Essential insights into the neuronal mechanism mediating attentional processes have been gained from research focusing on bottom-up versus top-down selection of stimuli. Bottom-up selection is a function of the intrinsic properties of the stimulus; stimuli compete and cooperate for detection and processing depending on their salience. Bottom-up, stimulus-driven attention is associated with increases in activity in sensory and sensory-associational regions representing the actual stimuli and their location. In addition, increased activity in frontoparietal networks indicates that stimulus-driven attentional control may also influence the executive management of attentional priorities and resources. In contrast, top-down selection is a function of experience, expectations, or instructions. It involves the tuning of receptive field properties, (sustained) anticipatory activity, and suppression of activity in irrelevant regions or modalities, all in order to optimize the detection and processing of expected targets. Top-down attentional control is generally thought to be executed by prefrontal modulation of parietal networks.

The actual mechanisms allowing prefrontal regions to initiate top-down effects, and the cognitive mechanisms and neuronal circuits mediating such top-down effects have remained largely unclear. Likewise, the neuronal circuitries mediating the bottom-up enhancement of stimulus processing, usually in a highly topographic fashion, are not known. As discussed further below, evidence on the role of neurotransmitter-specific cortical input systems provides the basis for hypotheses about the neuronal mechanisms modulating the detection of stimuli as a function of top-down, voluntary attention versus the bottom-up influences based on stimulus properties (see also **Figure 1**).

Evidence from recent fMRI experiments questioned the widely held view that the suppression of irrelevant information or modalities represents an important aspect of prefrontally controlled top-down regulation of attentional mechanisms. These studies demonstrated that prefrontal mechanisms act to amplify detection of task-relevant information and did not find consistent evidence for top-down suppression of irrelevant stimuli. However, other investigators have found evidence that instructions to ignore one stimulus set in order to more successfully memorize another caused brain activity associated with the ignored stimulus set to be suppressed below a perceptual baseline. As will be further discussed below, the view that selective detection is primarily mediated via enhancement of target stimuli, with little contribution of suppression of nontargets, corresponds with the attentional functions of the cortical cholinergic input system.

Intuitively, motivation is an important factor for engaging top-down mechanisms in order to combat fatigue- or distractor-related decline in attentional performance, to stabilize impaired performance, or to recover from performance impairments. The effects of motivational processes on top-down attention and the neuronal mechanisms via which motivation accesses the anterior attention system to facilitate top-down effects in challenging situations are emerging as an important theme. Increasing the incentives for attentional performance is associated with enhanced activity in frontoparietal attentional networks, and with activation in additional limbic regions involved in processing errors and response outcomes. Hypotheses concerning the interactions between motivational and attentional processes focus on the regulation of frontal–parietal attention systems via interactions with ventral striatal circuitry known to process reward, reward expectation, and prediction errors.

While motivation is a critical factor for top-down attention, stimuli associated with affective information exhibit superior potency for the bottom-up capture of attentional resources. For example, people in a crowded bar manage to ignore the TV until an emotionally charged symbol or action shifts their attention effectively from ongoing activities to the screen. The neuronal mechanisms allowing such stimuli to capture attentional resources and then drive the subsequent engagement of top-down mechanisms are not well known. However, it is safe to hypothesize, as illustrated in **Figure 1**, that such stimuli access the brain's main attention systems via reciprocal connections with prefrontal regions (not shown) and with ascending neuronal systems crucially involved in the mediation of attentional functions.

Neurotransmitter-Specific Projection Systems in Attention and Learning

Substantial evidence supports the hypothesis that the cortical cholinergic input system contributes

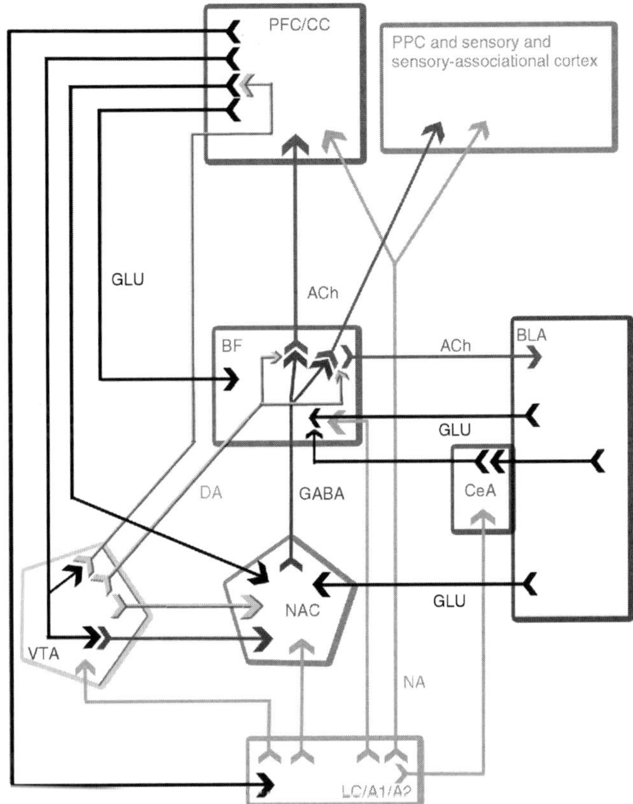

Figure 1 Schematic illustration of the main components of a neuronal network mediating attentional performance and the motivated activation of the cortical cholinergic input system in order to counteract the effects of challenges on attentional performance. The illustration depicts and emphasizes certain direct neuronal projections on the basis of anatomical evidence and importance in the present context. As discussed in the text, neurons using acetylcholine (ACh) as transmitter originate from basal forebrain (BF) regions and innervate all cortical regions, including the prefrontal cortex (PFC), cingulate cortex (CC), and somatosensory and posterior associational regions, including the posterior parietal cortex (PPC). Increases in cortical cholinergic activity contribute to the recruitment of anterior and posterior attention systems and the cholinergic amplification of input processing in sensory and sensory-associational regions. Cholinergic modulation of the PFC and CC is also involved in the implementation of top down mechanisms, and the cholinergic inputs to posterior cortical regions are a component of the prefrontal efferent circuitry mediating such top-down effects. Increases in top-down effects that are a result of challenges on attentional performance, as well as the subjects' motivation to stabilize residual performance or regain normal levels, depend in part on the regulation of BF neurons by direct projections from the dopaminergic (DA) ventral tegmental region (VTA) and indirectly, via the nucleus accumbens (NAC) and its GABAergic (GABA; γ-aminobutyric acid) projections to BF cholinergic neurons. These midbrain and ventral-striatal circuits mediate incentive information and, via feedback from the CC and PFC, information about errors and unpredicted reward contingencies. Therefore, cholinergic modulation by outputs from these regions forms the basis for the integration between motivational and attentional processes. Corresponding with this hypothesis is evidence indicating that control over cortical cholinergic activity by ventral-striatal regions is confined to prefrontal regions. In addition to signals predicting reward or reward loss, stimuli associated with salient affective qualities exhibit potent attention-capturing qualities. The cholinergic and glutamatergic (GLU) reciprocal connections between the basolateral amygdala (BLA), as well as additional projections from the amygdala to the BF via the central amygdaloid nucleus (CeA), are thought to be involved in the mediation of such processes. Finally, ascending noradrenergic (NA) projections originating from the locus coeruleus (LC) and the catecholaminergic cell groups in the medulla (A1/A2) innervate major components of this circuits and also receive afferent feedback from the PFC. Thus, ascending noradrenergic projections are hypothesized to contribute to specific aspects of attentional processing in parallel with those attributed to the BF cholinergic system.

essentially to the mediation of attentional performance. Cholinergic inputs contribute to both top-down and bottom-up modulation of detection processes, and represent a link between motivational systems and cortical attention systems. Originating from basal forebrain regions, cholinergic neurons receive main inputs from midbrain and telencephalic regions, including the prefrontal cortex, and innervate all cortical areas and layers.

Removal of cholinergic inputs results in persistent impairments in sustained, selective, and divided attentional abilities. Furthermore, attentional tasks selectively increase the release of acetylcholine (ACh) from cortical terminals. Evidence suggests that the right hemispheric cortical cholinergic input system is dominant for sustained attention performance; this finding corresponds with evidence from human fMRI studies and from patients with lateralized cortical damage (as described above).

Recent data indicate that in the prefrontal cortex, a transient cholinergic signal is elicited specifically by successfully detected targets, but not by targets that were missed. The temporal characteristics of these cholinergic signals confirm that essential aspects of the detection process are mediated via increases in cholinergic neurotransmission in the prefrontal cortex. These aspects include disengagement from noncontingent ongoing behaviors or from internal, associational processing, as well as the initiation of target-associated behavioral responses. These findings correspond with Posner's original hypothesis that the anterior attention system mediates the detection of attention-demanding targets (as described above).

The cortical cholinergic input system is involved both in the activation of the top-down attention system itself and in the implementation of its downstream effects. Cholinergic inputs to prefrontal regions, including cingulate cortex, specifically contribute to the activation of the anterior attention system, thereby enhancing target detection and activating top-down mechanisms. From there, cholinergic inputs to more posterior cortical regions, including parietal cortex, serve as a branch of the prefrontal efferent circuitry that implements top-down influences on input processing in sensory and sensory-associational regions.

The idea that cholinergic function can be separated into top-down and bottom-up components is supported by the dissociable interactions of these components with other brain systems. For example, ventral-striatal modulation of cortical cholinergic activity is limited to the prefrontal cortex. As described above, ventral-striatal modulation, particularly by the nucleus accumbens, is considered critical in situations characterized by the motivated, top-down increase in attentional effort. The modulation of cholinergic inputs to prefrontal regions corresponds with the role of those prefrontal cholinergic inputs in activating top-down effects.

In contrast, bottom-up, stimulus-driven recruitment of the cortical cholinergic input system is believed to involve recruitment of the entire cholinergic projection system, thereby directly influencing sensory processes while also allowing the stimulus to influence the executive management of attentional priorities. Such broad recruitment of the basal forebrain cholinergic system by salient stimuli is mediated in part by ascending noradrenergic projections targeting the cholinergic neurons in the basal forebrain. Noradrenergic neurons in the brain stem are wired to receive information about visceral correlates of salient stimuli and thus 'import' information about salience to forebrain regions. Support for the hypothesis that noradrenergic–cholinergic interactions are involved in bottom-up capturing of attentional resources by salient stimuli was generated by experiments demonstrating, for example, that the cortical processing of salient stimuli is attenuated by loss of cholinergic inputs to the cortex or blockade of receptors for noradrenaline in the basal forebrain.

However, the ascending noradrenergic system may exert additional and more specific contributions to attentional performance. There are direct prefrontal projections to noradrenergic neurons in the brain stem, and noradrenergic neurons of the locus coeruleus are activated by attended stimuli. Both of these findings indicate that this ascending system is involved in attentional functions that parallel, at least in part, the attentional functions attributed to the cortical cholinergic input system. The overlaps, interactions, and dissociations between the attentional functions of basal forebrain cholinergic and brain stem noradrenergic systems represent an important research topic.

Likewise, the interactions between ascending dopaminergic, cholinergic, and noradrenergic systems likely are essential mechanisms in the mediation of attentional processing. The processing of stimuli capable of predicting reward, including the processing of prediction errors, involves mesolimbic dopaminergic systems. Reward and error signals are capable of capturing significant attentional resources, particularly in response to prediction errors. Thus, interactions between dopaminergic systems and the two other ascending modulatory systems may be necessary to optimize arousal and attentional processing. The dopaminergic recruitment of basal forebrain cholinergic neurons is based on tegmental projections to the basal forebrain, and indirectly on dopaminergic projections to the prefrontal cortex and nucleus accumbens and the innervation of the basal forebrain by these regions (see **Figure 1**). The dopaminergic regulation of the cortical cholinergic input system supports the integration of motivation- and attention-related processing. The prefrontal regulation of brain stem noradrenergic neurons and noradrenergic–cholinergic links represents a second major branch of the neuronal systems which, in concert, regulate attentional processes and resources (see **Figure 1**).

Ascending Modulatory Systems Mediating Attention: Involvement in Learning

Failure to attend and thus to detect a stimulus involves a failure to produce a representation of this stimulus for encoding. Thus, it is not unexpected that the available evidence on brain regions involved in attention matches, at least partly, the prefrontal–parietal neuronal systems critical for L&M. Indeed, given the critical role of attention for effective encoding, efforts designed to dissociate brain regions involved in attention versus learning pose conceptual challenges. It appears that a system of cortical regions processes stimuli at levels giving rise to awareness about these stimuli; however, the source of such processing of stimuli, whether it is a result of attentional or mnemonic operations, is not indexed in these regions.

The overlapping roles of ascending modulatory systems in attention and L&M are less well documented. In fact, several animal studies on the effects of loss of cortical cholinergic inputs have suggested that L&M do not depend on the integrity of these neurons, and that therefore the neuronal circuitries mediating attention and L&M could be dissociated. However, the lack of effects of, for example, lesions of the basal forebrain cholinergic system on L&M in animals may reflect, at least in part, the limited degree to which conventional animal tasks for L&M assess attention-requiring encoding and retrieval of declarative information. By contrast, more recent studies using tasks that require involving attention to stimuli or attention shifts find that learning is readily impaired by manipulations of levels of cortical cholinergic neurotransmission. Recent studies in humans have begun to simultaneously measure the cognitive and hemodynamic effects of drugs modulating cholinergic neurotransmission ('pharmaco-fMRI'). These studies indicated that drug-induced increases in cholinergic transmission enhance attentional mechanisms and the selectivity of stimulus processing during encoding. These results confirm the overlapping role of the cholinergic system in attention and learning, at least in situations requiring the encoding of attended stimuli. Similar conclusions have been drawn based on data from experiments in animals and humans on the role of the noradrenergic system in attention and learning.

Attention and Learning: Relevance for Aging and Neurodegenerative and Neuropsychiatric Disorders

Normal and pathological aging, including mild cognitive impairments and the dementias, are characterized by coinciding impairments in attentional functions and learning.

In nondemented aging, reduced attentional function is typically thought to be the major source of age differences in forgetting. There is some debate as to the nature of age deficits in attention function, with some theories emphasizing age differences in the amount of attentional resources, whereas others emphasize age differences in the allocation of attention, particularly deficits in inhibition. Across these perspectives, there is broad agreement that the controlled, top-down aspects of attention are those that show the greatest declines, whereas more automatic, bottom-up influences are relatively spared. Decreases in top-down attention are often ascribed to atrophy and reduced function in prefrontal cortex and basal ganglia structures, the structures that typically show the largest volume reductions in both longitudinal and cross-sectional studies of normal aging. These changes are thought to be largely responsible for age differences in most areas of cognition, although recent longitudinal evidence suggests that changes in select medial temporal lobe structures may be greater than suggested by earlier cross-sectional studies. Moreover, age-related attentional impairments may be a result of dysregulation and eventual degeneration of basal forebrain cholinergic projections to cortical regions.

The idea that the reduced availability of attentional resources is a major contributor to age differences in L&M receives substantial support from studies showing that asking young adults to divide their attention between multiple tasks (thus reducing the attentional resources available to any single task) often leads to results similar to those of older adults under single-task conditions. This is especially the case when the performance measure is subsequent memory for material studied under divided attention. Like older adults under single-task conditions, young adults studying under divided attention conditions show less activity in left frontal brain areas associated with later successful memory than do young adults studying under single-task conditions. On behavioral tests, the memory costs of divided attention are often similar for young and older adults, but older adults show larger impairments on the secondary task.

On the positive side, reducing the demand for top-down control often improves both memory and brain function for older adults. For example, intentional memory instructions ('memorize the words') require participants to engage top-down control to choose and implement a strategy for processing words that will support their later memory. Older adults typically perform much worse than do young adults under these conditions, and show less activation in left prefrontal cortex areas involved in subsequent memory. By contrast, when given instructions that guide attention to the memory-supporting semantic aspects of a stimulus ("Does the word mean something abstract, or concrete?"), memory is improved, and older adults often show prefrontal activations that are at least as great as those shown by young adults.

While initial findings focused on age-related underactivations of frontal brain regions involved in controlled attention and memory, more recent data show that in many cases, older adults show more activation, or activate additional brain regions that young adults do not. In many cases, this additional activation is linked to better performance, especially on memory tests. Patterns of under- and overactivation of frontal brain regions by older adults may be related to failures of top-down, 'proactive' control, and later 'reactive' attempts to compensate.

A recent meta-analytic review suggested that reduced or disrupted activations may be more common in right anterior frontal regions (often thought to be involved in high-level controlled strategic processing), perhaps reflecting a failure to adequately engage top-down processing to organize efficient task execution. By contrast, left frontal regions were more often associated with greater activation by older adults, perhaps reflecting greater engagement of lower-level processes in an attempt to compensate. Further supporting the idea of an age-related shift to reactive control, memory-related frontal brain activations have an extended time course for older adults under conditions with high control demands (remembering words studied once), but equivalent time courses to young adults under conditions with low control demands (remembering words studied 20 times). This shift is specific to frontal regions; parietal brain regions involved in successful recognition do not show a similar sensitivity to control demand.

Whereas attention and dopamine function are the focus of most research on normal aging, deficits in memory and cholinergic function are the characteristic features of Alzheimer's disease (AD). However, AD is also associated with marked deficits in attention. For example, the ability to divide attention between two ongoing tasks is substantially impaired in AD, even when performance on the individual tasks has been matched with that of healthy controls.

Attention deficits are not easily detected in the earliest stages of the disease, which is primarily marked by memory deficits. However, difficulties with attention precede the breakdowns in language and visuospatial function that occur at the moderate and severe stages of the disease. It is not clear which aspect of attention (selective, divided, or sustained) is the first to deteriorate in AD. Several reports indicate that very demanding selective or divided attention tasks show declines early in the disease process, whereas simpler sustained attention tasks only show deficits at later stages or under conditions (e.g., stimulus degradation) that increase difficulty. However, there have also been reports of preserved performance on selective attention tasks in patients with reduced sustained attention performance.

Within a domain, the detection of AD-related deficits in attention may depend not only on disease severity but also on the specific processes being tested. In selective attention, patients are often able to shift and engage attention appropriately in response to a valid cue. However, they appear to be impaired at disengaging attention from an inappropriate location following an invalid cue, especially if the task involves discrimination of a target stimulus from nontargets rather than simple detection.

For both normal aging and AD, a heuristic description is that attention performance deficits become more obvious with increased complexity or control demand. Functions that require little or no top-down control generally show little or no deficit. Examples include the engagement of spatial attention by the sudden onset of a peripheral cue, or the inhibition of attention's return to a previously attended location.

Deficits can be especially large on so-called 'executive function' tests, which require top-down control in order to override automatic responses driven by bottom-up stimulus characteristics (e.g., moving one's attention away from a peripheral cue in the antisaccade task, responding to ink color rather than word identity in the Stroop task) or to maintain and rapidly switch between multiple response rules (e.g., dual-task procedures). The memory problems of AD may contribute to poor performance on tasks designed to measure attention, as patients may have difficulty both with remembering the response rule and with its execution.

The specific abnormalities in the regulation of integrity of neuronal systems responsible for the age- or dementia-related impairments in attention and encoding are still not well understood. However, structural and regulatory age differences in basal forebrain cholinergic projection have been extensively documented in brains of humans and animals. Furthermore, the development and maintenance of forebrain cholinergic neurons depend on nerve growth factor (NGF) signaling via several neurotrophic receptors expressed selectively by cholinergic neurons. The availability of such receptors is dramatically reduced in the brains of subjects with mild cognitive impairments. Given the central role of the cholinergic system in attention (as described above), these reductions support the hypothesis that the attentional and related cognitive impairments observed in these patients are due, at least to a significant extent, to dysregulation of forebrain cholinergic neurons. Subsequent loss of forebrain cholinergic neurons during the onset and progression of dementia contributes essentially to the severity of impairments in attention and memory.

Impairments in both the activation of relevant stimuli and the inhibition or filtering of irrelevant stimuli are among the fundamental cognitive dysfunctions of schizophrenia. These disruptions of attentional abilities are reflected in impaired L&M. For example, the exhaustion of attentional resources for encoding of relevant stimuli contributes to impaired maintenance and updating of patients' memory, thereby perhaps contributing to the development of aspects of positive symptoms. Abnormal metabolic responses to cognitive challenges have been observed in frontoparietal networks, although the specific neuronal mechanisms underlying the attentional dysfunctions of schizophrenia are not fully understood. However, available evidence strongly suggests an abnormally reactive dopamine system in schizophrenia. Given the role of dopaminergic–cholinergic interactions in the motivational regulation of attentional performance (as described above), both cortical cholinergic recruitment of the anterior attention system and the cholinergic mediation of input processing in sensory and sensory-associational regions are expected to be highly abnormal in schizophrenia. Evidence from animal models of this disease corresponds with this hypothesis, as does the demonstration of down-regulated muscarinic receptors in the cortex of schizophrenic patients. It is widely assumed that abnormalities in the development of cortical, particularly prefrontal, circuits represent a primary neuropathological foundation for schizophrenia. These abnormalities may in turn lead to the dysregulation of the ascending, bottom-up modulatory systems (as described above). Moreover, the dysregulated release of these neuromodulators interacts with defective cortical target circuits, collectively mediating the attentional and encoding dysfunctions characteristic for schizophrenia.

See also: Aging and Memory in Humans; Attentional Networks; Attentional Networks in the Parietal Cortex; Basal Forebrain and Memory; Cognition: An Overview of Neuroimaging Techniques; Cognitive Deficits in Schizophrenia; Executive Function and Higher-Order Cognition: Neuroimaging; Humans; Memory Representation; Prefrontal Cortex: Structure and Anatomy; Prefrontal Contributions to Reward Encoding; Psychophysics of Attention; Reward Systems: Human.

Further Reading

Aston-Jones G and Cohen JD (2005) An integrative theory of locus coeruleus-norepinephrine function: Adaptive gain and optimal performance. *Annual Review of Neurosciences* 28: 403–450.

Buckner RL (2004) Memory and executive function in aging and AD: Multiple factors that cause decline and reserve factors that compensate. *Neuron* 44: 195–208.

Cabeza R and Nyberg L (2000) Imaging cognition II: An empirical review of 275 PET and fMRI studies. *Journal of Cognitive Neuroscience* 12: 1–47.

Corbetta M and Shulman GL (2002) Control of goal-directed and stimulus-driven attention in the brain. *Nature Reviews Neuroscience* 3: 201–215.

Craik FIM and Byrd M (1982) Aging and cognitive deficits: The role of attentional resources. In: Craik FIM and Trehub S (eds.) *Aging and Cognitive Processes*, pp. 191–211. New York: Plenum.

Duclukovic NM and Wagner AD (2006) Attending to remember and remembering to attend. *Neuron* 49: 784–787.

Fernandes MA and Moscovitch M (2000) Divided attention and memory: Evidence of substantial interference effects at retrieval and encoding. *Journal of Experimental Psychology: General* 129: 155–176.

Kruschke JK (2003) Attention in learning. *Current Directions in Psychological Sciences* 12: 171–175.

Mesulam M (2004) The cholinergic lesion of Alzheimer's disease: Pivotal factor or side show? *Learning and Memory* 11: 43–49.

Mufson EJ, Kroin JS, Sendera TJ, and Sobreviela T (1999) Distribution and retrograde transport of trophic factors in the central nervous system: Functional implications for the treatment of neurodegenerative diseases. *Progress in Neurobiology* 57: 451–484.

Perry RJ, Watson P, and Hodges JR (2000) The nature and staging of attention dysfunction in early (minimal and mild) Alzheimer's disease: Relationship to episodic and semantic memory impairment. *Neuropsychologia* 38: 252–271.

Reuter-Lorenz PA and Lustig C (2005) Brain aging: Reorganizing discoveries about the aging mind. *Current Opinion in Neurobiology* 15: 245–251.

Sarter M, Bruno JP, and Givens B (2003) Attentional functions of cortical cholinergic inputs: What does it mean for memory? *Neurobiology of Learning and Memory* 80: 245–256.

Sarter M, Gehring WJ, and Kozak R (2006) More attention must be paid: The neurobiology of attentional effort. *Brain Research Reviews*. 51: 145–160.

Sarter M, Hasselmo ME, Bruno JP, and Givens B (2005) Unraveling the attentional functions of cortical cholinergic inputs: Interactions between signal-driven and top-down cholinergic modulation of signal detection. *Brain Research Reviews* 48: 98–111.

Sarter M, Nelson CL, and Bruno JP (2005) Cortical cholinergic transmission and cortical information processing following psychostimulant-sensitization: Implications for models of schizophrenia. *Schizophrenia Bulletin* 31: 117–138.

Wager TD, Jonides J, and Reading S (2004) Neuroimaging studies of shifting attention: A meta-analysis. *Neuroimage* 22: 1679–1693.

Attentional Mechanisms in Ventral Pathway

L Chelazzi, C Della Libera, and E Santandrea,
University of Verona, Verona, Italy

Introduction

Perhaps the most obvious form of visual selective attention is when individuals turn their gaze toward a salient or otherwise interesting object in their surroundings to align it with the high-resolution fovea of the retina. This allows more detailed processing of the fixated object at the expense of competing objects falling on peripheral regions of the retina. However, it is well established that selective attention can be aimed at extrafoveal locations and objects, thus effectively decoupling the high-resolution power of the fovea from enhanced central processing due to selective attention.

There appear to be several computational reasons why the brain implements selective attention mechanisms. First and foremost, selective attention can be viewed as the mechanism that mediates selection of the next target for preferential, foveal analysis. In this vein, selective attention primarily assists the oculomotor system to optimize sensory sampling of the visual environment, given the current goal. Second, motor systems in general, including those for reaching and grasping movements, are physically constrained and can act only on one (or a few) objects at any given moment. Therefore, selective attention is needed to focus processing onto a single object in order to plan coherent behavioral responses targeted at the selected object. Third, it is probably impossible, or perhaps simply disadvantageous, for the memory systems of the brain to store each and every single object and event occurring within a crowded environment. Therefore, selective attention is necessary to gate access of perceptual representations to memory systems. Finally, perceptual awareness is inherently limited in nature, and it unfolds serially, with a single perceptual representation gaining dominance at any instant in time. Therefore, selective attention is needed to allow entrance of the selected representation into working memory and conscious perception. On top of all the reasons above, students of vision and selective attention raise two further reasons why selective attention may be indispensable, and they are probably related. One reason is that processing of incoming retinal input must be focused on a single object at a time simply because, otherwise, processing and recognition of all objects simultaneously would overcome the limited processing capacity of the system. In addition, and more specifically, directing attention toward a single object at a time might serve the important function of aiding the correct conjoining of all its elemental features, therefore preventing the erroneous binding of features belonging to separate objects in a cluttered scene. In brief, selective attention appears to be a key mechanism aiding efficient object recognition, perceptual awareness, goal-directed behavior, and selective memory storage.

Given the key role of selective attention in visual processing, in particular its role in building and gating object representations, it comes as no surprise that much of the relevant experimental work over the past two decades has been devoted to the investigation of the neuronal correlates of selective attention along the ventral pathway of cortical visual processing. The ventral pathway originates at the level of primary visual cortex, or V1, and nearby secondary visual cortex, or V2, and further extends through extrastriate area V4 and posterior inferotemporal cortex, or area TEO, to culminate in a relatively vast cortical territory occupying the middle and anterior segments of the inferotemporal (IT) cortex. The ventral pathway represents a network of interconnected areas, largely organized according to a hierarchical scheme, whereby object representations are created with an ascending level of complexity and representational invariance. Ultimately, patterns of activity within IT cortex are now known to represent with remarkable speed and efficiency the various objects we are able to recognize. Key nodes along this pathway are represented by area V4 and the various sectors of IT cortex, and therefore this article will focus on these nodes of the pathway.

Studying the Manifestations versus the Control

In speaking of selective attention, one should distinguish between the manifestations and the causal control mechanisms. Specifically, one may use the term 'selective attention' to refer to the modulation of sensory processing along the ventral pathway in relation to concurrent changes in behavioral performance. In this case, the term would index the manifestations of visual selective attention at the neuronal, as well as at the behavioral, level. In contrast, one may use the term selective attention to refer to the signals that, within a given behavioral context, bring about the manifestations of attention considered above. The latter signals may or may not originate within the visual system, and the available evidence suggests that in most cases they do not. This article mainly concentrates on the manifestations of selective attention within the ventral pathway but also briefly discusses available evidence concerning the signals impinging on the ventral pathway to exert attentional control. Several forms of selective attention are distinguished, including enhanced processing of individual attended items, selective processing among competing items (or biased competition), feature-based guidance of target selection in visual search, and finally, feature-selective attention.

Enhanced Processing of Attended Objects: The Beneficial Effects of Spatially Directed Attention

Psychophysical studies of human observers have documented robust effects of attention on visual sensitivity at selected regions of space. Sensitivity has been shown to increase at attended versus unattended locations in the visual field, with relatively shorter reaction times to detect an item at the attended location, as well as greater accuracy. In particular, attentional facilitation entails better detection of faint, low-contrast stimuli and improved discrimination of their features, as if attention to the stimulus led to enhancement of signal strength. In turn, these effects are reminiscent of those produced by an increase in stimulus contrast, and it has been reported recently that indeed attention increases perceived stimulus contrast. Consistent with these behavioral results, single-unit recording studies in the behaving macaque have found enhanced neuronal responses (e.g., in area V4) to a single stimulus presented inside the receptive field (RF) of the recorded neuron when the animal's attention is aligned with the stimulus location, relative to when attention is directed elsewhere in the visual field. As a result, stimuli at an attended location engender stronger central representations than unattended stimuli do. These neural effects likely represent part of the mechanism underlying enhanced behavioral performance, as previously described. Overall, however, enhancement of neuronal responses to individual stimuli presented inside the RF is not very strong, typically on the order of 20%. Furthermore, the effect has not been found in all reported studies, and a possible account of this variability is offered below.

Recent studies of neuronal responses in area V4 have shed further light on the above modulation of responses to single RF stimuli as a function of attention. If the effects of attention are akin to those brought about by increased stimulus contrast, then one might predict that directed attention changes the contrast response function of neurons. Neurons at many stages of the visual system produce increasing responses as a function of stimulus contrast, up to a plateau, and the function takes the form of a sigmoid. If attention acts by increasing the effective contrast of the RF stimulus, then one predicts a leftward shift in the contrast response function of the neurons. In line with this prediction, it was found that attention directed to an RF stimulus causes a leftward shift of the sigmoid relative to when the stimulus is unattended. As a consequence, responses to an attended stimulus will not differ reliably from those to an unattended stimulus at or beyond the point of saturation in the contrast response function. Instead, effects of attention will be greatest within – or just below – the dynamic range of the contrast response function of the neuron. These findings may explain, at least in part, why not all single-cell recording studies have found enhanced responses to attended compared with unattended single RF stimuli along the ventral pathway, including area V4, since attentional effects may be minimal, if any, when stimuli of high contrast are employed. In summary, prevailing evidence indicates that stimuli presented at attended locations will elicit greater responses compared with stimuli at ignored locations. However, the effect is relatively large with stimuli of low contrast, whereas it tends to decrease with contrast of the stimulus.

Notice that there is an important difference between the effects of directed attention and contrast on responses of neurons in visual cortex, including area V4; namely, while attention mimics the effect of contrast in terms of response magnitude, it does not do so in terms of response onset latencies. Response latency has been shown to increase considerably for low-contrast stimuli, whereas no detectable change in response latency is associated with manipulations of attention. This imposes some caution in likening effects of attention to changes in effective stimulus contrast.

An important question is whether directed attention, in addition to changing the strength of neuronal responses, will modify neuronal tuning for the stimulus features, for example, stimulus orientation. This has been addressed in a number of studies, and the prevailing view is that tuning properties of neurons are relatively immune to the influence of directed spatial attention, although they may be modified as a result of extensive discrimination training with perceptual learning protocols. Instead, spatially selective attention has been shown to cause a multiplicative scaling of tuning curves. Responses throughout the tuning curve will be multiplied by a constant factor, with no appreciable changes in the filter properties of neurons. Again, this is similar to the known effect on tuning curves of varying stimulus contrast. Nonetheless, it is conceivable that at the population level, a gain modulation of tuning curves allows finer encoding of features at an attended location than at an unattended one, for instance by reducing the signal-to-noise ratio at the attended location.

Top-Down Control: Biases and Baseline Shifts

Given the distinction between manifestations of attention in sensory processing areas and control signals, researchers have sought evidence for control signals that may cause the manifestations of attention summarized previously. A key feature of these signals is that they ought to precede onset of task-relevant stimuli, that is, they should be present while the animal is attending to a given visual field location in preparation for performing a task on some relevant item. In practice, people have compared baseline activity of the neurons during the waiting period of the task between conditions in which the animal's attention was directed toward the RF of the studied neuron versus when attention was directed toward some location outside the RF. Single-unit recording studies have shown that neurons in area V4 (and V2) display elevated baseline firing during periods when the animal is attending to a location inside the RF of the neuron in anticipation of RF stimulus onset. It is interesting that analogous changes in baseline activity depending on the direction of spatial attention can be observed even when one compares attention to different locations inside the single RF, provided that the locations to be compared are not equally sensitive. Specifically, baseline activity has been found to covary with the strength of the visually evoked responses at any given location within the RF. Increases in baseline activity are typically small in absolute terms, on the order of a few spikes per second. However, in fractional terms, they can amount to a 50% increase in firing rate in the absence of visual stimulation. Therefore they represent a substantial percentage increment in neural activity over a relatively large population of neurons, those neurons with RFs encompassing the attended location.

The accepted account of elevated baseline activity due to spatial attention is that it reflects the influence of an incoming signal, originating in areas of the brain responsible for exerting control over spatially directed attention. In the case of area V4, these likely include areas in the posterior parietal and prefrontal cortices, although subcortical sources (e.g., the superior colliculus) have also been implicated. Recent evidence obtained with low-current electrical microstimulation has directly demonstrated that signals of this sort may originate at the level of the frontal eye fields, and they are capable of enhancing visual responses within area V4 at selected visual field representations. The same type of microstimulation was also shown to improve the animal's performance in a demanding stimulus detection task. Analogous effects on behavior have been obtained with electrical microstimulation of the superior colliculus, although it remains to be established whether microstimulation of the superior colliculus would also enhance neuronal responses in area V4 or other areas along the ventral pathway. In summary, the available data suggest that a number of cortical and subcortical regions are involved in delivering control signals for spatially directed attention, and they largely overlap with critical nodes of the circuit controlling saccadic eye movements. These signals are likely responsible for elevated baseline firing in areas along the ventral pathway when attention is directed to a location inside the RF of the recorded neuron. The elevated baseline firing, in turn, may be part of the mechanism that confers to the neurons increased sensitivity to visual stimulation.

Coherent Firing at the Population Level

Recent work has shown that attention to an RF location may entail, not only elevated baseline firing and enhanced responses to an RF stimulus, but also increased synchronization of firing among the relevant neurons. Increased synchronization may or may not take the form of oscillatory activity, but typically it does. Therefore evidence is rapidly accruing to indicate that when attention is directed to a given location in the visual field, neurons with RFs encompassing that location will entertain an enhanced coherent firing, usually in the gamma-band frequency range, around 50 Hz. In turn, increased synchronization of firing at the attended location may enhance synaptic transmission downstream of the considered neural population, effectively amplifying transmission of information in a spatially selective manner. It is interesting that this effect has also been observed under task conditions in which there was no consistent change in the magnitude of visual responses as a function of spatial attention. Therefore, enhanced processing and spike transmission at the attended location may take the form of increased firing, increased synchronization, or both. It remains to be established whether there are specific task parameters that lead preferentially to one or the other manifestation of attentional modulation.

Competitive Interactions among Multiple Visual Stimuli

A special problem for perceptual and attentional mechanisms to solve is one in which multiple stimuli are presented together (crowding) and an individual must select the relevant stimulus while at the same time discarding any potential distracter, in particular nearby distracters. In neurophysiological terms, this translates to conditions in which multiple stimuli impinge simultaneously onto the RF of an individual neuron and they compete for controlling the neuron's firing pattern. It has been demonstrated that neurons along the ventral pathway, including area V4 and the IT cortex, produce responses to two or more stimuli falling inside their RF that approximate the average of the responses elicited by the component stimuli presented in isolation. In other words, neurons in areas of the ventral pathway seem to be incapable of clutter invariance, a property that, if present, would allow neurons to encode the single most preferred stimulus inside the RF while automatically discarding other nearby stimuli, effectively implementing a MAX operation. In contrast, it appears that multiple stimuli falling inside a single RF, or in its immediate surroundings, compete for the encoding capacity of the neuron, and the neuron's firing is ambiguous as to which stimulus is encoded. It seems that competitive interactions among multiple RF stimuli are only weakly affected, if at all, by the specific nature of the stimuli involved, including the degree of their similarity (but see the discussion of luminance contrast in the section titled 'Top-down versus bottom-up in selective attention'), except that the greatest competitive interactions occur with stimuli far apart in their ability to drive a neuron's visual response, as when a highly preferred or a null stimulus is involved. Under these circumstances, the presence of the null or ineffective stimulus can drive the response to the preferred stimulus well below the level that it would have elicited if presented alone. An important notion that has emerged from these studies is that a stimulus, which causes only modest changes in firing rate when presented in isolation, can nevertheless exert a profound (suppressive) influence on the neuronal firing when presented in combination with an effective stimulus, thus demonstrating clear-cut decoupling between effectiveness of stimuli in driving a response from the given neuron and their effectiveness in determining the firing rate of the same neuron. In terms of the latter property, an ineffective stimulus can be no less effective than a highly preferred, or optimal, stimulus in exerting control over the neuron's activity. In area V4, competitive interactions of this sort have been shown to span a limited extent of visual space, covering the RF size and extending only a small distance beyond the boundary of a neuron's RF. In contrast, competitive interactions sometimes span a much larger extent of the visual field in IT cortex, including portions of the visual hemifield ipsilateral to the recorded hemisphere. However, it has been reported that competitive interactions in IT cortex are much weaker, or nearly absent, when competing stimuli are placed across the vertical meridian, as if competitive interactions could not come about at full strength when they involve the midline commissures (e.g., the corpus callosum). Selective attention mechanisms are needed to resolve these competitive interactions – the core notion of the biased competition model of attention.

Resolving the Competition: Selection and Filtering

The biased competition model of attention has been highly influential over the past decade, as it can account for a great deal of experimental observations obtained with a variety of approaches and techniques, in both human and animal studies of perception and attention. Mathematical and neural network implementations of the model have been developed. The model rests on two tenets. First, as discussed in the previous section, multiple stimuli falling within the RF of a given neuron (or in its immediate surround) compete for controlling the neuron's firing rate. The most compelling evidence of this takes the form of suppressed responses to an effective stimulus falling inside the RF of a cell when it is paired with a second, ineffective stimulus for the cell, with responses to the pair approaching an average of the responses elicited by each of the two stimuli in isolation. Second, competition among stimuli can be resolved when a signal biases the competitive interaction in favor of either stimulus in the pair, thus causing the cell's firing to be primarily determined by the favored stimulus. When this occurs, selective attention is enacted: one of the competing stimuli is selected; the other is filtered out of the RF, or ignored. In cell physiological terms, a neuron's firing to multiple stimuli impinging on its RF as if only one of them were present – the favored one – corresponds to selecting a salient or otherwise relevant stimulus while discarding distracters.

As already considered, the biasing signal for spatially directed attention may take the form of elevated baseline activity of the relevant neural population, but the proposal has been made that increased synchronization of firing across the population of neurons with RFs encompassing the attended location may as well bias competition in favor of the relevant stimulus location. It remains to be established to what extent increased baseline firing and enhanced synchronization are related phenomena in functional terms. Regardless of this, we have already mentioned that likely sources of signals biasing competition in favor of the attended location include cortical areas such as the frontal eye field and lateral intraparietal area, in the frontal and posterior parietal cortex, respectively, as well as subcortical structures, such as the superior colliculus. Future work might well reveal that other parts of the brain, at the cortical and subcortical level, play as important a role in controlling spatial attention.

Selection of a relevant object (or target) among competing stimuli can be achieved not only on the basis of its location in space, but also on the basis of its feature composition. For example, in visual search tasks, an observer is asked to find a target object among irrelevant distracters. Under some conditions, the target may be found easily, at no increasing cost as a function of the number of distracters, such as when it is characterized by some unique property (known as 'pop-out'). In contrast, under less efficient conditions, locating the target may take some effort and increasing time as a function of the number of distracters. By means of search tasks of the latter kind, it has been shown that neurons in areas V4 and IT may contribute significantly to the search process. In particular, as the search process unfolds, neurons in both areas come to encode the target but much less, or not at all, the distracters. Specifically, while neural activity shortly after search array onset to some extent represents all items in the array, later on, in anticipation of the behavioral response, only the target item activates the neural population which is selective for its constituent features, while neural populations activated by the features of the distracters are strongly suppressed. This form of selective attention has been shown to engage underlying mechanisms similar to those engaged by spatially directed attention, except that here, selection is guided by feature information. It has been further suggested that control signals for feature-based selection of a target object likely originate in at least partly different brain regions from those involved in delivering control signals for spatially selective attention. The proposal has been made that feature information specifying the target item and guiding its ultimate selection is represented within brain networks responsible for holding object feature information online during the execution of the task (working memory).

Behavioral evidence obtained following lesion or deactivation of area V4 (and/or TEO) in the monkey is in full agreement with the biased competition model of attention. This work has elegantly shown that, when selective attention mechanisms are knocked out, the animal is at the mercy of stimulus salience. In other words, when multiple stimuli are presented and the animal must select a high-salience target among low-salience distracters, behavior is largely unimpaired. Conversely, when the animal is required to select a low-salience target among high-salience distracters, performance shows a dramatic drop. Consistent with a key role of area V4 in the implementation of attention mechanisms, this deficit has been observed following lesion of area V4 in the macaque, as well as following damage to the homolog of area V4 in the human brain. These findings suggest that, when the mechanisms for cognitively mediated selection are compromised, such as can be obtained through damage to area V4 (and TEO), competitive mechanisms and selection are primarily controlled by the intrinsic salience of objects, the topic of the next section.

Top-Down versus Bottom-Up in Selective Attention

There is now evidence at the single-cell level that competitive interactions among multiple stimuli falling inside the RF of an individual V4 neuron are directly modulated by stimulus salience, such as can be obtained by varying the luminance contrast of the stimuli. As already noted, with attention directed well outside the RF of the recorded neuron (e.g., to the opposite visual hemifield), adding an ineffective stimulus reduces responses of V4 (and IT) neurons to a concurrently presented effective stimulus for the neuron. It has also been recently shown that the suppressive effect is progressively stronger as the luminance contrast of the ineffective stimulus is increased, with the contrast of the effective stimulus held constant at an intermediate level (40%). Although the suppressive effect increases with contrast of the ineffective stimulus, notice that at the same time, the ineffective stimulus presented alone elicits a progressively larger, albeit weak, visual response when its contrast is increased. This again indicates a remarkable dissociation between the efficacy of a stimulus to drive a visual response from a neuron and efficacy of the same stimulus to control the neuron's firing. A stimulus that, for its feature composition, may be largely ineffective in driving a visual response from a given neuron, can nonetheless be highly effective in determining the neuron's response, due to its salience, or strength, such as its high luminance contrast. Moreover, within the same experimental context, attention directed to the ineffective stimulus in the pair has been shown to further enhance the suppressive effect exerted by this stimulus to the point that attention to a high-contrast ineffective stimulus almost completely dominates the cell's firing, namely, it almost completely silences the cell. These findings indicate that competitive interactions are entertained automatically within visual cortex and that competition can be resolved in favor of a high-salience (e.g., high-contrast) stimulus in bottom-up, in the absence of top-down signals reflecting the current volitional control on selective attention.

Feature-Based Attention

As noted previously, selective attention can be directed toward a specific spatial location, or it can be guided by feature information specifying the target-defining properties. Furthermore, behavioral evidence in humans indicates that feature-based attention can affect processing throughout the entire visual field, in a parallel fashion. Consistent with this, single-unit recordings from area V4 of the macaque have revealed the correlates of this form of nonspatial selection. It has been discovered that neuronal responses to any potential target in the visual field – that is, any element that shares one or more of the target-defining features, including the target itself – are enhanced as the search process progresses, long before the animal actually locates the designated target. In other words, this form of feature-based attention is able to 'highlight' all the objects in the visual array that are potentially relevant for the task at hand. Essentially, the mechanism allows privileged processing of these objects, while other objects are effectively filtered out in parallel across the visual array. Although findings of this kind have come in slightly different flavors in the literature, perhaps related to specific characteristics of the experimental protocols, all converge to indicate that among the entire population of neurons in area V4 activated by the array elements, the neurons firing at the highest rate will be those directly stimulated by a feature in the RF that matches the feature preference of the neurons (e.g., red) while the animal is searching for a target item defined by the same feature (e.g., red). Evidently, depending on the currently relevant features, a specific control signal can target the neuronal populations with RFs anywhere in the visual field that are selective for the corresponding features.

Gating-Feature Information, or Feature-Selective Attention

Unlike the form of feature-based attention discussed in the previous section, feature-selective attention is engaged under task conditions in which an individual is asked to identify, or otherwise respond to, a specific object feature while at the same time ignoring other features of the same object. This form of feature-selective attention, therefore, entails that the unity of perceptual objects be broken down in order to cope with the current task. Feature-selective attention plays an important role in many real-life situations, for instance when an individual wishes to sort, or classify, objects on the basis of one elemental feature (e.g., color) and other features (e.g., shape and texture) must be ignored. In addition, this type of feature-selective processing is tapped by a number of classical neuropsychological tests, such as the Stroop test and the Wisconsin card sort test. In both cases, performance must be guided by selective feature information, and interference from the irrelevant feature or features must be blocked. The neuronal underpinnings of the latter form of feature-selective attention have been systematically explored in a recent single-unit recording study in which the activity of V4 neurons was recorded while an animal was attending to either one or the other feature of differently colored, oriented bars. It was found that, under these task conditions, responses of V4 neurons to otherwise identical stimuli are modulated depending on the component feature of the stimulus being currently attended. Most important, it turns out that a large fraction of the recorded neurons are able to cluster the attended features of the stimuli into one or the other of two behaviorally relevant response categories, indicating that area V4 may be important in the process of converting selected feature information into a categorical code available to guide the animal's behavioral responses.

Conclusions

Research over the past 25 years has allowed impressive progress in the understanding of the brain mechanisms underlying the ability to concentrate mental resources on a single location or object at any given time – an essential component of the ability to implement goal-directed behavior. Fundamental pieces of evidence have come from neurophysiological investigations in the awake, behaving macaque monkey. Science is very close to a full understanding of what it means at the single-neuron level to pay selective attention to a specific location or object, or object feature, including the fine details of the circuitry that brings about attentional modulation of firing in visual cortical areas, as well as the source and nature of the signals that control the same circuitry, thus initiating attention-related phenomena at the neuronal and behavioral level. The investigation of the neuronal correlates of visual selective attention along the ventral pathway of cortical visual processing has been particularly successful at identifying specific ways in which mechanisms for selective attention are intertwined with perceptual mechanisms for feature analysis and object recognition.

See also: Attention and Eye Movements; Attention: Models; Attentional Networks; Attentional Networks in the Parietal Cortex; Attentional Functions in Learning and Memory; Decision-Making and Vision; Neglect Syndrome and the Spatial Attention Network; Psychophysics of Attention; Vision for Action and Perception; Visual Attention.

Further Reading

Bichot NP, Rossi AF, and Desimone R (2005) Parallel and serial neural mechanisms for visual search in macaque area V4. *Science* 308: 529–534.

Chelazzi L, Duncan J, Miller EK, and Desimone R (1998) Responses of neurons in inferior temporal cortex during memory-guided visual search. *Journal of Neurophysiology* 80: 2918–2940.

Desimone R and Duncan J (1995) Neural mechanisms of selective visual attention. *Annual Review of Neuroscience* 18: 193–222.

De Weerd P, Peralta MR III, Desimone R, and Ungerleider LG (1999) Loss of attentional stimulus selection after extrastriate cortical lesions in macaques. *Nature Neuroscience* 2: 753–758.

Fries P, Reynolds JH, Rorie AE, and Desimone R (2001) Modulation of oscillatory neuronal synchronization by selective visual attention. *Science* 291: 1560–1563.

Luck SJ, Chelazzi L, Hylliard SA, and Desimone R (1997) Neural mechanisms of spatial selective attention in areas V1, V2, and V4 of macaque visual cortex. *Journal of Neurophysiology* 77: 24–42.

Maunsell JH and Cook EP (2002) The role of attention in visual processing. *Philosophical Transactions of the Royal Society of London, Series B: Biological Sciences* 357: 1063–1072.

Maunsell JH and Treue S (2006) Feature-based attention in visual cortex. *Trends in Neuroscience* 29: 317–322.

McAdams CJ and Maunsell JH (1999) Effects of attention on orientation-tuning functions of single neurons in macaque cortical area V4. *Journal of Neuroscience* 19: 431–441.

Mirabella G, Bertini G, Samengo I, et al. (2007) Neurons in area V4 of the macaque translate attended visual features into behaviorally relevant categories. *Neuron* 54: 303–318.

Moore T and Armstrong KM (2003) Selective gating of visual signals by microstimulation of frontal cortex. *Nature* 421: 370–373.

Motter BC (1994) Neural correlates of attentive selection for color or luminance in extrastriate area V4. *Journal of Neuroscience* 14: 2178–2189.

Reynolds JH and Chelazzi L (2004) Attentional modulation of visual processing. *Annual Review of Neuroscience* 27: 611–647.

Reynolds JH, Chelazzi L, and Desimone R (1999) Competitive mechanisms subserve attention in macaque areas V2 and V4. *Journal of Neuroscience* 19: 1736–1753.

Zoccolan D, Cox DD, and DiCarlo JJ (2005) Multiple object response normalization in monkey inferotemporal cortex. *Journal of Neuroscience* 25: 8150–8164.

Attentional Networks

N U F Dosenbach and S E Petersen, Washington University in St. Louis School of Medicine, St. Louis, MO, USA

Attention is the brain's ability to selectively allocate cognitive resources to those stimuli, responses, memories, and trains of thought that are behaviorally most relevant, at the expense of less relevant ones. As William James pointed out in 1890, "Each of us literally chooses, by his ways of attending to things, what sort of universe he shall appear to himself to inhabit."

Attention can have widespread effects on behavior. It has been known since the time of William James that attention can improve our ability to perceive, conceive, distinguish, remember, and respond. For example, attending to the spatial location at which a visual target will occur decreases the time it takes to respond to it, even when subjects only covertly shift their attention to the cued target location in the absence of overt eye or head movements.

Attention has been shown to alter neural activity. Single-unit recording studies in macaque monkeys placed stimuli in the receptive fields of single cells and compared two conditions: (1) when the monkey was attending to the stimulus and (2) when it was attending somewhere else in the visual field. The classical finding has been that selectively attending to a stimulus increases the neuronal response to it. Similar effects have been seen in neuroimaging studies of selective attention in humans. Selectively attending to the color, shape, and motion of an object, for example, increases activity in extrastriate visual regions specialized for processing these features.

The attention-driven modulation of neural activity is not believed to be inherent to early sensorimotor regions of the brain. Instead, it is thought that so-called biasing signals from higher order source regions influence moment-to-moment processing in sensorimotor regions such as extrastriate visual cortex.

The notion that anatomically separate brain regions may control the selective allocation of attention was initially driven by studies of neglect patients. Unilateral lesions, particularly in temporoparietal and frontal cortex, often cause patients to neglect the contralateral half of extrapersonal space, a condition known as spatial neglect. Such patients may only dress the ipsilesional half of their body, only eat the food on the ipsilesional half of their plate, and only attend to stimuli in the ipsilesional half of their visual field. Studies showed neglect to be a primary deficit of attention, not of sensorimotor processing.

Principles of the Human Attention System

The combination of connectional anatomy, electrophysiology, lesion research, cognitive psychology, and positron emission tomography (PET) imaging allowed Posner and Petersen to build a theoretical cognitive neuroscience model of human attention. This model proposed attention to be the emergent property of a network of functional areas. Posner and Petersen formulated three principles of attentional networks that still seem relevant: (1) The brain's attention system is anatomically separate from those downstream systems that process specific inputs independent of whether these inputs are being attended to or not; (2) attention is the emergent property of networks of distinct anatomical areas, not a single area; and (3) these areas and networks carry out separable attentional functions.

Posner and Petersen focused on three putative classes of attentional processes: alerting, orienting, and detecting targets for conscious processing. Much research since then has expanded and refined this initial set of proposed classes.

Alerting

Alerting is thought to constitute the most basic attentional function. It appears to consist of distinct subfunctions or processes. Intrinsic alertness describes the ability to maintain certain levels of arousal in the absence of cues. It is thought to reflect general increases in excitability, mediated by top-down control signals. Changes in intrinsic alertness can be assessed over longer periods of time (minutes to hours) by measuring simple reaction times to perceptual stimuli that occur without warning.

Alerting subjects to an upcoming target decreases reaction time and error rate. Phasic alerting effects can be documented by comparing reaction time and neural activity on uncued trials and trials for which a nonspecific warning cue provided temporal information about the upcoming trial (**Figure 1(a)**). Phasic alerting may ready task-specific processing pathways for the next stimulus.

Alerting is thought to be supported by the widespread cortical distribution of the brain's norepinephrine system arising in the locus coeruleus (LC-NE) of the midbrain. The reticular thalamus may relay the effect of LC-NE activity to the cerebral cortex. Imaging studies of phasic alerting indicate that the thalamus strongly responds to alerting cues. LC-NE neurons are most active during wakefulness and become silent during rapid eye movement sleep.

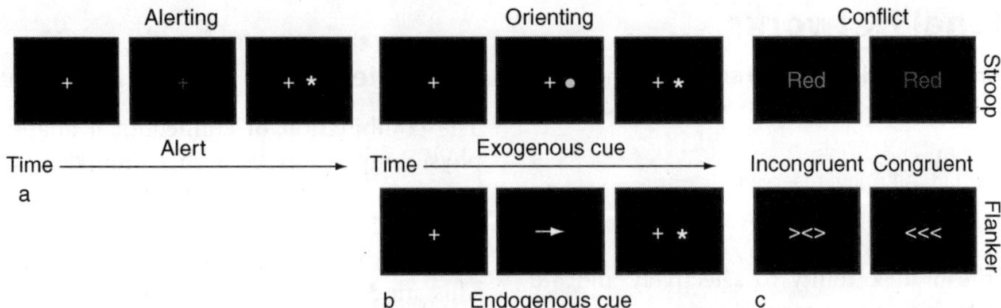

Figure 1 Examples of tasks commonly used to study attentional phenomena. (a) When asked to respond to a target (asterisk) by pressing a button, simple warning cues (e.g., color change of the fixation cross) that phasically alert subjects to an upcoming target can decrease reaction times and error rates. Such warning cues do not carry any spatial information about the target, only temporal information. (b) An exogenous orienting cue, such as a peripheral flash of light, will automatically capture selective attention and facilitate responses at the cued location, starting 50 ms after the cue. An endogenous orienting cue, such as a centrally placed arrow pointing to the right, will also facilitate responses at the cued location, but only after approximately 150 ms. Endogenous cueing effects are mediated by top-down mechanisms, whereas the effects of exogenous cues are thought to be entirely bottom-up or stimulus driven. (c) When the stimulus properties are incongruent, such that the task demands come in conflict with well-trained stimulus-driven responses, performance worsens. In the classic Stroop task, subjects are asked to report the ink color of words. When the word meaning (red) and ink color (green) are incongruent, the overtrained response of reading the word interferes with naming the ink color. In the Eriksen–Flanker task, subjects are asked to report the direction of a central arrow. Responses are faster when flanking arrows point in the same direction as the central arrow (congruent) than when they point in the opposite direction (incongruent). Since executive control processes are needed to overcome stimulus-driven responses, the Stroop, Eriksen–Flanker, and other conflict tasks have been used to study the brain's executive control networks. However, overcoming conflict from incongruent stimuli is only one of the many aspects of executive control.

Salient stimuli cause phasic LC-NE activations and norepinephrine release. LC-NE neurons project to parietal cortex, primary motor cortex, the pulvinar nucleus of the thalamus and the superior colliculus. Anterior cingulate cortex (ACC) and orbitofrontal cortex send strong projections to the LC. Therefore, it has been argued that LC activity might, in part, be controlled by the ACC.

Shifting Selective Attention: Cue Interpretation and Orienting

Attention can be selectively directed toward locations in space; intervals of time; features such as frequency, volume, color, and motion; semantic categories; abstract concepts; memories; and different output modalities. Although spatial attention has been the focus of many experimental studies, it may have its own specific mechanisms and represent a special case. It is important to keep in mind selective attention in its broader sense, which also includes selecting specific internal representations and response configurations.

In studies of spatial attention, the most commonly used analogy for focused selective attention is that of a spotlight. Although simple, this analogy captures the dynamics of selecting specific types of information initially proposed by Posner: disengaging attention from its current focus, moving attention, and engaging it at a new focus. Early PET and functional magnetic resonance imaging (fMRI) studies implicated regions in dorsal parietal and dorsal frontal cortex (DFC) under conditions of selective attention. Since then, lateral and medial parts of posterior parietal cortex (PPC), especially the intraparietal sulcus (IPS) and, more inferiorly, the temporoparietal junction (TPJ), have consistently been associated with shifts of selective attention. Regions in DFC, potentially constituting the human homologue of the frontal eye field, as well as parts of more ventral frontal cortex (VFC) are also widely believed to be important for selective attention.

A distinction can be made depending on whether the focus of attention is shifted involuntarily by a salient stimulus or voluntarily through top-down mechanisms. Stimulus-driven selective attention effects can be measured by flashing a cue on a screen (exogenous cue) and comparing how quickly subjects respond to targets at the cued location compared to a second location (**Figure 1(b)**). As early as 50 ms after the cue, reaction times are facilitated at the cued location. This is in contrast to situations in which cognitive or endogenous cues are used, such as a centrally placed arrow pointing toward one side of the visual field (**Figure 1(b)**) or the word 'right.' If the endogenous cue is valid and correctly predicts the location of the upcoming target, responses are also facilitated. However, these effects develop more slowly and are not measured until 150 ms after the cue.

Based largely on single-unit recording and event-related fMRI studies that can dissociate cue from target-related activity, Corbetta and Shulman proposed that stimulus-driven and goal-oriented shifts of selective attention might be mediated by partially distinct brain networks.

In this model, the right TPJ and parts of the right VFC appear to mediate stimulus-driven shifts of selective attention. The TPJ is relatively unresponsive to endogenous cues that provide information about an upcoming target, such as its likely location or direction of motion. Yet, the right TPJ and VFC are strongly activated by unexpected targets that are thought to automatically capture selective attention. This response to unexpected targets appears to be independent of the task's input and output modalities. Corbetta and Shulman have conceptualized the stimulus-driven attention control system as a circuit breaker that can disrupt the current attentional focus and redirect selective attention in the absence of voluntary control. This apparent right lateralization of stimulus-driven attention control is consistent with the clinical finding that neglect is most commonly due to right hemisphere lesions.

In contrast, bilateral regions in the IPS and DFC appear to be important for the voluntary engagement of selective attention. The IPS and DFC consistently show greater activity when subjects have been endogenously cued toward a specific target property or location than when they have been cued to passively view a display. Furthermore, the bilateral IPS and DFC show anticipatory pretarget activity that is time-locked to the presentation of the endogenous cue. This cue-related activity is more extended in duration than cue-related activity in occipital cortex, which likely reflects purely visual processing of the cue. It has been demonstrated that the IPS and DFC are also active when visuospatial attention is shifted based on long-term memory in the absence of cues.

Goal-directed selective attention signals in dorsal parietal and frontal cortex are not limited to visual tasks. Studies have demonstrated dorsal frontoparietal activity during endogenous shifts of selective attention between different locations in auditory space and different auditory features. Regions in PPC are also activated by voluntary shifts of selective attention between audition and vision. Furthermore, dorsal parietal and frontal regions are thought to covertly orient goal-directed selective attention toward specific movements. Such selective motor attention leads to reaction time facilitation analogous to selective visual attention.

In addition, DFC is thought to select specific movements in anticipation of a response. Single-unit recordings in adjacent parts of macaque PPC, as well as frontal cortex, have documented effector specific anticipatory activity triggered by endogenous cues. Dorsal frontoparietal regions may even be important for selectively attending to specific sensorimotor transformations or stimulus-response mappings, especially when they are simple and well practiced. This is consistent with task-switching experiments that show PPC and dorsal frontal regions to be active when subjects switch between different tasks while the attentional focus remains constant for both input and output.

Executive Control

Executive control of selective attention is believed to be the third major function of attentional networks. Executive control is composed of distinct processing classes related to the instantiation, maintenance, monitoring, and adjustment of attentional sets. The clearest evidence that humans have some voluntary control over the selective allocation of cognitive resources comes from the fact that we can choose to perform many different operations on a given stimulus. Top-down control is critically important for the flexibility of behavior because it allows us to implement arbitrary criteria for input and output selection, as well as stimulus categorization. Without executive control, humans would be automatons limited to a finite number of preset stimulus-response mappings.

The term executive implies that this system is informed about the current task goals. The brain's executive control system likely transmits top-down biasing signals to downstream moment-to-moment information processors, such as visual and sensorimotor cortex. The executive system should have some knowledge of the organizational states of downstream processors. Thus, executive control systems also include a bottom-up component. Executive control regions receive ongoing performance feedback signals that can be used to adjust top-down signals for improved task performance. Behavioral observations have provided insight into top-down and bottom-up signals related to executive control and their interplay. Task-switching paradigms, for example, have shown that under certain conditions reaction times increase on postswitch trials. It is thought that this response slowing reflects the time it takes executive control to clear the previous attentional set and implement a different one.

Despite the importance of executive control systems for behavioral flexibility, their control over the selection of processing pathways is incomplete. When voluntary task goals come in conflict with strong prepotent stimulus-response mappings, behavioral performance worsens. Several well-studied paradigms, such as the Stroop and Eriksen–Flanker tasks, demonstrate the behavioral decrements caused by such conflict (**Figure 1(c)**). For these tasks, reaction times increase when the stimulus properties are such that the task demands are incongruent with a well-learned prepotent response. In the Stroop task, for example, subjects are instructed to name the color of ink in which a word is written. Reaction times are slowest when the ink color and the meaning of the word are incongruent – for example, the word 'green' written in red ink. This response slowing is likely caused by competition between the voluntarily adopted task goals and the prepotent trained behavior of automatically reading the word.

Because top-down control over information processing is incomplete, executive systems are thought to receive feedback information about action outcomes so that top-down biasing signals can be adjusted as needed. The executive control system is thought to adjust the attentional set when performance, as indexed by slow reaction times or errors, is poor. Reaction time changes that are dependent on the nature of the previous trial are thought to reflect such trial-by-trial adjustments of control parameters. Often, reaction times will be systematically slower on the trial following an error, suggesting top-down adjustments of the attentional set. In the Stroop task, the average response time to an incongruent stimulus is faster if the preceding stimulus was incongruent than if it was congruent (**Figure 1(c)**). It has been proposed that adjustments of top-down biasing signals triggered by incongruent stimuli facilitate performance on subsequent trials.

Regions in dorsal anterior cingulate cortex/medial superior frontal cortex (dACC/msFC), dorsolateral prefrontal cortex (dlPFC), and anterior prefrontal cortex (aPFC) have been consistently associated with different executive control processes by a wide range of experimental approaches. The anterior insula/frontal operculum (aI/fO) has also been shown to play an important role in executive control. Although the brain's executive control network comprises all of these regions, each one of them likely carries out a slightly different executive control function.

The dACC/msFC is thought to play a central role in the exertion of executive control. It is believed to be essential for relating goal-oriented behavior to its outcomes. Evidence for the notion that the dACC/msFC carries out several important executive control processes comes from a variety of sources. Lesions of the dACC/msFC can lead to difficulties with the voluntary initiation and maintenance of complex behaviors, whereas more automatic stimulus-driven behavior is spared. In addition, dACC/msFC lesions can affect one's ability to correct task performance following an error.

Since executive control maintains the task goals, sustained neural activity is thought to be its hallmark feature. Maintenance activity has been measured in the dACC/msFC between a cue and the subsequent trial, as well as sustained across a whole block of trials. The dACC/msFC is activated by instructional cues that provide information about the task demands indicating that it is important for the instantiation of attentional sets. It also shows activity related to switching between tasks. Meta-analyses of neuroimaging studies have shown the dACC/msFC to be active for a wide variety of cognitive operations, which is consist with the idea that the dACC/msFC exerts executive control independent of the specific processing domain.

Besides signals thought to be related to the exertion of top-down control, a range of apparent feedback signals have also been measured in the dACC/msFC. Human neuroimaging studies have shown activation differences in the dACC/msFC related to errors, error likelihood, conflict, monetary loss and gain, pain, dread, social rejection, and expectancy violations. In addition, the dACC/msFC also carries domain-independent target detection signals.

Several experimental approaches besides human fMRI have shown that the dACC/msFC may help monitor behavior for errors. Event-related potentials (ERPs), for example, show a negative difference wave localized to the dACC/msFC when correct and error trials are compared. This effect, termed error-related negativity (ERN), is time-locked to the occurrence of the error. It has also been suggested that the dACC/msFC monitors conflict on a trial-by-trial basis. ERP studies have shown a difference wave when comparing congruent and incongruent stimuli localized to the dACC/msFC, labeled conflict-related-negativity (CRN; N450). Event-related fMRI studies have shown greater activity for high-conflict (incongruent) than low-conflict (congruent) trials in the dACC/msFC independent of input and processing domain.

It has been suggested that closely adjacent frontal midline structures may carry out different executive control functions. More posterior and dorsal msFC may implement attentional sets, whereas a slightly more anterior and ventral region in the dACC helps guide behavior by integrating actions and their outcomes. Imaging studies that compared self-guided actions to experimenter-guided ones showed greater activity for self-guided actions in the msFC. In contrast, the dACC did not show a preference for self-initiated movements. Instead, activity related to contingency-based learning and decision making has been documented in the dACC.

A region on the border of the anterior insula (aI) and frontal operculum (fO) has shown executive control properties very similar to the dACC/msFC. Imaging studies have shown the aI/fO to be coactivated with the dACC/msFC across a wide range of tasks.

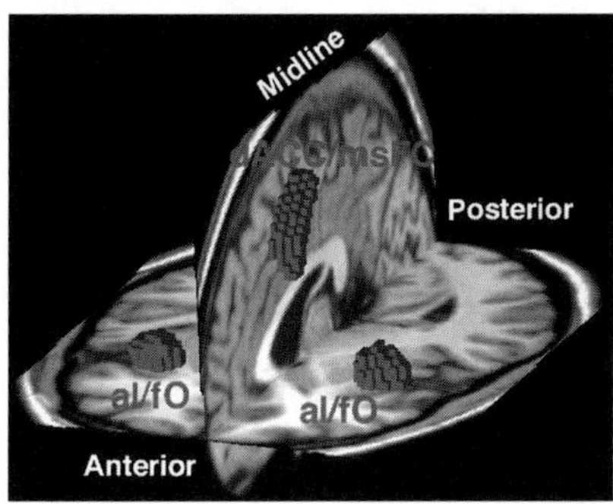

Figure 2 The dorsal anterior cingulate cortex/medial superior frontal cortex (dACC/msFC) has consistently shown activity related to attentional control. A cross-studies analysis of fMRI experiments documented attention-related signals in the dACC/msFC and bilateral anterior insula/frontal operculum (aI/fO). Across tasks, the dACC/msFC and aI/fO showed cue-related alerting/orienting as well as sustained task set-maintenance activity and error-related feedback signals important for executive control. Reproduced from Dosenbach NU, Visscher KM, Palmer ED, et al. (2006) A core system for the implementation of task sets. *Neuron* 50: 799–812, with permission from Elsevier.

Activation maps reveal that the bilateral aI/fO carries goal-maintenance and instantiation activity, as well as many of the same performance monitoring signals as the dACC/msFC (**Figure 2**). Similar to dACC/msFC lesions, strokes of the aI can lead to a reduction of self-initiated goal-directed activity.

It stands to reason that some brain regions may integrate executive control processes related to the instantiation, maintenance, monitoring, and adjustment of top-down biasing signals. Consistent with this notion, a cross-studies analysis showed that the dACC/msFC and aI/fO carried activity related to cue processing and the maintenance and monitoring/adjustment of attentional sets across a wide range of tasks. Therefore, it has been proposed that the bilateral aI/fO and dACC/msFC could form a domain-independent core of the human executive control network (**Figure 2**).

Regions in aPFC and dlPFC appear to support somewhat different executive control functions from the dACC/msFC and aI/fO. It is thought that the aPFC is especially important for the generation and maintenance of strategic plans, especially when they involve subgoaling and the integration of different types of information. It has also been proposed that aPFC neurons may adaptively code for different stimulus categorizations depending on the task goals. Humans with aPFC lesions often have difficulties solving complex tasks that require strategic planning. The maintenance of task contingencies, rules, and plans seems to be especially impaired by aPFC lesions. A series of fMRI experiments have documented sustained signals in the aPFC likely related to the maintenance of attentional sets and complex rules. However, this attentional set-maintenance activity was not common across all tasks. aPFC maintenance signals seem to be selectively recruited by more complex categorizations. Consistent with these findings, a meta-analysis of neuroimaging studies showed that the contrasts highlighting lateral aPFC had compared activity on trials with slow reaction times to activity on faster trials. In addition, neuroimaging studies have also shown activity related to switching between different task sets and stimulus categorizations in aPFC.

dlPFC may be specifically important for trial-by-trial adjustments of attentional control parameters. Consistent with this idea, an ERP study has shown that right dlPFC lesions increase errors and alter the ERN. Some dlPFC lesion patients fail to correct their errors and show no improvements during extended performance of complex cognitive tasks. Human fMRI studies have also shown greater dlPFC activity on error than correct trials. In contrast to the dACC/msFC, the dlPFC does not appear to carry conflict-related signals as measured by fMRI. According to the conflict-monitoring hypothesis, dlPFC functions as 'active memory in the service of control.' This hypothesis postulates that the dACC/msFC sends signals about needed adjustments in control parameters to the dlPFC, which helps to adjust attentional control parameters accordingly. In contrast, based on ERP data it has been argued that the dlPFC may be sending signals to the dACC/msFC, which in turn adjusts top-down biasing signals. Perhaps dlPFC maintains information about planned control adjustments from one trial to the next, whereas the dACC/msFC and aI/fO maintain the basic task parameters for the entire time period during which subjects are performing a specific task. The dlPFC may send adjustment-related signals directly to downstream processors, or it may transmit them to the dACC/msFC for downstream implementation.

Integration of Attentional Processes

The conceptual separation of attentional processes related to alerting, selective attention shifting (orienting), and executive control was initially based on differences in the behavioral effects of alerting, visuospatial cueing, and conflict. Although brain regions preferentially carry signals related to alerting, selective attention shifting, and executive control, these functions likely do not occur completely independently from each other. The brain's putative alerting, attention shifting, and executive control networks must communicate.

The executive control network needs to receive information about the meaning of sensory cues from both the alerting and the attention shifting networks so that it can implement the appropriate attentional settings. Conversely, the executive control network is thought to maintain the task goals according to which the attention-shifting network directs endogenous selective attention. It has even been shown that some stimulus-driven shifts in selective attention are contingent on the underlying attentional set. A stimulus that would not normally capture selective attention may do so if the subject is already searching for a feature shared by the stimulus. Voluntary changes in intrinsic alertness indicate that the executive control network can, at least indirectly, affect LC-NE activity.

Some data suggest that dACC/msFC and aI/fO may integrate several different executive control functions. It seems possible that dACC/msFC and aI/fO may also receive warning signals from the brain's alerting network, as well as information about the meaning of cues and attentional shifts from regions in PPC and frontal cortex. Perhaps specific nodes in each of the attentional networks form bridges between them that allow for an integration of attentional functions. Although distinct networks of brain regions support alerting, attention-shifting, and executive control functions, attention is likely a property that emerges from the interactions between these networks. One speculative idea is that the integration of attentional functions may be helped by the implementation of a basic goal-oriented task mode. This focused attention mode may stand in a mutually exclusive push–pull relationship with the brain's default mode.

See also: Attention and Eye Movements; Attention: Models; Attentional Functions in Learning and Memory; Attentional Mechanisms in Ventral Pathway; Attentional Networks in the Parietal Cortex; Decision-Making and Vision; Executive Function and Higher-Order Cognition: Definition and Neural Substrates; Frontal Lobe Syndrome; Neglect Syndrome and the Spatial Attention Network; Prefrontal Cortex: Structure and Anatomy; Psychophysics of Attention; Spatial Cognition and Executive Function; Visual Attention.

Further Reading

Aston-Jones G, Rajkowski J, and Cohen J (1999) Role of locus coeruleus in attention and behavioral flexibility. *Biological Psychiatry* 46: 1309–1320.

Braver TS, Reynolds JR, and Donaldson DI (2003) Neural mechanisms of transient and sustained cognitive control during task switching. *Neuron* 39: 713–726.

Bunge SA, Wallis JD, Parker A, et al. (2005) Neural circuitry underlying rule use in humans and nonhuman primates. *Journal of Neuroscience* 25: 10347–10350.

Corbetta M, Kincade MJ, Lewis C, et al. (2005) Neural basis and recovery of spatial attention deficits in spatial neglect. *Nature Neuroscience* 8: 1603–1610.

Corbetta M and Shulman GL (2002) Control of goal-directed and stimulus-driven attention in the brain. *Nature Reviews Neuroscience* 3: 201–215.

Corbetta M, Shulman GL, Miezin FM, and Petersen SE (1995) Superior parietal cortex activation during spatial attention shifts and visual feature conjunction. *Science* 270: 802–805.

Dosenbach NU, Visscher KM, Palmer ED, et al. (2006) A core system for the implementation of task sets. *Neuron* 50: 799–812.

Duncan J and Owen AM (2000) Common regions of the human frontal lobe recruited by diverse cognitive demands. *Trends in Neurosciences* 23: 475–483.

Eriksen CW and Hoffman JE (1973) The extent of processing of noise elements during selective encoding from visual displays. *Perception and Psychophysics* 14: 155–160.

Gehring WJ and Knight RT (2000) Prefrontal–cingulate interactions in action monitoring. *Nature Neuroscience* 3: 516–520.

James W (1890) *The Principles of Psychology.* New York: Holt.

Lau HC, Rogers RD, Haggard P, and Passingham RE (2004) Attention to intention. *Science* 303: 1208–1210.

Miller EK and Cohen JD (2001) An integrative theory of prefrontal cortex function. *Annual Review of Neuroscience* 24: 167–202.

Posner MI and Petersen SE (1990) The attention system of the human brain. *Annual Review of Neuroscience* 13: 25–42.

Posner MI, Snyder CRR, and Davidson BJ (1980) Attention and the detection of signals. *Journal of Experimental Psychology: General* 109: 160–174.

Raz A and Buhle J (2006) Typologies of attentional networks. *Nature Reviews Neuroscience* 7: 367–379.

Rushworth MF, Walton ME, Kennerley SW, and Bannerman DM (2004) Action sets and decisions in the medial frontal cortex. *Trends in Cognitive Science* 8: 410–417.

Sakai K and Passingham RE (2003) Prefrontal interactions reflect future task operations. *Nature Neuroscience* 6: 75–81.

Stroop JR (1935) Studies of interference in serial verbal reactions. *Journal of Experimental Psychology* 18: 643–662.

Weissman DH, Gopalakrishnan A, Hazlett CJ, and Woldorff MG (2005) Dorsal anterior cingulate cortex resolves conflict from distracting stimuli by boosting attention toward relevant events. *Cerebral Cortex* 15: 229–237.

Attentional Networks in the Parietal Cortex

G H Patel, B J He, and M Corbetta, Washington University School of Medicine, St. Louis, MO, USA

Introduction

The brain is continuously flooded with information from different senses: vision, audition, touch, smell, and taste. As the inflow of sensory information is much greater than what the brain can process at any given time, one of the fundamental interests of neuroscience is to understand which brain mechanisms are responsible for the selection of those few bits of information that are relevant to the ongoing goals of an individual, and how irrelevant information is filtered out. Attended objects tend to be perceived and remembered much better than unattended objects are, and only objects that are attended become the target of motor plans, such as when we look at and reach for an apple. Accordingly, attention is defined as the ensemble of psychological and neural operations that mediate selection of sensory stimuli and link them to response and memory systems.

The parietal lobe, from the Latin *paries*, or 'walls of a house,' is the part of the brain that sits between the occipital, temporal, and frontal lobes, and that includes the lateral superior part of each hemisphere. The parietal lobe is situated between sensory (visual, tactile, and auditory) areas and contains cells that respond predominantly to behaviorally relevant stimuli. The parietal lobe is also active when individuals prepare to look or move toward a stimulus, and is heavily connected with the frontal lobe, in which the actions are planned. The parietal lobe of the brain is therefore well suited to perform operations that are neither strictly sensory nor motor, but rather operations that integrate sensory and motor information. Because of the integrative nature of the parietal lobe, the functions of the cortical areas contained within it are complex and diverse, and damage to the parietal lobe often results in multifaceted deficits.

In this article we first describe the anatomical organization of the parietal lobe; next, we turn to what we know about the functional organization of parietal cortex, and finally, we consider some of the behavioral deficits that arise after it is damaged.

Organization and Connectivity

The parietal lobe is bordered on the posterior and ventral sides by visual and auditory cortex, respectively, and the anterior portion of the parietal lobe is occupied by somatosensory cortex. Anterior to the parietal lobe is the frontal lobe, much of which is devoted to the planning and execution of movements. The parietal lobe is divided into smaller parts based on gross anatomy. The most prominent anatomical feature of the parietal lobe is the intraparietal sulcus (IPS), which runs anterior–posteriorly along the lateral aspect of the parietal lobe. The IPS divides the parietal lobe into two lobules: the superior parietal lobule (SPL), which encompasses the lateral aspect of the parietal lobe dorsal to the IPS as well as the medial wall, and the inferior parietal lobule (IPL), which encompasses all of the parietal lobe ventral to the IPS. The part of the parietal lobe on the medial wall is also often called the precuneus.

Using histological techniques, investigators have subdivided the parietal lobe in several ways. Perhaps one of the best known schemes for subdividing parietal cortex was proposed by Brodmann in 1909. In this scheme, the human parietal cortex is subdivided into seven areas: areas 1–3, which comprise the anterior edge of the parietal lobe and cover somatosensory cortex; area 5, which is immediately posterior to area 2 and covers the anterior part of the SPL; area 7, which is posterior to area 5 and covers much of the lateral and medial SPL and some of the IPL; and areas 39 and 40, which cover much of the IPL (see **Figure 1(a)**). Beyond these coarse divisions, however, not much was known for many years about the anatomical organization of parietal cortex, in part because invasive techniques necessary to trace connections and study the function of this part of the brain in humans were not available. As a result, most of the detailed information that we have on the parietal lobe's organization and on other parts of the human brain comes from anatomical and physiological studies of nonhuman primates, especially macaques, the brains of which share many of the same sensory and motor functions of the human brain.

The gross and histological organization of macaque parietal lobe is similar to that of the human parietal lobe in many ways: an IPS separates the parietal lobe into an SPL and IPL, somatosensory cortex makes up the anterior edge of the parietal lobe, and visual areas lie along the posterior edge. Areas 1, 2, 3, 5, and 7 are also present in macaque; however, the relative position of areas 5 and 7 is more ventral, given that areas 39 and 40, which occupy the ventral part of the human IPL, are not present in the macaque (see **Figure 1(b)**). Despite these potential differences, the macaque continues to serve as a useful model of how human parietal areas may be involved in attention.

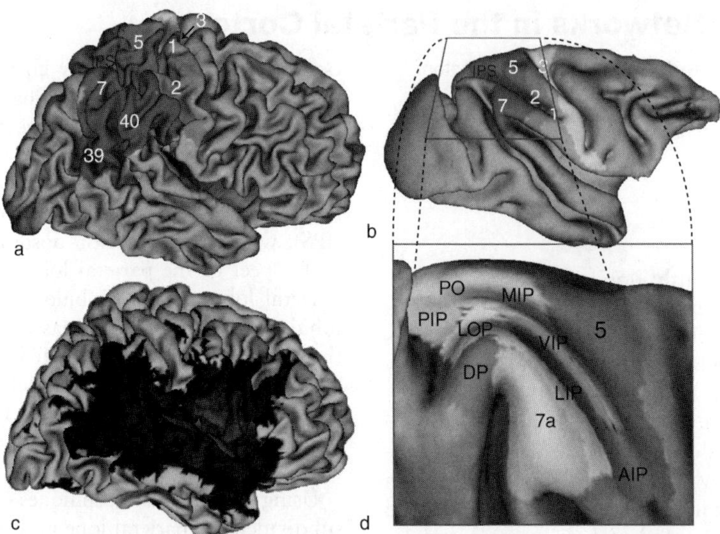

Figure 1 (a) Human Brodmann areas 1–3, 5, 7, 39, and 40, and the intraparietal sulcus (IPS). (b) Macaque Brodmann areas. (c) Cortical damage underlying neglect. (d) Areas in and around the macaque IPS (PO, parietal-occipital; MIP, medial intraparietal; PIP, posterior intraparietal; LOP, lateral occipitoparietal zone; VIP, ventral intraparietal; DP, dorsal prelunate; AIP, anterior intraparietal; 5, area 5; 7a, area 7a). Adapted from Lewis JW and Van Essen DC (2000) Mapping of architectonic subdivisions in the macaque monkey, with emphasis on parieto-occipital cortex. *Journal of Comparative Neurology* 428: 79–111.

In the 1970s, the advent of anatomical methods to trace connections between areas allowed for the partition of posterior parietal cortex into multiple areas based on their profile of feed-forward and feedback connections. Feed-forward connections refer to connections from lower to higher levels of a sensory hierarchy of cortical areas, whereas feedback connections refer to connections from higher to lower levels. There are several proposed schemes to divide the parietal cortex. Along the IPS, one common scheme divides the cortex into ten areas: dorsal prelunate (DP), posterior intraparietal (PIP), parietal-occipital (PO), the lateral occipitoparietal zone (LOP), medial intraparietal (MIP), ventral intraparietal (VIP; divided into medial and lateral), lateral intraparietal (LIP; divided into dorsal and ventral), anterior intraparietal (AIP), area 5, and area 7a (see **Figure 1(d)**). Other similar schemes have also been proposed. Tracer studies have shown that these areas receive input from other brain structures involved in the processing of vision, audition, and sensation, and may send output to the same sensory areas and/or to various motor and motor-planning areas. The IPS areas residing more posteriorly and laterally receive most of their input from visual areas and send output to oculomotor structures, whereas the more medial and anterior areas also receive input from somatosensory areas and send output to hand and arm motor areas.

For an area to be involved in the selective operations of visual spatial attention, it is likely to be connected to the visual areas responsible for the processing of incoming stimuli. It is also likely to be connected to areas involved in the planning and execution of saccades, since after the selection of a stimulus of interest, a saccade is often made to bring the stimulus into the fovea for further scrutiny. Area LIP in the macaque fits this description. It occupies the caudal half of the lateral bank of the IPS, and is demarcated histologically from surrounding parietal areas by increased myelination of layers 3–5. This area receives feed-forward connections from and sends feedback connections to many extrastriate visual areas, including areas V4, V3a, and middle temporal complex (MT), an area known to be involved in processing visual motion. LIP is also heavily interconnected with oculomotor structures, such as the superior colliculus in the midbrain, the pulvinar in the thalamus, and the frontal eye fields (FEFs) in prefrontal cortex.

Area 7a has a profile of connections with cortical areas similar to that of LIP, except rather than FEF, it is connected with area 46 in prefrontal cortex. Area 46 is an area known to be involved in spatial working memory, implying that 7a may also play a role in working memory and attention. Other posterior parietal areas, such as DP and PO, connect mainly with extrastriate areas and more anterior IPS areas, such as LIP, indicating that they play a role in relaying information from visual cortex to the higher level planning areas in IPS.

In general, the many anatomical studies of parietal cortex over the past several decades have shown that it appears to be divided into many areas, each of which appears to play a role in translating sensory information into motor plans. But what exactly this role entailed remained a mystery until the technology to study these areas *in vivo* was developed, first in macaques and then later in humans.

Function

In 1975 Mountcastle and colleagues first reported on electrophysiological recordings of macaque parietal cortex neurons while the monkey performed various tasks. They found that neurons in the IPS "appear[ed] to direct visual attention to objects of interest and motivational power, and to issue commands for maintaining directed fixation of the object when it [was] stationary, and to track it if it mov[ed]." In the decades since these early experiments, electrophysiological recordings of parietal cortex neural activity have determined that the SPL and IPL are subdivided into many smaller functional areas that appear to roughly correspond with the subdivisions determined by histological techniques.

Each of these areas appears to extract the spatial information from one or more sensory inputs, and then play some role in transforming that information into a general movement plan in the same spatial coordinates. Because of its involvement in spatial processing, the parietal cortex is said to be part of the 'where' pathway (as opposed to the ventral 'what' pathway, which appears to be involved in processing the identity of a stimulus regardless of spatial location). For instance, the area LIP is involved in the planning of upcoming saccadic eye movements. The neurons in this area respond transiently to visual stimuli presented within a specific part of the visual field, which is known as a receptive field. Moreover, if a saccade is to be performed to that stimulus at some point in the future, the neurons continue to fire until the saccade has been executed. In this way, they are said to represent the planned target of the saccade until the action is completed, even if the visual stimulus is no longer in the receptive field. This characteristic is often used to define the boundaries of LIP in electrophysiological recording experiments. LIP neurons have large visual receptive fields that cover on average a quarter of the visual field, and these receptive fields move with the position of gaze (gaze centered). They are also more likely to respond to stimuli in the contralateral visual hemifield than in the ipsilateral, and may contain a coarse but continuous map of the contralateral visual field (otherwise known as being retinotopically organized). LIP neurons, then, appear to represent the plan of an upcoming saccadic eye movement in a rough spatial map of the visual environment.

LIP neurons will also respond to a visual stimulus that is not the target of a planned saccade, but is otherwise task relevant. For instance, if the monkey is instructed to maintain fixation on a central point, and to indicate with his hand when a visual stimulus in the periphery dims just slightly, the LIP neurons representing the location of this stimulus continue to fire until the task is completed, and this increased level of firing is directly correlated to increased performance of whatever perceptual decision needs to be made at that location. Moreover, chemically deactivating LIP will result in the reduction of the monkey's ability to discriminate an oddball stimulus from other stimuli (such as a red circle among a field of green circles). It appears, then, that LIP neurons also represent the current locus of visuospatial attention.

Are these two purported functions of LIP neurons in conflict, or do they represent two ways of saying the same thing? The answer to this has been the source of a contentious debate. Thus far we have seen that LIP is involved both in covert shifts of attention (marking a location of interest so that processing of objects in that location can be enhanced) and in overt shifts of attention (making a saccade to a location so that it can be studied in more detail). One side of the debate holds that all covert shifts of attention represent potential saccades, and that the enhanced processing at that location is merely a side effect of planning a movement to that location. As evidence for this view, they point to other parietal areas, which appear to play the same planning role for other effectors, such as arm and hand movements. The 'intentional map,' then, might be a general principle of what the parietal cortex contributes to a sensorimotor transformation. The other side, however, contends that the LIP is a 'salience map' of the visual world, marking locations of interest for any number of systems to use, including the visual attention and oculomotor system. Part of the evidence for this view is that LIP neurons track the location of salient objects independently of stored oculomotor plans. While the differences between these two sides may seem minute, the resolution of this debate will give us insight into both what specific calculations parietal cortex neurons are performing on incoming information and in what terms the brain represents the external world – as a distorted version of reality, skewed toward the most interesting and relevant stimuli, or always in terms of a motor plan for interacting with the world?

Other parietal areas in the macaque may also play roles in selective attention, though these areas have not been as thoroughly investigated as LIP. Areas caudal to LIP, such as DP, appear to play a role in visuospatial processing, though probably at an earlier stage than LIP (again fitting with their profiles of connections). Area 7a, which covers much of the IPL lateral to LIP, also appears to be involved in visuospatial processing. Like LIP, its neurons have large receptive fields, though it appears to evenly represent both the contralateral and ipsilateral hemifields. The neurons in this area appear to respond to the novel appearance of behaviorally relevant visual stimuli, but not as many of the 7a neurons have presaccadic activity as compared to LIP cells. This may indicate that rather than representing the current focus of attention, 7a neurons may be involved in detecting novel but potentially relevant stimuli, a counterpart of sorts to LIP. How other macaque parietal areas are involved in spatial attention is less clear, as they have generally been studied under the rubric of motor planning. Another important organizing principle for thinking about parietal cortex is to consider how space is coded in this region of the brain. There is evidence that parietal cortex subregions may be specialized for coding spatial location away from the body (or extrapersonal space) or near the body (or peripersonal space).

This wealth of information about monkey's parietal cortex until recently did not have a counterpart in the human work, because studies were limited to clinical observations (see later). This state of affairs changed in the late 1980s with the advent of positron emission tomography (PET), and then again in the 1990s with the advent of functional magnetic resonance imaging (fMRI). These neuroimaging technologies allowed, for the first time, *in vivo* studies of neural activity with sufficient spatial and temporal resolution to discern areas of the brain that were active in different tasks. Early PET studies confirmed that in humans the parietal lobe is also part of the dorsal 'where' pathway and is involved in the control of both spatial attention and eye movements. Several subsequent fMRI studies have also shown that, like in the macaque, the parietal region activated during covert shifts of attention largely overlaps with the region activated during saccades. This region includes much of the cortex in and around the IPS. Parts of this region are also activated during nonspatial shifts of attention, such as changing the focus of attention from the direction of moving dots to the color of the moving dots. Because of this profile of activity, the region along the human IPS has been thought of as generally homologous to the macaque IPS.

However, due to the combination of relatively poor spatial resolution of fMRI and the high degree of variability in the location of sulci and gyri among human individuals, it has been difficult to subdivide this region into functional areas as has been done in the macaque. Two foci of neural activity are consistently activated in different tasks requiring shifting or maintenance of attention. The first is in the SPL, on the dorsal–medial bank of the IPS. Because it is thought to be homologous to the macaque LIP, it is sometimes called human LIP (hLIP). Like macaque LIP, hLIP appears to be gaze centered in its spatial reference frame, responds more strongly to stimuli in the contralateral visual hemifield than in the ipsilateral, and appears to be loosely retinotopically organized. This area is activated if there is an attention shift to a peripheral location, and activity is sustained in this area if either attention remains focused on, or a saccade is being planned to, the peripheral location. Activity in this area seems to track both the locus of visuospatial attention and the target of an upcoming eye movement, extending the debate about parietal function to the human parietal cortex. While much of the functional profile of hLIP appears to be broadly similar to that of macaque LIP, the lack of direct comparisons of histological data or neural activity during tasks requiring shifts of attention prevents a more thorough assessment of the homology of these areas.

Areas posterior to hLIP are also often activated in tasks requiring shifts of spatial attention. One of the most prominent is in the fundus of the caudal section of the IPS, and is variously termed ventral IPS (vIPS) or V7. This area is preferentially activated by attending to the contralateral hemifield, but appears to be more visual in nature than hLIP. V7 most likely represents an earlier stage of the 'where' pathway that probably relays visual information to hLIP, and is a potential homolog to one of the posterior parietal areas in the macaque.

While the aforementioned areas in the human SPL are activated during voluntary and involuntary shifts of attention, the IPL appears to play a different role in attention. Regions in the IPL are only activated in response to the appearance of a salient, behaviorally relevant object, and even more so if attention has to be reoriented from another location (known as stimulus-driven reorienting of attention). Moreover, while activity in the SPL areas is increased during sustained covert shifts of attention, activity in the IPL is suppressed. It has been proposed that these areas play a role in stimulus-driven attention, especially when the focus of attention is captured by a salient and relevant novel stimulus. In macaques, area 7a (on the macaque IPL) is one possible candidate for a homolog to the human IPL.

Another important feature of human parietal cortex is that it is anatomically and functionally asymmetrical. Several studies have now shown that functional regions of the supramarginal and angular gyrus at the temporoparietal junction (TPJ) in humans show hemispheric asymmetries of attention (right-dominant) or verbal memory (left-dominant) tasks. This asymmetry is even more dramatic when one considers the behavioral effects of stroke in the middle cerebral artery (MCA) distribution that feeds the parietal cortex. Whereas left MCA strokes commonly result in aphasia (language deficits), strokes of the right MCA commonly result in a syndrome termed 'neglect,' which is a collection of spatial attention–perception–premotor deficits (see **Figure 1(c)**).

An important goal for the future will be to reconcile monkey and human data in a common evolutionary framework that takes into account both commonalities and differences in functional organization. An important technological advance that will help this line of research is the development of fMRI studies in awake-behaving monkeys.

Lesions

Damage to the right IPL often results in spatial neglect, a common syndrome following stroke in which patients are biased toward attending to the right side of visual space more than to the left side. Neglect can leave patients unable to perform simple tasks requiring spatial attention, and occurs in about 30% of all stroke-affected individuals.

Patients with neglect often act as if part of the left side of their world does not exist. This inattention to the left side can occur in extrapersonal space or about the patient's own body, and can occur in different reference frames: gaze-centered frame (left with respect to the center of gaze), body-centered frame (left with respect to the midline of the body), or world-centered frame (left with respect to the environment). Less commonly, patients can manifest so-called object-centered neglect, where the left side of an object is ignored, no matter if it is presented in the left or right side of the visual space. For instance, if a page of text with three columns is presented, a patient with body-centered or world-centered neglect will miss the words on the left side of the page, whereas a patient with object-centered neglect will miss the left side of each column or the left side of each word.

Functionally, neglect patients may 'forget' to shave, groom, or dress the left side of body. They also have major problems with driving a car. Severely affected patients might also display a tonic rotation of the body or eyes toward the right, due to a coexisting motor imbalance. Some of these patients may still be able to detect a stimulus presented alone in the left hemifield, but when presented with stimuli simultaneously to both visual fields, patients tend to see only those in the right hemispace. This deficit is referred to as 'extinction.' Extinction is often tested by snapping fingers in one or both of the patient's visual fields and asking the patient to point to which hand they saw or heard snapping. When fingers are snapped simultaneously in both visual fields, neglect patients will inexorably point to the hand in their right visual field. This test is one of the many routine exams in clinical settings to assess the severity of neglect. Other commonly used neuropsychological tests for diagnosis of neglect include line bisection, in which patients with neglect bisect a horizontal line to the right of the true center; a series of cancellation tasks, in which neglect patients commonly miss marking targets on the left side of a paper; clock drawing, in which neglect patients may draw only the right half of a clock; and a baking-tray task, in which neglect patients usually cluster cookies on the right side of a baking tray.

In addition to the lack of awareness of the left side of space, neglect patients can also manifest deficits in planning hand or eye movements toward the left side of space. In this type of neglect, patients may not demonstrate a bias in awareness to either visual field, but will be less inclined to reach or look for objects located in the left visual field. This form of neglect is called motor or premotor neglect, or directional hypokinesia, to emphasize its relationship to action. In addition to lateralized (i.e., left worse than right space) deficits, a number of so-called nonlateralized deficits (i.e., similar across left and right visual fields) have also been described, including impairment of spatial working memory, sustained attention, and an overall lower level of alertness.

An important focus of current research is to assess the functional effect of different deficits, their importance for final outcome, their recovery over time, and their localization in the brain. Shall we think of neglect as a homogeneous or heterogeneous syndrome? What are the regions more responsible for one or another deficit? We know that spatial neglect can occur as a clinical syndrome for lesions in many parts of the brain, including parietal, temporal, frontal cortex, basal ganglia, thalamus, and in various white-matter tracts. It is still unknown how these different lesions may or may not cause different behavioral profiles of neglect, and how the effect of lesions in the brain relates to the functional organization observed in healthy individuals.

An alternative view considers neglect not to be the effect of damage to specific cortical areas, but rather the result of a distributed and combined anatomical–functional dysfunction of large parts of parietal and frontal cortices and their connections. In general, the areas that are damaged in neglect are located ventrally in the brain, including the IPL regions specialized for stimulus-driven attention. Conversely, damage to more dorsal IPS and SPL regions does not produce strong neglect; rather, these lesions produce primarily eye- or arm-movement planning problems, which is also consistent with the results of functional imaging studies in healthy volunteers. However, only a few patients with damage restricted to the SPL have been studied.

One model of neglect postulates that damage by stroke or trauma to the IPL in the region of the TPJ could give rise to both spatial and nonspatial deficits by interrupting input to the SPL attentional areas from the TPJ. This disruption would then reduce the brain's ability to detect important sensory events in both visual fields. In addition, this lack of input into ipsilesional dorsal areas may induce a relative interhemispheric imbalance in the dorsal attentional areas that code for spatial locations and eye and arm movements. The imbalance due to the competitive nature of interhemispheric processing will lead to a relative hyperorienting toward right space, with consequent problems of attention and detection in left space. This model of spatial bias based on interhemispheric competition is also supported by a number of animal studies in which neglect has been cured by inactivating homologous parietal regions of the intact hemisphere.

Conclusion

Parietal cortex is subdivided into different areas, based on both anatomical and functional criteria; these areas have connections with both sensory processing and motor planning regions of the brain. Some of these areas appear to be involved in the selection and representation of locations and objects of interest in the immediate environment. The spatial information in parietal cortex can then be 'read out' by other brain areas, both for the planning of movements and for the enhancement of sensory processing. Attention can be directed to a location or object by a premeditated plan, or by the appearance of a novel stimulus that may require additional processing. Area LIP in the macaque and its putative homolog in the SPL of humans appear to be involved in representing the locations of interest, whereas IPL areas appear to play the role of reorienting attention whenever a novel stimulus enters awareness. Damage to these areas results in the syndrome of neglect, which fundamentally involves a lack of awareness for spatial information, as well as problems with vigilance and motor planning.

See also: Attention and Eye Movements; Attention: Models; Attentional Functions in Learning and Memory; Attentional Mechanisms in Ventral Pathway; Attentional Networks; Decision-Making and Vision; Neglect Syndrome and the Spatial Attention Network; Parietal Cortex and Spatial Attention; Psychophysics of Attention; Visual Attention.

Further Reading

Andersen RA and Buneo CA (2002) Intentional maps in posterior parietal cortex. *Annual Review of Neuroscience* 25: 189–220.

Colby CL and Goldberg ME (1999) Space and attention in parietal cortex. *Annual Review of Neuroscience* 22: 319–349.

Corbetta M and Shulman GL (2002) Control of goal-directed and stimulus-driven attention in the brain. *Nature Reviews Neuroscience* 3: 201–215.

Desimone R and Duncan J (1995) Neural mechanisms of selective visual attention. *Annual Review of Neuroscience* 18: 193–222.

Egeth HE and Yantis S (1997) Visual attention: Control, representation, and time course. *Annual Review of Psychology* 48: 269–297.

Goldman-Rakic PS (1988) Topography of cognition: Parallel distributed networks in primate association cortex. *Annual Review of Neuroscience* 11: 137–156.

Hillis AE (2006) Neurobiology of unilateral spatial neglect. *Neuroscientist* 12: 153–163.

Husain M and Rorden C (2003) Non-spatially lateralized mechanisms in hemispatial neglect. *Nature Reviews Neuroscience* 4: 26–36.

Kastner S and Ungerleider LG (2000) Mechanisms of visual attention in the human cortex. *Annual Review of Neuroscience* 23: 315–341.

Lewis JW and Van Essen DC (2000) Mapping of architectonic subdivisions in the macaque monkey, with emphasis on parieto-occipetal complex. *Journal of Comparative Neurology* 428: 79–111. Avaliable at URL: http://sumsdb.wustl.edu:8081/sums/directory.do?id=679531.

Mesulam MM (1999) Spatial attention and neglect: Parietal, frontal and cingulate contributions to the mental representation and attentional targeting of salient extrapersonal events. *Philosophical Transactions of the Royal Society of London, Series B: Biological Sciences* 354: 1325–1346.

Mountcastle VB, Lynch JC, Georgopoulos A, et al. (1975) Posterior parietal association cortex of the monkey: Command function for operations within extrapersonal space. *Journal of Neurophysiology* 38: 871–908.

Orban GA, VanEssen D, and Vanduffel W (2004) Comparative mapping of higher visual areas in monkeys and humans. *Trends in Cognitive Science* 8: 315–324.

Pashler HE (1998) *The Psychology of Attention.* Cambridge, MA: MIT Press.

Posner MI and Petersen SE (1990) The attention system of the human brain. *Annual Review of Neuroscience* 13: 25–42.

Brain–Computer Interface

J R Wolpaw, New York State Department of Health and State University of New York, Albany, NY, USA

Introduction

In the nearly 80 years since Hans Berger first recorded electroencephalographic activity from the scalp, the electroencephalograph (EEG) has been used primarily for clinical diagnosis, for exploring brain function, and to a very limited extent for therapy. At the same time, many people have speculated that the EEG or other reflections of brain activity might be useful for another purpose as well: to serve as an alternative method for the brain to send messages and commands to the outside world. While the brain's normal communication and control capabilities depend on nerves and muscles, the existence of easily recordable brain signals, such as the EEG implied the possibility of establishing nonmuscular communication and control based on brain–computer interfaces (BCIs).

In spite of recurring scientific and popular interest in the idea of BCIs, and despite a few encouraging initial efforts, it is only in the past 20 years that sustained research has begun, and only in the past 12 years that a recognizable field of BCI research and development has emerged. The field is now populated by a large and rapidly growing number of research groups throughout the world. This new surge of interest and activity is due largely to the combination of four important elements.

The first element is greater appreciation of the needs and the abilities of people paralyzed by disorders such as cerebral palsy, spinal cord injury, brain stem stroke, amyotrophic lateral sclerosis (ALS), and muscular dystrophies. Life-support technology (e.g., home ventilators) now enables even the most severely disabled people to survive for many years. Furthermore, it is now clear that even people who have little or no voluntary muscle control, who may be nearly 'locked-in' their bodies, unable to communicate in any way, can have lives that they consider enjoyable and productive if they can be given even the most basic means of communication and control.

The second element is the greater knowledge of the nature and functional correlates of the EEG and other measures of brain activity that has come from animal and human research. Along with this new understanding have come improved methods for recording these signals, in both the short-term and the long-term. This increased knowledge and improved technology are directing and enabling more sophisticated and productive BCI research.

The third element is the easy availability of powerful, inexpensive computer hardware that supports the complex real-time analyses of brain activity important for successful BCI operation. Until quite recently, much of the online signal processing used in current BCIs was impossible or extremely expensive.

The fourth element contributing to the rapid growth of BCI research is new appreciation of the brain's remarkable adaptive capacities, both in normal life and in reaction to trauma or disease. The growing recognition of these adaptive capacities generates enormous excitement and interest in the potential for using them to create novel interactions between the brain and computer-based devices, interactions that can substitute for or even augment the brain's normal neuromuscular interactions with its external and internal environments.

Definition of a BCI

A BCI creates a nonmuscular output channel for the brain. Instead of being executed through peripheral nerves and muscles, the user's wishes are conveyed by brain signals (such as those detected by an EEG), and these brain signals do not depend for their generation on neuromuscular activity. (Thus, for example, a device that uses visual-evoked potentials in the EEG to determine eye-gaze direction is not a true BCI because it relies on muscular control of eye position and simply uses the EEG as a measure of that position.)

Like other communication and control systems, a BCI establishes a real-time interaction between the user and the outside world. The user gets feedback on the results of the BCI's operation, and that feedback influences the user's intent and the brain signals that encode that intent. For example, if a person uses a BCI to control the movements of a robotic arm, the arm's position after each movement affects the person's intent for the succeeding movement and the brain signals that convey that intent. Thus, a system that only records and analyzes brain signals, without providing the outcome of that analysis to the user in a real-time interactive fashion, is not a BCI. **Figure 1** shows the design and operation of any BCI.

Popular speculation and some scientific efforts have been based on the belief that BCIs are 'mind-reading' or 'wire-tapping' technology, devices that listen in on the brain, detect its intent, and then execute that intent. This is a misconception that ignores a central feature of the brain's interactions with the external world. The motor skills that accomplish a person's intent, whether it be to walk across a room, speak specific words, or play a particular piece on the

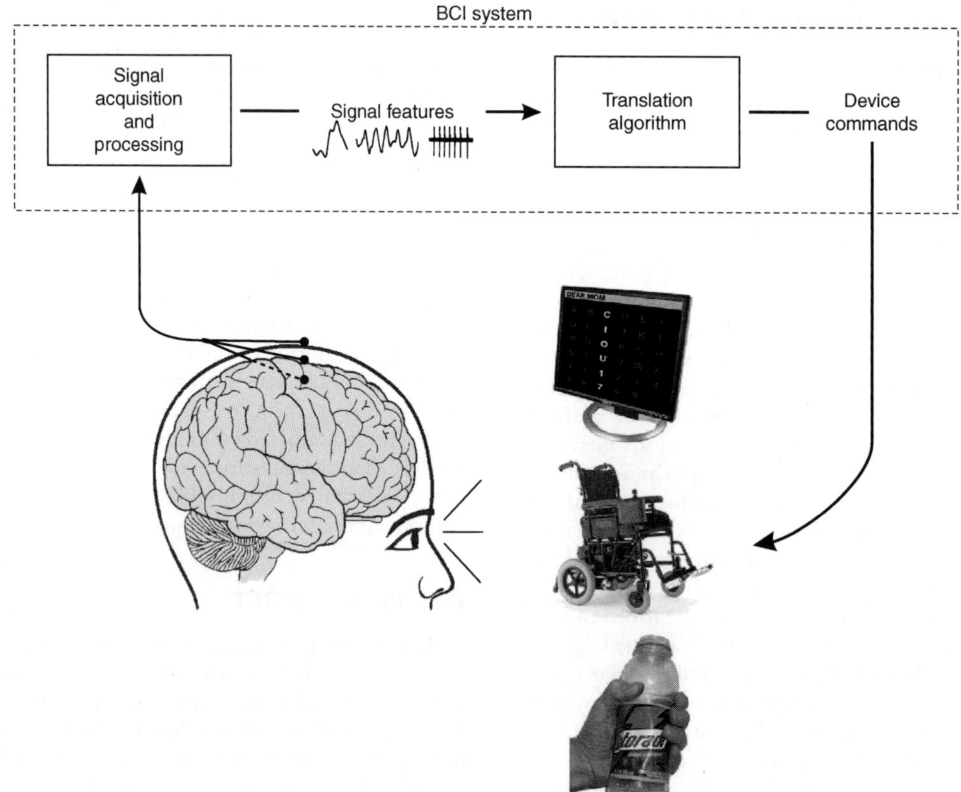

Figure 1 The basic design of any brain–computer interface (BCI) system. Signals reflecting brain activity are acquired from the scalp, from the cortical surface, or from within the brain and are analyzed to measure signal features (such as amplitudes of evoked potentials or electroencephalograph rhythms or firing rates of single neurons) that reflect the user's intent. These features are translated into commands that operate a device such as a word-processing program, a wheelchair, or a neuroprosthesis. Adapted from Wolpaw JR and Birbaumer N (2006) Brain–computer interfaces for communication and control. In: Selzer ME, Clarke S, Cohen LG, Duncan P, and Gage FH (eds.) *Textbook of Neural Repair and Rehabilitation; Neural Repair and Plasticity,* pp. 602–614. Cambridge: Cambridge University Press, with permission from Cambridge University Press.

piano, are mastered and maintained by initial and continuing 'adaptive changes' in brain function. In early development and throughout later life, central nervous system (CNS) neurons and synapses change continually to master new skills and to maintain those already mastered. This adaptive plasticity is responsible for basic skills such as walking and talking and for more specialized skills such as ballet, and it is guided by the results produced. Thus, as muscle strength, limb length, and body weight change with growth and aging, the CNS modifies its outputs so as to maintain its motor skills.

This requirement for initial and continuing adaptation exists whether the person's intent is carried out naturally, that is, by peripheral nerves and muscles, or through an artificial interface, a BCI, that uses brain signals instead of nerves and muscles. Successful BCI operation requires the effective interaction of two adaptive controllers: the user, who must generate brain signals that encode intent; and the BCI system, that must translate these signals into commands that accomplish the user's intent. Thus, BCI usage is essentially a skill that user and system work together to acquire and maintain. The user encodes intent in signal features that the BCI system can measure, and the system measures these features and translates them into device commands. This initial and continuing dependence on the mutual adaptation of user to system and system to user is a fundamental principle of BCI operation; its effective management is one of the principal challenges for BCI research and development.

Brain Signals That Could Be Used in a BCI

A variety of different methodologies can detect brain activity. These include methods for recording electrical or magnetic fields, functional magnetic resonance imaging (fMRI), positron emission tomography (PET), and functional near-infrared (fNIR) imaging. However, magnetoencephalography, fMRI, and PET are not currently suited for everyday use due to their intricate technical demands, high expense, and/or limited real-time capabilities. Only electrical field recording (and possibly fNIR imaging) are likely to be of value for practical applications in the near future.

The electrical fields produced by brain activity can be recorded at the scalp (electroencephalographic activity (EEG)), at the cortical surface (electrocorticographic activity (ECoG)), or within the brain (local field potentials (LFPs)) or neuronal action potentials (spikes). **Figure 2** shows these three recording alternatives. Each method has advantages and disadvantages. EEG recording is easy and noninvasive, but it has limited topographical resolution and frequency range and can be contaminated by electromyographic (EMG) activity from cranial muscles or electrooculographic (EOG) activity. ECoG has better topographical resolution and frequency range, but it requires implantation of electrode arrays on the cortical surface, which has been done as yet for only brief periods (a few days or weeks) in people. Intracortical recording, or recording within other brain areas, yields signals with the highest resolution, but it requires insertion of multielectrode arrays within brain tissue, and it faces as yet unresolved problems in reducing tissue damage and scarring and in achieving long-term recording stability.

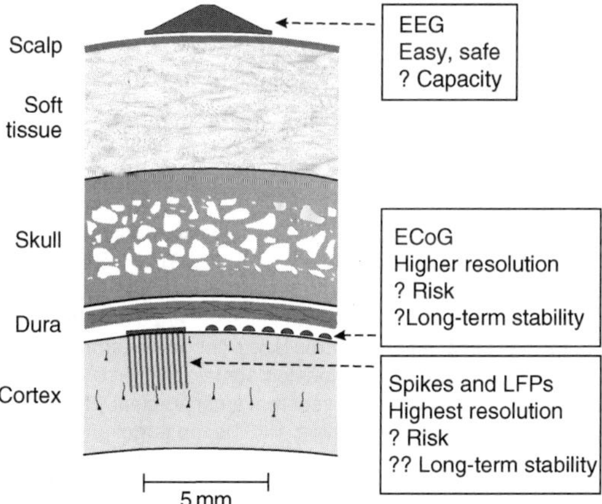

Figure 2 Recording sites for electrophysiological signals used by brain–computer interface (BCI) systems. Electroencephalographic activity (EEG) is recorded by electrodes on the scalp. Electrocorticographic activity (ECoG) is recorded by electrodes on the cortical surface. Neuronal action potentials (spikes) or local field potentials (LFPs) are recorded by electrode arrays inserted into the cortex. Each recording method has advantages and disadvantages. Adapted from Wolpaw JR and Birbaumer N (2006) Brain–computer interfaces for communication and control. In: Selzer ME, Clarke S, Cohen LG, Duncan P, and Gage FH (eds.) *Textbook of Neural Repair and Rehabilitation; Neural Repair and Plasticity*, pp. 602–614. Cambridge, UK: Cambridge University Press, with permission from Cambridge University Press.

The ultimate usefulness of each of these methods will hinge on the range of communication and control applications it can support and on the extent to which its disadvantages can be overcome. The question of the relative value of noninvasive methods (i.e., EEG), moderately invasive methods (e.g., ECoG), and more-invasive methods (e.g., intracortical recording) remains unanswered. It is conceivable that practical, stable, and safe techniques for long-term recording within the brain will prove relatively easy to develop. On the other hand, the information transfer rates possible with intracortical methods may turn out to be no greater than those achievable with less-invasive methods (e.g., ECoG, or even EEG). It is quite likely that different recording methods will prove useful for different applications and for different individuals. Comprehensive evaluations of the characteristics and capacities of each recording method are needed.

Present-Day BCIs

Human BCI experience to date consists largely of noninvasive EEG-based research. A few short-term ECoG studies have been reported, and limited data are available from a few people with intracortical implants. Most intracortical BCI data come from animals, primarily monkeys. EEG-based BCI methods can certainly support simple applications and seem to be able to support more complex ones. Invasive methods may be able to support more complex applications, but the issues of risk and long-term performance are not yet resolved.

Three different kinds of EEG-based BCIs have been evaluated in people. They are distinguished by the particular EEG features they use to derive the user's intent. **Figure 3(a)** illustrates a P300-based BCI. It focuses on the P300 component of the event-related brain potential, which appears in the EEG over central areas about 300 ms after a salient, or attended stimulus. In most P300-based BCIs described to date the stimulus is visual. Typically, letters, numbers, and/or other possible choices are arranged in a matrix, and the rows and columns of the matrix flash in rapid succession. Only the row and column that contain the item that the user wants to select produce P300 potentials. By detecting these P300 potentials, the BCI system can determine the user's selection. This BCI method is able to support operation of a simple word-processing program that enables users to

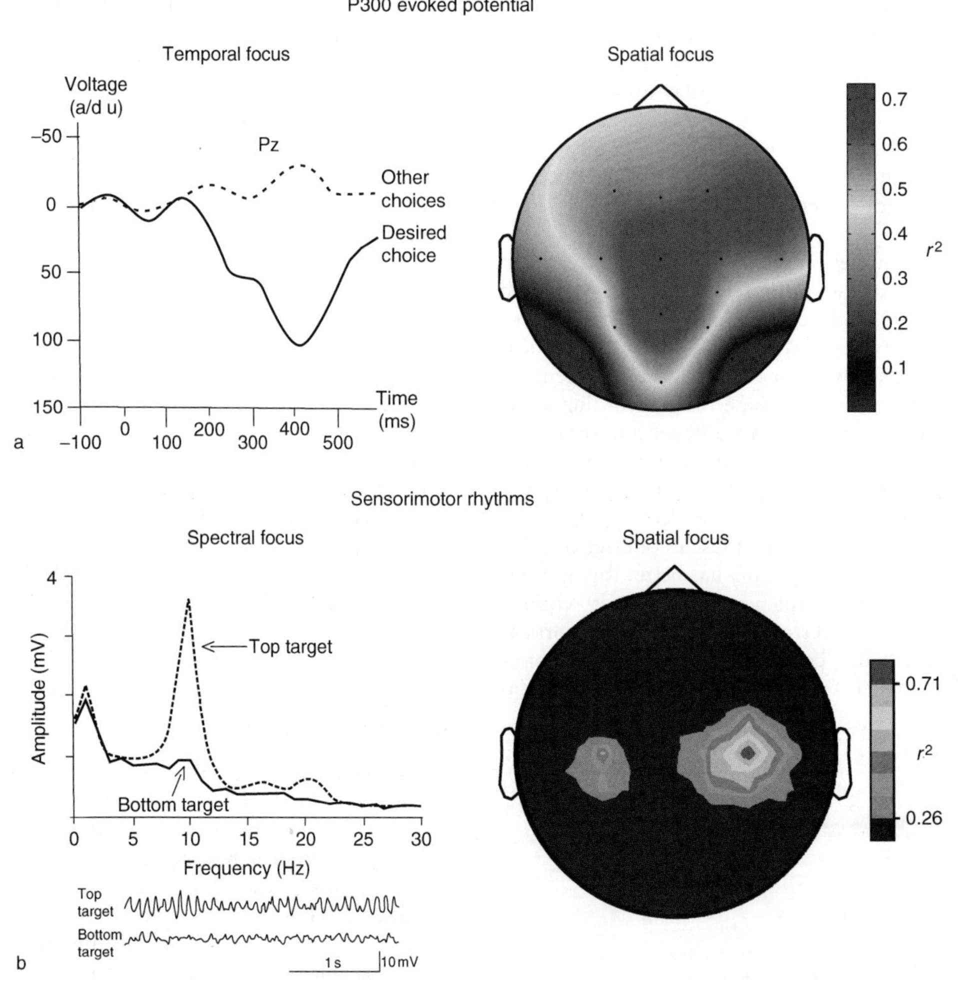

Figure 3 Noninvasive EEG-based BCI methods that use EEG recorded from the scalp. (a) P300 evoked potential brain–computer interface (BCI). A matrix of possible selections is shown on a screen. Scalp electroencephalographic activity (EEG) is recorded over centroparietal cortex (EEG recording location P_Z) while these selections flash in succession. Only the selection desired by the user evokes a large P300 potential (i.e., a positive potential about 300 ms after the flash). r^2 is the coefficient of variation; a/d u are the analog to digital conversion units. (b) Sensorimotor rhythm BCI. Scalp EEG is recorded over sensorimotor cortex. Users control the amplitudes of one or more 8–12 Hz mu rhythms or 18–26 Hz beta rhythms to move a cursor to a desired target located somewhere on a computer screen. Frequency spectra (top) for top and bottom targets indicate that this user's control of vertical cursor movement is clearly focused in the mu-rhythm frequency band. Sample EEG traces (bottom) also show that the mu rhythm is prominent with the top target and minimal with the bottom target. Trained users can also control movement in two dimensions. Adapted from Kübler A, Kotchoubey B, Kaiser J, Wolpaw JR, and Birbaumer N (2001) Brain–computer communication: Unlocking the locked-in. *Psychological Bulletin* 127: 358–375, with permission from American Psychological Association.

communicate at rates up to several words per minute. Improvements in signal analysis may substantially increase its capacities.

Figure 3(**b**) illustrates a BCI based on sensorimotor rhythms. Sensorimotor rhythms are 8–12 Hz (mu) and 18–26 Hz (beta) oscillations in the EEG recorded over sensorimotor cortices. Normally, changes in mu and/or beta rhythm amplitudes accompany movement and sensation, and motor imagery as well. BCI studies show that people can learn to control mu or beta rhythm amplitudes in the absence of any movement or sensation and that they can use this control to move a cursor to select letters or icons on a screen or to operate a simple orthotic device. Both one- and two-dimensional control are achievable. Sensorimotor rhythm-based BCIs, like P300-based BCIs, can support basic word-processing or other simple functions. They might also support multidimensional control of the movements of a neuroprosthesis or a device such as a robotic arm.

A BCI can also use slow cortical potentials (SCPs) in the EEG, which last from 300 ms to several seconds. In normal brain function, negative SCPs accompany preparatory depolarization of the underlying cortical network, and positive SCPs are thought to reflect cortical disfacilitation or inhibition. With appropriate training, people can learn to control SCPs to produce positive or negative shifts. With this control, they can perform basic word-processing and other simple control tasks such as accessing the Internet.

Current BCIs depend mainly on visual stimuli and visual feedback. However, people who are severely disabled may lack the vision or eye movements needed to perceive visual stimuli, especially if the stimuli change rapidly. Thus, BCI systems that employ auditory rather than visual stimuli would also be valuable – and are under investigation.

Figure 4(a) illustrates a BCI that uses sensorimotor rhythms in ECoG recorded by electrode arrays on the cortical surface. ECoG signals are much higher in amplitude than are scalp-recorded EEG signals, they have much higher spatial and temporal resolution, and they are much less susceptible to contamination by EMG or EOG. ECoG encompasses not only mu and beta rhythms but also higher-frequency gamma (>30 Hz) rhythms, which are very small or entirely lacking in EEG. With appropriate interelectrode spacing, ECoG can resolve activity limited to a few square millimeters of cortical surface. To date, ECoG studies have been confined to short-term experiments in people temporarily implanted with electrode arrays prior to epilepsy surgery. These studies reveal sharply focused ECoG activity associated with movement and sensation and with motor imagery. Furthermore, with only a few minutes of training, people can learn to use motor imagery to control cursor movement.

The speed of this learning, which appears to be faster than that usually found with sensorimotor rhythms in scalp-recorded EEG, together with ECoG's high topographical resolution, wide spectral range, and freedom from contamination, suggests that ECoG-based BCIs might provide communication and control superior to that possible with EEG-based BCIs. Widespread clinical use of ECoG-based BCIs will require development of fully implanted systems (i.e., systems that use telemetry and thus do not have wires passing through the skin) and clear evidence that they provide safe and stable recording for years.

Figure 4(b) shows a multielectrode array for intracortical recording and the locations of its implantation in human motor cortex. Intracortical BCI studies conducted in monkeys and to a limited extent in humans have shown that single-neuron activity recorded by such arrays can be used to control movement of a cursor in one, two, or even three dimensions. It appears that LFPs, which can be recorded by the same electrode arrays and reflect nearby synaptic and neuronal activity, might provide similar control. In these intracortical single-neuron and LFP studies, the usual strategy has been to define the neuronal activity associated with standardized limb movements, then to apply this activity to simultaneously control comparable cursor movements, and finally to demonstrate that the neuronal activity alone can continue to control cursor movements in the absence of actual limb movements. As **Figure 4(b)** shows, the relationships between neuronal activity and cursor movements change over time. Ideally, neuronal activity adapts over sessions so as to improve cursor control. This adaptation, like the adaptations seen with EEG- and ECoG-based BCIs, illustrates the need for initial and continuing adaptation of system to user and user to system.

The major questions that must be answered prior to clinical use of intracortical BCIs include their long-term safety, the stability and persistence of their signals in the face of cortical tissue reactions to the implanted electrodes, the long-term usefulness of these signals, and to what extent their capabilities in actual practical applications (e.g., in neuroprosthesis control) significantly exceed those of less-invasive BCIs. The first two websites listed provide videos that illustrate that a noninvasive EEG-based BCI using sensorimotor rhythms can provide cursor control comparable in speed and accuracy to that achieved to date with intracortical methods.

Signal Processing

A BCI records brain signals and analyzes them to derive device commands. This signal processing has two parts. The first part is feature extraction, the measurement of those features of the signals that encode the user's intent. These features can be relatively simple measures such as the amplitudes or latencies of particular evoked potentials (e.g., P300), the amplitudes or frequencies of particular rhythms (e.g., sensorimotor rhythms), or the firing rates of individual cortical neurons, or they can be more complex measures such as spectral coherences or weighted combinations of simple measures. To provide effective BCI performance, the feature-extraction part of signal processing needs to focus on features that actually do encode the user's intent, and it needs to extract those features accurately.

The second part of BCI signal processing is a translation algorithm that translates these features into device commands. Features such as rhythm

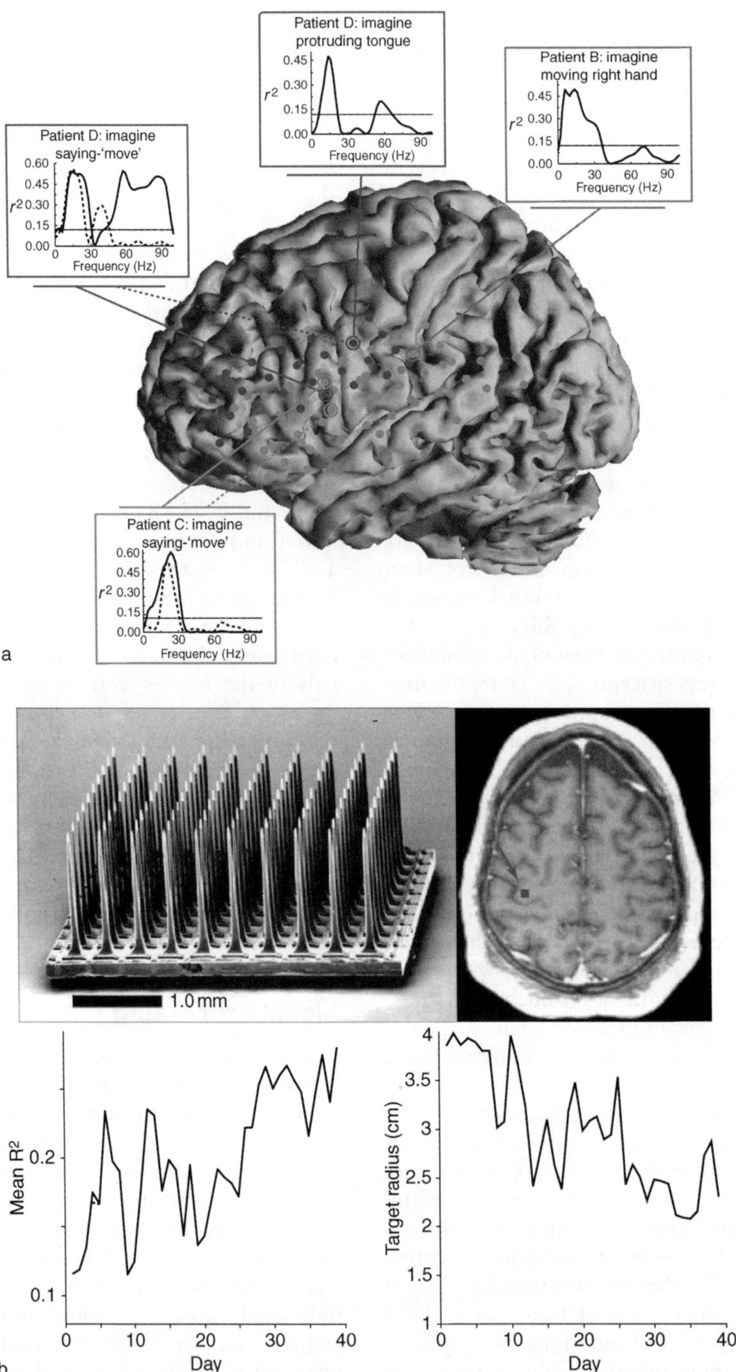

Figure 4 Invasive brain–computer interface (BCI) methods. (a) Human electrocorticographic (ECoG) control of vertical cursor movement using specific motor imagery to move the cursor up and using rest (i.e., no imagery) to move it down. The electrodes used for online control are circled, and the spectral correlations of their ECoG activity with target location (i.e., top or bottom of screen) are displayed. Electrode arrays for Patients B, C, and D are green, blue, and red, respectively. The specific imagined actions used are indicated. The substantial levels of control achieved with different kinds of imagery are apparent. (The dashed lines indicate significance at the 0.01 level.) For Patients C and D, the solid and dotted r^2 spectra correspond to the sites indicated by the dotted and solid line locators, respectively. Reproduced from Leuthardt EC, Schalk G, Wolpaw JR, Ojemann JG, and Moran DW (2004) A brain–computer interface using electrocorticographic signals in humans. *Journal of Neural Engineering* 1: 63–71, with permission from IOP Publishing Limited. (b) Top left: Array

amplitudes or neuronal firing rates are translated into commands that specify outputs such as cursor movements, icon selection, or prosthesis operation. Translation algorithms can be simple (e.g., linear equations) or complex (e.g., neural networks, support vector machines).

A successful translation algorithm ensures that the user's range of control of the chosen features supports selection of the full range of device commands. Suppose, for example, that the feature is the amplitude of a 21–24 Hz beta rhythm in the EEG over left sensorimotor cortex, that the user can vary this feature over a range of 1–5 μV, and that the application is horizontal cursor movement. In this case, the translation algorithm must ensure that the 1–5 μV range permits the user to move the cursor to both the right and left edges of the screen and at a rate consistent with the rapidity and maximum duration of the user's beta control. In addition, the algorithm must accommodate spontaneous variations in the user's range of control (i.e., variations due to diurnal change, fatigue, or other factors). Finally, the translation algorithm should be able to adapt to at least accommodate, and at best encourage, improvements in the user's control. Thus, if the user's range of control improves from 1–5 to 1–8 μV, the translation algorithm should take advantage of this improvement in order to increase the speed and/or precision of cursor control.

The need for ongoing adaptation of the translation algorithm to accommodate spontaneous and other changes in the signal features reflects the continuing importance of system–user and user–system adaptation and has important implications. First, it means that new algorithms cannot be evaluated adequately by off-line analyses alone. They must also be evaluated online, so that the effects of their adaptive interactions with the user can be determined. This online evaluation should be long-term as well as short-term since important adaptive interactions often develop gradually. Second, the need for ongoing adaptation means that simpler algorithms, for which adaptation is typically easier and more effective, have an inherent advantage. Simple algorithms (e.g., linear equations) should be replaced by more complex alternatives (e.g., neural networks) only after online as well as off-line evaluations demonstrate that the more complex alternatives give superior long-term performance without continual and laborious recalibration procedures.

Potential Users

In their current early stage of development, BCIs are likely to be of significant practical value primarily for people with the most severe neuromuscular disabilities, people for whom conventional assistive communication technologies, all of which require some measure of consistent voluntary muscle control, are not satisfactory options. These include people with ALS who decide to accept artificial ventilation (rather than to die) as their disease advances, children and adults with severe cerebral palsy who do not have useful muscle control, patients with brain stem strokes who have only minimal eye movement control, individuals with severe muscular dystrophies or peripheral neuropathies, and possibly people with acute disorders associated with extensive paralysis (such as Landry-Guillain–Barré syndrome). People with slightly less severe disabilities, such as those with high-cervical spinal cord injuries, may also find BCI technology preferable to conventional assistive communication methods that co-opt their remaining voluntary muscle control (e.g., methods that depend on gaze direction or EMG of facial muscles). The extent to which future BCIs prove useful to those with much less-severe motor disabilities will depend on the speed and precision of the control the BCI systems can provide and on the reliability and convenience of their use.

People with disabilities of different kinds may differ in the BCI methods that are most useful to them. For some, the CNS deficits responsible for their disability may impair their control of certain brain signals and not others. For example, the motor cortex damage that can accompany ALS or the subcortical damage of severe cerebral palsy could conceivably impair generation or control of sensorimotor rhythms or single neuron activity. In these individuals, other brain signals (e.g., P300 potentials or neuronal activity from other brain areas) might be good alternatives.

of 100 microelectrodes chronically implanted in human motor cortex to record neuronal action potentials and local field potentials to control a cursor or other device. Top right: Position of array in human motor cortex. Reprinted by permission from Macmillan Publishers Ltd: *Nature*, Hochberg LR, Serruya MD, Friehs GM, et al. Neuronal ensemble control of prosthetic devices by a human with tetraplegia. 442: 164–171; copyright 2006. Bottom: Control of three-dimensional cursor movements by single neurons in motor cortex of a monkey. The left graph shows the improvement over daily training sessions of the average correlation (r^2) between the firing rate of a single cortical neuron and target direction. The right graph shows the resulting improvement in performance (assessed as the mean target radius required to maintain a 70% target hit rate). As the firing rates of the neurons that are controlling cursor movement become more strongly correlated with target direction, the size of the target can be reduced. Adapted from Taylor DM, Helms Tillery SI, and Schwartz AB (2003) Information conveyed through brain-control: Cursor versus robot. *IEEE Transactions on Neural Systems Rehabilitation and Engineering* 11: 195–199 (© 2003 IEEE), with permission from IEEE.

In this regard, it is encouraging that people severely disabled by ALS appear to retain the ability to control sensorimotor rhythms or single-neuron activity in sensorimotor cortex.

Apparently trivial and prosaic factors are likely to have substantial impact on the practical success of BCI applications. Factors such as the steps required for donning and doffing electrodes or for accessing a BCI application, or the user's appearance while operating the BCI, may greatly affect the numbers and characteristics of the people who adopt the system and the degree to which they actually use it in their daily lives.

Applications

BCIs have an extensive range of possible practical applications, from very simple to very complex. Simple BCI applications have already been demonstrated in the laboratory and in limited clinical use. They include systems for answering Yes/No questions, managing basic environmental control (e.g., lights, temperature), adjusting a television, or opening and closing a hand orthosis. Such simple systems can be configured for basic word-processing, sending e-mail, or accessing the Internet. For people who are totally paralyzed (i.e., locked-in), these simple BCI applications could make it possible to lead lives that are pleasant and even productive. Indeed, many recent studies indicate that, with good supportive care and the capacity for basic communication, severely paralyzed people can enjoy what they consider to be a reasonable quality of life and are hardly more likely to be depressed than are people without physical disabilities. Thus, simple BCI applications seem to have a significant future in their capacity to improve the daily lives of those who are most severely disabled. Indeed, a few severely disabled people are already using EEG-based BCI systems for important purposes in their daily lives.

More-complex BCI applications could control devices such as a motorized wheelchair, a robotic arm, or a neuroprosthesis that provides multidimensional movement to a paralyzed limb. Although present efforts focus on development of invasive BCI systems for such applications, noninvasive EEG-based BCIs also offer the possibility of such control. The eventual practical importance of such BCI applications will hinge on their capacities, practicality, and reliability, on their acceptance by specific kinds of users, and on the extent to which they have important advantages over conventional methodologies.

Establishment of the clinical value and practicality of BCI applications will require thorough evaluation to demonstrate their long-term reliability, to show that people actually use the applications, and to document that this usage has beneficial effects on factors such as mood, quality of life, and productivity. Particularly in the first stages of their development, it will frequently be necessary to configure applications that match each user's unique needs, desires, and physical and social environments. Although the cost of BCI equipment is relatively modest, current systems need substantial and continuing expert oversight, which is extremely expensive and now obtainable only from a few research labs. As a result, these systems are not available to most potential users. Thus, the widespread dissemination of BCIs will also depend on the degree to which the need for such ongoing technical support can be minimized. BCI systems must be easy to set up, easy to use, and easy to maintain if they are to have significant practical impact on improving the lives of people with severe disabilities.

Nature and Needs of BCI Research and Development

BCI research and development is a multidisciplinary effort. It requires neuroscience, engineering, applied mathematics, computer science, psychology, and rehabilitation. The need to select useful brain signals, to record them reliably, to analyze them appropriately in real-time, to control devices that provide functions valuable for those with severe disabilities, to manage the intricate short-term and long-term adaptive interactions between user and system, and to integrate BCI applications into the daily lives of their users means that the expertise and efforts of all these disciplines are essential for success. Thus, each BCI research group must incorporate all the essential disciplines, or groups with different expertise must collaborate closely. Collaborative studies are being facilitated by the widespread adoption of the general-purpose BCI software platform BCI2000, which can readily accommodate a wide variety of different signals, processing methods, applications, operating protocols, and hardware (see third website address). Productive collaborations have also been encouraged by recent meetings drawing BCI researchers from all relevant disciplines and from all over the world, by numerous symposia and collections of BCI research presentations at larger general meetings, and by publication of extensive sets of peer-reviewed BCI articles.

See also: Amyotrophic Lateral Sclerosis (ALS); Axonal Transport and ALS; Corticomotoneuronal System; Corticospinal Development; Electroencephalography (EEG); Evoked Potentials: Recording Methods; Evoked Potentials: Clinical; Map Plasticity and Recovery from Stroke; Synaptic Mechanisms of Learning.

Further Reading

Birbaumer N, Ghanayim N, Hinterberger T, et al. (1999) A spelling device for the paralyzed. *Nature* 398: 297–298.

Donchin E, Spencer KM, and Wijesinghe R (2000) The mental prosthesis: Assessing the speed of a P300-based brain-computer interface. *IEEE Transactions on Rehabilitation Engineering* 8: 174–179.

Hochberg LR, Serruya MD, Friehs GM, et al. (2006) Neuronal ensemble control of prosthetic devices by a human with tetraplegia. *Nature* 442: 164–171.

Kübler A, Kotchoubey B, Kaiser J, Wolpaw JR, and Birbaumer N (2001) Brain–computer communication: Unlocking the locked in. *Psychological Bulletin* 127: 358–375.

Kübler A, Nijboer F, Mellinger J, et al. (2005) Patients with ALS can use sensorimotor rhythms to operate a brain-computer interface. *Neurology* 64: 1775–1777.

Leuthardt EC, Schalk G, Wolpaw JR, Ojemann JG, and Moran DW (2004) A brain–computer interface using electrocorticographic signals in humans. *Journal of Neural Engineering* 1: 63–71.

Pfurtscheller G and Lopes de Silva F (2005) Event-related desynchronization (ERD) and event related synchronization (ERS). In: Niedermeyer E and Lopes daSilva FH (eds.) *Electroencephalography: Basic Principles, Clinical Applications and Related Fields*, pp. 1003–1016. Baltimore: Williams and Wilkins.

Robbins RA, Simmons Z, Bremer BA, Walsh SM, and Fischer S (2001) Quality of life in ALS is maintained as physical function declines. *Neurology* 56: 442–444.

Schalk G, McFarland DJ, Hinterberger T, Birbaumer N, and Wolpaw JR (2004) BCI2000: A general-purpose brain–computer interface (BCI) system. *IEEE Transactions on Biomedical Engineering* 51: 1034–1043.

Taylor DM, Helms Tillery SI, and Schwartz AB (2003) Information conveyed through brain-control: Cursor versus robot. *IEEE Transaction on Neural System Rehabilitation and Engineering*. 11: 195–199.

Taylor DM, Tillery SI, and Schwartz AB (2002) Direct cortical control of 3D neuroprosthetic devices. *Science* 296: 829–832.

Vaughan TM and Wolpaw JR (eds.) (2006) *The Third International Meeting on Brain-Computer Interface Technology: Making a difference IEEE Transactions on Neural Systems Rehabilitation Engineering* 14(2): 126–127.

Wolpaw JR and Birbaumer N (2006) Brain–computer interfaces for communication and control. In: Selzer ME, Clarke S, Cohen LG, Duncan P, and Gage FH (eds.) *Textbook of Neural Repair and Rehabilitation; Neural Repair and Plasticity*, pp. 602–614. Cambridge, UK: Cambridge University Press.

Wolpaw JR, Birbaumer N, McFarland DJ, Pfurtscheller G, and Vaughan TM (2002) Brain–computer interfaces for communication and control. *Clinical Neurophysiology* 113: 767–791.

Wolpaw JR and McFarland DJ (2004) Control of a two-dimensional movement signal by a noninvasive brain–computer interface in humans. *Proceedings of the National Academy of Sciences of the United States of America* 101: 17849–17854.

Relevant Websites

http://www.bci2000.org – BCI 2000 (brain–computer interface research project).

http://www.nature.com – *Nature* Supplementary Information (Supplementary Video 1 download).

http://www.bciresearch.org – QuickTime video ('Two-Dimensional Cursor Control With Scalp-Recorded Sensorimotor Rhythms') from the BCI Group, Wadsworth Center, Albany, NY.

Cognition: An Overview of Neuroimaging Techniques

S A Bunge, University of California at Berkeley, Berkeley, CA, USA
I Kahn, Howard Hughes Medical Institute at Harvard University, Cambridge, MA, USA

Anatomical Techniques

Anatomical techniques are used in a variety of ways in the service of the study of cognition, for example, to localize neuropathies in patients with cognitive disabilities or to compare the size of specific brain structures between groups of subjects through volumetric analysis. Additionally, anatomical techniques are used in conjunction with functional techniques in order to localize brain activity.

The earliest technique for imaging brain structure was computed tomography (CT). Today, it has been largely replaced by the much more powerful technique of magnetic resonance imaging (MRI). MRI provides excellent detailed structural information and enables the naked eye to distinguish gray matter (neuronal cell bodies) from white matter (myelinated tracts). New anatomical techniques, such as diffusion tensor imaging, have been developed to specifically visualize myelinated tracts. These methods can be used to track the normal and abnormal development of neural pathways in childhood.

Functional Techniques

Functional techniques have been the dominant force in cognitive neuroscience because they enable us to determine when and where neural activity in the brain is associated with the ability to perform a particular cognitive task. These techniques allow us to examine the workings of the human brain throughout the life span, in sickness and in health.

It is common to design several task variants that differ slightly in terms of task requirements. On the basis of this approach, differences in brain activation between the task variants enable us to isolate brain structures that are implicated in hypothesized cognitive processes. For example, if one wanted to identify brain regions involved in actively maintaining information in mind (referred to as working memory), one might parametrically vary the number of items (or the load) that subjects needed to maintain and then identify brain regions in which the level of activation varied according to working memory load. Although parametric variation is arguably the most powerful functional brain imaging manipulation, a more standard approach is to compare two task variants that differ only in that task 1 but not task 2 is hypothesized to engage a specific cognitive process. This approach relies on the assumption of 'pure insertion'; that is, the assumption that the insertion of the new task requirement affects only the cognitive process of interest.

Classes of Functional Neuroimaging Techniques

A variety of noninvasive functional neuroimaging techniques are available for use in humans (**Figure 1**); these techniques are categorized into two main classes. The first consists of methods for directly measuring electrical activity associated with neuronal firing, such as electroencephalography (EEG) and magnetoencephalography (MEG). The second main class consists of methods for indirectly measuring neuronal activity, which operate under the principle that neural activity is supported by increased local blood flow and metabolic activity. These methods include positron emission tomography (PET), functional magnetic resonance imaging (fMRI), and near-infrared spectroscopy (NIRS). More information on each of these methods is provided in the following sections.

Direct measures of neural activity: EEG and MEG EEG is the oldest functional brain imaging technique, dating back to Berger's discovery in 1929 that brain electrical activity could be recorded from electrodes placed on the scalp. This technique is still widely used today because of its ability to provide real-time measurements of brain activity. EEG records transient electrical dipoles generated by the net flow of electrical current across the cellular membrane during neuronal depolarization associated with postsynaptic potentials. Global EEG is used to measure neural activity during different brain states, such as sleeping and waking. A more powerful tool for cognitive neuroscience than global EEG measurements consists of event-related potentials, which refer to EEG activity averaged over a series of instances (or trials) triggered by the same event (e.g., the presentation of a visual stimulus).

Whereas EEG records the electrical activity associated with neuronal depolarization, the newer technique of MEG records the magnetic field produced by this electrical activity. The signal measured by both techniques results primarily from the activity of pyramidal neurons, which constitute roughly 70% of cells in the neocortex and are oriented perpendicular to the cortical sheath. EEG records electrical activity oriented perpendicular to the surface of the brain,

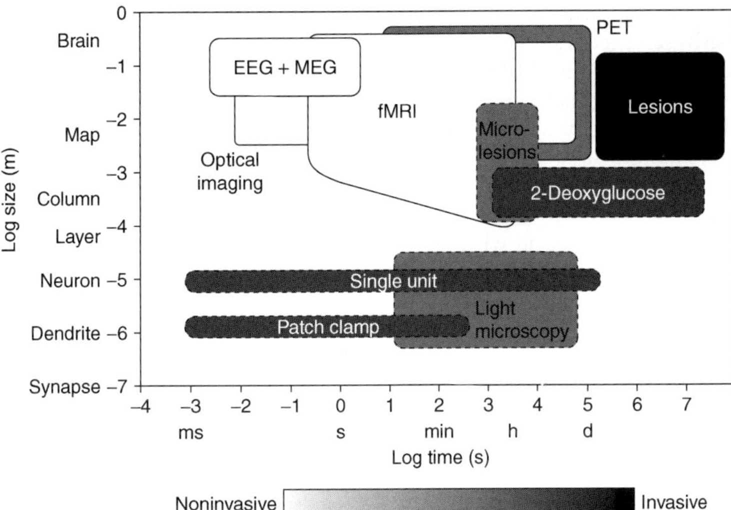

Figure 1 Relative spatial and temporal sensitivities of different functional brain imaging techniques. The level of invasiveness of each technique is indicated by a grayscale; more highly invasive techniques are shown in darker gray. Techniques used in animals only are outlined with a dashed line. Adapted from Cohen MS and Bookheimer SY (1994) Localization of brain function using magnetic resonance imaging. *Trends in Neuroscience* 17(7): 268–277.

whereas MEG records activity oriented parallel to the surface of the brain. Thus, EEG measures the activity of pyramidal cells in cortical gyri and the depths of the sulci, whereas MEG is sensitive primarily to the activity of pyramidal cells in the superficial parts of the sulci, and it is therefore more limited in its scope.

The major challenge with both EEG and MEG is referred to as the 'inverse problem,' which is the challenge of identifying the source of the underlying signal. This source can be a great distance from the point on the scalp at which it is measured, and it is affected by factors such as head shape and dipole location and orientation. Thus, it is necessary to build source localization algorithms to determine the likely source of a signal. One advantage of MEG over EEG is that the signal is less sensitive to factors such as head shape. Thus, the two techniques are complementary in that EEG samples from more neurons, but MEG is less sensitive to signal distortion. As such, some researchers take the approach of measuring EEG and MEG simultaneously to take advantage of what each technique has to offer.

Indirect measures of neural activity: PET Roy and Sherrington first showed in 1890 that brain stimulation led to a local increase in blood flow to active populations of neurons. Landau and others subsequently used radioactive tracers to measure regional cerebral blood flow (rCBF) in animals (1955), and in 1963 this technique was first applied to humans. The most widely used radioactive tracer is $^{15}O_2$, an oxygen molecule in which one electron has been removed from the atom to give an unstable form that will emit one positron to revert to the stable form $^{16}O_2$. In a PET scan, a small amount of radioactive tracer is injected into a vein. The tracer enters the brain after approximately 30 s, and in the following 30 s radiation in the brain rises to its maximal value; a picture of the rCBF is taken during this time frame.

The greatest advantage of PET over the more recent method of fMRI is the choice of radioactive tracer. Researchers can synthesize radiopharmaceutical compounds that bind to dopamine or serotonin receptors (C-11 or F-18 *N*-methylspiperone), opiate receptors (C-11 carfentanil), etc. PET is likely to continue to be important for understanding the role of various neurotransmitters in cognition. However, there are several disadvantages of PET that have led to its being surpassed by fMRI as the most widely used indirect measure of brain activity. The first of these is cost; PET facilities require not only a PET camera but also a cyclotron, which is used to produce the radioactive tracers. The second disadvantage is the poor temporal resolution – on the order of 1 min compared to 6–8 s for fMRI. Finally, PET is more invasive than fMRI, requiring the injection of a radioactive tracer (albeit one with a half-life of a few minutes), and thus it is not suitable for use in children or other special populations.

Indirect measures of neural activity: fMRI fMRI is currently the most widely used brain imaging technique for a number of reasons, including (1) widespread availability of MRI scanners and technology,

(2) relatively low cost per scan, (3) the lack of recognized risks for properly screened subjects, (4) good spatial resolution, and (5) better temporal resolution than other indirect neuroimaging methods.

In addition to observing that brain activity was associated with local changes in blood flow, Roy and Sherrington noted that the increase in total oxygenated blood delivered far exceeded the demand. It is this surplus of oxygen that is detected with fMRI, with what is known as the blood oxygen-level dependent (BOLD) contrast. Oxygenated hemoglobin, or oxyhemoglobin, has magnetic properties different from those of deoxyhemoglobin. Thus, the deployment of a strong magnetic field (typically 1.5–4 tesla when used in humans) enables one to measure changes in the ratio of oxy- to deoxyhemoglobin in local draining venules and veins. An increase in blood flow in response to a specific stimulus (be it brain stimulation or the presentation of a visual or auditory stimulus) is referred to as a hemodynamic response. This response is sluggish with respect to the underlying neural activity; for example, the hemodynamic response in visual cortex to a brief (e.g., 30 ms) visual stimulus peaks roughly 4–6 s after the onset of the stimulus.

Related Techniques

Perfusion fMRI enables direct measurement of the hemodynamic response, unlike BOLD fMRI, which relies on the comparison of hemodynamic responses under different conditions. This technique is less widely used than BOLD fMRI because of its much lower sensitivity. Magnetic resonance spectroscopy is used to measure the relative concentration and distribution of specific ions or compounds, such as hydrogen, phosphorus, or carbon.

Optical Brain Imaging

NIRS operates according to the same principle as optical brain imaging techniques that have been used in animals. Both techniques capitalize on the fact that changes in hemoglobin concentration in cortical tissue affect the absorption of infrared light by the tissue. However, NIRS is noninvasive, whereas optical imaging in animals is accomplished by exposing the surface of the brain. Because the cortical surface is not exposed in NIRS, light scattering by the skull leads to reduced spatial resolution.

During the past few years, Gratton, Fabiani, and colleagues have developed a new analytic approach to the analysis of optical data, known as the event-related optical signal (EROS). The EROS signal is based on measures of the optical properties of cortical tissue, which change when the tissue is active. The changes in these optical properties are likely to be due to changes in light scattering as a function of neuronal activity. Because this type of optical signal is directly linked to neural activity, rather than blood flow, it provides a much higher temporal resolution than the signal typically analyzed in NIRS studies. Additionally, the EROS signal has a high degree of spatial resolution, in that it can be localized to an area of less than 1 cm^3.

A drawback of all three optical imaging techniques noted previously is that they can only be used to measure activity on or near the surface of the brain (within 3–5 cm of the surface). However, these techniques are advantageous in that they are relatively inexpensive and completely noninvasive. Furthermore, because these techniques are not as sensitive to head movement as fMRI, they hold much promise for the study of clinical populations and children.

Trade-Offs between Temporal and Spatial Resolution

Direct measures of neural activity, such as EEG and MEG, have exquisite temporal resolution. They are sensitive to changes in neural activity on a millisecond resolution. However, these methods have poor spatial resolution in that it is difficult to pinpoint the precise origin of the signal. In contrast, indirect measures of neural activity have better spatial resolution than EEG or MEG but poor temporal resolution. The spatial and temporal characteristics of these various methods are shown in **Figure 1**. Thus, there is currently a trade-off between high temporal precision and high spatial precision. One solution to this problem is to use fMRI data to limit the possible sources of neural activity in EEG and MEG data; another – and even more challenging – solution is multimodal imaging, for example, the concurrent acquisition of fMRI and EEG data.

Advantages and Limitations of Neuroimaging Techniques

To date, much of what we know about the functions of different brain regions comes from neuropsychological studies in humans and lesion studies in animals. A distinct drawback of neuroimaging techniques is that, unlike neuropsychological and lesion techniques, they cannot demonstrate the necessity of a brain region for a specific cognitive process. However, neuroimaging techniques can demonstrate that humans without neurologic damage routinely recruit this region to perform the task. Moreover, it is possible to compare levels of activation across individuals and to state that greater activation of this region is associated with better performance on a task. Better yet, it is possible to compare activation between trials within an individual and to state that on trials in which the subject made an error, activation was lower in this region than on trials in which the subject performed correctly. Thus, functional brain imaging techniques can be used to characterize a region's contribution to specific cognitive processes. Moreover, brain imaging techniques can be paired with techniques for temporarily disrupting neural activity in a temporally and spatially precise manner (transcranial magnetic stimulation).

There are several important advantages of neuroimaging techniques over neuropsychological ones. First, neuropsychological studies necessarily rely on the output of behavior as the critical dependent measure, whereas neuroimaging studies can focus on cognitive processes that take place prior to – or are not associated with – a behavioral response. For example, it is impossible to determine whether lesions that result in a long-term memory impairment are associated with a deficit at encoding and/or retrieval. With brain imaging, however, one can identify brain regions associated with the effective encoding of memories separately from brain regions associated with effective retrieval.

Second, neuroimaging techniques enable us to identify the entire neural circuit underlying a cognitive process. Lesion studies in animals can accomplish this only piecemeal by lesioning each area in turn. Neuropsychological studies in humans would be hard-pressed to accomplish this at all, given the limited availability of patients with specific brain lesions. This point is an important one because with lesion studies it is possible to completely overlook – or instead to overestimate – the contributions of a specific region to cognitive function. For example, the hippocampus has long been thought to be the primary structure contributing to the encoding and retrieval of memories. However, brain imaging has demonstrated that in the healthy brain, prefrontal cortex routinely contributes to memory encoding and retrieval.

The third point is also related to the limited availability of neuropsychological patients: neuroimaging techniques enable one to examine the role of a given human brain region in cognition even if one does not have access to specific patient groups. Moreover, it can be very difficult (or next to impossible, depending on the brain region) to find a patient with a lesion limited to the region in which one is interested because most brain lesions are rather coarse. Furthermore, cortical reorganization can lead to recovery of function over time, which could lead one to assume mistakenly that a lesioned brain region is not normally involved in a specific cognitive process.

Finally, neuroimaging techniques with high temporal resolution, such as EEG and MEG, provide us with important clues about brain mechanisms. It is helpful to say that brain regions X and Y are involved in memory retrieval, but if we can say that brain region X is active a short time after region Y, we can begin to gain insight into the cascade of events leading to memory retrieval.

A common criticism of neuroimaging studies is that they can be highly unconstrained and atheoretical. Like any scientific tool, however, brain imaging can be used wisely or foolishly. Certainly, many exploratory brain imaging studies have been conducted, particularly in the initial phase of brain imaging, when it was important to validate the new techniques. However, the second generation of imaging studies, starting in the late 1990s, has been much more focused. On the whole, cognitive neuroscientists carefully devise experimental manipulations designed to test psychological theories or specific predictions about brain function. Brain imaging techniques are likely to be an important force in cognitive neuroscience for the foreseeable future.

Contributions to the Study of Cognition

Neuroimaging research has been used to enrich our understanding of the neural basis of a wide variety of cognitive abilities, including attention, language, and memory. In addition, neuroimaging techniques have been used to gain insight into the etiology of neurobehavioral disorders, for surgical planning, and to assess functional recovery after brain damage.

One area in which neuroimaging studies are making important contributions is that of memory. For example, studies of long-term semantic memory have begun to uncover the ways in which stored information is organized in the brain. These studies show that different attributes of an object are stored in a distributed manner across several brain regions, with visual form information stored in a region that processes form, and functional information stored near a region that processes motion. Furthermore, studies of memory encoding have been able to pinpoint the precise regions for which level of activation during stimulus processing predicts subsequent memory for that stimulus. Additionally, studies of memory retrieval are being used to adjudicate between models of episodic memory positing that recollection (i.e., distinct remembrance of an item and the context in which it was previously encountered) and familiarity (a vague sense that the item has previously been encountered) are either distinct processes or merely on a continuum of memory retrieval. These examples show how brain imaging studies can be used to test or adjudicate between psychological models.

Perhaps the most important contribution of neuroimaging to the field of cognition will be in the study of higher cognitive functions, which are not highly developed in nonhuman species and are therefore best studied in humans. Carefully designed brain imaging experiments have begun to fractionate the cognitive processes that underlie language, reasoning, problem solving, and other high-level mental functions, but further investigation is necessary.

See also: Cognitive Neuroscience: An Overview; Cognitive Control and Development; Electroencephalography (EEG); Event-Related Potentials (ERPs) and Cognitive Processing; Executive Function and Higher-Order Cognition: Neuroimaging; fMRI: BOLD Contrast; Magnetic Resonance Spectroscopy; Neuroimaging; Perfusion MRI; Single Photon Emission Computed Tomography (SPECT): Technique; Voxel Based Morphometry.

Further Reading

Andreassi JL (1995) *Psychophysiology: Human Behavior & Physiological Response*, 3rd edn. Hillsdale, NJ: Lawrence Erlbaum.

Cohen MS and Bookheimer SY (1994) Localization of brain function using magnetic resonance imaging. *Trends in Neuroscience* 17(7): 268–277.

Frith CD and Friston KJ (1997) Studying brain function with neuroimaging. In: Rugg M (ed.) *Cognitive Neuroscience*, pp. 169–195. Cambridge, MA: MIT Press.

Kutas M and Dale A (1997) Electrical and magnetic readings of mental functions. In: Rugg M (ed.) *Cognitive Neuroscience*, pp. 197–242. Cambridge, MA: MIT Press.

Levy I, Hasson U, Avidan G, Hendler T, and Malach R (2001) Center-periphery organization of human object areas. *Nature Neuroscience* 4(5): 533–539.

Raichle ME (1998) Behind the scenes of functional brain imaging: A historical and physiological perspective. *Proceedings of the National Academy of Sciences of the United States of America* 95(3): 765–772.

Rorden C and Karnath HO (2004) Using human brain lesions to infer function: A relic from a past era in the fMRI age? *Nature Reviews Neuroscience* 5(10): 813–819.

Wilkinson D and Halligan P (2004) The relevance of behavioural measures for functional-imaging studies of cognition. *Nature Reviews Neuroscience* 5(1): 67–73.

Cognition: Basal Ganglia Role

A R Aron, University of California, at San Diego, La Jolla, CA, USA
R A Poldrack, University of California at Los Angeles, CA, USA
S P Wise, National Institute of Mental Health, Bethesda, MD, USA

Published by Elsevier Ltd.

Introduction

The basal ganglia receive widespread input from the cerebral cortex and thalamus and return that projection through output to thalamocortical pathways. The basal ganglia also receive important neurochemical inputs, in particular a prominent dopaminergic projection from the midbrain. Because damage to the basal ganglia – in a broad range of neurological disorders – produces impairments in movement, expert opinion long held that the basal ganglia had an exclusively motor role. It is now clear, however, that these structures also contribute to a wide range of cognitive functions. These functions include learning, memory, skill, planning, switching, sequencing, timing, and the processing of rewards and other feedback. This article reviews evidence relating some of these cognitive functions to the basal ganglia.

Anatomical and Neurochemical Considerations

To understand how the basal ganglia contribute to cognitive functions, it helps to consider the pathways linking their component structures: the striatum, globus pallidus, substantia nigra, and subthalamic nucleus (STN) (**Figure 1**). Some of these pathways facilitate basal ganglia output, others inhibit it. In the next section, we discuss how different pathways engage in initiating, inhibiting, and switching behaviors, and also briefly mention a role in sequencing a series of behaviors.

In addition to the pathways illustrated in **Figure 1**, larger circuits – often called loops or modules – link different parts of cortex with distinct regions within the basal ganglia (**Figure 2**). Each of these circuits, which involve cortex, striatum, pallidum, and thalamus, carry different kinds of information. The terms often applied to the loops, such as associative (or complex), motor, oculomotor, and limbic, or, as illustrated in **Figure 2**, motor, spatial, visual, and affective, are not particularly significant. More important is the concept, which contrasts with earlier ideas about the anatomy of cortex–basal ganglia interactions, that many inputs and outputs of the basal ganglia involve cortical areas that have little direct sensory or motor function. The outputs of the basal ganglia do not, as previously believed, preferentially target motor areas of the cerebral cortex; instead, they target multiple sectors of cortex, including prefrontal cortical regions implicated in cognitive processing. This fact explains how damage to the striatum, such as occurs in Huntington's disease, can produce a range of cognitive and affective symptoms, even before motor performance deteriorates. The modules illustrated in **Figure 2** take the form of open rather than closed loops. That is, different loops share information, through corticocortical connections among others, so that diverse influences can contribute to the basal ganglia's final output. Most behaviors probably require cycling through multiple loops in an interactive fashion.

The neurochemical inputs to the basal ganglia also play a vital role in their function (**Figure 3**). In particular, prominent dopaminergic pathways originating in the substantia nigra pars compacta (SNc) and the ventral tegmental area (VTA) of the midbrain primarily innervate the dorsal and ventral striatum, respectively. As elaborated in the following discussions, several current models posit that the dopaminergic input to the dorsal striatum provides a reinforcing signal that binds the representations of stimuli and responses into stable associations, whereas the dopaminergic input to the ventral striatum plays a key role in rewarding or affective aspects of motivated behavior.

Overall, the cognitive function of the basal ganglia could be viewed as one of assigning behaviorally or biologically relevant feedback (**Figure 3**) to the computations performed by the various parallel loops involving the cerebral cortex, thalamus, and basal ganglia (**Figure 2**), with the basal ganglia's output controlled by the several different pathways converging on the pallidum (**Figure 1**). In the next section, these pathways are discussed in the context of preparing, initiating, inhibiting, and switching behaviors, while the subsequent two sections address the role of the basal ganglia in the processing of reward and feedback, and in the learning of new actions.

Cognitive Control: Preparing, Initiating, Inhibiting, and Switching Responses

Many lines of evidence in humans, nonhuman primates, and rodents implicate frontal cortex–basal ganglia loops in the control of responses, including both lower-order stimulus–response behaviors and the higher-order rules guiding such behaviors.

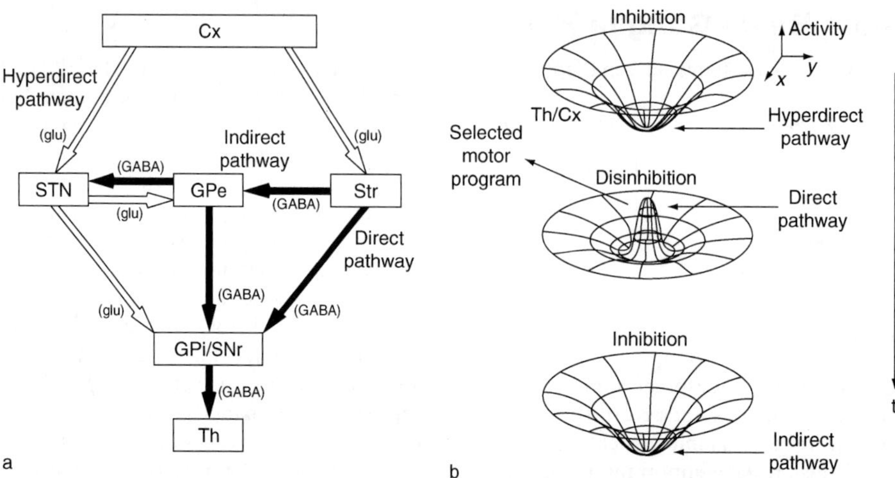

Figure 1 (a) Schematic diagram of hyperdirect, direct, and indirect pathways through the basal ganglia. Open arrows represent excitatory glutamatergic connections; filled arrows represent inhibitory γ-aminobutyric acid (GABA)ergic connections. Cx, cerebral cortex; STN, subthalamic nucleus; GPe, external segment of the globus pallidus; Str, striatum; GPi, internal segment of the globus pallidus; SNr, substantia nigra pars reticulata; Th, dorsal thalamus; glu, glutamatergic projections. (b) Schematic diagram showing the center-surround model of dynamic basal ganglia function, depicting activity changes in thalamus or cortical targets across time (vertical) caused by sequential inputs through the hyperdirect pathway (top), which inhibits all thalamocortical programs, the direct pathway (middle), which disinhibits some thalamocortical programs with concurrent suppression of alternatives, and the indirect pathway (bottom), which provides further inhibition of currently active programs to facilitate sequencing, among other functions. Reproduced from Nambu A, Tokuno H, and Takada M (2002) Functional significance of the cortico-subthalamo-pallidal 'hyperdirect' pathway. *Neuroscience Research* 43: 111–117, with permission from Elsevier.

Stimulus–Response Behavior

In some studies of stimulus–response behaviors, participants receive a cue that signals which task – of two or more tasks – they should perform once a stimulus appears. According to current thinking, this task cue evokes a top-down process by which the prefrontal cortex biases response channels within the basal ganglia. This bias could be understood to result from frontal inputs to the striatum, which excite a subpopulation of striatal cells and therefore prime the striatum for a particular type or class of sensory input (**Figure 4(a)**). If the expected stimulus appears, then the participants' reaction times will be quicker. Consistent with this model, individuals respond more quickly with adequately long intervals between the task cue and the subsequent stimulus, whereas they respond more slowly with shorter intervals. Functional imaging and neurophysiological data support these behavioral observations by showing that predictive cues lead to increased activation of striatum, compared to nonpredictive cues.

Response initiation begins once the stimulus appears. As illustrated in **Figure 5(a)**, this event engages the direct pathway of the basal ganglia, eventually leading to sufficient activation of motor cortex to generate the motor response or support an ongoing motor command initiated through other mechanisms. Inhibiting an already initiated response could occur via frontal activation of the STN, either via the hyperdirect or indirect pathways (**Figure 5(b)**; also see **Figure 1**). The STN, in turn, activates the internal segment of the globus pallidus (GPi), which inhibits thalamocortical output. Functional imagining has shown activation of the STN by response inhibition in humans. Further, patients with implanted STN stimulators (for treatment of Parkinson's disease) have improved response inhibition when the stimulator is turned on compared to when it is turned off, and rodents with lesions of the STN have impaired response inhibition.

In addition to their role in inhibiting already initiated responses, the basal ganglia may also be important for inhibiting incongruent or irrelevant responses or those recently performed as a movement sequence unfolds. For example, in performing a sequence of movements in which an action by the index finger is followed by a programmed movement of the thumb, the neural representation of the index-finger movement should be inhibited after the completion of the first part of the sequence. This kind of inhibition could also depend on the indirect pathway (**Figure 1(a)**).

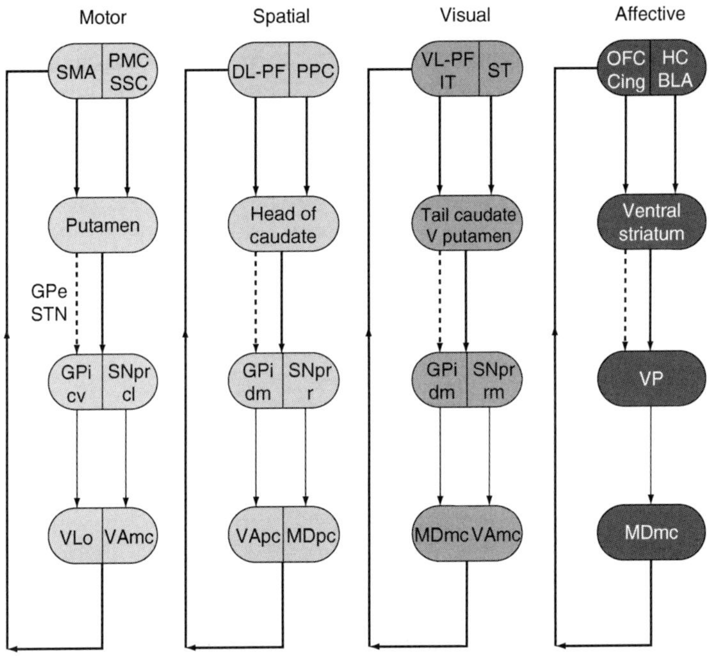

Figure 2 Cortical–basal ganglia loops, modified from the scheme of Alexander et al. Four parallel loops are shown, with possible functions labeled at the top. In the top row of rounded rectangles, the cortical areas in the left parts of bisected boxes are those that receive the thalamic projections indicated. The second row represents the striatum, the third row the pallidum, and the bottom row the dorsal thalamus. Dashed lines indicate net inhibitory influences of the indirect striatal output pathway. SMA, supplementary motor area; PMC, premotor cortex; SSC, somatosensory cortex; DL-PF, dorsolateral prefrontal cortex; PPC, posterior parietal cortex; VL-PF, ventrolateral prefrontal cortex; IT, inferior temporal cortex; ST, superior temporal gyrus; OFC, orbitofrontal cortex; Cing, anterior cingulate cortex; HC, hippocampal cortex; BLA, basolateral amygdala; V putamen, ventral putamen; GPe, external segment of globus pallidus; STN, subthalamic nucleus; GPi, internal segment of the globus pallidus; SNpr, substantia nigra pars reticulata; VP, ventral pallidum; VLo, oral (anterior) part of the ventrolateral thalamic nucleus; VA, ventral anterior nucleus of the thalamus, including the magnocellular (VAmc) and the parvocellular (VApc) parts; MDmc, magnocellular part of the mediodorsal nucleus of the thalamus. Subdivisions of the pallidum are labeled as follows: cv, caudoventral; cl, caudolateral; dm, dorsomedial; r, rostral; rm, rostromedial. Reproduced from Lawrence A, Sahakian BJ, and Robbins TW (1998) Cognitive functions and corticostriatal circuits: Insights from Huntington's disease. *Trends in Cognitive Sciences* 2: 379–387, with permission from Elsevier.

Task Switching

The same ideas that apply to stimulus–response behavior could contribute to understanding task switching, as well. A cardinal function of the basal ganglia involves switching between different tasks (or responses). Switching between tasks can be tested with a paradigm such as that shown in **Figure 4(b)**. On some trials, the experimenter cues the subject to respond according to the 'letter' task (say aloud the letter in the upcoming stimulus, and ignore the digit), whereas on other trials the cue instructs a response according to the 'digit' task (say aloud the digit, and ignore the letter). Individuals have a slower reaction time on trials in which the they switch to a different task compared to trials on which they repeat the same task, a phenomenon known as the switch cost (**Figure 4(c)**). Switching likely requires a combination of both facilitating (or preparing) some responses and inhibiting others. Many studies have shown that patients with Parkinson's and Huntington's disease are impaired at switching tasks, and neuroimaging studies in healthy persons have shown increased activation of the striatum for trials with switches, compared to trials lacking them.

In terms of the model shown in **Figure 4(a)**, frontostriatal inputs assist switching. As described earlier, the prefrontal cortex may bias the relevant response channels within the striatum in advance of the stimulus. If the expected stimulus later appears, then reaction time will be quick. If the respondent repeats the same task or response, reaction time will stay quick, because the relevant response channels remain primed, both by the top-down signal and by the just-performed response. However, if the respondent needs to switch tasks, the prefrontal cortex needs to activate or bias new response channels, and possibly inhibit previously

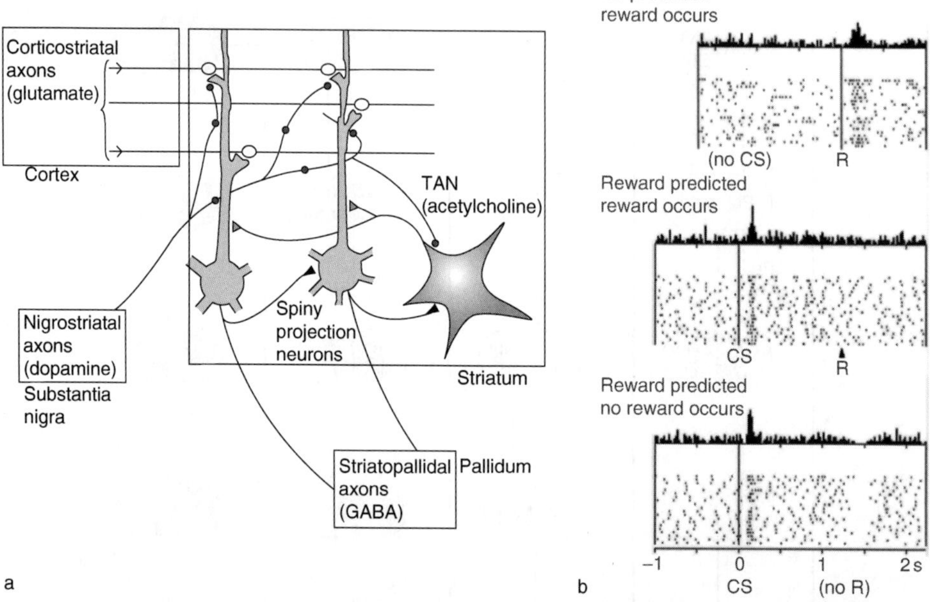

Figure 3 (a) Schematic diagram of striatal microcircuitry involved in reward-related motor learning. Corticostriatal axons make glutamatergic synaptic contacts (open circles) with the medium spiny projection neurons and cholinergic interneurons, thought to be the tonically active neurons (TAN). Nigrostriatal axons make dopaminergic synapses (filled circles) in the vicinity of corticostriatal synapses (as illustrated) and thalamostriatal synapses (not shown). Spiny projection neurons make γ-aminobutyric acid (GABA)ergic synapses (black triangles) on other spiny projection neurons and TANs, which, in turn, make cholinergic synapses (gray triangles) on spiny projection neurons. Phasic activity in the dopamine neurons produces pulses of dopamine able to act on corticostriatal and thalamostriatal synapses. This leads to strengthening of some synapses and weakening of others, which in turn facilitates selection of particular pathways. (b) Dopamine neurons convey an error in the prediction of reward. Each line of dots indicates a trial and each dot signifies the time that a single dopamine neuron fired an action potential in relation to the alignment event (middle vertical line). Top: No conditioned stimulus (CS). A drop of liquid reward (R) occurs unexpectedly, which constitutes a positive error in the prediction of reward, and the neuron increases its discharge rate. Middle: A learned, conditioned stimulus predicts a reward, and the reward occurs according to the prediction; hence, no error in the prediction of reward. The dopamine neuron does not respond to the predicted reward (at the time indicated by R), but instead increases its discharge rate following the reward-predicting CS (left). Bottom: Omission of predicted reward. The activity of the dopamine neuron decreases at the approximate time of an expected reward. (a) Adapted from Wickens JR, Reynolds JN, and Hyland BI (2003) Neural mechanisms of reward-related motor learning. *Current Opinion in Neurobiology* 13: 685–690, with permission from Elsevier. (b) Reproduced from Schultz W, Dayan P, and Montague PR (1997) A neural substrate of prediction and reward. *Science* 275: 1593–1599.

active ones. The interference between a currently relevant response and the recently primed one could partly explain the switch cost.

Rewards: Modulation of Striatal Signal Processing by Biological Feedback

Initiating, switching, inhibiting, and sequencing responses applies most to human behaviors in which task instructions are well understood or performance is relatively automatic. However, in many real-world situations the task to perform is not obvious and must therefore be learned or selected on the basis of biologically relevant feedback.

In many research settings with human participants and in nearly all studies with nonhuman ones, feedback is given in the form of primary reinforcers, such as water or food. Neurobiologically, feedback is coded by the firing rate of dopaminergic cells of the midbrain (**Figure 3**). In monkeys, this rate does not change significantly for highly overlearned behaviors, but, during the process of learning, these cells show significant modulation, which conveys to the basal ganglia either a reward signal or a signal that reflects an error in the prediction of reward. Therefore, as illustrated in **Figure 3(b)**, when an unpredicted reward occurs, the dopaminergic cells increase their discharge rates, but for highly predicted rewards they do not. When a predicted reward fails to materialize, these cells decrease their discharge rate. With repeated experience, the cells become unresponsive to rewards *per se*, but discharge in response to signals, such as

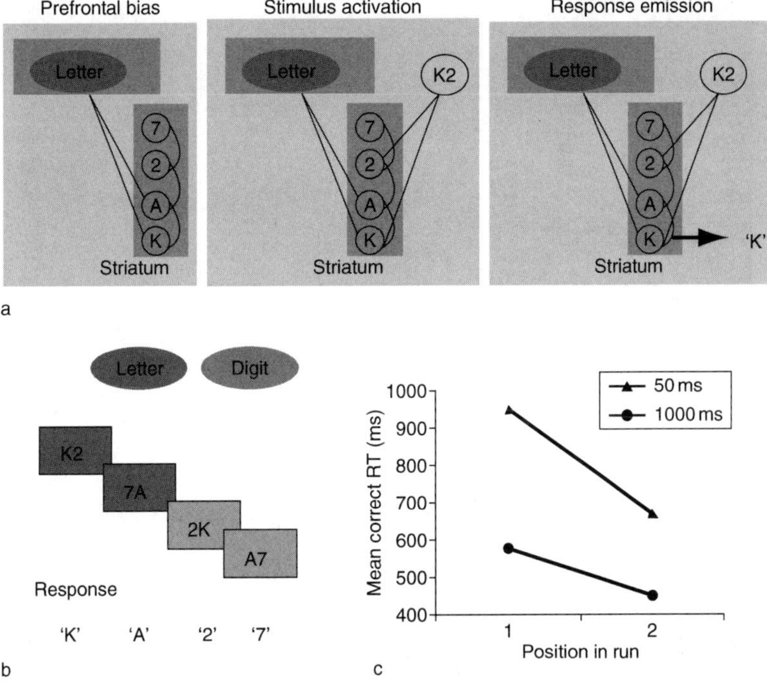

Figure 4 (a) A schematic model of how the prefrontal cortex could create top-down bias within the striatum to guide responding. The model is shown in three panels, representing different stages of task processing. Left panel: The person's knowledge of the upcoming task (letter task) creates bias over a subpopulation of striatal response channels by biasing 'A' and 'K.' Middle panel: The visual stimulus is shown ('K2'), which triggers striatal response channels for both a letter and a digit. Right panel: The striatal response channels are in mutual competition (e.g., via lateral inhibition), and the top-down prefrontal bias creates an advantage in favor of the letter channel, so that response is 'K.' (b) Illustration of a task-switching paradigm. On each trial the person responds as fast as possible to a stimulus such as 'K2' or '7A' by attending to the relevant task (letter or digit), which is cued (either 50 or 1000 ms) prior to the stimulus by means of a green- or yellow-colored rectangle. The third trial in the series is a switch trial because the subject must now attend to the digit, whereas previously the letter was relevant. In this paradigm, there are runs of two: the first position is always a switch (of task), the second position is always a repeat (of task). (c) Switching the task is associated with a longer reaction time (RT) than is repeating the task, and this effect is especially evident when the cue–stimulus interval is short (50 ms). This phenomenon is called the preparation effect.

conditioned stimuli, that predict reward. In accord with these findings in monkeys, studies in rats show that dopamine release increases as they approach a lever that they press to produce a reward. In rats trained to associate an initially neutral cue with the reward, the presentation of those cues also leads to an increase in dopamine release.

These data thus show that the dopaminergic signal to the basal ganglia provides feedback about response outcome in biologically significant terms. This feedback has the proposed function of strengthening some striatal synapses and weakening others. This synaptic plasticity, in turn, facilitates specific striatal output pathways, thus increasing the probability that a given input will trigger a given response. Empirical evidence provides support for this model. Neurons in the basal ganglia are highly sensitive to locations or movements associated with different levels of predicted reward. When monkeys choose to turn a handle leftward or rightward, and each choice leads to a different likelihood of reward, the activity of many striatal neurons correlates best with the predicted value of one of the two movements. Fewer neurons have activity that reflects the relative value of the two choices or the movements selected. Similar properties have been observed in the eye-movement part of the striatum, a part of the caudate nucleus. When monkeys make saccadic eye movement to either a left or a right target, and, for example, only saccades to the left target produce a reward for a given block of trials, neuronal activity is greater for leftward saccades than it is during a subsequent block of trials, when the same saccade fails to produce a reward. This higher level of activity correlates with quicker reaction times for the saccade target that will produce a reward. In terms of the model discussed earlier (**Figure 4(a)**), the higher

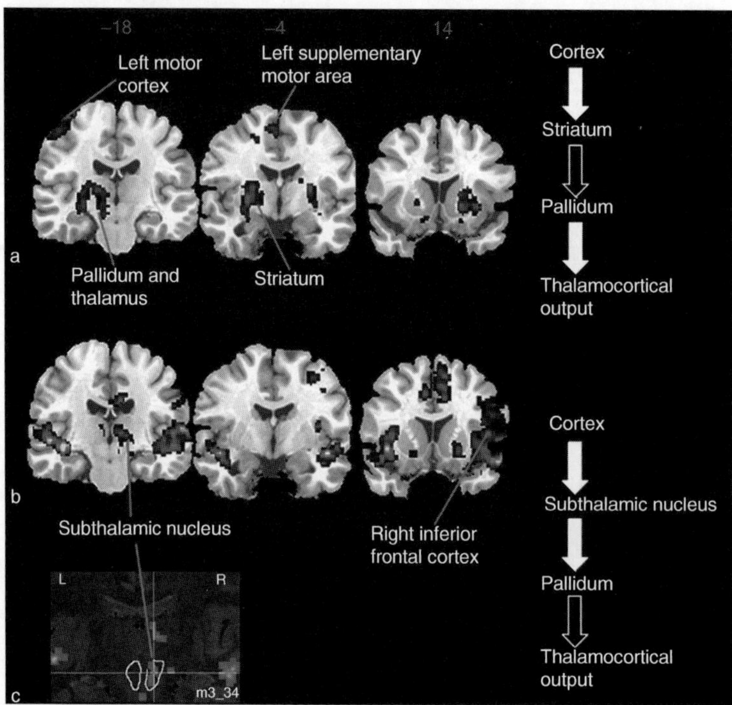

Figure 5 Functional imaging of executing a motor response and inhibiting an already initiated motor response. (a) Executing a motor response with the right hand. Activation is seen in the left (contralateral) supplementary motor area, striatum, pallidum, thalamus, and left motor cortex, consistent with the direct pathway through basal ganglia (right panel). (b) Inhibiting an initiated right-hand response activates the right subthalamic nucleus (confirmed by a high-resolution scan; see (c), in which the subthalamic nucleus is outlined by the white line, one in each hemisphere). This activation could result from inputs from the hyperdirect pathway (right panel), by which motor areas of the cortex excite the subthalamic nucleus, which, in turn, excites the pallidum and so suppresses thalamocortical output. Activation also occurs in the right inferior frontal cortex, consistent with the long-standing idea that the prefrontal cortex plays a key role in behavioral inhibition. At the top, the numbers in red denote Montreal Neurological Institute positions (in millimeters, posterior or anterior to the midpoint of the anterior commissure–posterior commissure line) of coronal slices through the brain. In the far right, unfilled arrows signify inhibitory projections, filled (white) arrows indicate excitatory ones. Adapted from Aron AR and Poldrack RA (2006) Cortical and subcortical contributions to Stop signal response inhibition: Role of the subthalamic nucleus. *Journal of Neuroscience* 26: 2424–2433.

level of activity reflects the current priming or bias for movements to that location, based on the prior probability of rewards.

Many functional imaging studies confirm a reward signal in the basal ganglia, especially in the ventral striatum. In some studies, activation in the striatum correlates with predicted reward; in others, it correlates with errors in the predicted reward or with negative reinforcement. Overall, it is thought that the response-channel biases described in the previous section occur in the striatum as a result of biologically relevant feedback from the midbrain dopaminergic system. In the aforementioned studies of eye movements, the striatum receives both cortical inputs bearing spatial and motor signals and dopaminergic inputs signaling reward or errors in reward prediction. This integrated signal, then, influences the motor system through its pallidal output. A key component of the basal ganglia's role in cognition thus involves the assignment of biologically relevant feedback to the computational operations of each of the loops illustrated in **Figure 2**, especially those involving the prefrontal cortex. In modulating the information processing of all cortical–basal ganglia loops at the striatal level, the dopaminergic inputs can influence a wide range of cognitive behaviors, including learning, memory, skills, and habits, the topics of the next section.

Learning, Memory, Skills, and Habits

Given its role in the adjustment of behavior based on feedback, it is not surprising that the basal ganglia play an important role in the learning of new skills and habits. For example, disorders of the basal ganglia impair learning of new motor skills, such as rotary pursuit, in which the individual attempts to keep a stylus positioned on a moving turntable. Because patients with basal ganglia disorders have impaired motor control, it can be difficult to interpret any deficits strictly in terms of an impairment in motor skill learning. However, it has been shown that these patients are impaired at motor learning even when the task is made easier, assuring that the patients and the controls start out at the same level of performance. Interestingly, some forms of motor skill learning, such as mirror tracing, are not impaired in patients with basal ganglia disorders. This can be explained based on the model that the basal ganglia may play a role in learning those tasks that require predictions generated internally (known as open-loop tasks, such as rotary pursuit), but not in tasks in which behavior is directly guided by external stimuli (known as closed-loop tasks, such as mirror tracing). This is consistent with the observation that patients with basal ganglia disorders are disproportionately impaired on tasks that require self-initiated movements, compared to visually guided ones.

The involvement of the basal ganglia in learning extends to perceptual and cognitive skills, as well. One paradigm that has been extensively investigated is probabilistic classification learning, in which an individual learns to classify stimuli into categories based on imperfect feedback (see **Figure 6(a)**). Patients with Parkinson's or Huntington's disease are impaired at this form of learning (**Figure 6(b)**), and neuroimaging studies have demonstrated activity in the striatum and dopaminergic midbrain areas during classification learning in normal persons (**Figure 6(c)**). This form of learning is often referred to as habit learning

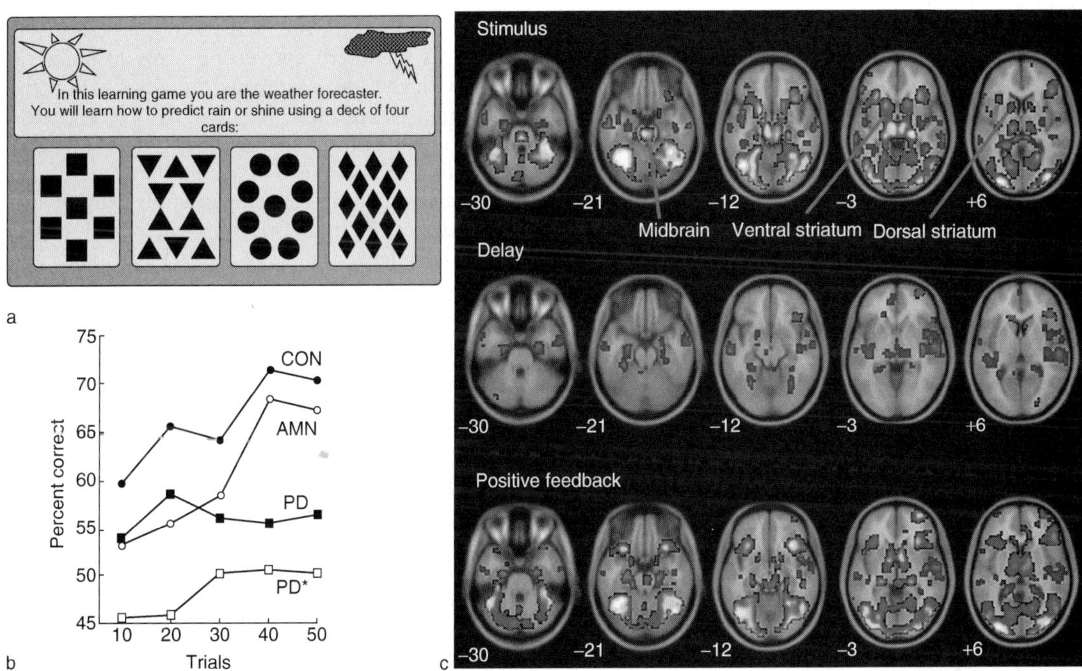

Figure 6 Probabilistic classification task. (a) The task involves the presentation of cards, which the person classifies as either predicting rain or sunshine. The stimulus is similar to a set of playing cards, and the feedback indicates a rain or sunshine outcome. (b) Patients with Parkinson's disease (PD) are impaired at learning the probabilistic classification task relative to controls (CON), particularly for advanced PD (PD$^+$), whereas patients with amnesia (AMN) due to medial temporal lobe damage have little or no impairment. It has been argued that the impairment in PD results from dysfunction of the basal ganglia. (c) Activation of basal ganglia and midbrain structures (putatively the substantia nigra and ventral tegmental area) during different phases of probabilistic classification in normal controls. Functional images are shown in axial format, starting at –30 mm beneath the anterior commissure–posterior commissure line, and rising dorsally to +6 mm above it. The stimulus (top row) and the feedback (bottom row) activate midbrain, as well as ventral and dorsal regions of the striatum, compared to a no-task baseline. This finding is consistent with the proposed role of the nigrostriatal system in mediating stimulus–response learning. The delay period (middle row) between the person's response and the outcome is associated with much less activation. Blue denotes 'deactivations' (i.e., regions of the brain where the functional magnetic resonance imaging signal is less for stimulus, delay, or feedback, compared to baseline); red/orange regions indicate the reverse. (b) Reproduced from Knowlton BJ, Mangels JA, and Squire LR (1996) A neostriatal habit learning system in humans. *Science* 273: 1399–1402, with permission. (c) Adapted from Aron AR, Shohamy D, Clark J, et al. (2004) Human midbrain sensitivity to cognitive feedback and uncertainty during classification learning. *Journal of Neurophysiology* 92: 1144–1152, with permission.

because it involves the gradual acquisition of stimulus–response associations without the necessity of conscious memory: this kind of probabilistic classification learning occurs normally in amnesic patients, who cannot consciously remember the details of the task.

As discussed in the previous section for stimulus–response learning, one important role of the basal ganglia in classification learning involves the processing of feedback. Neuroimaging studies have shown that learning with feedback more strongly engages the striatum than does learning without feedback. Patients with Parkinson's disease, who are impaired at learning the task with feedback, can learn the same information normally if they do not need to process feedback to do so. Thus, the role of the basal ganglia in some forms of learning may relate to a more general role in the integration of behaviorally relevant feedback with response selection and adjustments to ongoing behavior.

Learning is associated with changes in activity in medium spiny projection neurons (MSNs) and tonically active cholinergic interneurons (TANs) in the striatum. MSNs show changes as rats learn to run a maze. MSNs shift from firing throughout the behavior to firing selectively at the beginning and end of the behavior sequence. These patterns are also sensitive to extinction and reacquisition of the maze-running skill, and their firing is highly predictive of the animal's behavior. In primates, the observed learning-related changes in the putamen, as well as in the prefrontal cortex, closely mirror behavioral learning curves. In the caudate nucleus, similar changes appear earlier during the learning process, when cells appear to code for stimulus–response contingencies before they are fully reflected in behavior. These results are consistent with lesion studies which suggest that the caudate is responsible for learning of new stimulus–response relations (perhaps by quickly coding the reward associations of individual places or responses to those places), whereas the putamen is responsible for the learned expression of these relations. TANs in the striatum appear to be sensitive to the motivational relevance of stimuli regardless of their valence (appetitive or aversive).

The range of findings suggests that the striatum may in some cases compete with the medial temporal lobe to determine behavior. For example, in a cross-maze task, rats must learn to run from a particular starting point to a particular arm of the maze in order to receive food. The rat's response from a different starting point in the maze can be used to probe how it learns the task; early in training, rats will go to the same place in the maze (the place-learning strategy), which is dependent upon the hippocampus, whereas later in training they will make the same movements (a response-learning strategy), which is dependent upon the striatum. However, inactivation of the hippocampus or stimulation of the striatum early in training leads to the use of a response-learning strategy, whereas inactivation of the striatum or stimulation of the hippocampus late in training causes the animal to revert to a place-learning strategy. Thus, both systems appear to be able to drive behavior, and performance is determined by the relative balance of activity between the two systems. An alternative view is that early in training rats use external cues, such as those from vision, to determine the distance and direction to their next goal, whereas later in learning they use internal signals. These internal signals consist of efference copy, which matches the motor command that produces the response, and proprioceptive feedback that tells the motor system whether the current response is proceeding as planned. Thus, the place-learning strategy might be better construed as an exteroceptive strategy, and the response-learning strategy as an interoceptive one. This formulation agrees with the idea, expressed previously, that the basal ganglia's core function may involve a general role in the integration of behaviorally relevant feedback with response selection. Along these lines, functional imaging studies in human study participants show that activity in the striatum and medial temporal lobe correlates negatively across participants and across learning trials. Further, dysfunction of the basal ganglia is associated with a general increase in the engagement of the medial temporal lobe during the learning of tasks that are normally dependent upon the striatum. The mechanisms by which this competition occurs are not yet understood, but they could rely upon biasing signals from the prefrontal cortex (**Figure 4(a)**).

Synthesis

The basal ganglia play a nearly ubiquitous role in cognition. Their contribution can perhaps best be appreciated by considering them as a device that resolves the selection demands that confront a behaving organism. These demands require prioritizing, scheduling, planning, sequencing, and generally controlling the way in which context elicits behavior in accordance with external and internal constraints. Which behavior occurs depends on many factors: top-down biases from the prefrontal cortex that prime particular response channels, the salience and prior rewarding properties of stimuli, the prepotency of various alternatives, and the degree of competition from other cognitive systems. By integrating different information through the interconnections among parallel cortical–basal ganglia loops, moderating this flow according to the various pathways that influence basal ganglia output, and incorporating signals from neurotransmitter systems that monitor outcomes in biologically relevant terms, the basal ganglia can control systems of thought as well as action.

See also: Appetitive Systems: Amygdala and Striatum; Basal Ganglia: Functional Models of Normal and Disease States; Basal Ganglia and Oculomotor Control; Dopamine in Perspective; Dopamine – CNS Pathways and Neurophysiology; Dopamine: Cellular Actions; Executive Function and Higher-Order Cognition: Assessment in Animals; Motor Skill Learning; Procedural Learning: Striatum; Reward Systems: Human; Reward Processing: Human Imaging; Task Switching.

Further Reading

Aron AR and Poldrack RA (2006) Cortical and subcortical contributions to Stop signal response inhibition: Role of the subthalamic nucleus. *Journal of Neuroscience* 26: 2424–2433.

Aron AR, Shohamy D, Clark J, et al. (2004) Human midbrain sensitivity to cognitive feedback and uncertainty during classification learning. *Journal of Neurophysiology* 92: 1144–1152.

Barnes TD, Kubota Y, Hu D, et al. (2005) Activity of striatal neurons reflects dynamic encoding and recoding of procedural memories. *Nature* 437: 1158–1161.

Brasted PJ and Wise SP (2004) Comparison of learning-related neuronal activity in the dorsal premotor cortex and striatum. *European Journal of Neuroscience* 19: 721–740.

Hikosaka O, Nakamura K, and Nakahara H (2006) Basal ganglia orient eyes to reward. *Journal of Neurophysiology* 95: 567–584.

Jog MS, Kubota Y, Connolly CI, et al. (1999) Building neural representations of habits. *Science* 286: 1745–1749.

Knowlton BJ, Mangels JA, and Squire LR (1996) A neostriatal habit learning system in humans. *Science* 273: 1399–1402.

Lawrence A, Sahakian BJ, and Robbins TW (1998) Cognitive functions and corticostriatal circuits: Insights from Huntington's disease. *Trends in Cognitive Sciences* 2: 379–387.

Mink JW (1996) The basal ganglia: Focused selection and inhibition of competing motor programs. *Progress in Neurobiology* 50: 381–425.

Nambu A, Tokuno H, and Takada M (2002) Functional significance of the cortico-subthalamo-pallidal 'hyperdirect' pathway. *Neuroscience Research* 43: 111–117.

Packard MG (1999) Glutamate infused posttraining into the hippocampus or caudate-putamen differentially strengthens place and response learning. *Proceedings of the National Academy of Sciences of the United States of America* 96: 12881–12886.

Pasupathy A and Miller EK (2005) Different time courses of learning-related activity in the prefrontal cortex and striatum. *Nature* 433: 873–876.

Poldrack RA, Sabb FW, Foerde K, et al. (2005) The neural correlates of motor skill automaticity. *Journal of Neuroscience* 25: 5356–5364.

Redgrave P, Prescott TJ, and Gurney K (1999) The basal ganglia: A vertebrate solution to the selection problem? *Neuroscience* 89: 10009–10023.

Schultz W, Dayan P, and Montague PR (1997) A neural substrate of prediction and reward. *Science* 275: 1593–1599.

Shohamy D, Myers CE, Grossman S, et al. (2004) Cortico-striatal contributions to feedback-based learning: Converging data from neuroimaging and neuropsychology. *Brain* 127: 851–859.

Wickens JR, Reynolds JN, and Hyland BI (2003) Neural mechanisms of reward-related motor learning. *Current Opinion in Neurobiology* 13: 685–690.

Relevant Websites

http://web.mit.edu – Department of Brain and Cognitive Sciences, McGovern Institute for Brain Research.

http://en.wikipedia.org – Wikipedia: The Free Encyclopedia.

Cognition: Cerebellum Role

J E Desmond and C L Marvel, The Johns Hopkins Medical Institutions, Baltimore, MD, USA

Introduction

The cerebellum has been historically linked to the control of posture, gait, and skilled voluntary movement. Yet, numerous cases have been reported – dating back to the early 1800s – of nonmotor deficits, such as mental impairment, in patients with cerebellar degeneration and atrophy. Despite these reports, a distinct bias persists among many researchers and physicians that cerebellar-related cognitive deficits are attributed to some type of motor response or to lesion encroachment onto other brain regions. Indeed, some of the earliest functional neuroimaging studies used cerebellar metabolism as a baseline from which neocortical cognitive activation was compared because it was assumed that the cerebellum was silent during cognition.

A new wave of interest in nonmotor functions of the cerebellum began to emerge in the early 1990s. With functional neuroimaging in the hands of a rapidly increasing number of neuroscientists, increasingly more cerebellar activations that were difficult to explain in terms of simple motor processes were reported, and these results were seen to converge with results reported in the patient literature. This article reviews some of the relevant findings supporting a role for the cerebellum in executive function. Executive function refers to some of the highest levels of cognitive control, including planning, organization, decision making, problem solving, and logical analysis. Executive function is typically required when information needs to be coordinated or manipulated, or when prepotent or habitual responses need to be inhibited. Transynaptic neuroanatomical tracing studies have provided convincing evidence that lateral and posterior regions of the cerebellar cortex project through ventral portions of the dentate nucleus and the thalamus to connect with dorsolateral prefrontal regions implicated in executive control. Thus, an anatomical foundation exists by which cerebro-cerebellar networks can influence higher level cognition.

Functional Neuroimaging Studies

Functional neuroimaging methods such as positron emission tomography and functional magnetic resonance imaging (fMRI) are sensitive to regional metabolic changes in blood flow that occur as a result of increased neuronal activity. As summarized here, neuroimaging has revealed cerebellar activation in many investigations that focus on executive function.

Verbal Working Memory

Cerebellar activations have been consistently observed by a number of researchers in verbal working memory tasks. In their simplest form, these tasks require the online maintenance of verbal information via a 'phonological loop' – that is, the refreshment of phonological information through repeated articulatory rehearsal. For example, keeping a phone number in mind long enough to dial a telephone would typically require verbal working memory. Manipulation of the stored information is hypothesized to engage 'central executive' processes of working memory. For example, the n-back task entails sequentially presenting letters to the subject, whose task is to decide if the present letter matches the one that occurred n letters ago. Comparisons of activation in the n-back task relative to those observed in more maintenance-based tasks have shown that although the cerebellum responds to both kinds of working memory tasks, more lateral cerebellar activations are observed for the manipulation task, in conjunction with greater dorsolateral prefrontal activation.

Verbal Fluency

Verbal fluency is a frequently used measure of executive function. Common neuropsychological testing involves asking a subject to say as many words as possible in 60 s that begin with a specific letter. Usually, this procedure involves organizing output into meaningful clusters in order to speed responses. For example, if prompted with the letter S, one may first try to think of S words that begin with the letters S–E (set, settee, sell, self, seep, etc.). When neural activations during letter fluency are compared to a control condition (e.g., counting forward from 1), subjects increase activation in the left prefrontal cortex and right cerebellum.

Some of the earliest demonstrations of cognition-related cerebellar activations were reported for a particular type of verbal fluency task referred to as verb generation. This involves the presentation of a noun, such as 'ball,' and the subject responds with an appropriate action verb, such as 'throw.' As a control condition, the noun is simply read and repeated. This and other fluency tasks, such as word stem completion, are associated with robust right posterior cerebellar and left prefrontal activations. Interesting practice-related effects have been associated with these activations. If subjects are given a second run of the verb-generation task using the same set of nouns that they saw on the first run, left prefrontal and right cerebellar activation diminish concurrently and increase again when novel nouns are presented. These results demonstrate the close functional coupling of the cerebro-cerebellar network during cognitive operations. However, this coupling may reflect complementary rather than redundant functionality. For example, in the stem completion task, word stems with few possible completions (e.g., PSA__) elicit greater cerebellar activation compared to completion of stems with many possible completions (e.g., STA__), whereas the reverse is true for activation in left prefrontal regions. One possible explanation for this dissociation is that cerebellar activation during word stem completion is related to word search operations, whereas prefrontal activation is related to word selection.

Cognitive Flexibility

A popular neuropsychological test for assessing the ability to shift cognitive sets according to changes in stimulus contingencies is the Wisconsin Card Sorting Test (WCST). In the WCST, subjects are required to sort cards according to one of three possible dimensions: number, color, or shape. The subject must determine the correct sorting strategy on the basis of right/wrong feedback that is presented after the subject's response to each card. The experimenter can change the correct sorting strategy suddenly without warning, and the subject must then determine the new dimension for sorting. Impaired performance on the task is observed as a tendency to perseverate on the incorrect strategy in light of new information that contingencies have changed. As a neuropsychological test, the WCST appears to be sensitive to frontal lobe dysfunction, but the specificity of the test to the frontal lobes has been questioned. Indeed, neuroimaging studies have revealed a large network of cortical and subcortical activations, including bilateral cerebellum, when contrasting WCST performance with sensorimotor control tasks. Such control tasks effectively rule out simple visual- or response-elicited explanations for cerebellar activation, but they do not address whether the cerebellum may be responding to the nonexecutive working memory requirements of the task, such as the need to keep the current relevant dimension of the stimuli in mind. Recent investigations, however, have tried to separate higher order from lower order cognitive operations in the task. For example, by contrasting the WCST task with a task that cues the subject when a dimension change occurs, simple working memory maintenance operations are presumably subtracted out, and what remains are the most executive components of the task. Cerebellar activations have been shown to persist when such subtractions are performed.

Reasoning/Planning

A number of different studies have examined the neural substrates of higher order skills used in hypothesis testing and logical inference. These investigations have applied one of three main approaches. The first requires the subject to solve a puzzle, with the control condition attempting to equate the sensorimotor aspects of manipulating puzzle pieces in the absence of planning. The second requires the subject to form a hypothesis about features presented within a group of multidimensional stimuli (e.g., containing letters, numbers, shapes, and colors or composed of a large grid of squares, a subset of which are filled, whereas others are unfilled). On each trial, the subject determines which features of the stimuli are relevant or correct. Control conditions typically involve presenting identical stimuli but asking the subject to attend and respond to only one dimension. The third approach requires subjects to decide whether three-sentence syllogisms, presented with either semantic or nonsemantic content, are logically valid. An effective control condition for this type of study replicates much or all of the working memory requirements of the reasoning task. It entails reading three sentences, the first two of which are plausible premises, whereas the third contains unrelated content and therefore requires no reasoning. For each of these approaches, prominent cerebellar activation has been observed, suggesting a role for the cerebellum in reasoning and planning.

Dual Tasks

Patients with executive dysfunction often exhibit profound difficulties performing multiple tasks at once. In healthy subjects, performance typically declines for both tasks relative to performance in either task alone, but subjects are nevertheless able to perform both tasks to some degree. Dual-task performance has thus been used by neuroimagers to investigate whether there are specific neural correlates of cognitive coordination. Of particular interest are tasks that show unique regions of activation during dual-task performance relative to single-task performance. Such studies have shown that in cases in which neither prefrontal nor cerebellar activation are evident for either task alone, dual-task performance recruits new prefrontal, parietal, and cerebellar regions.

Random Number Generation

Random number generation (RNG) requires a subject to randomly generate numbers, usually 1–10, while suppressing the natural tendency to count in sequence or to repeat the same number habitually. Thus, RNG involves both fluency and inhibition. When subjects are forced to generate random numbers at increasing rates, numbers tend to become less random and more sequential. Neuroimaging investigations have thus used pacing stimuli to control the rate of RNG and have typically contrasted activation for this task with that obtained from counting in sequence. Medial portions of the cerebellum have been shown to increase activation with increasing rate of performance, consistent with either motoric or timing functions. However, more lateral portions of the cerebellar hemispheres have exhibited diminution of activation at faster rates of RNG compared to serial counting. These occur in parallel with similar diminutions seen in dorsolateral prefrontal and parietal regions. These results suggest that a cortical–subcortical executive network is involved in suppressing habitual responses and that at increasing rates, network activity and behavioral performance begin to break down.

Theory of Mind

The ability to infer intention or mental states in others is an important aspect of human social interaction and has been referred to as possessing a 'theory of mind.' Both verbal and nonverbal approaches have been used in neuroimaging investigations of theory of mind. An example of a nonverbal approach would be to present a subject with frames of a cartoon and ask the subject to choose an ending frame from two or three choices using a button press. For the theory of mind condition, the choice of the ending requires inferring the intention of the character depicted in the cartoon, whereas the control condition requires understanding physical causality but does not involve making inferences of motives. An example of a verbally based approach would be to ask subjects in the theory of mind condition to read a brief story describing the actions of a character and then to make up a story explaining the conditions that led to the character's behavior. As a control condition, subjects read aloud a story that requires no attribution of intentions, thereby equating the same amounts of reading and word production produced by the theory of mind task. In both approaches, strong cerebellar activation has been observed in the theory of mind condition relative to the control condition. For the nonverbal tasks, left cerebellar/right prefrontal activation has been observed, whereas the laterality of frontocerebellar activation is reversed for the verbally based approach.

Patient Studies

Evidence for cerebellar contribution to executive function can be drawn from neuroimaging and neuropsychological studies of cerebellar-affected clinical populations. In these cases, the cerebellum may be disrupted early on as a result of maldevelopment or during adulthood following years of normal function.

Neurological Disorders

Compelling evidence for the cerebellum's participation in executive function comes from studies of patients with neurological disorders confined to the cerebellum. These data have been derived from neuropsychological studies of patients with cerebellar stroke, tumor resection, cerebellar degeneration, and cerebellitis. In general, executive dysfunction seems to be most pronounced in cerebellar patients with large bilateral infarcts, followed by those with unilateral infarcts, and least in those with pancerebellar involvement. However, deficits are not always evident or as severe as might be expected given the size of the lesion. Heterogeneity of lesion type and time since lesion onset are two key factors that affect a patient's degree of impairment. Improved function has been noted in those with nonprogressive lesion types (e.g., stroke) after several months of recovery.

Relatively few studies have directly addressed the cognitive contributions of the cerebellum in clinical populations. This is due, in part, to the difficulty in acquiring patients with diseases confined to the cerebellum with an absence of disease elsewhere in the brain. However, one seminal study, conducted by Schmahmann and Sherman, tested 20 patients with cerebellar diseases on a variety of neuropsychological tests that involved executive skills. Patients were most impaired in working memory manipulation, verbal fluency, and complex figure copying. During complex figure copying, one is presented with a drawn design and asked to copy it while the figure is in plain view. Although this may appear to be a straightforward task, patients have difficulty copying the figure if they cannot develop a drawing strategy, such as where to begin. They may also be unable to organize and maintain a long-term plan for drawing so that the design is redrawn in sections. There may be a focus on details without consideration for the overall configuration. This results in a drawing of several geometric

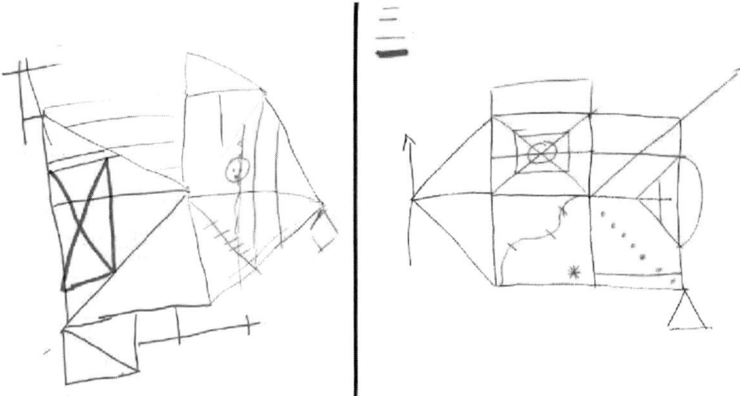

Figure 1 Copying complex figures relies on executive skills, such as planning, organizing, and maintaining a strategy for sequential actions. In these drawings, a copy of the Rey–Osterreith complex figure (ROCF; left) was drawn by a patient with a symptomatic postcerebellitis infection. The same patient copied the Taylor complex figure (TCF; right) 3 months later. Using the colored pencil lines as a key to the sequence of the patient's actions, one can see that the patient applied a part-based approach to the ROCF. She drew the figure piecemeal, completing the major sections of the right side first (black). Next, she drew the general composition of the left side (red) and then went back to fill in details on the right side (blue). Finally, she returned to the left side to add a few more details to complete the drawing (green). The final construction is awkward in design but includes all relevant pieces of the original figure. In sharp contrast, 3 months later the patient applied a highly organized copying strategy that included a configurational approach to the TCF. The patient began by drawing the general outline of the figure (black). She worked her way clockwise by filling in the upper left and right quadrants next (red). Finally, she filled in the bottom right and left quadrants (blue). This efficient strategy allowed her to complete the figure quickly before being asked by the experimenter to draw with the green pencil. In addition to improving her copying speed, the recovered patient drew neater, stronger lines that rendered a highly accurate depiction of the complex figure. Reproduced from Schmahmann JD and Sherman JC (1998) The cerebellar cognitive affective syndrome. *Brain* 121(Part 4): 561–579, by permission of Oxford University Press.

shapes that are not well integrated into a whole. Often, figure parts are misplaced or missing altogether. Without intact skills for creating and implementing a copying strategy, a patient can eventually produce a rough version of the figure but inefficiently and usually with errors. To illustrate such deficits, **Figure 1** shows two copies of complex figures drawn by a patient during the symptomatic phase of a postcerebellitis infection (left, Rey–Osterreith complex figure) and by the same patient 3 months later during recovery (right, Taylor complex figure). It is clear that during the symptomatic phase of the illness the patient was unable to appreciate the overall configuration, which resulted in an inefficient part-based approach to figure copying. After recovery, the patient was able to rely on her improved executive skills to use a configurational approach, which yielded a highly organized and accurate replication.

Although patients with cerebellar disease may exhibit executive dysfunction, the current opinion posits that disrupted communication between the cerebellum and the frontal lobe contributes to these deficits. A breakdown in the frontocerebellar network may result in an inability of the cerebellum to contribute to the frontal lobe's temporal organization of mental processes. Consequently, an otherwise coordinated sequence of cognitive events unravels, leading to a phenotype of cognitive impairment. The term dysmetria of thought has been given to describe this phenomenon in patients with cerebellar disease.

Developmental Disorders

There are a number of developmental disorders that involve the cerebellum. However, maldevelopment is not typically confined to the cerebellum and often influences additional areas of the brain. With increasing popularity in the use of neuroimaging tools, however, researchers have been able to associate structural and functional abnormalities of the cerebellum with executive dysfunction in several developmental disorders, as summarized here.

Attention-deficit/hyperactivity disorder Attention-deficit/hyperactivity disorder (ADHD) is characterized by inattention and hyperactive or impulsive behavior. Executive dysfunction is a prominent feature of ADHD and may be related to an underlying core disturbance in response inhibition. A fairly consistent finding in ADHD brain research is reduction in total cerebellar size, most markedly in the posterior vermis (lobes VIII–X). Although nearly all brain imaging research in ADHD has been conducted in children and adolescents, evidence suggests that cerebellar abnormalities are not progressive and are not related to medication treatment. Studies using fMRI in ADHD have reported decreased cerebellar activation during verbal working memory and response inhibition. However, the severity and consistency of cerebellar-related cognitive impairments in ADHD has not been firmly established. For example, several fMRI studies of executive-type tasks in ADHD children have implicated frontal–striatal rather than frontocerebellar pathways. It is possible that cerebellar disturbances in ADHD disrupt executive function through miscommunications with a larger neural network that includes the frontal lobe and basal ganglia.

Autism spectrum disorder Autism spectrum disorder (ASD) is marked by impaired interpersonal relations, poor communication skills, and reduced or repetitive interests and behaviors. It is believed that poor cognitive planning, flexibility, and inhibition underlie the social and behavioral abnormalities associated with ASD. The most consistent postmortem finding in ASD is decreased cerebellar Purkinje neurons in the absence of neurodegeneration. Genetic disturbances in cerebellar development may lead to a disruption in normal cerebellar functions and contribute to the onset of autistic symptoms. fMRI studies that target cerebellar functions in autism are beginning to emerge in the literature. For example, decreases in cerebellar activation have been reported in ASD subjects while observing (but not while imitating) emotional expressions. Attention-related decreases in cerebellar activation also have been reported. Cognitive and social deficits that are inherent to ASD may be attributed to maldevelopment of the cerebellum and/or its communication with other brain structures. However, there is an obvious need for future studies on this topic in order to better characterize the role of the cerebellum in autism.

Dyslexia Dyslexia is a developmental disorder identified in children who fail to attain reading and writing skills commensurate with their level of education and intelligence. Poor motor coordination and delayed motor milestones have also been noted in dyslexic children. Although there are several hypotheses regarding the fundamental disturbance in dyslexia, one view is that dyslexics have cerebellar-related difficulties with automatization of skills. Automaticity – the ability to perform a skill fluently and without conscious effort in doing so – is essential for multitasking. Impaired automaticity in dyslexia may contribute to difficulties in phonological processing, word recognition, verbal working memory, and, ultimately, fluent reading. It is generally accepted that the cerebellum plays a key role in automatization, and that cerebellar damage can force one to pay extra attention to skill sequences that never become automatic. Accordingly, dyslexics have difficulties performing tasks that require the blending of two or more skills. For example, balancing ability (e.g., standing on one foot) becomes disproportionately affected when dyslexics perform a counting task at the same time. Cerebellar structural abnormalities, such as decreased anterior lobe volume, have been reported in this population. Moreover, these abnormalities have been correlated with cognitive tests of verbal ability, such as spelling, word identification, and rapid letter naming. Although there is persuasive evidence to support cerebellar-related cognitive deficits in dyslexia, there has not been full agreement on this in the literature. Notably, some researchers maintain that the cerebellum is only secondarily related to dyslexic cognitive impairments, with primary deficits attributed to cortical areas. However, the cerebellar hypothesis provides an interesting and parsimonious explanation for both the motor and the cognitive deficits observed in this disorder.

Schizophrenia Schizophrenia is a psychiatric disorder that involves an array of perceptual, emotional, motor, and cognitive impairments. Cognitive deficits are widespread but are found in several important components of executive function, such as attention, working memory, sequencing, and problem solving. Data supporting cerebellar-related cognitive disturbances in schizophrenia have come from functional neuroimaging studies of working memory, verbal recall, and social cognition. In addition, structural imaging studies have found decreased cerebellar volume, especially of the vermis, although some reports have also noted increased cerebellar volume or normal cerebellar volume. Perhaps the most compelling study to date on this topic, conducted by Ho and colleagues, examined 155 neuroleptic-naive schizophrenia patients on a comprehensive cognitive battery. In addition, patients were examined for cerebellar soft signs (motor impairments referable to the cerebellum), including unsteady tandem gait, intention tremor, poor balance, and flaccid muscle tone. Thirty-two patients were identified as having cerebellar soft signs. Relative to the 123 patients without cerebellar soft signs, these 32 patients exhibited specific deficits of attention, working memory, problem solving, and figure copying in addition to having overall smaller cerebellar volume. These results suggest that decreased cerebellar volume in schizophrenia is related to impairments of motor coordination and higher order cognitive skills. Given that cerebellar abnormalities have been reported in many, but not all, regional brain volume studies of schizophrenia, this phenomenon may apply to only a subset of patients.

Individuals born very preterm Children born very preterm (i.e., <33 weeks of gestation) often show signs of putative cerebellar dysfunction, such as clumsiness and poor motor coordination. Although neuroimaging studies are only beginning to emerge on this topic, data suggest that total cerebellar volume is decreased in these individuals. Moreover, volumetric decreases in lateral cerebellar hemispheres have correlated with performance on tests of abstract reasoning and visuospatial construction. Functional neuroimaging of adolescents born preterm has revealed bilateral reductions in cerebellar activity during response inhibition, despite normal task performance. Because the pre-, peri-, and neonatal periods represent a vulnerable time for brain formation, individuals who are unable to complete the full gestation (approximately 38 weeks) run the risk of maldevelopment. This risk is not specific to the cerebellum, and indeed, abnormalities have been reported in multiple cortical and subcortical brain areas in this population. Therefore, cerebellar contributions to cognitive and motor deficits observed in preterm individuals may be further attributed to underlying factors, such as hypoxia, sepsis, or malnutrition around the time of birth.

Substance Abuse

A recent view on substance abuse holds that executive dysfunction is responsible for the loss of self-control that leads to drug and alcohol addiction. Evidence implicating the cerebellum in substance abuse suggests that the cerebellum may contribute to cognitive deficits (e.g., poor inhibition) that segue into drug-seeking behavior. Structural brain imaging of alcoholics has revealed volume reductions throughout the cerebellum, particularly in the anterior vermis. Similar cerebellar abnormalities have been reported in children exposed to high prenatal doses of alcohol. Functional neuroimaging has shown that activity in the left anterior cerebellum and cerebellar vermis increases during alcohol craving. Moreover, alcoholics have demonstrated excessive right anterior cerebellar activation while performing a task of verbal working memory. Studies have also shown that abnormal cerebellar blood flow is associated with the use of cocaine, marijuana, methylphenidate (Ritalyn), 3,4-methylenedioxymethampetamine (MDMA, or ecstasy), and amphetamine. For example, blood flow to the cerebellar vermis increases in cocaine users when viewing cocaine-related cues. Over-responsive activity in the left cerebellum of cocaine users has been associated with high demands on working memory and self-inhibition. A similar pattern of excessive left cerebellar activity has been observed in heavy marijuana users while performing a complex decision-making task. In nearly all cases, findings from the structural and functional imaging studies described previously have implicated the prefrontal cortex in conjunction with the cerebellum. This pattern suggests that a disrupted frontocerebellar circuit contributes to drug and alcohol addiction. However, specifying the contributions of the cerebellum to substance dependence first requires a deeper understanding of the cerebellum's role in cognition.

Cerebro-Cerebellar Interactions

Most complex behaviors require a response of some kind, and this inevitably invokes motor systems. Given the involvement of the cerebellum in motor control, it may be difficult to completely separate cognitive- and motor-related cerebellar functions. However, the results of Hulsmann et al. illustrate how cognitive and motor involvement of the cerebellum falls along a continuum, reflecting progressive activation of cerebro-cerebellar closed loops, rather than a dichotic absolute. **Figure 2** shows that for a self-paced finger response (button press), activations occurring close in time to the finger response, and soon thereafter, are observed in primary sensorimotor cortex as well as in medial spinocerebellar regions. In contrast, looking 3 or 4 s prior to the response, activations are observed in neocortical areas associated with motor planning, such as supplementary and premotor cortex, as well as in more lateral regions of the neocerebellum. This example is derived from a relatively simple behavior. However, it is not difficult to extrapolate from these results and hypothesize that as higher order planning is required – occurring even more remotely in time from the final motor response – neocortical regions, such as parietal and dorsolateral prefrontal regions, are in communication with the most lateral and posterior regions of the cerebellum during executive planning operations. As described in the introduction, anatomical studies have demonstrated the existence of these closed-looped cerebro-cerebellar circuits. The successive activation of these circuits during the time course of simple and complex behaviors gives us a beginning framework for understanding why the cerebellum is active in so many functions, from motor control to cognition.

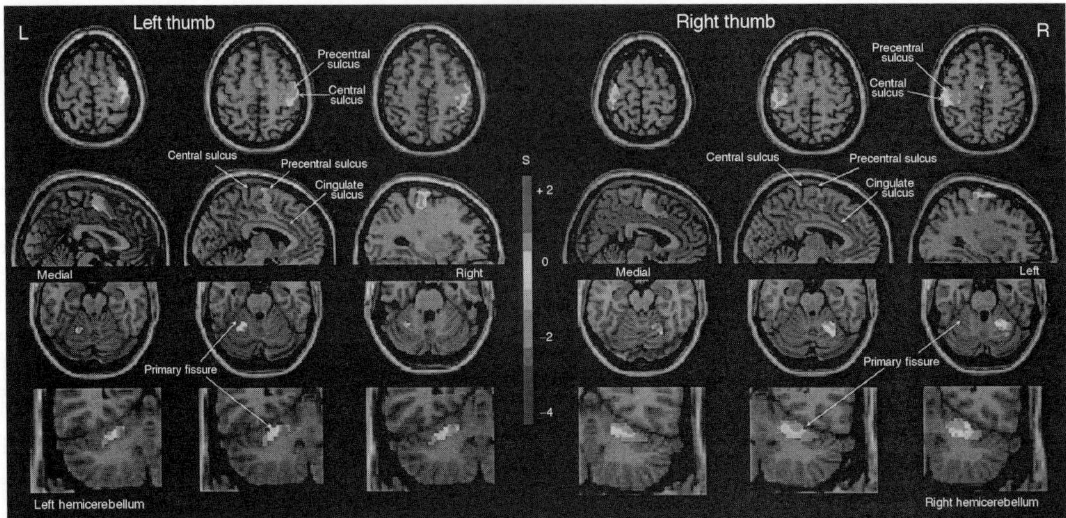

Figure 2 Color-coded map depicting the time course of maximum activation relative to a self-paced thumb movement. Earliest activations prior to movement are depicted in blue and green and occur in cingulate motor areas, supplementary motor, and premotor areas, as well in the lateral neocerebellar regions. Activations occurring at the time of movement and slightly thereafter are observed in primary sensory and motor cortex as well as in medial spinocerebellar regions. The sequential progression of regional activations during this simple motor behavior demonstrates how cerebro–cerebellar interactions could progress in similar closed-loop circuits during executive function. Reproduced from Hulsmann E, Erb M, and Grodd W (2003) From will to action: Sequential cerebellar contributions to voluntary movement. *NeuroImage* 20(3): 1485–1492, with permission from Elsevier.

See also: Cerebellum and Oculomotor Control; Cerebellum: Clinical Pathology; Cerebellum: Evolution and Comparative Anatomy; Cognitive Deficits in Schizophrenia; Executive Function and Higher-Order Cognition: Neuroimaging; Executive Function and Higher-Order Cognition: Definition and Neural Substrates; Frontal Lobe Syndrome; Procedural Learning: Cerebellum Models; Reasoning and Problem Solving: Models; Short Term and Working Memory; Substance Abuse and Dependence; Synaptic Plasticity: Cerebellum; Task Switching.

Further Reading

Calarge C, Andreasen NC, and O'Leary DS (2003) Visualizing how one brain understands another: A PET study of theory of mind. *American Journal of Psychiatry* 160(11): 1954–1964.

Chen SH and Desmond JE (2005) Temporal dynamics of cerebro-cerebellar network recruitment during a cognitive task. *Neuropsychologia* 43(9): 1227–1237.

Collette F, Olivier L, Van der Linden M, et al. (2005) Involvement of both prefrontal and inferior parietal cortex in dual-task performance. *Brain Research. Cognitive Brain Research* 24(2): 237–251.

Daniels C, Witt K, Wolff S, Jansen O, and Deuschl G (2003) Rate dependency of the human cortical network subserving executive functions during generation of random number series – A functional magnetic resonance imaging study. *Neuroscience Letters* 345(1): 25–28.

Dapretto M, Davies MS, Pfeifer JH, et al. (2006) Understanding emotions in others: Mirror neuron dysfunction in children with autism spectrum disorders. *Nature Neuroscience* 9(1): 28–30.

Desmond JE, Gabrieli JDE, and Glover GH (1998) Dissociation of frontal and cerebellar activity in a cognitive task: Evidence for a distinction between selection and search. *NeuroImage* 7: 368–376.

Goel V, Buchel C, Frith C, and Dolan RJ (2000) Dissociation of mechanisms underlying syllogistic reasoning. *NeuroImage* 12 (5): 504–514.

Ho BC, Mola C, and Andreasen NC (2004) Cerebellar dysfunction in neuroleptic naive schizophrenia patients: Clinical, cognitive, and neuroanatomic correlates of cerebellar neurologic signs. *Biological Psychiatry* 55(12): 1146–1153.

Hulsmann E, Erb M, and Grodd W (2003) From will to action: Sequential cerebellar contributions to voluntary movement. *NeuroImage* 20(3): 1485–1492.

Lie CH, Specht K, Marshall JC, and Fink GR (2006) Using fMRI to decompose the neural processes underlying the Wisconsin Card Sorting Test. *NeuroImage* 30(3): 1038–1049.

Nicolson RI and Fawcett AJ (2005) Developmental dyslexia, learning and the cerebellum. *Journal of Neural Transmission Supplementum* 69: 19–36.

Nosarti C, Rubia K, Smith AB, et al. (2006) Altered functional neuroanatomy of response inhibition in adolescent males who were born very preterm. *Developmental Medicine and Child Neurology* 48(4): 265–271.

Schmahmann JD and Sherman JC (1998) The cerebellar cognitive affective syndrome. *Brain* 121(Part 4): 561–579.

Sullivan EV, Harding AJ, Pentney R, et al. (2003) Disruption of frontocerebellar circuitry and function in alcoholism. *Alcoholism, Clinical and Experimental Research* 27(2): 301–309.

Valera EM, Faraone SV, Biederman J, Poldrack RA, and Seidman LJ (2005) Functional neuroanatomy of working memory in adults with attention-deficit/hyperactivity disorder. *Biological Psychiatry* 57(5): 439–447.

Cognition: Neuropharmacology

A B Hains and A F T Arnsten, Yale Medical School, New Haven, CT, USA

The prefrontal cortex (PFC) is instrumental in coordinating, controlling, and executing cognitive and emotional processes using appropriate judgment, flexibility, and attention. The ability to organize appropriate responses to a changing environment requires maintenance and updating of relevant information as well as control over the processing of new incoming information. This careful choreography allows the regulation of impulses, language, attention, decision making, and error correction and is commonly referred to as the executive functions. These abilities require the representation of information not currently in the environment (sometimes referred to as working memory) and are mediated by the PFC. The PFC receives ascending inputs from diverse areas of the brain. The dorsal and lateral surfaces of the PFC interconnect with the sensory and motor association cortices and are key for the regulation of behavioral responses and attention; the ventral and medial regions of PFC interconnect with brain regions involved with emotion, such as the amygdala, hypothalamus, and nucleus accumbens. The ventral surface is often referred to as the orbital frontal cortex (OFC) because it sits above the orbits of the eyes. In rodents, the PFC is much smaller; there is a medial portion (the prelimbic and infralimbic mPFC) that is needed for cognitive control and an orbital area more ventral-laterally that has functions similar to the OFC in primates. The homology of the mPFC in rodents to the dorsolateral PFC in primates is controversial. It is likely that it is more homologous to the mPFC in primates and involves a combination of affective and cognitive functions.

Single-unit recording studies in monkeys have shown that PFC neurons are able to hold modality-specific information online over a delay and to use this represented information to guide behavior in the absence of environmental cues. PFC neurons can also fire in relationship to an abstract rule that is used to govern action. A unique feature of PFC neurons is their ability to maintain information in the presence of distracting stimuli. Delay-related firing also can serve as the basis for behavioral inhibition (e.g., having to look away from a remembered visual stimulus or reverse reward contingencies). Neuromodulators can have powerful effects on the patterns of PFC neuronal response and on PFC cognitive functioning.

The PFC is highly sensitive to its neurochemical state. Evidence to date suggests that the dorsolateral PFC is particularly sensitive to catecholamines (dopamine (DA) and norepinephrine (NE)), whereas the ventromedial PFC is more influenced by serotonin (5-HT). This view has emerged from both lesion studies in nonhuman primates that selectively deplete catecholamines (vs. 5-HT) and from pharmacological studies in humans that preferentially block catecholamine (vs. 5-HT) transporters. However, there are critical exceptions to this generalization; for example, NE α2A-adrenoceptor stimulation can improve ventromedial PFC functions, and 5-HT2A receptor blockade can impair dorsolateral PFC function. Acetylcholine (ACh) also has powerful influences on PFC functions, although there has been little research on cholinergic mechanisms in the monkey PFC. Most of the research examining direct cholinergic mechanisms in PFC have been performed in rats using attentional tasks, and thus it is difficult to compare results across paradigms.

It is noteworthy that the PFC also projects back down to the monoamine and ACh cells, and thus it is positioned to regulate its own modulatory input. Interestingly, the NE and DA cells respond to informative cues and receive projections from the dorsolateral PFC, whereas the ACh cells respond to rewards and response choices, and these cells receive inputs from the OFC. Recent studies indicate that NE cells also receive projections from the OFC and anterior cingulate and that these projections may regulate their tonic firing rate rather than the response to specific stimuli. Thus, there is a coordinated interplay between the subregions of the PFC and their modulatory inputs.

Dopamine

The pioneering work of Goldman-Rakic first revealed the powerful influences of DA on the working memory functions of the dorsolateral PFC. This initial study found that depleting catecholamines in PFC was as destructive as removing the cortex itself. Although this first study focused on DA, it is now known that the depletion of both DA and NE may be especially deleterious.

The DA inputs to the PFC arise from the dorsal cells of the substantia nigra and from the ventral tegmental area in the midbrain. DA neurons project throughout the primate cortex, with highest levels in primary and secondary motor cortices. Within the PFC, the medial PFC actually has a denser innervation than the dorsolateral PFC, despite the established importance of DA to dorsolateral PFC function. Thus, the quantity of innervation cannot be equated with the importance of an input because it is possible that some delicate inputs may be relatively sparse because they are so powerful.

There are two families of DA receptors: the D1 family (D1 and D5) and the D2 family (D2, D3, and D4). There are currently no drugs available that distinguish between D1 and D5 receptors; thus, reference to D1 usually means D1 or D5. The highest levels of DA receptors in the PFC are the D1 family, and these receptors have been the focus of most research on DA mechanisms in the PFC. D1/D5 receptors can be found in both superficial and deep layers of the PFC, with D1 receptors concentrated on spines and D5 receptors on shafts of pyramidal cells. In contrast, the D2 receptor family is more concentrated in layer V, the cells that project to the basal ganglia. Thus, the D2 family may be especially involved with modulating the response output. D4 receptors are especially numerous on γ-aminobutyric acid (GABA)ergic interneurons in the PFC.

Most research on DA influences on PFC cognitive function has focused on spatial working memory. In monkeys, spatial working memory generally has been assessed using an oculomotor or classical delayed response task. This paradigm requires the monkey to remember a spatial location over a brief delay (seconds). The location changes on each trial so that memory must be continuously updated. Electrophysiological studies of PFC neurons record single units from monkeys performing the oculomotor version of this task. Many neurons in PFC exhibit spatially tuned firing during the delay period; that is, the cells fire more for a preferred than for a nonpreferred direction. This is considered the electrophysiological signature of spatial working memory. In rats, spatial working memory is often assessed in a spatial delayed alternation task, within a T-maze, or using automated operant procedures. Delayed nonmatch-to-position is often substituted for delayed alternation, but it is substantially easier due to diminished proactive interference. In humans, spatial working memory is tested in a variety of paradigms, including a search task on the CANTAB battery and N-back tasks developed from the monkey delayed-response task. In addition, human studies often use the Wisconsin Card Sorting task, Stroop Interference task, and Stop-Signal tasks, which emphasize the inhibitory functions of the PFC.

The D1 family of receptors has powerful effects on spatial working memory function. Either too little or too much D1/D5 receptor stimulation impairs working memory; that is, there is an inverted-U dose–response curve that occurs within normal physiological parameters (see **Figure 1**). Insufficient levels of DA D1 stimulation probably contribute to cognitive deficits in Parkinson's disease and may also contribute to normal age-related cognitive decline. Excessive levels of D1 receptor stimulation occur during stress exposure and contribute to stress-induced PFC dysfunction. This inverted U in working memory abilities has been observed in monkeys, rats, mice, and human subjects. In humans, an inverted U has been observed in relation to the COMT genotype, whereby the substitution of methionine for valine weakens enzymatic degradation of DA and shifts the U curve rightward. An inverted U is also observed in single-unit recordings of monkeys performing a spatial working memory task. D1 receptor stimulation is especially important for suppressing cell responses to nonpreferred spatial directions. These suppressive effects are mediated by the activation of cyclic adenosine monophosphate (cAMP) intracellular signaling. The effects of D1 receptor stimulation probably depend on the endogenous state of the neuron (e.g., whether it is broadly or narrowly tuned) and on the cognitive demands on the subject. This may explain why D1 receptor blockade or DA depletion has little effect on some kinds of executive function such as self-ordered tasks.

The influence of the D2 family is more complex and less well studied. There has been almost no research on D3 receptors mechanisms in the PFC, and drugs which distinguish between D2 and D3 receptors are scarce. Early studies showed that D2/D3 receptor blockade did not impair working memory, but rat studies suggest that D2/D3 receptor stimulation (e.g., during stress exposure) may impair

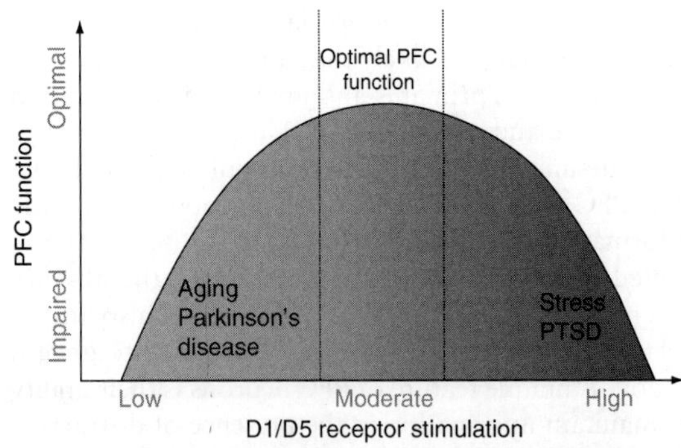

Figure 1 A schematic representation of the inverted-U relationship between D1/D5 receptor stimulation and PFC function; moderate levels of receptor stimulation produce enhanced delay-related firing in PFC neurons as well as optimal performance on working memory tasks, whereas insufficient or excessive D1/D5 receptor stimulation erodes spatial mnemonic tuning and impairs working memory. PFC, prefrontal cortex; PTSD, posttraumatic stress disorder.

working memory performance. Electrophysiological studies show that D2 receptor stimulation increases response-related firing, but not delay-related firing, of PFC neurons in monkeys performing a working memory task. Because some response-related firing occurs after the motor response is initiated, it may act as corollary discharge, informing the brain that a motor command has been initiated. This may have particular relevance to schizophrenia, in which hallucinations may involve weakened corollary discharge.

Recordings from rat PFC slices and from awake monkeys indicate that D4 receptor stimulation inhibits GABAergic interneurons via G_i inhibition of cAMP signaling. Thus, D4 receptor stimulation may have an overall excitatory effect on PFC circuits. However, D4 also appears to inhibit some pyramidal cells, and so the picture may be more complex. Behavioral studies of D4 antagonists may find an inverted-U dose–response curve on working memory, but these agents have not been studied extensively. It should be noted that NE has a higher affinity for D4 receptors than for adrenoceptors and thus that the D4 receptor should properly be considered a catecholamine receptor rather than a DA receptor.

Norepinephrine

It is now appreciated that NE has just as powerful an effect on NE function as DA. In contrast to DA D1, NE appears to dissociate its beneficial and detrimental effects at different types of adrenoceptors. Thus, these may be more practical targets for pharmacological treatment of PFC dysfunction.

The NE innervation of the PFC arises from the locus coeruleus (LC) in the pons. As with DA, there is a delicate innervation of both the supragranular and granular layers, with particular density in layer I. The superficial layers are the focus of cortical–cortical connections and have dense α1- and α2-adrenoceptor binding. There are three α2 subtypes; of these, the α2A subtype is particularly prominent in the monkey PFC. Electron microscopy studies have documented α2A receptors postsynaptically in the spines and dendrites of PFC pyramidal cells, as well as in presynaptic locations on NE axons and terminals. β-Receptor binding is densest in the middle layers (i.e., layer IV), which receives projections from the thalamus.

As with DA, NE has dual effects on PFC function depending on the amount of NE release. Moderate levels of NE release during normal waking have vital, beneficial effects on PFC function via higher-affinity postsynaptic α2A-adrenoceptors, whereas high concentrations of NE released during stress impair PFC function via lower-affinity α1-adrenoceptors and possibly β1-adrenoceptors (see **Figure 2**). In most parts of brain, NE has potent effects via β-adrenoceptors. In contrast, the PFC seems more dramatically altered by α-adrenoceptors. **Figures 3(a)** and **3(b)** illustrate the

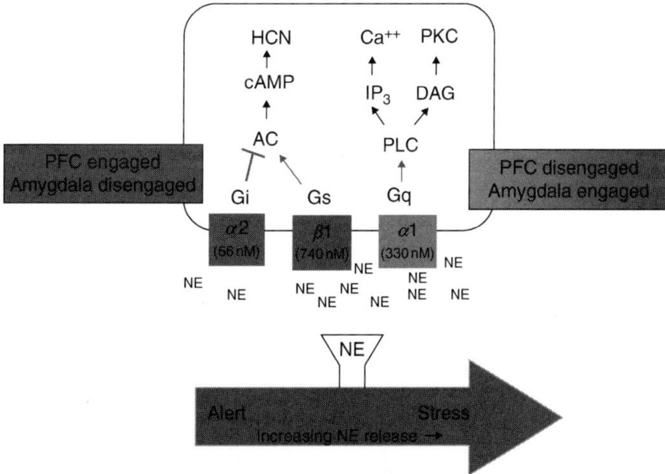

Figure 2 Levels of NE release determine the functional status of the PFC based on varying affinities for adrenergic receptors. Moderate concentrations of NE during the nonstressed, alert state lead to improved PFC function via binding to higher-affinity α2A-adrenoceptors (shown in blue). Higher concentrations of NE release in the PFC, which are observed in conditions of stress, lead to PFC impairment due to the binding to lower-affinity α1- and possibly β1-adrenoceptors. Recent studies have started to uncover downstream, intracellular signaling mechanisms that mediate these NE actions. In contrast, the amygdala is modulated in a manner opposite to the PFC, whereby α2-adrenoceptors impairs, and β- and α1-adrenoceptors strengthen, amygdala regulation of behavior. Thus, NE may act as a chemical switch to determine whether behavior is regulated by higher-order PFC operations or more primitive mechanisms mediated by the amygdala. AC, adenylyl cyclase; cAMP, cyclic adenosine monophosphate; DAG, diacylglycerol; IP_3, inositol triphosphate; NE, norepinephrine; PFC, prefrontal cortex; HCN, hyperpolarization-activated cyclic nucleotide-gated channels; PKC, protein kinase C; PLC, phospholipase C.

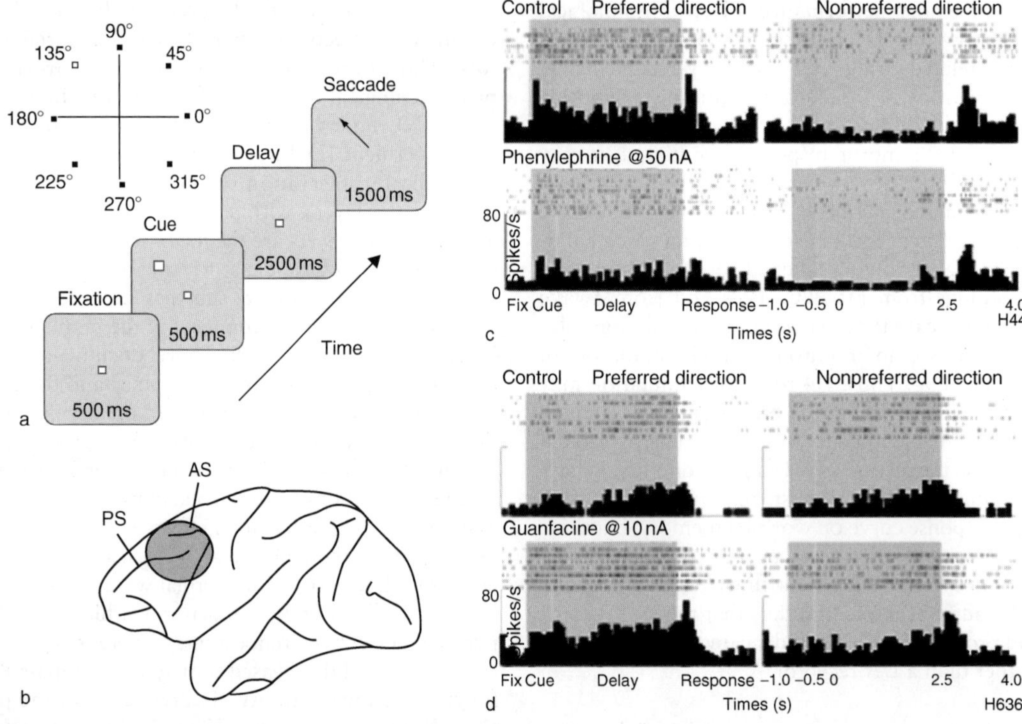

Figure 3 The delay-related activities of neurons of the monkey PFC provide a cellular representation of working memory: (a) the oculomotor delayed-response task often used for *in vivo* electrophysiological recordings; (b) an electrode is lowered into the monkey's dorsolateral PFC to record responses while the monkey is performing the task; (c) the response of delay-related neurons altered by the iontophoretic application of phenylephrine, an α1 agonist, acting on adrenoceptors; (d) the response of delay-related neurons altered by the iontophoretic application of guanfacine, an α2A agonist, acting on adrenoceptors. As shown in (a), following a cue at a specific orientation, there is a delay period during which the monkey must keep the previously presented cue in mind in order to guide the appropriate saccade (response). As shown in (c) and (d), cells show preferences for particular orientations (preferred vs. nonpreferred), and specific neurons fire selectively during either the cue, delay, or response periods. The iontophoretic application phenylephrine suppresses delay-related firing (c), whereas the application of guanfacine enhances delay-related firing (D). PS, principle sulcus; As, arcuate PFC, prefrontal cortex. This figure was generously supplied by Dr. Min Wang, Yale University.

influence of α1- versus α2-adrenoceptor stimulation on the delay-related firing of PFC neurons in monkeys performing an oculomotor delayed response task. Stimulation of α1-adrenoceptors with phenylephrine reduces delay-related cell firing for the preferred direction (**Figure 3(c)**), whereas stimulation of α2A-adrenoceptors with guanfacine enhances delay-related firing for the preferred direction (**Figure 3(d)**). However, β mechanisms are just beginning to be understood and may involve opposing actions at β1 versus β2 receptors that are obscured with nonselective compounds. The administration of α2A agonists improves spatial working memory in mice, rats, monkeys, and humans, especially in subjects with PFC dysfunction. In addition to working memory, the α2A agonist, guanfacine, has been shown to improve a number of other PFC functions, such as lessening distractibility, improving reversal performance and other measures of behavioral and cognitive inhibition (e.g., in humans, improving performance on the Stroop interference task), and strengthening conditional motor learning. It has little effect on posterior cortical functions and, indeed, can impair amygdala function. Conversely, the blockade of endogenous α2 receptors in the PFC with yohimbine impairs working memory, weakens no-go responding, and induces locomotor hyperactivity. Thus, this system is particularly relevant to attention-deficit hyperactivity disorder (ADHD). Recordings from PFC neurons in monkeys performing spatial working memory tasks show similar effects; α2A-adrenoceptor stimulation increases delay-related firing for the preferred direction (see **Figure 3(d)**), whereas yohimbine suppresses delay-related firing. These enhancing effects on working memory result from the stimulation of postsynaptic α2A receptors in the PFC, inhibiting cAMP production, closing HCN channels on dendritic spines, and strengthening the functional connectivity of PFC circuits. Based on research in animals, guanfacine is now in use for the treatment of ADHD, Tourettes syndrome, posttraumatic stress disorder (PTSD), and mild traumatic brain injury. Recent studies indicate that mutations on the Disordered In Schizophrenia 1 (DISC1) gene may lead to excessive cAMP signaling in patients with schizophrenia-like illnesses and that agents such as guanfacine may be useful in treating PFC deficits in these disorders as well.

In contrast to α2A-adrenoceptors, stimulation of α1-adrenoceptors impairs working memory. α1-Adrenoceptor antagonists have no effect on working memory when infused into the PFC during nonstress conditions, but they protect PFC cognitive function under conditions of uncontrollable stress. Conversely, infusions of α1-adrenoceptor agonists such as phenylephrine mimic the stress response and impair working memory. These detrimental actions are mediated by phosphotidyl inositol–protein kinase C intracellular signaling. Detrimental α1-adrenoceptor actions have been observed at the cellular levels as well, at which iontophoresis of phenylephrine onto PFC neurons decreased the delay-related cell firing necessary for working memory function (see **Figure 3(c)**). As with cognitive performance, this collapse in delay-related firing was reversed by a protein kinase C inhibitor. These mechanisms are especially relevant to PTSD, bipolar disorder, and schizophrenia, all of which are caused by, or worsened by, stress exposure. The α1-adrenoceptor antagonist prazosin is now used to treat patients with PTSD, and all atypical antipsychotic medications have α1 and 5-HT2 receptor-blocking properties. 5-HT2 receptors, like α1 receptors, are coupled to phosphotidyl inositol–protein kinase C intracellular signaling. Genetic and biochemical studies suggest that phosphotidyl inositol–protein kinase C intracellular signaling is overactive in bipolar disorder and schizophrenia (e.g., due to loss of function mutations in the genes encoding for DAG kinase or RGS4). Most antimanic agents reduce the activity of this signaling pathway. Thus, these agents may restore PFC regulation of behavior, thought, and affect by normalizing phosphotidyl inositol–protein kinase C intracellular signaling.

Serotonin

The raphe nuclei send widespread and dense 5-HT projections throughout the cortex, including the PFC. Electron microscopy studies indicate that these 5-HT projections make connections with both pyramidal cells and interneurons in the PFC. PFC neurons project back to the raphe nuclei, where they may have an inhibitory influence. There are a multitude of 5-HT receptor subtypes (at least 13); however, the localization and function of these receptors within the PFC are poorly understood. The 5-HT1 family appears to be more densely localized in superficial layers, whereas 5-HT2 receptors are more concentrated in middle layers.

It is well established that 5-HT plays a critical role in affective regulation by the OFC, whereas its effects on dorsolateral PFC function appear to be more complex. The most unambiguous evidence for the role of 5-HT in executive processes comes from studies of reversal learning in marmoset monkeys. In reversal learning, subjects are presented with two stimuli and initially learn to associate reward with one stimulus. After this pairing has been established, a subsequent reversal between stimulus and reward takes place, such that the animals must now make the previously unrewarded response in order to receive a reward. Studies in humans as well as lesion studies in nonhuman primates indicate that the performance of this task depends on the OFC as well as the ventromedial PFC. Selective reductions in 5-HT via injections of 5,7-dihydro-testosterone (DHT) directly into the OFC of marmoset monkeys impairs performance on serial discrimination reversal tasks. In contrast, performance is preserved on an attentional set-shifting task that requires subjects to reverse rules and learn new rules regarding a perceptual dimension of a stimulus (i.e., shape or color) or a specific feature of a percept (see **Figure 4**). Monkey studies have shown that set-shifting performance depends on the dorsolateral PFC. Similar results have been observed in humans, in whom rapid tryptophan depletion impairs reversal learning while preserving attentional set-shifting performance. Interestingly, studies in monkeys as well as rats have shown that OFC depletion of DA had no effect on performance of a serial reversal learning task.

In addition to regulating attentional set shifting, the lateral PFC inhibits inappropriate motor responses, which can be evaluated by performance on a stop-signal task. A study in humans found that increases in NE, via NE reuptake inhibition, led to faster reactions on a stop-signal task. Performance on a probabilistic learning task, an analog to reversal learning, was not affected by NE reuptake inhibition. Conversely, increased basal 5-HT levels produced impairments on a probabilistic learning task but did not influence stop-signal performance. These findings support the findings from depletion studies in humans and monkeys. Together, these data have led to the hypothesis that 5-HT and catecholamines have dissociable and specific roles in the modulation of PFC operations.

One significant barrier to interpreting studies using global depletions or enhancements of 5-HT action is

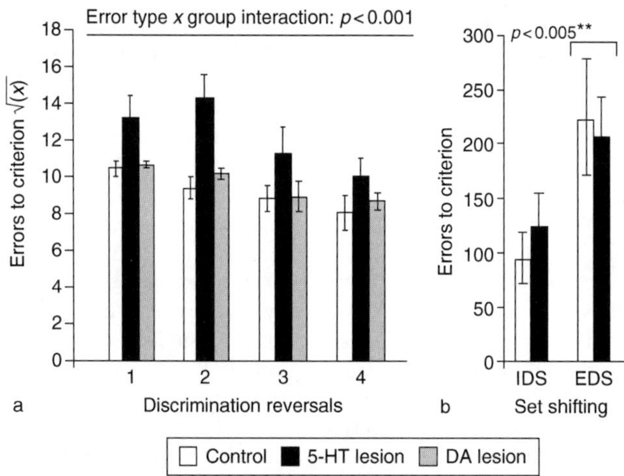

Figure 4 Effects of prefrontal serotonin depletions on learning and attention: (a) depletions of prefrontal serotonin (but not prefrontal dopamine) disrupt discrimination reversal learning; (b) prefrontal serotonin depletions have no effect on shifting an attentional set. In (b) note the greater number of errors made in performing a discrimination requiring a shift of attentional set (EDS) compared to one involving the maintenance of a previously acquired attentional set (IDS), in both groups. 5-HT, serotonin; DA, dopamine; EDS, extra-dimensional shift; IDS, intradimensional shift. Courtesy of Dr. Angela Roberts, Cambridge University, UK.

unraveling the heterogeneous actions of different receptor subtypes. Future studies need to examine the role of specific 5-HT receptor subtypes and determine whether dorsolateral PFC operations are altered when the 5-HT system is probed more selectively. For example, electrophysiological studies indicate that 5-HT2 receptors may influence spatial working memory operations, and these findings need to be pursued at the behavioral level.

In summary, 5-HT plays a distinct, if complicated role in the affective flexibility and the execution of primed behaviors and many of the activities of the mPFC and the OFC. Through its connections with limbic areas, the medial OFC is critical in connecting associative information regarding outcomes with the representational memory processes of the PFC. Ultimately, this positions the OFC to regulate the generation and use of outcome expectancies, which underlie the ability to make adaptive decisions. Thus, it is not surprising that studies of major depressive disorder in humans implicate dysfunction of the OFC as well as the dorsal raphe nucleus. Future studies using receptor-selective agents and behavioral paradigms probing a wide array of PFC-mediated cognitive functions will bring an improved understanding of the complex role of 5-HT in higher-order cognitive and affective processes.

Acetylcholine

Cholinergic neurons project from the basal forebrain to virtually all layers and all regions of the cortex, with approximately 75% of cholinergic cortical innervation originating from the nucleus basalis. Cholinergic axons make synapses in all layers of the monkey PFC, targeting pyramidal, and nonpyramidal cells. Most synapses on pyramidal cells target dendritic shafts, although there are some on spines and very few on the cell bodies. There are two general families of cholinergic receptors: muscarinic and nicotinic receptors. There are five muscarinic subtypes. Of these, the M2 receptor serves as both a presynaptic autoreceptor and a postsynaptic receptor on PFC pyramidal and nonpyramidal cells. In PFC pyramidal cells, M2 receptors are observed on dendritic spines receiving excitatory (asymmetric) inputs. The M1 receptor is also found postsynaptically on dendritic shafts and spines. Nicotinic receptors are often found presynaptically on the terminals of monoamine or ACh axons, where they can regulate transmitter release. They are most dense in layer I of the monkey PFC, which contains the highest levels of catecholamine fibers.

Although there have been detailed anatomical studies of the ACh inputs to the PFC, there has been little or no research on the function of these inputs in monkeys. Many studies have found alterations in working memory with systemic administration of muscarinic and nicotinic compounds, but these agents have powerful actions throughout the brain (e.g., in the thalamus), and thus alterations in cognitive performance cannot be necessarily attributed to PFC actions. In contrast, there has been a great deal of progress outlining ACh actions in the rodent mPFC, in which infusions of muscarinic blockers such as scopolamine directly into the mPFC induce working memory deficits. Much of this research has focused on the important role of ACh in attention, specifically vigilance. These effects are evident both in the early stages of sensory processing and in subsequent top-down processing, which is regulated by the PFC.

It is widely accepted that ACh-mediated enhanced processing of sensory information underlies the cognitive process of attention. Attention encompasses a variety of operations that together contribute to the detection and discrimination of stimuli; and the integrity of attention processes contributes to the efficacy of higher-order cognitive functions such as learning and memory. Numerous behavioral studies have implicated basal forebrain cortical cholinergic inputs in sustained attention functioning. Tasks measuring sustained attention, or vigilance, require an animal to distinguish signal trials, which typically use a panel of lights illuminated for a short duration of time, from nonsignal trials, in which no light is illuminated. Accuracy is measured by training the animals to make a designated response for both signal and nonsignal trials. A range of stimulus intensities, presentation intervals, and the introduction of distracters are often used to manipulate the difficulty of this task.

Performance on sustained attention as well as distracter tasks stimulates ACh release. Behavioral and electrophysiological studies have implicated the association areas of the cortex, most notably the mPFC, in the ACh facilitation of sustained attention. First, the PFC appears particularly sensitive to ACh. In rats, local administration of ACh stimulated mPFC neuronal activity. In addition, several studies have indicated that the mPFC requires ACh to effectively suppress the processing of irrelevant or distracting information. One study observed increases in ACh release in the frontal cortex of rats as they recovered from a distracter introduced in a sustained attention task. A separate study found rats with ACh depletion to be unimpaired on tasks of attention under normal conditions; however. the introduction of distracters into the task resulted in a significant decrease in performance as compared to their sham counterparts. These findings further support the importance of ACh to the maintenance of information and attention under challenging or unpredictable conditions, such as the presentation of distracters or the erosion of signal.

The modification of information processing and more complex operations by knowledge-driven or goal-oriented information is referred to as top-down regulation. Basal forebrain cortical cholinergic input is mediated by efferent projections from the PFC; thus, the PFC is well positioned to orchestrate cholinergic innervation throughout the brain. PFC-driven top-down control of signal processing is thought to be one mechanism through which the PFC filters distracting stimuli and directs thought and behavior appropriately. In primates, ACh cells probably receive information from the OFC regarding reward or other affective information that may motivate attentional state. It was recently shown in rodents that PFC cholinergic stimulation resulted in increased ACh release in the posterior parietal cortex, a region that has been implicated with attention. Thus, following stimulation, the PFC is positioned to deploy ACh release in other cortical regions.

Overactivity of ACh has been linked to attention performance deficits, specifically to an increased response to nonsignal stimuli. This impaired signal-to-noise processing results in overprocessing, leading to generically amplified and unfiltered information and ultimately to false-positive responses. However, underactive cholinergic input to the cortex may likewise contribute to cognitive and attention deficits. In Alzheimer's disease, cholinergic inputs from the basal forebrain deteriorate, and this loss of input is may contribute to impaired signal detection as well as subsequent impairments in the PFC-mediated or top-down regulation of attention. Although this ACh dysregulation appears to contribute to the symptoms of disorganized thought and behavior, at this time, no conclusive studies have distinguished the ramifications of ACh underactivity from gross impairments in executive centers that would otherwise direct this input. In sum, studies of dysregulated ACh processing in disease states reiterate that moderate levels of ACh are necessary for the appropriate signal-driven activation of cortical processing centers and for the subsequent regulation of attention via PFC-dictated ACh release.

Summary

The PFC subserves executive functions by organizing information required for future thought and action. A vast body of literature across species indicates that the cognitive tasks of the PFC are sensitive to a variety of neurochemicals and that different neurotransmitter systems have distinct roles in cognitive functions of the PFC. However, there are several formative obstacles to fully delineating the neurochemical modulation of executive functions, most notably, the myriad actions of specific receptors and the broad range of tasks regulated by the various subregions of the PFC. Understanding the intricacies of these powerful neurochemical influences on PFC function is key to our understanding of the etiology and treatment of many neuropsychiatric illnesses, including schizophrenia, ADHD, and PTSD, as well as the decline in PFC cognitive functions with advancing age.

See also: Acetylcholine Neurotransmission in CNS; Dopamine; Executive Function and Higher-Order Cognition: Definition and Neural Substrates; Norepinephrine: CNS Pathways and Neurophysiology; Prefrontal Cortex: Structure and Anatomy; Prefrontal Cortex; Serotonin (5-Hydroxytryptamine; 5-HT): Neurotransmission and Neuromodulation; Strategic Control of Memory; Working Memory: Capacity Limitations.

Further Reading

Arnsten AFT (2007) Catecholamine and second messenger influences on prefontal cortical networks of representational knowledge: A rational bridge between genetics and the symptoms of mental illness. *Cerebral Cortex* 17(Supplement 1): 16–17.

Arnsten AF and Li BM (2005) Neurobiology of executive functions: influences on prefrontal cortical functions. *Biological Psychiatry* 57: 1377–1384.

Arnsten AF and Robbins TW (2002) Neurochemical modulation of prefrontal cortical function in humans and animals. In: Stuss DT, and Knight RT (eds.) *Principles of Frontal Lobe Function*, pp. 51–84. Oxford: Oxford University Press.

Brozoski TJ, Brown RM, Rosvold HE, and Goldman PS (1979) Cognitive deficit caused by regional depletion of dopamine in prefrontal cortex of rhesus monkeys. *Science* 205: 929–932.

Chamberlain SR, Muller U, Blackwell AD, Clark L, Robbins TW, and Sahakian BJ (2006) Neurochemical modulation of response inhibition and probabilistic learning in humans. *Science* 311: 861–863.

Clarke HF, Walker SC, Dalley JW, Robbins TW, and Roberts AC (2007) Cognitive inflexibility after prefrontal serotonin depletion is behaviorally and neurochemically specific. *Cerebral Cortex* 17: 18–27.

Goldman-Rakic PS (1995) Cellular basis of working memory. *Neuron* 14: 477–485.

Robbins TW (2005) Chemistry of the mind: Neurochemical modulation of prefrontal cortical function. *Journal of Comparative Neurology* 483: 140–146.

Sarter M and Bruno JP (1997) Cognitive functions of cortical acetylcholine: Toward a unifying hypothesis. *Brain Research Reviews* 23: 28–46.

Sarter M, Hassemo M, Bruno JP, and Givens B (2005) Unraveling the attentional functions of cortical cholinergic inputs: Interactions between signal-driven and cognitive modulation of signal detection. *Brain Research Reviews* 48: 98–111.

Vijayraghavan S, Wang M, Williams GV, and Arnsten AFT (2007) Dopamine D1 receptor stimulation alters tuning of prefrontal cortical neurons during spatial working memory. *Nature Neuroscience* 10: 376–384.

Wang M, Ramos BP, Paspalas CD, et al. (2007) α2A-Adrenoceptors strengthen working memory networks by inhibiting cAMP-HCN channel signaling in prefrontal cortex. *Cell* 129: 397–410.

Wang M, Vijayraghavan S, and Goldman-Rakic PS (2004) Selective D2 receptor actions on the functional circuitry of working memory. *Science* 303: 853–856.

Cognitive Control and Development

D Amso and B J Casey, Sackler Institute for Developmental Psychobiology, Weill Medical College of Cornell University, New York, NY, USA

Immature cognition is characterized by a greater susceptibly to interference from competing inputs, representations, or responses. Cognitive control is the ability to reduce this interference. This ability has been included in a number of theories of attention and memory and referred to in a number of ways, including executive function, attentional bias, and supervisory attention. Each of these coined terms is suggestive of a mechanism that is required to direct or guide our attention or actions. The following question is addressed in this article: How is it that we gain this ability with development?

Measures of cognitive control across development are necessarily constrained by the changing repertoire of behaviors available at different points in development and by age-appropriate techniques. At the core of these tasks is the demand for selection of one target, action, location, or dimension in the presence of competing alternatives. While holding this defining feature constant, researchers have been able to manipulate aspects of cognitive control paradigms to be appropriate for use at different ages while still allowing valid examination of this one construct. We review findings from paradigms used across development.

Evidence of Cognitive Control in Infancy

In the context of the infant, the environment is full of sensory and perceptual information competing for attention. For learning to take place, there must be a developing control mechanism that allows for suppression of irrelevant information so that selection of information relevant for current learning or behavior is possible. Some of the earliest research targeting control over behavior in infancy made use of reaching paradigms and originally posited that cognitive control was not apparent until the end of the first postnatal year. However, research into the development of the oculomotor system has shed new light on control over behavior in infancy using an age-appropriate measure. Although it is clear that cortical influences on behavior are in place at birth, robust endogenous or voluntary control over eye movements is not apparent until approximately 3–4 months of age, with earlier behavior being largely reflexive and subcortically mediated. In this context, the developing ability to voluntarily suppress responses to one stimulus in order to select another reflects emerging components of cognitive control.

Infant eye-tracking studies have used negative priming paradigms to index cognitive control. In a negative priming paradigm, a distractor object or location that has previously been ignored on one trial becomes the target to be selected on the next trial. Typically, responses to it are slowed relative to a control stimulus. The simultaneous presentation of the target and distractor generates competition that needs to be resolved by inhibition of the distractor in favor of the target. Infants have been shown to have the capacity to suppress an irrelevant stimulus in order to select a competing salient alternative.

An attempt has been made to link observable changes in oculomotor control in infancy to the development of certain visual pathways. Endogenous control over eye movements indicates the development of the frontal eye fields and the strengthening of its projections to the oculomotor basal ganglia thalamocortical circuit. This circuit, one of several closed loops that project from cortex to the basal ganglia and subsequently back to cortex, receives projections from both the frontal eye fields and the parietal cortex and appears to be critical for the production of voluntary saccades. Infants as young as 4 months have been shown to be capable of inhibiting an automatic saccade to a peripheral flashing target, suggesting rudimentary functioning of this circuit early in life. Overriding an orienting response takes effort because the visual system is designed to orient to salient or novel stimuli in the environment.

By the end of the first postnatal year, manual dexterity (e.g., reaching for objects) provides another measure beyond simple looking behavior to document the development of cognitive control. The classic Piagetian A-not-B task that relies on reaching behavior has been used to document changes in cognitive control between 8 and 12 months. Infants watch a toy hidden in location A and are prompted to reach and retrieve it. After several trials of the toy being hidden at location A, the toy is hidden in location B in full view of the infant. Infants younger than 12 months show the A-not-B error (i.e., they perseverate and continue to search in location A). This error appears to be a failure in the ability to suppress a response to the salient competing location in favor of the correct one (i.e., cognitive control).

Nonhuman primate lesion studies suggest that the A-not-B task is dependent on development of the prefrontal cortex. Neural processes underlying this behavior in humans have been examined using a looking version of the task in combination with scalp electrode recordings. These recordings show an increase in frontal as well as posterior power values for only those infants who do not commit the A-not-B error, implicating the prefrontal cortex and related posterior circuitry in accurate performance of the A-not-B task.

Evidence of Cognitive Control in Early Childhood

Cognitive control paradigms in preschool children tend to focus on emerging proficiency in rule use and representational thought. In general, young children have difficulty if they are required to override a competing rule or dimension. Errors of cognitive control have been shown using tasks originally adapted from the adult neuropsychology literature, including the Stroop task and Wisconsin Card Sorting Task. In the Stroop task, subjects are required to name the color of the ink in which a word is written. The classic finding is a slowing of response times when the color of the ink is incongruent with the word (e.g., the word 'blue' written in red ink) relative to a color–word congruent example. Variations of this task have been developed for use with children, especially preschoolers who are nonreaders. For example, in the day–night Stroop-like task, subjects are asked to respond "day" to a card depicting a night scene and "night" to a card depicting a day scene. In both the adult and the child versions of the Stroop task, subjects must suppress the interfering salient information (color or image) in order to respond according to the appropriate rule. Children 3–5 years of age tend to have difficulty overriding the prepotent response, with performance not becoming more adultlike until later childhood. Manipulations that reduce the competing demands of the task or provide young children with more time to compute the answer result in even 4-year-olds performing well.

The Dimensional Change Card Sort is a simplified version of the Wisconsin Card Sorting Task and a more complicated version of the A-not-B task. Three- and 4-year-old children are presented with two cards that can be sorted in either of two ways (e.g., a red truck can be sorted by either color or shape). Children are generally able to sort the cards accurately by the preswitch dimension (e.g., color), but 3-year-olds perseverate on this dimension during the postswitch phase. That is, when the rules change such that they are required to respond based on the other dimension (e.g., shape), these children continue to sort by color, even though they can articulate the new rule. This behavior is consistent with the child not being able to suppress aspects of the situation that were previously relevant in the service of making the goal-appropriate action.

Evidence of Cognitive Control in Late Childhood and Adolescence

As children's fine motor skills improve, more precise measures of cognitive control, which index improvements in reaction time as well as accuracy across a wide age range, can be applied. Tasks used to measure cognitive control during this period of development include negative priming, Stroop tasks, go/no-go tasks, and Simon tasks. In all cases, children have a more difficult time ignoring or inhibiting irrelevant salient information or prepotent responses in favor of the relevant items or responses. In the Simon task, for example, a stimulus attribute is relevant for a response (e.g., left button press), whereas its location (e.g., right side of display) is interfering and irrelevant (e.g., a blue square appears on the left of the screen but requires a response with the right hand). The Simon effect is the difference in accuracy or reaction time between trials in which stimulus and response are on the same side and trials in which they are on opposite sides, with responses being generally slower and less accurate when the stimulus and response are on opposite sides. The size of the Simon effect decreases with age, suggesting that susceptibility to interference decreases with age.

Behavioral evidence from developmental studies of antisaccade tasks and go/no-go tasks in this age range provide similar results. In a go/no-go task, subjects are asked to respond to one stimulus (target) and withhold responding to a different stimulus (nontarget) as the stimuli are presented in succession. Both measures provide evidence of continued improvement in cognitive control into adolescence. Similarly, attention tasks that include distracting peripheral information, as in the case of the flanker task and stop signal tasks, show comparable developmental changes. Performance across these tasks continues to develop over childhood and does not reach full maturity until approximately 12 years (**Figure 1**). Importantly, these age-related differences are not observed on these tasks in the absence of interfering information.

Cortical Organization Underlying the Development of Cognitive Control

Advances in neuroimaging techniques have provided developmental scientists the opportunity to safely track cognitive and neural processes underlying

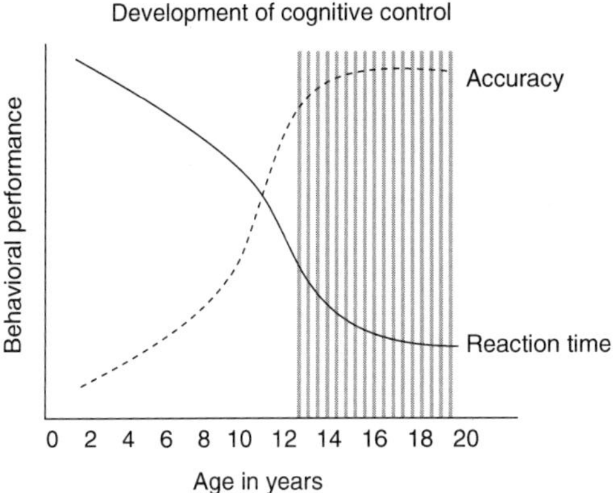

Figure 1 Model of developmental change in cognitive control with age as a function of accuracy and reaction time. From Casey BJ, Frontostriatal and frontocerebellar circuitry underlying cognitive control. In: Mayr U, Awh E, and Keele SW (eds.) *Developing Individuality in the Human Brain.* American Psychological Association, Washington, DC, 2005, reprinted with permission.

human development. These methods have advanced the field of developmental neuroscience by providing evidence of changes in cortical organization in the developing brain *in vivo*. Although these measures provide only an indirect index of a very dynamic process of regressive and progressive changes in brain structure and function across development (e.g., changes in myelination, dendritic pruning, and vascular, neuronal, and glial density), they provide information about regional changes in brain development.

One of the most influential magnetic resonance (MR) methods is functional magnetic resonance imaging (fMRI). This method provides *in vivo* measures of brain activity by indexing changes in blood oxygen levels in the brain. Studies using this method have begun to track developmental changes in patterns of brain activity that coincide with changes in cognitive control across childhood.

Prefrontal involvement in the development of cognitive control in children has been demonstrated most convincingly in fMRI studies that parametrically manipulate the salience of the competing information that must be suppressed. By definition, cognitive control is the ability to attenuate interference from competing sources and thus should be needed more when the interfering information becomes increasingly salient. For example, in the case of the go/no-go task, as the number of go trials preceding a no-go trial increases, so too do the number of errors (i.e., incorrectly responding on a no-go trial). The imaging data show that correctly withholding a response on a no-go trial is associated with activity in the ventral prefrontal cortex and basal ganglia, and activity in these regions correlates with successful task performance. Adults show a monotonic increase in prefrontal and parietal cortices as the number of go trials preceding a no-go trial increase. Children, on the other hand, maximally activate these regions regardless of whether they have to withhold a response following one, three, or five go trials (responses) and make significantly more errors. These findings provide evidence that susceptibility to interference is greater in children than adults but is attenuated with age. This increase in cognitive control with age is paralleled by maturational differences in the recruitment of underlying prefrontal and parietal cortices.

Many paradigms besides the go/no-go task have been used to study the neural development of cognitive control (e.g., antisaccade, Simon, flanker, and Stroop tasks). Children with effective cognitive control on these tasks typically recruit additional or larger portions of prefrontal cortex than those activated by adults, suggesting age-related differences in recruitment of this region. Children also recruit posterior parietal regions consistently activated in adults on these tasks, unless they have poor cognitive control, in which case they do not recruit these regions. These findings suggest that the improved ability to suppress irrelevant information may first require mature activation of posterior parietal regions prior to maturation of prefrontal regions. Tasks of lesser cognitive demand (e.g., selective attention tasks without response competition) do not appear to show age-related differences. This developmental pattern of brain activity parallels that of behavioral performance on cognitive tasks that do not require suppression of competing information, for which children also show an adultlike pattern.

Collectively, these imaging studies of cognitive control show that children recruit distinct but often more diffuse regions of prefrontal cortex than do adults. Based on cross-sectional and longitudinal studies, the pattern of activity within brain regions central to task performance becomes more focal or fine-tuned with increased activity, whereas regions not correlated with task performance show attenuation in activity with age. This pattern, observed across a variety of paradigms, has been suggested to reflect development within, and refinement of, projections to and from these regions.

Development of Brain Connectivity and Cognitive Control

Another MR method that has begun to be used in developmental research is diffusion tensor imaging (DTI). This method detects changes in white matter microstructure based on properties of diffusion.

Diffusion of water molecules in white matter tracts is affected by myelin and the orientation and regularity of fibers. As such, this method provides an index of regional brain connectivity and strengthening of connections among regions. Together with fMRI, this methodology has been used to track the refinement of cortical circuits involved in the fine-tuning of systems underlying the development of cognitive control.

Only a small number of studies have linked brain connectivity and cognitive development measures, although indirect measures of white matter suggest regional development in prefrontal cortex and presumably function. Across all these studies, strengthening of connections throughout the brain is shown to occur with development; however, connections between those regions implicated in cognitive control appear to be protracted and are also shown to correlate with behavioral performance. One such study showed that development of working memory was positively correlated with prefrontal–parietal connectivity consistent with imaging studies showing differential recruitment of these regions in children relative to adults. A second study examining the degree of connectivity between the prefrontal cortex and the basal ganglia and performance on the go/no-go task showed a tight association between connectivity and performance that was not present in a comparison corticospinal fiber tract that also showed changes with development.

Findings from the imaging literature suggest that development of cognitive control is paralleled by a fine-tuning of cortical systems, with protracted refinement of prefrontal regions relative to posterior cortical and subcortical regions. The reported shift in cortical architecture and function is presumably an experience-driven maturational process that reflects fine-tuning of neural systems with experience and development, and strengthening of cortico-cortical and cortico-subcortical connections. These imaging studies map onto findings from animal and human postmortem studies indicating that pruning and elimination of connections, in combination with strengthening of relevant ones, occur during this time period, and illustrate the subtle interplay between neuroanatomic and physiologic changes in neural circuitry and cognitive maturation.

A Developmental Model of Cognitive Control

The imaging literature on the development of cognitive control suggests that maturity of prefrontal regions is critical for the improvement of this ability with age. However, two other regions, the parietal cortex and basal ganglia, have been implicated repeatedly in directing or guiding attention and actions. Specifically, the basal ganglia have been implicated in signaling prefrontal cortex when competing actions require top-down adjustment of behavior, whereas the posterior parietal cortex has been implicated in signaling prefrontal cortex when competing stimuli require top-down biasing of attention in favor of one stimulus attribute or location over another. Both of these regions (basal ganglia and parietal cortex) are part of unique circuits that project both to and from prefrontal cortex, thus providing a means for signaling prefrontal regions to help impose top-down control of behavior (**Figure 2**).

Although these structures are neuroanatomically intact at birth, refinement of function and connectivity within and between these regions continues gradually across development. In this regard, each region has been suggested to have different developmental trajectories, whereby subcortical systems such as the basal ganglia develop before cortical systems. Within cortical systems, posterior regions (parietal cortex) have been suggested to develop before anterior ones such as the prefrontal cortex. The regional differences in functional development of brain regions may explain the protracted development of cognitive control. For example, intact signaling by subcortical regions, but immature top-down control due to

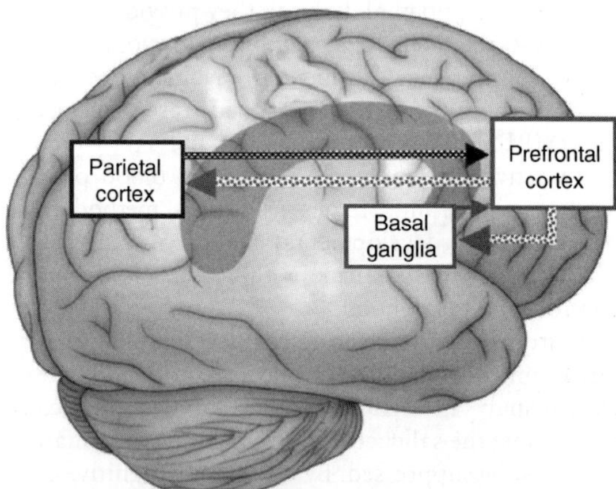

Figure 2 Simplified drawing of prefrontal circuits implicated in cognitive control. Each circuit has projections both to and from the prefrontal cortex. The basal ganglia and posterior parietal systems signal the prefrontal cortex when new or competing response or sensory information is encountered so that the prefrontal cortex can immediately adjust behavior to accommodate or suppress new or salient information during goal-oriented actions. Poor cognitive control early in development results from immature top-down control of prefrontal cortico-cortical and cortico-subcortical projections.

immature cortico-subcortical or cortico-cortical connections, could result in poor regulation of attention and behavior as seen in the review of studies of cognitive development. This developmental model of cognitive control suggests more of a refinement in the functional representations of intact brain regions as connections between brain regions are strengthened through experience over the course of development, as opposed to reorganization of brain circuitry with development or the development of new functional regions.

Conclusions

A hallmark of cognitive development is the ability to select information and actions from competing sources. Collectively, this article tracks this ability across development and shows how cognitive control emerges early in development and continues to be refined into adulthood. A recurring theme across all ages discussed in this article is the propensity to commit perseverative errors early in the development of cognitive control. For example, after frequent presentations of a toy at location A in the A-not-B task, infants cannot shift their response to a toy hidden at location B and continue to perseverate and search for the toy in location A. In the card sorting task, preschoolers have difficulty switching to a new rule after using another rule to sort cards. In the go/no-go task, increasing the number of go trials preceding a no-go trial increases the interference from a competing prepotent response and results in a decrease in the ability to withhold responding to the nontarget. Across the different tasks, the pattern of behavior suggests immature maintenance of relevant information (e.g., current hiding location and rule or task demands) from interference from the competing representation of a prior action.

Cognitive development is characterized as the growing ability to filter and suppress irrelevant information and actions in favor of more relevant ones as these neural systems develop. The prefrontal cortex has been shown to be involved in guiding actions by supporting representations of relevant information against interference from competing sources. Thus, developmental changes in prefrontal circuitry observed throughout childhood presumably contribute to the emergence of this ability.

See also: Adolescent Brain Development and the Risk of Psychiatric Disorders; Cognition: An Overview of Neuroimaging Techniques; Cognitive Neuroscience: An Overview; Diffusion Tensor Imaging (DTI); Executive Function and Higher-Order Cognition: Neuroimaging; Executive Function and Higher-Order Cognition: Definition and Neural Substrates; Functional Connectivity; Prefrontal Cortex: Structure and Anatomy.

Further Reading

Bunge SA, Dudukovic NM, Thomason ME, Vaidya CJ, and Gabrieli JD (2002) Immature frontal lobe contributions to cognitive control in children: Evidence from fMRI. *Neuron* 33: 301–311.

Casey BJ (2005) Frontostriatal and frontocerebellar circuitry underlying cognitive control. In: Mayr U, Awh E, and Keela SW (eds.) *Developing Individuality in the Human Brain.* Washington, DC: American Psychological Association.

Diamond A (1991) Neuropsychological insights into the meaning of object concept development. In: Carey S and Gelman R (eds.) *The Epigenesis of Mind: Essays on Biology and Knowledge*, pp. 67–110. Hillsdale, NJ: Lawrence Erlbaum.

Diamond A, Kirkham NZ, and Amso D (2002) Conditions under which young children can hold two rules in mind and inhibit a prepotent response. *Developmental Psychology* 38: 352–362.

Durston S, Davidson MC, Tottenham N, et al. (2006) A shift from diffuse to focal cortical activity with development. *Developmental Science* 9(1): 1–8.

Gogtay N, Giedd JN, Lusk L, et al. (2004) Dynamic mapping of human cortical development during childhood through early adulthood. *Proceedings of the National Academy of Sciences of the United States of America* 101: 8174–8179.

Hasher L and Zacks RT (1998) Working memory, comprehension, and aging: A review and a new view. *Advances in Research and Theory* 22: 193–225.

Johnson MH (2005) *Developmental Cognitive Neuroscience: An Introduction*, 2nd edn. Oxford: Blackwell.

Klingberg T, Forssberg H, and Westerberg H (2002) Increased brain activity in frontal and parietal cortex underlies the development of visuospatial working memory capacity during childhood. *Journal of Cognitive Neuroscience* 14: 1–10.

Liston C, Watts R, Tottenham N, et al. (2006) Frontostriatal microstructure predicts individual differences in cognitive control. *Cerebral Cortex* 16(4): 553–560.

Luna B and Sweeney JA (2004) The emergence of collaborative brain function: fMRI studies of the development of response inhibition. *Annals of the New York Academy of Sciences* 1021: 296–309.

Munakata Y (1998) Infant perseveration and implications for object permanence theories: A PDP mode of the AnotB task. *Developmental Science* 1: 161–184.

Ridderinkhof KR, van der Molen MW, and Band GPH (1997) Sources of interference from irrelevant information: A developmental study. *Journal of Experimental Child Psychology* 65: 315–341.

Schlaggar BL, Brown TT, Lugar HM, Visscher KM, Miezin FM, and Petersen SE (2002) Functional neuroanatomical differences between adults and school-age children. *Science* 296: 1476–1479.

Sowell ER, Thompson PM, Holmes CJ, Jernigan TL, and Toga AW (1999) *In vivo* evidence for post-adolescent brain maturation in frontal and striatal regions. *Nature Neuroscience* 2(10): 859–861.

Zelazo PD, Muller U, Frye D, and Marcovitch S (2003) The development of executive function. *Monographs of the Society for Research in Child Development* 68(3)Serial No. 274.

Cognitive Neuroscience: An Overview

C M Wessinger and E Clapham, University of Nevada, Reno, NV, USA

Understanding how brain enables mind is the goal of cognitive neuroscience. More broadly stated, cognitive neuroscience is concerned with understanding the neurobiological basis of mental processes – in other words, thinking about how the brain is involved in thinking. Thinking about thinking. There is little doubt that human brains can engage in the task of thinking about thinking and likely have been able to do so for some time. Unfortunately, throughout most of human history, more practical concerns necessarily occupied human thought. Humans were more concerned with thinking about and acting on behaviors that were related to their survival: storing enough food to enable them to survive the winter, killing the bear before the bear killed them, and finding shelter. They had to concentrate on understanding and working within their environment in order to survive to struggle another day. Anything that did not specifically contribute to their survival was a luxury. Thus, thinking about thinking would have been a luxury – a luxury that humans could not afford. However, as soon as civilization developed to a point that day-to-day survival did not occupy every waking thought, humans could afford to think about thinking. They began to think about how others thought and why they did what they did. Oedipus Rex, the ancient Greek play that deals with parent–child conflicts, as well as Mesopotamian and Egyptian theories designed to explain religion and the universe are excellent early attempts to understand why people act the way they do. Unfortunately, there are significant pieces of the equation missing. These thinkers and philosophers did not systematically explore the relationship between brain, behavior, and mind. This is where modern-day science and scientific methodology come into play. The notion that we must observe, manipulate, and measure the environment in order to understand the world and our place within it is central to scientific methodology. When we apply such techniques to understanding how the brain enables mind, we call that cognitive neuroscience.

Certainly, one could make a case that cognitive neuroscience has been around ever since scientists in different disciplines began exploring the common goal of understanding how brain enables mind. Such early explorations were quite illuminating and many have stood the test of time. Some early theories that specific areas of the brain gave rise to specific functions were put forth by the phrenologists Franz Joseph Gall and J G Spurzheim, who declared that the brain was organized around 35 distinct functions ranging from such basic cognitive functions as language and color perception to more philosophical concerns such as hope and self-esteem. Each of these areas was supported by a specific brain region, and with increased proficiency in one of these areas, the corresponding brain representation would grow in size, in turn causing a corresponding bump on the skull. However, once subjected to strict scientific methodology, phrenology was shown to be untrue. It took the great neurologist John Hughlings Jackson to again substantiate that a structure–function relationship between the brain and behavior existed. Rather than being associated with bumps on the skull, his hypotheses were based on careful clinical observations of patients. While seizing, some of his epileptic patients would move in characteristic patterns, almost with a systematic rhythm. This led him to propose a somatotopic organization – that is, a map of the body in the brain. Also at approximately this time, the French neurologist, Paul Broca, reported perhaps the most famous neurological case – one of his patients had suffered a stroke and now was unable to speak but was still able to understand speech. Postmortem examination showed damage in the left frontal area, which is now known as Broca's area and still believed to play a major role in language output. In contrast, German neurologist Carl Wernicke reported a patient who babbled incessantly following a stroke, but that is all it was – babbling – the words kept coming but made no sense. Wernicke's patient had a lesion in a more posterior region in the left hemisphere, which has become known as Wernicke's area, and it is still believed to play a major role in understanding language. Neuroanatomists were realizing similar divisions of the brain, but on a more cellular level. Perhaps the most famous is Korbinian Brodmann, who analyzed cellular organization of the cerebral cortex using a Franz Nissl developed stain to visualize the different layers of cortical neurons, dividing the cerebral cortex into more than 50 distinct regions. This method of looking at cellular differences in cortical layers is known as cytoarchitectonics. Many others contributed to this work, including Constantin Von Economo, Gerhardt von Bonin, and Percival Bailey. More recently, similar techniques have been used to demonstrate more than 30 different cortical areas in the visual system alone. Such early investigations still guide cognitive neuroscience today, particularly with regard to helping the field understand structure–function relations within the brain and how these combine to enable mind.

The formal birth of the field known as cognitive neuroscience was relatively recent. One story as to how the field developed involved a taxi ride shared by two eminent brain scientists – biopsychologist Michael S Gazzaniga and behavioral-turned-cognitive psychologist George Miller – on the way to a dinner meeting in the early 1970s. The dinner was being held so scientists from many different disciplines could discuss how to pursue a common goal: understanding how the brain enables the mind. Such a joining of forces deserved an appropriate name – not just a renaming of biopsychology or cognitive neuropsychology, well-respected disciplines already striving to understand the structure–function relations of the brain–mind problem, but a name that incorporated the investigations of information processing akin to cognitive science: one that reflected a merging of all of these many disciplines and more. After much discussion, the term 'cognitive neuroscience' seemed ideal. Another story concerning the birth of the field involves a similar meeting with other eminent brain scientists such as Larry Squire, a neuroscientist renowned for his research exploring the biological basis of memory, and Stephen Kosslyn, a cognitive psychologist well-known for his mental imagery research. However, the exact events that led to the adoption of the term cognitive neuroscience are not important. What is important is the fact that many scientists using quite varied methodologies are working together, and making headway, toward the common goal of cracking the code of the brain and understanding how this approximately 6-pound lump of soft, squishy, neuronal tissue allows us to think and feel and emote and cry and to dream – how the brain enables mind. Many of the varied methodologies that contribute to this exciting and rapidly expanding field are described here.

In order to help us understand the inherently multidisciplinary approach of cognitive neuroscience, we need to understand some of the key methodologies. Techniques ranging from exploring the molecular basis of the brain to exploring consciousness are utilized, combined, dissected, and manipulated by researchers in the quest to understand the neurobiological underpinnings of mental operations. However, cognitive neuroscience is more than a simple recombination of various methodologies and techniques. The field is extremely innovative in that it borrows the best techniques from the best disciplines in order to provide the best innovative insights into how brain enables mind. Such innovation can be more fully appreciated by exploring some of the key methodologies and techniques.

One key avenue in understanding how brain enables mind is grounded in understanding the relationship between brain anatomy and cognition. Many studies have tried to relate differences in intelligence to differences in brain size and structure. Differences in neuronal type, size, density, and connectivity have also been explored in trying to understand structure–function relations between brain anatomy and cognition. These explorations of brain structure can be loosely grouped under the term neuroanatomy. Formally, neuroanatomy is the study of structure of the nervous system. Primary questions of interest to neuroanatomy are identifying the various parts and components of the nervous system, as well as describing how these parts and components are interconnected. To further complicate matters, it is necessary to use specialized techniques and methods to ask these questions at multiple levels. Not only is it important to know the size and shape of a neuron but also it is important to know where that neuron connects. Where does the input come from and where does the output go? This very debate was truly a key development in the birth of neuroscience, and neuroscience is key to cognitive neuroscience. Two brilliant neuroanomists were debating the interconnectivity of the nervous system. Camillo Golgi invented a silver stain that permitted visualization of single neurons. Using Golgi's stain, Santiago Ramón y Cajal demonstrated that the neurons were discretely bound, individual entities that did not touch. This view was contrary to that of Golgi, who believed the whole brain was a continuous mass of tissue sharing a common cytoplasm, or syncytium. Cajal extended the field by being the first to identify the unidirectional (from axon to dendrite) nature of electrical transmission within neurons. These findings were elucidated with early microanatomical techniques. Microanatomy or fine anatomy has now developed to the point of exploring the organization of neurons and the connections. This is opposed to gross anatomy, which is concerned with the general structures and connections visible to the naked eye. Gross and microanatomical techniques continue to inform the field of cognitive neuroscience by providing essential knowledge concerning brain and neuronal structure and connectivity.

Another key technique employed by cognitive neuroscientists that is grounded in neuroscience is physiology. This is a branch of neuroscience that deals with the functions and processes of life, as well as the physical actions and reactions associated with these processes. Simply stated, physiology measures bodily responses such as blood pressure, heart rate, and neuronal electrical activity to the environment. One physiological measure of great import is neuronal electrical activity. Despite the fact that the electrical potential is extremely small, when large numbers of neurons are active simultaneously, they produce enough electrical signals that when summed can be measured by electrodes placed on the scalp. Electroencephalography (EEG) involves recording a continuous stream of overall brain activity while the person performs a variety of tasks, sometimes in an experimental setting and sometimes as part of everyday life. These continuous recordings of continuous activity have proven extremely useful clinically and have helped with epilepsy, sleep disorders, and anxiety.

EEG can only provide limited information when exploring cognitive processes because the recordings tend to reflect global brain activity, as opposed to specific cognitive or perceptual processes and functions. However, by synchronizing EEG collection with specific cognitive and perceptual events, it is possible to disentangle the brain waves and see changes in electrical activity associated with changes in cognitive and perceptual processes. This technique is called event-related potential (ERP) because the neuronal potentials are related to specific events. Given that neurons produce unidirectional electrical transmission and constraints of Faraday's law of induction (which states that a changing electric field produces a magnetic field orthogonal to the direction of flow of electricity), they produce miniscule magnetic fields. Magnetoencephalography (MEG) records these summed magnetic potentials at the scalp in a manner similar to ERPs.

One great advantage of these techniques is that millisecond accuracy is possible in terms of linking summed electrical signals specific to an event; thus, cognitive neuroscientists can understand exactly when and how the brain is responding to a specific event. One major drawback of these techniques is the very notion of summed electrical signals. Such summing results in limited spatial resolution. Furthermore, because the summed signals must be collected at the scalp, localization of depth is also problematic. It is difficult to determine where in the brain the signals occur.

This problem can be overcome by taking advantage of the inherently multidisciplinary nature of cognitive neuroscience by bringing other techniques to bear. One technique that can help inform EEG, MEG, and a variety of other cognitive neuroscience techniques is magnetic resonance imaging (MRI). Formally, MRI is a branch of neuroimaging that is a clinical specialty that uses noninvasive techniques to produce images of the brain. Interestingly, MRI also takes advantage of Faraday's law in that it uses a supercooled, superconducting electromagnet to produce a strong electrical field. This magnetic field is then systematically manipulated to produce images of the body. These images currently provide great detail concerning the gross anatomy, and even microanatomy, of the nervous system. Such information, when coupled with ERP and/or MEG techniques, can provide essential structure–function relations within the human brain. Such techniques can help surgeons understand not only tumor location but also functions compromised by the tumor and weigh them against functions that may be compromised by the surgery.

A recent interesting use of MRI in conjunction with other techniques involves trying to understand the biological basis of autism, an increasingly more problematic developmental disorder. Hutsler and colleagues showed that increases in dendritic spine density could be related to increases in autistic symptoms. Certainly, these data do not indicate that dendritic spine density is responsible for autism, just that there is some connection, and this connection needs to be investigated further. This is an excellent example of the utility of cognitive neuroscience: by combining neurology, neuropsychology, radiology, and microneuroanatomy, researchers are making tremendous strides in understanding the biological basis of autism.

Within the past 15 years, MRI has been extended to include a functional component. By taking advantage of what from a radiologist's viewpoint is noise, cognitive neuroscientists are able to see the brain in action – almost. It is well-known that changes in cognitive and perceptual activity result in localized changes in neuronal activity, which result in localized changes in metabolic needs, which result in localized changes in blood flow, which result in localized changes in blood oxygenation. The end of this cascade, the localized changes in blood oxygenation, can be visualized with functional magnetic resonance imaging (fMRI) in order to infer localization of function. Also, when MRI signals are time locked to cognitive and perceptual changes, localization of function, as well as localization of time, can be inferred. This is similar to positron emission tomography (PET), another neuroimaging technique that can image the blood flow change portion of the cascade to infer localization of function, except that PET uses ionizing radiation and fMRI does not. Another advantage that fMRI has over PET is greater spatial and temporal resolution. PET provides resolution in terms of minutes and centimeters for temporal and spatial properties, respectively. However, fMRI, particularly event-related fMRI, can provide temporal accuracy in seconds and spatial accuracy in millimeters.

So far, we have reviewed several biologically based techniques and have a greater understanding of the neuroscience part of cognitive neuroscience. But what about the cognitive part? Is there really a need for more when trying to understand how brain enables mind? Certainly. Without the 'cognitive,' there would be no true understanding of the mind portion of the equation.

Cognition can be defined as any form of information processing, mental operation, or intellectual activity such as thinking, reasoning, remembering, imagining, or learning. Thus, cognitive psychology, a major contributor to the field of cognitive neuroscience, is the study of behavior related to cognition. The principles and goals of cognitive psychology rest on two key concepts. First, mental operations depend on internal representations. Second, mental operations undergo transformations.

The notion that mental operations depend on internal representations is not that far-fetched; after all, by definition, if the operations are mental and taking place in the mind, then they are necessarily internal. It is also easy to accept and understand the notion that mental operations have to undergo transformations. After all, we do not directly perceive and act in the world; rather, our perceptions, thoughts, and actions depend on what our sensory systems are designed to detect within our environment, and our senses are not capable of translating everything in our environment into useable information. For example, we do not readily see infrared light or directly sense changing electrical and magnetic fields, but these physical properties do exist in the environment – they are just not detectable by our sensory systems. We need to use other physical-detection tools specifically designed to detect these aspects of our environment. Nonetheless, we still perceive, think about, and act within our environment reasonably well. This is because our brains take the information provided by our sensory systems and transform it into signals that can be understood, interpreted, and acted upon. Michael Posner and Richard Mitchell first conducted a classic study illustrating both of these key principles in the mid-1970s. Using a series of letters, they were able to clearly demonstrate that mental processes were internal and that these processes were necessarily manipulated and transformed when acting on them. The experiment is quite simple: it requires only that one present letter pairs to participants and ask them if the letters are the same or different. Why is it a classic experiment? Because of how the letters were paired and how the question of same or different was asked. In the simplest form, four different letters are used – two consonants and two vowels – and they are displayed in either upper or lower case. Using these stimuli, different levels of sameness can be asked. The lowest level is based on the physicality of the letters: are they physically the same? AA and aa are two examples of stimuli that would be judges as physically the same, Aa and aA are examples that would be correctly judged not the same. The next level of question involves identity, or the name of the stimuli. The previous four examples would all be judged the same based on name identity. AB and AE are examples of stimuli that would be judged as different. The next higher question involves judging if the letters are the same or different based on more detailed information concerning the letters – whether the letters are consonants or vowels. Reaction time data were collected during this experiment and clearly show that the mental processes cannot necessarily be overtly witnessed (they are internal) and various mental processes take various amounts of time, depending on the level of complexity involved in the process (or number of transformations necessary to perform the task). That is, the physical judgment was the easiest and fastest, the type judgment task was the most difficult and slowest, and the identity task (naming) was somewhere in between.

Another key technique that is often considered under the cognitive domain of cognitive neuroscience is neuropsychology. This is a science that seeks to integrate psychological observations of behavior and mind with neurological observations of the nervous system and the brain. This field is closely related to neurology, a branch of medicine concerned with understanding and treating disorders of the nervous system. One difference is that neuropsychology is specifically concerned with understanding and treating cognitive, perceptual, and other psychological deficits related to nervous system compromise. Such deficits can come in the form of vascular disorders such as strokes or bleeds, tumors, trauma, and disease.

These deficits of structure can also cause deficits of function, which is where cognitive neuroscience can benefit. The real strength of cognitive neuroscience is the ability to take a variety of seemingly disparate technologies and bits of data and integrate them into a coherent explanation of how brain enables mind. One of the most fruitful paradigms in cognitive neuroscience that depends on converging data involves the effects of brain lesions on behavior. Fundamental concepts, such as the notion that language resides primarily in the left hemisphere and the fact that the left hemisphere controls the right side of the body (and vice versa), are grounded in such a combination of techniques. The logic is pretty straightforward. If mental processes and behavior depend on processing within a certain brain region, then damage to this region should impact the processes and behavior. Unfortunately, it is not that straightforward. Just because behaviors are disrupted following brain damage does not necessarily mean that the region damaged is responsible for the disrupted process, only that it is involved in the processes.

This is why cognitive neuroscientists often design research paradigms that involve at least two tasks, and two different types of brain compromise. Such a combination of techniques provides the most information because it is useful in dissociating structure–function issues. This notion of separating or dissociating various mental processes into relatively independently functioning units is quite attractive. A classic example of this approach can be illustrated by considering the findings of Broca and Wernicke. Broca's patient had trouble with speech output, but his language comprehension was intact. Wernicke's patient has problems with language comprehension, but his speech output was intact. These were two different language disorders in two different people. Behaviorally, these two language functions are dissociable. By adding the component of neuroanatomy – what part of the brain is compromised – the dissociation is strengthened. A modern example of a similar double dissociation can be illustrated with the phenomenon of blindsight. Blindsight is extremely interesting because it allows cognitive neuroscientists to pursue what is perhaps the highest level of cognition possible by the human brain – consciousness – in an established patient model. Blindsight comes about following damage to cortical regions of the primary visual pathway. Such damage results in corresponding regions of blindness in the visual field. Under certain testing conditions, some patients demonstrate residual vision within this area of blindness – residual vision without awareness. That is, they can respond correctly to some stimuli while denying actually having 'seen' the stimuli. Hence the term blindsight.

Interestingly, few patients with such damage demonstrate blindsight, and those who do so demonstrate the phenomenon differently. A study by Wessinger and colleagues showed this in terms of a dissociation: one participant (FN) can detect direction of motion but cannot detect differences in shape, whereas another participant (CLT) can detect differences in shape but not differences in motion. These data suggest a dissociation of motion and shape processing in blindsight. Interestingly, MRIs demonstrate differences in the location and extent of their damage. FN has greater damage in his inferior occipital lobe and CLT has greater damage in his parietal lobe – both have limited sparing around the calcarine fissure. These data suggest that it is not the damage to primary visual cortex that results in differences in blindsight; rather, it is compromise of higher order visual processing (i.e., extrastriate) modules. CLT's motion module is damaged, and thus does not have motion blindsight, but it does have shape blindsight because his form regions are less damaged. The opposite is true for FN: his form processing capabilities are too damaged to provide any useful form processing data, but his motion processing capabilities still provide some limited information – information that is sufficient to drive motion blindsight. Overall, these data indicate that blindsight may depend on surviving remnants of primary visual cortex and vestiges of connections to surviving, albeit severely compromised, extrastriate visual modules.

Blindsight is not the only interesting exploration of consciousness undertaken by the multidisciplinary approach of cognitive neuroscience. In an extremely interesting combination of philosophy and neuroscience, Benjamin Libet has made a career of investigating consciousness.

In a groundbreaking and often controversial series of experiments, Libet investigated the neural time factors in conscious and unconscious processing. These experiments are the basis for his 'backward referral hypothesis.' Libet and colleagues conclude that awareness of a neural event is delayed ~500 ms following the onset of the stimulating event, and more important, this awareness is referred back in time to the onset of the stimulating event. Thus, we are not aware of the event until after it occurs, although we often think we are aware of the event from the onset. Fortunately, backward referral of our consciousness is not so delayed that we act without thinking. The actual beginning of the act occurs sufficiently after the awareness of the intent to act, giving us time to override inappropriately triggered behavior. This ability to detect and correct errors is what Libet believes is the basis for free will. Cognitive neuroscience is investigating consciousness and free will and making headway.

Certainly, this is not an exhaustive review and explanation of the methods that converge to form the field of cognitive neuroscience. In fact, there are a whole host of animal techniques not covered. By definition, the field of cognitive neuroscience – a multidisciplinary science that borrows from many seemingly disparate fields in order to develop coherent explorations of the neurobiological underpinnings of cognition – is dynamic. The field is in constant flux, always expanding and growing and exploring new questions related to furthering our understanding of how brain enables mind. To some, such constant change may seem disconcerting, but to others it is what makes cognitive neuroscience exciting. Such constant change is in fact why cognitive neuroscience came about in the first place. By combining the best of many disciplines, cognitive neuroscience is asking and answering interesting questions about how the brain enables mind, putting the field at the forefront of helping humans understand their place within the world.

Given that scientists from many seemingly disparate fields were already pursuing the common goal of understanding how brain enables mind, why was it necessary to formally define a multidisciplinary approach that has now become known as cognitive neuroscience? It is hoped that by raising exciting issues ranging from the development of the neuron doctrine to the use of cytoarchitectonics to relate brain morphology to autism, from the collection of behavioral data in cognitive paradigms to the integration of converging data in dissociation paradigms, and the combination of philosophy and neuroscience to understand consciousness, this article helps you understand why cognitive neuroscience emerged as a new multidisciplinary field of study. In sum, it was to accurately represent the merging of many different brain sciences, ranging from a neuroscientific and structural approach to a cognitive and functional approach. A neuroscientific approach is concerned with understanding the basic mechanisms of neural action that result in processing and communication of information within neuronal assemblies. It is also necessary to consider the anatomical substrates or structures that are composed of these neuronal assemblies. A cognitive approach is concerned with characterizing the cognitive processes that lead to specific functions or behavior. Cognitive neuropsychology is concerned with similar characterizations with the added dimension of trying to understand what structures are necessarily involved in various cognitive processes. Similarly, cognitive science is concerned with characterizing the computational algorithms necessary for such cognitive processes. By incorporating the concerns of these wide-ranging disciplines, cognitive neuroscience is more than just a sum of its parts; rather, it is a stronger, more comprehensive approach to understanding how the brain enables the mind – one that begins at the molecular level and continues to the problem of understanding human conscious experience.

See also: Cerebral Cortex; Cognition: An Overview of Neuroimaging Techniques; Cognitive Control and Development; Contextual Interactions in Visual Perception; Electroencephalography (EEG); Executive Function and Higher-Order Cognition: Neuroimaging; fMRI: BOLD Contrast; History of Neuroscience: Early Neuroscience; Neuroanatomy Methods in Humans and Animals; Neuroimaging; Phrenology; Positron Emission Tomography (PET).

Further Reading

Banich MT (2004) *Cognitive Neuroscience and Neuropsychology*, 2nd edn. Boston: Houghton Mifflin.

Farah MJ and Feinberg TE (eds.) (2000) *Patient Based Approaches to Cognitive Neuroscience*. Cambridge: MIT Press.

Finger S (1994) *Origins of Neuroscience: A History of Explorations into Brain Functions*. New York: Oxford University Press.

Gazzaniga MS (2000) (editor-in-chief) *The New Cognitive Neurosciences*. Cambridge: MIT Press.

Gazzaniga MS, Ivry RB, and Mangun GR (2002) *Cognitive Neuroscience: The Biology of the Mind*, 2nd edn. New York: Norton.

Hutsler JJ, Love T, and Zhang H (2007) Histological and magnetic resonance imaging of cortical layering and thickness in autism spectrum disorders. *Biological Psychiatry* 61: 449–457.

Kandel ER, Schwartz JH, and Jessell TM (1991) *Principles of Neural Science*, 3rd edn. New York: Elsevier.

Kosslyn SM and Koenig O (1992) *Wet Mind: The New Cognitive Neurosciences*. New York: Free Press.

Libet B (2005) *Mind Time: The Temporal Factor in Consciousness*. Cambridge, MA: Harvard University Press.

Posner MI and Mitchell RF (1967) Chronometric analysis of classification. *Psychological Review* 74(5): 392–409.

Rains GD (2002) *Principles of Human Neuropsychology*. Boston: McGraw-Hill.

Wessinger CM, Fendrich R, and Gazzaniga MS (1999) Variability of residual vision in hemianopic subjects. *Restorative Neurology and Neuroscience* 15: 243–253.

Wessinger CM, Fendrich R, and Gazzaniga MS (2005) Cognitive neuroscience: What is it and why? In: Adelman G and Smith BH (eds.) *Encyclopedia of Neuroscience*, 3rd edn. (on CD-ROM). Oxford: Elsevier.

Emotion and Vigilance

F C Davis, J A Oler, and P J Whalen, Dartmouth College, Hanover, NH, USA

Introduction

A common strategy invoked by scientists who aim to understand the neural substrates of emotion is to focus on one emotion exemplar. For instance, we have learned much about the role of the amygdala and its interaction with reciprocally connected prefrontal cortical regions by studying their reactivity during fear states. Emotional states such as fear have lasting impacts on neural organization, as plastic changes in brain regions such as the amygdala, hippocampus, and prefrontal cortex subserve memories that allow us to avoid fear-inducing stimuli in the future.

Fear states also serve to protect us in the moment. For example, a scared organism often initially 'freezes' its movement, a behavioral response that is orchestrated by the amygdala. In addition to being the quintessential manifestation of a state of fear, somatomotor arrest is also useful if the organism believes that it has more to learn before resuming action. Such a response in the face of a cue that predicts a biologically relevant outcome allows an organism to physically orient sensory organs (e.g., eyes, ears) toward a stimulus, thereby optimizing sensory information processing. This strategy is particularly adaptive if the outcome predicted by this cue is not entirely clear, as it aids in processing additional environmental information that might facilitate the interpretation of a predictively ambiguous cue. Thus, a state of fear includes amygdala responsivity, which influences nonspecific attentional systems that support learning about the environment in order to facilitate behavioral responses now and in the future. A critical question currently under investigation concerns whether an extreme state of fear is necessary to engage amygdala modulation over this sort of acute information gathering. Research on this topic suggests that the amygdala is involved along a continuum of state changes, from subtle changes in the state of vigilance, to more punctate moments of surprise, to a full-blown state of horror.

The purpose of this article is to review data demonstrating that a partially shared prefrontal–amygdala neural circuit subserves more subtle fluctuations in vigilance as well as more extreme fear states. This network is responsible for monitoring the environment for biologically relevant events, learning about the cues that predict those events, and modifying behavior in order to appropriately react to those cues in the future. Thus, affective information processing is part of a greater system that facilitates biologically relevant learning, especially when learning contingencies are uncertain. This system is capable of, but does not necessitate, the generation of extreme emotional states.

The Amygdala

The anatomy of the amygdala is not detailed here. Rather, we focus on three important aspects of amygdala anatomical organization relevant to the ensuing discussion (see **Figure 1**). First, the heaviest feedback projections from sensory and prefrontal cortical regions are received by the basolateral amygdala (BLA). This design allows for the convergence of multimodal cortically processed information with the latest sensory stimuli being detected. Second, in addition to the known role of the central nucleus (CN) in modulating autonomic and motor responsivity, the CN also projects to all major neuromodulatory centers (e.g., cholinergic, dopaminergic, serotonergic, and noradrenergic source neurons). It is these connections that can more globally modulate the 'readiness' of cortical and subcortical sensory neurons, thereby setting an appropriate level of vigilance. Third, whether BLA activity will provoke activity within the CN (thereby affecting vigilance) is largely controlled by the gamma-aminobutyric acid (GABA)ergic intercalated cell masses (ICMs), which also receive direct prefrontal input. Thus, the functional role of the ICMs provides an answer to a long-standing conundrum concerning amygdala function: how can a detection system (e.g., BLA) effectively continue to represent the present value of a predictive stimulus (e.g., in terms of valence) without necessarily calling the action system (e.g., CN) into action? The answer lies in the ICMs. By acting as a sort of 'moat' the ICMs provide an inhibitory barrier between the BLA and the CN. In this way, the BLA can continue to represent potential threats, while the ICMs inhibit CN output, thereby inhibiting overt responses to potentially threatening stimuli that have proved to pose no threat in the present context (i.e., habituation). Thus, habituation of responsivity of the amygdaloid complex to repeated presentation of biologically relevant stimuli is an active process. It does not necessitate a time-limited role for the amygdala, but instead represents the conservation of resources (e.g., responsivity of the CN), while the BLA continues

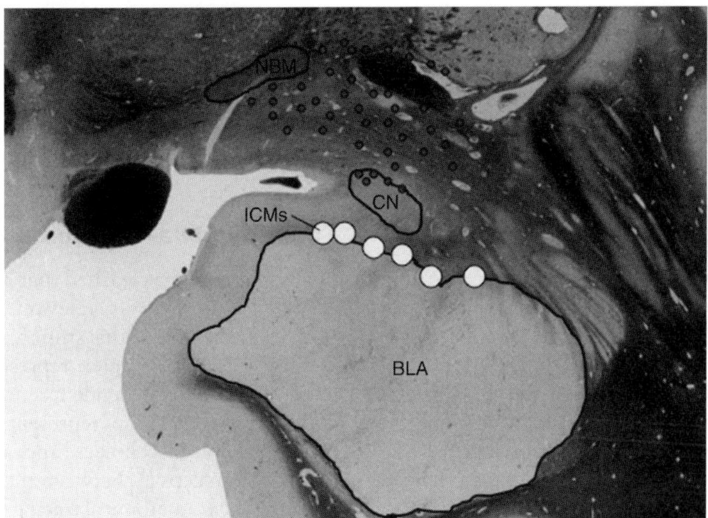

Figure 1 Coronal depiction of the human amygdala: BLA, basolateral amygdala; ICM, intercalated cell masses; CN, central nucleus; NBM, nucleus basalis of Meynert. Adapted from Mai JK, Assheuer J, and Paxinos G (2004) *Atlas of the Human Brain*. Amsterdam: Elsevier Academic press.

to represent the present, potential, and/or future significance of these stimuli.

Nonspecific Arousal Facilitates Attention

The CN serves two primary functions. The most widely recognized role of the CN is that of an output station for the amygdala. With direct connections to the hypothalamus and numerous brain stem motor neuron targets, the CN can drive autonomic nervous system reactivity and affect the coordination of behavioral responses to biologically relevant stimuli. However, the CN also serves another primary purpose during biologically relevant learning, which is to enhance nonspecific arousal and facilitate attention to allow the animal to detect and appropriately respond to stimuli in its environment. Indeed, stimulation of the CN enhances reflexes such as the nictitating membrane reflex, startle reflex, pupil dilation, eye widening, and somatomotor arrest; all responses that indicate that an organism is gathering information. During Pavlovian conditioning, an animal is first exposed to a surprising event (e.g., shock), which automatically and nonspecifically enhances this group of attentional reflexes. This enhanced level of vigilance allows the animal to detect any additional environmental events that may be related to the occurrence of shock, specifically, another event that may aid in predicting its reoccurrence. One CN projection that aids in producing this increased level of vigilance is the projection from the CN to the nucleus basalis of Meynert (NBM). The NBM is directly superior to the CN within the substantia innominata (SI) region of the ventral basal forebrain. While the NBM comprises a compact, 'nucleus-like' portion medially, this nucleus also includes a more distributed lateral portion where individual NBM neurons can be found immediately superior to and even within the CN (see **Figure 1**). NBM neurons provide the primary source of acetylcholine (ACh) for the entire cortex. ACh release from the NBM serves to potentiate neuronal responsivity (i.e., decrease response thresholds) and thereby facilitates information processing throughout cortical systems. Stimulation of the CN in the rabbit produces activation of cortical neurons (as measured by cortical EEG), and cholinergic antagonists can block this effect. Driven by inputs from the BLA signaling the detection of important sensory stimuli, the CN can directly influence the NBM, thereby augmenting sensory information processing by increasing ACh release throughout the cortex. An organism in this heightened state of vigilance becomes a more efficient processor of information. Any new information collected during this state of arousal can then be communicated back to the BLA via cortical feedback projections. Such feedback serves to update information stored in the BLA, which impacts the response of the animal the next time a similar activating stimulus is encountered.

The BLA–CN Connection

Lesion data from appetitive learning paradigms support a role for the BLA in assigning motivational significance to neutral stimuli and for the CN/SI in influencing widespread attentional mechanisms. While neither BLA nor CN/SI lesions impair the ability to associate rewarding outcomes with conditioned stimuli, more subtle deficits have been observed that help to elucidate the differential roles of these amygdaloid subregions during biologically relevant learning. For example, during second-order appetitive conditioning a neutral stimulus (e.g., a light) initially predicts a reward (e.g., food). Once the animal has learned this association, the light becomes rewarding because of its predictive value. Subsequent pairing of the light with a tone results in second-order associative learning, as the animal learns that the tone will also predict a reward. Lesions of the BLA block acquisition of this second-order association, suggesting that the light never becomes reinforcing in BLA-lesioned animals. Another phenomenon that has helped to elucidate the role of the BLA during associative learning is that BLA-lesioned animals do not show stimulus devaluation. In intact animals, it is possible to devalue a food reward by mixing it with a toxin, and later presentation of the light (conditioned stimulus – CS) no longer elicits a conditioned response, suggesting that the light has also been devalued. However, BLA-lesioned animals do not show this type of learning. Taken together, these data suggest that the BLA is necessary to assign reinforcing value to a CS, such that the light assumes some of the reinforcing qualities of food.

Lesions of the CN have no effect on second-order conditioned responding or stimulus devaluation, but do impact attentional mechanisms during appetitive learning. Intact animals orient to novel stimuli (e.g., a light), and this orienting reflex habituates as the animal learns that the novel stimuli are not biologically significant. However, if you then pair light with a food reward, orienting to the light returns. This sort of orienting is referred to as 'associative' orienting. CN-lesioned animals do not show potentiated associative orienting to light-food pairings, even though they still show basic orienting responses to novel stimuli. Thus, the CN is necessary for associative orienting, a process that facilitates attention to predictive stimuli in anticipation of a biologically relevant event.

The aforementioned research emphasizes projections from the CN/SI in increasing cortical ACh release, which lowers neuronal response thresholds, thereby facilitating attention during associative learning paradigms. However, it is important to note that other neurotransmitter systems are also modulated by amygdala function and play a role in behaviors such as associative orienting. For example, CN modulation of the nigrostriatal dopaminergic pathway is necessary for the acquisition and expression of conditioned orienting responses. This same pathway is also implicated in enhancement of attention to surprising (i.e., unpredictable) stimuli during associative learning tasks. Thus, the amygdala's influence on attention during biologically relevant learning is diffuse and likely involves multiple neurotransmitter systems.

The Amygdala–Prefrontal Connection

Once an animal has learned that a particular stimulus predicts a biologically relevant event, the motivational significance of this stimulus can be represented in the BLA. But complex representations of stimuli (e.g., contextually dependent representations) and the coordination of these representations with appropriate behavioral choices appear to be subserved through connectivity between the amygdala and prefrontal cortex. Anatomical tracing studies in nonhuman primates document reciprocal connections between the BLA and the medial prefrontal cortex (mPFC), and functional data in both animals and humans suggest that these connections support fundamental context-dependant valence calculations. Moreover, stimulation studies in the rat show that BLA stimulation inhibits mPFC, and that mPFC stimulation has inhibitory effects on both the BLA and the CN. These effects could be mediated by direct inhibition of the BLA, and/or via direct mPFC projections to GABAergic ICMs, which exert inhibitory control over CN output. Indirect routes could also support modulatory effects between these regions. For example, the amygdala projects to ventral tegmental brain stem neurons that provide the mPFC with dopamine. Interestingly, activation of these dopaminergic neurons inhibits mPFC activity, suggesting that similar effects seen following BLA stimulation could be mediated indirectly via the brain stem.

The animal literature documents that the mPFC provides an important regulatory input to the amygdala, communicating cortical valence representations as they relate to predicted outcomes. Much information about this circuitry has been elucidated through the study of the extinction process following Pavlovian conditioning, which indicates that a specific ventral portion of the mPFC (vmPFC) is necessary for the consolidation and expression of extinction memories (i.e., tone now predicts no shock). This region is referred to as the infralimbic cortex (IL) in the rat but will be generally referred to as vmPFC as we discuss data in rats and humans here. Lesions of the vmPFC do not disrupt initial extinction learning, but on the day following extinction, vmPFC-lesioned animals show no memory for their previous extinction training (i.e., continue to freeze in response to the tone, though it now predicts no shock). Single-unit recording studies indicate that vmPFC neurons respond to conditioned stimuli, and their responses are positively correlated with extinction memory (i.e., reductions in conditioned freezing). Stimulation of vmPFC neurons during extinction training accelerates learning, and evidence suggests this active inhibition of conditioned responding works via a vmPFC–ICM–CN pathway. Thus, vmPFC inputs to the amygdala can dynamically inhibit amygdala activity, signaling either a new, more positive interpretation of a once negative predictive stimulus, or, perhaps, a more general override message that the valence of the outcome predicted by the cue has changed.

Initial neuroimaging studies of the extinction process in humans have reported results consistent with these data in animals. While amygdala activation predicts expression of a conditioned response during both conditioning and extinction training (while stimulus contingencies are changing), activity in the vmPFC only predicts a conditioned response during extinction trials 1 day later. Moreover, recent work indicates that the cortical thickness of the vmPFC is significantly correlated with retention of extinction memory. These data are consistent with the notion that the amygdala is involved in biologically relevant learning while stimulus contingencies are changing, but that the vmPFC is involved in the consolidation and expression of extinction memories via regulatory inputs to the amygdala.

Thus, consistent with the modulatory role the vmPFC appears to play during extinction, interactions between the vmPFC and amygdala may be especially important for producing appropriate responses to changes in the predictive meaning of stimuli, especially when these changes include a shift in predicted valence. These animal and human findings resonate with observations of clinical patients with vmPFC lesions, who show intact psychophysiological responses to positive and negative outcomes (e.g., GSR responses), but lack the ability to choose advantageously when these situations are subsequently encountered.

Amygdala–vmPFC Interactions to Predictive Uncertainty

Thus far we have summarized just a small portion of what we have learned about amygdala–prefrontal function through paradigms that necessarily induce a strong fear state in animal subjects. However, many neuroimaging studies in humans have also sought to assess the role of the amygdala in processing more innocuous biologically relevant predictive stimuli that likely induce more subtle fluctuations in attention. For example, static pictures of facial expressions of emotion consistently activate the amygdala during human neuroimaging studies. This is because facial expressions are salient, biologically relevant stimuli that have predicted important events for you in the past. In other words, facial expressions are conditioned stimuli. A happy facial expression likely predicts reinforcing or affiliative behavior from a conspecific, whereas an angry facial expression predicts social threat. Fearful facial expressions are of particular interest to the amygdala, presumably because they tell the viewer that something important and potentially dangerous is happening in the environment, but, unlike angry faces, do not reveal the source of this threat.

A recent neuroimaging experiment in humans delineates a functional spatial dissociation in the amygdala using facial expressions of emotion that differ in their predictive value. In an experimental environment, static pictures of facial expressions have no biological relevance to viewers, but, because of the past predictive nature of the expressions, the amygdaloid system does respond to these conditioned stimuli, at least initially. As predicted by the animal data outlined thus far, both fearful and angry facial expressions activate the BLA, which represents these faces as negatively valenced. However, these two facial expressions differ on one important dimension: angry faces are inherently embody of negativity, while in the case of fearful faces, more information is needed to determine the exact nature of the source of threat. Such a model predicts that angry expressions can be handled via BLA outputs related to the enactment of an appropriate response plan (e.g., are you going to fight or flee?). In contrast, the meaning of a fearful facial expression is context dependent and thus requires the CN and its connections to neuromodulatory centers, such as the corticopetal cholinergic neurons of the NBM, to call upon the cortex to process additional information in the environment. This assertion was validated recently in a neuroimaging study showing that both fearful and angry faces activate the ventral amygdala where the BLA is located, but only fearful faces activate the dorsal amygdala/SI region where the CN and NBM are located. Thus, facial expressions call for parallel processing across a number of different dimensions, as two different circuits through the amygdaloid complex simultaneously compute valence (fear and anger are both clearly negative and activate the ventral amygdala) and uncertainty (only fear requires greater processing of contextual information and is related to dorsal amygdala/SI activation) processes. These data predict that information processing should be enhanced following the presentation of fearful facial expressions. Indeed, recent data show that humans show enhanced perceptual discrimination abilities following presentations of fearful faces.

One way to further understand amygdala response to fearful facial expressions would be to test an expression that, like fear, was ambiguous in terms of its eliciting event but, unlike fear, could predict either a negative or positive event. Facial expressions of surprise are similar to facial expressions of fear both configurally (e.g., wide eyes) and in terms of their information value in that they tell you that something important is happening in your environment, but you need more information to determine what it is and how to react to it. However, they differ from fearful facial expressions on one important dimension: surprised expressions can predict both positive and negative outcomes. When viewers are asked to rate surprised faces using a valence scale (see **Figure 2**), some viewers interpret the expression positively, while others interpret it negatively. Consistent with the previously discussed data comparing amygdala response to fear and anger, surprised faces produce greater ventral amygdala activation only in viewers who interpret them negatively. Further, this effect within the amygdala appears to depend on inputs from the prefrontal cortex. In this same study amygdala activity was inversely correlated with vmPFC activity. That is, viewers with a more positive interpretation of

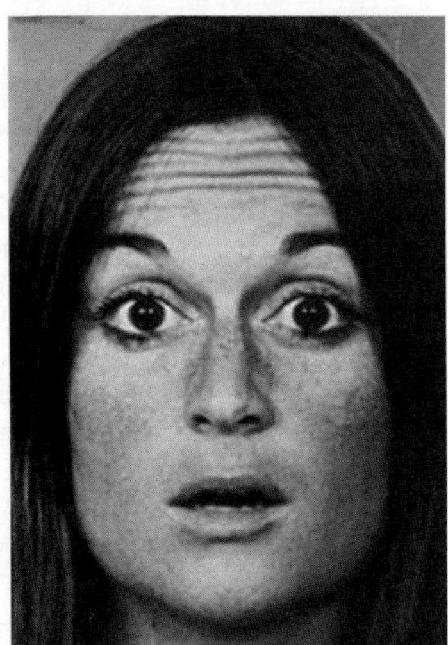

1-------2-------3-------4-------5-------6-------7-------8-------9
VP P NN N VN

Figure 2 Valence scale. Study participants view surprised facial expressions and are asked to rate how positive or negative the expression on the face is: VP, very positive; P, positive; NN, neither negative nor positive; N, negative; VN, very negative. Reproduced from Ekman P and Friesen WV (1976) *Pictures of Facial Affect.* Palo Alto, CA: Consulting Psychologists Press. Face image used by permission from PaultEkman.com.

surprised faces show greater vmPFC and lower amygdala activity. Thus, viewers showing a stronger vmPFC reaction in an area known to send inhibitory projections to the amygdala interpret the ambiguous facial expressions more positively.

Linking Amygdala–vmPFC Response and Surprised Faces to the Fear Extinction Literature

The amygdala is necessary for the acquisition and expression of learned fear associations. Typically, animals learn to fear a CS (e.g., tone) that predicts an unconditioned stimulus (US; e.g., shock). Thalamic and cortical afferents communicate CS and US information to the BLA, where CS–US associations are thought to be formed. As described earlier, the behavioral and autonomic expression of conditioned fear, however, is thought to result from excitatory influences of the BLA on the coordinated efferent systems of the CN.

As already discussed, extinction involves the attenuation of a conditioned response when a tone CS is repeatedly presented in the absence of a US. Behavioral studies have demonstrated that extinction does not expunge the CS–US association, but rather a new memory trace is formed that inhibits the previously established conditioned response. After extinction, therefore, the CS is inherently ambiguous, potentially predicting either shock or the absence of shock.

Relevant to the present discussion, lesions of the vmPFC in the rat affect the ability to use this new information learned about the CS during extinction, when the CS is subsequently encountered. For example, while neurons of the vmPFC are not responsive to a tone CS during conditioning or extinction training, these same cells show robust CS-evoked firing when the animal is recalling extinction the following day. In addition, electrical stimulation of the vmPFC is sufficient to inhibit the expression of freezing, mimicking the effects observed following extinction training. This suggests that the vmPFC can regulate the response of the amygdala to extinguished tones that now have ambiguous predictive value.

It is hoped that the reader sees the parallel between this discussion (vmPFC control of the amygdala to extinguished tones in rats) and the preceding discussion (vmPFC–amygdala response to surprised faces) (see **Figure 3**). Like extinguished tones, surprised faces also have an inconsistent reinforcement history, predicting both positive and negative outcomes. Viewers who show strong vmPFC activation to extinguished tones, or surprised faces, are readily able to recall the more positive interpretation of the presented stimulus. While these effects have been shown to be causal in

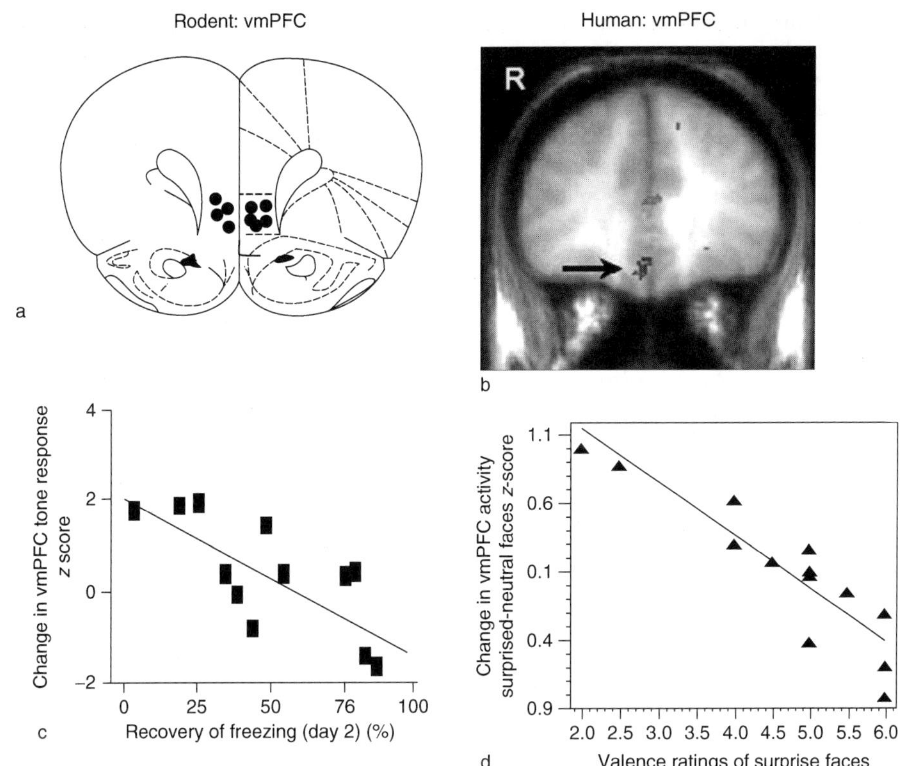

Figure 3 Ventromedial prefrontal cortex (vmPFC) activity and behavior are inversely correlated in the rodent and human. (a) Single-cell recording sites in the rodent vmPFC. (b) Functional magnetic resonance imaging data in the human; blue color indicates surprised < neutral faces. (c) Scatter plot showing that less activity in vmPFC is related to increased recovery of freezing on day 2 (i.e., reduced extinction memory) in rats. (d) Scatter plot showing that less activity in vmPFC is related to more negative interpretations of surprised facial expressions in humans. Study participants view surprised facial expressions and are asked to rate how positive or negative the expression on the face is (see **Figure 2**; higher ratings indicate more negative interpretations). Adapted from Milad MR and Quirk GJ (2002) Neurons in medial prefrontal cortex signal memory for fear extinction. *Nature* 420: 70–74; and Kim H, Somerville LH, Johnstone T, et al. (2003) Inverse amygdala and medial prefrontal cortex responses to surprised faces. *NeuroReport* 14: 2317–2322.

the animal model and necessarily remain correlational in the human model, we believe a vmPFC–amygdala circuitry similar to that which extinguishes conditioned fear accounts for subjective interpretations of valence in humans who encounter an ambiguously valenced facial expression (such as surprise).

The animal and human data lead us to the following working hypothesis: upon encountering the expression of surprise, the amygdala initially sends out a 'first pass' message, identifying the uncertain nature of these faces with respect to valence, and likely categorizes these faces as 'potentially threatening' in all viewers. The vmPFC, based upon additional inputs from multiple brain regions providing information about past experiences or present context, could then communicate alternative hypotheses back to the amygdala, including the 'potential positivity' of these faces. Individual differences in the strength of this vmPFC 'override' message would account for the observed differences in valence ratings. This scenario is consistent with numerous models and examples of inverse amygdala–vmPFC interaction, and suggests a mechanism by which complex representations of valence, communicated via the vmPFC, can influence the amygdala's representation of the predictive value of a stimulus. These valence representations are used to calculate appropriate behavioral responses within a given environmental context and can change the way that the amygdala influences cognitive functions such as attention and memory.

The notion that the amygdala is sensitive to environmental uncertainty *per se* and that it will first test whether this uncertainty is potentially negative was demonstrated in a recent study using mice and humans. The amygdala was shown to be more active during segments of time when unpredictable tones were played compared to segments when tones were played in a predictable pattern. Critically, unpredictable tones also biased the study participants to treat other biologically relevant environmental events as potentially threatening. Thus, unpredictablity *per se*, even for events that are not biologically relevant, is enough to engage the amygdala. This activity creates a vigilance state that augments an animal's reaction to subsequent potential danger.

Role of the Amygdala in Vigilance: Resolving Associative Ambiguity

Resolving associative ambiguity is a complex process requiring access to memory, temporal contexts, spatial contexts, and visceral contexts in order to make a probabilistic 'guess' as to the best course of action. More than simple uncertainty, when one does not yet have a working hypothesis about predicted outcomes, the term 'associative ambiguity' very specifically refers to a situation in which a predictive stimulus has more than one potential meaning (based upon prior learning) that must be selected in a given situation. Here we consider the role of vmPFC–amygdala interactions in determining which valence representation (positive or negative) will be invoked in a particular circumstance. Stimuli with inconsistent reinforcement histories (such as extinguished tones and surprised faces) are inherently ambiguous, potentially predicting either a positive or negative outcome, and this vmPFC-amygdala circuit appears to subserve the calculation and/or retrieval of this information.

The vmPFC is ideally situated for this function, given its access to working memory, spatial (hippocampal) function, and visceral inputs, as well as to outputs able to override subcortical fear expression centers. Each of the divergent brain stem autonomic and somatic targets of the amygdala CN also receives a projection from these medial prefrontal areas, most of which are inhibitory. This arrangement, in a healthy human brain, effectively gives the vmPFC 'veto power' over subcortical conditioned responses, allowing the organism to respond appropriately based on recent experience.

Failure to resolve associative ambiguity appropriately can lead to pathological outcomes, and the vmPFC has been implicated in a variety of affective disorders, as well as the genetic predisposition to inappropriate or pathological expression of affect. For example, posttraumatic stress disorder (PTSD) is characterized by an inability to suppress fear responses to stimuli that were once associated with trauma but now no longer predict danger. Consistent with impaired cortical regulation of the amygdala, PTSD patients show decreased volume and decreased activity in vmPFC, coupled with increased amygdala activity. As mentioned previously, a similar area of the vmPFC was recently shown to correlate (in thickness) with memory for fear extinction in normal study participants, suggesting that PTSD patients may be deficient in the neural circuitry underlying extinction. Thus, similar to those persons showing a negative bias in the interpretation of surprised faces, persons with smaller vmPFC volume tend to interpret conditioned stimuli that had been extinguished (and were therefore ambiguous) as dangerous.

Conclusions

The amygdala coordinates emotional responses and also modulates cognitive functions such as attention that affect subsequent learning and memory. The amygdala is consistently implicated in learning about, and assigning emotional meaning to, biologically relevant events and the stimuli that predict those events. Interactions between the amygdala and vmPFC provide flexible, context-dependent representations of emotional valence. If a stimulus predicts a certain aversive or appetitive event, then the amygdala can coordinate an appropriate behavioral response to that stimulus. If the predictive value is uncertain, because more contextual information is needed, or perhaps because of a stimulus' inconsistent reinforcement history, vigilance networks are recruited to gather additional information from the environment. Here we have highlighted the amygdala's influence over this process through the NBM cholinergic system. But the amygdala projects to all major neuromodulatory centers. Indeed, amygdala projections to substantia nigra dopaminergic corticopetal neurons have been specifically implicated in response to surprising outcomes. Through these networks, the amygdala influences cognition in the service of protecting us from danger or leading us toward reward. This not only happens in extreme emotional circumstances, but it also happens on a more subtle, moment-by-moment basis. By constantly monitoring the environment for biologically relevant cues, the amygdala maximizes our ability to avoid danger or avail ourselves of reward.

The complementary animal and human findings discussed in this article are consistent with a role for the vmPFC in the regulation of amygdala responsivity during the subjective interpretation of ambiguous stimuli. Indeed, these results join a diverse list of experimental paradigms implicating the vmPFC in regulatory control when stimuli are associatively ambiguous. Associative ambiguity is high following extinction, when conflicting facts about a CS have been learned. Associative ambiguity is also high during reversal learning, set-shifting, and other situations requiring behavioral flexibility. Taken together, these studies support the more generalized involvement of frontotemporal interactions in behavioral flexibility. As more unified theories of limbic function advance, such theories must include a role for vmPFC–amygdala integration and regulatory control of biologically relevant information processing, particularly when contingencies are ambiguous.

See also: Amygdala: Structure and Circuitry in Primates; Amygdala: Structure and Circuitry in Rodents and Felines; Amygdala: Contributions to Fear; Emotion: Neuroimaging; Emotion: Computational Modeling; Emotional Influences on Memory and Attention; Pharmacology of Fear Extinction; Posttraumatic Stress Disorder: Overview; Social Emotion: Neuroimaging.

Further Reading

Aggleton JP and Saunders RC (2000) The amygdala – what's happened in the last decade? In: Aggleton JP (ed.) *The Amygdala: A Functional Analysis,* 2nd edn., pp. 1–30. New York: Oxford University Press.

Amaral DG, Price JL, Pitkanen A, et al. (1992) Anatomical organization of the primate amygdaloid complex. In: Aggleton JP (ed.) *The Amygdala: Neurobiological Aspects of Emotion, Memory, and Mental Dysfunction*, pp. 1–66. New York: Wiley-Liss.

Bouton ME (1994) Context, ambiguity, and classical conditioning. *Current Directions in Psychological Science* 3: 49–53.

Davis M and Whalen PJ (2001) The amygdala: Vigilance and emotion. *Molecular Psychiatry* 6: 13–34.

Ekman P and Friesen WV (1976) *Pictures of Facial Affect.* Palo Alto, CA: Consulting Psychologists Press.

Heimer L and VanHoesen GW (2006) The limbic lobe and its output channels: Implications for emotional functions and adaptive behavior. *Neuroscience & Biobehavioral Reviews* 30: 126–147.

Herry C, Bach DR, Esposito F, et al. (2007) Processing of temporal unpredictability in human and animal amygdala. *Journal of Neuroscience* 27: 5958–5966.

Holland PC and Gallagher M (1999) Amygdala circuitry in attentional and representational processes. *Trends in Cognitive Sciences* 3: 65–73.

Kapp BS, Wilson A, Pascoe JP, et al. (1990) A neuroanatomical systems analysis of conditioned bradycardia in the rabbit. In: Gabriel M and Moore J (eds.) *Learning and Computational Neuroscience: Foundations of Adaptive Network*, pp. 53–90. Cambridge, MA: MIT Press.

Kim H, Somerville LH, Johnstone T, et al. (2003) Inverse amygdala and medial prefrontal cortex responses to surprised faces. *NeuroReport* 14: 2317–2322.

LeDoux JE (1987) Emotion. In: Blum F, Geiger SR, and Mountcastle VB (eds.) *Handbook of Physiology, Section 1, The Nervous System,* vol. 5, pp. 419–459. Bethesda, MD: American Physiological Society.

Likhtik E, Pelletier JG, Paz R, et al. (2005) Prefrontal control of the amygdala. *Journal of Neuroscience* 25: 7429–7437.

Mai JK, Assheuer J and Paxinos G (2004) *Atlas of the Human Brain.* Amsterdam: Elsevier Academic Press.

Milad MR and Quirk GJ (2002) Neurons in medial prefrontal cortex signal memory for fear extinction. *Nature* 420: 70–74.

Phelps EA, Ling S, and Carrasco M (2006) Emotion facilitates perception and potentiates the perceptual benefits of attention. *Psychological Science* 17: 292–299.

Weisz DJ, Harden DG, and Xiang Z (1992) Effects of amygdala lesions on reflex facilitation and conditioned response acquisition during nictitating membrane response conditioning in rabbit. *Behavioral Neuroscience* 106: 262–273.

Whalen PJ (1998) Fear, vigilance, and ambiguity: Initial neuroimaging studies of the human amygdala. *Current Directions in Psychological Science* 7: 177–188.

Emotional Influences on Memory and Attention

E A Phelps, New York University, New York, NY, USA

Introduction

The interaction of emotion and cognition is obvious to most people. It is not uncommon for traffic to slow because the attention of the drivers ahead is distracted by the view of an accident. It is also not uncommon for someone to proclaim that his or her memory for an event is vivid or detailed because the event is highly emotional, or what is often called 'memorable'. In spite of the common recognition that emotion and cognition are intertwined, the study of emotion in the scientific investigation of cognitive processes, such as memory and attention, has only recently blossomed. The reasons for this have to do with both the philosophical foundations of the discipline of cognition within psychology and the emergence of cognitive neuroscience as a dominant approach in understanding cognitive functions. When one examines brain function, it is apparent that the neural systems of emotion and cognition are intertwined from perception to reasoning and decision making. This recent emphasis on understanding the neural representation of human behavior has resulted in a new appreciation of the important role of emotion in cognitive functions.

One brain region that plays a prominent role in the interaction of emotion and cognition is the amygdala. The amygdala is a small structure in the medial temporal lobe that sits adjacent and anterior to the hippocampus (see **Figure 1**). The amygdala is known to be important in a range of emotional behaviors, most notably the ability to learn that stimuli in the environment predict potential aversive consequences, referred to as fear conditioning. The amygdala is critical for the acquisition, storage, and expression of fear conditioning. In addition to its role in emotional learning, the amygdala is widely connected to other brain regions that mediate a range of cognitive functions. It has been suggested that through these connections, the amygdala can influence cognition in the presence of potentially important stimuli. This additional role for the amygdala in the tuning of cognition by emotion helps assure that events that may be important for our survival receive priority in processing. This article reviews what has been learned from the study of the amygdala concerning the interaction of emotion, attention, and memory.

Emotion's Influence on Attention and Perception

Attention and perception are the first stages of stimulus processing. Factors that influence these processes will also influence downstream cognitive functions, such as memory. An early example of emotion's impact on attention is the classic 'cocktail party effect' described by Cherry in 1953. This effect gets its name from the observation that when we focus our attention on one stream of information and ignore others, such as paying attention to a single conversation at a cocktail party, we might inadvertently pick up on some of the unattended information if it is salient or important, such as when one's own name is mentioned in another conversation at the party. This finding and others suggest that emotion can facilitate awareness for emotionally salient stimuli in situations in which attention is limited.

Recent cognitive neuroscience research indicates the amygdala may mediate the facilitation of attention with emotion. This was investigated using a paradigm that tests the temporal limitations of attention, called the attentional blink. In this paradigm, stimuli, such as words, are presented in rapid succession – so quickly it is difficult to identify any words. However, if participants are told that they can ignore most of the words presented and selectively attend to a few target words, such as those printed in a different color ink, they can usually identify the target words. However, this ability to selectively attend to and identify specific words in the rapid stream of words is limited by the temporal relation between the targets. If the second target word is presented a few items after the first target word, participants will often miss it. It is as if noticing and encoding the first target word results in a temporary refractory period during which it is difficult to notice and encode a second target. When this occurs, it is as if attention 'blinked'. However, if the second target word is emotional and arousing, this temporal limitation of attention is not as great. During the 'blink' period, when attentional resources are limited, arousing words are more likely to be identified than are neutral words. This attenuation of the attentional blink effect is not apparent for patients with damage to the amygdala. Unlike normal controls, patients with damage to the left amygdala experience a similar decrement in the ability to report emotional and neutral words. This finding is consistent with previous studies indicating that in situations when one has limited attentional resources, emotional stimuli are more likely than neutral stimuli to reach

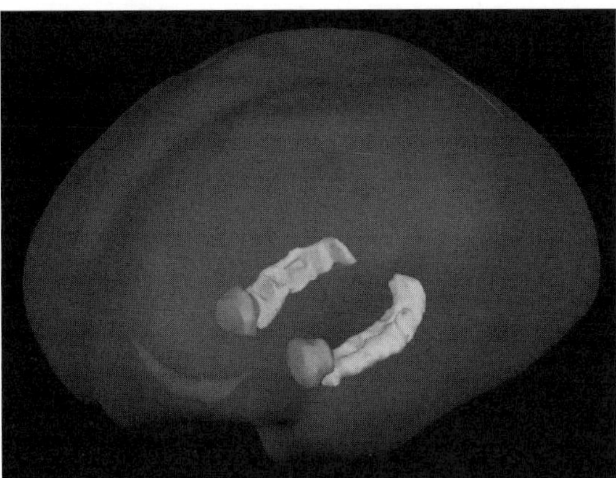

Figure 1 The human amygdala (blue) and the hippocampus (green).

awareness. It also indicates that the amygdala plays a critical role in this facilitation of attention with emotion.

It is suggested that the amygdala has its influence on attention by modulating processing in brain regions known to mediate perception. Two distinct mechanisms have been explored that may explain the amygdala's facilitation of attention. The first was proposed by Weinberger and colleagues, who demonstrated that fear conditioning can tune the representation of emotional stimuli in sensory cortices. In studies with rats, they showed that the representation of simple tones in the auditory cortex is changed through fear conditioning when a tone is paired with, and comes to predict, an aversive shock. This change in the cortical representation creates a heightened sensitivity to the tone that predicts shock. This sensory tuning with emotional learning depends on the amygdala. If the amygdala is damaged, fear learning does not occur, and the representation of the tone in the auditory cortex is unchanged. It is interesting that once fear learning has occurred, this change in the auditory cortex will last, even if new learning diminishes the fear response to the tone or the amygdala is damaged and the learned fear is no longer expressed. In other words, the amygdala is needed to create this change in the auditory cortex to an emotional stimulus, but it is not required to maintain it. A recent study that used functional magnetic resonance imaging (fMRI) in humans showed a similar lasting change in the auditory cortex in response to a tone that predicted a shock. Although it has been suggested that a change in the cortical representation of stimuli in the visual cortex might also occur with emotional learning, this has yet to be explored. It is clear, however, that one way that emotion can influence attention is by creating a lasting change in the cortical representation of stimuli that have acquired emotional properties through learning.

The second mechanism that has been proposed to underlie emotion's influence on attention is more transient and has been demonstrated primarily in studies of visual processing. Anatomical studies have shown that there are reciprocal connections between the amygdala and the sensory cortices, including the visual cortex. It is proposed that early in stimulus processing, the amygdala receives input about the emotional significance of a stimulus and, through projections to the visual cortex, modulates further attentional and perceptual processes. Three lines of evidence from brain imaging studies in humans support this model: (1) studies demonstrating that emotional stimuli are processed automatically, (2) findings of enhanced responses in visual cortical regions for emotional stimuli, and (3) findings demonstrating that the amygdala mediates this enhanced cortical response.

The idea that emotional stimuli are processed automatically is consistent with suggestions in the psychological literature that the emotional qualities of stimuli are detected quickly and prior to awareness. Similarly, it is proposed that the amygdala receives input about the emotional significance of a stimulus quickly and prior to awareness. In support of this hypothesis, fMRI studies have demonstrated robust amygdala activation in response to subliminally presented images of faces with fear expressions, in contrast to the response to neutral expressions. In addition, a number of studies have shown that attention and awareness have little impact on the amygdala's response to fearful stimuli. It is suggested that this early, automatic amygdala response to fear or threat stimuli is an important factor in the amygdala's ability to modulate further cognitive processes and responses to potential danger.

One of the first brain imaging studies to examine emotion demonstrated that visual cortical regions show enhanced activation to novel emotional scenes compared with novel neutral scenes. This finding has also been observed in comparisons of responses in the visual cortex to faces with fear versus faces with neutral expressions. The studies of facial expression have also demonstrated an enhanced amygdala response to fearful versus neutral faces, the magnitude of which is correlated with the enhanced visual cortex activation to these same stimuli. This line of research is consistent with the proposed mechanism by which the amygdala detects the emotional significance of a stimulus quickly and modulates further perceptual and attentional processing. However, one drawback of these studies is that most brain imaging findings are correlational in nature and thus cannot determine the precise function of a given brain region or the direction of the communication between two regions. In an effort to demonstrate that the amygdala's input mediates the enhanced response observed in the visual cortex to emotional stimuli, Vuillimier and colleagues combined functional imaging and lesion methodologies. During brain imaging, patients with varying degrees of damage to the amygdala were shown pictures of faces with fear and neutral expressions. The amount of amygdala damage predicted the magnitude of the response in the visual cortex: the more damage to the amygdala, the smaller the enhanced visual cortex response to fear faces. This finding strongly supports the suggestion that the amygdala mediates the enhanced response in the visual cortex.

If the amygdala is responding to the emotional significance of a stimulus in the environment quickly and prior to awareness, and modulating further processing in the visual cortex, then certain properties of emotion's influence on attention should emerge. First, any enhanced visual response should be transient and evoked by the presence of an emotional stimulus. Second, the enhanced response with emotion should be apparent in perception, since this is the job of the visual cortex. This enhanced perception may underlie the observed facilitation of attention in that it requires less attentional resources to detect something that is easier to perceive. Finally, the enhanced processing with emotion is not necessarily tied to the emotional stimulus itself, but should extend to neutral stimuli that are cued by emotional stimuli and presented close in time.

To explore whether these properties emerge, researchers have used a psychophysical paradigm to examine the effect of a fearful face cue on sensitivity to changes in contrast – that is, the subtle gradations of gray that help us differentiate edges of lines. The ability to detect contrast is an early perceptual function that has been linked to primary visual cortex. In this study, a fear or neutral face cue was presented in one or four quadrants of a computer screen. Then 40 ms later, four patches with lines appeared in the corners of the screen (adjacent to the location of faces). The lines in one of the four patches were tilted, and the participants had to indicate whether the lines were tilted to the right or to the left. If only one face was presented, then the patch with tilted lines was presented in the same quadrant as the face. This single-face condition allowed participants to covertly attend to the location of the subsequent patch. Across trials, the contrast in the patches varied so that the ability to detect the orientation of the lines was easier or harder. Two effects for the emotional expression of the face cue were observed. First, irrespective of whether the face cue directed covert attention, a fear face enhanced contrast sensitivity. That is, less contrast was needed to detect the orientation of the lines if the lines were preceded by a fear face rather than by a neutral face. Second, if a fear face cue directed covert attention, contrast sensitivity was enhanced more than would have been predicted by the independent effects of a fear face cue and covert attention on perception. In other words, emotion potentiates the perceptual benefit of covert attention. These psychophysical results are consistent with a model in which the emotion, via the amygdala, modulates processing in early visual regions in a transient manner for stimuli cued by emotion.

The amygdala, through its extensive connectivity with sensory processing regions, is ideally situated to influence perception. The existing evidence supports two independent means by which emotion influences perception, one of which is long lasting and affects perception of an emotional stimulus that predicts an aversive outcome, and the other of which is transient and can affect the perception of stimuli cued by emotion. It is suggested that the amygdala's influence on perception may underlie emotion's facilitation of attention. Discussions of the adaptive function of emotion's facilitation of attention emphasize the preferential detection of stimuli that signal potential importance or threat and suggest a primary role for the amygdala is the modulation of vigilance in the presence of these stimuli. The current evidence of emotion's influence on attention and perception is largely consistent with this interpretation.

What is less clear at this point is whether these mechanisms that lead to the facilitation of perception with emotion also play a role in any perceptual cost that may emerge for other stimuli. It has been suggested that emotion can capture attention. When attention is captured by emotion, there is impaired processing of nonemotional aspects of the stimulus or event. A number of behavioral studies have demonstrated the capture of attention with emotion, and it is suggested that this effect is due to difficulty disengaging attention from the emotional qualities of a stimulus. Only a few studies have examined the neural systems underlying the capture of attention with emotion, and these suggest that emotion may decrease activity in regions of the parietal lobe thought important for the allocation of attention. It is not known how this effect may or may not be related to the facilitation of attention and perception observed when people are processing emotional aspects of a cue or stimulus.

Emotion's Influence on Memory

"An impression may be so exciting emotionally as almost to leave a scar upon the cerebral tissues." This phrase is attributed to William James in his classic textbook, *Principles of Psychology*, which was first published in 1890. Although James did not have the benefit of experimental research to support his claims, his intuition was that emotion should strongly influence how impressions are remembered. This intuition has been largely supported by scientific research since 1890. The questions remain, how does the brain enable this 'scar' to form, and what are its qualities?

Memory can be broken down into a series of stages. The first, called encoding, occurs when a stimulus is first encountered. After the encoding stage, the memory is stored. Although storage may seem like a passive stage, it is known that during storage, processes occur over time that allow the memory to become more or less stable. This time-dependent storage process is called consolidation. Finally, when a memory is called to mind, it is retrieved. There is evidence that emotion might influence all three of these stages of memory processing. Although episodic memory critically depends on other brain regions, most notably the hippocampus and surrounding cortices (see **Figure 1**), the amygdala appears to play an important role in modulating the neural circuitry of memory with emotion.

To start with the first stage, emotion can influence the encoding of to-be-remembered stimuli through its modulation of attention and perception. Research has indicated that manipulations of attention will significantly affect memory encoding. Therefore, the changes in attention and perception that occur with emotion, outlined earlier, should lead to differences in memory performance. In support of this hypothesis, a recent study found that patients with amygdala damage show impairments only in memory for details of emotional scenes that are central to the event, with intact memory for details that are more peripheral. This study suggests that the amygdala may be involved in highlighting and narrowing attention around central, emotional details, leading to enhanced encoding of these details in normal study participants. However, most studies to date have failed to differentiate the amygdala's influence on encoding and consolidation. In fact, with many studies, it is not clear how to differentiate emotion's impact on encoding and consolidation since both are assessed with retrieval and occur close in time. Although a number of brain imaging studies have demonstrated that amygdala responses during encoding can predict later recognition or recall for emotional stimuli, these studies often attribute this effect to emotion's influence on the modulation of memory storage rather than on attention and perception.

The primary neural mechanism that has been explored in an effort to understand emotion's influence on episodic memory is the amygdala's modulation of consolidation. Evidence across species suggests that the consolidation of episodic memory critically depends on the hippocampus. Emotion, specifically arousal, is proposed to enhance hippocampal-dependent consolidation. Research by James McGaugh and colleagues conducted in rats has identified the neural mechanisms underlying the effect of arousal on memory consolidation. These studies have shown that physiological arousal results in activation of β-adrenergic receptors in the amygdala. The amygdala, in turn, modulates hippocampal processing, resulting in enhanced consolidation or storage for events that elicit an arousal response. Damage to the amygdala does not impair episodic memory for a stimulus, but it eliminates any enhancement observed with physiological arousal. Evidence that this effect is due to the modulation of consolidation, as opposed to encoding, comes from studies demonstrating that manipulations of amygdala function after stimulus encoding will alter arousal's influence on episodic memory. McGaugh suggests that one adaptive function of having a slow consolidation process is to allow for the emotional reaction to a stimulus, which occurs after presentation, to influence memory strength. In this way, events that result in an emotional response, and are more likely to be important for future survival, are less likely to be forgotten.

Consistent with the proposed mechanisms outlined by McGaugh and colleagues, a number of studies in humans have reported that arousal enhances the retention of episodic memories so that they are less likely to be forgotten over time. Evidence that the human amygdala plays a role in this enhanced memory with arousal comes from studies using a range of cognitive neuroscience techniques. As mentioned earlier, brain imaging studies have reported that activation of the amygdala at encoding can predict later retention for emotional stimuli. The amygdala has direct projections to the anterior portion of the hippocampus. A recent study found that the activation of the amygdala and anterior hippocampus is correlated during the encoding of emotional scenes that were later remembered. In addition, patients with amygdala damage fail to show the normal enhancement of episodic memory with arousal. Consistent with a role for the amygdala in modulating storage or consolidation, patients with amygdala damage show similar forgetting curves for arousing and neutral stimuli, in contrast to normal controls, who show enhanced retention for arousing stimuli. In addition, pharmacological manipulations in humans that block β-adrenergic receptors also block arousal's impact on episodic memory, consistent with animal models. Taken together, these studies provide strong support for the mechanism proposed by McGaugh and colleagues suggesting the amygdala modulates hippocampal consolidation with arousal.

Although there is substantial evidence that emotion can influence later memory accuracy, a few limitations should be mentioned. First, the magnitude of the effect of emotion on episodic memory varies depending on the paradigm. It can be quite subtle and is not always observed. Second, in addition to arousal, other factors that vary with emotion, such as the similarity of to-be-remembered stimuli, can also influence later memory. These other factors most likely achieve their influence on memory through different neural mechanisms. Finally, more-extreme stress can have an opposite effect; that is, an impairment of hippocampal function and episodic memory accuracy. In spite of these caveats, there is robust evidence that the human amygdala, through its modulation of hippocampal consolidation, plays a critical role in situations in which physiological arousal leads to enhanced episodic memory.

The final stage of memory is retrieval, when the stored information is called to mind. Processes that occur at retrieval reflect the outcome of encoding and storage, as well as additional functions related to judgment and memory monitoring. Although most studies investigate memory accuracy, there is also research indicating that the retrieval of emotional stimuli may be marked by a difference in subjective quality. Studies of episodic memory of real-life, public, emotional events have suggested that emotion may influence the subjective experience of memory retrieval, irrespective of memory accuracy. These studies examining 'flashbulb' memories have found that for highly emotional, public events, the confidence that a memory is accurate and the sense that it is detailed and vivid may not reflect actual accuracy for details. One of first examples of this effect examined memory of the explosion of the space shuttle *Challenger.* Within a few days of this tragedy, study participants were asked to record their memory for the circumstances in which they become aware of this event. Two and a half years later, the participants were asked to report the same memory. Even though the participants gave detailed recollections and were highly confident in their accuracy, most of these memories were inaccurate. More recently, a study examining memory for the terrorist attack of September 11, 2001, found that accuracy for memories of learning about this event did not differ from other, nonemotional events that occurred around the same time. However, memories of the terrorist attacks, in comparison to the more mundane events, were rated as more confident, vivid, detailed, and recollected. These studies of flashbulb memories suggest that emotion has an independent effect of enhancing the subjective sense of remembering during retrieval.

In an effort to explore the mechanisms underlying the enhanced subjective sense of remembering with emotion, laboratory studies have used the 'remember–know' paradigm. Recognition memory judgments are thought to rely on two independent processes: recollection, which includes the retrieval of contextual details, and familiarity, which is a sense that a stimulus is familiar in the absence of contextual details. The remember–know procedure is a subjective measure of these two processes. During recognition judgments, study participants view old and new stimuli and are asked to judge whether each stimulus is 'new' (not presented before), 'known' (familiar, but there is no specific recollection of details for the encoding context), or 'remembered' (recollected with details of the encoding context). For neutral stimuli, it has been demonstrated that the subjective judgment of 'remember' is correlated with accuracy for memory of the contextual details of the stimulus, suggesting that the accurate recollection of details and the subjective judgment of remembering rely on the same processes. For emotional stimuli, it has been found that the subjective judgment of remembering is enhanced, but this subjective judgment of recollection is not as closely linked to a corresponding increase in accuracy of memory of the contextual details. In other words, emotion may enhance the feeling of remembering independent of its impact on memory accuracy.

Using a similar paradigm with fMRI, researchers have demonstrated that different neural mechanisms underlie the subjective judgment of remembering for pictures of emotional as opposed to neutral scenes. Consistent with previous studies, responses in a part of the hippocampal complex, the posterior parahippocampus, differentiated 'remember' and 'know' judgments for neutral scenes. In contrast, signals in the amygdala differentiated 'remember' and 'know' judgments for emotional scenes. The posterior parahippocampus has previously been linked to memory accuracy for details of visual scenes, which is the type of information that might be expected to result in a judgment of 'remember' if this subjective judgment reflects accurate memory for scene details. However, responses in this region were not similarly enhanced for 'remembered' emotional stimuli. These results suggest that the neural mechanisms underlying the subjective judgment of recollection differ between emotional and neutral scenes. The amygdala is specifically linked to judgments of recollection for emotional scenes.

In a recent study, a similar pattern was observed when participants who were in Manhattan on September 11, 2001, retrieved autobiographical memories from that day or the summer of 2001. Although memory accuracy could not be verified in this study, it was found that those participants who were closer to the World Trade Center (WTC) on that day reported September 11 memories that were rated as more vivid, detailed, and confident. Proximity to the WTC was not only correlated with the subjective sense of remembering but also increased activation of the amygdala and decreased activation of the posterior parahippocampus during memory retrieval. These findings are consistent with previous studies of flashbulb memories, which indicate that unique processes may underlie the judgment of recollection during the retrieval of highly emotional events.

Studies of memory retrieval suggest that for emotional stimuli, judgments of the subjective sense of remembering may be influenced by the emotional qualities of the stimulus, with less emphasis on mnemonic details. Consistent with behavioral reports of flashbulb memories suggesting emotion enhances the feeling of retrieval accuracy irrespective of actual accuracy, brain imaging results indicate emotion may alter the neural mechanisms underlying the subjective judgments of remembering. The impact of emotion on subjective quality of memory retrieval likely reflects emotion's influence on processes that occur at encoding and storage, as well as retrieval.

Although there is significant evidence that emotion interacts with episodic memory, and that the amygdala plays an important role in this interaction, an understanding of the complexity of this relationship is just beginning to emerge. Most studies in humans examining the neural systems underlying emotion's influence on episodic memory have emphasized arousal's impact on memory consolidation, perhaps inspired by the elegant animal models outlining this mechanism. However, only a few studies have clearly documented arousal's specific influence on memory consolidation in humans, independent of its effect on encoding. Disentangling the range of mechanisms by which emotion interacts with episodic memory will be a challenge for future studies. An exploration of the underlying neural systems will aid in determining the complex components of the "scar upon the cerebral tissues" that characterizes emotion's impact on human memory.

Conclusions

This article has reviewed what is known about two cognitive processes, attention and memory, that are influenced by emotion. What is clear from this limited review is that the relation between emotion and cognition is complex and nuanced. One topic that was not mentioned is the complexity of the conceptualization of emotion. Although emotion is often described as a single construct, this is clearly an oversimplification. Not only does emotion influence cognition at several stages of stimulus processing, but different facets of emotion likely have different effects on cognitive functions. In the psychological literature, the relation between emotion and cognition has often been described as two separate processes that interact at specific stages of processing. Emerging evidence from studies of human neuroscience suggest this distinction may not be sufficient. When brain function is examined, it is difficult to identify a clear dividing line between the representation of processes that are generally referred to as either emotion or cognition. Emotion affects cognition at every stage of stimulus processing, and the neural mechanisms of emotion and cognition appear to be inherently intertwined.

See also: Amygdala: Structure and Circuitry in Primates; Amygdala: Structure and Circuitry in Rodents and Felines; Amygdala: Contributions to Fear; Attention: Models; Attentional Functions in Learning and Memory; Cognition: An Overview of Neuroimaging Techniques; Emotion and Vigilance; Emotion: Neuroimaging; Emotional Hormones and Memory Modulation; Hormones and Memory; Neuroimaging; Social Emotion: Neuroimaging.

Further Reading

Amaral DG (2003) The amygdala, social behavior, and danger detection. *Annals of the New York Academy of Science* 1000: 337–347.

Davis M and Whalen PJ (2001) The amygdala: Vigilance and emotion. *Molecular Psychiatry* 6: 13–34.

Dolan RJ and Vuilleumier P (2003) Amygdala automaticity in emotional processing. *Annals of the New York Academy of Sciences* 985: 348–355.

Hamann S (2001) Cognitive and neural mechanisms of emotional memory. *Trends in Cognitive Sciences* 5: 394–400.

LeDoux JE (1996) *The Emotional Brain.* New York: Simon and Schuster

McEwen BS and Sapolsky RM (1995) Stress and cognitive function. *Current Opinions in Neurobiology* 5: 205–216.

Phelps EA (2004) Human emotion and memory: Interactions of the amygdala and hippocampal complex. *Current Opinion in Neurobiology* 14: 198–202.

Phelps EA (2006) Emotion and cognition: Insights from studies of the human amygdala. *Annual Review of Psychology* 57: 27–53.

Phelps EA and LeDoux JE (2005) Neural systems underlying emotion behavior: From animal models to human function. *Neuron* 48: 175–187.

Pourtois G and Vuilleumier P (2006) Dynamics of emotional effects on spatial attention in the human visual cortex. *Progress in Brain Research* 156: 67–91.

Whalen PJ (1998) Fear, vigilance, and ambiguity: Initial neuroimaging studies of the human amygdala. *Current Directions in Psychological Science* 7: 177–188.

Executive Function and Higher-Order Cognition: Assessment in Animals

J D Schall, Vanderbilt University, Nashville, TN, USA

General Issues for Animal Testing

Any use of animals in research is governed by laws interpreted by regulatory agencies and local institutions with which researchers must be conversant and compliant. Studies of cognition of necessity require measurements of behavior, and the behavior must be controlled in the context of the experiment. Verbal instructions are not effective, so animals must be coaxed to perform a task. The motivation to perform the task can be appetitive or aversive. Appetitive control occurs through pairing an event or behavior with a food or fluid reinforcement. Aversive control occurs through pairing an event or behavior with an undesirable stimulus such as electric shock or a brief loud noise. Aversive control can be used only if scientifically justified as, for example, in studies of anxiety.

Classical (Pavlovian) conditioning is accomplished by repeatedly pairing a conditioned stimulus (e.g., a tone) with an unconditioned stimulus (e.g., a puff of air) that reliably elicits an unconditioned response (e.g., an eye blink). The sensitivity of the animal to the conditioned stimulus can then be assessed by measuring the occurrence or magnitude of the unconditioned response as some characteristic of the conditioned stimulus (intensity, frequency, etc.) is varied systematically. Operant (instrumental) conditioning is accomplished by reinforcing an emitted behavior (e.g., looking at a spot of light) with a reward (e.g., a food item or fluid) or a punishment (e.g., a mild electric shock). Behaviors followed by positive reinforcements are more likely to be emitted in the future by an organism motivated to receive the reward. Behaviors that are followed by a negative reinforcement are less likely to be emitted in the future. Decades of research has detailed many principles and nuances of operant conditioning that the interested student can learn from a textbook on learning and memory. Also, detailed procedures for various species and situations can be found in the methods sections of peer-reviewed publications. Finally, we should also note the obvious specializations of behavior and associated cognition across the phylogenetic scale.

Taxonomy of Cognition

Stimuli can be presented and overt responses measured. However, to explain orderly and arbitrary relationships between responses and stimuli, it is now regarded as useful, if not necessary, to hypothesize certain covert processes mediating the encoding, selection, and categorization of stimuli and preparation of responses.

Before reviewing methods used to investigate higher order cognition in animals, we should begin by determining how to distinguish cognition from simple sensation and movement. We can also formulate at least a provisional minimal taxonomy of cognition. Reflexes are the most direct link between sensory and motor processes. It could be argued that any behavior that is not a reflex must include some cognitive component. It could also be argued that only behaviors that arise from or are concomitant with conscious mental content qualify as cognition. For the purposes of this article, we can be satisfied with an intermediate position that only holds that processes that intervene between or adaptively adjust sensation and movement constitute cognition. If so, then we can ask, how many cognitive processes can be distinguished reasonably? We will work with the following list:

- Perception, including categorization
- Attention
- Memory, including long-term and working memory
- Response selection and preparation
- Emotion
- Executive control

We are also interested in more complex activities that involve all of the processes listed previously:

- Decision making
- Problem solving
- Communication

Less space is devoted to processes that are described elsewhere in detail, and more space is devoted to less well-studied processes.

Methods to Study Perception

Discrimination and Categorization

Distinguishing the characteristics of stimuli for the purpose of guiding behavior has been investigated in many species. The testing requires designing alternative stimuli appropriate for the sensory apparatus of the particular animal and is based on the principle that two (or more) physically distinct stimuli can be rendered indistinguishable from one another by manipulation of the magnitude of their physical differences. Thus, a natural component of an animal's behavior is placed under control of the stimulus and then the characteristics of the stimuli are varied to determine how sensitive the animal is to the variation of the stimulus. For example, monkeys can be trained to shift gaze or press bars to signal whether a visual stimulus has a particular color, shape, or pattern of motion. Similarly, rats can be trained to perform tactile discriminations with their whiskers, such as judging the width of an aperture, the texture of a surface, or the distance of a gap, or also to signal their discrimination of mixtures of odors. Animals are capable of making more complex sensory discriminations. For example, animals as diverse as monkeys and pigeons can learn rapidly to discriminate among color photographs of different categories of objects, such as trees, humans, fish, and water, and these discriminations are generalized to novel examples from the categories of objects.

Awareness

A fruitful line of inquiry in the past decade has investigated neural correlates of awareness in monkeys. This has been accomplished by presenting a single ambiguous stimulus that can be perceived as either of (usually) two alternatives to macaque monkeys trained to report which of the alternatives they perceive. One way to dissociate the presentation of a stimulus from the phenomenal awareness of that stimulus is to employ binocular rivalry. Binocular rivalry occurs when markedly different stimuli are presented to the two eyes (e.g., horizontal stripes to the left eye and vertical stripes to the right). The perception is not of some plaid combination but instead of the stimulus in one eye and then the other, alternating randomly until one or both stimuli are removed.

Another means of dissociating presentation from report is through visual masking. This is accomplished by presenting a stimulus that may be weak in some respect but not below threshold to detect and then rapidly thereafter presenting a stronger stimulus at the same or nearby location. The presence of the subsequent stronger stimulus results in a lack of awareness of the earlier stimulus; this is referred to as backward masking. Critical to these studies is some objective measure of how the sensory system registers the stimuli because animals are very likely to respond in a biased and stereotyped manner to ambiguous stimuli unless reinforcement contingencies prevent this.

Methods to Study Attention

To study the allocation of attention, the most common procedure is to present a cue that informs the animal that a response is required for a subsequent stimulus at the same location. In a fraction of trials, the test stimulus is presented at an uncued location. The difference in response time or discriminability of the test stimulus at the cued versus the uncued location is taken as a measure of the allocation of attention. Alternatively, multiple stimuli can be presented simultaneously with one of the stimuli distinguished by sensory properties, a prior cue, or a memory template to guide the response. The quality of response to the target in the presence versus the absence of distractor stimuli is taken as a measure of the allocation of attention. The more diverse the distractors' appearance and the more similar the distractors are to the target, the more attention demanding the task becomes. In addition, a stimulus with multiple attributes (e.g., color and shape) can be presented following a cue that instructs the animal to respond according to one of the attributes. The demand for attention can be manipulated by making the cued attribute more or less difficult to discriminate and by making the noncued attribute more or less potent. Note that in studies of the allocation of visual attention in space, it is essential to monitor gaze to prevent confounds introduced by movements of the eyes.

Attention has been investigated predominantly with nonhuman primates, but procedures have also been devised for rodents and even birds such as pigeons. Procedures to assess attention in a less specific sense have been formulated to study mouse models of attention deficit disorder. For example, mice can be trained to poke their nose into a hole to receive a reinforcement in response to a visual stimulus. By offering multiple alternative holes signaled by different lights turned on for short durations, the mice must attend to the stimuli to respond quickly enough to receive reinforcement. The attention capacity of the mice can then be assessed by manipulations of target light presentation rate, duration, salience, and temporal predictability.

Methods to Study Memory

Memory can be inferred by persistent and consistent changes in behavior following learning. An overview of classical and operant conditioning learning procedures was provided previously. Memory can be divided into short-term working memory and long-term procedural and declarative memory.

Short-Term Working Memory

Short-term memory has been studied using delayed-response tasks in which a stimulus or set of stimuli are presented briefly but a response cannot be produced until after a retention interval typically lasting approximately 1–10 s. Animals can guide their responses by the location or identity of the stimuli. The task has been elaborated in various ways. Delayed alternation requires monkeys to select the object at the location that was not selected in the previous trial (delayed spatial alternation) or to select the object that was not selected in the previous trial (delayed object alternation). This task requires working memory retention across as well as within trials. Delayed match to sample exposes monkeys briefly to an object and then after an interval presents the target object plus a distractor object. Monkeys are reinforced for selecting through a gaze shift or a reaching movement the target object that they had observed previously. Delayed nonmatch to sample reverses the logic, requiring monkeys to select the object they had not observed previously. It is important to note that delayed-response tasks require not only working memory but also response inhibition to prevent premature movements and may also invoke response preparation if the monkey can anticipate the termination of the retention interval when it can respond.

Long-Term Memory

Memory persisting over days or months must be tested in a species-specific manner. For example, rats are commonly tested using spatial navigation through locomotion in a maze to locate a reinforcement. Also, the water maze was developed to assess spatial learning and memory in rats. It is commonly used with mice, but species and strain idiosyncrasies must be recognized in the interpretation of the results. A platform is placed at a particular location beneath the surface of a round pool of murky water. When placed in the pool, mice swim to locate the hidden platform, and learning can be measured by a reduction in the amount of time taken to locate the platform as the mice or rats encode orienting cues in the environment. Contrasting performance when the platform is hidden with that when it is visible permits resolving confounds of sensory or motor impairments.

Implicit in the description of all the complex tasks monkeys can be trained to perform is the fact that they have long-term memory. The nature and capacity of that memory has been probed largely through tests of categorization of stimuli and of relations among stimuli. More evidence for long-term memory is derived from learning sets (learning to learn), an improvement in the speed of acquisition of successive discriminations between arbitrary objects or of reversing responses when reinforcement changes. Learning set has been demonstrated in nonhuman primates as well as in dogs, rats, and some birds.

Methods to Study Response Selection and Preparation

All motor responses can be explained in terms of causes (the muscle contracted because the neuron fired), but some responses can be explained also in terms of reasons (the bar was pressed to obtain the food to satisfy the hunger). This section considers movements that can be explained in terms of reasons and not just causes.

Response Selection

Requiring an arbitrary response to a particular stimulus invokes a process referred to as stimulus response mapping. A wealth of studies of human subjects can inform the design of experiments with animals; however, it should be clear that different species are incapable of producing more or less complex mappings. The capacity of rodents to learn arbitrary responses through operant conditioning is more limited than that of macaque monkeys, for example. Studies with macaque monkeys have explored progressively more complicated degrees of mapping a response onto a stimulus so that we can say that monkeys are encoding instructions and following rules or even strategies.

At the lowest level, monkeys can produce an arbitrary response not directed toward a stimulus – for example, a shift of gaze to a location directly opposite a target (antisaccade). At the next level, macaque monkeys can be trained to produce arbitrary responses to specific cues on successive trials and to change the mapping if the reinforcement contingencies change (conditional motor learning). Monkeys can also be trained to produce an arbitrary sequence of a few movements guided by particular cues. Perhaps the greatest expression of this ability is seen in apes that learn sign language. In studies with humans, evidence for response selection is an increase in the latency to initiate the first movement with an increase in the number of movements in the sequence. Unfortunately, animal studies have not performed this simple test. Beyond producing sequences of movements in response to sequences of stimuli, monkeys can be trained to produce self-ordered sequences of responses in which successive responses are guided by previous responses.

At perhaps the highest level, macaque monkeys can be trained to respond according to alternative strategies that require flexibility in applying rules with no fixed stimulus–response mapping. For example, monkeys can switch between repeat-stay and change-shift strategies. To perform a task such as this, monkeys must remember the previous response, remember the stimulus or stimulus–response pair preceding that choice, use that memory to evaluate whether the stimulus on the current trial was different from that on the previous trial, and apply the strategy to choose the same target when the stimulus repeated and to reject that target when the stimulus changed.

Response Preparation

The time of an overt response to a given stimulus is variable and unpredictable. Within that unpredictability, however, certain trends have been observed. For example, when given a warning ('ready') before an imperative trigger signal ('go'), subjects respond earlier and more reliably than when no warning is given. The interval between the warning and trigger signals is referred to as a foreperiod. Response time can also be influenced by repetition of stimuli or responses or by success in previous trials. To explain this variation, one can hypothesize a process that transpires after an instruction or warning signal and is influenced by events in preceding trials to influence the readiness to initiate a movement. Such a covert process may be called response preparation.

The influence of foreperiod on response time varies according to the statistical properties of the foreperiod. If the foreperiod is a fixed value of the appropriate interval, then the animal can learn to anticipate when it will elapse. If the foreperiod is too short (e.g., <100 ms), response time is unaffected because some time is needed for response preparation to engage. If the foreperiod is too long (e.g., >2000 ms), response time is unaffected because it is not possible to sustain response preparation indefinitely. Thus, foreperiods ranging from 100 to 1000 ms afford the largest reduction of response time. The reduction of response time occurs because the passage of time allows a sense of expectation, permitting preparation before the trigger signal so that sometimes the movement might occur before the trigger signal (jump the gun). In fact, such self-generated responses are clear evidence of a covert response preparation process.

Foreperiods can be randomized to reduce predictability. For example, the foreperiod on a given trial could be sampled with equal probability from the range 100 to 1000 ms. This does introduce some variability in response time, but response time tends to decrease as foreperiod increases, and anticipatory responses are often generated especially at the longest foreperiods. This occurs because although the foreperiods are selected randomly across trials, they have a maximum value (i.e., a deadline that the animal can learn through experience). The more time that elapses from the warning stimulus, the higher the probability that the trigger stimulus will occur given that it has not yet. This conditional probability is referred to as the hazard rate of the foreperiod. If the hazard rate increases, the foreperiod is referred to as aging. A nonaging distribution of foreperiods has a flat hazard function; in other words, the passage of time conveys no predictability about when the foreperiod will elapse. Nonaging foreperiod distributions have many short values and exponentially decreasing probability of progressively longer values. Response times obtained with nonaging foreperiods decrease little, if at all, as a function of foreperiod and anticipatory responses are produced rarely.

Further evidence for response preparation is the fact that partially prepared responses can be withheld if an imperative 'stop' signal occurs. This ability can be explained by hypothesizing another covert process that prevents movements. The stop signal or countermanding task has been introduced in the past decade into animal studies. The countermanding paradigm probes a subject's ability to control the initiation of movements by infrequently presenting an imperative stop signal in a response time task. The subjects' task is to cancel the planned movement if a stop signal is presented. Performance on this task can be accounted for by a race between a process that generates the movement (go process) and a process that cancels the movement (stop process). This race model provides an estimate of the stop signal reaction time, which is the time needed to cancel the planned movement. The stop signal reaction time can be used in tests of neural processes and manipulations.

Intention

The disposition to perform some act is a central feature of an intention, but intention cannot be identified entirely with response preparation. A statement of intention must also answer the question, 'Why was that done?' An answer about the causal path through neurons to muscles is not as satisfying as an explanation addressing the reasons for the action based on preferences, goals, and beliefs. In other words, to judge whether a movement was intended, one must refer to the agent's beliefs about which action must be performed in what circumstances to bring about the desired object of the intention.

These concepts about intention have been formulated in the domain of human interactions, but research describing communication and deception, for example, indicates that the attribution of intention to monkeys at least seems justified. A particular form of intention involves reasoning about the relation between observations of events in the environment and actions in that environment – in other words, about how actions result in consequences. In fact, some have concluded that guiding actions based on reasoning about the causes of events is uniquely human. However, research has shown that rats can make correct inferences guiding responses for reinforcement on the basis of purely observational learning of causal relations between events. Comparable results have been obtained from nonhuman primates.

Methods to Study Emotion

Other articles should be consulted for details on emotion, and this article does not debate whether animals have emotions like humans. Most studies of animal emotion involve fear, anxiety, and depression. Being aversive, the procedures used in these studies deserve special scrutiny and oversight to ensure animal welfare in the pursuit of scientific information.

Fear in animals has been studied most effectively using classically conditioned fear responses. Fear conditioning is a form of learning in which fear is associated with a particular neutral stimulus (e.g., a tone) by pairing the neutral stimulus with an aversive stimulus (e.g., an electric shock, loud noise, or unpleasant odor). Ultimately, the neutral stimulus elicits the state of fear. Fear conditioning has been studied in numerous species, from snails to humans. In animals, conditioned fear can be measured as a period of attentive immobility (freezing), a potentiated startle reflex, as well as changes in heart rate, respiration rate, or muscle tension.

Learned helplessness occurs when an animal is exposed to inescapable aversive stimulation (e.g., electrical shock) and learns that it cannot control its environment. This is regarded as a useful model of human depression.

Anxiety has been investigated by putting mice in an open area and measuring how much time they explore in the exposed interior of the area; more anxious mice spend more time close to the walls.

Methods to Study Executive Control

When the environment is ambiguous or presents competing demands, or the mapping of stimulus onto response is complex or contrary to habit making performance prone to errors, then executive control is required to perform the task. Such executive control over the perception, selection, and response systems is seen as a central component of human cognition, and it can be investigated in animals, particularly nonhuman primates, in a variety of ways. The basic approach is to study how performance changes according to the history of trials. For example, if a particular movement is called for in response to a given stimulus on repeated trials, and then in a subsequent trial a different movement is called for in response to the same stimulus, then a cost will be observed in the accuracy and latency of that response. Such experimental paradigms are referred to as task switching. The cost for switching tasks can arise at least in part because of the conflict between producing the rehearsed response and producing the new response.

Response conflict can be investigated by training macaque monkeys extensively to respond to objects with multiple features such as color and shape with alternative responses cued by different features (e.g., red or circle means go and green or square means nogo). Once the mapping is mastered, testing proceeds by presenting congruent (e.g., red circle) stimuli that cue the same response and incongruent stimuli (e.g., red square) that cue the opposite responses. Evidence of conflict evoked by the incongruent features is slowed response times and increased error rates. Response conflict can be elicited in rats by training them to associate a response lever with a particular reinforcement (e.g., food pellet vs. sugar water). Conflict is induced by rewarding the correct responses with the reinforcement opposite the discriminative stimulus. In other words, by correctly pressing the bar associated with the food pellet stimulus, rats receive sugar water reinforcement and vice versa.

When performing in conditions that require executive control, errors are often produced. A cognitive process of error monitoring is believed to be a component of executive control. In human studies of choice responses, a sign of error monitoring is slowing of response time on the trial after errors.

Decision Making

This process has many aspects, most of which have been summarized. If we define a choice as an action performed in the context of alternatives to achieve a goal, we can appreciate that decision making occurs when the alternatives are vague or the payoffs are unclear. Accordingly, one approach to studying decision making requires animals to perform particularly challenging sensory discriminations; this can be done in any sensory modality. Another approach is to manipulate reinforcement amount or probability in a more or less predictable manner. A classic finding is that animals will produce alternative responses (e.g., bar presses) in direct proportion to the amount or probability of reinforcement for the alternative responses; this is referred to as matching law.

A popular area of inquiry in the past few years has applied concepts and procedures formulated in game theory and economics to the study of animal behavior. For example, monkeys are trained to perform tasks resembling games such as rock–paper–scissors or matching pennies. These mixed strategy games allow investigators to explore whether theories developed to explain human decision making in games and economic settings apply to animal behavior. All of these approaches result in behavior that is more or less stochastic but amenable to analysis in terms of quantitative models of the processes hypothesized to produce the responses. This approach has shown that animals express in at least a rudimentary manner many of the biases that characterize human decision making. For example, monkeys show aversion to inequity by refusing a lower valued reinforcement if they observe another individual obtaining a higher valued reinforcement.

Problem Solving and Tool Use

Animal cognition is perhaps nowhere more evident than in the solution of problems, especially through the use of tools as highlighted by Kohler's pioneering studies of the use of tools by apes. Although several species learn to use tools in the wild as well as in the laboratory, it remains unclear to what extent animals understand the physical processes by which these tools are effective. In fact, some of the most interesting evidence to date that animals understand the causal properties of physical objects comes from birds, particularly the corvids (crows and ravens). For example, a New Caledonian crow spontaneously bent a piece of ineffective straight wire into an effective hook tool for retrieving food, and another species of corvid learns rapidly to avoid maneuvering food into a clearly visible and inaccessible trap. Chimpanzees do not fashion tools or avoid such traps without considerable training, but they do keep objects used as tools for future use.

Communication

None doubt that animals communicate in rich and diverse manners. For example, vervet monkeys in the wild exhibit a very advanced system of communication, but it is believed to be instinctive, not learned. What is more contentious is whether animals such as great apes can be said to learn language. Investigators have trained chimpanzees, bonobos, gorillas, and orangutans to communicate through symbols on a keyboard or sign language. Individual chimpanzees have acquired vocabularies of at least 200 words or signs and have demonstrated the capacity to respond appropriately and produce meaningfully different sentences.

Learning to produce words is not limited to primates. African gray parrots have gained notoriety through a phenomenal ability to learn words or even phrases, in some cases as complicated as songs. One individual bird has been trained to use English speech to label dozens of objects, features, and categories as well as use commands and requests.

See also: Anxiety Disorders; Binocular Rivalry; Cognitive Control and Development; Episodic Memory: Assessment in Animals; Game Theory and the Economics of Animal Communication; Games in Monkeys: Neurophysiology and Motor Decision-Making; Operant Conditioning of Reflexes; Pharmacology of Fear Extinction; Procedural Learning: Classical Conditioning; Reasoning and Problem Solving: Models; Referentiality and Concepts in Animal Cognition; Reward Decision-Making; Short Term and Working Memory; Spatial Memory: Assessment in Animals.

Further Reading

Blake R (1999) The behavioural analysis of animal vision. In: Carpenter RHS and Robson JG (eds.) *Vision Research: A Practical Guide to Laboratory Methods*, pp. 137–160. Oxford: Oxford University Press.

Crawley JN (2000) *What's Wrong with My Mouse? Behavioral Phenotyping of Transgenic and Knockout Mice.* New York: Wiley-Liss.

Emery NJ and Clayton NS (2004) The mentality of crows: Convergent evolution of intelligence in corvids and apes. *Science* 306: 1903–1907.

Griffin D (2001) *Animal Minds.* Chicago: University of Chicago Press.

Hanes DP and Schall JD (1995) Countermanding saccades in macaque. *Visual Neuroscience* 12: 929–937.

Karl T, Pabst R, and von Horsten S (2003) Behavioral phenotyping of mice in pharmacological and toxicological research. *Experimental Toxicology and Pathology* 55: 69–83.

Logothetis NK and Schall JD (1990) Binocular motion rivalry in macaque monkeys: Eye dominance and tracking eye movements. *Vision Research* 30: 1409–1419.

National Research Council (1996) *Guide for the Care and Use of Laboratory Animals, Institute of Laboratory Animal Resources.* Washington, DC: National Academy Press.

Panksepp J (2004) *Affective Neuroscience: The Foundations of Human and Animal Emotions.* New York: Oxford University Press.

Pearce JM (1997) *Animal Learning and Cognition: An Introduction.* Hove, UK: Psychology Press.

Terry WS (2005) *Learning and Memory: Basic Principles, Processes, and Procedures.* New York: Allyn & Bacon.

Tomasello M and Call J (1997) *Primate Cognition.* Oxford: Oxford University Press.

Wahlsten D, Rustay NR, Metten P, and Crabbe JC (2003) In search of a better mouse test. *Trends in Neuroscience* 26: 132–136.

Whishaw IQ and Kolb B (2004) *The Behavior of the Laboratory Rat: A Handbook with Tests.* Oxford: Oxford University Press.

Executive Function and Higher-Order Cognition: Computational Models

J W Brown, Indiana University, Bloomington, IN, USA
T S Braver, Washington University in St. Louis, St. Louis, MO, USA

Introduction

Executive functions include a range of processes that impact attention, working memory, goal setting, action selection and sequencing, and problem solving. Theories of higher cognitive function aim to account for how complex cognitive processes are carried out in the brain and may offer conceptual-level mechanistic explanations. Yet all too often, the mechanisms proposed to explain higher functions suffer from an implicit dependence on unspecified higher level control processes so that the actual neural mechanisms subserving the cognitive phenomena remain mysterious. This problem is called the homunculus problem. The term homunculus means 'little man' and refers to the unspecified higher level controller that is implicitly required by some theories of cognition. There has been much discussion about how to banish the homunculus – that is, to provide an explicit and mechanistic description of how control functions emerge and interact so that unspecified high-level controllers will not need to be invoked. Computational models of executive function provide critical tools in this effort. When conceptual theories are fleshed out in working computational models, accounts that claim to overcome homunculus problems are more compelling for several reasons. First, a viable computational model must work; it must actually perform a task and account for data. Second, all components of the model are explicit, which makes it easy to identify any control signal components of the model that are less well specified. Third, when a computational model does exhibit properties and behavior associated with executive function, it is easier to trace, specify, and quantify the origin and nature of the computational mechanisms that produce such cognitive properties and behavioral patterns.

Computational models of executive function include a range of formalisms from production systems to neural networks. Whereas production system models are typically more abstract, and involve symbolic processing, neural network models are more closely tied to neurobiological principles and constraints. Both types of models have focused on understanding the functions subserved by specific brain regions thought to be critical for executive control, such as the prefrontal cortex (PFC), anterior cingulate cortex (ACC), and basal ganglia (BG). Work since the late 1990s has developed a distinction between performance monitoring and control processes related to executive function, and this distinction provides a useful framework for delineating components of executive function. This article discusses computational models of distinct brain centers in executive function, and it concludes with a discussion of more abstract production system models of executive function.

Prefrontal Cortex and Control

Active Goal Maintenance

The lateral PFC is important for actively maintaining information via sustained neural firing that is robust in the face of potentially distracting information. The standard neural model of PFC has cells that reciprocally excite each other so that activity is self-sustaining: active neurons send excitation to other neurons that then send excitation back, creating a self-sustaining activity pattern that constitutes a stable attractor state. Once a particular population of PFC neurons is activated in this attractor state, it suppresses other populations via lateral inhibition. The state is maintained even when the inputs that activated the PFC are no longer present (i.e., working memory), and it is robust in the sense that activity persists despite other distracting inputs. *N*-methyl-D-aspartate (NMDA) channels may provide a cellular mechanism by which PFC cells that are more active become more easily excitable. As cells become active and depolarize, NMDA channels lose their Mg^{2+} block, thus increasing their conductivities at higher levels of depolarization. In a population of cells that reciprocally excite each other, this has the effect of enhancing self-perpetuating activity.

Neural network models of PFC are generally implemented as either rate-coded or spiking models. Rate-coded models quantify the cell activity as the instantaneous average firing rate of a local population of cells. Mathematically, a population of such rate-coded cells can exhibit bistable activity if the equilibrium output activity signal increases faster than linearly within a certain range. For example, if the input signal to a cell is doubled, the output signal from the cell would need to be greater than double at equilibrium in order for reciprocal excitatory activity to be self-sustaining. Models of PFC have been developed to account for a range of empirical data, including healthy human and monkey performance of tasks that involve working memory, as well as executive control deficits in clinical populations such as individuals with schizophrenia and individuals with focal lesions of PFC.

Spiking models of PFC attempt to simulate the actual spikes generated by individual PFC cells. Typically, these models use a simplified integrate-and-fire scheme (which simulates action potentials as a point process) rather than a more sophisticated and computationally expensive Hodgkin–Huxley formalism (which simulates actual ionic channel kinetics and thus the full time course of the action potential). Spiking models have been developed to account for the data from single-unit recordings in awake, behaving monkeys performing a variety of tasks, including delayed match to sample, sequence learning, and various types of rule-based decision making. Other more biophysically detailed models have accounted for complex interactions among specific neurotransmitters and receptor types in mediating sustained activity, especially dopamine, NMDA, α-amino-3-hydroxy-3-methyl-4-isoxazole propionic acid (AMPA), and γ-aminobutyric acid (GABA) receptors. These models make specific predictions regarding the effects of different kinds of pharmacological manipulation on executive control.

An important computational problem involves the mechanisms that enable PFC networks to maintain information in the face of interfering input while at the same time appropriately updating stored information when relevant signals arrive. Various solutions have been proposed to solve this problem, and all of them involve an input gating mechanism. Opening the gate essentially involves making the attractor states become less stable by amplifying new inputs. The result of the open gate is that PFC is rapidly updated with the new input. In contrast, when the gate is closed, input signals do not disrupt maintained states. Some models of PFC gating depend on the neuromodulator dopamine. Cells in the ventral tegmental area (VTA) provide dopaminergic signals to the PFC. According to these models, transient increases in the level of VTA firing release more dopamine in PFC, which switches the PFC between fast updating and stable maintenance. The interactions among PFC cells and various D_1 and D_2 dopamine receptor subtypes are complex, and computational modeling has clarified how these elements work together functionally. In one model, dopamine D_1 receptor activation effectively stabilizes PFC states, whereas D_2 receptor activation leads to destabilizing effects. Others have argued that PFC stability follows an inverted U pattern, such that stability is greatest for a baseline level of dopamine but falls off rapidly for either too little or too much dopamine.

The dopamine-based gating models suffer from a limitation. The gating signal is global and nonspecific, so with these models, it is not possible to update certain areas of PFC while maintaining others. To address this issue, another class of gating mechanism has been proposed based on the strong reciprocal connections between the PFC and the BG complex. Neurons in the direct pathway of the BG drive a net disinhibition of the thalamus, which may in turn allow fast updating of selected parts of PFC. Conversely, neurons in the indirect pathway of the BG drive a net inhibition of the thalamus, which may effectively close the PFC gate and maintain stable representations against distractors in selected parts of PFC. Both the dopaminergic and BG gating mechanisms have included learning mechanisms, which allow the system to discover the appropriate signals and timing for opening the gate.

Biased Competition

Most computational models of executive control cast the PFC as serving a biasing function that regulates activity in other brain areas involved in domain-specific processing and behavior. The Stroop is the best known experimental task for illustrating the need for control biases. In the task, subjects view a color word (e.g., the words 'red' or 'blue') printed with an ink color that may be the same as (congruent) or different from (incongruent) the word (**Figure 1**). Subjects are asked to respond according to the ink color (the color-naming task) but to avoid responding based on the semantic meaning of the word (the word-reading task). For example, the word red presented in green ink (**Figure 1**) should elicit the correct response green, not red. This is a difficult task because for literate individuals, the automatic tendency to read a word is stronger than the process of indicating which color ink is used to write the word.

According to conceptual framework known as biased competition, activity in PFC representing the color naming task (the task demand units in **Figure 1**) strongly activates other areas in the brain responsible for generating specific responses based on the ink color. The PFC control signal does not directly determine the response but only enhances activity in other areas that determine the response according to the current rule. In the model of **Figure 1**, there are two task pathways, one for word reading and one for ink color naming. Each pathway can work in isolation from the other to produce task-appropriate processing and responses without executive control signals. However, control is critical when both the word-reading and color-naming pathways are simultaneously engaged. Under such conditions, there is competition during processing between the two dimensions of semantic meaning and ink color. In **Figure 1**, the thicker arrows from the word-reading units to the response

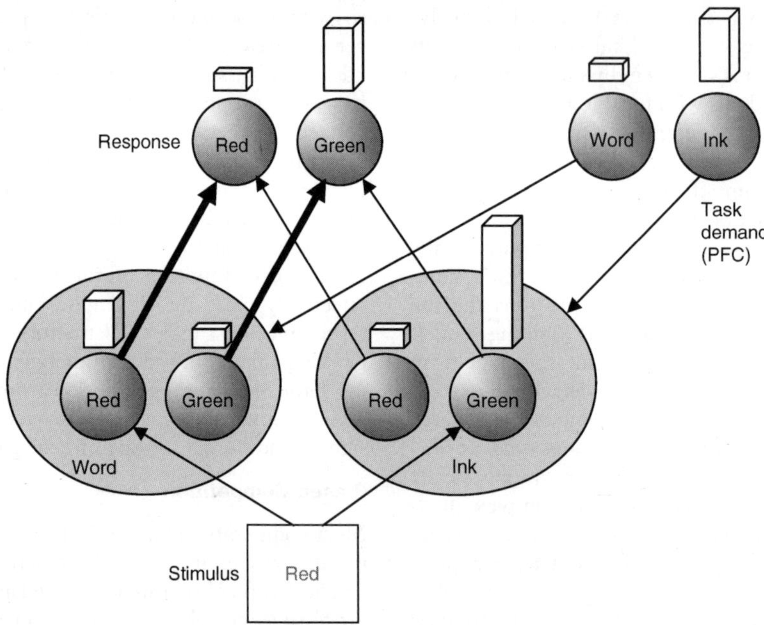

Figure 1 Executive control enables correct performance of the Stroop task.

units represent the stronger connection weights due to the effects of more learning and practice of reading words. The word-reading pathway will dominate processing competition in the absence of executive control. Thus, to be successful during execution of the color-naming task, the color pathway needs additional support to counteract the stronger weights on the word pathway. This support comes in the form of top-down biasing control, carried by a task demand unit (reflecting PFC), that represents the color-naming tasks. This task demand unit sends a signal that provides an additive source of activation to the entire input color dimension. When this control signal is present, the color pathway can successfully compete with the otherwise stronger word pathway to control responding. Conversely, without the strong biasing signal from PFC, the incorrect default response of word reading would prevail. Models of PFC that implement such control biasing signals have been found to account for human behavioral performance in a range of cognitive tasks that have Stroop-like properties of competition and interference from automatic processing tendencies.

Anterior Cingulate Cortex and Performance Monitoring

A key question in understanding goal-driven or top-down executive control is how and when it is engaged. Executive control mechanisms direct behavior, but what controls the executive? This question of what controls the controller relates to the homunculus problem discussed previously. In the case of executive control, there must be a mechanism that indicates when top-down attentional control is needed. The kinds of mechanisms that determine when control must be implemented do so by monitoring performance of the behaving cognitive system to detect the need for control.

Conflict Theory

One hypothesis that has received widespread interest is the so-called conflict monitoring account. For the purposes of executive control, conflict is defined as the coactivation of mutually incompatible response processes. This hypothesis takes as its starting point the theoretical idea that control is primarily required as a means of managing the cross-talk interference that can arise between concurrent and overlapping processing pathways in the brain. A measure of conflict provides a quantitative index of the degree of cross-talk between response pathways, and therefore the degree of executive control that must be exerted to resolve the interference. The critical addition of the conflict monitoring hypothesis is the adoption of an explicit mechanism which detects the presence and level of cross-talk interference and which conveys this information as an output signal that is used to regulate the engagement of top-down control signals. In some formulations, the conflict signal is computed as the Hopfield energy of the response system. Essentially, this reduces to the multiplicative product of activity in two mutually incompatible response pathways. In the case of the Stroop task stimulus word red written in green ink (**Figure 1**), the conflict signal would be computed as the product of activity in the red and green response units. Various models have used other formalisms instead of the multiplicative model, but all compute a measure of coactivation such that two incompatible response pathways must be simultaneously coactive for a conflict signal to be generated.

Neuroanatomy

Based on an accumulating literature – primarily arising from human neuroimaging studies examining conflict-based interference effects – the area surrounding and including the ACC was identified as the neural locus of a conflict monitoring mechanism. The conflict monitoring hypothesis states explicitly that ACC implements the calculation of an online index of the conflict between competing representations, particularly at the response level. In computational models of conflict monitoring, fluctuations in ACC activity index ongoing fluctuations in conflict, and this information is then conveyed to the PFC, which in turn implements control strategies and maintains representations of the ongoing behavioral context. According to this hypothesis, more cognitive control is needed when conflict is high, but less is needed when conflict is low. The system is postulated to function as a closed loop, whereby the detection of conflict (in ACC activity) serves to engage control (in the PFC), which then acts to reduce the conflict experienced in similar future situations. Thus, the ACC has been identified as a mechanism that determines when executive control is needed and in turn activates the PFC to implement executive control. Models of the role of ACC in executive control have accounted for a variety of data from functional neuroimaging studies of cognitively demanding tasks in healthy individuals and clinical populations.

Conflict and Errors

In addition to the monitoring of response conflict, ACC also appears to be critical for situations of error commission. This brain region transiently activates both when conflict is high and when errors are actually committed. Computational modeling work reflects an ongoing controversy over the ultimate nature of performance monitoring functions in ACC. Much of the empirical data have come from studies using the event-related potential technique and focused on a specific scalp activity pattern known as the error-related negativity (ERN), which occurs at the time of error commission or at the time of explicit error feedback if the error was not predictable. There have been alternative computational models developed which postulate a specific and distinct role for the ACC in error detection rather than conflict monitoring, and these models make somewhat different claims about the function of ACC outputs in regulating behavioral performance. One class of models assumes that dopaminergic error signals drive or train the ACC to respond to errors. These models have accounted for the timing of error signals in ACC, such as whether the ERN occurs before or after receipt of feedback confirming that an error has been committed. The models have also addressed the greater magnitude of ERN signals in contexts in which errors are less frequent.

Work has also suggested that many of the phenomena originally thought to be uniquely captured by the error-detection models can also be successfully explained by the conflict monitoring account. Nevertheless, there has been a growing appreciation of the idea that the ACC may play a more general role in performance prediction and action outcome monitoring than just detecting the presence of errors or conflict. One computational model proposes that since errors are more likely when conflict is present, the ACC may generally compute the likelihood of an error based on previous learning. Despite some differences in implementation and focus, computational models of ACC primarily serve as a mechanism for evaluating the level of executive control needed in a given task situation.

Time Course of Executive Control

According to the conflict model, ACC monitors performance and then drives PFC to implement executive control. Early models suggested that control is implemented quickly, but there may be distinct timescales in which monitoring and control signals are effective. In particular, some kinds of control mechanisms may be implemented rapidly enough to detect and resolve conflict within a single trial, whereas others may use conflict detected in one trial to implement control in subsequent trials. A model of the Stroop task postulates a dual form of conflict detection: one acting in the short (i.e., subsecond) timescale and another in the long (i.e., several second/multiple trial) timescale. These different conflict measures in turn activate two separate forms of cognitive control, respectively called reactive and proactive control. Thus, a temporally extended period of high conflict will push the system toward a state of preemptive attentional control in which goal-relevant context is actively maintained across trials to bias target-relevant aspects of attention, before stimuli are actually presented. In contrast, in situations of low conflict, this type of proactive control is not engaged. Instead, the actual detection of conflict within a trial (i.e., poststimulus presentation) rapidly engages a transient goal reactivation mechanism which can do rapid biasing of the target-relevant dimension. This computational model was able to successfully account for behavioral and brain imaging data from the Stroop task under conditions involving either a high percentage of incongruent trials or a high percentage of congruent trials. It should be noted that individuals may not be explicitly aware of changes in the frequency of conflict occurrence, and therefore the adjustments in attentional control may occur even in the absence of conscious intervention.

Multiple Kinds of Control

In the event that the need for greater control is detected, the PFC must determine what kind of control to implement. Different kinds of executive control signals have been dissected using task-switching paradigms. Task switching involves interleaved performance of two different cognitively demanding tasks. For example, the previously mentioned Stroop task might be modified so that subjects must perform the ink color-naming and the word-reading tasks on alternating trials. The most basic finding of task-switching studies is the switch cost, meaning that task performance is slower and more error-prone when a new task is performed than when an old task is repeated. The origin of the switch cost is controversial. In some models, the switch cost is due to the time needed for an executive controller to reconfigure the system to perform the new task. In other models, the switch cost is simply due to the lack of priming in the new task pathways, and therefore no executive control need be invoked to explain the switch cost.

Computational models of task switching provide insight into executive function by dissociating attentional and motor control processes. Returning to the Stroop task example, stimuli may be either congruent (e.g., the word red written in green ink) or incongruent (e.g., the word red written in red ink). Incongruent stimuli require more focused attention on the color of the ink while excluding the semantic meaning of the word from further cognitive processing. In contrast, when a task switch occurs, executive control may be required to implement the new task. Alternatively, as suggested by a more recent computational model, executive processes may not implement the task switch directly but may slow responding to enable the system to adequately process the new task prior to generating a response. Regardless of the particular form of motor control implemented, a distinction can be seen between attentional control driven by incongruency and motor control associated with the task switch.

Basal Ganglia and Action Selection

When multiple completing behavioral plans are formed and activated, an action selection mechanism allows one to be executed and suppresses or defers the remaining incompatible plans. This constitutes an executive control function. Some models posit a role of ACC in action selection, but a number of models of executive function have suggested that the BG play the main role in action selection. Of note, action selection may include control of external actions as well as internal manipulations such as deciding when and how to update the PFC state.

The BG consist of several subcortical nuclei. The striatum (caudate nucleus and putamen) receive projections from a number of frontal cortical structures. The striatum provides two main output projections. The first is known as the direct pathway, by which the striatum inhibits the internal pallidum, which in turn inhibits the motor thalamus. Computational models have suggested that the net effect of direct pathway activity is to facilitate action execution because striatal inhibition of the internal pallidum results in a net disinhibition of the thalamus, which may allow actions to be executed. In contrast, activity in the second output projection from the striatum (known as the indirect pathway) results in a net increased inhibition of the motor thalamus, which may prevent other actions from being executed. In this way, computational models suggest that the BG can actively allow some motor plans to be executed while simultaneously suppressing others. A related BG structure known as the subthalamic nucleus may further prevent multiple competing plans from being simultaneously executed. Thus, according to several computational models, these components of the BG apparently monitor ongoing activity in PFC in order to control which plans are executed.

In terms of performance monitoring, a number of BG models have focused on the substantia nigra pars compacta (SNC), which includes a dense population of dopaminergic cells that project widely to the other parts of the BG, especially the striatum. These SNC cells respond transiently to unexpected rewards and unexpected cues that predict reward, and they transiently pause their firing when an expected reward is not received. As posited by several computational models, these performance-monitoring signals train other parts of the BG to select the actions that are most likely to lead to reward.

Models of executive control by the BG have addressed a wide range of empirical data. Several models of action selection in the BG have focused on neurophysiology. These have simulated and accounted for a variety of cell types found in the BG and connected areas of awake, behaving macaque monkeys performing cognitive tasks. Cognitive-level models generally employ a connectionist framework and have accounted for behavioral data in healthy and clinical populations, such as those with schizophrenia, Parkinson's disease, and Huntington's disease. These models have accounted for specific kinds of errors, both random and perseverative, on tasks thought to involve executive control, such as the Wisconsin Card Sort Task. These models have been applied to the domain of decision making and have been extended to include other structures such as the orbitofrontal cortex, which may serve to actively maintain (in working memory) reward prediction errors over an extended delay.

Production System Models

In contrast with neural network models, production system computational models do not explicitly simulate neural activity. Instead, they are often referred to as cognitive architectures. They rely on abstract formalisms from the field of machine intelligence, using a set of if–then conditional rules. A cognitive processor regularly evaluates the environment to determine whether a particular rule is applicable. When the conditions required for a particular rule are satisfied, then the operation specified by that rule is executed. In this way, external stimuli and internal goals lead to actions. Notably, multiple rules can be active simultaneously. Some models include specific assumptions about the time needed for a conditional rule to be activated and execute an action, and this allows production systems to make specific predictions about response time for comparison with human data, such as the psychological refractory period. Such models can also make predictions about reaction time in high-level tasks involving nested goals, such as planning tasks like the Tower of London, and the comprehension and production of complex sentences. These tasks have been traditionally difficult for neural network models to simulate. Executive control in a production system is needed to mediate among multiple rules and tasks that would otherwise interfere with each other when executed simultaneously. Such control may include lockout scheduling or interleaved scheduling. In lockout scheduling, the executive processes detect when two or more rules compete for simultaneous access to the same resource and allow only one to have access at a given time. Interleaved scheduling involves switching back and forth between the two processes. When executive control is explicitly specified, it is generally implemented as a set of rules that manipulate the internal state of the production system, such as the current goal state and working memory contents.

See also: Cognition: Basal Ganglia Role; Consciousness: Theoretical and Computational Neuroscience; Executive Function and Higher-Order Cognition: Assessment in Animals; Executive Function and Higher-Order Cognition: Neuroimaging; Prefrontal Cortex: Structure and Anatomy; Prefrontal Cortex.

Further Reading

Anderson JR, Bothell D, Byrne MD, Douglass S, Lebiere C, and Qin Y (2004) An integrated theory of the mind. *Psychological Review* 111(4): 1036–1060.

Botvinick MM, Braver TS, Barch DM, Carter CS, and Cohen JC (2001) Conflict monitoring and cognitive control. *Psychological Review* 108: 624–652.

Braver TS and Cohen JD (2000) On the control of control: The role of dopamine in regulating prefrontal function and working memory. In: Monsell S and Driver J (eds.) *Attention and Performance XVIII*, pp. 713–738. Cambridge, MA: MIT Press.

Brown JW, Bullock D, and Grossberg S (2004) How laminar frontal cortex and basal ganglia circuits interact to control planned and reactive saccades. *Neural Networks* 17(4): 471–510.

Brunel N and Wang XJ (2001) Effects of neuromodulation in a cortical network model of object working memory dominated by recurrent inhibition. *Journal of Computational Neuroscience* 11(1): 63–85.

Cohen JD, Dunbar K, and McClelland JL (1990) On the control of automatic processes: A parallel distributed processing account of the Stroop effect. *Psychological Review* 97(3): 332–361.

Durstewitz D, Seamans JK, and Sejnowski TJ (2000) Dopamine-mediated stabilization of delay-period activity in a network model of prefrontal cortex. *Journal of Neurophysiology* 83(3): 1733–1750.

Grossberg S (1982) *Studies of Mind and Brain*. Boston: Reidel.

Holroyd CB and Coles MG (2002) The neural basis of human error processing: Reinforcement learning, dopamine, and the error-related negativity. *Psychological Review* 109(4): 679–709.

Meyer DE and Kieras DE (1997) A computational theory of executive cognitive processes and multiple-task performance. Part 1. Basic mechanisms. *Psychological Review* 104(1): 3–65.

Miller EK and Cohen JD (2001) An integrative theory of prefrontal cortex function. *Annual Review of Neuroscience* 21: 167–202.

Norman DA and Shallice T (1986) Attention to action: Willed and automatic control of behavior. In: Davidson RJ, Schwartz GE, and Shapiro D (eds.) *Consciousness and Self-Regulation*, vol. 4, pp. 1–18. New York: Plenum.

O'Reilly RC and Frank MJ (2006) Making working memory work: A computational model of learning in the prefrontal cortex and basal ganglia. *Neural Computation* 18(2): 283–328.

Rougier NP, Noelle DC, Braver TS, Cohen JD, and O'Reilly RC (2005) Prefrontal cortex and flexible cognitive control: Rules without symbols. *Proceedings of the National Academy of Sciences of the United States of America* 102(20): 7338–7343.

Yeung N, Cohen JD, and Botvinick MM (2004) The neural basis of error detection: Conflict monitoring and the error-related negativity. *Psychological Review* 111(4): 931–959.

Executive Function and Higher-Order Cognition: Definition and Neural Substrates

E K Miller, Massachusetts Institute of Technology, Cambridge, MA, USA
J D Wallis, University of California at Berkeley, Berkeley, CA, USA

Cognitive, or executive, control refers to the ability to coordinate thought and action and direct it toward obtaining goals. It is needed to overcome local considerations, plan and orchestrate complex sequences of behavior, and prioritize goals and subgoals. Simply stated, you do not need executive control to grab a beer, but you will need it to finish college.

Executive control contrasts with automatic forms of brain processing. Many of our behaviors are direct reactions to our immediate environment that do not tax executive control. If someone throws a baseball toward our face, we reflexively duck out of the way. We have not necessarily willed this behavior; it seems as if our body reacts and then our mind 'catches up' and realizes what has happened. Evolution has wired many of these reflexive, automatic processes into our nervous systems. However, others can be acquired through practice because learning mechanisms gradually and thoroughly stamp in highly familiar behaviors.

For example, consider a daily walk to work. If the route is highly familiar and if traffic is light, our mind can wander. Before we know it, we may have gone a considerable distance and negotiated street crossings and turns with little awareness of having done so. In these cases, the control of our behavior occurs in a 'bottom-up' fashion: it is determined largely by the nature of the sensory stimuli and their strong associations with certain behavioral responses. In neural terms, they are dependent on the correct sensory conditions triggering activity in well-established neural pathways.

Suppose, however, that during our walk to work something unexpected happens or we encounter difficulty. For example, we might encounter a busy street that we need to cross. Then, the executive system takes over and we need to 'take charge' of our actions. We pay attention to the people and cars around us to anticipate and accommodate their actions, or we may decide to take an alternate route. Now, straightforward stimulus–response associations are insufficient to govern our behavior. We must use knowledge of our current objective (arriving at work on time and intact) and results from previous experiences to weigh the alternatives and consequences. During this 'controlled mode,' we also engage the basic sensory, memory, and motor processes that mediate automatic behavior. Only now, the environment is not simply triggering these processes. Instead, we use our current goals to shape and control these processes in a 'top-down' fashion.

Figure 1 summarizes these ideas by illustrating a widely accepted view of the architecture of cognition. At the lower level are the automatic processes, which include sensory analysis, memories, details of motor acts, and well-learned skills. The system is in automatic mode when processing flows through the lower level, from input to output, along established pathways without any hindrance or modification. However, at any given instant the executive system can step in and modify this flow should it detect that the automatic processes are no longer sufficient to obtain our goals. In understanding the neuronal mechanisms that underlie this process, the prefrontal cortex (PFC), the brain area directly behind our forehead, seems especially critical.

The Prefrontal Cortex

PFC has dramatically expanded in size and complexity across evolution, and its development correlates with the complexity of the behavioral repertoire exhibited by an organism. It has reached its pinnacle in humans, in which it accounts for approximately 30% of the total cortical area. It consists of a collection of cortical areas that differ from one another in terms of the size, density, and distribution of their neurons. **Figure 2** shows the major PFC divisions of the monkey PFC, although anatomists have subdivided these further, describing at least 18 distinct areas. The subdivisions have partly unique, but overlapping, patterns of connections with the rest of the brain, which suggests some regional differences in function. As in much of the neocortex, however, there are local connections between different PFC areas that can result in an intermixing and synthesis of the disparate information needed for cognitive control.

PFC is anatomically in a good position for a central role in executive control. Collectively, the various PFC areas have interconnections with brain areas processing external information, including all sensory systems and cortical and subcortical motor system structures, as well as internal information from limbic and midbrain structures involved in affect, memory, and reward. Indeed, neuronal activity in PFC reflects the multimodal nature of its inputs. PFC neurons

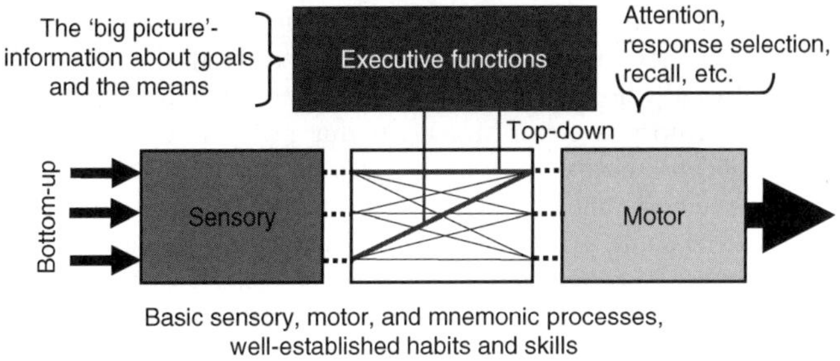

Figure 1 Two levels of cognitive processes. Specialized functions that acquire information about goals and means (top) select and coordinate among innate and well-established routines (bottom). Inputs from the environment are 'bottom-up,' whereas signals based on knowledge about goals and task demands are 'top-down.' Active processing lines are shown in blue.

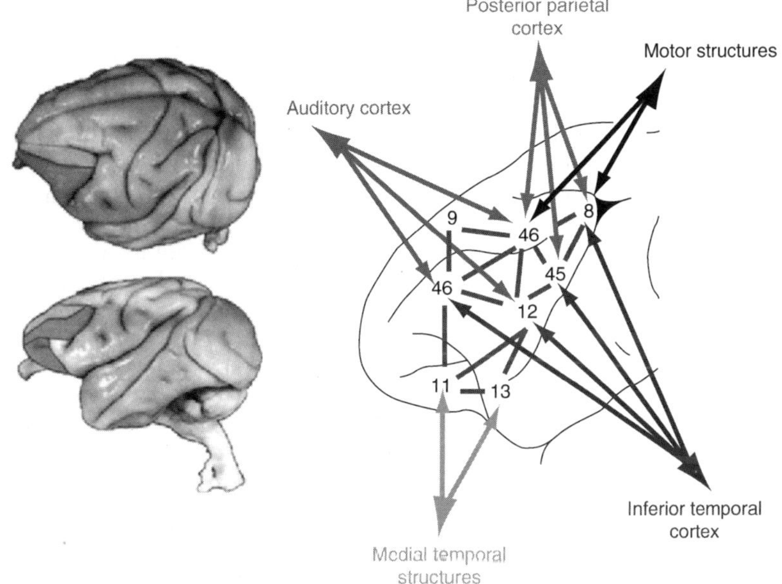

Figure 2 The monkey prefrontal cortical areas with some connections. (Left) Dorsal is yellow, dorsolateral is red, ventrolateral is green, and orbital is blue. The medial PFC is not pictured. (Right) Some extrinsic and intrinsic connections. Not all connections are illustrated; this figure is meant to convey how the PFC can synthesize and integrate diverse inputs from other brain structures.

encode visual, auditory, tactile, olfactory, and gustatory cues, as well as recalled memories and behavioral responses such as voluntary limb and eye movements. In short, the functional and morphological anatomy of PFC is consistent with its role in synthesizing diverse information about the external and internal world in order to produce goal-directed behavior.

PFC Contributions to Executive Control

PFC damage does not result in simple deficits; there is relatively little overt impairment, at least with superficial examination. Patients with PFC damage have intact sensory capabilities, they can remember events and facts, and they appear remarkably normal in casual conversation. However, despite the superficial appearance of normality, PFC damage devastates a person's life. Patients have trouble staying employed, married, or even completing simple daily errands. Furthermore, they often seem to act without any apparent consideration to future consequences. Careful testing of PFC patients has revealed a number of underlying cognitive deficits that might explain their impairments.

Inhibition

PFC damage often produces 'stimulus-bound' behavior. Patients engage in whatever habitual behaviors happen to be triggered by cues in the immediate environment. For example, when they see a glass of water, they may drink it regardless of whose glass it is. Because other learning and memory systems are intact, they can learn to respond to specific cues in specific ways. However, they then become stuck in that behavioral rut, producing the same response to the cue even when it is no longer appropriate – a phenomenon called 'perseveration.'

Planning

After PFC damage, the basic units of behavior remain intact. What is lacking is the ability to organize them toward a goal. For example, one patient, when making coffee, first stirred and then added milk. Another example is a patient who had been an excellent cook until she had a large tumor removed from her frontal lobes. Her basic skills remained but she seemed unable to organize them. She would move haphazardly from preparing one part of the meal to another so that some parts of the meal would burn, whereas others had hardly been started.

Evaluating Consequences

Goal-directed behavior depends on our capacity to evaluate the consequences of our actions so that we can choose an optimal plan. Evidence that certain types of PFC damage impair this process comes from a gambling task. The subject has to choose cards from four different decks. Some cards win the subject some money, but others cause the subject to lose money. Unbeknownst to the subject, cards from two of the decks will occasionally win large amounts of money but are also occasionally associated with very large losses. Thus, consistently choosing from these decks will lead to a net loss. In contrast, if the subject chooses from the other two decks, he or she will win smaller amounts, but the losses are also smaller, so that overall the subject will obtain a net profit. Control subjects quickly learn to limit their choices to the profitable decks, whereas patients with PFC damage, particularly of the orbital region, continually choose from the decks associated with large rewards and larger losses until they lose all their money.

This led to the hypothesis that the orbital PFC is responsible for labeling cues or situations with an affective significance or 'somatic marker.' It associates memories of past, affect-laden events with a representation of the state of the autonomic nervous system that the event evoked. Similar events in the future can then evoke a 'gut feeling' of the appropriate course of action by recall of the somatic marker. This is particularly helpful in very complex situations in which it is difficult to evaluate rationally and deliberatively all the pros and cons of a choice.

Further evidence that PFC neurons participate in this process comes from studies showing that a large proportion of them encode information about expected rewards. For example, some neurons encode the delivery of a reward, whereas others respond when a reward does not occur as expected. After training, many PFC neurons will show responses to visual cues that signal whether a reward will or will not be forthcoming and reflect the identity, size, and preference of an expected reward.

Working Memory

The importance of a short-term memory buffer for cognition is apparent to anyone who has tried to do math in their head; intermediate answers and operations must be buffered in a way that allows them to be kept 'in mind.' The pattern of deficits following PFC damage might be sequelae of an underlying deficit in working memory. Patients may have difficulty planning or appear disinhibited because without working memory, goal-relevant information is lost over all but the briefest delays and thus their behavior takes its cue from the immediate environment.

This hypothesis stems from observations that PFC damage in monkeys impairs a spatial delayed-response task that requires them to remember the location of a stimulus or behavioral response over a brief delay of several seconds. In addition, there are many studies illustrating that PFC neurons sustain their activity over several seconds to bridge short delays imposed between a cue and a response – observations that Fuster, Niki, and colleagues first made in the 1970s. Goldman-Rakic and colleagues used a more controlled version of the task using an oculomotor response to a visual target presented in the periphery of the visual field. They demonstrated that dorsolateral PFC neurons have precise tuning for memories of particular visual field locations.

In humans, a similar task, called the 'two-back' task, is sensitive to PFC damage or dysfunction. Subjects observe a sequence of sample stimuli and must respond if a current sample stimulus matches one seen two samples ago. Because this involves matching to a specific stimulus, it may rely on working memory rather than other, more passive, forms of immediate memory, such as those that automatically detect repetition.

PFC activity sustains brief memories of a wide range of behaviorally relevant cues: objects, colors, the frequency of a vibration to the hand, and forthcoming movements. Similar activity is also evident in the sensory and motor systems. This is not surprising; sustained activity is evident in many brain structures and must play a role in many neural processes from sensory afterimages to holding a motor state. However, specificity and robustness are what separates more 'cognitive' short-term memory processes, such as working memory processes, from such lower level processes. Working memory selectively retains task-relevant information, rather than just any stimulus, and does so over potential distractions. PFC neurons have this ability. For example, when monkeys are required to sustain the memory of a sample object across a delay period filled with visual distractors that require attention and processing, sustained activity within the PFC can still maintain a memory of the sample object. By contrast, sustained activity in visual cortical areas seems more labile; it is disrupted by the presence of distractors.

Learning and Using Rules

The PFC is important when we need top-down processing – that is, when our internal states or intentions guide behavior. It is critical in situations in which the mapping between sensory inputs, thoughts, and actions is weak relative to other existing ones or when the mapping is rapidly changing. In such circumstances, we often rely on previously constructed models of regularities in our environment and our expectancies of future events – the so-called 'rules of the game.'

Conditional learning tasks are a laboratory test of rule learning. They require learning of associative relationships that are arbitrary and extend beyond the simple one-to-one mappings that underlie reflexive reactions. Whether or not a given response is the correct response to a given cue constantly changes because it depends on additional information. For example, reaching for a beer can be rewarding, but only if one considers other information. If the beer belongs to another patron, the result could be disastrous. Monkeys with PFC damage are impaired at a variety of conditional learning tasks. When monkeys learn associations between, for example, three visual cues and three directional movements of a joystick, simply moving the joystick is not enough to produce reward. Rather, the specific movement direction is dependent on the specific cue. One means 'up,' the other 'down,' etc. Following PFC damage, monkeys have difficulty acquiring this task. Furthermore, PFC neurons encode multiple aspects of conditional tasks, including the sensory cues, the motor responses, and the specific associations between the cues and responses (**Figure 2**).

PFC is also essential in enabling the control of behavior by abstract, high-level rules. Consider, for example, dining in a restaurant. We are not born knowing how to act in this situation. Instead, after several experiences in restaurants we begin to abstract the common features of importance. For example, we learn the important sensory information deserving our attention (e.g., the wine list), typical events, appropriate actions, and expected consequences (e.g., paying the bill). The rules underlying ordering a meal in a restaurant are essentially networks of predictive relationships between immediate cues, internal and external context, and actions and consequences long divorced from the details of the individual restaurants in which we have dined. We can then use these abstract rules to order a meal in any subsequent restaurant, even those in which we have never dined before. Several investigators have argued that the encoding of rule information is a cardinal function of the PFC.

One task that directly tests this ability is the Wisconsin Card Sorting Test (WCST). The patient is required to sort a deck of cards on which there are a number of colored shapes. The patient has to determine by trial and error the correct property by which to sort the cards. For example, if the 'color' rule were in effect, the subject would have to sort the cards according to the color of the shapes. Unbeknownst to the subject, the experimenter can switch which is the correct rule, and the subject needs to detect this and modify his or her behavior accordingly. Patients with PFC damage, particularly lateral PFC, have difficulty doing this. Using more focal, experimentally induced lesions in monkeys, experimenters have confirmed that lateral PFC is the most important PFC region for rule or strategy implementation. Furthermore, studies show that single PFC neurons are capable of encoding abstract rules. For example, monkeys saw two pictures appear successively separated by a delay. At the start of the trial, a cue instructed the monkeys to release a lever if the two pictures were either the same or different. Thus, to solve the task the monkeys had to maintain in working memory both the picture and the currently relevant abstract rule (same or different) during the delay. Many PFC neurons, more than one-third, encoded the abstract rule.

What function does the ability to abstract a rule serve? Abstraction is a type of generalization that permits a shortcut in learning, allowing us to apply what we have learned in similar situations to novel circumstances. Without the ability to abstract the general principles behind related situations, we would have to learn the correct behavior on each new occasion by trial and error. The problem with such trial-and-error learning is that errors necessarily occur. This is a less efficient way of dealing with novelty since errors frequently lead to lost opportunities for reward. Consistent with these ideas, PFC seems to be most important when subjects must deal with novel situations.

Neurobiological Models of Executive Control

Note that the pattern of deficits following PFC damage seems to reflect a selective loss of the higher level functions from the bipartite cognitive architecture pictured in **Figure 1**. Well-established automatic routines on the lower level are intact and available to be triggered by the appropriate sensory cues. However, without the higher level functions specialized to acquire and represent goals and means, the system would be at the mercy of the environment, ruled by whatever sensory inputs happen to flow into the system and by whatever thoughts, emotions, and actions are strongly associated with these inputs. Thus, behavior would seem impulsive and disinhibited and reactions inappropriate because they would be emitted reflexively without any consideration of the future. Furthermore, without the influence of predicted goals to continually drive task-appropriate processes, individuals would be distractible and would easily go 'off track' when there are temporal gaps between sensory inputs or between those inputs and the individual's responses. The system might be capable of learning to react to cues, but this learning would be inflexible. Without the ability to predict goals and means, the system would be stuck in a behavioral rut, always reacting to a cue with whatever behavior it was first associated.

This architecture is also apparent in neurobiological models of executive control. Network models of Dehaene and Changeux include an executive layer of 'rule-coding' units, thought to correspond to the PFC, that controls the flow of information between the input and output layers (**Figure 3(a)**). Arthur Shimamura proposed a dynamic filtering model of PFC function in which patterns of information sustained by the PFC select and reroute the flow of activity in posterior association cortex (**Figure 3(b)**). Miller and Cohen proposed that the cardinal PFC function is to acquire and actively maintain patterns of activity that represent goals and the means to achieve them (rules) in terms of a map of the cortical pathways needed to perform the task (hence 'rulemaps') (**Figure 3(c)**). Under this model, activation of a PFC rulemap sets up bias signals that propagate throughout much of the rest of the cortex, affecting sensory systems as well as systems responsible for response execution, memory retrieval, emotional evaluation, etc. The aggregate effect is to guide the flow of neural activity along pathways that establish the proper mappings between inputs, internal states, and outputs to best perform the task. In short, rule information is acquired by the PFC, which provides support to related information

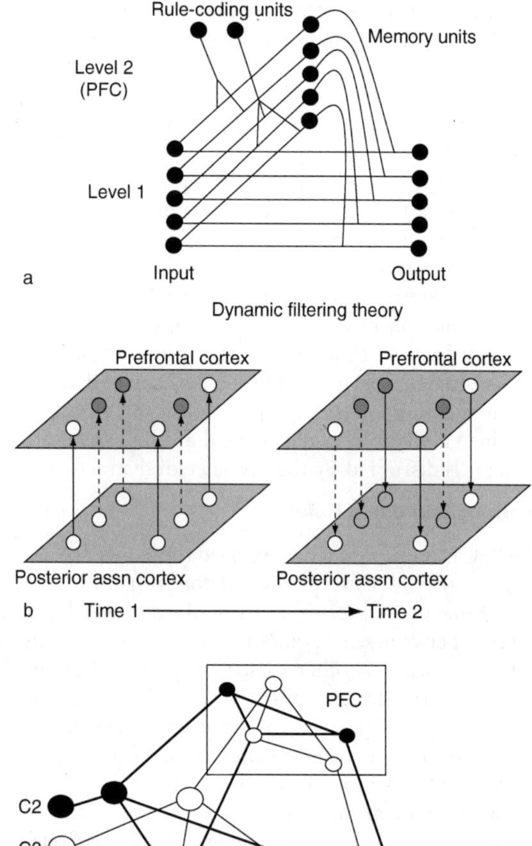

Figure 3 Models of PFC function. (a) The models of Changeux and Dehaene include an executive level (level 2, thought to correspond to the PFC) with rule-coding units and working memory units that gate the flow of activity along lower level input–output lines. (b) Shimamura's dynamic filtering model. At time 1, a region in PFC is activated by feed-forward (i.e., bottom-up) projections from posterior cortex. This activity, along with influences such as task demands, sets up a pattern of activation in PFC (light circles, activation; dark circles, inhibition). At time 2, posterior cortex is modulated by PFC via feedback (i.e., top-down) projections that enable both selection of task-relevant and inhibition of task-irrelevant neural activity. Figure provided by Arthur Shimamura. (c) In the Miller and Cohen model, a task model is formed in the PFC when reward signals link together neurons activated by the events that led to reward. A subset of cues can then activate the entire representation. Bias signals resulting from the maintenance of this pattern guide the flow of activity along neural pathways that establish the task-relevant mappings between representations of inputs (C1, C2, C3), internal states, and outputs (R1, R2) in posterior cortex. Thick lines and solid circles denote active processing lines. Reproduced from Miller EK and Cohen JD (2001) An integrative theory of prefrontal function. *Annual Review of Neuroscience* 24: 167–202.

in posterior brain systems, effectively acting as a global controller or 'traffic cop.'

A key issue is to understand how PFC acquires these high-level representations. One possibility is that they develop through the action of reinforcement signals on multimodal PFC circuitry. During learning, when a behavior meets with success, reward signals augment the unique pattern of PFC activity evoked by that situation, action, and consequence by strengthening connections between the neurons activated by those events. These representations might begin quite modestly, but with time and repeated iterations of the process, the PFC representation can 'bootstrap' into further elaboration as combinations of events and contingencies between them and the requisite actions are learned. Midbrain dopaminergic neurons have ideal properties for the reinforcement signal. Early in learning, rewards activate dopamine neurons, but later in learning the cues that predict those rewards activate dopamine neurons rather than the rewards. Furthermore, there is an inhibition of the firing rate of the dopamine neurons when an expected reward does not occur. This 'reward prediction error' signal is ideal for instructing when and what the system should learn and consequently enables the organism to acquire the representations necessary to achieve reward.

The resulting pattern of PFC activity reflects the task's contingencies and in neural terms amounts to a 'map' of the pathways between inputs, internal states, and outputs needed to perform the task successfully. The ability to construct this map arises from the intermingling of diverse information that takes place within PFC. Although the PFC may be critically involved in acquisition of this information, other parts of the brain may be responsible for its consolidation in long-term memory. The PFC, however, would retain the requisite links to retrieve the appropriate pattern and bring it online to guide behavior.

Summary

Executive control refers to the ability to take charge of one's actions and direct them toward unseen aims. Virtually all theories of cognition posit that executive control requires making predictions about available goals and what means might achieve them. This knowledge can then be used to select and coordinate among a myriad of lower level, automatic sensory, memory, and motor functions.

The PFC, a brain structure that reaches its greatest complexity in the primate brain, seems to play a central role in executive control. It has access to all major forebrain systems, as well as the means to influence them. Individuals with PFC damage seem capable only of emitting habitual or innate reactions to the immediate environment without any consideration or anticipation of future consequences and unseen goals. Neurophysiological studies indicate that PFC neurons seem to mediate the mechanisms essential for a cognitive control system: They are multimodal, they acquire and signal the formal demands of tasks, and they can sustain their activity to keep task-relevant information online and available during behavior.

Different theories of PFC function emphasize different contributions to cognitive control: maintenance and/or manipulation of information in working memory, the assignment of affective tags on events and choices, and the acquisition and online representation of task rules. These theories are not mutually exclusive; each may reflect different facets of a system that is necessarily multivariate because of its role in guiding many different behaviors and interfacing with many other brain systems. However, in the healthy individual, the different processes work in harmony and enable the organism to behave flexibly and cope efficiently with novel situations, which are hallmark features of PFC function.

See also: Cognitive Control and Development; Cognitive Deficits in Schizophrenia; Congenital Muscular Dystrophy; Executive Function and Higher-Order Cognition: Neuroimaging; Executive Function and Higher-Order Cognition: Computational Models; Frontal Lobe Syndrome; Prefrontal Cortex: Structure and Anatomy; Short Term and Working Memory.

Further Reading

Damasio AR (1994) *Descartes' Error: Emotion, Reason, and the Human Brain.* New York: Putman.

Fuster JM (1995) *Memory in the Cerebral Cortex.* Cambridge, MA: MIT Press.

Miller EK and Cohen JD (2001) An integrative theory of prefrontal function. *Annual Review of Neuroscience* 24: 167–202.

Schultz W and Dickinson A (2000) Neuronal coding of prediction errors. *Annual Review of Neuroscience* 23: 473–500.

Executive Function and Higher-Order Cognition: EEG Studies

L Y Deouell, The Hebrew University of Jerusalem, Jerusalem, Israel
R T Knight, University of California at Berkeley, Berkeley, CA, USA

Introduction

Multiple goals, from survival to pleasure, coexist at every given moment, and internal needs as well as external events act in a push–pull manner to bias behavior. To maintain optimal goal-directed behavior, a control ('executive') system is needed that will dynamically prioritize the processing of information as well as the planning of actions and their execution. In addition to direct motor planning, major components of this executive system are working memory, attention, and conflict/error monitoring. Working memory would allow maintaining a goal across time, as well as information required to achieve the goal. Selective attention ('voluntary' or 'endogenous' attention) would facilitate the processing of one stream of input and suppress another while involuntary attention mechanisms allow for changes in the environment, as well as changes in internal drives, to interfere with ongoing behavior in a rapid and flexible manner. A monitoring module is needed to assess the efficiency of the executed behavior so that behavior can be adjusted in an optimal way. Consequently, the executive system needs to interact with multiple sensory regions of the brain, as well as with motor output regions involved in orientation, locomotion, and speech. Event-related brain potentials (ERPs), recorded on the scalp (and recently also intracranially) have established scalp-recorded signatures of executive functions. The effect of brain lesions on these measures of electrical brain activity provides a window into the networks supporting the executive system. This article describes ERP studies conducted specifically with patients suffering from well-circumscribed brain lesions involving mainly the lateral prefrontal cortex (LPFC), a major hub of the executive system.

Selective Attention

Patients with LPFC damage are frequently unable to suppress inappropriate reaction to objects and events in their environment (so-called environmental dependency syndrome) or to suppress prepotent responses. Whereas some of these effects may be at the level of response selection, ERP studies of these patients suggest that LPFC is essential for normal suppression of information processing at the level of unimodal sensory cortices.

Knight and coworkers delivered auditory stimuli (clicks or tone bursts), or brief electric shocks to the median nerve, to patients with damage to LPFC and to patients with comparably sized lesions in the temporoparietal junction or the lateral parietal cortex, as well as to age-matched controls. Both types of stimuli were distractors, not relevant to the task. Lesions in posterior association cortex, sparing primary sensory regions, had no effects on the amplitudes or latencies of the primary cortical evoked responses. Lesions invading either the primary auditory or somatosensory cortex reduced early latency (20–40 ms) evoked responses generated in these regions. In a distinct contrast, LPFC damage resulted in enhanced amplitude of both the primary auditory and somatosensory evoked responses generated 20–40 ms poststimulation. Spinal cord and brain stem potentials were unaffected by prefrontal damage, indicating that the amplitude enhancement of primary cortical responses was due to abnormalities in either prefrontal-thalamic connectivity or direct interactions between LPFC and sensory cortex. Selectively attending to a sensory stream and maintaining the goal of behavior requires not only enhancement of processing of some sensory stimuli or motor plans, but also suppression, or inhibition, of competitive stimuli or plans ('biased competition'). Apparently, a signal from LPFC to upstream sensory cortices provides such a biasing signal. Failure to produce such a signal may impair selective attention.

The failure to inhibit irrelevant sensory input indeed affects the patients' performance. Chao and Knight showed that patients with LPFC lesions are impaired in an auditory delayed-match-to-sample task when the delay period is filled with irrelevant tone pips. In the same task, the irrelevant tones elicited abnormally augmented primary auditory potentials (Na, Pa) in the patients, and the performance decrement directly correlated with the Pa enhancement. Similarly, in patients with right prefrontal damage, sounds presented to an unattended ear in a dichotic paradigm abnormally reduced the attentional enhancement (see the section titled 'Novelty and deviance detection and involuntary attention shift') of subsequent to-be-attended sounds. In agreement with these findings, patients with prefrontal lesions show reduced or even reversed negative priming effects, which suggests that processing of stimuli that should be outside the focus of attention is not properly suppressed.

The role of the LPFC in biased competition is not limited to inhibition. In fact, LPFC may also provide the excitatory signal. This excitation may be implemented through three distinct mechanisms: (1) through a tonic excitatory influence on ipsilateral posterior areas, affecting attended and nonattended sensory inputs alike; (2) by enhancement of extrastriate cortex response to attended information; and (3) by a phasic excitatory influence on ipsilateral posterior areas' response to correctly perceived task-relevant stimuli (targets). This was shown in a series of ERP studies conducted by Knight and colleagues in patients with LPFC damage (centered on Brodmann's areas 9 and 46), in which the patients were asked to detect rare (odd ball) targets (inverted triangles) in a series of distractors (upright triangles). This paradigm is referred to below as the triangles task.

When the stimuli in the triangles task were presented at fixation, the patients showed a diminished extrastriate N1 component (at 170 ms) relative to controls. A similar reduction of N1 was observed in another experiment, which used visual word stimuli. Even more revealing were conditions in which targets and nontargets were lateralized and could appear in either visual field. In one of these conditions, the patients were instructed to attend to all stimuli regardless of location. The extrastriate P1, immediately preceding the N1 component, was reduced for all stimuli presented to the contralesional hemifield. Moreover, when the patients' attention was directed to one of the fields at a time, this reduction of P1 over ipsilesional extrastriate cortex was observed for attended and nonattended contralateral stimuli alike, and can thus be considered attention independent. Thus, LPC seems to exert a modulatory, tonic, attention-independent facilitation over processing at ipsilateral extrastriate cortex. A similar effect of reduced association cortex activity ipsilateral to LPFC damage has been reported for auditory-induced N1 potentials.

Directing attention to one hemifield in a target detection task normally elicits a sustained negativity (known as 'selection negativity' or 'negative difference'), starting at around 100 ms, for all stimuli presented at this hemifield. When attention was directed to the contralesional visual field of LPFC patients, this attention effect on extrastriate cortex was normal in the first 200 ms after stimulus onset but was significantly disrupted thereafter. This finding suggests that LPFC exerts attention-dependent selective facilitation starting around 200 ms after stimulus onset. Other cortical areas are probably responsible for attention-dependent regulation of extrastriate cortex in the first 200 ms. It is conceivable that inferior parietal cortex is responsible for the early reflexive component of attention whereas LPFC is responsible for more-controlled and sustained aspects of visual attention beginning later on. The effect of LPFC lesion on the selection negativity is not limited to visual areas. In an auditory selective attention task, prefrontal lesion patients generated reduced selection negativity as well. Notably, this diminished attention effect depended on the side of the lesion. Patients with left hemisphere lesions showed a mildly reduced attention effect regardless of which ear was attended. In contrast, patients with right prefrontal damage showed reduced effect mainly when the contralateral ear was to be attended. Posterior association cortex lesions in the temporoparietal junction had comparable effects on the selection negativity regardless of ear of stimulation.

Target detection in the visual oddball paradigm described above is normally associated with a prominent late response, starting at 200 ms and continuing for the next 500 ms, including the N2–P3b complex. Since this component is elicited only by detected targets, it is considered to be a manifestation of phasic top-down effects contingent on the identity of the stimulus. Following LPFC lesions, the N2, a component which likely reflects postselection processing of the target in the inferior temporal lobe, was not observable over the lesioned hemisphere in response to targets in either visual field. The P3b was reduced over the temporo-occipital electrodes but not at parietal sites, attesting to the fact that the P3b most likely reflects multiple distinct cortical processes related to target detection. The patients' performance in this study, producing more errors, was concordant with this electrophysiological evidence of impaired top-down effects following LPFC lesion. A spatially limited reduction of target P3 was recently reported also by Daffner et al., although in that group of LPFC patients, the main reduction of target P3 was reported to be in anterior electrodes. Thus, in addition to both attention-dependent and attention-independent tonic facilitation, the LPFC is critical in establishing a phasic, stimulus-dependent facilitation.

Novelty and Deviance Detection and Involuntary Attention Shift

Task requirements in an experimental setting, as well as the ongoing goals in natural settings, require that a subset of the sensory stream and a subset of motor plans be preferentially processed and, at least in humans, be available for conscious awareness and deliberation. However, such biased selection may be perilous as events outside the focus of attention might pose either dangers (e.g., an approaching predator) or opportunities (e.g., prey). Such events may be slight perturbations of an established sensory regularity, such as an intensity decrement in background noise, or grossly unexpected ('novel') events, such as the sound of screeching brakes. This need calls for a surveillance mechanism that automatically detects deviant events.

Automatic response to slight changes in acoustic regularity outside the focus of attention bears the electrophysiological signature of the 'mismatch negativity' (MMN), a frontal scalp negative potential accompanied by lower temporal positivity, with a peak latency of 100–250 ms following the deviation. The MMN presumably reflects an 'error signal' generated automatically in the secondary auditory cortex by a neural mechanism comparing a perceived stimulus to a sensory 'memory trace' formed by the regular stimuli or the process of updating the existing model of the environment. The MMN is elicited when participants attend to a primary task and ignore the stream of sounds in which the pertinent deviations occur. Although it might be somewhat attenuated outside the focus of attention, it is completely suppressed only under very specific circumstances of competition for processing a specific feature between two auditory streams. Moreover, whereas attention-related components of the ERP are largely absent when deviation is predictable (e.g., when a deviation occurs regularly in the stream), the MMN is immune to this manipulation. Thus, the MMN is considered to represent a nonintentional, largely preattentive process. This signal may be a trigger for an ensuing shift of attention toward the deviant event. These shifts are reflected on the scalp as a positivity following the MMN, called P3a.

The P3a is a positive frontoparietal scalp potential peaking around 300 ms following the onset of a rare, task-irrelevant distractor in an oddball sequence. The novelty P3a is similar in response to either novel sounds or visual stimuli. The P3a is considered a marker of attention orienting, elicited by a distributed multimodal corticolimbic system. Both the MMN and the novelty P3a components were shown to be reduced in patients with PFC lesions.

In paradigms designed to study the MMN, patients and controls watched silent movies or were engaged with a visual reaction time paradigm and were instructed to ignore series of repetitive sounds. Infrequently, the regularity of the sound stream was broken by the occurrence of a deviant stimulus. The MMN in response to pitch and pattern changes was reduced in patients with PFC lesions, indicating an early deficit in automatic detection of deviance outside the focus of attention. Whereas temporoparietal lesions caused an MMN reduction mainly to contralesional stimuli, LPFC lesions elicited comparable deficits regardless of stimulus side in one study, and more to ipsilesional sounds in another. In addition, there was a tendency for right prefrontal lesions to be associated with larger MMN reductions than left prefrontal lesions were, but no such asymmetry was found for the temporoparietal lesions. These results suggest different contributions of the temporoparietal region and the prefrontal region to the MMN. Further research will be needed to determine whether the reduced MMN following prefrontal damage reflects a weakened memory trace of the previous regularity due to disinhibition of irrelevant information, reduced frontal facilitation of a comparator mechanism in the secondary auditory cortex (which is the main generator of scalp MMN), a failure to initiate an attention switch following the detection of the change, or damage to a postulated frontal generator of MMN. In addition, it is still unclear whether the effect of LPFC damage is independent of the dimension of the regularity which is disturbed (e.g., spatial location, pitch, or more-abstract dimensions of the sound).

Novelty P3a responses generated over prefrontal scalp sites to unexpected novel stimuli are reduced by prefrontal lesions, with reductions observed throughout the lesioned hemisphere. Comparable P3a decrements have been observed in the auditory, visual, and somatosensory modalities in humans with prefrontal damage. Reductions appear to be more severe after right prefrontal damage. In most studies of novelty P3a, the novel stimuli are completely task irrelevant, and the response is considered to reflect an 'involuntary' orienting response toward the salient event. Accordingly, galvanic skin response, a peripheral marker of the orienting response, is also reduced by damage to the prefrontal as well as posterior association cortex. LPFC damage caused a dramatic reduction in P3a amplitude even in a paradigm in which the novels where relevant to one of two tasks the patients were involved with. In the paradigm used by Daffner et al., patients had to self-pace a succession of visual stimuli while also looking for a designated (non-novel) target. LPFC patients not only showed a significantly attenuated P3a response to novel visual stimuli but also spent less time than controls did looking at novels, suggesting a more general decrement of 'novelty seeking.' Taken together, these findings converge with both clinical observations and animal experimentation supporting a critical role of prefrontal structures in the processing of novel stimuli, probably as part of a prefrontal-hippocampal network.

Monitoring

In demanding task situations, it is important to detect when actions may be erroneous and to adjust behavior to avoid additional mistakes. Evidence from electrophysiological and neuroimaging studies suggests that the anterior cingulate cortex (ACC) and the LPFC are active in situations demanding such monitoring activity. Evidence linking the ACC to action monitoring derives from studies of error-related negativity (ERN), an ERP that occurs at the moment of an error in cognitive reaction time tasks. Dipole localization studies of ERN suggest that it is generated by a medial frontal structure, most likely the ACC. Functional magnetic resonance imaging (fMRI) studies examining error processing confirm the presence of ACC activation associated with errors or with situations prone to errors. A rare single unit recording in a human patient showed that dorsal ACC is associated with the use of rewards to guide action and further that ablation of the dorsal ACC increases errors in a situation requiring reward processing. Also, fMRI studies demonstrate that in addition to the ACC, activation may occur also in LPFC in conflict situations. Some of these studies suggest that activation in the ACC and LPFC is not related to errors *per se* but rather to the need to avoid errors or losses in more-demanding situations. Co-occurrence of prefrontal and cingulate activity related to error processing has been observed also in single-neuron recordings from nonhuman primates, as well as in intracerebral recordings from implanted depth electrodes in epileptic patients. These observations have not determined, however, whether the ACC and the LPFC interact or are independent.

The question of the interaction of the ACC and the LPFC was investigated by Gehring and Knight, who measured ERN in a group of patients with unilateral circumscribed lesions of the LPFC. A normal pattern of ERN activity in these individuals would indicate that the medial frontal regions operated independently of the LPFC in generating the ERN. In contrast, an absence or reduction of ERN activity in these individuals would indicate that the LPFC was either necessary for generation of the ERN in the ACC, or was itself a generator of the ERN. Other disruptions in the pattern of ERN activity would suggest that LPFC modulated the generation of the ERN, perhaps by supplying information or activation that was critical for ACC processing.

Six patients were studied, four with left and two with right LPFC damage. They were compared to ten age-matched controls and ten younger individuals. Participants made a squeezing response to a pair of letters, one of which was designated as a target letter. One letter appeared in red and the other in green. At 1 s before the letter pair, a precue (the word 'red' or 'green') indicated which letter was the target letter. The task was to respond with one hand if the target letter was 'H' and with the other hand if the letter was 'S'. On half of the trials, the irrelevant flanking letter was identical to the target letter; on the other half of the trials, the irrelevant flanking letter signaled the incorrect response (a manipulation that provoked erroneous responses).

The patients were slower than the control groups but did not perform with more errors than the control groups did. However, they showed less online corrective action in error trials. While controls showed reduced squeezing force during error trials, suggesting online inhibition of response, patients showed a reduction in this effect. In addition, the patients corrected their error less frequently than controls did. The pattern of the patients' electrophysiological response was also dramatically different from that of the control groups. Whereas in the young and age-matched controls, the response-locked negativity was significantly larger during error trials than during correct trials (i.e., it was an ERN), there was no difference between the error and correct trials in the patients with LPFC lesions. However, this did not result from absence of negativity. Rather, an ERN was seen for correct trials just as often as for incorrect trials, and this ERN was not different in amplitude from the response elicited by the controls during incorrect trials.

This pattern suggests an interaction or interdependence between the LPFC and the ACC in error or conflict monitoring. However, it is not consistent with a simple serial model in which the LPFC detects the need for executive control during high-conflict situations and signals the ACC, which performs the actual control function. Nor is it compatible with a serial model in which the ACC detects conflicts and transmits to the LPFC, which exerts its executive control functions. Since the most conspicuous observation was the lack of differentiation between correct and error trials, one possible account suggested by Gehring and Knight was that the damaged LPFC failed to represent or transmit the contextually appropriate stimulus–response mapping. As a consequence, the ACC may not have been able to confirm a correct response and thus elicited an ERN by default for every trial. Alternatively, the impaired stimulus–response representation in the LPFC might have created an additional conflict in each trial, detected by the ACC. In both cases, the ACC would produce an unreliable cue for errors, reflected in the disruption of corrective responses.

Conclusion

The behavior of patients with LPFC lesions suggests an interruption of executive and attentional control at multiple levels. Thus, in everyday life, patients may inadequately respond to environmental stimuli, be disproportionately distracted by irrelevant information, and be unable to focus on a task, on the one hand, and unable to flexibly shift from one goal to another (perseveration), on the other hand. The data from electrophysiology reveal the role of LPFC in automatic processes such as maintaining an adequate level of responsiveness to all stimuli, detecting change, and processing novelty, as well as controlled processes such as inhibition of irrelevant information, enhanced processing of relevant information, phasic responses to targets, and conflict monitoring. Moreover, the electrophysiological data reveal that LPFC implements some of these functions through interaction with remote regions of the brain, including unimodal sensory cortices, the hippocampus, and the ACC. All these effects are evident early (100–300 ms) in the course of neural processing.

See also: Attention: Models; Attentional Functions in Learning and Memory; Cognitive Control and Development; Electroencephalography (EEG); Electrophysiology: EEG and ERP Analysis; Executive Function and Higher-Order Cognition: Assessment in Animals; Executive Function and Higher-Order Cognition: Definition and Neural Substrates; Working Memory: Capacity Limitations.

Further Reading

Alain C, Woods DL, and Knight RT (1998) A distributed cortical network for auditory sensory memory in humans. *Brain Research* 812: 23–37.

Barcelo F, Suwazono S, and Knight RT (2000) Prefrontal modulation of visual processing in humans. *Nature Neuroscience* 3: 399–403.

Boller F and Grafman J (eds.) (2002) *Handbook of Neuropsychology: The Frontal Lobes.* Amsterdam: Elsevier.

Chao LL and Knight RT (1998) Contribution of human prefrontal cortex to delay performance. *Journal of Cognitive Neuroscience* 10: 167–177.

Daffner KR, Scinto LFM, Weitzman AM, et al. (2003) Frontal and parietal components of a cerebral network mediating voluntary attention to novel events. *Journal of Cognitive Neuroscience* 15: 294–313.

Desimone R and Duncan J (1995) Neural mechanisms of selective visual-attention. *Annual Review of Neuroscience* 18: 193–222.

Gehring WJ and Knight RT (2000) Prefrontal-cingulate interactions in action monitoring. *Nature Neuroscience* 3: 516–520.

Knight RT, Hillyard SA, Woods DL, and Neville HJ (1981) The effects of frontal cortex lesions on event-related potentials during auditory selective attention. *Electroencephalography and Clinical Neurophysiology* 52: 571–582.

Knight RT, Scabini D, Woods DL, and Clayworth C (1988) The effects of lesions of superior temporal gyrus and inferior parietal lobe on temporal and vertex components of the human AEP. *Electroencephalography and Clinical Neurophysiology* 70: 499–509.

Lhermitte F (1986) Human autonomy and the frontal lobes. Part II: Patient behavior in complex and social situations: The "environmental dependency syndrome." *Annals of Neurology* 19: 335–343.

Metzler C and Parkin AJ (2000) Reversed negative priming following frontal lobe lesions. *Neuropsychologia* 38: 363–379.

Miller EK (2000) The prefrontal cortex and cognitive control. *Nature Reviews Neuroscience* 1: 59.

Ramnani N and Owen AM (2004) Anterior prefrontal cortex: Insights into function from anatomy and neuroimaging. *Nature Reviews Neuroscience* 5: 184.

Stuss DT and Knight RT (eds.) (2002) *Principles of Frontal Lobe Function.* Oxford, UK: Oxford University Press.

Williams ZM, Bush G, Rauch SL, Cosgrove GR, and Eskandar EN (2004) Human anterior cingulate neurons and the integration of monetary reward with motor responses. *Nature Neuroscience* 7: 1370–1375.

Executive Function and Higher-Order Cognition: Neuroimaging

S A Bunge and M J Souza, University of California at Davis, Davis, CA, USA

Executive Function

The terms executive function and cognitive control refer to cognitive processes associated with the control of thought and action. Putative control functions include the ability to (1) selectively attend to relevant information while filtering out distracting information (selective attention and interference suppression), (2) work with information that is currently being held in working memory (manipulation), (3) flexibly switch between tasks (task switching), (4) inhibit inappropriate response tendencies (response inhibition), and (5) represent contextual information that determines whether a thought is relevant or whether an action is appropriate (e.g., task-set representation).

Although a number of control processes have been proposed, it is unclear which of these putative processes are distinct from one another. Thus, an important challenge in cognitive control research is to identify a set of elemental control processes and to understand the brain mechanisms underlying each of these processes. One approach that has proven useful for dissociating cognitive processes is the study of patients with various forms of neurological disease and damage. This approach, however, is not without its limitations. As such, convergent evidence from brain imaging techniques is proving increasingly useful.

Probing Executive Function with Neuroimaging Techniques

Functional magnetic resonance imaging (fMRI) has proven useful for identifying brain regions involved in cognitive control. As such, this technique allows us to test whether tasks involving putatively distinct control processes recruit separable brain networks. On the other hand, fMRI allows us to determine whether different tasks that involve a common control process recruit some of the same brain regions.

Prefrontal cortex (PFC) has long been implicated in executive function. Indeed, in 1895, the Italian physiologist Bianchi observed that experimental ablations of the frontal lobes destroyed the ability to synthesize incoming percepts together and to integrate these with outgoing motor commands. Since this early work more than a century ago, countless experiments have been conducted with a variety of techniques to better understand how PFC exerts control over other brain regions.

It is now clear that PFC should not be considered a monolithic structure; indeed, this expansive region constitutes roughly one-third of the human brain and consists of a number of different subregions. Each of these subregions is thought to provide a distinct contribution to cognition via different cellular characteristics and anatomical connectivity. As such, the use of a technique with high spatial resolution, such as fMRI, is essential for determining whether two executive tasks rely on the same or different PFC subregions.

Additionally, it is clear that if we want to understand cognitive control mechanisms, we must examine how PFC interacts with other brain regions. Some information about these interactions can be gleaned from functional connectivity analyses of fMRI data, although fMRI provides little information about the timing of these interactions. For several decades, event-related potential (ERP) data from electroencephalography (EEG) studies have contributed to our knowledge about the timing of control mechanisms. The ERP research of Robert Knight, involving patients with PFC lesions and healthy controls, demonstrated that PFC is necessary for top-down enhancement of relevant information in primary sensory regions.

Tasks Used to Study Executive Function

The most common type of executive task requires participants to override a prepotent response tendency. In the widely used Stroop task, one must override the impulse to read a word out loud and instead indicate the name of the color in which the word is printed (**Figure 1a**). In the go/no-go paradigm, one must press a button in response to a series of rapidly presented visual stimuli but must inhibit responding to a particular stimulus (**Figure 1b**). The continuous performance test known as AX-CPT is similar to go/no-go but additionally has a monitoring component because one must respond to an X followed by an A, but not to an X followed by a B. In the flanker paradigm, one must press one of two buttons in response to a central target stimulus while overriding the response specified by distracters on either side of the target (**Figure 1c**). In a task-switching paradigm, one must switch abruptly from one task rule to another (**Figure 1d**). This type of paradigm is thought to involve both suppression of the prior task rule and retrieval of the new rule. Here, several experimental paradigms are discussed in-depth.

Selective Attention

Goal-directed behavior hinges on the ability to focus on relevant information and ignore distracters, a

Say the name of the color that the word is 'printed' *in*

Stimulus	Response	Trial type
GREEN	'Green'	Congruent
GREEN	'Blue'	Incongruent

a

Press the button for every letter 'except' 'X'

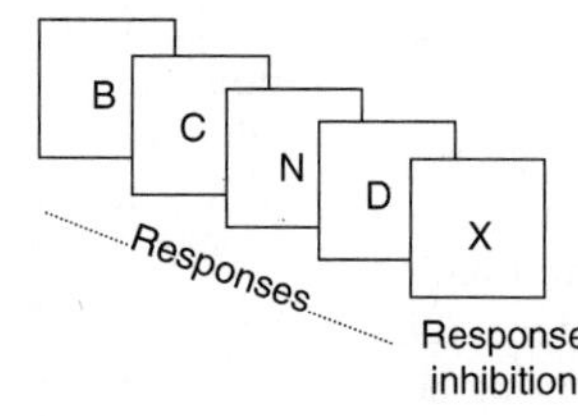

b

Press the left or right button according to the direction of the 'central' arrow

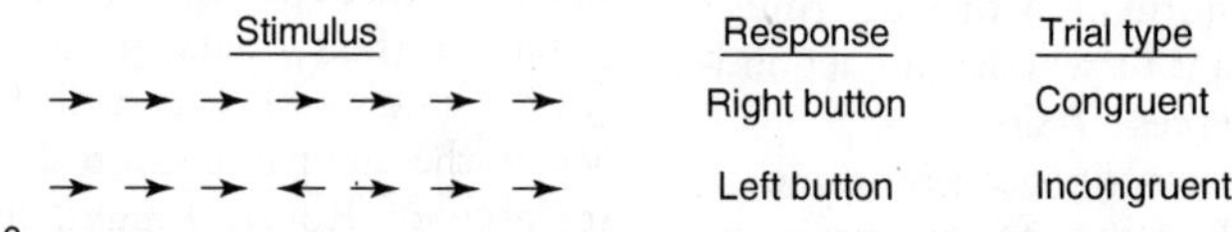

c

'Light borders': press left button for consonants, right button for vowels
'Dark borders': press left button for even numbers, right button for odd numbers

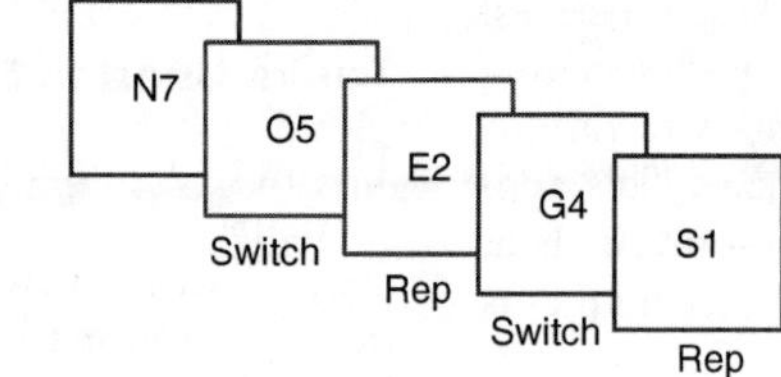

d

Figure 1 Standard versions of several tasks commonly used to study executive function: (a) the Stroop task, (b) the go/no-go task, (c) the Flanker task, and (d) an example of a task-switching paradigm. Variants of these basic paradigms have been used in a number of brain imaging studies.

function referred to as selective attention and/or interference suppression. Although the neural mechanisms are not yet fully understood, a widely accepted model proposed by Desimone and Duncan postulates that selective attention relies on top-down biasing mechanisms. The model proposes that long-range excitatory projections from PFC to posterior cortical regions enhance the activation of relevant representations, which in turn serve to suppress irrelevant representations through local inhibitory interactions. Herd et al. adapted this model in such a way that it can better account for performance and brain activation data from the Stroop task.

Building on earlier behavioral and fMRI work by Lavie and collaborators, Gazzaley and colleagues have conducted fMRI and ERP studies that provide compelling evidence for separable top-down enhancement and suppression effects in a selective attention paradigm. In their task, participants viewed a series of pictures of faces and scenes pseudorandomly intermixed. They were instructed to (1) remember the faces and ignore the scenes, (2) remember the scenes and ignore the faces, (3) remember both, or (4) passively view the stimuli.

The researchers found that a region involved in processing faces – the fusiform face area (FFA) – exhibited enhanced activation relative to the other conditions when participants selectively attended to faces. They further showed that FFA activation was lower relative to the passive view condition when participants ignored faces and attended to scenes instead. The opposite pattern of results was found for the parahippocampal place area (PPA), a region involved in processing scenes (**Figure 2**).

An ERP study involving the same paradigm also showed an enhancement of face processing-related neural activity (the face-selective N170 component)

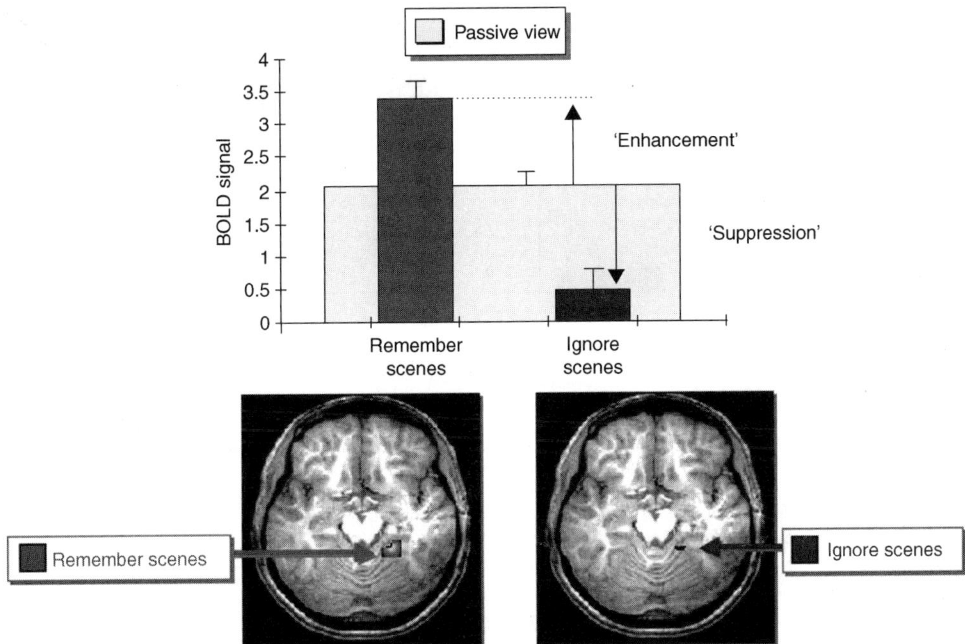

Figure 2 Data from 18 adults aged 19–30 years in an fMRI study on selective attention by Gazzaley and colleagues. These data show that the PPA was more active when participants selectively attended to scenes rather than faces than when they passively viewed both scenes and faces. Additionally, the PPA was less active when participants selectively attended to faces (ignored scenes) than in the passive viewing condition. Participants view the same number of scenes across tasks, and therefore the modulation observed in PPA must be mediated by top-down mechanisms. BOLD: Blood-oxygen level dependent. Courtesy of Adam Gazzaley.

when subjects were instructed to selectively attend to faces. The ERP data further revealed that attention to faces led to faster face processing: indeed, the peak latency of the N170 component was shifted 10 ms earlier for the 'remember faces' condition than for 'ignore faces.' Taken together, these fMRI and ERP results provide strong evidence for top-down modulation of posterior cortical representations as a function of goal relevance.

A large behavioral literature suggests that older adults have difficulty ignoring irrelevant information, but it is unclear from these data whether this deficit is rooted in a specific deficit in top-down suppression of irrelevant information, top-down enhancement of relevant information, or both. As such, Gazzaley and colleagues used the paradigm discussed previously to study selective attention in older adults. Their fMRI data revealed that in older adults, the PPA was not suppressed in the 'ignore scenes' condition relative to the 'passive view' condition (**Figure 3**). In contrast, the PPA did exhibit enhancement for the 'remember scenes' condition relative to 'passive view.' These data indicate that older adults showed a specific deficit in top-down suppression. In addition to providing insight into cognitive changes during aging, this finding lends credence to the idea that suppression and enhancement mechanisms are neurally separable.

Response Inhibition

The ability to inhibit a contextually inappropriate response tendency is central to goal-directed behavior. Numerous brain imaging studies have been conducted in an effort to identify the brain structures that mediate response inhibition. In the go/no-go paradigm, participants must respond to the presentation of each of a rapidly presented stream of visual stimuli, thereby building up a prepotent response tendency. Participants are also instructed to withhold their response to a particular stimulus (the 'no-go' stimulus), which will be presented without warning from time to time (**Figure 1b**). fMRI studies involving the go/no-go paradigm have revealed a network of largely right-hemispheric brain regions associated with successful response inhibition, including right ventrolateral PFC. The go/no-go paradigm has been used not only to study inhibitory control in healthy young adults but also to probe the neural basis of inefficient inhibitory control in children and in patient populations.

Another paradigm used to study response inhibition is the stop-signal task. In the most common variant of this paradigm, participants press a button in response to visual stimuli but must on some occasions (e.g., if they hear a tone) inhibit their response at the last moment (**Figure 4a**). This task is thought to tax

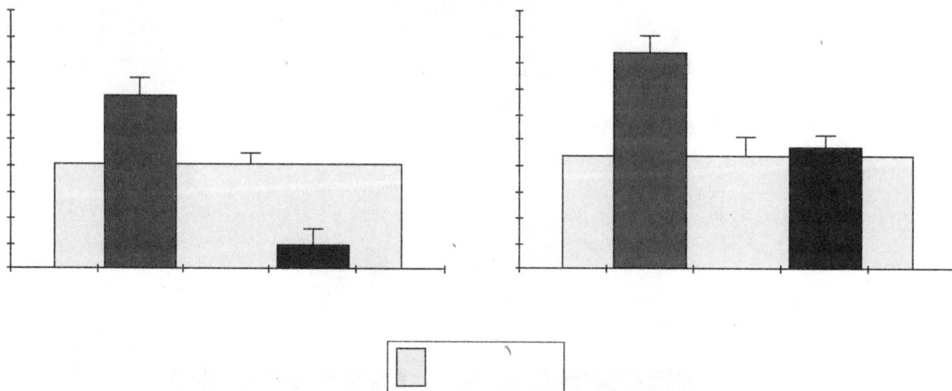

Figure 3 The data from younger adults in **Figure 2** are replotted here as a point of comparison for PPA activation in 16 older adults, aged 60–77 years. For the older adults, like the younger adults, activation in PPA was greater during selective attention to scenes than during passive viewing. In contrast, PPA activation for older adults did not differ between the ignore scenes condition and the passive viewing condition. Thus, the older participants exhibited top-down enhancement of PPA activation but failed to demonstrate top-down suppression. Blood-oxygen level dependent. Courtesy of Adam Gazzaley.

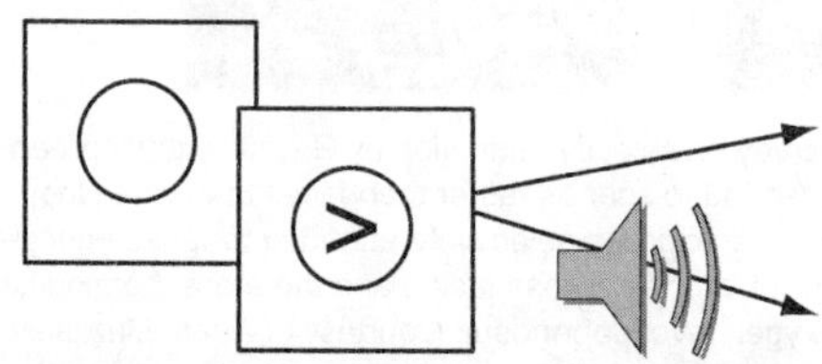

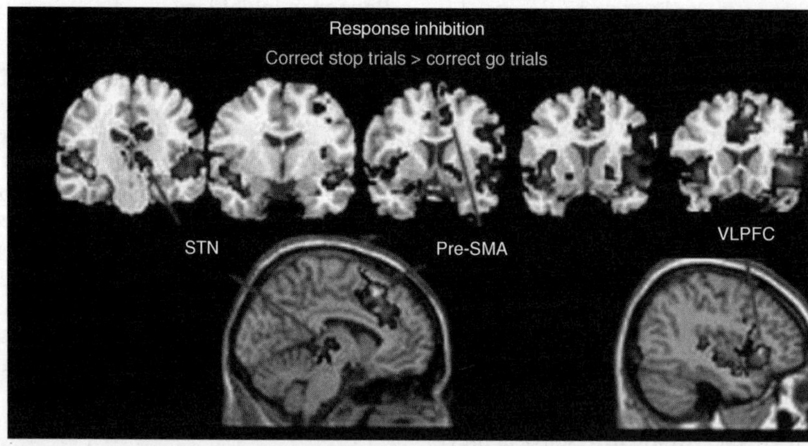

Figure 4 (a) A simplified illustration of the stop-signal paradigm used by Aron and Poldrack. (b) The neural correlates of successful inhibition of motor programs are shown in these activation maps. In particular, three regions – all in the right hemisphere – have been associated with stopping: the subthalamic nucleus (STN), pre-supplementary motor area (pre-SMA), and ventrolateral prefrontal cortex (VLPFC). This pattern of activation suggests that stopping behavior relies on the hyperdirect pathway from PFC to the STN.

response inhibition more heavily than the go/no-go paradigm because participants must override a motor response that they have already initiated. The stop-signal paradigm has an advantage over other response inhibition paradigms for use in clinical and developmental brain imaging studies: the task difficulty varies dynamically on a trial-by-trial basis to ensure a fixed level of performance across participants. As such, differences in brain activation between groups cannot simply be attributed to differences in performance.

In an fMRI study involving the stop-signal paradigm, Aron and Poldrack proposed that stopping is achieved through excitation of the subthalamic nucleus by PFC (**Figure 4b**). From prior work in animals, it is known that the subthalamic nucleus is inhibitory, and that excitation of this nucleus should result in a dampening of activity in the thalamus and cortex. This fMRI study provides evidence in humans for hyperdirect inhibition, bypassing the slower, indirect loop through the basal ganglia. It is likely that some response inhibition paradigms engage the hyperdirect pathway, whereas others engage either the indirect pathway through the basal ganglia or cortico-cortical projections that result in top-down biasing of posterior representations. Further brain imaging research is needed to determine whether various types of response inhibition are indeed neurally separable.

Task-Set Representation

The majority of research on cognitive control focuses on the issue of how PFC controls thought and behavior. An equally interesting question is how PFC 'knows' which thoughts and behaviors to facilitate or suppress. Until we have a satisfactory answer for this question, we will continue to treat PFC as a homunculus – a little man inside the brain who mysteriously knows everything and can direct our thoughts and actions accordingly.

Computational modelers have attempted to decompose or decentralize the homunculus. However, more neuroanatomically detailed computational models will be needed to account for the roles of distinct PFC subregions and other parts of the brain. Such models await a larger body of research on context representations – that is, the information that is used to decide on an appropriate course of action. Context representations could include information about current goals, motivational state, the current situation, rules for behaving in this situation, etc.

The type of context representation that can perhaps be most readily operationalized and studied is the representation of a currently relevant task rule. Research in our laboratory is focused on understanding how rules for behavior are stored in long-term memory, retrieved, maintained online during task preparation, and implemented. Along the same lines, Sakai and Passingham have conducted several elegant studies examining the role of anterior prefrontal cortex (APF; lateral Brodmann area 10) in task preparation.

In these studies, Sakai and Passingham provide evidence from functional connectivity analyses that APF interacts with different brain regions during task preparation, depending on the type of task to be performed. Their first study, in 2003, showed that when participants prepared to perform either a challenging verbal or spatial working memory task, APF activation was strongly correlated with regions involved in verbal or spatial working memory, respectively. Their second study, in 2006, focused exclusively on the verbal domain, and it showed that when participants prepared to perform either a semantic or phonological task, APF was correlated with distinct regions in ventrolateral PFC that have been associated with either semantic or phonological processing. These studies show that APF coordinates task performance by interacting with brain regions that are needed to perform an upcoming task.

Current and Future Directions

During the past decade of brain imaging research, the emphasis has been on using fMRI to localize individual brain regions engaged in various tasks. These endeavors have given us a fairly good idea of the key players in cognitive control and have allowed us to test specific hypotheses regarding their contributions. Furthermore, fMRI studies focusing on adult-individual differences have shown that task performance can be tightly correlated with level of engagement of specific brain regions. Similarly, developmental and clinical fMRI studies have identified brain regions for which differences in level of activation across groups may underlie performance differences.

The next generation of brain imaging techniques will need to combine high-resolution spatial and temporal information. Additionally, further research is needed to better characterize neuropharmacological and genetic influences on brain activation. Several methods that hold promise for the next wave of studies probing executive function are discussed here.

Combined fMRI and EEG Methodology

fMRI and EEG are complimentary techniques in that the former allows for the precise spatial localization of active brain regions, and the latter provides exquisite timing information about the onset and offset of neural activity. To push our understanding of cognitive control mechanisms to the next level, it will be necessary to acquire data with high spatial and temporal resolution.

One approach is to acquire fMRI and EEG data on the same group of participants, in separate sessions. The set of brain regions identified from the fMRI data can then be used to constrain the source localization of the ERP data. Another, more technically challenging, approach is to simultaneously acquire fMRI and EEG data from the same participants. This latter approach has been used successfully in a study on performance monitoring by Debener and colleagues. Several groups are working on multimodal imaging approaches, including combined fMRI/EEG, and the further development of these methods should provide new insights into the neural mechanisms of executive function.

Event-Related Optical Signals

Gratton and Fabiani and their colleagues have developed an optical imaging technique with high spatial and temporal resolution known as EROS, or the event-related optical signal. The standard analytic approach for optical imaging data analysis is to focus on changes in optical properties of the cortical brain tissue associated with changes in blood flow, which are only indirectly related to changes in neural activity. Given the sluggish blood flow response to neuronal activity, optical imaging – like fMRI – typically has poor temporal resolution. In contrast, with EROS, the optical changes that are being analyzed are directly related to neural activity. In addition to having high temporal resolution, the EROS signal also has a high degree of spatial resolution; it can be localized to an area of less than a cubic centimeter. The main drawback of this method is that it can only be used to measure activity within 3–5 cm of the surface of the brain.

The developers of EROS have used it to study response competition in a Stroop task. They showed that both left and right motor cortices were active in response to an incongruent Stroop stimulus, even though participants were instructed to respond to the stimulus by pressing a button with only one hand. In contrast, congruent Stroop stimuli, which did not elicit response competition, elicited activation of only the contralateral motor cortex. Since this validation study was performed approximately 5 years ago, the technique has been further fine-tuned and validated. Although only a few published studies have employed EROS thus far, the use of this technique may spread as more researchers become aware of its potential.

See also: Attentional Networks; Cognition: An Overview of Neuroimaging Techniques; Cognitive Control and Development; Electroencephalography (EEG); Event-Related Potentials (ERPs) and Cognitive Processing; Executive Function and Higher-Order Cognition: Assessment in Animals; fMRI: BOLD Contrast; Neuroimaging; Optical Imaging of Intrinsic Signals; Prefrontal Cortex: Structure and Anatomy.

Further Reading

Aron AR and Poldrack RA (2006) Cortical and subcortical contributions to Stop signal response inhibition: Role of the subthalamic nucleus. *Journal of Neuroscience* 26: 2424–2433.

Braver TS and Barch DM (2002) A theory of cognitive control, aging cognition, and neuromodulation. *Neuroscience & Biobehavioral Reviews* 26: 809–817.

Bunge SA, Dudukovic NM, Thomason ME, Vaidya CJ, and Gabrieli JD (2002) Immature frontal lobe contributions to cognitive control in children: Evidence from fMRI. *Neuron* 33: 301–311.

Casey BJ, Trainor RJ, Orendi JL, et al. (1997) A developmental functional MRI study of prefrontal activation during performance of a go-no-go task. *Journal of Cognitive Neuroscience* 9: 835–847.

Collette F, Hogge M, Salmon E, and Van Der Linden M (2006) Exploration of the neural substrates of executive functioning by functional neuroimaging. *Neuroscience* 139: 209–221.

de Fockert JW, Rees G, Frith CD, and Lavie N (2001) The role of working memory in visual selective attention. *Science* 291: 1803–1806.

Debener S, Ullsperger M, Siegel M, et al. (2005) Trial-by-trial coupling of concurrent electroencephalogram and functional magnetic resonance imaging identifies the dynamics of performance monitoring. *Journal of Neuroscience* 25: 11730–11737.

Desimone R and Duncan J (1995) Neural mechanisms of selective visual attention. *Annual Review of Neuroscience* 18: 193–222.

DeSoto MC, Fabiani M, Geary DC, and Gratton G (2001) When in doubt, do it both ways: Brain evidence of the simultaneous activation of conflicting motor responses in a spatial Stroop task. *Journal of Cognitive Neuroscience* 13: 523–536.

Durston S, Tottenham NT, Thomas KM, et al. (2003) Differential patterns of striatal activation in young children with and without ADHD. *Biological Psychiatry* 53: 871–878.

Frith CD and Friston KJ (1997) Studying brain function with neuroimaging. In: Rugg M (ed.) *Cognitive Neuroscience*, pp. 169–195. Cambridge: MIT Press.

Garavan H, Ross TJ, and Stein EA (1999) Right hemispheric dominance of inhibitory control: An event-related functional MRI study. *Proceedings of the National Academy of Sciences of the United States of America* 96: 8301–8306.

Gazzaley A, Cooney JW, McEvoy K, Knight RT, and D'Esposito M (2005) Top-down enhancement and suppression of the magnitude and speed of neural activity. *Journal of Cognitive Neuroscience* 17: 507–517.

Gazzaley A, Cooney JW, Rissman J, and D'Esposito M (2005) Top-down suppression deficit underlies working memory impairment in normal aging. *Nature Neuroscience* 8: 1298–1300.

Goethals I, Audenaert K, Van de Wiele C, and Dierckx R (2004) The prefrontal cortex: Insights from functional neuroimaging using cognitive activation tasks. *European Journal of Nuclear Medicine and Molecular Imaging* 31(3): 408–416.

Goldberg TE and Weinberger DR (2004) Genes and the parsing of cognitive processes. *Trends in Cognitive Science* 8(7): 325–335.

Gratton G and Fabiani M (2001) Shedding light on brain function: The event-related optical signal. *Trends in Cognitive Science* 5: 357–363.

Gratton G and Fabiani M (2003) The event-related optical signal (EROS) in visual cortex: Replicability, consistency, localization, and resolution. *Psychophysiology* 40: 561–571.

Herd SA, Banich MT, and O'Rei RC (2006) Neural mechanisms of cognitive control: An integrative model of Stroop task performance and fMRI data. *Journal of Cognitive Neuroscience* 18: 22–32.

Knight RT, Grabowecky MF, and Scabini D (1995) Role of human prefrontal cortex in attention control. *Advances in Neurology* 66: 21–36.

Kutas M and Dale A (1997) Electrical and magnetic readings of mental functions. In: Rugg M (ed.) *Cognitive Neuroscience*, pp. 197–242. Cambridge: MIT Press.

O'Reilly RC, Noelle DC, Braver TS, and Cohen JD (2002) Prefrontal cortex and dynamic categorization tasks: Representational organization and neuromodulatory control. *Cerebral Cortex* 12: 246–257.

Sakai K and Passingham R (2006) Prefrontal set activity predicts rule-specific neural processing during subsequent cognitive performance. *Journal of Neuroscience* 26: 1211–1218.

Sakai K and Passingham RE (2003) Prefrontal interactions reflect future task operations. *Nature Neuroscience* 6: 75–81.

Executive Functions: Eye Movements and Neuropsychiatric Disorders

A B Sereno, S L Babin, A J Hood, and C B Jeter,
The University of Texas Health Science Center at Houston, Houston, TX, USA

What Are Executive Functions?

Executive functions are complex, higher order processes moderated primarily by the frontal lobe, specifically the prefrontal cortex. The complexity of executive function has made a universally accepted definition elusive, but attention (focusing on relevant information and ignoring distractors), working memory (maintaining information until execution), and motor planning (goal-directed motor planning and programming) are generally considered key executive functions. Executive functions influence social, emotional, intellectual, and organizational aspects of one's life. Life can be devastated when executive functions are disrupted. Unfortunately, such disruptions occur in many human disorders.

Eye Movements and Executive Functions

Eye movements are any shift of position of the eye in its orbit. There are many different kinds of eye movements, which are defined in the next section titled 'Classes of eye movements.' Eye movements determine what information reaches our retina, visual cortex, and most important, higher cortical centers. Hence, eye movements are critically important for vision, attention, and memory; they determine what we see, attend to, and remember about our surroundings. They are thus central to executive functions. Much scientific work also suggests that the brain circuitry subserving certain executive functions, such as that for spatial attention and spatial working memory, overlaps parts of the brain circuitry subserving control of eye movements. Thus, better understanding of eye movements provides a valuable window into executive functions.

Classes of Eye Movements

There are several classes of eye movements, with, for the most part, distinct neural circuitry. Eye movements serve to stabilize images on the retina and to keep objects of interest on the fovea, the retinal area that has the greatest visual acuity and the greatest representation in visual cortices. Without compensatory eye movements during self-motion (locomotion) or head movement, images of the visual world would blur and slip across the retina with each movement. Two classes of eye movements, vestibulo-ocular and optokinetic reflexes, evolved to stabilize images on the retina during such head and body perturbations. In the case of the vestibulo-ocular reflex, when the head moves to the right, 'vestibular' sensors in the inner ear are triggered and signal nuclei in the horizontal and vertical gaze centers of the brainstem to create an equal and opposite eye velocity signal. The result is that the vestibulo-ocular reflex initiates a rapid eye movement to the left (within about 15 ms) to compensate for the head movement, keeping the retina stable with respect to the world. The second mechanism, the optokinetic reflex, complements the first by using full-field 'visual' information about self-movement to compensate for the perturbation of the visual world on the retina. That is, as a result of self-motion to the right, the entire visual image will move across the retina in a leftward direction. The speed of the image drift on the retina triggers nuclei in the brainstem to create an equal leftward eye velocity signal. The result is the optokinetic reflex, an eye movement in the same direction as the retinal slip to keep the retina stable with respect to the world.

A third class of eye movements serves to rapidly shift gaze (up to $900°s^{-1}$) to bring a new object of interest to the fovea. These saccades are often further subdivided into two general subclasses: reflexive and voluntary. Reflexive saccades are elicited in response to a sudden movement, flash, or change in the environment. The latency (onset of movement) of a reflexive saccade to a visual target is typically about 200–250 ms, but it can be as short as 70–80 ms. Voluntary saccades are more complex, involve executive functions, are thought to critically involve frontal cortex, and have latencies as long as 400 ms. In real life, for instance, the same environment can result in different voluntarily controlled saccadic eye movements, depending on what information is sought or needs to be remembered. This was elegantly demonstrated by Yarbus in 1967 when he presented the same picture to participants several times but each time asked a different question. Depending on the question, the participants scanned the picture with a strikingly different set of voluntary saccades to acquire the pertinent information. In a similar fashion, **Figure 1** illustrates an example of the scanpaths of a naïve participant viewing a Vermeer painting.

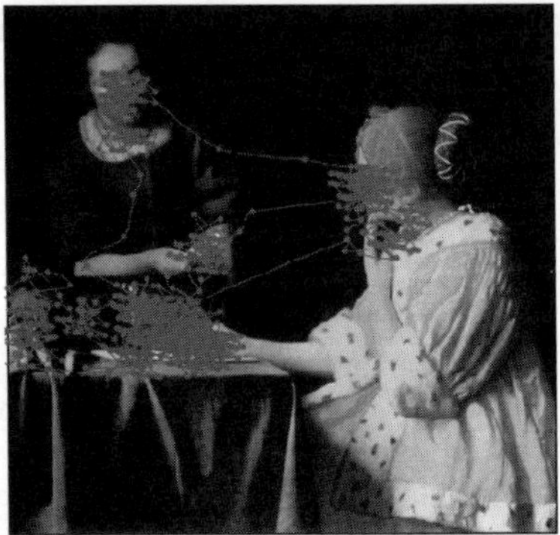
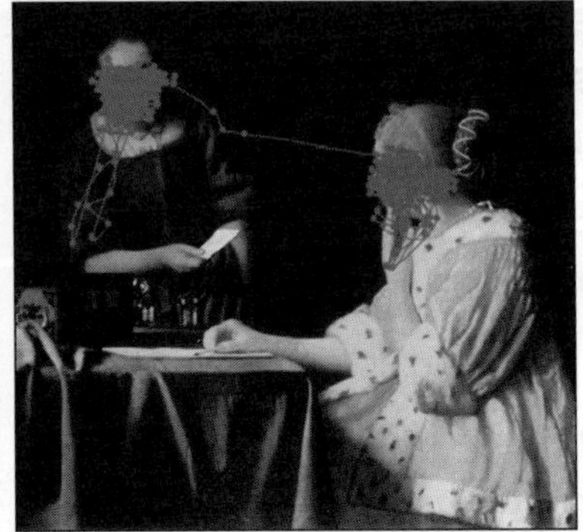

Figure 1 Scanpaths of a naïve individual viewing Vermeer's *Mistress and Maid.* This person was told that two pictures would be presented sequentially for 5 s each and that before each picture, a question would be asked. The person was told to look at the picture for the answer and reply after the viewing finished. (Left) The first question asked was, "What are they doing?" The picture was then presented, and the person's scanpath was recorded for 5 s. The individual then replied, "delivering and receiving a letter." (Right) The second question asked was, "How old are they?" The same picture was presented again and the scanpath recorded for 5 s. The person then replied "35." The scanpaths for the same picture were very different based simply on the context of what the individual was asked.

The first panel illustrates the scanpath when the picture was preceded with the question, "What are they doing?" The participant made saccades that followed the gaze of the two women in the picture and then dwelled on the hands, the table, and the objects on the table. The second panel illustrates the scanpath when the same picture was preceded with the question, "How old are they?" In this context, the participant looked almost exclusively at the women's faces.

In the research lab or clinic, a prosaccade task is frequently used to elicit reflexive saccades (see **Figure 2**). In this paradigm, the participant fixates a center spot, a visual target appears to the left or right of center, and the participant is instructed to look at the target. Voluntary saccades can be elicited by many different eye movement paradigms (see also **Figure 2**). In an antisaccade task, a peripheral target is presented (as in the prosaccade task), but the correct response is to look to the opposite side of the screen, away from the target. The antisaccade task requires a person to (1) inhibit the reflexive inclination to look at the target and (2) generate a voluntary saccade to the correct location opposite the target. Abnormal responses in the antisaccade task include increased latency and directional errors (looking to the target). A delayed saccade task also requires a voluntary saccade. This task is similar to a prosaccade task in that the person is required to make an eye movement to the target. However, the person is also instructed to wait until a go signal is given (a tone or change in fixation cue). Therefore, the person must inhibit the reflexive tendency to look at the target immediately and generate a voluntary saccade when the go signal is presented. A third commonly used voluntary saccade paradigm is a memory-guided saccade task. This task is identical to the delayed saccade task, except that the target is removed from the screen during the delay period. Now, the person must inhibit the eye movement until the go signal and also remember where the target was presented. Hence, this task also demands working memory.

Smooth pursuit eye movements (SPEMs) function to keep a small moving stimulus on the fovea and are typically much slower than saccades, with a maximum velocity of about $100\,°\mathrm{s}^{-1}$. Smooth pursuit is a voluntary task requiring both motivation and attention. Hence, if one chooses to track a mosquito, when the mosquito takes off, one's eyes would initiate smooth pursuit 100–150 ms later, an onset of movement that is generally shorter than that for a saccade. Thus, the eyes would first begin to pursue but lag a bit behind the mosquito. After about another 100 ms, this is remedied by a 'catch-up saccade' that repositions the moving eyes directly on the mosquito. SPEMs are the result of a complex transformation from visual motion signals at the fovea to an oculomotor signal. Cortical input to the smooth eye movement generation centers in the brainstem is required to enable smooth tracking motion. At the same time, however, there must be suppression of the optokinetic reflex and, if the eye movement is accompanied by head tracking, the vestibulo-ocular reflex. SPEM paradigms are used frequently to measure executive function in clinical populations. One measure of accuracy in SPEM paradigms is pursuit gain (the ratio between eye velocity and target velocity). Gain values below 1.0 indicate that the pursuit system is not matching the velocity of the target. Errors in gain can be amended with catch-up saccades (when

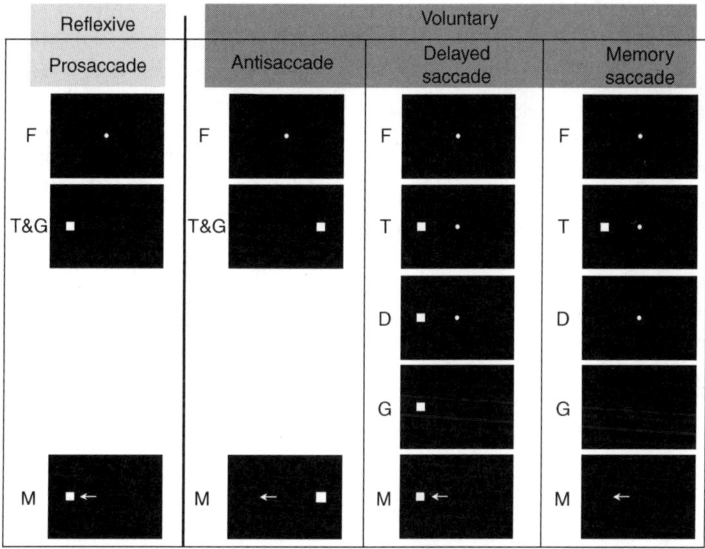

Figure 2 Examples of four saccade tasks. All tasks are presented sequentially from top to bottom, and the arrows indicate the direction of the correct eye movement. Prosaccade: This is a reflexive task in which an individual begins by fixating the center point (F). Once fixation is maintained, a target light appears, and the person makes an eye movement to the light (T&G). Antisaccade: An individual begins by fixating the center point (F). The target light then appears (T&G), and the person is to make an eye movement to the equal and opposite position of the target. Delayed Saccade: The individual begins by fixating the center point (F). Next, the target light appears (T), followed by a delay period (D), during which the person must continue fixating the center point. At some variable time, the fixation light disappears, which serves as a go signal (G) for the person to begin an eye movement to the target. Memory Saccade: The individual fixates the center point (F). The target light then flashes on the screen (T), followed by a delay period (D), during which the individual must continue fixating the center point. At some variable time, the fixation light disappears, which serves as the go signal (G) for the person to begin an eye movement to the remembered location where the target had previously flashed. F, fixation screen; T, target onset; G, go signal to begin an eye movement; D, delay period, when the participant must wait for the go signal; M, eye movement.

smooth pursuit lags behind the target) and backup saccades (when tracking gets ahead of the target). Further, there can be intrusive saccades, which interrupt smooth pursuit tracking and are indicative of inhibitory failures or inappropriate activations.

Vergence is the only disconjugate eye movement; that is, the eyes move simultaneously in opposite directions. Vergence movements occur reflexively in order to focus and reduce disparity between the locations of an image on the retina of each eye.

Eye Movements in Human Disorders

Voluntary eye movements as a general class can be used to tease out specific deficits in different aspects of executive function in clinical populations. By careful comparison of performance on voluntary eye movement tasks, a 'deficit in executive function' (as generally classified, for example, by a neuropsychiatric test) can be broken down into separable aspects of executive function, including the voluntary planning, generation, and accuracy of a response, the ability to inhibit or control impulse responding, and working memory. Voluntary eye movements have been linked to different anatomical circuitry and can be used to characterize subtypes within some patient populations.

Neurological

Tourette's syndrome and Parkinson's disease are movement disorders involving the basal ganglia. Both disorders show deficits in executive function with evidence of disrupted prefrontal–basal ganglia circuits. Voluntary eye movement deficits are consistent with these documented impaired executive functions. Both groups show increased antisaccade latency and antisaccade errors. The effect of medication on voluntary eye movements in Tourette's syndrome is not clearly known. On the other hand, dopaminergic medications, routinely given to treat Parkinson's disease, do improve voluntary eye movement performance. Further, voluntary saccade performance differentiates between subtypes of Parkinson's disease patients such that akinetic-rigid Parkinson's disease patients have more difficulty on voluntary eye movement tasks than do tremor-dominant patients.

Developmental

Autism is a developmental behavioral disorder marked by abnormal language and social communication resulting from deficits in limbic and cortical structures. Numerous studies have investigated voluntary eye movement performance in children and adults with autism as a means of understanding the etiology and social implications of this disorder. For instance, voluntary eye movements (saccades and SPEMs) have been used to show that executive function abilities are delayed in autistic patients; their voluntary abilities seem to mature to a lower level and at a slower rate. Likewise, results from voluntary saccade tasks suggest that deficits in autistic individuals critically involve the prefrontal cortex.

Psychiatric

Eye movements have been studied most extensively in schizophrenia, as is discussed in the next section. Attention-deficit/hyperactivity disorder (ADHD) is characterized by symptoms (sometimes beginning before age 7) of inattention, hyperactivity, or impulsivity that cause impairment at school, home, or work. ADHD patients have been shown to be impaired on a countermanding task (similar to a delayed saccade task, but a stop signal may be presented on some trials to indicate the response should be withheld), which suggests that their impairment mainly consists of increased impulsivity. In addition, voluntary eye movement deficits have shown subtype differences within the ADHD population. Specifically, patients classified as ADHD-Inattentive have better motor planning and are less impulsive than ADHD patients with both inattentive and impulsive characteristics. Interestingly, methylphenidate improves the voluntary eye movement performance of both ADHD subtypes. Bipolar disorder is a disturbance in mood marked by cycling periods of mania and/or depression. Bipolar patients have been shown to have an inhibition problem but to date no deficit in working memory on voluntary eye movement paradigms. Bipolar patients, as well as lithium-withdrawn manic patients, have been shown to perform more poorly than normal controls on a SPEM task.

Eye Movement Deficits in Schizophrenia

What Is Schizophrenia?

Schizophrenia is the most prevalent mental illness in the world, occurring in about 1% of the population. It is also considered the most costly and debilitating mental disorder and is among the top causes of disability in developing countries. In 2002, it cost the United States approximately $\$65 \times 10^9$, and this estimate accounted only for patient hospitalizations, loss of work, and cost of disability. Schizophrenia is a psychiatric disorder that is usually characterized by hallucinations, delusions, blunted affect, alogia (i.e., poverty of speech), and avolition. Numerous cognitive functions in areas such as executive control, working memory, and attention are disturbed. These disrupted executive functions are more persistent than psychotic symptoms. More robust measures of cognitive deficits are crucial, given that there is a strong positive correlation between improved cognitive functioning and long-term prognosis. Classically, neuropsychological tests have been used to investigate cognitive dysfunctions in schizophrenia, but recently, eye movement tasks have been shown to be a more sensitive and reliable measure of these deficits. Eye movements are also more easily mapped to specific neural structures and hence may be a more specific biological marker for differentiating subtypes. For these reasons, the study of eye movements is an important research tool that will shed light on both executive functions and debilitating human disorders such as schizophrenia.

Eye Movement Deficits

Nearly a hundred years ago (1908), using a photographic technique, Diefendorf and Dodge were the first to report that SPEMs were impaired in schizophrenia. They found that pursuit was commonly interrupted by saccades. With the advent of new techniques for measuring eye movements, as well as renewed interest, much is now known about SPEM deficits in schizophrenia.

There seem to be two basic deficits in the SPEMs of people with schizophrenia: (1) reduced gain of smooth pursuit and (2) increased saccadic events. Pursuit gain is a measure of the accuracy of the smooth eye movement, and people with schizophrenia show reduced gain, that is, their eyes do not keep up with the target, and they often fall behind. As a result, schizophrenic patients often exhibit increased saccadic activity (catch-up saccades) during smooth pursuit. These saccades are automatic and compensatory in nature and serve to quickly refoveate the target on the retina. Other increased saccadic events observed in schizophrenia are saccadic intrusions. These eye movements are not compensatory and are thus inappropriate. Common examples of saccadic intrusions are square-wave jerks and anticipatory saccades. A square-wave jerk is a small pair of saccades whose initial direction takes the eyes off the target. After a 100–250 ms intersaccadic interval, during which pursuit continues, a second saccade returns the eyes to the target. Anticipatory saccades overshoot the location of the target. These saccades have larger amplitudes than those of square-wave jerks and longer intersaccadic intervals, and they do not maintain continuous pursuit during the intersaccadic period. Both these types of intrusive saccadic eye movements are rarely found in young controls (although they are sometimes found in older people) and indicate inappropriate activation or lack of inhibition of the saccadic system during smooth pursuit.

In addition to smoothpursuit deficits, a number of saccadic eye movement dysfunctions have been identified in schizophrenia. Numerous studies have shown deficits in various voluntary saccade tasks, including delayed, remembered, or predictive saccades. In an antisaccade task, schizophrenic participants typically are slower to generate a saccade to the correct location and make more errors (i.e., eye movements to the target) compared with normal controls. In contrast, many studies have demonstrated that schizophrenic participants perform normally or in some cases faster than controls on a prosaccade task. This pattern of saccade task performance has in some studies been related to the participant's performance on SPEMs. That is, schizophrenic patients with smooth pursuit deficits make significantly more errors on the antisaccade task than schizophrenic patients without eye tracking deficits.

Biological Basis of Eye Movement Deficits

Schizophrenic patients with SPEM deficits do not show abnormal slow phases of vestibulo-ocular and optokinetic responses. This dissociation suggests that the smooth pursuit abnormalities in schizophrenia are due to cortical deficits rather than deficits in common brainstem motor output pathways. Evidence for a prefrontal cortex dysfunction model of schizophrenia has also gained support. One key piece of evidence for such a model came from the similarity between symptoms of blunted affect, avolition, and inattention seen in schizophrenic patients and symptoms exhibited by neurological patients with a loss of frontal lobe function. A further piece of evidence in support of frontal lobe dysfunction in schizophrenia came from eye movement research. It was already well established that frontal regions, especially the frontal eye fields, play a role in saccades. Further research also demonstrated that lesions in the frontal eye fields disrupt SPEMs. Hence, frontal dysfunction could account for both pursuit deficits and saccadic deficits.

It is interesting to note that between 50% and 85% of individuals with schizophrenia exhibit SPEM dysfunction, in contrast to only about 8% of normal controls. Similarly, about 60% of individuals with schizophrenia exhibit antisaccade eye movement deficits. People with schizophrenia are heterogeneous in terms of both smooth pursuit deficits and voluntary saccade deficits. This division of impaired and nonimpaired patients (for either pursuit gain or voluntary saccade performance) may prove to be more useful than the classic clinical subtypes in characterizing homogeneous subgroups of patients.

Genetics of Eye Movement Deficits

In the late 1970s and early 1980s, a series of studies investigated the genetics of smooth pursuit deficits in monozygotic and dizygotic twins who were discordant for schizophrenia. These studies found that a larger proportion of monozygotic twins than dizygotic twins exhibited abnormal smooth pursuit eye tracking. Moreover, about half of clinically well first-degree relatives of schizophrenic patients exhibit SPEM deficits, a prevalence much greater than recurrence risk for schizophrenia in first-degree relatives, which is about 6.5%. In addition, some recent reports suggest that 25–50% of nonsymptomatic first-degree relatives of schizophrenic patients exhibit antisaccade deficits. Within the last several years, linkage has been reported for both smooth pursuit deficits and anti-saccade deficits in genetic studies of schizophrenia. Endophenotypes such as eye movement dysfunctions may be a more penetrant expression of a schizophrenia susceptibility gene than schizophrenia.

Importance of Subtypes and Genetics for Outcome

Eye movement monitoring is an important research tool because it affords the opportunity to use a quick, easy, and noninvasive technique to help identify behaviors that may indicate susceptibility for schizophrenia. Since it is possible that people with schizophrenia who exhibit eye movement deficits are genetically differentiable from those who do not, eye tracking may provide more reliable and robust criteria for the classification of different groups of people with schizophrenia. Such a biologically based classification system may allow us to investigate particular antipsychotic medication effects across different subgroups of schizophrenic patients. For example, it is possible that task-impaired patients will show a greater benefit from a specific medication. Such a finding has been reported with nicotine and schizophrenia: patients impaired on an antisaccade task showed a greater benefit from nicotine than did nonimpaired patients and controls. A similar subtype-specific medication effect has also been demonstrated in Parkinson's disease. It was found that akinetic-rigid patients are poorer than tremor-dominant patients on voluntary eye movement tasks, such as the antisaccade task, and that only tremor-dominant patients were able to significantly improve their performance on this task after dopaminergic medications were administered. A better understanding of subtype-specific medication effects would be pivotal in assigning the most effective medication to the patients who would benefit the most.

In summary, eye movements provide invaluable information about executive functions and provide an efficient, noninvasive way to study the role of abnormal brain processes in a variety of human disorders. Their study may afford the development of more effective and efficient treatments of executive dysfunction.

See also: Attention Deficit Hyperactivity Disorder; Attention and Eye Movements; Attention: Models; Autism; Brainstem Control of Eye Movements; Cognitive Deficits in Schizophrenia; Cortical Control of Eye Movements; Eye Tracking and Mental Illness; Eye and Head Movements; Eye Movement Disorders; Frontal Eye Fields; Prefrontal Cortex: Structure and Anatomy; Psychophysics of Attention; Saccades and Visual Search; Saccadic Eye Movements; Schizophrenia: Epidemiology, Clinical Features, Course and Outcome; Visual Attention.

Further Reading

Büttner U and Büttner-Ennever JA (1988) Present concepts of oculomotor organization. *Reviews of Oculomotor Research* 2: 3–32.

Calkins ME and Iacono WG (2000) Eye movement dysfunction in schizophrenia: A heritable characteristic for enhancing phenotype definition. *American Journal of Medical Genetics* 97: 72–76.

Clementz BA and Sweeney JA (1990) Is eye movement dysfunction a biological marker for schizophrenia? A methodological review. *Psychology Bulletin* 108: 77–92.

Hanisch C, Radach R, Holtkamp K, Herpertz-Dahlmann B, and Konrad K (2006) Oculomotor inhibition in children with and without attention-deficit hyperactivity disorder (ADHD). *Journal of Neural Transmission* 113(5): 671–684.

Klein C, Fischer B, and Hartnegg K (2002) Effects of methylphenidate on saccadic responses in patients with ADHD. *Experimental Brain Research* 145: 121–125.

Levin S (1984) Frontal lobe dysfunctions in schizophrenia. II. Impairments of psychological and brain functions. *Journal of Psychiatric Research* 18: 57–72.

Levy DL, Holzman PS, Matthysse S, and Mendell NR (1993) Eye tracking dysfunction and schizophrenia: A critical perspective. *Schizophrenia Bulletin* 19: 461–536.

Reuter B and Kathmann N (2004) Using saccade tasks as a tool to analyze executive dysfunctions in schizophrenia. *Acta Psychologica* 115: 255–269.

Schiess MC, Zheng H, Soukup VM, Bonnen JG, and Nauta HJ (2000) Parkinson's disease subtypes: Clinical classification and ventricular cerebrospinal fluid analysis. *Parkinsonism and Related Disorders* 6: 69–76.

Sereno AB (1996) Parsing cognitive processes: Psychopathological and neurophysiological constraints. In: Matthysse S, Levy DL, Kagan J, and Benes FM (eds.) *Psychopathology: The Evolving Science of Mental Disorder*, pp. 407–432. New York: Cambridge University Press.

Sweeney JA, Takarae Y, Macmillan C, Luna B, and Minshew NJ (2004) Eye movements in neurodevelopmental disorders. *Current Opinions in Neurology* 17: 37–42.

Frontal Lobe Syndrome

D T Stuss, Rotman Research Institute, Baycrest, Toronto, ON, Canada; and University of Toronto, Toronto, ON, Canada
M P Alexander, Harvard Medical School, Beth Israel Deaconess Medical Center, Boston, MA, USA and Rotman Research Institute, Baycrest, Toronto, ON, Canada

Introduction

This article describes the functions associated with the frontal lobes, particularly as demonstrated by studies of patients with focal brain lesions. Modern neuroscience is overwhelmingly dominated by functional imaging studies in normal subjects, but functional imaging can only demonstrate, or in some cases only imply, a role for a region in a particular, often very narrowly defined cognitive task. Lesion studies are an essential counterbalance to functional imaging as the only mechanism to identify areas that are necessary for specific functions. Lesion studies have, however, often been hampered by sweeping up an amorphous and varied group of deficits, including cognitive, affective, comportment, and personality changes, under the term 'frontal lobe syndrome' as though there were a single frontal lobe syndrome that only varied in severity. The notion of a unitary frontal lobe syndrome, based solely on the coarsest anatomical distinctions, evolved at a time when lesion location was not easily specified and often in patients who were examined at a later stage of disease. The unitary syndrome notion was not strongly influenced by the observations that it could include diametrically opposite properties: patients could be impulsive or apathetic, distractible or perseverative, restless or bradykinetic, and so on. In recent years, the clinical research focus has changed from a concentration on the anatomical basis of the disordered cognition or behavior to an emphasis on the functional nature of those impairments under the supraordinate label of 'dysexecutive' disorder, but attribution of the dysexecutive syndrome to lesions of the frontal lobes has always been clear, although usually only implied and not demonstrated. This switch to a functional definition has its own problems. It, too, was often seen as a unitary disorder, and many, possibly most, patients with executive impairments did not have lesions restricted to frontal structures. In fact, many had disorders such as depression, sleep apnea, concussions, chronic pain, and other problems not easily tied to a structural injury of the frontal lobes. Although clinical neurology and neuropsychology are still quite tied to the concepts of frontal lobe syndrome and dysexecutive disorder, clinical research has increasingly demonstrated that specific, highly differentiated cognitive, motivational, behavioral, and attentional deficits are associated with discrete regional frontal injuries.

Our analysis suggests that frontal lobe functions fall into four distinct categories, each associated with a different frontal region. Only one of these categories is truly 'executive.' The other three categories cannot be subsumed under the common understanding of executive functions. Executive functions are best understood within a model of higher level attentional abilities. The executive functions are associated with discrete regions within the frontal lobes. We conclude that there is no single frontal system and not even a single frontal executive system and, thus, no undifferentiated frontal lobe or dysexecutive syndrome. There are domain general executive functions, each with a specific regional frontal basis, that are recruited over time in response to contextual demands.

There are four sections to this article. The first summarizes the anatomy and pathophysiology of the frontal lobes to provide a context for understanding research in frontal lobe functions. The second defines the proposed four categories of frontal lobe functions, with an emphasis on the one category most consonant with the term executive. The third section describes the interactive relationship between the executive functions and between executive functions and the other categories of frontal functions, emphasizing the organization of networks of processes and the unfolding of processes in time. We conclude with a brief description of the potential treatment of patients with frontal lobe damage.

Anatomy and Pathophysiology

The frontal lobes are the regions anterior to the Rolandic fissure and superior to the Sylvian fissure. They constitute one-fourth to one-third of the human brain. This article focuses on the prefrontal cortex, the area rostral to primary motor (Brodmann area 4, generation of movement) and premotor (Brodmann area 6, programming of sequential movements) cortex. The prefrontal cortex can be roughly subdivided into regions in which adjacent Brodmann area regions have similar connectivity patterns: lateral (dorsolateral: 9, 46, and perhaps 8; ventrolateral: 44, 45, and lateral 47/12), orbitofrontal (11–14; and orbital 47/12), polar (area 10), inferior medial (ventral anterior cingulate and paracingulate 24, 25, and 32), and superior medial (8, 9, dorsal anterior cingulate 24, 32, and perhaps including supplementary motor

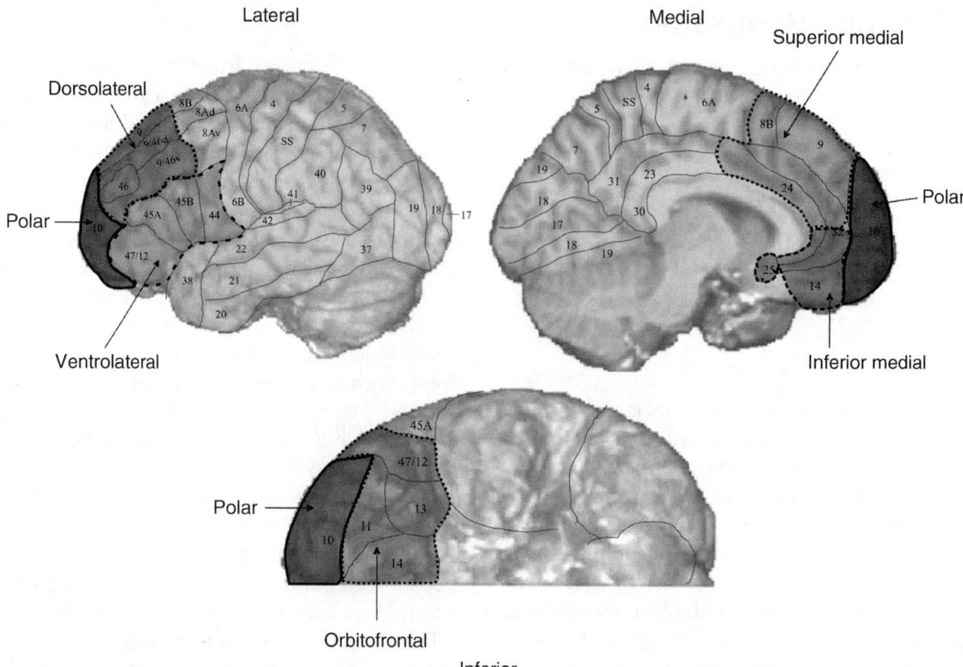

Figure 1 Depiction of the different regions within the frontal lobes.

area 6) (**Figure 1**). Only the lateral regions show strong functional hemispheric asymmetry.

The prefrontal cortex has strong reciprocal connections with virtually all other cortical regions. The specific patterns of connectivity determine the roles of different prefrontal regions in integrating and influencing all types of mental operations, cognitive and affective. In addition to functionally relevant cortico-cortical connections, there are parallel but independent frontal–subcortical circuits. The circuits are functionally distinct, and damage to any part of a circuit may produce similar discrete functional impairments. These may be more pervasive than suggested by cortical lesion alone and may be significant even in the absence of cortical lesions.

With the possible exception of early frontal–temporal lobe degeneration, there is no natural clinical condition in which pathology only involves the frontal lobes, but almost any neurological disease may preferentially affect the frontal lobes. Each has specific advantages for illuminating frontal functions.

Infarction is most common. Because infarcts are almost always unilateral and lesion boundaries are sharp, infarcts have always been the 'preferred' pathology for clinical–anatomical studies. Anterior cerebral artery (ACA) territory infarction can involve the orbital cortex, the frontal pole, the anterior cingulate, and/or the supplementary motor area. Bilateral lesions may be more frequent with ACA infarction since both ACAs may originate from a common internal carotid artery. Involvement of the anterior corpus callosum aggravates deficits caused by damage to the medial frontal cortex. Rupture of an ACA aneurysm is a common cause of ACA infarction. The perforator branches of that vessel supply the septal nuclei, and infarctions may cause significant limbic dysfunction including memory impairment. The vascular territory of the recurrent artery of Heubner includes the 'limbic caudate' and the inferior anterior limb of the internal capsule, which contains thalamofrontal connections. Middle cerebral artery (MCA) territory infarcts can involve significant regions of the dorsolateral and ventrolateral frontal convexity. Since MCA infarcts are not often restricted to the frontal lobes, care must be taken to demonstrate lesions restricted to frontal regions when studying the effects of MCA infarcts. If the lenticulostriate branches of the MCA are affected, the dorsolateral caudate, dorsolateral anterior limb of the internal capsule, and the putamen may also be damaged. Deep frontal white matter lesions can also affect the interconnection between prefrontal cortex (undamaged) and connected regions (e.g., posterior cortex and fibers of passage from ipsilateral medial frontal lobe and the contralateral frontal lobe).

Intracerebral hemorrhages do not necessarily follow vascular territories, potentially resulting in more anatomical variability than infarctions. Hemorrhages may also complicate behavior–lesion studies because of mass effects, secondary herniation damage, and hydrocephalus. Nevertheless, the potential involvement of combinations of structures not involved in infarctions indicates that hemorrhage cases can be of importance for brain–behavior studies.

Tumors can unilaterally infiltrate the frontal lobe, and as with hemorrhages they may produce a much wider range of combinations of regional injury than infarcts. Not all types of tumors are suitable for brain–behavior correlation study (e.g., rapidly growing intracerebral tumors (gliomas)) because of mass effects and uncertain margins of lesion. Relatively benign primary tumors (ependymomas, oligodendrogliomas, cystic astrocytomas, etc.) that have been excised may provide useful correlations. Extracerebral tumors (meningiomas) may cause considerable cortical impairment by compression and vascular compromise. Both of these tumor types are most informatively studied after resection, and only postoperative neuroimaging can define the areas of damaged brain.

Traumatic brain injury results in two broad categories of brain damage: diffuse axonal injury (DAI) and focal cortical contusions (FCCs). Although much DAI pathology is located in the deep frontal white matter, the widespread nature of DAI hinders demonstration of specific frontal–behavioral relationships. FCCs, on the other hand, may be appropriate for analysis of specific frontal–behavioral relationships provided that there is strong evidence that DAI is relatively modest (e.g., short duration of posttraumatic amnesia). Indeed, inclusion of such patients may be the only way to assess involvement of basal/polar frontal regions. Gunshot or other penetrating head wounds almost routinely produce unusual patterns of brain damage. Diffuse effects may be difficult to measure.

Many other disorders may affect the frontal lobes directly or disrupt the subcortical connections of frontal systems. Herpes simplex encephalitis and frontotemporal dementia commonly involve discrete frontal regions, but usually with extensive temporal injury as well. Large vessel and small vessel vascular diseases, hydrocephalus, and multiple sclerosis produce considerable white matter damage but rarely restricted to the frontal lobes. There are degenerative diseases with a predilection for subcortical structures that are critical components of frontal systems – Parkinson's disease, Huntington's disease, and progressive supranuclear palsy – but pathology is not restricted to these structures and is difficult to specify in life. Since many of these disorders involve multiple brain regions, they are not optimal for analysis of specific functions of the frontal lobes.

For much of the history of neuropsychology, strategies for lesion localization were fairly primitive, often analyzing case material only by frontal/posterior or right–left–bilateral frontal distinctions. In recent years, a variety of different procedures have evolved that sharpen frontal functional/anatomical correlations. Dividing the patients into those with and those without impairment in comparison to the control group and analyzing lesion site differences, either by simple overlaps or by lesion size within site correlations, have been fruitful. The classification and regression tree is a technique that can be used to divide patients based on their performance on a dependent variable into anatomically diverse groups. The performance groups are then analyzed for lesion region differences. 'Hotspotting' requires mapping the lesion of each patient onto an architectonic map. Then, for a defined dependent measurement (e.g., performance on a specific task), all individuals who have damage in a specific architectonic region are compared to all those who do not have damage in that area. This effectively identifies which region (or regions) results in most impairment of that particular process. This procedure requires experimental isolation of the specific process being studied and evaluation of a relatively large number of patients with focal lesions. The end result of fractionation of frontal processes is not phrenology but the identification of specific regions involved in simpler processes as a first step in understanding the unfolding of these abilities in more complex tasks and in real time.

Functional Domains within the Frontal Lobes

The existence of distinct functional domains within the frontal lobes is supported by evidence from developmental, anatomical connectivity, and lesion effects. The human cortex develops from two discrete sources. The lateral prefrontal cortical cortex (LPFC) has developed from hippocampal, archicortical sources. It determines spatial and conceptual reasoning processes. The ventral (medial) prefrontal cortex (VPFC) has evolved from paleocortical sources. It is associated with emotional processing, including the acquisition and reversal of stimulus–reward associations. These two broad developmental divisions form the two major (executive cognitive and behavioral/emotional self-regulatory) functional divisions within the frontal lobes and map onto two of the three proposed frontal–subcortical circuits involved in cognitive and/or emotional processing. Another frontal system is determined by the unique convergence of sensory and limbic input combined with a distributed frontal output. This characterizes the medial frontal structures that are uniquely placed for regulating energization of all cognitive activities. The final category of frontal functions (metacognitive) is suggested by research on higher order integrative functions of the frontal polar area 10. Some authors use the term 'executive' for all four of these functional domains, but, as described later, we consider this inappropriate.

Regulating Energization

Energization of cognitive functions is important for adequate performance of any function. (This is commonly called activation, but this term has come to have multiple meanings – psychological, vascular, imaging, etc. – and we prefer energization.) Extensive damage to more superior medial (anterior cingulate and superior) frontal pathology results in abulia or severe apathy or, at its worst, akinetic mutism. This lack of energization of activity, defined by a diminished capacity to generate and maintain actions of mental processes, can be demonstrated even in much less clinically obvious cases. Patients with damage in this region are slow in generating lists of words (particularly in the first 15 s); have notably slower reaction time (RT), particularly if tasks are more demanding; are deficient in maintaining over time the benefit of a warning stimulus; and have problems maintaining a selected target such as in the Stroop interference test. RT speed is correlated with functional activation in the same superior medial region. Verbal fluency and the Stroop task are commonly used in the clinical setting to assess energization, but they do not isolate this deficit because they are not specific and require other cognitive (often executive) abilities. Perhaps the best measures to evaluate impaired activation are demanding reaction time tests.

Executive Cognitive Functions

Executive cognitive functions are defined as, and the definition is limited to, those high-level cognitive functions that require control and direction (e.g., planning, monitoring, activating, switching, and inhibiting) of lower level, more automatic functions. Much of the research on executive functions in neuropsychological studies has demonstrated deficits in patients with primarily LPFC damage. Tests commonly used by many clinicians as measures of frontal lobe executive functioning include the Wisconsin Card Sorting Test, Trail Making Test Part B, the Stroop Interference subtest, and specific measures within verbal fluency tasks. These tests are indeed more sensitive in general to focal LPFC (and also not generally to orbitofrontal/ventral medial) pathology and fall within the classification of tests of 'executive cognitive' processes. However, the tests are complex and multifactorial, and individuals can fail for many reasons.

Significant efforts have been made to develop and evaluate tests that more precisely isolate specific executive processes. Structured RT tasks that isolate discrete performance measures have identified specific dissociations of executive cognitive functions. Two major dissociations of executive cognitive functions within the dorsolateral prefrontal regions have been demonstrated. Impaired task setting has been related to left lateral frontal lobe damage, particularly ventrolateral. This has been shown as impaired bias in a feature integration task (errors are primarily false positives) and as significantly increased errors in the first block of 100 trials in a concentrating task requiring rapid stimulus–response matching. This deficient task setting is domain general; that is, deficits can be seen in any task, not just in RT tasks. For example, in a word list learning task, patients with left frontal damage had increased false positive errors in memory recognition.

The right lateral frontal area, on the other hand, is important in monitoring. Damage in this region results in several types of deficits that are attributable to deficient monitoring: as increased errors of all types in a complex feature integration task, indicating a problem in monitoring the difference between targets and nontargets (i.e., impaired sensitivity); as an abnormal foreperiod effect – that is, an increase in RT with longer interstimulus intervals, rather than the normal decrease in RT, suggesting a deficiency in monitoring the occurrence of stimuli over time; and as significantly increased variability of timing performance in a tapping task.

The mechanisms behind this top-down within-subject (intra-individual) variability of performance both within a testing session and across sessions appear to be the same attentional mechanisms evidenced by other RT measures – that is, task setting, monitoring, and energization. As would be expected of impairment in domain general abilities, such intra-individual variability can be seen in other tasks such as memory.

There are efforts to bridge the gap between laboratory tasks of executive cognitive functions and everyday functioning with the investigation of naturalistic actions under controlled conditions. Since 'real-life' measures are more complex and require the involvement of multiple functional systems, these measures overlap with behavioral/emotional self-regulatory measures.

Behavioral/Emotional Self-Regulatory Functions

The VPFC region is involved in emotional processing. An important, and natural, role for the VPFC, because of its involvement in reward processing, is behavioral self-regulation required in situations in which cognitive analysis, habit, or environmental cues are not sufficient to determine the most adaptive response. Patients with damage to the inferior medial frontal cortex have difficulty in understanding the emotional consequences of their behavior, despite intact performance on commonly used neuropsychological tests of executive functioning. Assessments of these abilities tend to be more experimental in nature, and they include gambling tasks and naturalistic multiple subgoal tasks.

Because of the role of the ventral prefrontal cortex in emotional processing (basic drives and rewards that inform and direct high-level decision making), tests assessing the acquisition and reversal of stimulus–reward associations can be used. This reversal learning (interpreted as affective) is dissociable from the impairment in attentional (extradimensional) set shifting found after LPFC lesions, reinforcing the distinction between executive attentional and affective/emotional behavioral measures.

The VPFC is also involved in higher level decision-making tasks involving reward processing in unstructured situations, such as the gambling task that has been suggested as both sensitive and specific to VPFC lesions. However, as with many neuropsychological tests, further evaluation suggests that these tests may also be multifactorial in nature, and the true behavior/anatomy specificity remains to be determined. Decision-making performance on the gambling task has been dissociated from deficits in working memory and inhibition.

A broad term to encompass the type of deficits observed on the gambling task is 'self-regulatory disorder,' defined as the inability to regulate behavior according to internal goals and constraints particularly in less structured situations. Qualitative descriptions with naturalistic multiple subgoal tasks, and paper-and-pencil laboratory versions, have been developed. There are also efforts to develop various scales of behavioral dyscontrol or assessment of frontal lobe personality characteristics.

Metacognitive Processes

The fourth category of frontal function is related to the frontal polar region, Brodmann area 10, although there is still debate as to how much this functional category is associated with damage to a more general area including the anterior medial regions. This frontal region appears to be maximally involved in the metacognitive aspects of human nature: integrative aspects of personality, social cognition, autonoetic consciousness, theory of mind, humor appreciation, and self-awareness. Self-awareness implies a meta cognitive representation of one's own mental states, beliefs, attitudes, and experiences. This self-reflection is key to understand the relationship of one's own thoughts to external events and, from this self-knowledge, to understand the mental states of others. This ability to make inferences about the world, and to empathize with others, allows correct interpretation of events and correct social judgments. Family reports often precisely describe the changes in behavior that have occurred: lack of empathy, unconcern, and inability to appreciate humor that requires self-reflection (appreciation of slapstick humor may be intact).

Because area 10 is among the most recently evolved of human brain regions, it may be uniquely positioned to integrate the higher level executive cognitive functions and emotional or drive-related inputs. This bridging of behavioral self-regulatory and executive cognitive functions may be the neural basis for their role in metacognitive functions. There is evidence, however, that there are potential dissociations within this domain, and that metacognitive processes are not reducible to these other functions.

The neuropsychological assessments in this category of frontal lobe functions are generally experimental. They include reactions to verbal and cartoon humor, visual perspective-taking tasks, and comparison of performance on remember–know memory tasks. For some individuals, however, these tasks can be solved on the basis of factual knowledge, not inference. Moreover, the relationship of process to anatomy is not certain, and it may depend on the differential demand of different tests within the overall 'metacognitive' rubric.

The general localization of the four separable frontal lobe processes is depicted in **Figure 2**.

Networks and Integration in Time

The evidence for fractionation of the functions of the frontal lobes does not imply that frontal lobes are simply a series of independent processes. Depending on task demands, there is the fluid recruitment of different processes anywhere in the brain into different networks. Lesion research demonstrates the effect of impairment in the networks; functional imaging demonstrates the recruitment of processes. For some task demands, one or more anatomically distinct frontal processes may be recruited. In tasks with simple demands, the more automatic nonfrontal processes function independently; as task demands increase or

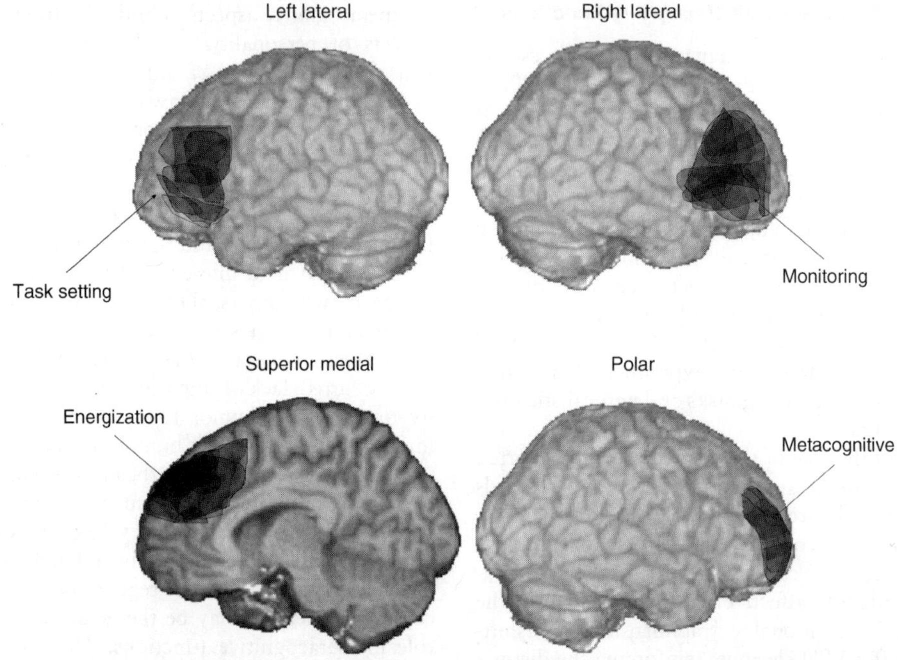

Figure 2 Illustration of three of the four major anatomical regions within the prefrontal cortex related to the different functional categories within this brain region. The four categories are energization (superior medial), executive (lateral), behavioral/self-regulatory (inferior medial; not illustrated), and metacognition (polar). Two executive processes are illustrated, one related with the left lateral region (task setting) and the other with the right (monitoring).

alter, there may be increased involvement of different frontal (more 'strategic') regions, even to the point where it appears all frontal regions are involved. In other demands the network may function 'top-down.'

These networks function in real time. Language provides one example. To request an object, answer a simple question, or tell a familiar story require essentially no control or monitoring and these presumably occur with no executive processes required. To give a complicated response to a difficult question will require more control. To tell a complex narrative – deciding what to include, what the listener may already know of the story, what is socially appropriate to include for a particular audience, and to keep track of the goal of the story while adding a critical digression – will require substantial executive control. Setting the task goal, monitoring the content and the listener, and sustaining and maintaining intention are essentially dependent on the several functions described previously. They are recruited at different levels, at different times across the task, and they in turn recruit a variety of posterior cognitive operations, each at a specific point in the narrative. Multiple executive processes, each primarily dependent on a specific frontal region, must be knitted together in real time.

Rehabilitation

There are no class I randomized controlled trials of executive rehabilitation in focal frontal patients, although there are a few studies on patients with traumatic brain injury, primarily DAI. Clinical treatments have been targeted at the disability level of rehabilitation, not at specified frontal lobe impairment. Three types of treatments have been utilized, individually or alone, with some success:

Drugs. Stimulants may help patients with low arousal states or who are easily distracted. Dopaminergic agents may help patients with poor activation (energization).

Cognitive. A few theoretically sound programs addressing 'executive dysfunction' have demonstrated some possible efficacy. These techniques often rely on training patients to stop before they begin a task (inhibit impulsive responses), then explicitly define goals (set task requirements), check off performance as they progress (monitor subgoals), and confirm appropriate completion (compare goal to outcome). Each step in this treatment would appear to be directed at a specific executive or self-regulatory factor of frontal function, but no study has yet assessed the specificity of treatment effectiveness.

Behavioral self-regulation/self-awareness. There have been successful efforts to improve self-awareness. It is uncertain how much of this is dependent on the environmental support provided to the patient.

Compensatory. Commonly, environmental compensation has focused on a limiting disability or handicap, resulting in greater functional independence. These programs make, appropriately, no claims for directly treating executive dysfunction.

Conclusion

Prior to the availability of computed tomography scans, patients with frontal lobe lesions were often not identified until clinical signs were well advanced, and by the time of identification, many patients had lesion extension into brain regions outside the frontal lobes or had extremely large frontal lesions or both. Patients' deficits were often characterized only with behavioral descriptions or with multidimensional tests that have high sensitivity but low specificity for frontal injury. The historical notions of the frontal lobe syndrome come from observations of such patients. In the past 25 years, early diagnosis, precise lesion definition, and a broad range of specific and sensitive tests of regulation of attention, discrete executive functions, self-regulatory behaviors, and empathy and social awareness have combined to provide a much more precise understanding of the many consequences of specific frontal injuries and have made it clear that there is little evidence of a single frontal lobe or dysexecutive syndrome.

See also: Brain Trauma; Executive Function and Higher-Order Cognition: Neuroimaging; Executive Function and Higher-Order Cognition: Definition and Neural Substrates; Humans; Prefrontal Cortex: Structure and Anatomy; Prefrontal Cortex.

Further Reading

Bechara A, Tranel D, and Damasio H (2000) Characterization of the decision-making deficit of patients with ventromedial prefrontal cortex lesions. *Brain* 123: 2189–2202.

Cicerone KD, Dahlberg C, Malec JF, et al. (2005) Evidence-based cognitive rehabilitation: Updated review of the literature from 1998 through 2002. *Archives of Physical Medicine and Rehabilitation* 86: 1681–1692.

Corbetta M and Shulman GL (2002) Control of goal-directed and stimulus-driven attention in the brain. *Nature Reviews Neuroscience* 3: 201–215.

Cummings JL (1993) Frontal–subcortical circuits and human behavior. *Archives of Neurology* 50: 873–880.

Grafman J, Holyoak KJ, and Boller F (eds.) (1995) *Structure and Functions of the Human Prefrontal Cortex*. New York: New York Academy of Sciences.

Lhermitte F (1986) Human anatomy and the frontal lobes. 2. Patient behavior in complex and social situations: The environmental dependency syndrome. *Annals of Neurology* 19: 335–343.

Miller EK (2000) The prefrontal cortex and cognitive control. *Nature Reviews Neuroscience* 1: 59–65.

Norman DA and Shallice T (1986) Attention to action: Willed and automatic control of behavior. In: Davidson RJ, Shwartz GE, and Shapiro D (eds.) *Consciousness and Self-Regulation: Advances in Research and Theory*, vol. 4, pp. 1–18. New York: Plenum.

Pandya DN and Yeterian EH (1996) Comparison of prefrontal architecture and connections. *Philosophical Transactions of the Royal Society of London, Series B: Biological Sciences* 351: 1423–1432.

Passingham R (1995) *The Frontal Lobes and Voluntary Action.* New York: Clarendon.

Petrides M (2005) Lateral prefrontal cortex: Architectonic and functional organization. *Philosophical Transactions of the Royal Society, Series B: Biological Sciences* 360: 781–795.

Rolls ET (2004) The functions of the orbitofrontal cortex. *Brain and Cognition* 55: 11–29.

Siegal M and Varley R (2002) Neural systems involved in 'theory of mind.' *Nature Reviews Neuroscience* 3: 463–471.

Stuss DT and Knight RT (eds.) (2002) *Principles of Frontal Lobe Function.* New York: Oxford University Press.

Stuss DT and Levine B (2002) Adult clinical neuropsychology: Lessons from studies of the frontal lobes. *Annual Review of Psychology* 53: 401–433.

Functional Amnesia

M Kritchevsky, San Diego VA Healthcare System, San Diego, CA, USA

Published by Elsevier Ltd.

Introduction

Functional amnesia is an uncommon condition in which patients develop severe retrograde amnesia in the absence of significant anterograde amnesia and without any known brain injury or disorder. This nonneurological syndrome is variously referred to as psychogenic amnesia, hysterical amnesia, dissociative amnesia, and functional retrograde amnesia. Functional amnesia is easily distinguished from the neurological amnesic syndrome that is commonly seen with dysfunction of bilateral medial temporal lobe or bilateral medial diencephalic structures important for memory, in which patients have severe anterograde amnesia with variable retrograde amnesia. In contrast, functional amnesia may be indistinguishable from malingered amnesia. Functional amnesia is the disorder of memory that is most commonly popularized in literature and film, and it appears to be the condition that the majority of lay persons regard as amnesia.

Early descriptions of functional amnesia included large numbers of cases that were characterized primarily by a loss of personal identity. Memory for previously known facts and personal events sometimes was noted to be impaired as well. In 1982 the first case of functional amnesia that had been formally studied with neuropsychological testing was published. Subsequently many additional case studies have been described. In 2004 the first series of patients with functional amnesia who had been studied clinically and neuropsychologically in a systematic fashion was reported. The increasing understanding of functional amnesia has facilitated diagnosis of this condition, but treatment of many patients with functional amnesia has remained difficult.

Clinical Characteristics of the Patient with Functional Amnesia

The Clinical Picture of the Patient

The typical patient with functional amnesia presents with the sudden onset of retrograde amnesia without clinically significant anterograde amnesia. Most commonly, the retrograde amnesia affects all of the memories that occurred prior to the onset of amnesia, including memory for personal identity. Thus, the patient reports that he or she cannot remember their past. They do not know their name, where they were born, or where they were raised. They can not recall where they went to school, when or to whom they were married, where they live, or by whom they are employed. Once their identity is discovered, they do not recognize their name. When they meet their friends and family, they do not recognize them. In general, the loss of past memories affects public as well as personal material. For example, the patient will not recall or recognize previously known public figures such as sports figures, movie stars, and political leaders. They will not recall or recognize previously known public events such as wars or national disasters. Because the person with functional amnesia has no significant anterograde amnesia, they are able to relearn past memories. However, these newly learned memories typically have no sense of familiarity to them.

Uncommonly, the patient with functional amnesia has retrograde amnesia that affects only a period of time before the onset of memory loss. For example, if the period of amnesia is 2 years, then the patient will not recall or recognize memories that occurred during the 2-year period before the onset of amnesia. The patient will know their name and will have normal recollection of memories that occurred more than 2 years ago. However, he or she will give the year as 2 years earlier than the correct year, and will report their marital status, place of residence, and workplace as they were 2 years previously despite any significant changes that may have occurred since. The patient can relearn past memories, but the new memories will not have a sense of familiarity.

The patient with functional amnesia most often will report a complete loss of memories from the period of retrograde amnesia. However, on occasion a patient will be aware of one or more vague and incomplete memories from the period of amnesia.

At about the time of onset of functional amnesia, many patients have one or more abnormalities, in addition to the amnesia, that also appear to be psychogenic. These have included inability to name objects, inability to name numbers, difficulty with calculations, loss of ability to read and write, inability to move the eyes voluntarily during formal testing, bilateral leg weakness with inability to walk independently, weakness on one side of the body, and an inability to carry out previously familiar activities such as using a telephone or driving a car with a manual transmission. One patient has reported that he had to relearn the English language by reading a dictionary during the first 2 days of his amnesia. Another has reported that she could no longer remember the Spanish language, though she had been bilingual prior to the onset of her amnesia. With regard to anterograde amnesia, patients characteristically have good memory for events that occurred after the onset of amnesia. One patient has reported difficulty with new learning, and on neurological examination was poor at learning new verbal, but not nonverbal, material. However, like other patients with functional amnesia, he did not appear to be forgetful.

Occasionally, a patient with functional amnesia will present immediately after a period of sudden and unexpected travel during which they appear to have exhibited normal behavior. The period of travel is termed a fugue state, and whatever occurred during the fugue state will be included in the period of retrograde amnesia.

Risk and Precipitating Factors

Many patients with functional amnesia have significant premorbid psychiatric histories, including one or more of the following: alcohol abuse, other substance abuse, previous conversion symptoms, anxiety disorder, posttraumatic stress disorder, schizophrenia, depression, history of suicide attempt, and histrionic or borderline personality disorder. Many patients with functional amnesia have one or more of the following possible precipitating factors at the onset of amnesia: intoxication with alcohol, mild closed head injury, active depression, psychological stress, and involvement or alleged involvement in illegal activity.

Clinical Course

The clinical course of patients with functional amnesia is highly variable. Some patients appear to have a full recovery of their retrograde amnesia. In these cases the recovery most often occurs gradually over days to weeks. The recovery most often appears to consist of the gradual return of memories from throughout the period of amnesia. Rarely, the amnesia appears to resolve suddenly. Many patients have only a partial recovery of their lost memories. Sometimes this involves partial but incomplete recovery of memories from throughout the period of memory loss. In contrast, at times the initially extensive retrograde amnesia appears to shrink over a period of months to a shorter period of retrograde amnesia for a period of time (e.g., 6 months) immediately preceding the onset of amnesia. Some patients with functional amnesia report that they experience little or no recovery of their lost memories over an interval as long as 42 months. Patients who experience no significant recovery of memory occasionally appear to have established new personalities. It appears to be very uncommon for functional amnesia to suddenly and completely resolve in association with a mild head injury or a psychological catharsis.

The recovery of lost memories sometimes appears to have been facilitated by reacquainting the patient with their past, or by addressing and initiating treatment for ongoing psychological stressors. Also, sometimes hypnosis or an amobarbital interview appears to facilitate the recovery of lost memories. Memories initially remembered with these therapies sometimes are again inaccessible immediately following the session, but then rapidly return in the following days.

Recovery from retrograde amnesia should be distinguished from relearning lost memories. The patient with functional amnesia usually will report with confidence that a particular memory was relearned. They sometimes will recall the event of relearning and usually will report that the memory feels new and is unassociated with the familiar feel of an old memory.

Additional psychogenic cognitive deficits that are associated with the retrograde amnesia often resolve within hours to days of onset. General neurological deficits, particularly weakness, of psychogenic origin may persist throughout the course of the amnesia.

Laboratory Tests

In patients with functional amnesia, structural neuroimaging tests such as computed tomography (CT) and magnetic resonance imaging (MRI) brain scans are usually normal, though they occasionally show abnormalities unrelated to the functional amnesia. Electroencephalography also is usually normal, but may show abnormalities that are unrelated to the amnesia. Functional neuroimaging tests such as single-photon computed tomography (SPECT), positron emission tomography (PET), or functional MRI brain scans have been reported to show abnormal findings related to the retrograde amnesia in some patients. The findings have not been consistent in the different patients studied. Although the demonstrated functional abnormalities may be related to the patients' retrograde amnesia, the presence of such abnormalities does not imply that functional amnesia is due to or associated with brain injury or disorder.

Differential Diagnosis

Malingered (intentionally feigned) amnesia also can present with the sudden onset of retrograde amnesia without clinically significant anterograde amnesia. In fact, it may be that a patient with malingered amnesia only can be distinguished from a patient with functional amnesia with certainty if the malingerer confesses. One clue that a patient has malingered amnesia may be the absence of a significant past psychiatric history. The precipitating factors for malingered amnesia may be similar to those for functional amnesia. One malingerer hit himself in the head with a bottle so there would be evidence of an appropriate precipitating factor for his amnesia.

Rare neurological patients have been reported to have significant retrograde amnesia with a lesser degree of anterograde amnesia. This may be associated with bilateral damage to the anterior or inferior temporal lobes. Personal identity probably is preserved, the retrograde amnesia covers a period of several years to several decades, and there is some degree of anterograde amnesia. Neuroimaging typically will reveal the responsible brain injury.

The neurological amnesic syndrome that is commonly seen with dysfunction of bilateral medial temporal lobe or bilateral medial diencephalic structures important for memory is easily distinguished from functional amnesia. Patients with the neurological amnesic syndrome have significant anterograde amnesia with variable retrograde amnesia.

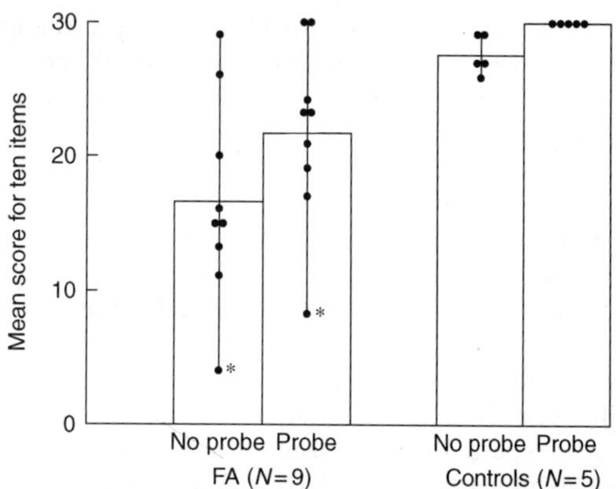

Figure 1 Patients with functional amnesia (FA) and controls were asked to recollect ten autobiographical episodes. Responses were scored (0–3) before (no probe) and after (probe) encouragement by the examiner to elicit as specific a recollection as possible. Each filled circle indicates the score for one subject. The asterisk indicates the score for the patient who later confessed that he had malingered his amnesia. Kritchevsky M, Chang J, and Squire LR (2004) Functional amnesia: Clinical description and neuropsychological profile of 10 cases. *Learning and Memory* 11: 213–226.

Neuropsychological Findings in Patients with Functional Amnesia

In 2004, a series of ten patients who had initially been diagnosed with functional amnesia was published. The patients had been studied clinically and neuropsychologically in a systematic fashion. Nine of the patients presented with loss of past memories that extended into childhood and included loss of personal identity. One had retrograde amnesia that was limited to 2–3 years. Eight of the ten patients were thought to have definite functional amnesia. One of the patients (whose performance is noted by an asterisk in the figures) subsequently confessed that he had malingered his amnesia. The final patient was considered to be a possible malingerer. The patients ranged in age from 28 to 54 years (mean, 37 years). For the eight patients for whom the data were known, education ranged from 9 to 16 years (mean, 13 years). Eight patients were men and two women. Seven were tested neuropsychologically 1–14 days after the onset of amnesia. Three were tested 10 weeks to 9 months after the onset of amnesia. Five patients were tested between 1982 and 1985. The other five were tested between 1992 and 1995. Four men and one woman, matched to the patients with respect to age and education, served as controls. They were tested in 1996. The neuropsychological data presented in this section are from these patients and controls.

Retrograde Amnesia

Figure 1 shows the performance of nine of the ten patients on a test of past autobiographical memory. This test was not administered to the patient who had retrograde amnesia of only 2–3 years. Ten common words (e.g., bird, clock) were presented one at a time with the instruction to recall a specific personal event from any time in the past that involved the stimulus word. Subjects were asked to describe the memory in as much detail as possible and then to date the memory. When recall was not clearly specific to time and place, the examiner probed to elicit the most specific memory possible. Responses were scored on a 0–3 scale, with 3 representing a well-formed episodic memory. The patients performed more poorly than the controls, both without ($t\,[12] = 3.2, p < 0.01$) and with probing ($t\,[12] = 2.7, p < 0.05$) by the examiner. The two patients who obtained the best scores were tested 3 and 9 months after the onset of the amnesia. Their good performances resulted from their ability to recall memories from the period after the onset of their amnesia. On neurological examination, both of these patients exhibited significant loss of autobiographical memories for events that had occurred before the onset of amnesia.

Figure 2 shows the percentage of well-formed episodic memories that were recalled from different past time periods (0 days to > 20 years) on the test of past autobiographical memory. One patient, the malingerer, was unable to produce any well-formed recollections and was not included in this analysis. The remaining patients each recalled from three to ten memories. The patients differed markedly from the controls in that they recalled most of their memories from the most recent time period (patients, 78%; controls = 24%; $t\,[11] = 3.1, p < 0.01$) and very few

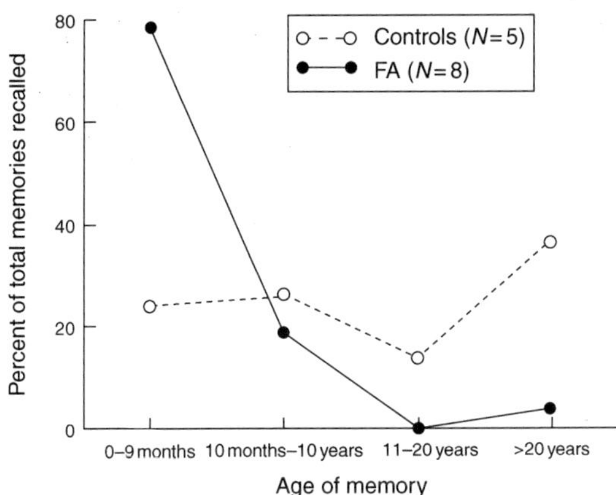

Figure 2 Percentage of memories that were recalled from the indicated time periods for patients with functional amnesia (FA) and controls. The data are based only on those recollections given a maximum score of 3 on the ten-item test of past autobiographical memory (**Figure 1**). The patient who later confessed that he had malingered his amnesia had no recollections that were given a three-point score. For the eight patients, all the memories from the 0–9 months time period were taken from the period after the onset of amnesia. Kritchevsky M, Chang J, and Squire LR (2004) Functional amnesia: Clinical description and neuropsychological profile of 10 cases. *Learning and Memory* 11: 213–226.

of their memories from the most remote time period (patients, 3%; controls, 36%; $t\,[11]=3.2$, $p<0.01$). It was notable that all of the memories recalled by the patients from the most recent time period were drawn from the time after the onset of amnesia. Thus, compared with the controls, the patients had a striking tendency not to recall remote memories, but rather to draw their memories from the period after the onset of the amnesia.

Figures 3(a) and **3(b)** show the performance of four of the patients on a test of recall and recognition of public events. These patients were tested between 1992 and 1994. Twenty-four questions about public events that had occurred from 1970 to 1985 were asked. This test first was administered in a recall format (e.g., Who killed John Lennon?) and then, for each item that was not recalled or was incorrectly recalled, in a four-alternative, multiple-choice format (John Hinkley, Sara Jane Moore, David Roth, and Mark Chapman). The recognition score was based on the items that were recalled correctly plus the items that were recognized correctly. The four patients were impaired both at recall (16.7% correct for patients; 39.2% correct for controls; $t\,[7]=4.2$, $p<0.01$) and at recognition (44.8% correct for patients; 76.6% correct for controls; $t[7]=4.2$, $p<0.01$). One of these patients, who had retrograde amnesia of only 2–3 years, performed better than the other three. However, he still performed at the low end of the control range on recall (29.2%) and poorer than the controls on recognition (62.5%). The six other patients took a similar test consisting of 17–26 questions about the two most recent decades before the onset of their amnesia. They also scored poorly at recall (16.3% correct; one patient did not take the recall test) and at recognition (48.3% correct). One of these patients, the possible malingerer, had a score of 0% on the recall test and 11% on the recognition test (chance = 25%).

Figures 3(c) and **3(d)** show the performance of four of the patients on a test of recall and recognition of famous faces. These patients were tested between 1992 and 1994. Nineteen photographs of famous people who came into the news from 1970 to 1989 were shown. The test first was administered in a recall format and then, for each item that was not recalled or was incorrectly recalled, in a recognition format. For recognition, half the items were yes/no questions (e.g., Is this person's name Liza Minelli?) and half were three-alternative, multiple-choice questions (e.g., Liza Minelli, Ann Margaret, Helen Reddy). The recognition score was based on the items that were recalled correctly plus the items that were recognized correctly. As a group, the four patients were impaired both at recall (40.8% correct for patients; 64.2% correct for controls; $t\,[7]=5.7$, $p<0.01$) and at recognition (80.2% correct for patients; 94.7% for controls; $t\,[7]=4.2$, $p<0.01$). The six other patients took a similar test consisting of 20–27 faces from the two most recent decades before the onset of their amnesia. They also scored poorly as a group at recall (39.1% correct) and at recognition (77.8% correct; one patient did not take the recognition test). There was marked variability in the individual scores of the ten patients. Thus, both the recall and recognition scores of two patients (one of these was the malingerer) were as good as or better than the control scores. Also, the patient who had retrograde amnesia of only 2–3 years performed just below the controls at recall and obtained a perfect score at recognition. A fourth patient scored well enough on the recognition test to reach the low end of the control range. A fifth patient scored 0% correct at recall but nearly reached the control range at recognition. Finally, a sixth patient (the possible malingerer) scored 0% correct at recall and 18.5% correct at recognition (chance = 41.7%). His overall score on the public events and famous faces recognition tests was 2.75 standard deviations below the score that would have been expected from guessing.

Figure 4 shows the performance of nine of the ten patients on tests of identification of US and southern California cities. First, each subject was read the names of 16 real and 16 plausible US cities and associated

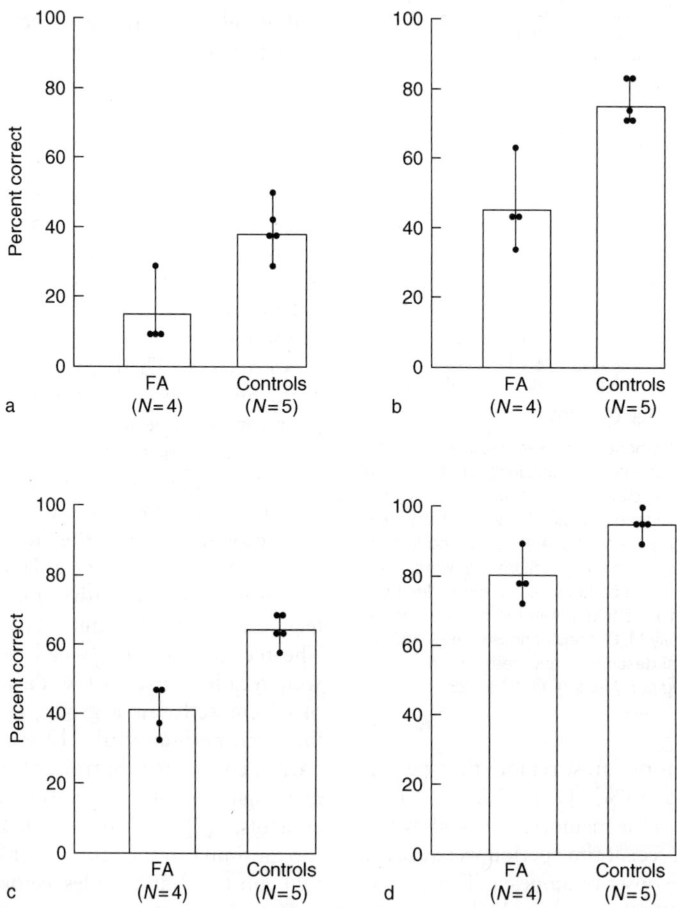

Figure 3 Performance on tests of remote memory for public events and famous faces. Patients with functional amnesia (FA) and controls were asked 24 questions about public events that had occurred during the two decades prior to testing (a) and then took a four-alternative, multiple-choice test about the same events (b). Subjects also were asked to identify 19 photographs of famous people who came into the news during the two decades before testing (c) and then to recognize the names that they could not recall (d). The recognition scores were based on the number of items recalled correctly plus the items that were recognized correctly. Chance = 25% for public events, 41.7% for famous faces. Each filled circle indicates the score for one subject. Kritchevsky M, Chang J, and Squire LR (2004) Functional amnesia: Clinical description and neuropsychological profile of 10 cases. *Learning and Memory* 11: 213–226.

states (e.g., Phoenix, Arizona, or Nelander, Michigan) and asked to identify whether each city name was real or fabricated. Then each subject was read a list of ten real and ten plausible southern California cities (e.g., Oceanside or Palmville) and again asked whether each city name was real or fabricated. The score on each test was the number of cities correctly identified. Overall, the patients performed similarly to the controls (US cities; $t[12] = 1.8, p = 0.09$; southern California cities, $p > 0.10$). However, two patients scored more than two standard deviations below the control mean on both tests. One of these, the possible malingerer, scored 47% correct on the US cities test and 30% correct on the southern California cities test (chance = 50% for each test).

In summary, all patients were impaired in their ability to recall autobiographical memories of specific events from their past. In contrast, there was marked variability in their performances on tests of their ability to recall and recognize public events and famous faces from the two decades before the onset of their amnesia. Thus, the possible malingerer scored significantly below chance on the recognition tests, and it is possible that he intentionally chose the wrong answers. Also, three patients (one was the malingerer) performed particularly well on the famous faces tests despite performing poorly on the public events tests. Another patient was unable to recall a single item on the famous faces test, but then did well on recognition of the faces. There was less variability in the patients'

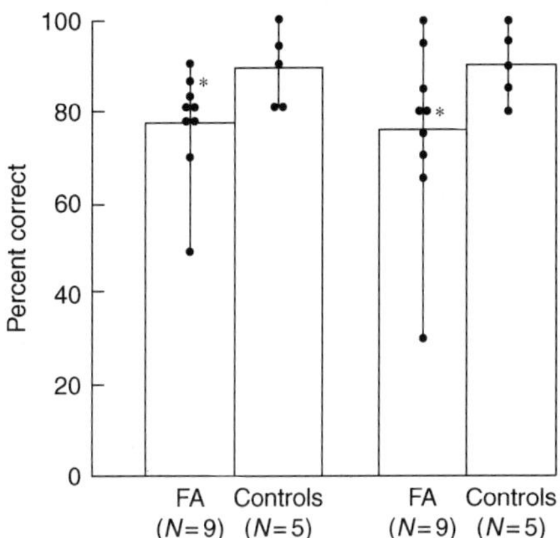

Figure 4 Patients with functional amnesia (FA) and controls were asked to identify the names of cities in the United States (left two bars) and the names of cities in southern California (right two bars) from lists of real and fictitious city names. Chance = 50%. Each filled circle indicates the score for one subject. The asterisk indicates the scores for the patient who later confessed that he had malingered his amnesia. Kritchevsky M, Chang J, and Squire LR (2004) Functional amnesia: Clinical description and neuropsychological profile of 10 cases. *Learning and Memory* 11: 213–226.

ability to distinguish names of real cities from the names of fictitious cities. Two patients, one the possible malingerer, performed abnormally on these tests.

Anterograde Amnesia

Figure 5(a) shows the performance of the ten patients with functional amnesia on a test of story recall. A short prose passage was read to the patient. Recall was tested immediately and again after a 10–20 min delay. The score was the number of story segments correctly recalled. Overall, the patients were marginally impaired at immediate recall (t [13] = 2.1, $p < 0.06$) but similar to controls at delayed recall ($p > 0.10$). Nonetheless, there was considerable variability in the performance of individual patients. Six of the patients (including the malingerer and the possible malingerer) had immediate recall scores that were more than two standard deviations below the control mean. Only the malingerer had a delayed recall score that was more than two standard deviations below the control mean.

Figure 5(b) shows the performance of the ten patients on a test of paired associate learning. A series of ten noun–noun word pairs was presented verbally and visually on each of three study trials. After each study trial, the patient was shown the first word of each pair and asked to recall the second word. The score was the number of words correctly recalled on each trial. Patients and controls performed similarly overall (F [1,13] = 2.7, $p > 0.10$) and improved at a similar rate across the three trials (F [2,26] = 0.5, $p > 0.10$). There was some variability in the scores,

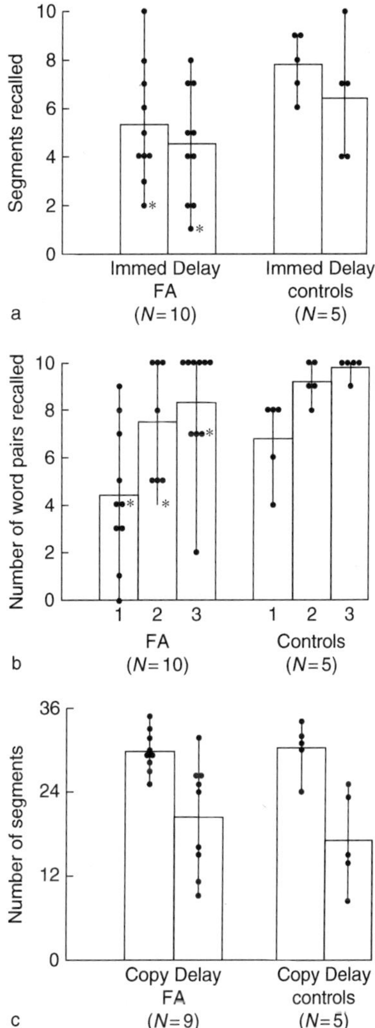

Figure 5 Performance of patients with functional amnesia (FA) and controls on tests of anterograde amnesia. (a) Story recall. Recall was tested immediately (Immed) and again after a delay of 10–20 min (Delay). (b) Paired-associate learning. Ten word pairs were presented on each of three study trials. (c) Copy of a complex diagram and reconstruction of the diagram from memory after 10–20 min (Delay). Maximum score = 36. Each filled circle indicates the score for one subject. The asterisk indicates the scores for the patient who later confessed that he had malingered his amnesia. He did not receive the diagram recall test. Kritchevsky M, Chang J, and Squire LR (2004) Functional amnesia: Clinical description and neuropsychological profile of 10 cases. *Learning and Memory* 11: 213–226.

with four of the patients (including the malingerer) having total number of words recalled across the three trials more than two standard deviations below the overall control mean.

Figure 5(c) shows the performance of nine of the patients on a test of recall of nonverbal material.

This test was not administered to the malingerer. Each patient copied a complex diagram. After a 10–20 min delay and without forewarning, they were asked to reproduce the diagram from memory. The score was the number of parts of the diagram correctly recalled. The patients scored similarly to the controls, both when they copied the diagram and when they reconstructed it from memory ($p > 0.10$). No patient obtained a score on this test that was below the lowest score obtained by the controls.

In summary, the patients as a group performed well on tests of anterograde amnesia for verbal and nonverbal material. However, there was some variability among patients. Some appeared to have abnormal performances on immediate verbal memory for a prose passage or on paired associate learning. Despite these abnormal performances, no patient exhibited any difficulty learning and remembering day-to-day events after the onset of amnesia.

Etiology of Functional Amnesia

Functional amnesia is a nonneurological, conversion symptom-like disorder. The model for the amnesia is the amnesic syndrome that is popularized in literature and film, namely a loss of past memories that usually includes a loss of personal identity. Each patient has their own individual conception of what past memories should be lost, which leads to the striking variability in the clinical and neuropsychological findings of patients with functional amnesia. In functional amnesia, as in a conversion disorder, the patient is not intentionally producing the deficits. It has been proposed that posthypnotic amnesia might serve as a laboratory model of functional amnesia, and self-hypnosis is one possible mechanism of conversion disorder and of functional amnesia.

Evaluation and Treatment of the Patient with Functional Amnesia

The evaluation of the patient should begin with neurological and psychiatric histories. The patient may be able to provide some of this information, but early in the course of evaluation most of the history will come from family members, friends, and healthcare or legal professionals. Neurological and psychiatric examinations should be performed. Laboratory investigations usually are not required, but may be obtained in selected patients.

The patient should be treated in the same manner as a patient with a conversion disorder. They should be reassured that there is no evidence of serious or significant brain problem. Significant psychological stressors should be identified and treated. They should be informed that their memories may begin returning within days of the onset of the amnesia. Contact with friends and family members should be encouraged unless there is a contraindication. If there has been little or no return of past memories within about a week, then treatment with hypnosis or an amobarbital interview should be considered if the treating psychiatrist agrees. If psychologically painful memories are remembered during hypnosis or an amobarbital interview, then the patient will require careful observation to be sure that these memories do not lead to undue distress or even to a suicide attempt. Despite the best possible therapy, some patients have only partial recoveries and some patients do not appear to have any recovery from their functional amnesia.

See also: Cognition: An Overview of Neuroimaging Techniques; Cognitive Dysfunction in Psychiatric Disorders; Declarative Memory System: Anatomy; Episodic Memory; Humans; Memory Consolidation: Systems; Memory Disorders.

Further Reading

Abeles M and Schilder P (1935) Psychogenic loss of personal identity. *Archives of Neurology and Psychiatry* 34: 587–604.

American Psychiatric Association (2000) Dissociative amnesia. In: *Diagnostic and Statistical Manual of Mental Disorders*, 4th edn., pp. 520–523. Arlington, VA: American Psychiatric Association.

Barnier A (2002) Posthypnotic amnesia for autobiographical episodes: A laboratory model of functional amnesia? *Psychological Science* 13: 232–237.

Kanzer M (1939) Amnesia: A statistical study. *American Journal of Psychiatry* 96: 711–716.

Kapur N (1993) Focal retrograde amnesia in neurological disease: A critical review. *Cortex* 29: 217–234.

Kritchevsky M, Chang J, and Squire LR (2004) Functional amnesia: Clinical description and neuropsychological profile of 10 cases. *Learning and Memory* 11: 213–226.

Kritchevsky M, Zouzounis J, and Squire LR (1997) Transient global amnesia and functional retrograde amnesia: Contrasting examples of episodic memory loss. *Philosophical Transactions of the Royal Society of London B* 352: 1747–1754.

Schacter DL, Wang PL, Tulving E, and Freedman M (1982) Functional retrograde amnesia: A quantitative case study. *Neuropsychologia* 20: 523–532.

Yang JC, Jeong GW, Lee MS, et al. (2005) Functional MR imaging of psychogenic amnesia: A case report. *Korean Journal of Radiology* 6: 196–199.

Hemispheric Specialization and Cognition

M T Banich, University of Colorado at Boulder, Boulder, CO, USA

Hemispheric Differences in Cognition

Discovery of Hemispheric Differences in Cognition

Paul Broca, a French neurologist and anthropologist, is generally considered the first person to have clearly illustrated hemispheric differences in cognitive function. As such, he is often said to have discovered the phenomenon. His critical insight derived from his visit with a patient who demonstrated an interesting dissociation in language abilities. Although able to understand what was said to him, the man had an inability to produce speech, being able only to utter the syllable 'tan.' Broca's postmortem analysis of his brain showed that damage was localized to the third convolution of the inferior frontal gyrus in the left hemisphere. Broca then went on to examine other patients who exhibited a similar cognitive profile – an inability to produce speech in the face of a retained ability to comprehend speech. In all cases, the damage was localized to the same region but, most important, always in the left hemisphere – a region now known as Broca's area. As a result of these findings, Broca proposed in 1863 that the left hemisphere is specialized, or dominant, for speech output. Thus, Broca's paper was the first systematic and compelling demonstration of hemispheric specialization of function. In fact, unlike most other aspects of hemispheric specialization, this one is absolute: the right hemisphere has no ability to control speech output in practically all right-handed individuals.

Evidence from Patients with Unilateral Brain Damage

As a result of Broca's discovery, the idea of cerebral dominance was overgeneralized. Probably because language was considered synonymous with thought, his work was interpreted to mean that the left hemisphere was dominant for all aspects of cognitive function. This idea only began to erode gradually over the next century as studies of patients with unilateral brain damage demonstrated different consequences depending on which hemisphere was damaged. As apparent to any neurologist or clinical neuropsychologist, left hemisphere damage usually results in deficits in the domains of verbal, sequential, and analytic processing. For example, aphasia is a common consequence of left hemisphere damage. In contrast, right hemisphere damage typically yields deficits in nonverbal, holistic, and Gestalt processing. For example, deficits in visuospatial processing are more often observed after right hemisphere damage.

Evidence from Split-Brain Patients

In the 1960s, research by Nobel laureate Roger Sperry and colleagues with split-brain patients dramatically demonstrated the relative specialization of the cerebral hemispheres. In these split-brain patients, the main nerve fiber tract connecting the cerebral hemispheres, the corpus callosum, is severed for the treatment of intractable epilepsy. As a result, higher order information, such as that about an item's identity (e.g., a car, the letter 'A,' and the face of Bill Clinton), cannot be transferred from one hemisphere to the other. Thus, information directed to a single hemisphere is functionally isolated to that hemisphere. This situation provides a unique opportunity to examine the relative specialization of the cerebral hemispheres because each hemisphere's capabilities can be examined in isolation from those of its partner. As a result, research with split-brain patients has yielded much important information about hemispheric specialization. Absolute differences have been demonstrated only for a couple of functions, namely speech output and phonological processing, which are under sole control of the left hemisphere. Both hemispheres can perform all other tasks, albeit with differing levels of ability and in different manners. Whereas the left hemisphere has a rich ability to perform most all language tasks, the vocabulary of the right hemisphere is much more limited, as is its ability to process complicated grammatical functions. On the other hand, the right hemisphere is superior at processing most types of spatial relationships, especially those involving three-dimensional relations or complicated geometries.

Perceptual Asymmetries in Neurologically Intact Individuals

The relative specializations of the cerebral hemispheres can also be demonstrated in neurologically intact individuals through the use of methods that essentially pit the hemispheres against one another. These methods, which include tachitoscopic presentation, dichotic listening, and dichaptic presentation, all take advantage of the neuroanatomical wiring of the human brain that transfers information from sensory receptors to the contralateral sensory cortex. In these methods, information is presented laterally so it is received either solely or predominantly by one hemisphere. Then behavioral performance, with regard to either reaction time or accuracy, can be examined depending on which hemisphere initially received the sensory information. These behavioral measures are often referred to as perceptual asymmetries because they reflect the asymmetry in the perception of information depending on the hemisphere to which information was initially directed. Even though the corpus callosum in neurologically intact individuals contains more than 250 million fibers by which the hemispheres can communicate, differences in performance are nonetheless observed. Typically, these effects are in the range of a 10% difference in accuracy in performance or a 20–50 ms difference in reaction time. These studies provide converging evidence with data obtained from patients with unilateral brain damage and from split-brain patients. Myriads of studies have confirmed a left hemisphere superiority for processing verbal information and a right hemisphere superiority for processing nonverbal material, regardless of sensory modality – visual, auditory, or tactile.

Neuroimaging Studies of Hemispheric Specialization

The surge in neuroimaging during the past decade has also served to emphasize that the specializations of the hemispheres are more relative than absolute. These studies have shown that for most all tasks, activation is bilateral, although not necessarily of equal extent nor intensity. Even classic language tasks, such as verbal word reading, activate both hemispheres, although the activation is more left-sided than right-sided. In addition, the complimentarity of the hemispheres is revealed by these studies. For example, single-word processing leads to greater left than right hemisphere activation, but understanding the nonliteral meaning of language, such as analogy or the moral of a story, leads to greater right than left hemisphere activation.

Asymmetries Related to Emotion and Emotional Processing

Hemispheric specialization is not limited to cognitive function; it is found for emotional processes as well. The majority of evidence suggests that the right hemisphere is specialized for the interpretation of emotional information, including information contained in tone of voice and facial expression. Moreover, it is also specialized for the production of emotional cues that serve a communicative function (e.g., a smile that sends a communicative signal to someone else letting him or her know you are happy or pleased).

In contrast, lateralization of mood – that is, the subjective experience of one's internal emotional state – appears to rely on a pattern of brain activation across prefrontal and parietal regions. A large body of research has indicated that asymmetry of activation of frontal regions of the brain is linked to mood states. Greater activation of left than right frontal regions is associated with positive mood and approach behaviors. In contrast, greater activation of the right than left frontal regions is associated with negative mood and avoidance behavior. Moreover, individual differences in these asymmetries have been linked to differences in temperament in infants and to susceptibility to depression in later life. Overlaid on these effects of valence (positive and negative) are differences in activation of right parietal regions, which are linked to arousal. Depressed mood is associated with decreased activity of right parietal regions, whereas the panic associated with heightened anxiety is associated with increased activity of right parietal regions.

Models of Hemispheric Specialization

The broad body of work – from patients with unilateral brain damage, split-brain patients, and studies of perceptual asymmetries with neurologically intact individuals – was originally framed with regard to differences in the type of material that each hemisphere is specialized to process. Initially, the left hemisphere was considered specialized for processing verbal materials, whereas the right hemisphere was considered specialized for processing nonverbal materials. However, in a series of studies in the late 1960s and early 1970s, studies with split-brain patients clearly demonstrated that in many cases both hemispheres were capable of processing a given type of material. What differed, however, was the manner in which they processed that material. This led to a new rubric for understanding hemispheric specialization. The left hemisphere was conceptualized to analyze information in an analytic, piecemeal, and local manner, whereas the right hemisphere was conceptualized to analyze information in a holistic and Gestalt manner. For example, although the right hemisphere of a split-brain patient is superior to the left at identifying a previously viewed face, both can do so. The right hemisphere appears to analyze the overall configuration of the face, such as whether the face is long and narrow or wide and round, and whether the eyes are wide set compared to the width of the face. In contrast, the left hemisphere processes the features or local details, such as the shape of the chin or the eyes. This shift in conceptualizing hemispheric specialization was important because it explained a potential advantage of a specialized brain, namely the ability of simultaneous dual processing. Practically all information can be processed independently and in a distinct manner by each hemisphere at the same time, providing two distinct ways of simultaneously understanding and interpreting the world.

With this conceptual shift, researchers began to explore hemispheric differences from a computational perspective, with the goal of determining the fundamental differences in computations performed by each hemisphere. One early theory suggested that the hemispheres differed in their ability to process low-level sensory information. In particular, the right hemisphere was conceived as being specialized for processing information of low visual spatial frequency – that is, information that does not shift from dark to light within a small degree of visual space. This information generally provides the general contours and outline of visual forms but not the details. In contrast, the left hemisphere was conceived as being specialized for processing information of high spatial frequency – that is, information that shifts quickly, within a given amount of visual space, from dark to light. Such information provides the detail in visual forms. Moreover, asymmetries in higher order cognitive function were posited to emerge from these sensory asymmetries. For example, the overall configuration of a face would be provided by visual information of low spatial frequency, whereas the detailed information would be provided by visual information of high spatial frequency.

This theory was highly influential and has been subsequently modified. Further research demonstrated that the hemispheres appear to be specialized not for the absolute frequency of sensory information but, rather, for the relative frequency, an effect that holds across different sensory modalities. For example, when individuals are presented with information of high auditory frequency, the left hemisphere exhibits a performance advantage for processing the higher half of those high auditory frequencies and the right hemisphere for processing the lower half of those high auditory frequencies. Findings such as these have been expanded to be accounted for by the double-filtering hypothesis, which argues that hemispheric differences arise from an attentional bias in the information that each processes. It is argued that the right hemisphere employs a low pass filter on incoming information, whereas the left hemisphere employs a high pass filter.

Other researchers have focused on why there might be a need to have distinct ways of processing information in each of the cerebral hemispheres. These theories have focused on how the hemispheres might insulate conflicting or independent processes from one another. For example, in the spatial domain it has been argued that the right hemisphere is specialized to coordinate spatial relationships, considered those that provide information about the distance between objects. In contrast, the left hemisphere is specialized for categorical spatial relations that describe the relationship between items (e.g., above, below, to the right of, and to the left of). These two ways of describing information are considered orthogonal to each other because knowing the coordinate information, such as that one item is 3 ft from another, provides no information about categorical information, such as if one item is behind the other. Computational models suggest that these two types of spatial processing are best supported by independent insulated processing systems because the representations required are mutually incompatible and/or create interference. Performance on spatial tasks is superior in a split rather than unitary computational model, suggesting that the hemispheres are specialized to allow for noninterference of processing.

Similar arguments have been made with regard to language processing. Even though the left hemisphere alone has control over speech output and phonological processing, its specialization for language is also relative. Whereas the left hemisphere has been found to be superior to the right hemisphere in aspects of grammar and syntax, the right hemisphere is superior at processing the nonliteral aspects of language, such as discourse, metaphor, and analogy. These differences may arise from incompatible means of semantic access and/or organization. The left hemisphere appears to access words in a very specific, precise, and local manner, whereas the right hemisphere accesses words in a more diffuse manner that allows activation for more far-flung associates. For example, if a paragraph was about gardening, the left hemisphere would quickly hone in on the particular meaning of 'bug' related to insects, whereas the right hemisphere would hold onto a more diffuse set of meanings, including not only the meaning related to insects but also that related to spying devices. As such, the right hemisphere would be better equipped to make connections across sentences and phrases that would allow for discourse and for nonliteral aspects of language comprehension.

Origins of Hemispheric Asymmetry

Although there was once speculation that cerebral asymmetry is a unique feature of the human brain, hemispheric asymmetry is observed in other species, including not only mammals but also fishes, reptiles, and amphibians. The asymmetries observed in behaviors range from those involved in courtship and copulation to escape behavior and limb use (i.e., 'handedness'). These asymmetries are found not only for an individual organism (i.e., a right-sided limb preference in a given animal) but also at the population level. For example, apes tend to use the left hand for stabilizing objects and the right hand for fine motor manipulation. Likewise, 59% of certain species of toad prefer to use their right paw to remove an object affixed to their head.

Because hemispheric asymmetries are observed in many other species, much theorizing has focused on how language processing becomes lateralized. Some theories posit that the association of fine motor coordination of the right hand associated with tool use served as the platform for the fine motor control that is associated with the vocalizations that underlie human language. Other theories posit that a lateralized gestural system, when linked to vocalizations, led to language lateralization. Cross-species support for such an idea is provided by research showing that cells in area F5 of the macaque monkey brain, a region homologous to Broca's area in humans, fire when a monkey sees someone else perform a grasping action similar to one which it has just performed. It has been argued that these 'mirror' neurons underlie the ability to form, through gesture, a common communicative system between individuals. Such a common communicative system would then have evolved to include vocalization. Supporting this idea, gestures linked to speech are produced with much more frequency by the right hand in humans and chimpanzees, whereas gestures that do not have a communicative value (e.g., straightening one's clothes) are not produced asymmetrically.

Developmental Issues and Hemispheric Specialization

Given the evidence for an evolutionary history of lateralization of functioning, it is not surprising that hemispheric asymmetries exist at birth. That is not to say, however, that this pattern cannot be modified by environmental factors. Evidence for an inborn pattern of asymmetry comes from numerous sources. First, gyral and sulcul patterns, which differ between right- and left-handers (who, as discussed later, differ in behavioral asymmetry) are present before birth and not modified thereafter. Second, the effects of hemispherectomy at birth differ depending on whether the left or right hemisphere is removed. Although individuals with only one hemisphere acquire both verbal and nonverbal skills, the degree to which these skills are acquired varies by the hemisphere removed. Individuals with only a right hemisphere perform, on average, better on spatial tasks than those with only a left hemisphere, whereas individuals with only a left hemisphere perform better on verbal tasks than those with only a right hemisphere. Third, asymmetries can be observed in the newborn. These include motoric asymmetries, behavioral asymmetries, and asymmetries in brain responses. For example, a larger evoked response is recorded over the left hemisphere to verbal materials and over the right hemisphere to nonverbal materials.

Thus, it appears that the basic blueprint of hemispheric specialization exists at birth. However, the nature of that blueprint can be altered by environmental factors. For example, it has been well documented that after damage to the left hemisphere during approximately the first 2 years of life, the right hemisphere can acquire the ability to control speech. Somewhat more ambiguous are findings that experience can influence the degree of perceptual asymmetry that is observed. For example, a greater left visual field advantage is observed for holistic processing of faces from a racial group with which one is familiar than for faces of a group with which one is not familiar. Whether this result indicates that the nature of hemispheric specialization is changed by experience, or whether more experience tends to engage more specialized processors in the brain, remains unclear.

The Effect of Handedness

One individual difference, that of handedness, has been clearly linked to patterns of hemispheric specialization for cognitive and emotional function. The relative specializations of the cerebral hemispheres described previously appear to hold only for individuals who are right-handed. In contrast, left-handed individuals, who comprise approximately 10% of individuals worldwide, can have a diverse pattern of lateral organization. This difference is well-known by neurologists and neuropsychologists who have long observed that handedness is an important factor in predicting the types of deficits and the amount of recovery that is likely to be observed after unilateral brain damage. However, there is much variability among left-handers regarding the type of lateralized brain organization they display. In some cases, it is similar to that of right-handers, with the left hemisphere specialized for verbal functions and the right for nonverbal functions. In other cases, it is the opposite, with the right hemisphere specialized for verbal function and the left for nonverbal function. It is estimated that such a brain organization is found in only 1% or 2% of right-handers. Finally, other left-handers exhibit a pattern in which both hemispheres appear to be able to process both verbal and nonverbal information, including speech output. Although much research has attempted to isolate a factor that can predict the type of brain organization a given left-hander will exhibit, for the most part, these efforts have failed. Currently, the leading model of the genetic basis of handedness and its relationship to lateralized brain organization suggests that handedness (and hence brain organization) is randomly distributed, unless one inherits a right-shift allele, which shifts handedness to the right hand and language to the left hemisphere. Such a model assumes that it was evolutionarily advantageous to have motor control of the right hand and control of language co-lateralized to the same hemisphere.

Interhemispheric Integration

After the explosion of research examining hemispheric specialization in the 1970s and 1980s, recent work has examined how the processing of the hemispheres is coordinated and the effects of integration of information between the cerebral hemispheres.

Interhemispheric integration occurs mainly via the massive bundle of nerve fibers connecting the cerebral hemispheres, the corpus callosum. Because information from the peripheral nerves is directed contralaterally, at least for vision, motor, and somatosensory information, integration of information across the hemispheres allows information from each sensory half-field to be bound together. For example, in the visual domain, information is represented contralaterally in V1, V2, and V3a/VP. In fact, there are few, if any callosal connections in BA 17. Representation of information from the ipsilateral visual field first appears at the level of V3a and V4v, which are brain regions whose cells have receptive fields that span the midline. This critical role of the callosum in fusing the sensory worlds is made apparent by split-brain patients who cannot bind information from different sensory fields. For example, if fixated on a central point and shown two items, one on each side visual midline so that they are projected to opposite hemispheres, a split-brain patient cannot determine if they are the same or different.

Although the callosum acts as a mechanism to transfer information between the hemispheres, this transfer involves time costs as well as degradation of information. Transfer of information via the corpus callosum takes approximately 5 ms via the large myelinated fibers that connect sensory and motor areas and 20–50 ms for small unmylineated fibers. The fidelity costs are apparent in old/new memory paradigms. If an item is presented in one visual field, correctly recognizing of that item as previously viewed is poorer if presented to the hemisphere that did not initially view the item as compared to the hemisphere. Such findings are consistent with theorizing that the representations supported by each of the hemispheres are different and are not completely interchangeable.

Integration of information across the cerebral hemispheres plays an additional role above and beyond that of binding together the visual world – that of attentional control. Evidence suggests that the cerebral hemispheres dynamically couple and decouple to meet task demands. When tasks involve relatively low attentional demands, performance is better when all the critical information needed for a decision (e.g., are these two items physically identical?) is directed to a single hemisphere compared to divided between them. It has been proposed that under such conditions, the processing capacity of a single hemisphere is adequate to meet the demands and the cost of interhemispheric communication takes a toll on performance. In contrast, when attentional demands are high, dividing processing between the hemispheres enables more resources to be brought to bear and the advantage provided by these additional resources more than outweighs the cost of callosal transfer. Such an outcome can occur because, as described previously, the specialization of the hemispheres is not absolute but relative, allowing both hemispheres to process almost all types of information. Thus, the additional resources provided by the partner hemisphere, even if not specialized for the task, can nonetheless have a major impact on performance. These findings are consonant with data from individuals in whom the corpus callosum is severed or damaged, such as occurs in multiple sclerosis. A common consequence of callosal damage or insufficiency is problems in attentional control. Although the neural mechanisms that allow the callosum to play such a role remain somewhat obscure, connectionist modeling suggests that the advantage afforded by dividing processing between the hemispheres is an emergent phenomenon of having two somewhat insulated and distinct processors.

Summary

Each of the human cerebral hemispheres has a distinct manner of processing information, with the left hemisphere more adept at attending to and processing more fine-grained information and the right hemisphere more adept at attending to and processing more coarse-grained information. This distinction holds for all types of information, whether verbal or spatial. The complimentarity of these modes of processing means that the human brain contains two processors, each of which provides a unique manner of understanding and interpreting the world.

Moreover, this dichotomy and isolation of processing also provides for a system that can dynamically reconfigure to act in isolation or in tandem depending on attentional demands.

See also: Brain Asymmetry: Evolution; Cognition: An Overview of Neuroimaging Techniques; Dichotic Listening Studies of Brain Asymmetry; Emotional Hormones and Memory Modulation; Memory: Genetic Approaches; Multisensory Convergence and Integration; Split-Brain Patients.

Further Reading

Annett M (2002) *Handedness and Brain Asymmetry: The Right Shift Theory.* New York: Psychology Press.

Banich MT (1998) The missing link: The role of interhemispheric interaction in attentional processing. *Brain and Cognition* 36: 128–157.

Beeman MJ and Chiarello C (1998) Complementary right- and left-hemisphere language comprehension. *Current Directions in Psychological Science* 7: 2–8.

Corballis MC (2003) From mouth to hand: Gesture, speech, and the evolution of right-handedness. *Behavioral and Brain Sciences* 26: 199–260.

Davidson RJ (1992) Anterior cerebral asymmetry and the nature of emotion. *Brain & Cognition* 20: 125–151.

Hellige JB (2001) *Hemispheric Asymmetry: What's Right and What's Left.* Cambridge, MA: Harvard University Press.

Hugdahl K and Davidson RJ (eds.) (2003) *The Asymmetrical Brain.* Cambridge: MIT Press.

Ivry RB and Robertson LC (1998) *The Two Sides of Perception.* Cambridge: MIT Press.

Keller J, Nitschke JB, Bhargava T, et al. (2000) Neuropsychological differentiation of depression and anxiety. *Journal of Abnormal Psychology* 109: 3–10.

Kosslyn SM (1987) Seeing and imagining in the cerebral hemispheres: A computational approach. *Psychological Review* 94: 148–175.

Levy J, Trevarthen C, and Sperry RW (1972) Perception of bilateral chimeric figures following hemispheric deconnexion. *Brain* 95: 61–78.

Monaghan P and Pollmann S (2003) Division of labor between the hemispheres for complex but not simple tasks: An implemented connectionist model. *Journal of Experimental Psychology: General* 132: 379–399.

Sergent J (1985) Influence of task and input factors on hemispheric involvement in face processing. *Journal of Experimental Psychology: Human Perception and Performance* 11: 846–861.

Trevarthen C (1996) Lateral asymmetries in infancy: Implications for the development of the hemispheres. *Neuroscience & Biobehavioral Reviews* 20: 571–586.

Zaidel E and Iacoboni M (eds.) (2003) *The Parallel Brain: The Cognitive Neuroscience of the Corpus Callosum.* Cambridge: MIT Press.

Human Methods: Psychophysics

B A Schneider, University of Toronto at Mississauga, Mississauga, ON, Canada
S Parker, The American University, Washington, DC, USA

Introduction

Psychophysical methods have been developed by researchers in an attempt to determine how the mind encodes and represents environmental events – that is, to determine the relationship between the mind ('psycho') and the world ('physics'). To investigate such relationships, methods were developed in which observers were required to make judgments concerning the presence or absence of stimuli, or the sensory relationship of one stimulus to another (e.g., whether stimulus one is brighter than stimulus two). These judgments were then used to determine how the stimulus is encoded and represented in the minds of the observers. Note that the nature of this representation is inferred from behavioral judgments. Hence psychophysical methodology is a way of indirectly investigating how information about the physical world is organized and represented in the nervous system.

Although these methods were initially used to investigate the relationship between a physical aspect of the stimulus and how it is experienced by the observer (e.g., how the loudness of a sound is related to its physical intensity), they are now used to investigate how information in general is encoded and represented. Hence, psychophysical methodology can be, and is, used not only to investigate how a psychological attribute varies as a function of some physical variable, but also to determine, among other things, the psychological utility of objects, the prestige of various occupations, or the discriminability between classes of words previously presented to observers and semantically related words that were not previously presented. Note that in these latter three examples, the psychological property under investigation is not directly related to any specific physical aspect of the stimulus.

In approaching psychophysical methodology we begin here by describing the theory upon which many of these methods are based. We then describe the range of psychophysical methods that have been developed to assess how information is encoded and represented, along with examples of their application.

Theoretical Concepts

Representation of Information

Psychophysical methodologies assume that the activity a stimulus evokes in the nervous system can be represented as a point in an n-dimensional space. Consider, for example, a pure tone, which has four physical dimensions, intensity, frequency, duration, and phase. If each of these dimensions had a psychological counterpart, we would need four dimensions to represent the manner in which an observer experiences that tone. However, because observers are not sensitive to monaural phase, it is likely that there are only three dimensions to the psychological experience: loudness, pitch, and perceived duration. In **Figure 1**, the loudness, pitch, and perceived duration evoked by single presentations of each of three tones are indicated as points in a three-dimensional (3-D) space. Because a stimulus will not give rise to exactly the same experience each time it is presented (because of the presence of external noise or intrinsic variability in the nervous system), repeated presentations of a stimulus are depicted as giving rise to a cloud of points clustered around a mean position in this 3-D space.

To better illustrate the degree of variability in the evoked experience, **Figure 2** plots the probability density functions that result when three pure tones having different intensities and frequencies, but identical durations, are presented repeatedly to an observer. (Because the mean perceived duration is the same for all three tones, variation along the perceived duration dimension is not illustrated.) As in **Figure 1**, variations in loudness and pitch are assumed to be independently and normally distributed with standard deviations of 1.0. In this example, because the tones are closely spaced together, the distributions exhibit some degree of overlap.

It is important to note that, theoretically, we could assume any two-dimensional probability function for the stimuli in this space, and we need not assume that all probability density functions are equally variable. However, the default assumption is usually that the distributions are normal or Gaussian in shape, and that the variation of stimuli along any one dimension is constant. (In **Figure 2** the variances are shown as equal across the two dimensions.) In addition, in the vast majority of cases in which psychophysical methods are employed, it is assumed or shown that the stimuli being judged can be represented along a single

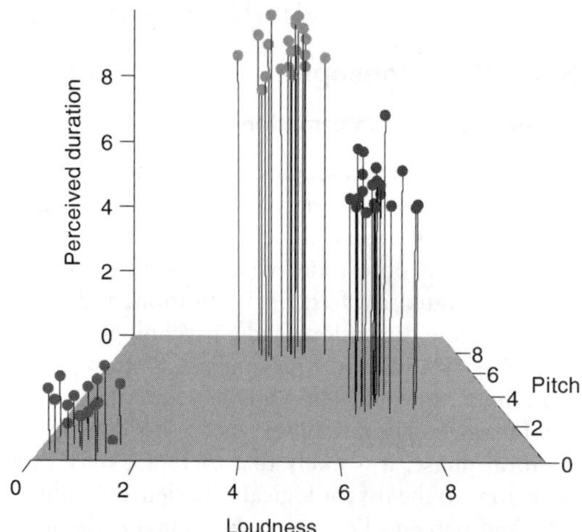

Figure 1 Each tone is presumed to evoke a sensation of loudness, pitch, and perceived duration. The subjective experience corresponding to a tone presentation is represented as a point in a 3-D perceptual space with axes of loudness, pitch, and perceived duration. Because of variability in the stimulus, and the presence of internal noise, the location of a point varies from trial to trial, even when the stimulus remains the same. In generating a cluster of points for a tone, it was assumed that the loudness, pitch, and perceived duration values were independently and normally distributed with a standard deviation equal to 1.0. Shown here are hypothetical clouds of points resulting from 20 repetitions of three tones. The mean locations of the three tones, for loudness (L), pitch (P), and perceived duration (PD), are depicted as follows: red ($L=1$, $P=1$, PD $=1$), green ($L=5$, $P=8$, PD $=8.5$), and purple ($L=7$, $P=4$, PD $=4.5$).

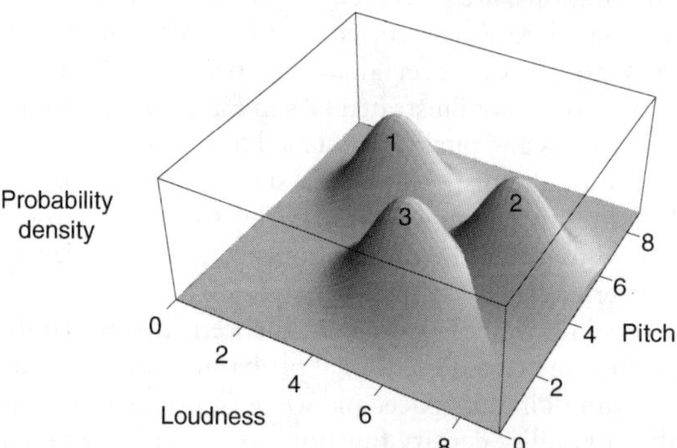

Figure 2 Probability density functions for three tones having identical perceived durations but different loudness and pitch values. Loudness (L) and pitch (P) values are as follows: tone 1 ($L=3$, $P=6$), tone 2 ($L=7$, $P=5$); and tone 3 ($L=5$, $P=3$). The loudness and pitch values for each of the tones are assumed to be independently and normally distributed with standard deviations equal to 1.0.

psychological dimension. For example, were we to restrict our set of pure tones to have the same mean pitch and perceived duration, so that they differed reliably only in loudness, we would choose to represent their density functions along a single psychological dimension, such as the one shown in **Figure 3**. Here, the Gaussian probability density functions for all tones have the same variance, and differ only in their mean values. We refer to this situation as the unidimensional, normally distributed, equal-variance case. In describing the various psychometric methods, we restrict our discussion herein to this case.

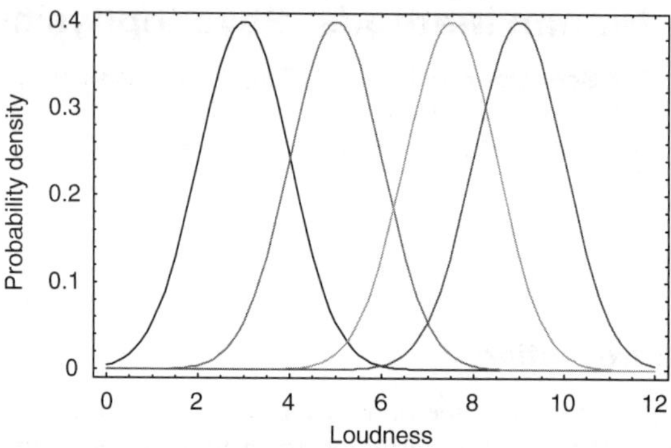

Figure 3 Hypothetical distributions of loudness values for four pure tones in the equal-variance Gaussian model.

Relationship to the Goal of Psychophysics

As mentioned in the Introduction, psychophysical methods were developed to explore how sensory information is structured in the mind, and to relate this structure to the physical world. For instance, if **Figure 3** truly represented how the loudness of four different tones was experienced, then one could relate the mean loudness values of these stimuli to their physical intensities, thereby establishing a psychophysical relationship. Psychophysical methods, based on observers' judgments, were developed to establish how the physical properties of stimuli were experienced, so that psychophysical relationships, such as the one between loudness and sound intensity, could be established. However, these methods can be used to determine how other psychological phenomena are represented, such as the utilities of a collection of objects, even though it may be difficult to determine exactly how the utility of an object is related to its physical properties. In all cases, these psychophysical methods are based on judgments about relationships among stimuli. Here we consider different types of judgments and what can be learned from them.

Psychophysical Methodologies

Detection Experiments

In many instances, the experimenter wants to know the minimum value of a stimulus that can be detected. For example, a vision scientist might want to know the smallest degree of contrast that can be detected in a sinusoidal grating (see **Figure 4**, top row), and the simplest way of determining this is to ask the observer to report the presence or absence of contrast on a trial. There are two classes of psychophysical methods that have been developed for the detection experiment, the Yes/No method and the *m*-interval forced-choice method.

The Yes/No method In the simplest version of this method there are *n* trials and a single stimulus. The occurrence of a trial is signaled in some fashion, and there are two types of trials: those in which a stimulus appears and those in which no stimulus is presented. For example, consider an experiment in which the stimulus is a low-contrast sinusoidal grating (**Figure 4**, top row), and the observer's task is to detect the presence of this stimulus when it is added to a field of Gaussian noise (**Figure 4**, middle row). The occurrence of a trial is signaled by the presentation of a fixation cross in the middle of the screen, and a trial of fixed duration begins either shortly after the fixation cross occurs, or shortly following a button press by the observer. The trial consists of a presentation of the noise field alone (N trial; **Figure 4**, middle row), or the sum of the sinusoidal grating (S) and the noise field (signal + noise, or SN, trial; **Figure 4**, bottom row). The probability of an SN trial, *p*(SN), is fixed throughout the session, and the observer's task to indicate whether there is a signal present (a Yes response) or not (a No response). Correct detection of a signal is typically referred to as a Hit (H); responding Yes when there is no signal is referred to as a False Alarm (FA). If there are *n*(N) noise trials and *n*(SN) signal trials, the critical data in this experiment are the proportion of Hits, *n*(H)/*n*(SN), versus the proportion of False Alarms, *n*(FA)/*n*(N). These two proportions are used to estimate the detectability of the sinusoidal grating, assuming that the N and SN stimuli give rise to two different distributions of events along a unidimensional decision axis (e.g., perceived contrast). As mentioned previously, it is usually assumed that these two distributions are Gaussian and have equivalent standard deviations (see **Figure 5(a)**).

Interpretation of the results of this experiment, however, depends on whether or not one assumes that the threshold for detecting a grating is fixed or variable. **Figure 5** illustrates what we would expect if the threshold was fixed. Here, the observer would report the presence of a grating whenever the occurrence of a trial produced an event along the decision

Figure 4 Images of signals and noises. (Top row): Signals; vertically oriented sine wave gratings (four cycles/image). The leftmost image has a contrast of 0 (no grating, i.e., uniform gray); the contrasts of the other images in the row increase from left to right. (Middle row): Noises; five independent samples of Gaussian noise. (Bottom row): Signal + noise; here, the gratings in the top row have been added to independent samples of noise. Note that there is no sinusoidal grating in the leftmost square of this row. Hence, this is technically a noise trial. The other four squares constitute signal + noise events.

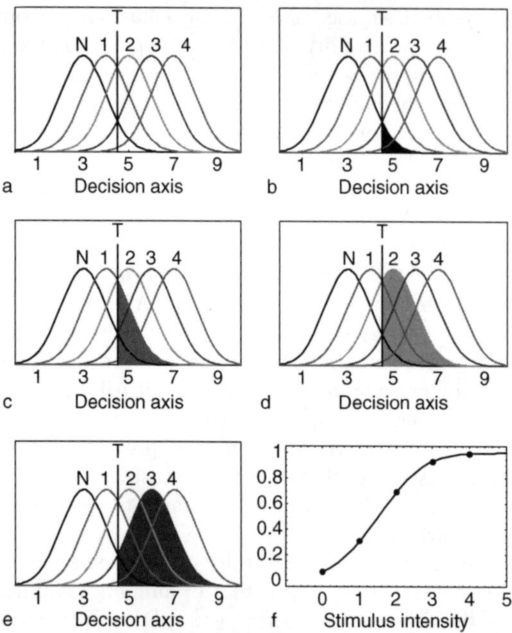

Figure 5 (a) Noise (N) and four signal + noise distributions (1, 2, 3, 4) along a unidimensional decision axis; T represents the point on the decision axis corresponding to a fixed threshold. (b) The portion of the N distribution that exceeds threshold. (c–e) The corresponding portions of the first three signal + noise distributions (1–3) that exceed threshold. (f) Probability of a Yes response as a function of stimulus intensity. This function assumes that the mean location of a stimulus event along the decision axis is linearly related to stimulus intensity. If the relation mapping stimulus intensity onto the decision axis is nonlinear, the shape of this function will change accordingly.

axis (the neural representation of contrast) to the right of the threshold, T. The area under an SN distribution to the right of the threshold would correspond to the probability of a Hit in an SN trial. Increasing the degree of contrast would shift the mean of the SN distribution to right, thereby increasing the proportion of the distribution to the right of T (compare areas to the right of T for **Figures** 5(**b**)–5(**e**)). Hence, by presenting different stimulus contrasts over successive experimental sessions one could map out a psychometric function relating the proportion of Yes responses to the degree of visual contrast as indicated in **Figure** 5(**f**). Note that as visual contrast approaches 0, p(H) approaches p(FA). The reason for this is that the N distribution extends to the right of T, so occasional events occur along the decision axis that exceed this fixed threshold even in the absence of a stimulus. Hence, p(FA) provides a floor for p(H), as stimulus contrast becomes smaller and smaller.

Note that if the threshold is fixed, the probability of a False Alarm will be independent of the stimulus contrast in the signal. Therefore, rather than varying stimulus contrast across sessions (where each session consists of N and SN trials), it would be more efficient to simply vary stimulus contrast within a session, with one of the several contrast values being zero (an N trial). This method is called the 'method of constant stimuli,' and the asymptotic value of the psychometric function obtained when stimulus magnitude approaches zero is sometimes referred to as the 'probability of guessing.' Under fixed-threshold theory, it would be interpreted as a measure of the location of the threshold relative to the null event (no stimulus presentation).

Assuming a fixed threshold and a unidimensional decision axis, one can measure the location of each of the stimuli along the decision axis with reference to the null event, measured in standard deviation units. Assume for the moment that we use the method of constant stimuli (in which one of the stimuli was the null stimulus) to map out a psychometric function relating p(Yes) to stimulus contrast. To do this we first rescale the x axis so that all distributions have a standard deviation of 1.0. Second, we determine the z-score corresponding to the location of the threshold T with respect to the mean, μ_N, of the N distribution ($z_{N,T} = \mu_N - T$). Third, we determine the z-score for T relative to the mean for an SN stimulus (e.g., $z_{SN1,T} = \mu_{SN1} - T$). Note that p(FA) (see **Figure 5(b)**) is the probability that an event elicited on an N trial, $z_{N,}$, exceeds $z_{N,T}$ – that is, $p(FA) = p(z_N > z_{N,T})$ – and that p(H) on an SN_1 trial (see **Figure 5(c)**) is the probability that an event elicited on an SN_1 trial, z_{SN1}, exceeds $z_{SN1,T}$ – that is, $p(H) = p(z_{SN1} > z_{SN1,T})$. Hence, p(FA) and p(H) can be used to find $z_{N,T}$ and $z_{SN1,T}$, respectively. Now if we subtract $z_{N,T}$ from $z_{SN1,T}$ we obtain $(\mu_{SN1} - T) - (\mu_N - T) = \mu_{SN1} - \mu_N$. Hence, the difference between the z-transformation of p(H) when SN_1 is presented, and the z-transformation of p(FA), is an estimate of the distance between the means of the two distributions when the abscissa has been rescaled so that all distributions have a standard deviation of 1.0. This difference between the two means is called d' (d prime). Therefore, we can determine the separation between the means of the signal distributions with respect to the mean of the N distribution in units of d'. Note that to do this, we need to assume that the decision axis is unidimensional and that the distributions corresponding to different stimuli are equal-variance normal distributions. Increasing the separation between the distributions in **Figures 5(a)–5(e)** will increase d' and the rapidity of the growth of the function in **Figure 5(f)**. An individual who has a large value of d' has good resolving power – a good ability to discriminate between presentations of N and of SN.

Note that up to this point we have assumed a fixed threshold. A number of experiments have suggested that the location of the decision point along the decision axis is variable and can be set by the observer. For example, in a simple Yes/No experiment, we can vary the probability of an SN trial across sessions and/or we could create variable rewards for Hits and penalties for False Alarms. If the threshold is truly fixed, then p(FA) and p(H) should be independent of both p(SN) and the payoff structure of the experiment. However, in general they are not, and there is every indication that observers can adjust location of the decision point (the 'criterion') to improve outcomes in the experiment.

Consider the case in which the probability of an SN trial is 0.5, and the observer is penalized \$2.00 for every False Alarm, and rewarded with \$1.00 for every Hit. Assume that the N and SN distributions are separated by 1.5 standard deviation units ($d' = 1.5$). **Figure 6** shows five different possible locations (panels a–e) of the criterion along the decision axis. Each of these criterion locations will give rise to different proportions of False Alarms and Hits in an experiment. Assume 1000 (500 N and 500 SN) trials. The amount of money that a person will earn is \$1.00 × n(H) – \$2.00 × n(FA), where n(H) and n(FA) are the numbers of Hits and False Alarms. The amount of money earned for each of the criterion locations is also shown in **Figures 6(a)–6(e)**. **Figure 6(f)** shows how the expected payoff for this experiment varies as a function of criterion location. Observers in this experiment will maximize their payoffs if they locate their criterion approximately 5/6 of the way between the mean of the N distribution and the mean of the SN distributions. Clearly, if possible, observers should position their criterion to maximize payoff. A similar argument holds when p(SN) is varied.

By convention, the unbiased condition occurs when the observer locates the criterion midway between the two distributions. Under these conditions, p(FA) will equal $1 - p$(H). Changing the location of the criterion away from the unbiased location will change p(FA) and p(H) in a systematic way, but will not change d'. A plot of p(H) versus p(FA) for a constant d' is called a 'receiver operating characteristic' (ROC). **Figure 7** shows ROCs for $d' = 0$ (the diagonal line), $d' = 0.5$, $d' = 1$, $d' = 1.5$, and $d' = 2.0$.

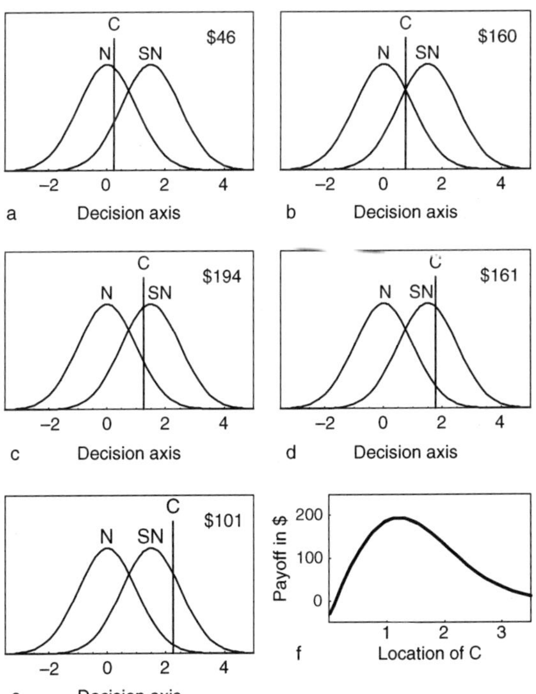

Figure 6 (a–e) Different criterion (C) locations for detecting a signal in noise, where d' between the noise (N) and signal + noise (SN) distributions is 1.5. The dollar amount is the expected payoff if the observer is given \$1 for each hit and penalized \$2 for each false alarm (number of trials = 1000). (f) The expected payoff for this experiment as a function of criterion location.

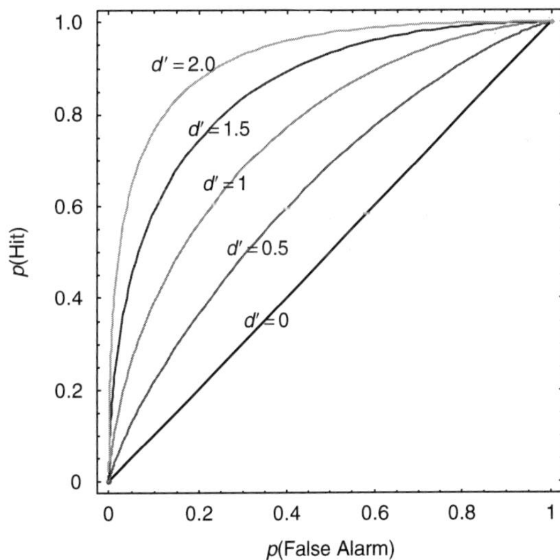

Figure 7 Receiver operating characteristics for a Yes/No paradigm, assuming that repeated presentations of noise give rise to a normal distribution of events along a decision axis, and that repeated presentations of signal + noise give rise to another normal distribution of events along the decision axis with the same variance as that of the noise distribution. The probability p of a Hit is plotted as a function of the probability of a False Alarm in this paradigm for four different values of d'. Each curve is generated by determining and plotting p(Hit) and p(False Alarm) as the location of the criterion is swept along the decision axis.

It is important to note that signal-analysis techniques based on the Yes/No paradigm can also be applied to neural data. For instance, suppose a researcher is measuring the response rate of a single unit in visual cortex that is sensitive to luminance contrast. Using the method of constant stimuli, the researcher could repeatedly present the each of the five gratings shown in the top row of **Figure 4** an equal number of times, and record the response rate during that presentation period. Distributions of response rates could then be determined for each of the stimuli, and a threshold response could be set by the experimenter. This would be equivalent to setting the location of T in **Figure 5**. The experimenter could then determine the area under each distribution to the right of the threshold criterion and then plot this area (proportion of times threshold is exceeded) as a function of stimulus contrast, thereby mapping out a function like the one shown in **Figure 5(f)**. In this way, the experimenter can determine the shape of the function relating d' to physical contrast. Note, however, that in this kind of application, it is the experimenter, rather than the subject of the experiment, who is setting the location of the criterion.

The advantage of a signal-detection analysis of a Yes/No experiment is that it allows the experimenter, in analyzing the data, to separate shifts of criterion location (also referred to as response biases) from sensitivity. Both changes in d' and shifts of criterion location will affect both p(H) and p(FA) – the observer's performance will be sensitive to both. However, to estimate both accurately requires the collection of enough data to plot an ROC curve. Often, experimenters are primarily interested in sensitivity measures (such as d') and not interested in determining response criteria. In such circumstances, an m-interval or m-alternative forced-choice paradigm is typically used.

m-Interval forced-choice method In an m-interval forced-choice paradigm, a trial consists of the presentation of m intervals separated by a short but constant interinterval time period. Most experimenters prefer to use two intervals only, and two stimulus values (N and SN), so that this method is referred to as a two-interval, two-alternative, forced-choice (2I2AFC, or sometimes just 2IFC) procedure. In a 2IFC paradigm, SN is randomly assigned to one of the two intervals, with N occurring in the other. Hence, there are two types of trials, N_SN and SN_N, with the probability of each trial type typically being set to 0.5. The observer's task is to decide which type of trial it is. The ideal strategy is for the observer to note the value of the event that occurs along the decision axis in each of the intervals and subtract one from the other. Let the difference between the means of the N and SN distributions be d'. Suppose the observer subtracts the observation in interval one from the observation in interval two. On N_SN trials, this strategy will give rise to a normal distribution with a mean of d' and a standard deviation $= \sqrt{2}$. On SN_N trials, this strategy will give rise to a distribution with a mean $= -d'$ and a standard deviation of $\sqrt{2}$. If these two distributions are then normalized so that their standard deviations are 1.0, the separation between the means of these two distributions is $\sqrt{2}d'$. The distribution of this difference score is shown for N_SN and SN_N presentations in **Figure 8**, where the d' value separating the original N and SN distributions in the Yes/No task is 1.0. Note that if the observer chooses to respond that the signal is in interval 2 if the observation in interval 2 is greater than the observation in interval 1, this places the location of the criterion, C, for deciding which type of trial type occurred, midway between the distributions for N_SN and SN_N (i.e., the decision is unbiased). Provided that the two types of trials occur equally frequently and the payoff for correct identification of both kinds of trials is unbiased, there is every reason to believe that observers will set their criterion to zero, i.e., to the unbiased position. Hence, the 2IFC is said to minimize the possibility of the occurrence of response biases. Because the expectation in a 2IFC experiment is that the observer is unbiased, d' values

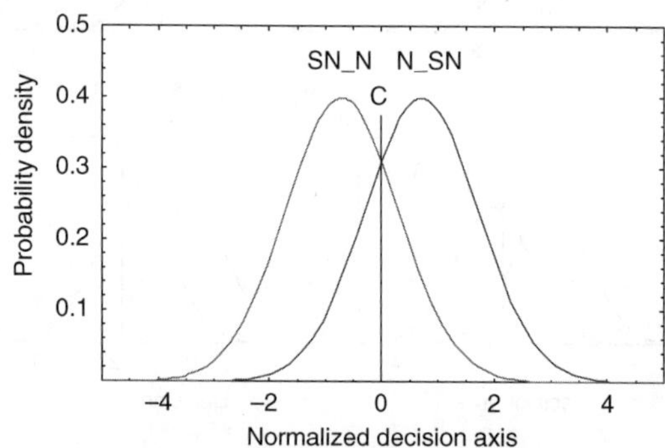

Figure 8 Shown here are hypothetical distributions of events along a normalized decision axis in a two-interval forced-choice experiment. For noise (N) and signal + noise (SN), both the SN_N distribution (signal in first interval, noise in the second interval) and the N_SN distribution (noise in the first interval, signal in the second) were generated by assuming that the observer subtracts an observation along the decision axis during the first interval from an observation along the decision axis during the second interval on both kinds of trials. In other words, the observer responds that the signal is in the second interval when this difference observation is >0. The two distributions of difference judgments corresponding to the two types of trials (SN_N and N_SN) have been normalized to have unit variances, with the separation between the means of the N and SN distributions along the original decision axis being equal to 1 ($d'_{Yes/No} = 1$); C, criterion location.

are typically not computed, and experimenters usually plot percent correct identification as a function of stimulus intensity.

A very significant advantage of the 2IFC procedure is that it is amenable to adaptive techniques in which the intensity of the signal is changed from trial to trial in an attempt to rapidly converge to the stimulus intensity corresponding to a particular point on the psychometric function relating percent correct to stimulus intensity. Consider the following rule for adjusting the stimulus contrast on successive trials in a 2IFC task. If the observer is correct on three successive trials, lower the contrast. However, if the observer makes a mistake on a trial, increase the contrast. Typically, the amount by which the contrast is increased or decreased becomes smaller each time there is a reversal in direction. **Figure 9** plots the performance of an observer in such a task when the initial stimulus contrast was set to 50%, and the first step size is a 10% change in contrast, with the step size decreased by one-half with each reversal of direction, until a minimum step size is reached. The session is usually terminated after a certain number of reversals have occurred, and the threshold is estimated by averaging the last few reversals in intensity. For an attentive observer this '3 down, 1 up' rule will converge on the 79% point of the psychometric function.

Many different algorithms have been developed, including some based on maximum-likelihood procedures, to achieve efficient and unbiased convergence on the targeted point on the psychometric function using the 2IFC procedure. In general, the algorithms that provide the most rapid convergence are sensitive

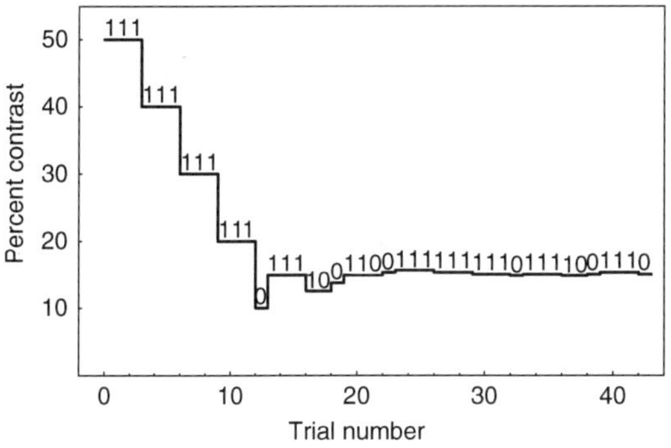

Figure 9 Performance of a hypothetical observer in a method of adjustment paradigm employing a '3 down, 1 up' procedure in a two-interval forced-choice experiment paradigm. In this procedure, three correct responses in a row (a correct response is denoted by the numeral 1) reduce the contrast by a fixed amount on the next trial. If an incorrect response (0) occurs, the contrast is incremented on the next trial. On each reversal of direction of change, the size of the increment is halved on the next trial until a minimum step size for a contrast change is reached. The session is terminated when performance has stabilized.

to lapses in attention. Therefore, the appropriate method to choose will depend on the motivation and attentiveness expected of the observers.

Vigilance paradigm In Yes/No and 2IFC methods, the trial periods are discrete and usually short. In the vigilance paradigm, there is usually one long trial period, during which stimuli are occasionally and infrequently presented. In order to perform well on this task, the observer has to remain focused on the task (i.e., remain vigilant). The dependent measure is the proportion of times the observer detects the presentation of the signal. The vigilance paradigm is typically employed in an attempt to simulate situations in which constant monitoring is required, and the occurrence of signals is unpredictable and infrequent (e.g., monitoring a radar screen to detect intruder aircraft).

Tracking techniques In the techniques just described, stimulus presentations are usually brief, intermittent, and under the control of the experimenter. One can determine the threshold value of a stimulus, however, by using a tracking technique in which stimulus intensity is controlled by the observer. For instance, observers can be told that as long as they press down on a button, the intensity of a tone will continue to decrease and will increase only when the button is released. They are then told to hold down the button when they can hear the tone and to release it when the tone becomes inaudible. In this way, the threshold can be tracked during the course of a session.

Discrimination Experiments

In addition to determining the detectability of a stimulus, one often wants to determine how discriminable pairs of the stimuli are. Here, rather than having a no-signal condition (with or without external noise) versus a signal condition (again, with or without noise), the two conditions become stimulus 1 versus stimulus 2 (S1 and S2). Because of inherent variability in the nervous system, repeated presentations of the two stimuli are assumed to give rise to dispersions of events along a decision axis (even in the absence of external noise), presumably with Gaussian distributions. Hence, by simply substituting S1 for N, and S2 for SN, stimulus discriminability can be investigated using either the Yes/No or the 2IFC method.

Scaling Experiments

In many cases the experimenter would like to know how a dimension of stimulus experience is represented in the nervous system. Two classes of procedures exist for determining this: direct scaling methods and indirect scaling methods. In direct scaling methods the observer is asked to directly report, say, on the loudness of a sound by assigning a number to it, or by indicating where the loudness of that sound would lie along some scale. The most commonly used direct methods require observers to assign numbers to the stimuli that reflect the magnitude of a sensory property of a stimulus. For example, one could present observers with pure tones ranging from 40 to 100 dB, and ask them to assign numbers to these tones such that the numbers are directly proportional to the loudness they experience (magnitude estimation). Or, one could ask them to assign a number that represents the ratio of the loudness of one tone to another (ratio estimation), or the difference in loudness between two tones (interval estimation), or one could ask them to rate loudness on a 1 to 10 scale (category estimation). The assumption in such techniques is that observers can assign numbers in such a way that they are proportional to sensory experience – that is, $N_L = k \times L$, where N_L is the numerical estimate of loudness generated by the observer, and L is the magnitude of the psychological loudness experience evoked by the stimulus. These techniques are easy to employ, require relatively few trials, and typically generate reliable and replicable relationships between numerical estimates and stimulus intensity. Their weakness is that they assume that observers can accurately, and without bias, assign numbers to reflect stimulus qualities.

Indirect scaling methods derive sensory scales without assuming that the observer can directly assign numbers to sensory experience. For example, consider a set of 12 pure tones differing only in intensity. Suppose each tone gives rise to a value along a unidimensional loudness scale, these 12 tones form $12 \times 11/2 = 66$ distinct pairs. Suppose the observer is asked, when presented with two pairs of tones, to indicate whether the loudness difference between the tones in pair 1 was larger or smaller than the loudness difference between the tones in pair 2, and these judgments are based on a comparison of the psychological distance between the tones in pairs 1 and 2. It turns out that there is sufficient information in the comparisons of pairs to permit the experimenter to recover the location of the tones along this subjective dimension such that the recovered locations, P, are related to the loudnesses of the tones, L, by $P = k \times L + b$. In **Figure 10**, 12 points were randomly chosen along the line segment from 0 to 1. The 66 interpoint differences between the points were then computed and used to decide which of two intervals was larger. These binary comparisons of intervals were used to recover the location of the original points along a line segment from 0 to 1. **Figure 10** plots the recovered locations of the points as a function of their original values, and shows that a comparison of intervals contains sufficient information to recover the original points, such that $y = k \times x + b$, where y is the recovered value of the point, and x is the original value of the point. When 12 stimuli are involved, and the observer can accurately judge which interval is larger, agreement between the recovered and original points is almost perfect.

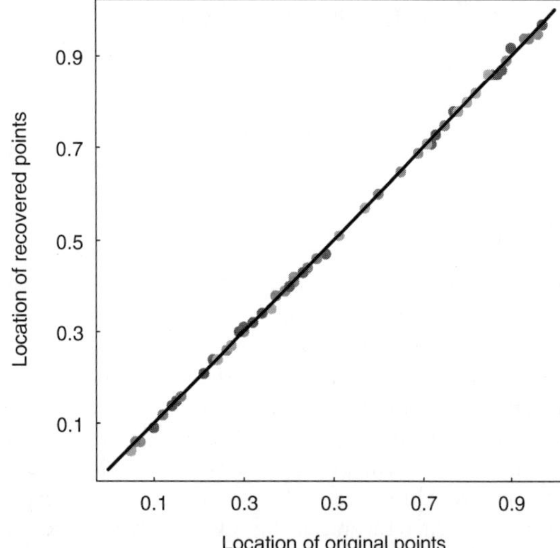

Figure 10 Five simulations of the application of a nonmetric scaling procedure to recover the location of a set of 12 points, randomly sampled from the line segment (0, 1), from comparisons of the intervals between pairs of points. Different colors are assigned to the five different sets of 12 points. In each simulation, all pairwise distances were determined among the set of 12 points. These distances were then used to determine whether the interval between a pair of points (a, b) was greater than, equal to, or less than the interval between another pair of points (c, d). These inequality judgments served as input to a nonmetric scaling program, which returned the best fitting locations of the points along the line segment (0, 1). These recovered points are plotted as a function of the original points. The squared correlation coefficients between the recovered and original points exceed 0.999 in all five cases.

See also: Decision-Making and Vision; Ideal Observer Theory; Information Coding; Statistical Tests and Inferences.

Further Reading

Bissett RJ and Schneider B (1991) Spatial and conjoint models based on pairwise comparisons of dissimilarities and combined effects: Complete and incomplete designs. *Psychometrika* 56: 685–698.

Dunn-Rankin P, Knezek GA, Wallace S, et al. (2004) *Scaling Methods*, 2nd edn. Mahwah NJ: Lawrence Erlbaum Associates.

Gescheider G (1997) *Psychophysics: The Fundamentals*, 3rd edn. Mahwah, NJ: Lawrence Erlbaum Associates.

Goldstein EB (2005) Cross-talk between psychophysics and physiology in the study of perception. In: Goldstein EB (ed.) *Blackwell Handbook of Sensation & Perception*, pp. 1–23. Malden, MA: Blackwell.

Macmillan NA (2001) Psychometric functions and adaptive methods [Special issue]. *Perception & Psychophysics* 63(8).

Macmillan NA and Creelman CD (2005) *Detection Theory: A User's Guide*, 2nd edn., Mahwah NJM: Lawrence Erlbaum Associates.

Marks LE and Gescheider GA (2002) Psychophysical scaling. In: Pashler H and Wixted J (eds.) *Stevens' Handbook of Experimental Psychology: Volume 4. Methodology in Experimental Psychology*, 3rd edn., pp. 91–138. New York: Wiley.

Schneider B, Parker S, and Stein D (1974) The measurement of loudness using direct comparisons of sensory intervals. *Journal of Mathematical Psychology* 11: 259–273.

Taberner AM and Liberman MC (2005) Response properties of single auditory nerve fibers in the mouse. *Journal of Neurophysiology* 93: 557–569.

Wickens TD (2002) *Elementary Signal Detection Theory*. New York: Oxford University Press.

Humans

A P Shimamura, University of California, Berkeley, CA, USA

The frontal lobes comprise roughly a third of the human cerebral cortex. Through evolution this brain region has increased disproportionately, and as a result of this expansion it has been viewed as the basis for human intellect and thought. Studies of individuals with brain injury have suggested that frontal lobe damage affects many aspects of cognition, including attention, memory, language, problem solving, emotion, and decision making. Yet, its role as the seat of human reasoning and thought became suspect, as findings indicated that frontal lobe damage did not grossly affect measures of general intelligence. Now, there is general consensus that the frontal lobes – or more specifically the anterior portion of the frontal lobes identified as the prefrontal cortex (PFC) – contributes to the regulation or control of mental processing.

The PFC can be parceled into five general regions – the dorsolateral (dlPFC), ventrolateral (vlPFC), posterior (pPFC), anterior (aPFC), and ventromedial (vmPFC) prefrontal regions. These first four regions are spatially located as north, south, east, and west regions within the PFC when the left hemisphere is viewed from the side (i.e., laterally). The fifth region, vmPFC, refers to the lowest and medial (i.e., inner) portions of the PFC. These regions are intricately connected to regions outside the PFC (i.e., in the posterior cortex) and also have interconnections among themselves. These regions are distinct both in terms of anatomical and functional characteristics. In particular, functional neuroimaging techniques, such as functional magnetic resonance imaging (fMRI) and positron emission tomography (PET), have been successful in demonstrating that these brain regions play different roles in the control of cognitive (and emotional) processes. With respect to memory, the dlPFC, vlPFC, and aPFC have been most associated with control processes associated with encoding, organizing, and retrieving memory.

Consider the following question: What did you eat for dinner 3 days ago? It is unlikely that you were able to answer this question immediately. However, with some time and searching through your memory, you may have been able to retrieve the information. Most of us would begin by trying to figure out the day of the week. "Let see, today is Wednesday, three days ago would be Tuesday, Monday, Sunday…yes Sunday, what was I doing on Sunday…." If you ultimately retrieved the information – or even if you tried but were unsuccessful – you likely engaged in a variety of mental processes, particularly those involved in selecting, maintaining, organizing, and ultimately retrieving the desired memory. These processes enabled you to guide and control your mental path toward successful retrieval. In psychological terms, these functions enabled executive control, a process that is critically dependent on the PFC. By analogy, the PFC is your brain's chief executive – it functions to select information, monitor its use, disregard irrelevant information, make decisions, and initiate actions. Without it, your memory – just like a poorly run business – is disorganized, inefficient, and more susceptible to disruptions.

Stimulus Overload and Working Memory

One reason for the necessity of executive control is that we cannot possibly hold in mind everything that we know or perceive. Indeed, it would be an inordinate load on our cognitive system if we even attempted to consider everything that we experienced at any given moment. Because of this stimulus overload, we need to select certain information to be analyzed. Other information is filtered or ignored. For instance, at this moment you are reading and presumably paying attention to this sentence. Yet, pause briefly and pay attention to other sensory information. Perhaps, you can now hear surrounding noises such as a fan or people talking. You can direct your attention to other things, such as the rhythmic changes of pressure on your chest as you breathe. Clearly, at any given moment we experience a multitude of sensations. Not only can we select aspects from the environment, we can select and consider a plethora of memories. It almost seems incredible that in the midst of this information overload, we are able to select, maintain, and control what to bring into our realm of consciousness. The term working memory is used to describe the information that we choose to keep in mind at any given moment. Working memory is transient, and executive control is the dynamic process by which information is selected, maintained, updated, and organized in working memory.

Patients with damage to the PFC (more specifically damage to dlPFC and vlPFC) exhibit a syndrome in which executive control is severely impaired. These patients have problems in paying attention, holding things in mind, organizing thoughts, and retrieving memories. They experience particular problems when confronted with multiple sensations or choices and must decide which ones to select and which ones to disregard. One particular problem concerns their ability to hold information in mind. A simple task to test this ability is the digit span test, in which individuals are asked to report a short string of digits immediately after presentation. Most individuals can hold about six or seven digits in mind, just as we might when we have to hold a phone number in mind before placing a call. Patients with PFC damage have reduced digit span – they have difficulty keeping information in mind. This deficit pervades many domains, including the ability to maintain locations, colors, or sounds in mind.

Neuroimaging studies have confirmed the role of the PFC in working memory. When individuals must hold or maintain information in mind for a brief delay, prefrontal activity is increased. Interestingly, different prefrontal regions appear to be responsible for maintaining different kinds of information. For example, increased activity in left vlPFC is observed when individuals are asked to hold names of objects in mind, whereas increased activity in right vlPFC is observed when individuals are asked to keep spatial locations in mind. In many instances, these prefrontal activations are linked to activations in posterior regions of the brain, suggesting that the holding of information in working memory involves a brain circuit that includes the information to be activated (presumed to be stored in posterior cortex) and the executive control process that keeps the information active (presumed to be established by PFC).

In addition to its role in maintaining information in mind, the PFC is also involved in updating and manipulating information in working memory. In many everyday situations, it is necessary to rearrange or update information in mind. In laboratory studies, this aspect of working memory has been investigated by asking individuals to reorganize information, such as putting a random string of letters in alphabetical order. Another manipulation task is called the self-ordered pointing task in which individuals are presented with an array of stimuli (e.g., eight objects) and asked to point to one of the stimuli. On subsequent trials, the same objects are shown in different positions, and individuals are asked to point to a different object on each presentation. This task not only requires the holding of objects in mind but also remembering which objects have already been selected. Thus, after each presentation, the contents in working memory must be updated or reorganized to include another item. Patients with PFC damage have difficulty performing this task. Also, neuroimaging studies suggest that the dlPFC is particularly active during such manipulations of information in working memory compared to conditions in which only the maintenance of information is required. Taken together, findings suggest that the mere maintenance or holding of information involves the vlPFC, whereas the manipulation of that information additionally recruits the dlPFC.

Encoding Memories

Executive control is also critical for efficient learning – that is, the encoding of new memories. For example, how would you learn the following series of words: peach, bus, shirt, car, apple, socks, train, shoe, pear? Perhaps, you continually repeated the words in your mind. Alternatively, you may have noticed that the words could be grouped into three meaningful categories: vehicles, fruits, and clothing. In fact, when learning such word lists, many people organize words during encoding and then report the words by grouping all of the words in each category – such as reporting the vehicles first, then fruits and clothing. This kind of organizational strategy would involve maintaining, manipulating, and updating items while they are being presented. Thus, efficient encoding of memories would depend critically upon the kind of executive control processes involved in working memory tasks, such as digit span and the self-ordered pointing task.

Patients with frontal lobe lesions exhibit poor organizational strategies during learning. They fail to elaborate information, such as grouping information into meaningful categories. Moreover, long-lasting memory formation requires the integration of the new information with existing knowledge. This interchange between new and existing information is called elaborative encoding and depends upon the PFC for efficient analysis. Neuroimaging studies corroborate the role of the PFC in elaborative encoding. For example, the left vlPFC has been shown to be particularly active when individuals are asked to consider the meaning of items, such as determining whether a word is concrete (e.g., dollar) or abstract (e.g., freedom) compared to conditions in which they determine superficial features, such as the number of vowels in a word.

The extent of PFC activity during encoding can predict the success of later retrieval. In neuroimaging studies, activations during the initial encoding of items were analyzed separately on the basis of whether the items were later remembered or forgotten. Remembered items were associated with greater prefrontal activity (generally in left vlPFC) during encoding compared to forgotten items. That is, if you recruited PFC during the encoding of an item, you increased your chances of later remembering that item. These findings further support the notion that efficient encoding depends upon prefrontal activation during learning. The method of backsorting brain activations during learning in terms of whether items are subsequently remembered or forgotten offers a useful means by which to relate efficient encoding strategies to long-lasting memory retrieval.

Another aspect of executive control is related to the suppression of distracting or irrelevant information. In such situations, multiple activations of information place heavy demands on updating and manipulating information in working memory. Proactive interference is the term used to describe instances when earlier information impedes or interferes with the encoding of new information. For example, in memory tests individuals are asked to learn word associates, such as thief–crime, which are then tested by presenting the first word in a pair and asking for the second word, such as theif– ? Proactive interference is assessed by presenting a second learning phase involving the same cues but different responses (e.g., thief–bandit). Patients with PFC damage exhibit particular impairment when they try to recall the second set of responses. That is, they exhibit heightened proactive interference due to the learning of the first set of associates. Evidence for interference is demonstrated by the fact that these patients make many intrusion errors – that is, they use words from the first set during testing of the second set. These problems can be explained by a lack of inhibiting or suppressing the activation of related but now irrelevant information. With respect to executive control, the mitigation of proactive interference requires selecting and updating relevant information. The importance of the PFC in inhibitory control of distracting information has also been demonstrated in fMRI analyses using similar learning paradigms. For example, when individuals are asked to learn word associates such as dog–boxer then later dog–Labrador, they exhibit increased left dlPFC activity when attempting to learn the second related word pair.

Selecting Semantic Memory

A hallmark feature of PFC damage is a problem in searching through memory and selecting specific information. This deficit can be demonstrated in the verbal fluency task, in which individuals are given a minute to retrieve words from a specific semantic category (e.g., 'animals') or retrieve words that begin with a specific letter (e.g., 'A'). This task requires a search through semantic memory – that is, our database of memory for facts and knowledge. Similar to tasks involving the manipulation of working memory or the encoding of new information, efficient retrieval involves the development of strategies to control what words are generated. For example, after trying to come up with just any animal, it would be useful to consider subcategories of animals, such as pets, farm animals, or reptiles. Such strategies are efficient because they facilitate the selection of different words and prevent the report of words already generated. Patients with PFC damage have difficulty controlling their memory searches on this task. They report only 10–12 animal names in a minute, whereas most individuals would be able to retrieve twice as many animal names. Moreover, patients with PFC damage tend to repeat words over and over, as if they have difficult in suppressing the activation of words that were already selected.

The verbal fluency task appears to be a rather easy one, though it is important to appreciate the role of executive control in selecting and updating such information. Not only is it necessary to generate and select information, it is also necessary to monitor responses so that one avoids repeating the same word. Thus after each response all prior responses must be kept in mind so that they will not be repeated. As such, this task has some similarities with the self-ordered pointing task and tasks associated with proactive interference, in which prior information interferes with current performance. In these tasks, it is necessary to monitor and control the activation of previously relevant but currently irrelevant information.

In neuroimaging studies, vlPFC is particularly active during the generation and selection of semantic knowledge. One often-used task to assess retrieval from semantic memory is the verb generation task, in which individuals are presented a noun cue (e.g., 'nail') and asked to generate an associated verb (e.g., 'pound'). As in the verbal fluency task, verb generation requires a search and selection process through one's semantic database. Also, it is necessary to control competing or interfering items during retrieval. In fact, vlPFC activity increases to the extent that there are many competing responses from which to choose. Such regulation of semantic retrieval extends to other linguistic tasks, such as making decisions about the conceptual relatedness between items or interpreting difficult or ambiguous sentences.

The retrieval of general factual knowledge can be assessed by tests of remote pubic events (e.g., "Who shot John Lennon?" [answer: Chapman]). In one study, patients with PFC lesions and control subjects were asked to recall public events or faces of famous people. These tests assessed recent to very remote semantic knowledge. Thus, exposure to these events and people occurred well before the onset of neurological damage. As such, it can be presumed that deficits in performance are due to problems in retrieval rather than encoding. Patients with PFC damage exhibited recall impairment that was similar across all time periods tested. However, the patients were not impaired on tests of recognition memory, in which they selected the correct answers from several choices. The disproportionate impairment on tests of recall compared to recognition memory suggests that the PFC is involved in controlling the search through semantic memory rather than impairment in the knowledge itself. That is, selecting, updating, and manipulating information in working memory play a significant role in strategic retrieval of information, such as recalling a public event or a famous face. Such retrievals require searching through semantic knowledge, generating relevant information, and disregarding irrelevant information. Recognition memory can be based on a familiarity judgment. That is, on recognition tests it is simply necessary to determine which choice seems most closely related or familiar.

Another example of the distinction between impaired in control of semantic memory and damage to semantic memory itself can be demonstrated in other analyses of recognition versus recall. Consider again the verbal fluency task, in which patients are asked to generate animal names. This task requires recall of information, and patients with PFC damage are impaired. Yet, these patients exhibit intact semantic knowledge of animals when asked to make recognition judgments of animal characteristics. In one study, patients were shown three animal names, such as dog, cow, and pig, and asked to determine which two animals go together. They were told that there were no correct answers and to simply make decisions based on which two go together. The patients exhibited intact semantic memory ability in that they based their decisions on appropriate subcategories of animals, such as associating farm animals (e.g., indicating that cow and pig go together in the example above). In such studies, executive control is minimized by having individuals make simple choice decisions rather than searching, updating, and organizing self-generated retrievals.

Retrieving Autobiographical Memories

Another aspect of memory that requires extensive executive control is the retrieval of autobiographical memory – that is, recollecting an event or experience from the past. The opening exercise of remembering what you had for dinner 3 days ago is an example of retrieving autobiographical memory. Closely related to this form of memory is the notion of source recollection, in which individuals are asked to recollect specific time and place features of an event, such as when an event occurred or who was present during an event. Remembering such information requires executive control in that it is likely that you will have to make a guided analysis to reconstruct an autobiographical memory.

Neuropsychological studies have also demonstrated a prominent role of the PFC in mediating aspects of autobiographical retrieval. Although patients with PFC damage do not exhibit severe amnesia, they are impaired when asked to recollect past experiences. As in the retrieval of semantic knowledge, patients with PFC damage exhibit a particular impairment of recall compared to recognition memory. With respect to source recollection, patients with PFC damage exhibit particular impairment in remembering details of a learning event, such as where and when some information was presented. Such findings are consistent with disorders in memory for the temporal order of events, a common disorder in patients with PFC damage.

In neuroimaging studies, the dlPFC and aPFC are particularly involved in retrieval of autobiographical memory. Studies of autobiographical memory have assessed brain activity during the reminiscence of life experiences, reexperiencing spatial locations in virtual realities, and recognizing photographs taken by oneself or others. Such retrieval tasks have implicated both right and left PFC along with a host of other brain regions, including parietal cortex, medial temporal cortex, and retrospenial cortex. Similarly, studies of source recollection have shown similar brain activations. In such studies, individuals are asked to recollect features of a learning event, such as the color a stimulus, its spatial location, or its temporal order. In studies of source recollection, left PFC appears to be more active than right PFC.

To the extent that the PFC is involved in the control of autobiographical retrieval – rather than in the actual storage of such information – it is necessary to demonstrate that this kind of retrieval places particular demands on executive control. That is, it must be demonstrated that the selecting, maintaining, updating, and organizing of memory is particularly important for retrieval of details about one's past experiences. This issue was addressed with a task that facilitated executive control in patients with PFC damage. Individuals were presented objects and were asked to perform an action with each one (e.g., bounce the ball). This manipulation was presumed to increase sensorimotor activation during encoding and thereby increase the distinctiveness of stimuli. Memory for the temporal order of items was assessed by presenting pairs of objects and asking individuals to determine which of the two was presented more recently. Performance by patients with PFC damage did not differ from performance by control subjects on this test. However, the patients exhibited significant impairment on a control task in which they were presented the objects but did not manipulate them. This benefit appeared to be rather selective to patients with PFC damage because performance by amnesic patients with temporal lobe lesions was not facilitated by the manipulation condition.

A Board of Executives

How can one interpret the role of the PFC in memory processes? As described here, the PFC monitors and controls information processing thus enabling executive or 'top-down' control. Top-down control refers to the manner in which thoughts and knowledge control lower levels of analysis. In one view of top-down processing, called metacognitive control, basic processes – such as object recognition, speech analysis, and semantic memory access – are defined as 'object-level' processes, which are controlled by 'meta-level' processes. Meta-level processes monitor object-level processes, and – as a result of this monitoring – initiate control (see **Figure 1**). The PFC fits well in this model as it can serve as the meta-level processor to basic processors. It is presumed that top-down control is implemented by reciprocal neural pathways between PFC and posterior regions. Control occurs as a result of selecting and maintaining task-relevant activity (activation) and by filtering irrelevant activity (inhibition).

As suggested by findings presented above, different PFC regions serve different control functions, such as selecting information from the environment, maintaining information in working memory, accessing semantic knowledge, and retrieval. Thus, rather than one executive controller, there appear to be numerous controllers that monitor and control different aspects of information processing. By analogy, one could view the brain as having a board of executives, with each one assigned to a specific function. Executives interact with each other, though each one is responsible for monitoring and controlling a particular part of a business. It is known that different PFC regions are connected to distinct regions in the posterior cortex. By way of these reciprocal interconnections, PFC has the capability of influencing many object-level processes in posterior cortex.

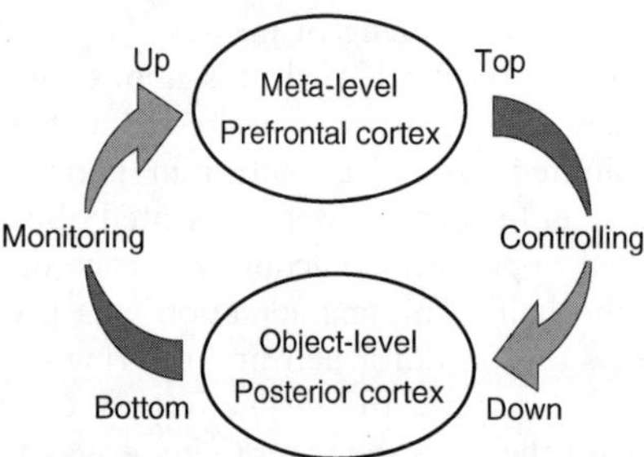

Figure 1 Metacognitive model of executive control. Monitoring of object-level processes is achieved by bottom-up pathways from posterior cortex to PFC. Meta-level processors in the PFC initiate control by top-down pathways to object-level processes. Control of memory is enabled in this model by the role of the PFC in selecting, maintaining, accessing, and retrieving object-level processes for efficient learning and memory.

Physiological evidence exists for the role of the PFC in metacognitive control of neural activity. Studies using electroencephalogram (EEG) scalp recordings assess neural activity in response to stimulus presentations. Patients with PFC lesions exhibit abnormal increases in neural response in posterior cortex. Thus, as a result of PFC damage, bottom-up neural signals are disinhibited due to a failure to modulate or control posterior cortical activity. In PET and fMRI studies of normal individuals, increased activity in the dlPFC is often correlated with decreased activity in posterior cortical regions, as if PFC can not only select posterior activity, but it can also suppress irrelevant activity.

In summary, the frontal lobes play a significant role in human memory. Rather than being the storehouse of semantic knowledge or autobiographical memories, the PFC monitors and controls processes associated with accessing, encoding, and retrieving memories. PFC initiates and channels information so that it can be held in working memory and efficiently manipulated or updated. PFC facilitates encoding and organization during learning, and access and recall during retrieval. Without it, thoughts are disorganized, and memories are poorly learned and retrieved. Executive control, top-down processing, and metacognitive control are terms used to describe how PFC monitors and controls information processing. In the service of memory processes, PFC is critical for efficient access to and retrieving from our storehouse of knowledge, as well as adding new knowledge to it. It is as critical for memory as an efficient librarian is for a library.

See also: Cognition: An Overview of Neuroimaging Techniques; Episodic Memory; Executive Function and Higher-Order Cognition: Neuroimaging; Frontal Lobe Syndrome; Memory Representation; Memory Consolidation: Systems; Memory Disorders; Prefrontal Cortex: Structure and Anatomy; Recognition Memory; Semantic Memory; Short Term and Working Memory.

Further Reading

Baddeley A (1986) *Working Memory.* Oxford: Oxford University Press.

D'Esposito M, Postle BR, and Rypma B (2000) Prefrontal cortical contributions to working memory: Evidence from event-related fMRI studies. *Experimental Brain Research* 133: 3–11.

Duncan J (2001) An adaptive coding model of neural function in prefrontal cortex. *Nature Reviews Neuroscience* 2: 820–829.

Johnson MK, Hashtroudi S, and Lindsay DS (1993) Source monitoring. *Psychological Bulletin* 114: 3–28.

Luria AR (1973) *The Working Brain.* New York: Penguin Books.

Maguire EA (2001) Neuroimaging studies of autobiographical event memory. *Philosophical Transactions of the Royal Society of London B* 356: 1441–1451.

Miller EK and Cohen JD (2001) An integrative theory of prefrontal cortex function. *Annual Review of Neuroscience* 24: 167–202.

Paller KA and Wagner AD (2002) Observing the transformation of experience into memory. *Trends in Cognitive Science* 6: 93–102.

Roberts AC, Robbins TW, and Weiskrantz L (eds.) (1998) *The Prefrontal Cortex: Executive and Cognitive Function.* Oxford: Oxford University Press.

Rugg MD, Otten LJ, and Henson RNA (2002) The neural bases of episodic memory: Evidence from functional neuroimaging. *Philosophical Transactions of the Royal Society B* 357: 1097–1110.

Shimamura AP (2000) The role of the prefrontal cortex in dynamic filtering. *Psychobiology* 28: 207–218.

Squire LR and Schacter DL (eds.) (2002) *Neuropsychology of Memory,* 3rd edn. New York: The Guilford Press.

Teuber H-L (1964) The riddle of frontal lobe function in man. In: Warren JM and Akert K (eds.) *The Frontal Granular Cortex and Behavior,* pp. 410–444. New York: McGraw-Hill.

Thompson-Schill SL, Bedny M, and Goldberg RF (2005) The frontal lobes and the regulation of mental activity. *Current Opinion in Neurobiology* 15: 219–224.

Wagner AD (2002) Cognitive control and episodic memory. In: Squire LR and Schacter DL (eds.) *Neuropsychology of Memory,* 3rd edn., pp. 174–192. New York: The Guilford Press.

Inhibitory Control over Action and Memory

M C Anderson and C Weaver, University of Oregon, Eugene, OR, USA

Functions of Inhibitory Control

The ability to suppress strong habitual (prepotent) responses supports at least two broad computational functions necessary for the effective control of behavior: selection and stopping. Selection refers to the act of isolating one representation among competitors vying for the control of behavior or thought. Selection is necessary at all stages of cognitive activity. In memory, selection must occur to retrieve a target memory trace in the face of many competing memories activated by the cues guiding retrieval. In action, a stimulus may initiate multiple compatible physical actions, only one of which should guide behavior. Stopping refers to the need to either preempt or override a mental or physical activity that is inappropriate in a certain context or that, in the course of execution, has become undesirable. For instance, reflexively reaching to catch a falling object might be abruptly stopped when it is realized that the falling object is a hot pan or a potted cactus. The general models of both functions are depicted in **Figures 1(a)** and **1(b)**.

In both selection and stopping, the ability to limit the influence of unwanted representations is mediated by a top-down control process acting directly or indirectly on this entity, rendering it temporarily less accessible. In this article, we refer to the brain structure originating the top-down control signal as the source of the inhibitory control and the area representing the to-be-controlled representation or process as the site of inhibition. Broadly, research indicates regions in the lateral prefrontal cortex (either the ventrolateral prefrontal cortex (VLPFC), Brodmann's area 44/45, or the dorsolateral prefrontal cortex (DLPFC), Brodmann's area 9/46) as likely candidates for the source of control, whereas differing cortical and subcortical targets constitute control sites, depending on the content to be controlled.

Paradigms Used to Study Inhibitory Control

Behavioral paradigms used in research with human subjects have taken two approaches to measuring inhibitory control. Many studies measure subjects' ability to implement control by quantifying the accuracy or speed with which selection or stopping is achieved. This approach provides a straightforward measure of behavioral control. Other studies, however, focus on the aftereffects of selection or stopping on the stopped representations. If a response is suppressed, there should be measurable consequences on the ability to subsequently access the representation, reflecting persisting inhibition. For instance, if a motor action is inhibited, people should be slower to emit that same response later, or if a memory has been inhibited, it should become more difficult to retrieve. Methods that measure the inhibitory aftereffects of response override have the advantage of not presupposing inhibition as the mechanism. For example, although inhibition may be engaged to stop a motor action, stopping may instead be achieved by facilitating an antagonistic response that precludes the execution of the to-be-stopped action. Measures based on the first approach cannot conclusively confirm that inhibition is involved in stopping the rejected representation. Examples of both methods are discussed here.

Inhibitory Control of Action

Inhibitory control of actions has been studied in the contexts of selection and stopping, and it is typically measured with functionally oriented tasks. The use of these paradigms, accompanied by various imaging and electrophysiological techniques has established that inhibitory control engages the lateral prefrontal cortex (LPFC). Further, inhibitory control depends on the integrity of this region, as revealed by studies of patients with LPFC damage, studies using transcranial magnetic stimulation (TMS), and lesions in nonhuman primates.

Inhibitory Control in Selective Responding

A variety of paradigms have focused on the role of inhibitory control in selecting one response in the face of interference from prepotent competitors. One approach used to investigate response selection across a variety of stimulus modalities and response types is to manipulate the compatibility of perceived stimuli and their associated responses. Tasks measuring stimulus–response (S–R) compatibility effects have two conditions: (1) trials in which S–R mappings (i.e., associations) are compatible and exploit innate biases, and (2) trials characterized by incompatible S–R mappings which require that the tendency to make the natural response be overcome and the task-appropriate response selected. For example, subjects might see an arrow in the center of a screen pointing left or right and be required to indicate

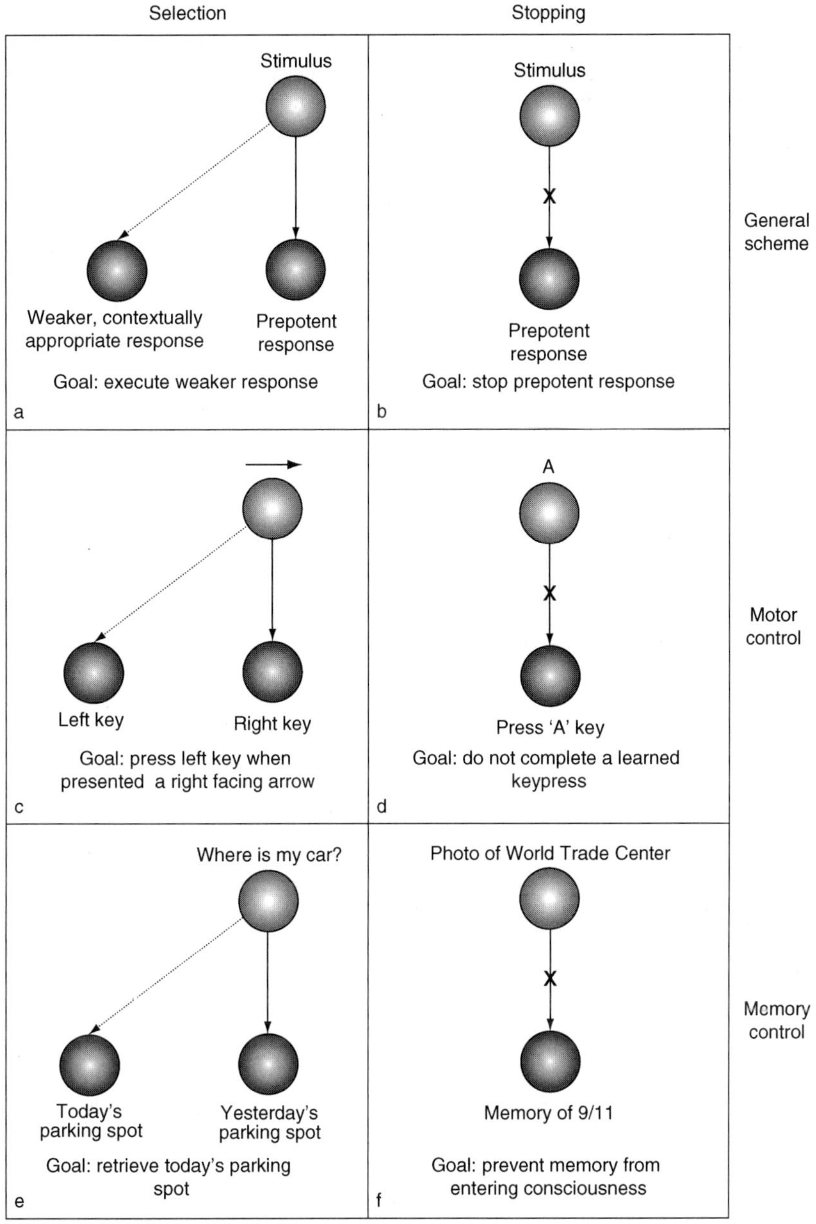

Figure 1 Two situations that require response override in human action and thought and commonly used paradigms: (a) selection; (b) stopping; (c) S–R compatibility paradigm; (d) stop-signal paradigm; (e) selection to inhibit the interference of a memory; (f) stopping the retrieval of a memory. The top row represents a schematization of these two situations. In each instance, a stimulus is associated with one or more responses, such that when the stimulus appears, the responses become active in proportion to their associative connection to the cue (represented by thickness of the line). In selection (a), the weaker response must be made, despite the existence of a strong competitor that becomes more active and threatens to capture control of behavior. In stopping (b), there is only one response, but it must be prevented. As shown in (c), sometimes the prepotent action is not the correct response, and a nondominant movement must instead be made (e.g., S–R compatibility and antisaccade tasks). As shown in (d), if no alternative response is warranted, the movement can simply be canceled (e.g., go/no-go, stop-signal, and countermanding saccade tasks). As shown in (e), sometimes inhibition must be initiated to selectively retrieve a memory with a weaker association to a cue that is shared by another trace (e.g., retrieving today’s parking spot and suffering interference from the memory of yesterday’s; RIF). In other circumstances (f), confronting a cue may activate an unwanted memory, leading the person to stop retrieval. For instance, when the sight of the World Trade Center initiates retrieval of the memory of the events of 9/11, retrieval might be stopped. This process can be assayed by TNT tasks. RIF, retrieval-induced forgetting; S–R, stimulus–response; TNT, think/no-think.

which direction the arrow is pointing by pressing one of two keys. If the instructions require subjects to press a key with their left hand in response to left-pointing arrows and a key with their right hand in response to right-pointing arrows, the S–R mappings are compatible. If, however, subjects must press a key with their right hand in response to a left-pointing arrow (doing the converse for the right-pointing arrow), the S–R mappings are incompatible. In a nonspatial variant, subjects are presented two consecutive color patches and asked to judge and report whether they are the same or different. In the incompatible mapping condition, subjects are instructed to say 'same' when the colors actually differ. The response selection requirement of such tasks is illustrated in **Figure 1(c)**. The reduced accuracy and increased reaction time (RT) of stimulus-incompatible responses are the measurable costs of resolving the interference created by the prepotent compatible response.

Human imaging work suggests that the LPFC contributes to the resolution of this interference. Response selection appears to be subserved by both the DLPFC and VLPFC, together with a network of regions often observed in attentional control tasks, including the superior parietal cortex, anterior cingulate cortex (ACC), and lateral premotor cortex. A number of imaging studies have sought to differentiate the contributions of these areas, and converging evidence from S–R compatibility and other response selection designs is consistent with the view that the ACC contributes to the detection of response conflict, signaling the need for greater top-down control to the LPFC. In contrast, the LPFC – specifically, BA46 within the DLPFC – is thought to be instrumental in achieving response selection. Consistent with this, lesions and TMS of the human DLPFC compromise response selection. Intriguingly, cellular and neuroimaging studies in nonhuman primates emphasize the VLPFC over the DLPFC as the principal source of response selection. There is also conflicting evidence for the generality of response selection. Considerable behavioral evidence from dual-task interference indicates that response selection constitutes a central processing bottleneck spanning varied stimulus and response modalities. These findings are corroborated by neuroimaging findings that reveal overlapping neural activation across many stimulus and response demands. However, response selection appears in some situations to be lateralized according to stimulus characteristics, with spatial tasks associated with increased activation in the right hemisphere and nonspatial stimuli causing left lateralized activations. Thus, it is unclear whether response selection is a unitary process across all input and output modalities, although most research points to the importance of the LPC in achieving this function.

Inhibitory control over motor action has also been studied in the context of oculomotor response selection. In human subjects, saccade termination similarly appears dependent on the DLPFC. In oculomotor inhibition paradigms, subjects intentionally try to override a reflexive foveal orientation to a stimulus, and the number of failed suppressions is measured. For example, in antisaccade tasks, subjects are instructed to look away from visual targets when they abruptly appear instead of toward them. This requires the inhibition of the visually triggered saccade that ordinarily orients subjects' eyes to the onset stimulus. Although the DLPFC is not necessary to execute accurate saccades, numerous lesion studies show that damage to this area, and to BA46 in particular, markedly increases antisaccade errors, suggesting its importance in their cancellation. Similar patterns of errors have been reported in nonhuman primates following lesions of the DLPFC homolog (dorsal bank of the principal sulcus). Further, substantial neurophysiological work done in nonhuman primates has identified neurons within the DLPFC and frontal eye field (FEF) that show preferential activity during antisaccade trials. In human neuroimaging studies, increased activation for antisaccade trials has been found bilaterally in the DLPFC. Based on these findings, the DLPFC is believed to originate a top-down signal that acts on the FEF and possibly the superior colliculus (SC), which serve as the sites of the inhibition.

Taken together, research from these paradigms and others, including task-set switching, Stroop, and flanker tasks, consistently implicate the LPFC in implementing the top-down signal by which prepotent responses are suppressed to achieve selective motor response. Additional work is required to ascertain the relative involvement of the DLPFC and VLPFC, their respective roles, and the extent to which response selection is general or lateralized by content.

Inhibitory Control in Motor Stopping

Intended actions can be stopped, and some cognitive process must support this function, perhaps inhibition. To study stopping, many paradigms ask subjects to occasionally prevent a response they have been trained to complete, and then they measure the effectiveness or efficiency with which this is done. In the go/no-go (GNG) task, participants are presented with a stimulus to which they must make a motor response. On a minority of trials, a special no-go stimulus is presented, for which subjects must prevent their response. For example, people might be presented with a series of letters on a screen. For every letter, they might be asked to press the same key as quickly as possible, unless they see the letter X, for which they must withhold their response. The percentage of no-go trials successfully withheld is a metric of inhibitory control ability. Another approach used to study motor stopping is the stop-signal paradigm developed by Gordon Logan, illustrated in **Figure 1(d)**. In this paradigm, subjects typically perform a simple perceptual discrimination (e.g., deciding whether a letter is X or O), to which they must make a motor response (e.g., pressing the key corresponding to X or O) as quickly as possible. On a minority of the trials, a stop signal (typically a tone, but visual and tactile signals are sometimes used) occurs at some point after the stimulus, indicating that subjects should withhold their motor response (commonly a key press, although hand, arm, and eye movements; verbalization; and hand squeezes have been used). Over trials, the delay between the appearance of the stimulus and the stop signal is modulated by a dynamic tracking algorithm that adjusts the stop-signal delay (making it longer or shorter, depending on subjects' accuracy) until stopping performance is at chance. Using the average go trial RT and the average stop-signal delay latency required for an equal probability of successful and failed inhibition, the stop-signal RT (SSRT) can be computed. The SSRT, which is approximately 200 ms for manual responses, quantifies the speed of the stopping process itself and is commonly used as a measure of inhibitory control ability. Stop signal and GNG paradigms have been used to study inhibitory control across the life span, in neuropsychological patients, and as a way to study the neural basis of inhibitory control in nonhuman subjects such as monkeys and rats.

Considerable evidence from motor-stopping paradigms indicates that response inhibition is mediated by the VLPFC and DLPFC, with a right lateralization tendency, at least in humans. For example, work by Aron and colleagues showed that, in patients with damage to the right VLPFC or DLPFC (and not the left), SSRT is significantly slowed and the degree of slowing is correlated with the lesion volume. Work with a variety of other techniques yielded similar conclusions. For example, TMS over the right VLPFC disrupts motor stopping in human subjects, and lesions to a VLPFC homolog (the inferior frontal convexity) in nonhuman primates disrupts performance on GNG tasks. Electrophysiological studies in nonhuman primates have demonstrated a no-go potential originating in the dorsal bank of the principal sulcus (homologous to the DLPFC in humans) and in the rostroventral corner of the PFC (see **Figure 2**). The no-go potential is an electrical signature of the behavioral no-go response. Strikingly, when stimulation is applied during go trials in which the monkey should respond, the response is cancelled or delayed, concomitant with reduced electrical activity in the motor cortex. The strength of the suppressive effect depends on the stimulation timing, with the maximal suppressive effect observed when the no-go potential would have peaked (75–125 ms), and occurs exclusively in the regions of the PFC in which the no-go potential is generated. As might be predicted from the foregoing findings, response inhibition activates the DLPFC and VLPFC in neuroimaging studies, very often right laterally, although sometimes bilaterally, and frequently accompanied by a network of areas implicated in attentional control. Further, direct comparisons of the neural correlates of three inhibitory tasks (the GNG and two response selection tasks, a S-R compatibility task and a flanker task) within-subjects revealed the DLPFC to be a region activated by these distinct cognitive control tests. Taken as a whole, these findings indicate that both the DLPFC and VLPFC contribute to a top-down signal for inhibiting prepotent motor responses, although some investigators have emphasized the primacy of the right VLPFC.

Although the lateral PFC appears to be the source of a top-down signal that suppresses prepotent motor responses, the site of action, and the circuit through which that site is influenced depends on the nature of the response. In the case of manual motor responses, stopping activates the expected control areas of the VLPFC and dorsomedial PFC, and the regions on which that control is exerted within the motor system. Subcortically, the control of movement within the basal ganglia is conceptualized using the brake–accelerator model. The accelerator is the direct pathway in which the cortex acts on the striatum and internal pallidum, increasing the activation of the motor cortex by the thalamus. Braking is accomplished by the same structures with the critical addition of the subthalamic nucleus (STN), which indirectly inhibits the thalamus and hence the motor cortex. Recent work suggests that a faster inhibitory mechanism, the cortico-subthalamo-pallidal hyperdirect pathway, may be contributing to response stopping. In this conception, the VLPFC interprets the stop signal and (circumventing the striatum) increases the activation of the STN, and thus the internal pallidum, resulting in the inhibition of the thalamus and, consequently, the motor cortex. Consistent with this possibility, a recent stop-signal neuroimaging study conducted by Aron and Poldrack revealed that the amount of activation in the STN (and not the striatum) predicted SSRT. Thus, in the case of manual motor response inhibition, the VLPFC may control action by exciting structures that inhibit motor cortex.

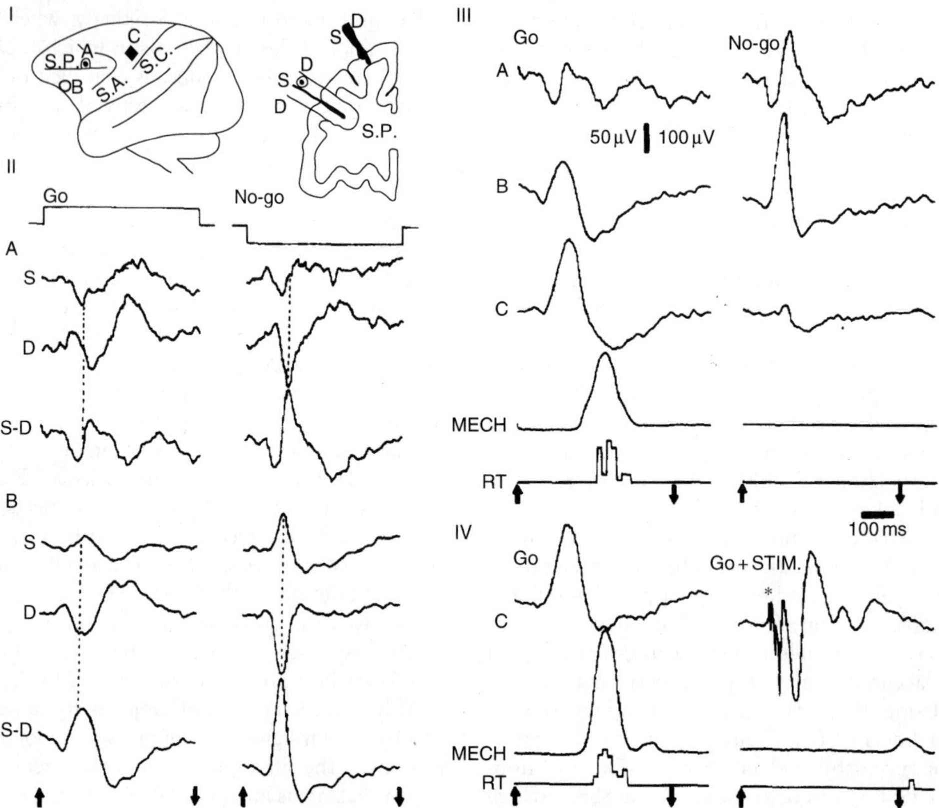

Figure 2 Stimulation of the DLPFC and VLPFC homologs suppresses motor responses in nonhuman primates. Monkeys were rewarded for completing manual responses to a light stimulus and learned to respond accurately. Responses to another light stimulus were unrewarded, and the monkeys learned to withhold their responses. No-go activity coincides with no-go behavior and is characterized by surface-negative, depth-positive field potentials generated 110–150 ms after presentation of the visual stimulus. Emergence of no-go potential is contingent on learned discrimination of light stimuli. Moreover, stimulation of specific lateral PFC loci induces no-go behavior. **(I)** Lateral (left hemisphere) and coronal (right hemisphere) views of the frontal lobe illustrate electrode localization. Surface (S) and depth (D) electrodes were placed in the monkey homologs of the DLPFC (dorsal bank of the principal sulcus; A, open circle with central dot), VLPFC (rostroventral corner of the prefrontal cortex; B, open circle), and forelimb area of the motor cortex contralateral to responding hand (C, filled diamond). (II) Field potentials consistent with no-go potential at S and D electrodes and S-D at prefrontal loci A and B during go (left column) and no-go (right column) trials for a single monkey. (III) S-D field potential data for each of the three recording regions across both conditions; A, B, and C in go (left column) and no-go trials (right column). Specificity of no-go potentials to regions and A and B, illustrated by lack of potential in area C. In addition to field potentials, movement (as measured by mechanogram (MECH)), and reaction times (RT) are also reported for each condition. (V) Presentation of go stimulus produces typical field potentials, movement, and reaction times, whereas the go stimulus coupled with bilateral stimulation of areas A and B prevented response, as is typical of no- to trials (compare to III). Arrows indicate onset and offset of visual stimulus. DLPFC, dorsolateral prefrontal cortex; PFC, prefrontal cortex; S.A., sulcus arcuatus; S.C., sulcus centralis; S.P., sulcus principalis; VLPFC, ventrolateral prefrontal cortex. Reproduced from Sasaki K, Gemba H, and Tsujimoto T (1989) Suppression of visually initiated hand movement by stimulation of the prefrontal cortex in the monkey. *Brain Research* 495(1): 100–107, with permission from Elsevier.

Suppressing unwanted eye movements, like suppressing manual responses, engages the LPFC, and in particular the DLPFC, as noted in the discussion of antisaccade research. The site acted on by LPFC, however, is different than in the case of manual responses. For instance, research on the cellular dynamics of motor inhibition with nonhuman primates points to the importance of the FEF. An adaptation of the stop-signal paradigm, called the countermanding saccade task, is often used. The monkeys learn a saccade RT task and are subsequently trained to stop their saccadic eye movements whenever an infrequent stop signal is administered. Thus, the performance of this task requires two processes: (1) initiation of the intended saccades and (2) revocation of the to-be-cancelled saccade. Both of these processes are believed to be supported by the FEF, although movement cancellation is also supported by the SC and the supplementary eye fields. In particular, within the FEF and SC, movement neurons drive go processes, whereas fixation neurons are implicated in stop processes. Whether a saccade is executed or not depends on the relative activity of these types of neurons. Increasing activation and the rate of that increase in movement neurons are predictive of commitment to saccade initiation and the timing of the initiation, respectively. In contrast, fixation neurons demonstrate activity that is reciprocal to that of movement neurons; their activity is gradually reduced before saccade initiation and increases with saccade suppression. Thus, movement and fixation neurons implement saccade initiation and termination in the FEF. Together with the work on antisaccade performance in human subjects, this suggests that inhibitory control of eye movements is implemented by an interaction between the DLPFC and regions of the FEF involved in initiating and canceling eye movement responses.

Thus, whereas the source of inhibitory control in LPFC may well be shared across different motor-stopping tasks, the site of action depends on the effector system being controlled. Next we discuss evidence indicating that this principle is not limited to the control of physical actions but also applies to the control of internal cognitive acts, such as long-term memory retrieval.

Inhibitory Control in Long-Term Memory

Inhibitory control over memory retrieval provides a model system for the role of inhibitory control in cognition; it has also been studied in selection and stopping. Human behavioral studies have revealed that overcoming the influence of prepotent traces in long-term memory retrieval yields an inhibitory aftereffect such that suppressed traces are subsequently less accessible. Neurobiological research indicates that retrieval suppression, like motor stopping, engages the LPFC, which modulates the activation in the hippocampus and other medial temporal regions associated with memory and emotion. The similarities between the systems engaged by memory and action control suggest that the same or perhaps isomorphic computational solutions may exist for solving response-override problems for physical and cognitive actions.

Inhibitory Control in Selective Retrieval

One procedure that has been designed to study inhibitory control is known as the retrieval–practice paradigm, developed by Anderson and colleagues. In a typical version of this procedure, subjects encode six exemplars from each of eight taxonomic categories (e.g., fruits-orange, fruits-banana, and drinks-gin) in a study phase. Following the initial study, subjects perform directed retrieval practice on a subset of exemplars from some of the studied categories (e.g., three of the six fruits) via category-plus-stem cued recall tests (e.g., fruit or___). Subjects are then tested on all exemplars from all categories. On the final test, subjects can either be cued with the category name and asked to recall all studied exemplars or be given a recognition memory test on all items. Of interest are the effects of practicing some category exemplars on the ability to recall the remaining unpracticed exemplars of those categories. Repeatedly retrieving some exemplars of the category impairs the subjects' ability to recall the remaining unpracticed exemplars, relative to their performance on baseline categories that were also studied, but none of whose exemplars were retrieved in the interim. This effect, known as retrieval-induced forgetting (RIF) is thought to reflect the consequences of an inhibitory process that suppresses unpracticed competitors during retrieval practice, causing enduring impairment of those items on subsequent tests. RIF has been induced with verbal and visuospatial stimuli, and across levels of complexity ranging from simple word pairs to complex factual knowledge and even eyewitness events. RIF affects episodic, semantic, and implicit memory as measured by conceptual fluency and lexical decision. Further, RIF appears on tests of episodic recall and recognition memory. Thus, RIF may be an example of inhibitory control aiding in the function of selection during the retrieval process by suppressing interfering items during retrieval of a target. The selection requirements of RIF are illustrated in **Figure 1(e)**.

RIF exhibits functional properties that firmly establish the involvement of an inhibitory control process that overcomes interference. First, it is retrieval-specific; repeated study of some associates of a cue does not impair the recall of related items, even when repeated retrieval of those same items does. Further, RIF is interference-dependent, with larger RIF effects observed for competitors that cause interference during retrieval, consistent with the view that inhibitory control is engaged to suppress interfering competitors. Finally, RIF is cue-independent; the impairment of a competing memory item generalizes to novel cues used to test the inhibited items, indicating a generalized reduction in the accessibility of the suppressed trace. Thus, in the domain of memory control, theoretically focused behavioral research based on inhibitory aftereffects has firmly established the involvement of inhibition.

A large body of work establishes the role of the VLPFC in selective retrieval of verbal semantic knowledge under conditions of interference. Moreover, patients with LPFC damage show heightened susceptibility to proactive interference in long-term episodic memory retrieval, as revealed in work by Shimamura and colleagues. Nevertheless, only recently has work begun to tie the LPFC to inhibitory aftereffects measured in RIF. Consistent with executive control literature, the ACC appears central to the detection of conflict between competing memories associated with a cue, signaling the need for top-down control to resolve competition; in contrast, the VLPFC appears to initiate control processes that resolve that conflict through inhibition. These principles can be seen in a study by Kuhl and colleagues, who hypothesized that because RIF is a consequence of resolving interference from competing items during target retrieval, inhibited items should cause less interference on later retrievals of the target items. Indeed, more activation was observed in the bilateral VLPFC and right DLPFC during early than during late retrieval practice trials, and the more activation decreased over trials in the right VLPFC and ACC, the more memory inhibition was found. Moreover, subjects showing higher inhibition exhibited elevated activation in the ACC and hippocampus during early trials that gradually diminished with repeated retrievals; low-inhibition subjects did not show this pattern. Thus, subjects who experience the greatest initial competition between the medial-temporal representations of the target and competitors (as indexed by medial temporal lobe (MTL) and ACC co-activation) show the greatest engagement of control and, consequently, the greatest RIF.

Similar conclusions have been reached using other techniques, such as electrophysiology. For example, more positive going event-related potentials (ERPs) are observed over frontal electrode sites during selective retrieval of target items than in a passive practice condition with the same targets. The magnitude of this retrieval-specific ERP effect on the PFC predicts the amount of RIF observed on the final test. These findings indicate that some functional requirement uniquely associated with retrieval, such as the need to resolve competition, engages the PFC and induces RIF, as before. Mounting evidence points to the involvement of the LPFC in the induction of RIF and the importance of this process in achieving selective retrieval, echoing the role of inhibitory processes in selective motor responding.

Inhibitory Control in Retrieval Stopping

Another method used to study inhibitory control of memory is known as the think/no-think (TNT) procedure, developed by Anderson and colleagues. Modeled after the GNG task, TNT measures the inhibitory aftereffects of stopping memory retrieval. Subjects learn a collection of cue-target pairs, so that whenever they are presented with the cue, they can recollect its associated target item. Following encoding, subjects participate in the TNT phase, during which a single cue item from one of the earlier pairs is presented on each trial. For some of these cues, the subjects are directed to think of the associated target memory and keep it in mind for as long as the cue is on the screen. For other cues, subjects are directed to not think about the associated target memory, keeping it out of mind for as long as the cue is on the screen. The latter no-think task requires that the subject override the retrieval process and prevent the associated declarative memory from entering awareness, despite the tendency for the cue to elicit that memory (see **Figure 1(f)** for an example of memorial stopping). Subjects are then tested on their memory for all cue–target pairs. In the typical design, one-third of the original pairs participate in the think trials in the TNT phase, one-third in the no-think trials, and one-third are reserved as baseline items against which to measure the effects of retrieval and retrieval suppression on later memory performance.

Repeatedly presenting participants with reminders of an event and asking them to stop retrieval of that event has several notable effects. First, it eliminates the normally beneficial effects of reminders in enhancing a memory's later accessibility, so that reminders can be presented over a dozen times with little apparent benefit in accessibility of the associated traces. Second, stopping retrieval very often impairs the ability to recall the associated trace, relative to other baseline cue–reminder pairs that were trained at the same time but that did not have their reminders presented in the interim during no-think or think trials. Thus, repeated exposure to reminders coupled with an effort to stop declarative memory retrieval impairs access to the associated trace. Third, the impairment of the excluded trace occurs even when that trace is tested with a novel cue, indicating a generalized impairment of the trace, consistent with the idea that the trace has been inhibited. Most of these effects have been observed with both verbal cue–target pairs and visual pairs such as face–scene pairs, and the effects appear to generalize to target items with emotional content. Thus, stopping unwanted retrievals appears to be effected in part by suppressing the associated memory, consistent with inhibitory control. As such, the TNT paradigm provides an example of the role of inhibitory control that is analogous to the GNG and stop-signal paradigms.

Neuroimaging studies have established several key findings about the neural systems involved in stopping long-term memory retrieval. First, as can be seen in **Figure 3**, suppressing retrieval of an episodic memory in response to a reminder engages the LPFC, including the VLPFC and DLPFC, often bilaterally,

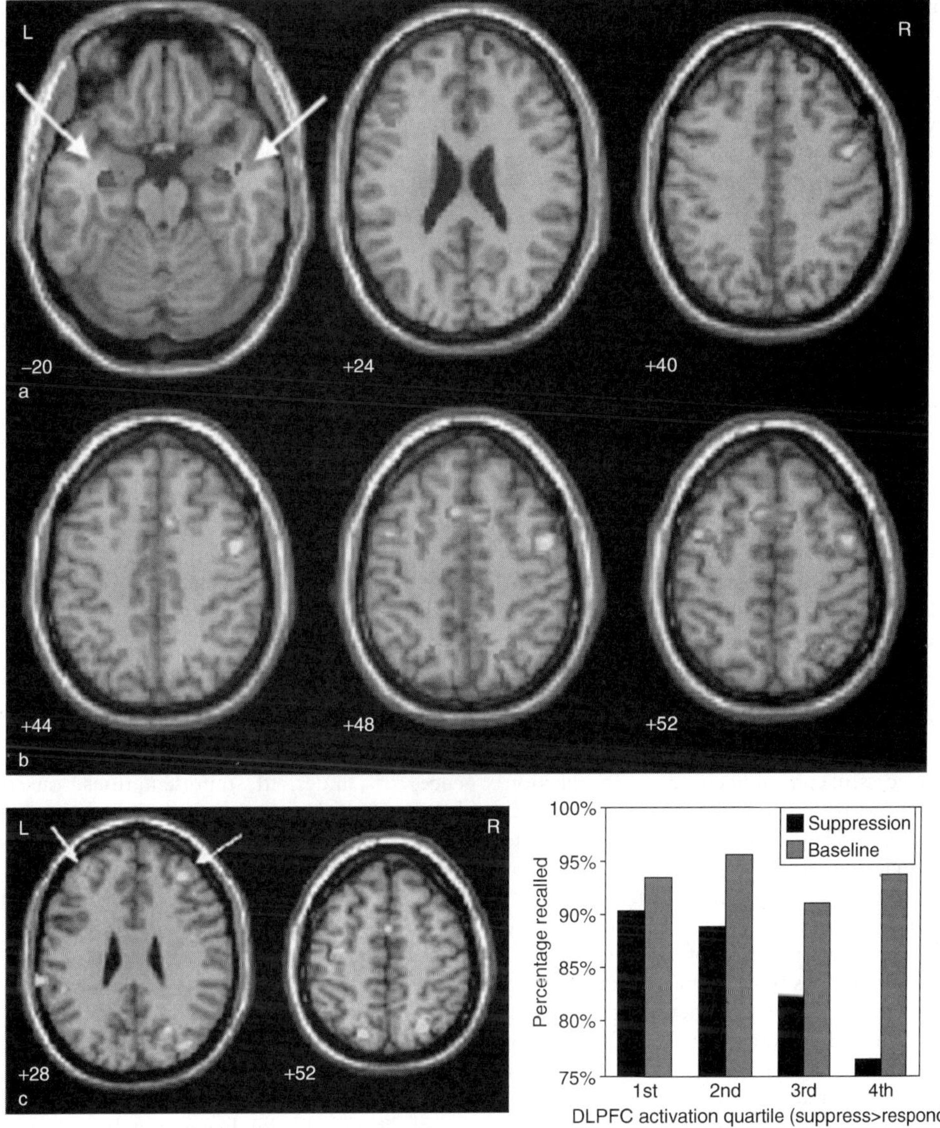

Figure 3 fMRI results during no-think trials and think trials: (a) brain regions that significantly differed in activation between the no-think trials and think trials during the TNT phase ($n = 24$); (b) successful recruitment of the DLPFC, which predicts individual differences in memory inhibition (the inhibitory aftereffect of stopping retrieval); (c) inhibitory aftereffects for four subject groups, differing in DLPFC activation. In (a), areas in yellow were more active during no-think trials than during think trials, whereas areas in blue were less active during no-think trials ($P < 0.001$). The white arrows highlight the reduced hippocampal activation in the no-think condition. In (b), plotted in warm colors are the regions that predict the magnitude of the inhibitory aftereffect observed on the final memory tests (the white arrows indicate the DLPFC; VLPFC was also observed in this study but not in a later study involving photographs). In (c), the greater the DLPFC activity shown by a subject group, the more impaired was the later recall of no-think items on the final test, compared to the recall of baseline items that were learned at the same time but that did not appear during the TNT phase. DLPFC, dorsolateral prefrontal cortex; fMRI, functional magnetic resonance imaging; TNT, think/no-think; VLPFC, ventrolateral prefrontal cortex. From Anderson MC, Ochsner KN, Kuhl B, et al. (2004) Neural systems underlying the suppression of unwanted memories. *Science* 303(5655): 232–235.

although sometimes with right lateralization. VLPFC engagement parallels the activations observed for RIF and for motor-response suppression, although the DLPFC appears to be more consistently engaged in retrieval stopping. Second, individual differences in the engagement of the DLPFC (and sometimes the VLPFC) during suppression predict memory inhibition, with inhibition increasing with increasing activation, as might be expected if the DLPFC originated a top-down signal responsible for memory impairment. Third, suppressing retrieval reduces activation in the hippocampus, compared to engaging retrieval, suggesting that inhibitory control modulates functional activity in structures involved in declarative memory. Recent work indicates that activation is reduced below the levels observed during passive fixation, with the extent of this reduction predicting memory failure. Finally, retrieval suppression engages the full network of regions associated with endogenous attention, including the lateral premotor cortex, ACC, and intraparietal sulcus, indicating common brain systems may support controlled attention during perception and memory tasks. With emotional memories, suppression also significantly reduces amygdalar activation, probably reflecting control over emotional aspects of the negative memories. Taken together, these findings indicate that functional interactions between the LPFC and MTLs support inhibitory control over memory retrieval.

As already discussed, imaging studies indicate that suppressing retrieval of an episodic memory significantly reduces activation in the hippocampus, compared to retrieval and a passive fixation baseline. The hippocampus has widely acknowledged involvement in episodic memory, and many studies indicate that it is also involved in the recollection of recently encoded events. As such, reduced hippocampal activation may reflect the successful control of conscious recollection by inhibitory control processes. Electrophysiological studies using the TNT procedure also support the conclusion that conscious recollection (as measured by an ERP component, the parietal old/new effect) may not merely be reduced, but may be eliminated by retrieval suppression. The extent of the modulation of this component predicts subsequent forgetting of no-think items, consistent with the view that regulating recollection induces later forgetting. Thus, both hemodynamic and electrophysiological measures converge on the conclusion that inhibitory control can be engaged to modulate the neural machinery responsible for generating episodic recollection.

The foregoing research illustrates the strong functional and neurobiological similarities between the control of action and memory. Both engage a common frontal region – the LPFC – to override the influence of unwanted neural activity in support of selection and stopping. What differs between motor and memory control (and, indeed, between different forms of motor control) appears to be the sites of control and, perhaps, the means of achieving that control (see the section titled 'Neural architecture of inhibitory control'). The work on memory control adds the unique and theoretically significant contribution of showing that both selection and stopping induce inhibitory aftereffects on rejected representations, verifying and quantifying the involvement of inhibition in achieving control. To the extent that memory control may be used as a model system for cognitive control, these findings suggest the existence of a domain general system for controlling action and thought via inhibition. Consistent with this possibility, the LPFC is engaged in an extraordinarily diverse collection of cognitive tasks, and Duncan and colleagues have shown that it predicts individual differences in fluid intelligence (gF, or psychometric g). A common theme running throughout these tasks appears to be the management of interference, consistent with the putative role of this region in inhibitory control. Nevertheless, it remains possible that there is not one mechanism of control in the LPFC but many content-specific ones, localized similarly, the differences between which cannot yet be ascertained in the absence of direct comparisons between cognitive and motor control. Even, so, lateral prefrontal-posterior interaction remains a valid organizing principle that characterizes our understanding of the networks underlying inhibitory control.

Neural Architecture of Inhibitory Control

Many investigators agree that inhibitory control supports the regulation of behavior by limiting the influence of undesired representations on ongoing behavior by functionally altering the state of the undesired representation. Although the brain clearly solves the computational problems of stopping and response selection, there is not yet widespread agreement on how they are solved or on whether they are solved in a unitary manner. There are two general views on how inhibition may be achieved: direct inhibition and biased competition. Direct inhibition hypothesizes that an inhibitory process targets the unwanted representation or system (either directly or by exciting inhibitory interneurons), degrading its control over behavior. In contrast, biased competition hypothesizes that attentional control signals facilitate the representations of desired actions and that, as a result, competing representations are inhibited through local reciprocal inhibitory projections. The evidence base for biased competition is well developed, and Miller and Cohen have argued that this computational principle may be a primary means of implementing executive control. It is established, however, that both types of inhibitory control take place in the nervous system. For example, as reviewed by Sotres-Bayon and colleagues, excitatory projections from the medial frontal cortex terminate on inhibitory interneurons in the amygdala that modulate the functioning and output of that structure and, correspondingly, suppress conditioned emotional responding. Similarly, the frontal cortex excites inhibitory neurons in the reticular nucleus of the thalamus, which inhibit the thalamus, gating sensory input to the cortex. The fronto-subthalamic circuitry underlying motor-response suppression (discussed earlier) may be another such example. Thus, inhibitory control may often be accomplished, not by facilitating a competing response but by inhibitory modulation of the brain system underlying the undesired process. The types of situations in which these mechanisms of control operate are an interesting area for future study.

Concluding Comments

The capacity to override unwanted actions and memories is a fundamental component of the effective control of behavior and thought. The pervasiveness of selection and stopping as computational problems has led to the proposition that individual variation in the efficiency with which people inhibit may underlie differences in intellectual functions of many sorts (e.g., attention, working memory, long-term memory, reading, reasoning, and behavioral control) and may even be an important contributor to some psychological disorders. When a population exhibits perseverative tendencies, difficulties managing interference, or distractibility, investigators often consider the potential contribution of frontal lobe dysfunction (and, consequently, inhibitory dysfunction). These proposals, often referred to as inhibitory deficit theories, have been advanced to explain a range of phenomena. For example, because of the late development and early decline of the PFC in the life span, alterations in inhibitory control efficiency have featured prominently in theories of cognitive development and cognitive aging. Clinically, it has been proposed that inhibitory deficits contribute to psychopathologies, including obsessive–compulsive disorder, depression, schizophrenia, attention deficit/hyperactivity disorder, addiction, and chronic posttraumatic stress disorder. It seems unlikely that these diverse conditions are produced by the same deficit and, indeed, that even the various deficits within each population are produced by a single underlying deficiency. Nevertheless, the overlap between systems engaged during motor and memory inhibition suggests that generalized inhibitory control deficits are possible. If so, elucidating the neural systems that subserve inhibitory control is not merely of theoretical interest but has the potential for broad impact on problems of clinical importance.

See also: Computational Approaches to Motor Control; Cortical Control of Eye Movements; Episodic Memory: Assessment in Animals; Episodic Memory; Prefrontal Cortex: Structure and Anatomy; Prefrontal Cortex; Saccadic Eye Movements; Semantic Memory; Strategic Control of Memory.

Further Reading

Anderson MC and Green C (2001) Suppressing unwanted memories by executive control. *Nature* 410(6826): 366–369.

Anderson MC, Ochsner KN, Kuhl B, et al. (2004) Neural systems underlying the suppression of unwanted memories. *Science* 303 (5655): 232–235.

Aron AR (2007) The neural basis of inhibition in cognitive control. *Neuroscientist* 13(3): 214–228.

Aron AR, Robbins TW, and Poldrack RA (2004) Inhibition and the right inferior frontal cortex. *Trends in Cognitive Sciences* 8(4): 170–177.

Bergstrom ZM, Velmans M, de Fockert J, and Richardson-Klavehn A (2007) ERP evidence for successful voluntary avoidance of conscious recollection. *Brain Research* 1151: 119–133.

Boucher L, Palmeri TJ, Logan GD, and Schall JD (2007) Inhibitory control in mind and brain: an interactive race model of countermanding saccades. *Psychological Review* 114(2): 376–397.

Bunge SA, Ochsner KN, Desmond JE, Glover GH, and Gabrieli JD (2001) Prefrontal regions involved in keeping information in and out of mind. *Brain* 124(part 10): 2074–2086.

Carlson SM and Moses LJ (2001) Individual differences in inhibitory control and children's theory of mind. *Child Development* 72(4): 1032–1053.

Dagenbach D and Carr TH (1994) Inhibitory Processes in Attention Memory and Language. San Diego, CA: Academic Press.

Depue BE, Curran T, and Banich MT (2007) Prefrontal regions orchestrate suppression of emotional memories via a two-phase process. *Science* 317: 215–219.

Diamond A (1990) Developmental time course in human infants and infant monkeys, and the neural bases of, inhibitory control in reaching. *Annals of the New York Academy of Sciences* 608: 637–669 [discussion 669–676].

Duncan J and Owen AM (2000) Common regions of the human frontal lobe recruited by diverse cognitive demands. *Trends in Neuroscience* 23(10): 475–483.

Garavan H, Ross TJ, Murphy K, Roche RA, and Stein EA (2002) Dissociable executive functions in the dynamic control of behavior: inhibition, error detection, and correction. *Neuroimage* 17(4): 1820–1829.

Goldman-Rakic PS (1987) Circuitry of primate prefrontal cortex and regulation of behavior by representational memory. In: Mountcastle VB and Plum F (eds.) *Handbook of Physiology, Sec. 1: The Nervous System, Vol. 5: Higher Functions of the Brain, Pt. 1*, pp. 373–417. Baltimore, MD: American Physiological Society.

Gorfein DS and MacLeod CM (eds.) (2007) *Inhibition in Cognition.* Washington, DC: American Psychological Association.

Jiang Y and Kanwisher N (2003) Common neural substrates for response selection across modalities and mapping paradigms. *Journal of Cognitive Neuroscience* 15(8): 1080–1094.

Johansson M, Aslan A, Bauml KH, Gabel A, and Mecklinger A (2007) When remembering causes forgetting: electrophysiological correlates of retrieval-induced forgetting. *Cerebral Cortex* 17(6): 1335–1341.

Jonides J and Nee DE (2006) Brain mechanisms of proactive interference in working memory. *Neuroscience* 139(1): 181–193.

Knight RT, Staines WR, Swick D, and Chao LL (1999) Prefrontal cortex regulates inhibition and excitation in distributed neural networks. *Acta Psychologica (Amsterdam)* 101(2–3): 159–178.

Levy BJ and Anderson MC (2002) Inhibitory processes and the control of memory retrieval. *Trends in Cognitive Sciences* 6(7): 299–305.

Logan GD (1994) On the ability to inhibit thought and action: A users' guide to the stop signal paradigm. In: Dagenbach D and Carr TH (eds.) *Inhibitory Processes in Attention, Memory and Language*, pp. 189–239. San Diego, CA: Academic Press.

Lustig C, Hasher L, and Toney ST (2001) Inhibitory control over the present and the past. *European Journal of Cognitive Psychology* 13(1–2): 107–122.

Miller EK and Cohen JD (2001) An integrative theory of prefrontal cortex function. *Annual Review of Neuroscience* 24: 167–202.

Munoz DP and Everling S (2004) Look away: The anti-saccade task and the voluntary control of eye movement. *Nature Reviews Neuroscience* 5(3): 218–228.

Proctor RW and Vu KL (2006) Stimulus-Response Compatibility Principles: Data, Theory, and Application. Boca Raton, FL: CRC Press.

Rowe JB, Toni I, Josephs O, Frackowiak RS, and Passingham RE (2000) The prefrontal cortex: response selection or maintenance within working memory? *Science* 288(5471): 1656–1660.

Sasaki K, Gemba H, and Tsujimoto T (1989) Suppression of visually initiated hand movement by stimulation of the prefrontal cortex in the monkey. *Brain Research* 495(1): 100–107.

Schumacher EH and Jiang Y (2003) Neural mechanisms for response selection: Representation specific or modality independent? *Journal of Cognitive Neuroscience* 15(8): 1077–1079.

Shimamura AP (2000) The role of the prefrontal cortex in dynamic filtering. *Psychobiology* 28(2): 207–218.

Sotres-Bayon F, Bush DE, and LeDoux JE (2004) Emotional perseveration: An update on prefrontal–amygdala interactions in fear extinction. *Learning & Memory* 11(5): 525–535.

Thompson-Schill SL, D'Esposito M, Aguirre GK, and Farah MJ (1997) Role of left inferior prefrontal cortex in retrieval of semantic knowledge: A reevaluation. *Proceedings of the National Academy of Sciences of the United States of America* 94(26): 14792–14797.

Neglect Syndrome and the Spatial Attention Network

M-M Mesulam, Northwestern University Feinberg School of Medicine, Chicago, IL, USA

Damage to the right side of the brain can trigger a debilitating impairment known as the left hemineglect (selective inattention) syndrome. Patients with this syndrome minimize the salience of events in the contralesional side of the environment, display a reluctance to shift attention in a leftward direction, and cannot effectively search for targets embedded within the left hemispace. The left hemineglect syndrome is assumed to reflect damage to a large-scale frontoparietal network that normally sustains the adaptive distribution of spatial attention.

In this context, the term 'spatial attention' designates a set of interrelated sensory, motor, and cognitive processes that collectively enable the selective allocation of neural resources to motivationally relevant parts of the environment. The spatial representation of events according to their emotional salience, their targeting for oculomotor fixation or manual grasp, the anticipatory biasing of regions where interesting events are expected to occur, and the search for objects embedded among distractors are components of spatial attention.

Experiments in monkeys traced the two major nodes of an analogous spatial attention network to posterior parietal cortex (e.g., 7a in the inferior parietal lobule (IPL) and lateral intraparietal (LIP) in the intraparietal sulcus) and a premotor/prefrontal area that includes the frontal eye fields (FEF). These two areas are reciprocally interconnected and contain neurons that encode spatial coordinates in multiple reference frames, represent extrapersonal space in terms of salience rather than object characteristics, and direct orientating and search behaviors toward salient events. They collectively provide a coarse mapping of salient extrapersonal events and encode the intent to generate saccadic eye movements or arm reaching movements toward behaviorally relevant events. Both of these areas receive peristriate information and project to the superior colliculus in a way that would allow them to exert a top-down modulation of oculomotor and visual areas involved in the motor and sensory aspects of spatial attention.

In general, area 7a has more sensory properties and may play the major role in encoding a salience-based representation of the extrapersonal events, whereas areas LIP and FEF tend to have a closer relationship to the programming of saccades in the direction of behaviorally relevant targets. Although Chafee and Goldman-Rakic have shown that neuronal firing is greater in the FEF just before a memory-guided saccade and in the LIP just after the onset of a salient spatial cue, these two areas are functionally interdependent and display relatively few differences in response patterns. They collectively represent an advanced state of sensorimotor synthesis in which perception can be represented as salience rather than sensory features, and action as intent rather than movement.

Axonally transported tracer experiments in the monkey brain showed that area 7a/LIP and the FEF are reciprocally interconnected not only to each other but also to the cingulate gyrus. Cingulate neurons in the awake animal respond to behaviorally relevant extrapersonal events and may participate in the remapping of salience following saccadic eye movements. Through its connections with the amygdala and parahippocampal complex, the cingulate gyrus provides a limbic component of the spatial attention network.

The complexity of this network and the heterogeneity of lesion sites associated with the neglect syndrome account for the large variety of clinical manifestations and explanatory theories. Research in this field has proceeded in two major directions: investigation of patients with the hemispatial neglect syndrome and functional imaging of neurologically intact subjects performing tasks of spatial attention that are impaired in these patients. This research has led to exciting new insights but has also generated two major questions. The first is related to hemispheric asymmetry. Although severe contralesional neglect is far more common after right than after left hemisphere lesions, functional imaging has not yet revealed a consistent asymmetry of neural activity during tasks of spatial attention in normal subjects. The second question concerns the location of neglect-causing lesions. Although functional imaging highlights the engagement of dorsal frontoparietal cortex in spatial attention tasks, clinical evidence links the neglect syndrome to more ventral lesions of the inferior parietal lobule and temporoparietal junction. This review summarizes clinicoanatomical correlates of the neglect syndrome and functional imaging experiments on spatial attention. The two questions discussed previously will not be resolved, but the facts that generate them will be reviewed.

The Neuropsychology of Neglect

Contralesional neglect is more lasting and severe after lesions in the right side of the brain. This asymmetry is consistent with a neural model postulating that the left hemisphere directs attention primarily to the contralateral hemispace, whereas the right hemisphere directs attention to both hemispaces or, alternatively, serves a more global orienting function. According to this model, left hemisphere lesions do not cause prominent neglect because the right hemisphere continues to direct attention to either side of space. When neglect is severe, the patient with a right hemisphere lesion may behave almost as if one-half of the universe had abruptly ceased to exist in any meaningful form. One patient may shave, groom, and dress only the right side of the body; another may fail to eat food placed on the left side of the tray; another may omit to read the left half of each sentence or even the left side of every word printed anywhere on the page; still another may fail to copy detail on the left side of a drawing and may show a curious tendency to leave an uncommonly wide margin on the left side of the paper when asked to write.

Neglect behavior has perceptual, motor, and motivational components. Perceptual aspects of neglect can be probed with tests of extinction, line bisection, and covert attentional shifts. Extinction is said to exist when patients who respond accurately to unilateral stimulation from either the left or the right side consistently ignore the stimulation on the left under conditions of bilateral simultaneous stimulation. If extinction occurs in only one modality, it can conceivably reflect a subtle disruption of relevant sensory pathways or even a callosal disconnection syndrome. Multimodal extinction, however, almost always reflects the representational aspect of neglect. In the traditional version of the line bisection task, patients are asked to mark the midpoint of a horizontal line drawn on a sheet of paper. Patients with left hemineglect tend to place their mark substantially rightward of center, suggesting that the representational impact of the left side becomes diminished and that it takes a longer segment on the left to balance the salience of a shorter segment on the right.

A rightward skewing of mental representations was demonstrated by Bisiach and colleagues in experiments in which patients were asked to mentally retrieve prominent features along the Piazza del Duomo in Milan as they imagined themselves looking toward the cathedral. Patients with left neglect were more accurate in listing details situated on the right side of the square as viewed from that vantage point. Upon being asked to imagine looking at the square while facing away from the cathedral, the same patients showed better recall of the items that had been omitted when assuming the former vantage point. Thus, the impaired evocation of left-sided details in the first part of the experiment was not due to an obliteration of the information but to an inability to activate the part of the representation which fell to the left of the imaginary perspective. In addition to this difficulty in activating the left side of previously encoded mental representations, patients with left neglect also display a relative deficit in encoding the left side of sensory experience during the compilation of new representations.

A task developed by Posner and colleagues has played an influential role in this field of investigation. No eye movements are allowed, central fixation is required at all times, and the attentional orientation is shifted covertly within a mental representation of the ambient visual scene. These shifts can be triggered exogenously through sensory priming or endogenously through centrally presented arrows which induce directional expectancy. Patients with left hemineglect but no hemianopia show much longer reaction times when responding to targets in the left. They also display an excessive difficulty disengaging attention from a cue in the right hemispace when the task requires a subsequent leftward shift of covert orientation to targets on the left. This resistance to disengagement is partially analogous to the phenomenon of extinction.

Patients with neglect can also display a reluctance to scan and explore the left hemispace even in the absence of obvious gaze or limb paresis. The resultant impairments of search behaviors are readily elicited by tasks which require the patient to circle or check targets on a sheet of paper. Patients omit many more targets on the left, need more time to find left-sided targets, use a disorganized scanning strategy, make fewer and lower amplitude eye movements to the left, and have longer visual fixation times on right-sided targets. The use of a 90° mirror, which reverses the direction of a manual movement needed to mark a target from the direction of the shift in visual attention that leads to its detection, shows that target cancellation impairments reflect a failure to look left in some patients and a failure to reach to the left in others. The frequent observation that targets oriented randomly on the page are far less efficiently detected than targets organized into rows and columns implies that an inability to endogenously impose an orderly scanning strategy contributes to the severity of the neglect.

Patients with left unilateral neglect also display difficulties in manual search. Blindfolded search for small objects by manual palpation is intact on the right side of the table not only with the right hand but also with the left hand, whereas it becomes ineffective on the left side of the table even when the intact right hand is being used. These observations show that left neglect is associated with impaired tactile exploration within the left hemispace regardless of the limb that is being used. Thus, motor programs involved in exploration appear to be organized not according to the muscle groups that are being activated but, rather, according to the hemispace within which the movement is to be discharged.

A major role of any attentional system is to shift the attentional spotlight toward extrapersonal events of emotional and motivational significance. Patients with unilateral neglect devalue the left side of the world and behave not only as if nothing is actually happening in the left but also as if nothing of any importance could be expected to emanate from that side. The influence of this factor can be probed by varying motivational valence. For example, a patient showed marked improvement in detecting targets on the left when he was promised one penny for each accurate detection. Another patient with severe left hemineglect failed to reach for food on the left side of a tray and would bitterly complain that his tea had been left out. On a day when the nurse was instructed to withhold breakfast, the patient became unusually hungry by noontime but did not show any change in the severe neglect of left-sided targets in a letter-cancellation task. When his lunch tray was brought, however, he had no reluctance to reach for his tea on the left side of the tray. These anecdotal observations suggest that a devaluation of sensory events on the left may contribute to the emergence of neglect and that the relationship between neglect and motivation may be material specific so that hunger decreases the spatial distribution of neglect for edible items but not for letters on a test sheet.

Many aspects of neglect are based on top-down processes that impose a spatial bias on the encoding of a percept or the reactivation of its representation. In patients with extinction, for example, reaction times to unilateral right-sided stimuli are longer than those to bilateral stimuli. Since both conditions are reported as unilateral right-sided stimulation by the patient, the extinguished stimulus appears to gain access to the central nervous system and exert a covert influence on behavior. According to a case report by Marshall and Halligan, a patient with left hemineglect who was shown line drawings of two houses, one of which had flames coming out of the left side, judged the two drawings to be visually identical but chose the one without flames when asked to select the house she would prefer to live in.

In the preceding account, the word 'left' has deliberately been used without further qualification, as if it constituted a fixed attribute such as color or texture. This is clearly not the case since there is no left or right without a specific frame of reference. At least four frames of reference define the leftness of an extrapersonal event: egocentric (defined with respect to the observer), allocentric (defined with respect to another extrapersonal event), world-centered (defined with respect to a fixed landmark in the environment), and object-centered (defined with respect to a principal axis in the canonical representation on an object). Since the eyes, head, and trunk can rotate and tilt with respect to each other, the egocentric frame of reference contains retinocentric, cephalocentric, somatocentric, and gravitational coordinates so that an event which is in the left according to one egocentric coordinate could be on the right according to another. Furthermore, perceptual and conceptual factors influence the segmentation of the stimulus field into individual clusters with their own left and right sides. Left hemineglect is defined as a behavioral state in which a location in one of the egocentric lefts, in the environmental left, in the canonical or object-centered left, in the allocentric left, and in the segmentational left is endowed with less perceptual salience and becomes less likely to attract attentional capture through search and orienting behaviors.

Spatial Attention Network in the Human Brain

Contralesional neglect can arise in patients with parietal, frontal, cingulate, or subcortical lesions. In the group of patients with parietal lesions, some investigators point to the IPL (or temporoparietal junction) as the critical site, whereas others emphasize the importance of the superior temporal gyrus, an opinion that is difficult to reconcile with the auditory functions of the superior temporal gyrus. A study by Hillis and colleagues based on the remote cortical dysfunction caused by subcortical lesions suggested that interference with IPL function may cause the egocentric (observer-centered) aspects of neglect, whereas interference with superior temporal gyrus function may cause its allocentric and object-centered aspects. Reaching deficits, extinction, and extinction-like phenomena (e.g., a slowing of attentional disengagement in tasks of covert attentional shifts) may be associated with superior parietal lobule (SPL) lesions, whereas the distortions of spatial representation may be associated with IPL lesions. In the frontal lobes, some studies show that the critical lesion site is in the FEF, whereas others implicate the inferior frontal gyrus. It is also not clear if subcortical lesions cause neglect because of the tissue they destroy or because of the remote cortical dysfunction they induce. A relatively attractive hypothesis involves the possibility that 'parietal neglect' might be predominantly perceptual, whereas 'frontal neglect' might be predominantly motor. In support of this possibility, several studies have shown that 'perceptual' tasks such as extinction and line bisection are more likely to be associated with parietal lesions, whereas 'motor' tasks such as target cancellation are more likely to be associated with frontal lesions. Ingenious experiments with pulleys and mirrors have shown that errors in line bisection and target-detection tasks can be attributed to representational biases in patients with parietal lesions and to directional hypokinesia in patients with frontal lesions. Other studies, however, have not been able to confirm the presence of a relationship between directional hypokinesia and frontal lesions.

The strong interconnectivity between the frontal and parietal components of this network raises the possibility that damage to one may induce distal hypometabolism in the other through the process of diaschisis. It therefore seems unrealistic to expect a strict behavioral dissociation between the manifestations of neglect that result from parietal versus frontal lesions since these two components of the attentional network collectively subserve a level of sensorimotor integration in which the boundaries between action and perception become blurred.

Functional Imaging of Spatial Attention

In neurologically intact volunteers, numerous tasks of attentional shifts in the visual or auditory modalities, with or without eye movements, guided by exogenous or endogenous cues, and entailing variable components of manual or oculomotor search, have elicited conjoint activations in the FEF and in the banks of the intraparietal sulcus (IPS), together with additional but more variable clusters of activity in other posterior parietal, temporoparietal, cingulate, and prefrontal regions. These experiments have supported the contention that the FEF and posterior parietal cortex exert a top-down modulation of the superior colliculus and visual areas of the cerebral cortex so that the representation of significant events and the actions necessary for their attentional capture can be promoted. It is interesting to note that spatial attention tasks most commonly activate the IPS and FEF, whereas the clinical observations suggest that the lesions responsible for neglect tend to be more ventral in location.

According to functional imaging experiments, frontal components of the spatial attention network (FEF, supplementary eye fields, and middle frontal gyrus) are more closely related to the compilation of a prospective motor code for overt search, whereas the parietal components (IPS, SPL, and IPL) are more closely related to the maintenance of the underlying spatial representations that guide the search. The IPL/SPL region may also mediate the cue-induced voluntary reorientation of spatial attention and the remapping of the attentional landscape based on the spatial distribution of salience.

The FEF has an internal functional segregation characterized by a partially overlapping mosaic of areas mediating saccadic eye movements, visual search, working memory, and covert shifts of attentional orientation. Functional heterogeneity is also emerging within the cingulate component of the network where an anterior sector seems to mediate processes related to cognitive control, target detection, vigilance, conflict resolution, and response selection, whereas a posterior sector seems to mediate the anticipatory allocation of attention toward locations where relevant events are expected to occur. As shown by Small and colleagues, posterior cingulate activations linked to anticipatory spatial biasing are further enhanced by monetary incentive, supporting the contention that posterior cingulate neurons mediate the motivational modulation of spatial attention.

Some functional imaging experiments have yielded results consistent with right hemisphere specialization, whereas others have not. The critical role of the right hemisphere for spatial attention, so convincingly illustrated by clinical observations on neglect patients, is therefore not obvious in functional imaging experiments.

Conclusions

It is becoming increasingly clear that neglect cannot be attributed to a unitary deficit of orientation, representation, or intention. Instead, it represents an outcome of interacting perturbations in each of these processes. As in the case of aphasia and amnesia, neglect is a 'network syndrome.' It represents damage to one or more interactive components of the distributed network shown in **Figure 1**, in which each component has a different pattern of physiological and anatomical specialization.

The spatial attention network revolves around cortical epicenters in the posterior parietal cortex, FEF, and the cingulate gyrus. Each of these macroscopic components serves a dual purpose: it provides a local network for regional neural computations and also a nodal point for the linkage of distributed information. Although each component displays a relative specialization for specific behaviors, spatial attention as a whole is the emergent property of the entire network. Compiling a salience map of the extrapersonal space and transforming spatial coordinates into targets for reorienting attention can be included among the relative specializations of the parietal component; translating representations into systematic search behaviors reflects one of the relative specializations of the FEF, and calibrating spatial expectancy according to motivational valence represents one of the specializations of the cingulate component. The coherent

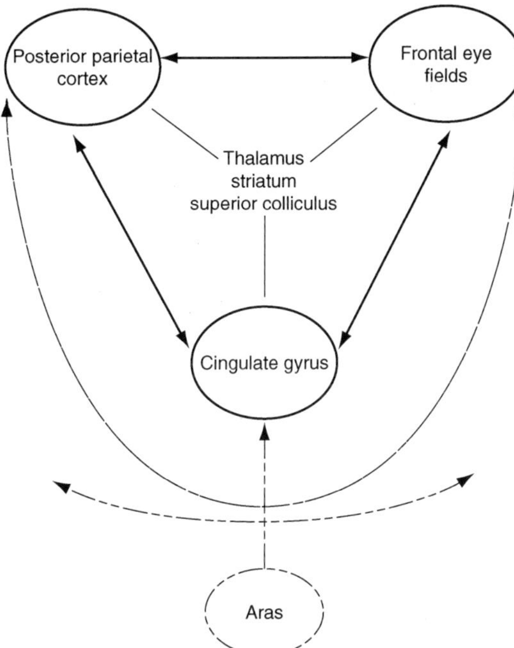

Figure 1 A large-scale network for spatial attention.

engagement of this network as a whole enables motivationally relevant extrapersonal events to become the selective targets of attentional behaviors.

Although much has been learned about the spatial attention network shown in **Figure 1**, many crucial questions remain. In particular, the computational features of the network, its interactions with other partially overlapping networks, the internal functional heterogeneity of its major components, and the physiological basis of right hemisphere specialization are among the major questions that will be attracting new and exciting insights.

See also: Attention and Eye Movements; Attentional Networks; Attentional Networks in the Parietal Cortex; Frontal Eye Fields; Neural Coding of Spatial Representations; Parietal Cortex and Spatial Attention; Spatial Cognition and Executive Function; Spatial Cognition; Visual System: Multiple Visual Areas in Monkeys; Visual Attention.

Further Reading

Andersen RA, Snyder LH, Bradley DC, and Xing J (1997) Multimodal representation of space in the posterior parietal cortex and its use in planning movements. *Annual Review of Neuroscience* 20: 303–330.

Bisiach G, Geminiani G, Berti A, and Rusconi M (1990) Perceptual and premotor factors of unilateral neglect. *Neurology* 40: 1278–1281.

Chafee MV and Goldman-Rakic PS (2000) Inactivation of parietal and prefrontal cortex reveals interdependence of neural activity during memory-guided saccades. *Journal of Neurophysiology* 83: 1550–1566.

Corbetta M, Kincade JM, Ollinger JM, McAvoy MP, and Shulman GL (2000) Voluntary orienting is dissociated from target detection in human posterior parietal cortex. *Nature Neuroscience* 3: 292–297.

Curtis CE, Rao VY, and D'Esposito M (2004) Maintenance of spatial and motor codes during oculomotor delayed response tasks. *Journal of Neuroscience* 24: 3944–3952.

Daffner KR, Ahern GL, Weintraub S, and Mesulam MM (1990) Dissociated neglect behavior following sequential strokes in the right hemisphere. *Annals of Neurology* 28: 97–101.

Gitelman DR, Parrish TB, Friston KJ, and Mesulam M-M (2002) Functional anatomy of visual search: Regional segregations within the frontal eye fields and effective connectivity of the superior colliculus. *NeuroImage* 15: 970–982.

Gottlieb JP, Kusunoki M, and Goldberg ME (1998) The representation of visual salience in monkey parietal cortex. *Nature* 391: 481–484.

Heilman KM, Watson RT, and Valenstein E (1985) Neglect and related disorders. In: Heilman KM and Valenstein E (eds.) *Clinical Neuropsychology*, pp. 279–336. New York: Oxford University Press.

Hillis AE, Newhart M, Heidler J, Barker PB, Herskovits EH, and Degaonkar M (2005) Anatomy of spatial attention: Insights from perfusion imaging and hemispatial neglect in acute stroke. *Journal of Neuroscience* 25: 3161–3167.

Hopfinger JB, Buonocore MH, and Mangun GR (2000) The neural mechanisms of top-down attentional control. *Nature Neuroscience* 3: 284–291.

Karnath H-O, Ferber S, and Himmelbach M (2001) Spatial awareness is a function of the temporal not the posterior parietal lobe. *Nature* 950–953.

Marshall JC and Halligan PW (1988) Blindsight and insight in visuo-spatial neglect. *Nature* 336: 766–767.

Mesulam M-M (1999) Spatial attention and neglect: Parietal, frontal, and cingulate contributions to the mental representation and attentional targeting of salient extrapersonal events. *Philosophical Transactions of the Royal Society B* 354: 1325–1346.

Nobre AC, Coull JT, Maquet P, Frith CD, Vandenberghe R, and Mesulam M-M (2004) Orienting attention to locations in perceptual versus mental representations. *Journal of Cognitive Neuroscience* 16: 363–373.

Posner MI (1980) Orienting of attention. *Quarterly Journal of Experimental Psychology* 32: 3025.

Small DM, Gitelman D, Simmons K, Bloise SM, Parrish T, and Mesulam M-M (2005) Monetary incentives enhance processing in brain regions mediating top-down control of attention. *Cerebral Cortex* 15: 1855–1865.

Summerfield JJ, Lepsien J, Gitelman DR, Mesulam M-M, and Nobre AC (2006) Orienting attention based on long-term memory experience. *Neuron* 49: 905–916.

Vallar G (1993) The anatomical basis of spatial hemineglect in humans. In: Robertson IH and Marshall JC (eds.) *Unilateral Neglect: Clinical and Experimental Studies*, pp. 27–59. Hillsdale, NJ: Erlbaum.

Weintraub S and Mesulam M-M (1988) Visual hemispatial inattention: Stimulus parameters and exploratory strategies. *Journal of Neurology, Neurosurgery & Psychology* 51: 1481–1488.

Yantis S, Schwartzbach J, Serences JT, et al. (2002) Transient neural activity in human parietal cortex during attentional shifts. *Nature Neuroscience* 5: 995–1002.

Neural Coding of Spatial Representations

N M Bentley and E Salinas, Wake Forest University School of Medicine, Winston-Salem, NC, USA

Neuronal Signals That Encode Spatial Location

In mammals, spatial information is derived primarily from three sensory modalities: vision, audition, and somatosensation. In many regions of the neocortex, and across sensory modalities, individual neurons fire action potentials at high rates only when objects to which they are sensitive appear in a particular region of space – the neuron's receptive field. For example, a neuron in the primary visual cortex (V1) responds vigorously only when a stimulus to which it is sensitive stimulates a particular region of the retina of approximately 1° of visual angle. Similarly, in primary somatosensory cortex, neurons respond only when a particular part of the body is touched, and tactile receptive fields on the fingertips are typically only a few millimeters wide. In the auditory system, some neurons respond only when a sound originates at some particular angle in space relative to the head. This case is special, however, because, unlike visual and somatic primary receptors on the eyes and skin, primary receptor neurons in the cochlea are not space-specific; the neurons that become selective for sounds from specific regions in space are constructed in a series of computational steps. In all of these cases, however, spatial information is conveyed basically through a labeled-line code, which means that the stimulus location can be inferred from the identity of the activated neuron or neurons. So, to determine where is the stimulus, one needs to know which neurons are responding.

As these examples illustrate, in general, spatial information is carried by firing rate distributions, and it is widely held that brains rely on such distributions to track object location. Cortical microstimulation experiments have largely corroborated this hypothesis. For instance, eye movements toward specific points in space can be elicited with high reliability by microinjecting electrical current at specific points in the cortex, a manipulation that increases the firing rate of a restricted population of neurons around the electrode. It remains possible, however, that brains also rely on other aspects of neural activity to encode object location, for example, correlations between the activity of different neurons or precise spike-train sequences. That firing rates carry a large amount of spatial information is an important premise on which many of the conclusions discussed here depend.

Receptive Field Properties

Receptive field sizes vary widely across regions of the cortex. Consider, for example, the visual system. From the thalamus, visual information first reaches the cortex in the back of the head, in the occipital lobe, where the V1 is located. Receptive fields in V1 are small, typically covering on the order of 1° of visual angle, and they are topographically arranged, meaning that neighboring neurons have receptive fields that overlap or are close to one another in visual space. From V1, visual information is transmitted to a number of different areas in the parietal, occipital, and temporal lobes. In general, the closer a visual area is to the front of the brain, the larger the receptive fields become and the less ordered their topography. The largest visual receptive fields can be almost as large as the whole visual field, as may be found, for example, in the inferotemporal cortex (IT). In general, receptive fields not only increase in size toward more central structures but also become more complex; for instance, V1 neurons are selective for small oriented bars or gratings (stripes), whereas IT neurons respond most strongly to highly complex images such as faces or whole objects.

Areas That Specialize in Spatial Processing

Cortical visual areas have traditionally been divided into two groups, which lie along the ventral and dorsal pathways. The distinction rests both on anatomical grounds and on functional evidence based on brain-damaged patients and lesioned primates, both of whom show consistent kinds of deficits depending on which pathway is affected. Damage to the ventral pathway, which includes areas V2, V4, and IT, generally leads to problems in object recognition (agnosias), whereas damage to the dorsal pathway, which includes V3, the middle temporal area (MT), and several parietal regions, such as areas 7a and the lateral intraparietal area (LIP), leads to problems in navigation and the perception of space (ataxias and visual neglect). The response properties of neurons in these areas also reflect their differing functional roles. Neurons in the ventral pathway are often highly selective for specific objects, but their responses to those objects are relatively invariant to their color, size, position, or perspective, among other properties. On the other hand, neurons in the dorsal pathway are typically not as selective for object identity, but their activity often depends on the spatial relation between the viewed object and the organism's body. The general conclusion here is that parts of the brain are specialized for processing spatial information. Why this separation of function has evolved remains unclear. It should also be emphasized that the dorsal pathway is not exclusively involved in vision. Rather, it processes auditory and somatosensory signals in addition to visual signals and appears to be important for spatial processing and movement planning in general.

The Precision of Spatial Representations in the Brain

How precisely can we locate an object in space, and what determines this precision? First, spatial accuracy depends on the modality and the species in question. For example, auditory localization acuity varies tremendously across mammals, from hundreds of degrees in subterranean species to approximately 1° in humans and elephants. Second, acuity can depend on the form of the stimulus itself. For example, a person's ability to discriminate between fine-grained textures or Braille letters through touch depends on whether and how those stimuli move across the skin. Third, accuracy also typically depends on where an object is located. For example, spatial acuity in humans is much lower in the periphery than in the center of the visual field (i.e., the fovea), and somatosensory spatial acuity is much higher on the fingertips than on the palm of the hand. Physiologically, in both cases the differences are due to differences in the densities of primary receptors and cortical neurons dedicated to cover each region of space. Touch mechanoreceptor density is approximately four times higher at the fingertips, where acuity is high, than at the palm, where acuity is lower. Differences in photoreceptor numbers across the retina impose similar limits on acuity across the visual field. Discrimination performance in difficult perceptual tasks is often limited by such fundamental constraints as the density of primary receptors.

Tuning Curve Width and Optimal Sensory Coding

Naively, we might also expect receptive field sizes in a population of cortical neurons to limit the precision with which the population can represent an object's position. After all, if only one neuron is firing, the larger its receptive field, the larger is the uncertainty about the location of the stimulus that triggered the response. This intuition, however, is not always correct. First, information about stimulus location is typically spread out across a population of neurons with overlapping receptive fields, in which case spatial accuracy depends not only on the receptive field width but also on the density of neurons and their variability. An array of narrow tuning curves may be extremely ineffective if they leave gaps between them (a tuning curve here is the mean response of a neuron plotted as a function of stimulus location). On the other hand, an array of neurons with wide and overlapping receptive fields may be highly accurate if their variability is low. Some of these possibilities are illustrated in **Figure 1**.

A second and more profound factor that affects spatial accuracy was identified by Zhang and Sejnowski. They used a measure of accuracy known as the Fisher information to characterize the efficiency of populations of model cortical neurons with tuning curves of different widths. They found that the relationship between tuning width and Fisher information depends on the dimensionality of the stimulus to be represented. That is, whether narrow or wide curves are better depends crucially on the number of parameters that the neurons are representing. Recent work along similar lines by Brown and Bäcker showed that, when an infinite number of neurons cover one dimension (say, distance to a target) or two dimensions (say, target location on a surface), encoding accuracy always increases with decreasing tuning width – narrower curves are always better. However, for three dimensions or higher, the advantage of narrow curves goes away; there is an optimal tuning width in terms of Fisher information, even though the number of neurons remains infinite.

Another theoretical study, by Pouget and colleagues, demonstrated that whether wide or narrow tuning curves are better also depends on the mechanisms that generate those tuning curves. In many models, tuning curve width is determined by the strength of lateral interactions between neurons in a population, such that stronger interactions are needed to generate narrow tuning than wide tuning. Strong lateral interactions, however, also tend to produce strong noise covariations across neurons; that is, the random response fluctuations of pairs of neurons become more similar to one another. In practice, this may limit information transmission quite severely, and therefore, a population with wide tuning curves may be much more informative than a population with narrow curves if the narrowing involves traditional mechanisms that increase noise covariations. This result suggests that generating arrays of narrow tuning curves from arrays of wide ones is probably a rather inefficient strategy, even if the encoded stimulus is one- or two-dimensional, because narrowing mechanisms effectively increase the noise.

In summary, then, in terms of the accuracy for encoding an object's position, the optimal tuning curve width depends on the number of neurons in

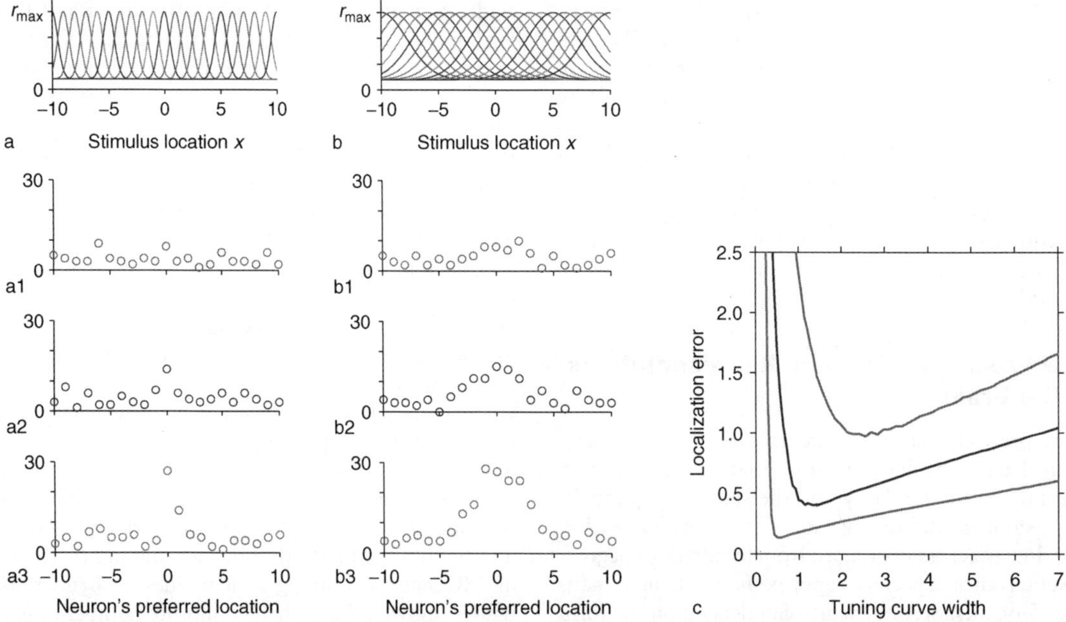

Figure 1 Encoding of spatial location by populations of neurons with Gaussian tuning curves: (a) a population of narrowly tuned neurons, tuning curve width = 0.5; (b) a population of widely tuned neurons, tuning curve width = 2.3; (c) localization error as a function of tuning curve width. In (a), each curve represents the mean response of a neuron as a function of the location of a stimulus *x*. There are 21 neurons, and *x* may be between −10 and 10 (arbitrary units). The tuning curves are narrow (width $\sigma = 0.5$), so only one or two neurons fire significantly above the baseline in any trial (a trial is one stimulus presentation). The graphs (a1)–(a3) show the responses of the 21 neurons in three single trials with low (red points), medium (blue points), and high (magenta points) signal-to-noise ratios. Variability across trials was modeled as a Poisson process, so the variance of each response was equal to the mean. The signal-to-noise ratio was controlled by varying the maximum response of the neurons: $r_{max} = 10$, 15, and 30 spikes s^{-1} for the red, blue, and magenta points, respectively. Background firing was constant at 4 spikes s^{-1}. (b) As in (a), but for wide tuning curves (width $\sigma = 2.3$). In this case, approximately eight neurons typically fire above baseline in each trial. (c) Localization error as a function of tuning curve width for the three signal-to-noise ratios in (a) and (b). The error is the average deviation between the true stimulus location, *x*, and the location that is estimated from the responses of the 21 neurons in each trial, x_{est} (more specifically, $E^2 = \langle (x - x_{est})^2 \rangle$, where *E* is the localization error and the brackets indicate an average over trials and over all values of *x*). The width that is optimal for representing stimulus location depends on the signal-to-noise ratio. If it is high (magenta curve), narrow tuning curves are better because they generate smaller localization errors; in contrast, if the signal-to-noise ratio is low (red curve), broader tuning curves are more accurate.

the population, their noise properties, and the number of dimensions of the encoded position vector.

Tuning Curve Width and Motor Constraints

An interesting and perhaps counterintuitive observation about the neural activity that encodes spatial location is that it should not be more accurate than required by the animal's behavior. Just as commuting between home and school in a Formula 1 race car would be costly and inefficient, localizing objects with greater accuracy than necessary would waste resources. A recent theoretical study by Salinas highlighted the crucial role that motor constraints play in determining optimal sensory representations, and an impressive data set collected by Heffner and colleagues illustrated the point. Based on the analysis of more than 30 species of mammals, Heffner and collaborators found that sound localization capacity varies tremendously in this group – discrimination thresholds range from approximately 1°in humans and elephants to approximately 25°in gerbils and horses. Discrimination threshold in this case corresponds to an angular separation between two sound sources, such that a subject can distinguish with 75% accuracy which source generated a short noise burst. According to Heffner's analysis, the measured differences across species are not accounted for by variations in sound environment, interaural distance, or animal lifestyle. Rather, sound localization acuity in mammals seems to depend on the precision required for the visual orienting response to sound. The logic is as follows. The primary function of sound localization is to produce an orienting response, that is, to bring the sound source into the most sensitive part of the field of view (the fovea) for visual inspection. Therefore, species that have small areas of best vision (e.g., humans and elephants) need to make highly precise movements, whereas species that have large areas or streaks of optimal vision (e.g., gerbils and horses) do not. This is an important observation because it means that when behavior does not require high accuracy, the sensory representation should be correspondingly coarse, even if, in principle, it could be made more precise.

Reference Frames in the Cortex

References for Sensory Responses

Because there are no absolute spatial coordinates, an object's position in space can only be specified relative to a landmark that serves as reference. A crucial question therefore is: relative to which reference or references does the neocortex represent object locations? Experiments suggest that different parts of the cortex use different references, and some neurons seem to combine multiple ones. Those regions of cortex that receive sensory information most directly often use the topography of peripheral sensory organs themselves as references. For example, in the early visual cortex the reference is the retina – V1 neurons are said to encode visual information in retino-centered or eye-centered coordinates. In the early somatosensory cortex, the reference is the skin. Audition is different because firing rate distributions among the inner ear's sensory neurons do not depend in a straightforward way on where in space a sound originates. Thus, early auditory neurons do not represent spatial information in an ear-centered coordinate frame. Further downstream, however, through a series of computations involving the combination of interaural level differences, monaural spectral cues, and interaural time differences, cortical neurons create a representation of sound-source location in a head-centered or eye-centered reference frame.

References for Motor Responses

Just as sensory neurons require a reference for encoding the position of objects that are seen, heard, or touched, the motor system requires one or more references in order to move a limb to a desired position. In more central areas, the reference frames of cortical neurons that contribute to generating behavior are more complex than those of traditional sensory neurons. In a series of landmark papers, Gross, Graziano, and their colleagues showed that in the premotor cortex of monkeys many neurons fire strongly only when an object is seen at a particular place relative to a specific body part; that is, they have body-part-centered reference frames. For example, many premotor neurons are bimodal, in that they respond to both visual and somatosensory stimuli, and their visual receptive field is typically a three-dimensional region of space near the somatosensory receptive field. The key finding is that both of these receptive fields move where the body part moves. Neurons with receptive fields anchored to the arms, upper body, and head are especially prevalent. This multiplicity of reference frames suggests that neurons in the motor system rely on reference points specific to and convenient for the types of behavior they help to generate. Visual receptive fields attached to the foot may be useful for playing soccer, visual receptive fields attached to the mouth may be useful for biting an apple, and so on. Thus, the responses of such neurons may allow a sensory signal to act directly as a motor signal. Another implication is that sensory processing is not limited to sensory cortex, traditionally conceived. In fact, sensory processing seems to occur all over the cortex and to be inseparably intermingled with motor planning.

Changing Reference Frames

That sensory and motor cortical areas exhibit different sets of reference frames indicates that information about object location must be transformed from one set of reference frames to another as it propagates between brain regions. This operation is known as a coordinate transformation. According to the work of Richard Andersen and collaborators, the posterior parietal cortex (part of the dorsal pathway, not surprisingly) is largely responsible for coordinate transformations in the cortex. Many posterior parietal neurons are multimodal, and many represent locations in mixed reference frames, which means that receptive fields are partially anchored to more than one body part. For example, parietal neurons often have receptive fields that are sensitive to the position of the eyes in the orbit as well as to the position of the head relative to the body. Several theoretical studies have demonstrated that such mixed representations can underlie coordinate transformations. Lesion studies also suggest that the parietal cortex is crucial for coordinate transformations. Parietal lesions famously lead to neglect, a condition wherein a person loses awareness of a region of space. The condition consists not merely of blindness or of a failure to locate objects within a region but of a total lack of awareness of the region's existence. Neglect does not have one characteristic reference frame; rather, it depends on the nature of the task at hand (and of the lesion). The neglected region of space may be defined relative to the eye, the arm, the body, or even an object in the environment. These observations support the idea that the parietal cortex represents the location of objects in many different reference frames.

As an example, consider the problem of reaching for an object, say, a teacup. To grasp the teacup, the brain must compute the difference between the position of the hand and the position of the cup (with positions specified by vectors). To compute this motor error, the two positions can be defined with respect to a number of reference frames. It is thought, however, that at some point in the visuomotor cascade the two locations must be encoded in the same reference frame and that the corresponding neural signals should be combined to produce the motor error. Indeed, neurons in a cortical area called the parietal reach region respond to both target and current hand positions in an eye-centered reference frame. Let us call these E neurons. For E cells, there is a special point in the visual field (the preferred target location) such that their activity is strongest when the target is located there; but there is also another point (the preferred hand location) such that their activity is strong when the hand is seen there. When the subject moves his eyes, each E neuron changes its firing rate by some amount, but as a population the E responses still encode the hand and target positions (if these have not changed). In contrast, neurons in another parietal area, area 5, seem to encode the displacement vector explicitly, independently of eye position. We call these M neurons. They have a preferred displacement vector, so their activity can be described as signaling target position in hand coordinates. The key difference it that, when the subject moves his or her eyes, the activities of all M neurons remain unchanged. This resembles much more closely a motor command. There is yet another type of parietal neuron that seems to use a mixed or intermediate representation. The activity of those intermediate cells signals target location and is sensitive to both hand and eye positions, but the dependence is more complicated than for E and M neurons. Their properties are similar to those observed in intermediate layers of artificial network models that are trained to transform object location from one reference frame to another, so they are thought to be an important link for constructing M neurons out of E neurons.

How exactly such coordinate transformations occur remains unclear, but experimental and modeling studies indicate that an important component is a mechanism called gain modulation. Gain modulation is observed when the sensitivity of a neuron to a stimulus changes as a function of another variable or parameter. For example, when the response of a parietal neuron is plotted as a function of the position of a spot of light, the resulting curve typically has a bell shape. For a neuron that is gain modulated by, say, eye position, the amplitude of the curve varies as a function of eye position. Andersen and colleagues documented the modulation of visual responses depending on a variety of parameters, such as eye and head position, arm position, and eye velocity, in many parts of the parietal cortex. This particular way to integrate information from multiple sources is powerful because populations of gain-modulated neurons do not represent spatial information in a fixed reference frame; rather, by combining those responses appropriately, different groups of downstream neurons can extract spatial information in the reference frame that best suits their function.

Keeping Objects Separate

As previously mentioned, evidence suggests that separate parts of the cortex are specialized for processing information about object identity and location. Psychophysics corroborates this idea because brain damage can destroy a person's ability to locate an object in space while leaving relatively intact his ability to identify it, or vice versa. Therefore, it has been suggested that there must be some mechanism by which the brain can keep track of which visual features appear in which parts of visual space; otherwise, it would be impossible for an organism to avoid confusing the attributes of multiple objects in different locations. This is often referred to as the binding problem. Evidence that such a mechanism exists comes from studies of patients with Balint's syndrome, which can occur following bilateral damage to the parietal lobes. A Balint's patient is capable of seeing only one object at a time. When there is more than one object in the visual field, the patient often claims that the object he or she sees has some of the attributes of other objects that he or she does not see, such as color, even though it does not. It is unknown whether such patients actually see objects or just jumbles of features, but it is undeniable that they somehow lose track of the locations of different features in space, suggesting that they have lost some mechanism by which normal brains avoid such problems.

One of the earliest and most influential attempts to explain our ability to keep track of object attributes in space is called feature integration theory, developed by Anne Treisman. The theory posits that, when the brain directs attention to an object, the neural representations of its features and its location are selectively enhanced (the firing rates of responding neurons are increased); this allows these representations to be singled out from those of other features and locations, so that there is no longer an ambiguity regarding which belongs with which. Although this is a powerful theory and it is consistent with known effects of attention on neural activity, a number of objections have been raised over the years. For example, numerous studies suggest that a person can attend to multiple objects simultaneously, without confusing their attributes. Standard feature integration theory does not specify how the brain resolves location ambiguities in such cases.

Another theory, which was popularized by von der Malsburg, Singer, and Gray, among others, is based on binding by neural synchrony. The idea is that the neurons representing an object's features and location fire spike trains in synchrony with one another and out of synchrony with neurons representing the features and locations of other objects. The synchrony between neurons tags the encoded features as belonging together. Unlike in feature integration theory, in this mechanism features and locations of multiple objects can be simultaneously grouped. Although there is substantial evidence that is consistent with this hypothesis, in recent years important violations of its predictions have also appeared, so its validity remains an open question.

It should also be pointed out that the binding problem may not be quite as difficult as it seems at first. Although it is true that we rely on different areas of the cortex to track object identity and location, those areas are not totally devoid of information regarding their conjunction. For example, inferotemporal neurons, thought previously to be largely insensitive to object location, can be very sensitive to location when the visual field contains multiple objects. However, because the brain does not rely directly on this spatial information to locate an object in space (we know it relies on mechanisms in the dorsal pathway, and the parietal regions in particular), object representations in the ventral pathway may still have to be matched to spatial representations in the dorsal pathway. The conjunction information in IT could provide a basis for this match.

See also: Attentional Networks in the Parietal Cortex; Balint Syndrome; Information Coding; Motor Psychophysics; Natural Images: Coding Efficiency; Neglect Syndrome and the Spatial Attention Network; Neural Synchrony and Feature Binding; Parietal Cortex and Spatial Attention; Spatial Transformations for Eye–Hand Coordination; Spatial Cognition.

Further Reading

Avillac M, Deneve S, Olivier E, Pouget A, and Duhamel JR (2005) Reference frames for representing visual and tactile locations in parietal cortex. *Nature Neuroscience* 8: 941–949.

Brown WM and Bäcker A (2006) Optimal neuronal tuning for finite stimulus spaces. *Neural Computation* 18: 1511–1526.

Buneo CA and Andersen RA (2006) The posterior parietal cortex: Sensorimotor interface for the planning and online control of visually guided movements. *Neuropsychologia* 44: 2594–2606.

Cohen YE and Andersen RA (2002) A common reference frame for movement plans in the posterior parietal cortex. *Nature Reviews Neuroscience* 3: 553–562.

Deneve S, Latham PE, and Pouget A (2001) Efficient computation and cue integration with noisy population codes. *Nature Neuroscience* 4: 826–831.

Graziano MSA, Hu TX, and Gross CG (1997) Visuospatial properties of ventral pre-motor cortex. *Journal of Neurophysiology* 77: 2268–2292.

Heffner RS (1997) Comparative study of sound localization and its anatomical correlates in mammals. *Acta Otolaryngological (Stockholm)* 532(supplement): 46–53.

Johansson RS and Vallbo AB (1979) Tactile sensibility in the human hand: Relative and absolute densities of four types of mechanoreceptive units in glabrous skin. *Journal of Physiology* 286: 283–300.

Knudsen EI (2002) Instructed learning in the auditory localization pathway of the barn owl. *Nature* 417: 322–328.

Palanca BJA and DeAngelis GC (2005) Does neuronal synchrony underlie visual feature grouping? *Neuron* 46: 333–346.

Pouget A and Sejnowski TJ (2001) Simulating a lesion in a basis function model of spatial representations: Comparison with hemineglect. *Psychological Review* 108: 653–673.

Salinas E (2006) How behavioral constraints may determine optimal sensory representations. *Public Library of Science, Biology* 4(12): e387.

Series P, Latham PE, and Pouget A (2004) Tuning curve sharpening for orientation selectivity: Coding efficiency and the impact of correlations. *Nature Neuroscience* 7: 1129–1135.

Singer W and Gray CM (1995) Visual feature integration and the temporal correlation hypothesis. *Annual Review of Neuroscience* 18: 555–586.

Xing J and Andersen RA (2000) Models of the posterior parietal cortex which perform multimodal integration and represent space in several coordinate frames. *Journal of Cognitive Neuroscience* 12: 601–614.

Zhang KC and Sejnowski TJ (1999) Neuronal tuning: To sharpen or broaden? *Neural Computation* 11: 75–84.

Neuropsychological Testing

D C Delis, University of California at San Diego, La Jolla, CA, USA; and San Diego veterans Affairs Healthcare System, San Diego, CA, USA

Introduction

The psychometric assessment of cognitive and motor functions has proved to have considerable utility in the diagnosis of neurological and psychiatric disorders. Many insidious disorders that evade early identification using the most advanced medical technologies (e.g., neuroimaging; electroencephalography, EEG) can often be effectively diagnosed using neuropsychological testing. Following are examples of neurological conditions that depend heavily on neuropsychological assessment for accurate diagnosis:

- Individuals with early Alzheimer's disease often have normal neurological examinations, magnetic resonance imaging (MRI) and computed tomography (CT) brain scans, and EEG findings. However, studies have found that neuropsychological testing has proved to be one of the most effective procedures for the earliest diagnosis of this pervasive disorder.
- Some elderly patients with severe depression present with memory complaints and low scores on mental status exams that are comparable to those of patients with early Alzheimer's disease, thereby making it difficult to distinguish between these two conditions. However, neuropsychological tests can differentiate between the qualitatively different memory profiles of depressed individuals versus those of early Alzheimer's patients with approximately 95% accuracy.
- Children with fetal alcohol syndrome (FAS), who often have significant deficits in cognitive development, are typically first identified by their facial dysmorphic features. However, many children who are exposed to alcohol *in utero* have normal facial features but go on to develop levels of cognitive impairment that are comparable to those of children with FAS. Neuropsychological testing is important for identifying children who were prenatally exposed to alcohol but who do not have the facial dysmorphic features in order to determine if they should receive early educational interventions for cognitive impairments.
- Some individuals who have had serious head traumas suffer brain damage and cognitive impairments and yet have normal findings on neuroimaging. Other individuals can have head trauma without brain damage, but exaggerate cognitive deficits for external incentive. Neuropsychologists have developed empirically based methods for distinguishing between head-injured individuals with bona fide cognitive deficits secondary to brain damage versus head-injured individuals without permanent brain damage who attempt to feign cognitive impairment on cognitive testing.

Historical Perspective

The field of clinical neuropsychology evolved in the 1940s through the 1960s primarily as a tool to aid in addressing the very broad question of whether a patient had organicity or brain damage. The need to address this general question was important at that time, because CT and MRI brain scans had not yet been developed. In addition, the primary focus of the neurological examination has always involved testing of reflexes and senses, both of which are mediated by the sensorimotor cortex and connecting pathways. This focus leaves vast regions of the brain that can be damaged but without altering sensorimotor functions. Instead, neuropathology in these other regions often affects cognitive skills. When brain damage is subtle to moderate, the decline in cognitive functions can also be mild to moderate. Neurologists and other physicians often conduct a 'mental status exam,' which is a cursory assessment of cognitive skills, such as asking the patient to remember three words. Such brief, nonstandardized exams usually are capable of identifying patients with severe brain damage, but they frequently fail to identify patients with mild to moderate neurocognitive dysfunction.

The need to identify individuals with mild to moderate brain damage outside the sensorimotor circuitry was one of the primary reasons why psychologists began studying neurological patients. Since the early 1900s, psychologists have been armed with powerful methodologies for rigorously measuring subtle differences in mental abilities. The fields of psychometrics and IQ testing, two of the most important contributions in the history of psychology, have long provided clinicians with the means for reliably measuring the development of intellectual and cognitive functions in children and adolescents. In the hands of the neuropsychologist, these methodologies offer the ideal procedures for gauging even subtle declines in intellectual and cognitive functions in individuals with brain dysfunction.

The pioneers in this area were a handful of psychologists during the 1940s through the 1960s; working at a time before there was a field of clinical neuropsychology, these psychologists had the vision to see the tremendous utility of adapting psychometric tests to the assessment of cognitive decline in brain-damaged patients. These early leaders included, among others, Arthur Benton, Kurt Goldstein, Harold Goodglass, Ward Halstead, Donald Hebb, Edith Kaplan, Alexander Luria, Brenda Milner, Ralph Reitan, Andre Rey, Hans-Lukas Teuber, Elizabeth Warrington, and David Wechsler. In administering a wide variety of cognitive tests to patients with focal brain damage, psychologists soon discovered another vital contribution of their methodologies: more accurate characterizations of neuropsychological syndromes with different profiles of cognitive strengths and weaknesses. This work resurrected the importance of the early writings (late 1800s and early 1900s) of neurologists on the aphasias, agnosias, apraxias, and other syndromes, and brought a psychometric rigor to the descriptions of these syndromes. In addition, the emergence of cognitive science in the 1960s also brought more sophisticated experimental procedures for isolating and studying the integrity of specific cognitive processes in patients with focal brain lesions.

In modern times, the need for neuropsychologists to identify organicity or brain damage *per se* has decreased with the development of more sensitive structural and functional neuroimaging techniques. Although there continues to be some neurological disorders (e.g., Alzheimer's disease) that begin with such microscopic lesions that neuropsychological testing is still required for early detection, neuroimaging will likely soon be capable of detecting these insidious disorders as well. However, with advances in the detection of more subtle neurological conditions, and with such diverse individual differences in how similar levels of brain damage can affect cognitive functions, there continues to be growing need for clinical neuropsychologists to document each patient's profile of cognitive and motor strengths and weaknesses. In this context, clinical neuropsychology has become a flourishing field of practice.

The Basic Premise of Neuropsychological Testing

As a general rule, cognitive and motor functions tend to fall within the normal range of the bell curve in an individual with a healthy brain, with some relative strengths and weaknesses. However, when one or more regions of the brain have been damaged by injury or disease, the cognitive and motor functions that are mediated at least in part by those regions often will become significantly impaired. Accordingly, the clinical neuropsychologist will typically administer to a patient with known or suspected brain damage 20–30 different tests assessing attention, language skills, math abilities, visual–spatial functions, new learning and memory, problem solving, abstract thinking, and other cognitive and motor skills. In past research, these tests were administered to large numbers of neurologically intact individuals (the normative group) and to patients with different types of brain damage; the neuropsychologist uses these normative and clinical data to draw conclusions about whether a patient's raw scores on the tests fall within the expected or impaired ranges. This determination is not an exact science, since many neurologically normal individuals will have some test scores that fall in the impaired range, and some brain-damaged patients, especially if they have relatively high premorbid cognitive skills, may have few scores in the impaired range. Nevertheless, by examining the patient's profile of cognitive and motor strengths and weaknesses, the neuropsychologist can make inferences about the integrity of different brain regions and can begin to formulate hypotheses about the presence or absence of different neurological disorders.

What Comprises a Neuropsychological Evaluation?

The typical neuropsychological evaluation takes 6–8 h. For most teenagers and adults, the examination can be completed in a day, with ample breaks. For younger children, older adults, or patients whose endurance has been significantly compromised by a neurological, medical, or psychiatric condition, the examination can be conducted across two or three sessions.

In the morning and early afternoon hours of a 1-day exam, patients are typically administered the cognitive and motor tests when they are usually more alert. Some neuropsychologists administer the tests themselves, whereas others employ a trained psychological technician to administer the tests; both approaches are acceptable in the field, since the tests have standardized administration procedures. In the afternoon, patients who have adequate cognitive skills are often administered a psychological inventory designed to assess their self-reported emotional functioning. In addition, a comprehensive clinical interview is also typically conducted. In this era of managed care, many patients are first given neuropsychological screening exams, which usually vary from 30 min to 3 h in duration. If a patient exhibits some evidence of cognitive impairment on the screening exam, then more extensive neuropsychological testing may be conducted.

Selection of Tests

Neuropsychologists typically select tests that have empirically documented reliability and validity;

adequate, updated normative data; and empirically demonstrated utility in identifying neurocognitive deficits in brain-damaged patients. Modern neuropsychological tests often contain improvements over their predecessors by the incorporation of constructs from cognitive science, thereby making the tests more sensitive to the assessment of specific cognitive processes. Some neuropsychologists use a 'battery approach,' meaning that they will administer all tests or subtests that comprise a particular battery or scale (e.g., all subtests of the Wechsler Memory Scale-III). Other neuropsychologists use an 'eclectic approach,' meaning that they will pick and choose only certain tests or subtests from different batteries or scales (e.g., many psychologists administer only two subtests of the Wechsler Memory Scale-III: the Logical Memory subtest and the Visual Reproduction subtest). In addition, some neuropsychologists adopt a 'fixed approach,' meaning that they try to give the same tests to all patients, whereas other neuropsychologists use a 'flexible approach,' meaning that they will tailor the selection of tests administered to each patient based on the patient's presenting problems and referral question. These different approaches are all acceptable in the field, provided that the major domains of cognitive, motor, and behavioral functions are adequately covered by the tests selected. **Table 1** lists a number of tests that are commonly used by neuropsychologists to assess cognitive and motor functions in children and adults.

The Clinical Interview

A critical part of the neuropsychological evaluation is the clinical interview. A comprehensive survey of possible risk factors for brain damage should be explored in the interview. In addition, many factors beyond brain damage *per se* can affect performance on rigorous psychometric tests of cognitive and motor skills, and these factors should also be covered in the interview. Important areas to explore in the interview include early developmental problems (e.g., pregnancy and delivery complications; prenatal exposure to alcohol, drugs, or other teratogenic agents; delays in achieving developmental milestones as an infant or toddler); cultural factors (e.g., English as a second language, being raised in another country); educational history (e.g., level and type of education obtained, history of learning disability or attention problems); occupational history (e.g., the degree to which an individual's work requires higher level thinking skills); history of medical illnesses that are risk factors for brain dysfunction (e.g., hypertension, diabetes); history of head injury or loss of consciousness; past and current psychiatric disorders; past and current alcohol and drug use; current medications (e.g., narcotic analgesics); current emotional state; current physical state (e.g., headaches and other pain symptoms, which can affect performance on psychometric tests); and family history of medical and psychiatric disorders (e.g., a family history of Alzheimer's disease is a risk factor for this disorder). Based on information gathered in the clinical interview, the neuropsychologist attempts to identify which risk factors may be present in an individual and how they may affect the person's performances on the cognitive and motor tests.

Another step in the clinical interview is to ask the patient, and family members if they are available, about their perceptions of the patient's cognitive complaints, the onset of the problems, and whether the problems have changed over time. Sometimes this information can be helpful in evaluating, for instance, whether a patient's cognitive difficulties started abruptly, as with a stroke, or gradually, as in Alzheimer's disease. However, the self-reported cognitive difficulties of patients and their family members often fail to correlate with objective test results. For example, depressed patients sometimes report severe memory difficulties when their actual scores on objective tests of memory may be normal or near normal.

Finally, the clinical interview allows the neuropsychologist to observe directly patients' emotional demeanor and behavioral functioning at a time when they are discussing their problems and symptoms. These observations can be valuable for identifying whether a psychiatric component is contributing to a patient's presentation.

Test-Taking Effort

Scores on difficult cognitive and motor tests are valid only if the examinee exerts adequate effort in taking them. An important part of the neuropsychological evaluation is the assessment of the individual's motivation to perform well on the tests. Some individuals exert minimal effort on neuropsychologist tests for secondary gain. For example, an inmate may intentionally perform poorly on memory tests to support his or her claim of amnesia for the accused crime. As another example, an individual involved in litigation related to a car accident may claim that he or she suffered a brain injury in the accident. When this individual undergoes a neuropsychological evaluation, he or she may fail to exert adequate effort on the tests, with the hope of looking 'brain damaged' and obtaining a large settlement. The frequency with which individuals have been found to exaggerate cognitive problems on neuropsychological tests has been reported to be as high as 30% of cases referred in the context of forensic evaluations.

Table 1 Examples of commonly used neuropsychological tests for adults and children

Domain	*Representative test*
Adults	
Intellectual functions	Wechsler Adult Intelligence Scale-III
Learning and memory	California Verbal Learning Test-II
	Rey Auditory Verbal Learning Test
	Rey Osterrieth Complex Figure Test
	Warrington Recognition Memory Test
	Wechsler Memory Scale-III
Visuospatial abilities	Block Design Subtest (WAIS-III)
	Hooper Visual Organizational Test
	Judgment of Line Orientation
	Rey Osterrieth Complex Figure Test
Language	Boston Diagnostic Aphasia Exam
	Boston Naming Test
	Controlled Oral Word Association Test
	Token Test
	Vocabulary Subtest (WAIS-III)
Executive functions	Category Test
Abstraction ability	Delis–Kaplan Executive Function System
	Similarities Subtest (WAIS-III)
	Trail Making Test
	Verbal Fluency Tests
	Wisconsin Card Sorting Test
Attention	Digit Span Subtest (WAIS-III)
	Digit Vigilance Test
	Spatial Span (WMS-III)
Motor Functions	Finger Tapping Test
	Grooved Pegboard Test
	Grip Strength (Hand Dynamometer)
Emotional/behavioral functions	Beck Depression Inventory
	Hamilton Depression Scale
	Millon Clinical Personality Inventory
	Minnesota Multiphasic Personality Inventory-II
Screening instruments	Kaplan Baycrest Neurocognitive Assessment
	Mattis Dementia Rating Scale
	MicroCog
	Repeatable Battery for the Assessment of Neuropsychological Status
Academic achievement	Wechsler Individual Achievement Test
	Wide Range Achievement Test-III
Children	
Intellectual functions	Cognitive Assessment System
	Wechsler Intelligence Scale for Children-IV
	Woodcock–Johnson Tests of Cognitive Ability
Specific neuropsychological domains	California Verbal Learning Test–Children's Version
	Children's Memory Scale
	Delis-Kaplan Executive Function System
	NEPSY Neuropsychological Battery
	Peabody Picture Vocabulary Test-III
	Wide Range Assessment of Memory and Learning
	WISC-III as a Neuropsychological Instrument
Emotional/behavioral functions	Child Behavior Checklist
	Personality Inventory for Children

Neuropsychologists have developed a number of tools for evaluating an individual's test-taking effort, including specific cognitive 'malingering' tests, analysis of typical and atypical profiles of neurocognitive dysfunction, consistency of test findings and profiles across repeat evaluations, and examination of whether a patient's low scores on neuropsychological tests are consistent with how he or she is functioning in everyday life. Even with these procedures, however, it is sometimes difficult to identify a clever patient who is feigning cognitive difficulties, especially if he or she does so to a mild degree (more blatant forms of exaggeration are easier to detect). As reported in the literature, some individuals have admitted to having been 'coached' by their attorneys as to which tests are designed to detect malingering, prior to their neuropsychological evaluations. In addition, individuals can learn about malingering tests on the Internet. For these reasons, neuropsychologists strive to use different methods for the detection of inadequate effort and to stay one step ahead of public knowledge by developing new effort-testing techniques.

Premorbid Level of Cognitive Functioning

The most common reason that patients are referred for a neuropsychological evaluation is to determine whether they have acquired brain damage from some neurological insult, and, if so, whether they have experienced a decline in their level of cognitive functioning from a premorbid (preexisting) state. However, inferences about declines in cognitive functioning must include estimates of the individual's level of cognitive functioning before the onset of the insult. Neuropsychologists employ several techniques for estimating or correcting for premorbid level of cognitive functioning, including the following approaches:

- Testing overlearned cognitive skills that tend to be resilient to the effects of more diffuse brain damage and that correlate significantly with preexisting IQ (e.g., tests of individual word reading or vocabulary level are good predictors of premorbid verbal IQ).
- Developing normative test data that are corrected not only for age but also for education level, a strong predictor of premorbid IQ.
- Obtaining prior scholastic test scores from the individual's school records, since these scores correlate robustly with an individual's verbal IQ as an adult.
- Using regression analyses based on key demographic variables, such as education and occupation levels, to derive formulas for estimating premorbid IQ.

The estimation of premorbid level of cognitive functioning is a difficult task. Each method should be considered as a tool that may or may not be useful or even appropriate for a particular patient. For instance, the use of education-corrected norms can be invaluable for one patient and misleading for another. Following are three case examples that illustrate this point:

- A physician with 20 years of education and a premorbid IQ of 130 suffers a left hemisphere stroke. While her postinjury scores on language tests are within the average (normal) range for her normative age group, these scores fall in the impaired range for her education group (i.e., compared to age-matched individuals with approximately 20 years of education). In this case, the education-corrected norms are warranted because they provide an empirically based method for documenting evidence of acquired cognitive decline in this individual.
- A self-made businessman has a premorbid IQ of 130 but left high school after his sophomore year because his father was killed in a car accident and he had to begin working to help support his family. As an adult, this individual suffers a left hemisphere stroke and obtains scores on language tests that fall in the average (normal) range using both age- and education-corrected norms (i.e., compared to age-matched individuals with approximately 10 years of education). However, these standardized scores are likely misleading, because they are obtained from a normative reference group that likely has a lower mean premorbid verbal IQ than that of the patient. For this individual, it would have been more appropriate to use one or more of the other methods to estimate the patient's premorbid level of cognitive functioning (e.g., obtain school records to see if scholastic test scores are available for this individual; administer a single-word reading test).
- At birth, an individual suffers a brain insult secondary to delivery complications. In school, he is found to have an IQ that falls in the borderline mentally retarded range. He completes only 8 years of education. As an adult, he is evaluated by a neuropsychologist who scores the test findings using education-corrected norms (i.e., his raw scores are compared to age-matched individuals with approximately 8 years of education). The patient's standardized scores using these norms fall in the low-average range and the neuropsychologist claims that the patient does not have brain damage. However, the use of education-corrected norms is inappropriate for this case. The patient's relatively low education level was likely one of the 'effects' of his early brain insult (not the cause), and to correct his scores for a low level of education essentially negates one of the main effects of his brain damage. For this individual, age-corrected norms would be more appropriate to document that the patient shows evidence of cognitive impairment (i.e., borderline mental retardation) relative to his age-matched peers.

As a general rule, prior scholastic or IQ test scores that are obtained from a patient's school records when he or she was around 10 years of age or older are often the best method for estimating premorbid level of intellectual functioning, because achievement and IQ scores tend to be relatively stable across the life span. In addition, each person's premorbid functioning should be estimated individually, given that there are significant individual differences in IQ level among people with similar levels of education. Other factors that contribute to discrepancies in IQ among people with similar levels of education include motivation to achieve in school (e.g., a person with average IQ and high motivation may achieve a high level of education, whereas a person with superior IQ and low motivation may drop out of school early); differences in the quality of the education (e.g., university-based graduate school versus private professional graduate school); and English as a second language (e.g., a highly educated person may have learned English as a second language and, as a result, obtain only average scores on English-based verbal tests, despite achieving a relatively high level of education). Unfortunately, for the majority of patients evaluated, school test results are not accessible, necessitating the use of one of the other methods for estimating premorbid functioning. Finally, it is important to note that the different methods for estimating premorbid mental abilities may apply to certain domains of cognitive functioning but not to others. For example, the ability to read individual words of varying difficulty has been found to be a significant predictor of verbal IQ. However, verbal IQ tends to have relatively low correlations with executive functions and memory skills (accounting for 0–16% of the variance). Thus, while current reading ability can be a useful predictor of premorbid verbal IQ, it tends to be less effective in predicting premorbid level of executive functions and memory skills.

Analysis of Test Performance

After the neuropsychological tests have been administered, raw scores are summed for each test and converted to standardized scores. In addition to these quantitative scores, many neuropsychologists also examine test performance for qualitative features that may be pathognomonic of brain dysfunction. For instance, a patient may speak primarily in content words and omit the little grammatical words of language (e.g., the patient says, "Hospital . . . Monday" when trying to say that he came into the hospital on Monday). This qualitative feature of the patient's language, when seen consistently, is pathognomonic of a type of language disorder called Broca's aphasia, and likely reflects a brain injury in the posterior region of the left frontal lobe. As another example, a patient may omit most details and features from the left side of his drawings (see **Figure 1**); this neurobehavioral syndrome, known as left hemi-inattention, typically occurs following brain damage to posterior regions of the right hemisphere.

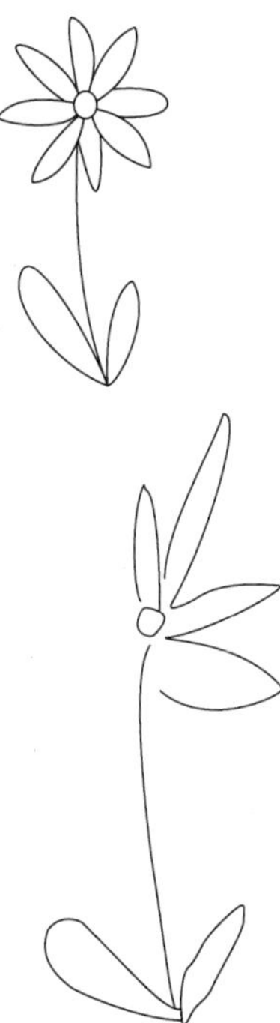

Figure 1 An individual who suffered a cerebral vascular accident in the right parietal lobe was asked to copy a model drawing of a daisy (top). The patient's drawing (bottom) illustrates left hemi-inattention.

Emotional, Behavioral, and Personality Testing

The neuropsychological evaluation typically goes beyond the assessment of cognitive and motor skills, and also includes psychometric testing of emotional, behavioral, and personality functioning. Many neuropsychologists administer tests such as the Minnesota Mutiphasic Personality Inventory-2 (MMPI-2) or the Beck Depression Inventory as part of their standard evaluation, given that the patient has the cognitive capacity to take them. These tests assist the neuropsychologist in determining whether a patient has a psychiatric disturbance, which, in turn, may be affecting his or her performance on the neuropsychological tests. Most practicing neuropsychologists obtain their doctoral degrees in clinical psychology before receiving specialized training in neuropsychology, and this training enables them to conduct general psychodiagnostic assessments as part of their neuropsychological evaluations.

Final Interpretations and Recommendations

The heart of the neuropsychological evaluation, and the most difficult part, is drawing final conclusions about the presence, nature, extent, and causes of a patient's cognitive, motor, and behavioral difficulties and, if necessary, formulating recommendations for helping the patient. Just because a patient obtains test scores that fall in the impaired range does not mean that he or she has brain damage.

The first step in the interpretation process is to determine whether a patient's test scores are valid (using techniques discussed earlier) and internally consistent (e.g., if a patient has a word-finding deficit, then he or she should exhibit difficulty on any task that places extensive demands on precise naming ability). If the test scores appear valid and consistent, the neuropsychologist then attempts to characterize the patient's profile of cognitive–motor strengths and weaknesses. Based on an estimate of the patient's premorbid level of cognitive functioning, the neuropsychologist opines whether the patient's weaknesses represent acquired deficits. Next, the neuropsychologist, drawing upon his or her knowledge of brain–behavior relationships, tries to decide whether the patient's profile of cognitive–motor strengths and weaknesses is typical of particular types and locations of brain dysfunction. The neuropsychologist then must weigh all of the patient's risk factors for acquired brain damage, such as a recent head trauma or stroke, history of medical illnesses that may compromise brain functioning, history of serious psychiatric disorder, past alcohol or drug abuse, or a family history of a genetically based neurological disorder (e.g., Alzheimer's disease). In considering these different risk factors, the neuropsychologist tries to determine whether the patient's cognitive–motor profile is more likely to be associated with one risk factor than another, or with multiple risk factors.

Before a final conclusion can be reached about the presence of neurocognitive dysfunction, the neuropsychologist must rule out all possible explanations for the patient's low test scores, going beyond brain damage *per se*, such as educational and cultural factors, current medications, current emotional and physical state, and level of motivation to perform well on the tests. In addition, the neuropsychologist must conduct a psychodiagnostic evaluation to determine whether the patient has a psychiatric disorder and, if so, whether this disorder is contributing to the patient's cognitive difficulties. After integrating, analyzing, and synthesizing this extensive and varied body of information, the neuropsychologist is then in a position to proffer his final impressions about the presence or absence of brain dysfunction and its sequelae. If the neuropsychological data strongly implicate a neurological disorder, such as Alzheimer's disease, then it falls within the neuropsychologist's purview to make those diagnoses.

At the end of the report, the neuropsychologist will typically offer recommendations for the patient. Common areas of recommendations include the following approaches:

- Additional neurological, medical, or psychiatric examinations, consultations, or procedures (e.g., MRI brain scan; psychotropic medication consultation).
- Speech therapy or cognitive rehabilitation.
- Individual or family psychotherapy or other behavioral interventions.
- Educational interventions and programs (especially for children and young adults).
- Vocational testing and counseling.
- Social work consultation to address the patient's living situation and the need for various levels of assistance and supervision with activities of daily living.
- Repeat neuropsychological evaluation in the future to determine the status of the patient's cognitive functioning over time.

When feasible, the neuropsychologist often will meet with the patient and his or her family to discuss the findings of the evaluation and the need for the various recommended interventions.

Repeat Neuropsychological Testing

The readministration of the same or similar neuropsychological tests to a patient at a later time can serve several clinically useful purposes. As an example, for patients suspected of having a progressive dementia such as Alzheimer's disease, the first neuropsychological testing provides baseline data. The repeat testing, which usually is done 9–12 months later, affords an objective measure of whether the patient exhibits a decline in cognitive functions typical of a progressive disease. Some neuropsychological tests may show practice effects on repeat testing, which is an improvement in performance from having taken the same or similar tasks at an earlier time. However, the inexorable progression of a disorder such as Alzheimer's disease typically overrides any improvement in scores related to practice effects.

Repeat testing also is helpful for charting the recovery of neurocognitive functions over time following a brain insult, such as a stroke or brain injury. Recovery of brain functions tends to occur relatively slowly, with a 1-year time period often used as the benchmark for the vast majority of the recovery to have occurred. By comparing a patient's test scores obtained a few months after an injury with those obtained a year or more postinjury, the neuropsychologist, after factoring in practice effects, can provide objective data about the patient's recovery process. Other important reasons for conducting repeat testing include monitoring improvement in cognitive functions following various interventions, such as cognitive rehabilitation and pharmacological treatment, and determining the validity of an individual's test scores by examining the consistency of his or her profile of cognitive and motor strengths and weaknesses over time.

Common Referral Questions for Adults

Adult patients typically are referred for a neuropsychological evaluation by neurologists, neurosurgeons, clinical psychologists, psychiatrists, primary care physicians, speech pathologists, other health professionals, and attorneys. The following examples of consult questions illustrate some of the reasons why adult patients undergo neuropsychological testing:

- To assist in evaluating whether a patient with increasing cognitive difficulties, as reported by the patient, family members, or health professionals, has an insidious neurological disorder. Examples of these disorders include multiple sclerosis, brain tumor, idiopathic hydrocephalus, white-matter ischemic changes, and Alzheimer's disease.
- To evaluate whether a patient who has had a risk factor for brain damage does, in fact, exhibit cognitive–motor deficits or emotional–behavioral changes consistent with brain dysfunction. Examples of these risk factors include head trauma, chronic alcohol or drug abuse, certain medical illnesses (e.g., hypertension, diabetes, kidney failure, HIV infection), certain psychiatric disorders (e.g., schizophrenia), and exposure to neurotoxic agents.
- To assess the presence, nature, and extent of cognitive–motor deficits and emotional–behavioral changes in patients with known brain pathology. These patients are referred after it has been determined, usually from the neurological examination and neuroimaging, that they have had, for instance, a cerebral vascular accident or have a brain tumor, Parkinson's disease, probable Alzheimer's disease, or MRI- or CT scan-confirmed brain damage following a head trauma. The question for these patients is not whether they have brain damage, but rather the presence, nature, and extent of cognitive, motor, and behavioral sequelae of their brain dysfunction.
- To assist neurosurgeons in several ways, such as in evaluating whether a patient with intractable seizures and in need of resection of the epileptogenic focus has language skills localized in this general brain region (this testing usually involves a Wada procedure, where one cerebral hemisphere at a time is anesthetized during cognitive screening); in conducting pre- and postsurgery evaluations to determine whether a neurosurgical procedure (e.g., insertion of a shunt tube to relieve hydrocephalus; resection of a brain tumor) alters cognitive–motor functions for better or worse; and in reevaluating cognitive functions over a period of several years in a hydrocephalus patient who has received a shunt in order determine if the shunt has continued to function normally.
- To evaluate the cognitive functions of individuals with more serious psychiatric disorders that often have a neurological component (e.g., schizophrenia).
- To provide recommendations regarding the patient's capacity to return to work or to receive vocational retraining in a new occupation that would be best suited for the patient, given his or her profile of cognitive strengths and weaknesses.
- To offer recommendations for cognitive rehabilitation (e.g., teaching the patient memory compensatory strategies).
- To assist in determining whether a patient with brain dysfunction has the cognitive, motor, and behavioral capacity to perform important activities of daily living (e.g., ability to drive a car, handle finances, prepare meals, live independently, comply with medication regimens, care for self).
- To make recommendations regarding the best living situation for the patient in light of his or her cognitive, motor, and behavioral deficits (e.g., independent, assisted-living, or nursing-home placement).

Common Referral Questions for Children

Neuropsychological evaluations are generally more difficult to conduct for children than for adults. Just as children differ in their physical growth rates, they also differ in the development of their cognitive and motor functions. It is sometimes difficult to determine whether a 'cognitive deficit' in a child represents a permanent impairment or simply a lag or delay in the development of that ability. In addition, the classic brain–behavior relationships that have been documented in adults do not always apply to children, making it difficult to localize cognitive deficits to particular brain regions. For example, a lesion in the left superior temporal gyrus can result in a Wernicke's (fluent) aphasia in an adult and in a nonfluent aphasia in a child. Finally, some children present with pronounced attention problems, hyperactivity, or other behavioral disturbances that make it difficult for the child to focus on the psychometric tests and provide valid test responses.

Despite the challenges inherent in child neuropsychology, this area of practice has become one of the fastest growing disciplines within the field. Referrals for child neuropsychological evaluations usually are made by pediatricians, pediatric neurologists, clinical psychologists, school psychologists, speech therapists, educators, and sometimes parents. Many of the referral questions for children are similar to those for adults, such as assessing whether the apparent onset of new cognitive difficulties reflects an insidious neurological disorder (e.g., brain tumor); evaluating whether a known risk factor for brain damage (e.g., birth complications, head trauma, lead exposure) has, in fact, resulted in cognitive, motor, or behavioral dysfunction; and assessing the presence, nature, and extent of cognitive, motor, and behavioral changes in patients with known brain pathology (e.g., childhood seizure disorder). Following are examples of other specific reasons why children are referred for neuropsychological testing:

- To determine whether a child who is struggling academically in school has a learning disability. Neuropsychological research has documented different types of learning disabilities (e.g., verbal vs. nonverbal) that may reflect neurodevelopmental abnormalities in distinct brain regions.
- To assess whether a child whose mother abused alcohol or drugs or consumed other teratogenic agents during her pregnancy (e.g., certain medications) exhibits cognitive, motor, or behavioral deficits suggestive of prenatal brain damage (e.g., FAS).
- To assist educators in developing the best educational program for a child based on the child's profile of cognitive and behavioral strengths and weaknesses.
- To assess recovery of function in a child who has suffered a documented traumatic brain injury and to provide recommendations for cognitive remediation and educational assistance.

Conclusions

Clinical neuropsychology has become one of the fastest growing disciplines in psychology. Neuropsychological testing not only provides an empirically rigorous method for assisting in the diagnosis of neurological, medical, and psychiatric patients, it also enhances our scientific understanding of one of the great mysteries of life, namely, the generation of mental processes from brain structures.

See also: Aging of the Brain and Alzheimer's Disease; Cognition: An Overview of Neuroimaging Techniques; Cognitive Neuroscience: An Overview; Human Methods: Psychophysics; Magnetic Resonance Spectroscopy; Neuroimaging; Neuropsychology: Theoretical Basis; Psychophysics of Attention.

Further Reading

Benton AL (1980) Psychological testing for brain damage. In: Kaplan HI, Freedman AM, and Badock BJ (eds.) *Comprehensive Textbook of Psychiatry,* vol. 1, ch. 12. Baltimore, MD: Williams & Wilkins.

Delis DC, Kaplan E, and Kramer JH (2001) *The Delis-Kaplan Executive Function System.* San Antonio, TX: The Psychological Corporation.

Delis DC, Kramer JH, Kaplan E, et al. (2000) *The California Verbal Learning Test,* 2nd edn. San Antonio, TX: The Psychological Corporation.

Goodglass H and Kaplan E (1983) *The Assessment of Aphasia and Related Disorders.* Philadelphia, PA: Lea & Febiger.

Grant I and Adams K (eds.) (1996) *Neuropsychological Assessment of Neuropsychiatric Disorders,* 2nd edn. New York: Oxford University Press.

Heaton RK, Grant I, and Matthew CG (1991) *Comprehensive Norms for an Expanded Halstead–Reitan Battery.* Odessa, FL: Psychological Assessment Resources.

Heilman K and Valenstein E (eds.) (1993) *Clinical Neuropsychology,* 3rd edn. New York: Oxford University Press.

Kaplan E, Fein D, Morris R, et al. (1991) *WAIS-R as a Neuropsychological Instrument.* New York: Psychological Corporation.

Larrabee GL (ed.) (2005) *Forensic Neuropsychology.* New York: Oxford University Press.

Lezak MD, Howieson DB, Loring DW, et al. (2005) *Neuropsychological Assessment,* 4th edn. New York: Oxford University Press.

Luria AR (1980) *Higher Cortical Functions in Man,* 2nd edn. New York: Basic Books.

Massman PJ, Delis DC, Butters N, et al. (1992) The subcortical dysfunction hypothesis of memory deficits in depression: Neuropsychological validation in a subgroup of patients. *Journal of Clinical and Experimental Neuropsychology* 14: 687–706.

Mattson SN, Riley EP, Gramling L, et al. (1997) Heavy prenatal alcohol exposure leads to IQ deficits with or without all of the features of fetal alcohol syndrome. *Journal of Pediatrics* 131: 718–721.

Spreen O and Strauss E (1998) *A Compendium of Neuropsychological Tests: Administration, Norms, and Commentary,* 2nd edn. New York: Oxford University Press.

Squire L and Butters N (eds.) (1992) *Neuropsychology of Memory,* 2nd edn. New York: Guilford Press.

Parietal Cortex and Spatial Attention

M E Goldberg, Columbia University, New York, NY, USA

Introduction

The brain has a problem: sights, sounds, smells, and touches bombard our sensory apparatus constantly, and the primate brain cannot possibly deal with all of them simultaneously. Instead, it chooses among the myriad objects in our intense sensory world those most relevant to its behavior for further processing. This act of selection is called attention. In 1890, William James described attention as "the taking possession by the mind in clear and vivid form, of one out of what seem several simultaneously possible objects or trains of thought... It implies withdrawal from some things in order to deal effectively with others." James then described two different kinds of attention:

> It [attention] is either passive, reflex, non-voluntary, effortless or active and voluntary. Voluntary attention is always derived; we never make an effort to attend to an object except for the sake of some remote interest which the effort will serve. In passive immediate sensorial attention the stimulus is a sense-impression, either very intense, voluminous, or sudden...big things, bright things, moving things...blood. (William James (1890), *The Principles of Psychology*)

The attention you are now paying to this article is voluntary. Your momentary distraction by a thunderclap or a flash of lightning would be involuntary. Recently, these two kinds of attention have been described as endogenous, or 'top-down' attention, and exogenous, or 'bottom-up' attention, respectively.

Studies of attention have relied upon a number of different methods to establish the locus of attention. The simplest, but least precise, is *post hoc*: if a person has responded to something, then at some point he/she attended to it. There are three other precisely measurable effects of attention. (1) Attention lowers reaction time: if a cue flashes in the visual field, for the next 300 ms an individual has a faster reaction time to respond to a second stimulus that appears at the position of the cue, and a longer reaction time to respond to a second stimulus that appears away from the cue. (2) Attention improves perception: when for some reason an individual attends to a position in space (e.g., if a cue flashes there), the contrast sensitivity – how different the stimulus must be from the background – improves at the attended location relative to another part of the visual field. (3) Attention limits the effect of distractors: it is easier to pick out a searched-for object among cluttering distractors at the locus of attention.

The posterior parietal lobe, Brodmann's area 7, has long been thought to be important in the neural mechanisms underlying spatial attention. This concept arose from the study of patients with lesions of the parietal lobe, who exhibit two different sorts of deficits. The most severe deficit is a neglect of the contralateral world: patients with right parietal lesions do not recognize that the paralyzed contralateral limb is theirs, nor do they recognize that they are ill. Although they cannot see the left visual field, or the left side of their egocentric space, they are unaware of the deficit. As this extreme deficit recovers they begin to perceive their own contralateral space and limbs, but can have three types of milder deficits. One is a residual neglect: these patients have difficulty constructing the contralateral side of objects. When they are asked to draw a clock they cram the numbers into the right half of the clock (**Figure 1**). When they are asked to bisect a line they place the midline far to the right of the true midpoint. When they are asked to strike out lines on a page they begin at the far right and often leave out a few lines at the far left. The second deficit is extinction: these patients have an inability to see an object in the affected visual field when a similar object appears in the unaffected visual field, although they can see a single object in the affected field perfectly well. Extinction can be tactile as well – a patient who can appreciate a light tap on his left hand may not perceive the same tap when his right hand is tapped simultaneously. These patients behave as if objects in their unaffected field grab their attention, so they neglect objects in the affected field. The third deficit is in making accurate visually guided movements: patients with parietal lesions often misreach. All of these clinical observations suggest that the parietal lobe is important for three interrelated functions – attention, spatial perception, and the generation of accurate movements to visual stimuli.

Although introspectively we tend to think of perceptual space as being unitary, a homogeneous sphere of which we are at the center, neuropsychological studies have questioned this idea. Thus, certain patients who can bisect a line accurately when they shine a laser pointer at a distant light cannot use a pencil to bisect the same line when it is within arm's reach. Thus, neural mechanisms of spatial attention must distinguish more than the azimuth and elevation of the attended object, but also its distance. One way to explain this multiplicity of attentional spaces is to view them as

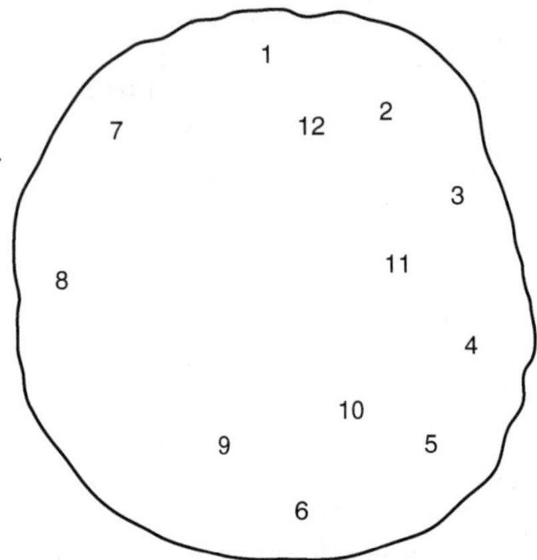

Figure 1 A clock drawn by a parietal patient. The examiner draws the circle and asks the patient with a right parietal lesion to write in the numerals of the clock phase in their proper position. The patient places 1 through 6 in their proper position, but fails to place the remaining numbers properly, putting them on the right side of the clock rather than the left. Adapted from Critchley M (1953) *The Parietal Lobes.* London: Edward Arnold.

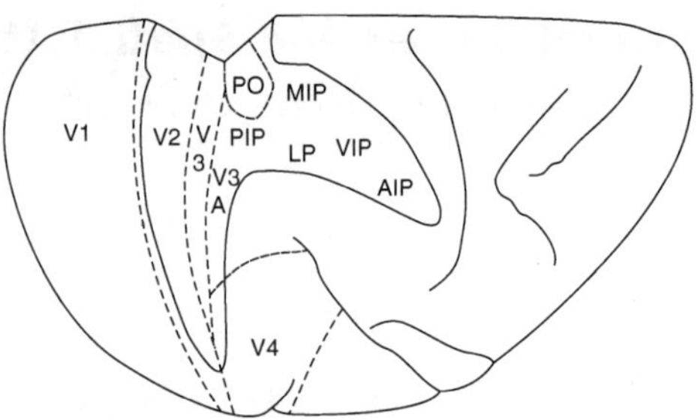

Figure 2 Location of visually responsive areas in rhesus monkey cortex. In this dorsal view of the right hemisphere, the lunate and intraparietal sulci are opened up to show the locations of several extrastriate areas and visually responsive areas within the intraparietal sulcus. Visual areas V2, V3, and V3A are shown in the lunate sulcus. Other areas: PO, the parieto-occipital area; PIP, the posterior intraparietal area; MIP, the medial intraparietal area; LIP, the lateral intraparietal area; VIP, the ventral intraparietal area; AIP, the anterior intraparietal area. Area 7a lies on the surface of the prelunate gyrus. Adapted from Colby CL, Gattass R, Olson CR, et al. (1988) Topographic organization of cortical afferents to extrastriate visual area PO in the macaque: A dual tracer study. *Journal of Comparative Neurology* 269: 392–413.

related to motor workspaces. Thus, attention for far space ranges through the part of space uniquely explored by eye movements. Attention for near space ranges through the workspace for reaching movements.

A second major function of the posterior parietal lobe is to describe the world for action. When you reach out to grab a thick object such as an apple, you open your hand so that when your fingers reach the apple they are opened wider than the apple, and you easily close your hand around the apple. When you reach out to grasp a pencil, you open your fingers much less widely than you did when you grasped the apple. Patients with parietal lesions cannot do this: they cannot use visual information to set their grasp, even though they can tell you whether the apple or the pencil is wider.

Physiological studies of parietal function have emphasized both of these major functions of the parietal lobe: generating spatial attention and analyzing the visual world for action. Most of our understanding of the neurophysiology of the posterior parietal lobe comes from studies of the parietal lobe of the rhesus monkey. Brodmann described the posterior parietal cortex as a single area, area 7, on the basis of its cellular morphology. Recent studies have shown that area 7 is divided into a number of different regions, with differing anatomical projections and physiology. Many of these subdivisions lie within the intraparietal sulcus (**Figure 2**). Each of the areas in the intraparietal sulcus has neurons which respond to the appearance of visual stimuli. These neurons do not respond to the appearance of stimuli everywhere in the visual field; instead, they respond only to stimuli which appear in a limited part of the visual field. The part of the visual field which can excite the neuron is called its receptive field, and the receptive fields of parietal neurons usually lie in the visual field opposite the hemisphere in which the neuron lies – the contralateral visual field. The properties of each individual area make them suitable for representing objects which can be the target for a specific set of movements – a 'motor workspace'.

Each area in the intraparietal sulcus sends projections to premotor areas which define the actual movements in that workspace. Thus, the ventral intraparietal (VIP) area has neurons which represent the near space around the mouth, and the tactile areas on the face. The neurons have congruent responses: neurons which represent the upper visual field also represent the upper face (**Figure 3**). Many VIP neurons respond to visual stimuli close to the face, but not to stimuli with the identical visual angle further away. The VIP area projects to area F4 in premotor cortex, which represents movements of the face and head. The medial intraparietal (MIP) area has neurons responding to tactile stimulation of the arm and discharges when the monkey reaches to targets. The MIP area projects to F2 in premotor cortex, which represents movements of the arm. The anterior intraparietal (AIP) area has neurons which respond to visual stimuli which can be grasped, and which discharge when a monkey makes a grasping movement in the dark. The AIP area projects to area F5 in premotor cortex, which is important in the generation of grasping movements.

The most extensively studied area in the intraparietal sulcus is the lateral intraparietal (LIP) area. This area has reciprocal connections with two areas important in

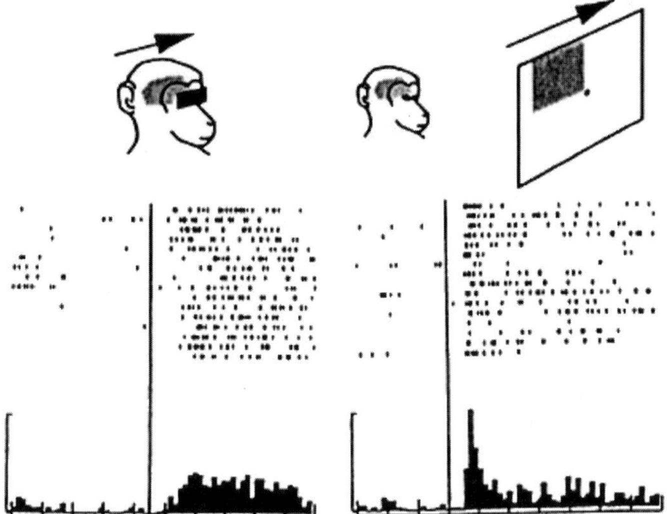

Figure 3 Correspondence of visual and tactile receptive fields in the ventral intraparietal area of the monkey. The top of each column has a drawing depicting the experiment, and the raster diagram of the activity of a single neuron in the ventral intraparietal area under different circumstances is below, showing the individual neuronal response. Each dot is an action potential; each line is a single trial. Successive lines are synchronized on a single event – on the left when the experimenter began to stroke the animal, and on the right when the visual stimulus appeared. The vertical lines show when the synchronizing event began. Histograms beneath the rasters sum the activity of the rasters. Each tick in the raster is 200 ms. The raster in the left column shows the tactile responses and that in the right column shows the visual responses of a neuron in ventral intraparietal area. The receptive fields correspond if one considers the mouth to be analogous to the fovea. Each depicted neuron was directionally selective: Visual and tactile stimuli moving in the opposite direction had little or no effect on the neuron (not shown here). Reproduced from Duhamel J-R, Colby CL, and Goldberg ME (1998) Ventral intraparietal area of the macaque: Congruent visual and somatic response properties. *Journal of Neurophysiology* 79: 126–136, with permission.

the generation of rapid eye movements (saccades), the frontal eye field (FEF) and the superior colliculus (SC). The projection from the SC to the LIP area is disynaptic via the thalamus; the projections to and from the FEF are monosynaptic. The LIP area also has reciprocal connections with areas important for the analysis of patterns in the visual world: prestriate area V4, and TEO and TE in the inferior temporal cortex. Activity in the LIP area is consistent with providing information both for generation of eye movements and for pinning attention in the visual field.

LIP neurons do not respond to every object in the visual field. Most of the objects in the visual field, especially those that are stable and irrelevant to an individual's behavior, are not represented by activity in the LIP area. Instead, only those objects which can be the object of voluntary or involuntary attention are represented. The same object can evoke little or no response when it appears in the receptive field of neuron, or a very strong response, depending upon the behavioral significance of the object. LIP neurons are closely related to the neural mechanisms for the control of saccadic eye movements. When a monkey plans a memory-guided saccade to the spatial location of a recently vanished stimulus in a LIP neuron's receptive field, the neuron discharges in response to the appearance of the stimulus, during the delay period, and before the saccade itself. This activity is consistent with saccade planning, and also voluntary attention, because attention, as measured by an improvement in perceptual threshold, lies at the goal of the memory-guided saccade. However, LIP neurons also respond to the abrupt onset of a distractor which appears in the receptive field when the animal is planning a saccade elsewhere. Attention lies at the goal of the planned saccade unless a distractor appears elsewhere in the visual field, at which point the mechanisms for involuntary attention overwhelm the voluntary attention induced by the eye movement, and attention shifts away from the goal of the saccade to the location of the distractor. The activity of the LIP area in this case parallels the location of the monkey's attention. The time at which attention returns from the distractor to the saccade goal is predicted by the time at which the activity evoked by the distractor falls below that evoked by the saccade plan (**Figure 4**). Under the circumstances of this experiment, although LIP reflects a saccade plan, its activity does not necessarily correlate with when, where, or if the monkey will make a saccade – the distractor has no effect on the monkey's eye movements. Instead, its activity correlates with the

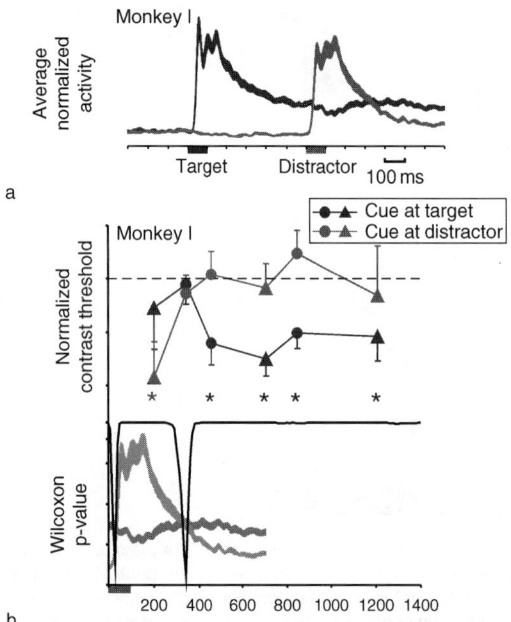

Figure 4 Top-down and bottom-up attentional activity in the lateral intraparietal area. (a) Average activity of 23 lateral intraparietal neurons during the delayed saccade task. Blue trace: the saccade target appears briefly in the receptive field (blue bar). The normalized neuronal spike density is calculated with a sigma of 10 ms (ordinate) plotted against time (abscissa). The thickness of the line is the standard error of the mean of the activity, Note the onset transient in response to the target appearance, followed by delay period activity well above the background activity, despite the fact that the target is no longer present. The delay activity continues until the monkey makes the saccade (not shown). Red trace: distractor appears in the receptive field (red bar) while the monkey is planning a saccade away from the receptive field. Note the brisk onset transient and decay of activity beneath the level of the saccade delay period activity. (b) Relationship of the monkey's attention to neuronal activity in the lateral intraparietal area. The top trace shows the monkey's perceptual performance during the task. The normalized contrast threshold for a stimulus flashed for one video frame (abscissa) is plotted against time from the appearance of the distractor (ordinate). A significant decrement in contrast threshold denotes that the monkey's attention lies at the spatial location of the stimulus. Before the distractor appeared, the perceptual threshold was lower at the saccade goal (not shown). At 200 ms after the distractor appeared, the perceptual threshold was significantly lower at the distractor site but not at the saccade goal. The bottom trace shows the neuronal activity during this epoch. Note that when the neuronal activity was greater at the distractor site (red trace) than it was at the saccade goal (blue trace), the distractor site was the locus of attention. When there was no difference between the activity at the distractor site and the saccade goal (the black line shows the Wilcoxon p value of the difference between the two points), there was no attentional advantage at either site. When the neuronal advantage became significant again at the saccade goal, the attentional advantage returned to the saccade goal and remained there throughout the delay period.

location of the monkey's attention on a millisecond-by-millisecond basis, including the attention that is pinned to a location in space by the plan to make a saccade there. In contrast, when a monkey is exploring the visual field in a search task, activity in the LIP area predicts the goal and reaction time of the saccade. Thus activity in the LIP area is best understood as representing a map of the salient locations in the visual field in the far space explored by eye movements. The visual system presumably uses this representation to pin attention at the peaks in the salience map; the oculomotor system can drive the eyes to the peak of the salience map when a saccade is appropriate.

Neurons in the LIP area have retinotopic receptive fields. The visual, memory, and saccade-related signals carried by these neurons describe stimuli in terms of the distance and direction of the stimulus or saccade location relative to the center of gaze. This retinotopic organization presents a paradox: how can accurate spatial information be derived from retinotopic input? Every time we move our eyes, each object in our surroundings activates a new set of retinal neurons. Despite these changes, we experience the world as stable and move accurately in it. This perceptual stability has long been understood to reflect the fact that what we see is not a direct impression of the external world but an internal image of it. The brain must construct a representation that can compensate for changes in eye position. Neurons in the LIP area compensate for eye movements: if a stimulus flashes outside the receptive field of a neuron, but an eye movement brings the spatial location of the vanished stimulus into the receptive field, neurons in the LIP area will respond, after the eye movement, to a stimulus which never appeared in their receptive field, but would do so if it were still illuminated after the eye movement (**Figure 5**). Some neurons respond to stimuli which will be brought into their receptive fields by an impending saccade even before the saccade. Thus, LIP neurons update their representation of the visual world, compensating for eye movements, so that there is a continuously spatially accurate representation of the visual world in the LIP area despite a moving eye. Neurons in the MIP area, which describe the workspace for reaching movements, also describe the world in retinal coordinates and compensate for saccades in a similar way. In keeping with this, patients with right parietal lesions cannot make this compensation: they cannot make a saccade to a stimulus which appears and disappears before an intervening saccade. This suggests that without an intact parietal lobe they cannot compensate for

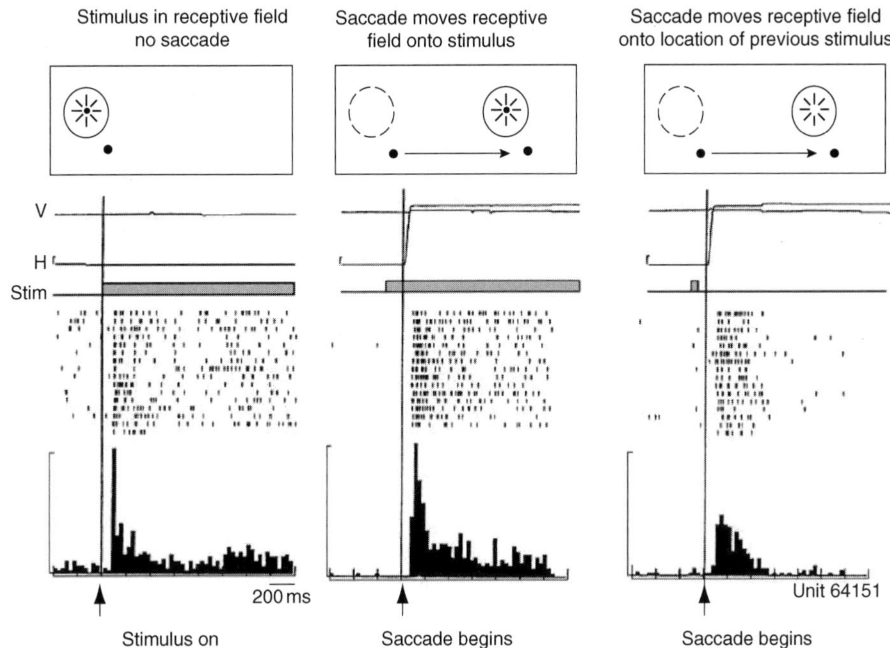

Figure 5 Remapping of visual activity in the lateral intraparietal area. Diagrams show the arrangement of the fixation point, receptive field, stimulus location, and saccade. (Left) In the fixation task, the neuron responds to the onset of a stimulus in the receptive field. (Middle) The same neuron responds when a saccade moves the receptive field onto the location of a recent stimulus. (Right) Response after a saccade moves the receptive field onto a previously stimulated location. The stimulus is flashed on for only 50 ms and is extinguished before the saccade begins. The neuron is responding to the remapped memory trace of the previous stimulus. Control experiments (not shown) indicate that neither the stimulus alone nor the saccade alone can drive the neuron. Adapted from Duhamel J-R, Colby CL, Goldberg ME, et al. (1992) The updating of the representation of visual space in parietal cortex by intended eye movements. *Science* 255: 90–92.

their own eye movements. Thus, the neural activity in the LIP area reflects the three functions described by lesions in patients: attention, spatial perception, and describing the visual world for movement. Whether the other areas in the intraparietal sulcus perform the same functions for the motor workspaces they describe will be the subject for future research.

See also: Attentional Networks in the Parietal Cortex; Neglect Syndrome and the Spatial Attention Network; Neural Coding of Spatial Representations; Spatial Memory: Assessment in Animals; Spatial Cognition and Executive Function; Spatial Cognition; Spatial Cognitive Maps; Vision for Action and Perception; Visual–Vestibular Interactions.

Further Reading

Colby CL, Gattass R, Olson CR, et al. (1988) Topographic organization of cortical afferents to extrastriate visual area PO in the macaque: A dual tracer study. *Journal of Comparative Neurology* 269: 392–413.

Colby CL and Goldberg ME (1999) Space and attention in parietal cortex. *Annual Review of Neuroscience* 23: 319–349.

Critchley M (1953) *The Parietal Lobes*. London: Edward Arnold.

Duhamel J-R, Colby CL, Goldberg ME, et al. (1992) The updating of the representation of visual space in parietal cortex by intended eye movements. *Science* 255: 90–92.

Duhamel J-R, Colby CL, and Goldberg ME (1998) Ventral intraparietal area of the macaque: Congruent visual and somatic response properties. *Journal of Neurophysiology* 79: 126–136.

James W (1890) *The Principles of Psychology*. New York: Holt.

Perception and Eye Movements

L S Stone and B R Beutter, NASA Ames Research Center, Moffett Field, CA, USA
M P Eckstein, University of California at Santa Barbara, Santa Barbara, CA, USA
D B Liston, San Jose State University Foundation, NASA Ames Research Center, Moffett Field, CA, USA

Published by Elsevier Ltd.

The study of eye movements has long enjoyed a special status in biomedical research. First, compared to other sensorimotor systems, quantitative visual stimuli are relatively easy to create and quantitative eye movement measurements are relatively easy to acquire. Second, prior to the development of advanced imaging technologies, eye movements were the most important noninvasive diagnostic tool to localize brain pathology. Third, the eyeball has a constant rotational inertia and does not lift anything; thus, eye movements can be made largely independent of the on-line proprioceptive feedback needed to calibrate the force–displacement relationships of other motor systems. In summary, oculomotor control was perceived to be a straightforward, simple model system for understanding human sensorimotor control.

On the motor side, the 1960s brought about a revolution in oculomotor research, driven largely by the work of David A Robinson and Robert Wurtz. These researchers pioneered the combined use of the rigorous analytical tools of linear systems theory and of the powerful new experimental capability to reliably and precisely monitor eye movements while recording for extended periods of time from single visuomotor neurons of monkeys performing oculomotor tasks. In the subsequent half century, by systematically tracing, recording from, lesioning, stimulating, and ultimately modeling the major oculomotor pathways in cortical and subcortical structures, their two laboratories and those of their scientific progeny and colleagues made amazing progress in extending our understanding of how visual signals are transformed into eye movement motor commands.

On the vision side, the 1960s brought a similar revolution with John Robson, Fergus Campbell, Christina Enroth-Cugell, and others applying linear systems theory to visual perceptual performance. The 1980s brought a second revolution in vision science driven by David Marr and others, who applied a machine vision, computational perspective to human vision. Their synthetic approach of seeking biologically inspired (and constrained) solutions to real-world engineering and robotics problems by emulating the information processing within the human brain served to highlight the full complexity of the visual processing needed for the effective control of motor actions.

During approximately the past two decades, it has become increasingly clear that the initial hope of the 1960s – that quasi-linear feedback models that transform a retinal position signal (and its derivatives) into an eye position signal (and its derivatives) might explain the critical aspects of voluntary oculomotor behavior – was overly optimistic. Indeed, recent results have highlighted that highly complex and nonlinear aspects of visual perception play a critical role in guiding both voluntary smooth pursuit and saccades. Decades of research using small-spot visual stimuli that were nearly infinitely detectable, identifiable, and localizable revealed much about the motor factors and circuits that limit human oculomotor performance; however, much less was learned about the visual mechanisms that both limit and enrich oculomotor performance. A number of laboratories have begun to measure human saccadic and pursuit performance under more realistic visual conditions in order to examine how visual processing shapes oculomotor behavior.

Action and Perception

In 1982, Ungerleider and Mishkin made a major contribution to our understanding of primate visual information processing by identifying two major ascending processing streams through extrastriate cortex: a dorsal stream through parietal cortex with a hierarchical set of areas that focus on static and dynamic spatial characteristics of the stimulus (the 'where' pathway) and a ventral stream through the inferotemporal cortex with a hierarchy of areas that focus on identifying features of the stimulus (the 'what' pathway). Later, based largely on clinical observations, Goodale and Milner pushed this dichotomy a step further by proposing that the dorsal and ventral streams represent separate, largely independent, visual pathways supporting action and perception, respectively. They argued that object shape information from the ventral stream used for perception is not available to motor systems, and that spatial information from the dorsal pathway was not available to support perception. The critical finding from Newsome's laboratory that local microstimulation of the middle temporal (MT) or medial superior temporal (MST) areas generates spatially localized and directionally specific biases in visual motion discrimination performance demonstrates that the dorsal pathway does play a major causal role in perception. However, these findings do not rule out the possibility that ventral stream information may be inaccessible to motor systems.

A careful reexamination of early reports of dissociations of visual responses for perception and action used to support the Goodale–Milner hypothesis has shown that the purported failure to find a vulnerability to visual illusions for motor actions could be accounted for by subtle differences in the visual demands of the perceptual and motor tasks or by offsetting effects of a misperceived target location and of a distorted motor reference frame that obscure the visual impact of the illusion on motor action. When perception and motor actions are tested either simultaneously or using carefully matched conditions and tasks, both are similarly vulnerable to illusions and other properties of the visual stimulus, undermining the view that visual information for perception is not shared with those systems controlling motor actions.

This article reviews key findings in the recent literature examining the extent to which the visual signals supporting perception are also used to drive voluntary human smooth pursuit and saccadic eye movements.

Smooth Pursuit and Visual Motion Perception

The linear systems view of pursuit has been dominated by retinal image motion models (**Figure 1(a)**). In this view, pursuit is essentially a simple, quasi-linear,

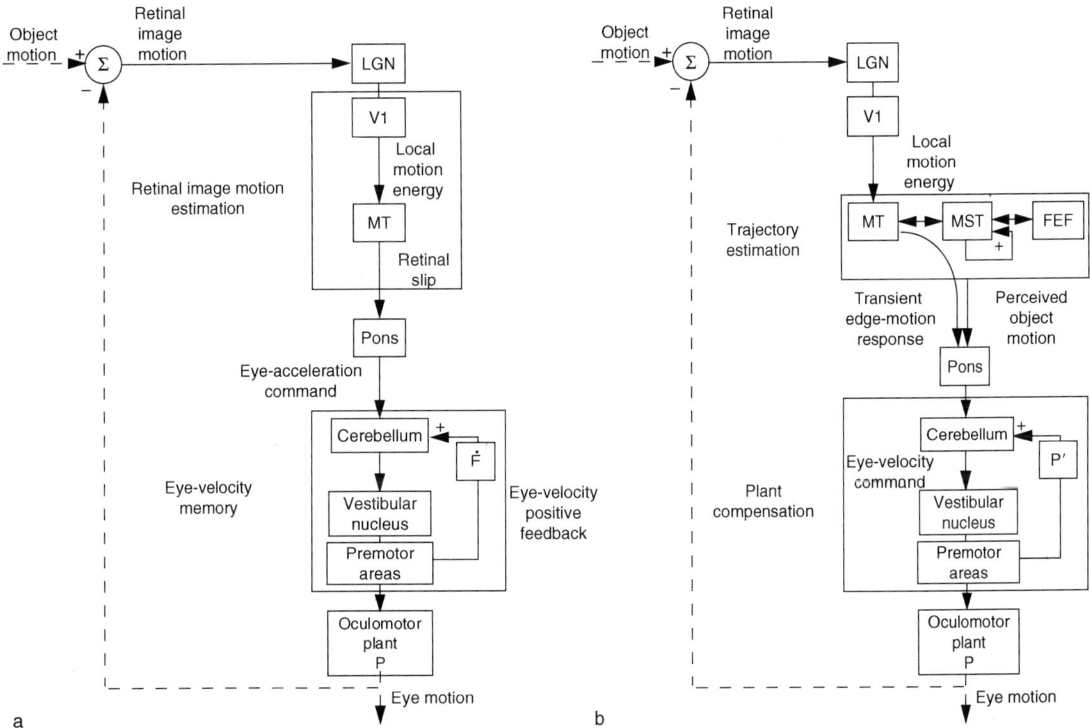

Figure 1 Pursuit models. (a) Retinal image motion models. In this framework, retinal image motion is analyzed in area MT (and associated extrastriate cortical areas in the superior temporal sulcus) to generate retinal position, velocity, and acceleration error signals. Weighted versions of these signals are summed and then sent to the brain stem–cerebellar structures as a command for pursuit eye acceleration. A positive feedback loop between the brain stem and cerebellum sustains ongoing eye velocity and integrates the eye-acceleration commands to generate changes in eye velocity. (b) Object motion models. In this framework, retinal image motion is first segmented in order to identify local edge motions which are subsequently selectively integrated to yield a measure of object motion. To attempt to resolve the inherent ambiguities in this problem, bottom-up retinal motion data, top-down cognitive assumptions and expectations, and either feed-forward or feedback signals related to ongoing eye motion are combined in a sluggish process that involves at least parietal and frontal cortex. The resulting visual object–motion signal is then sent to brain stem–cerebellar premotor circuits that prefilter the object-motion signal to compensate for the oculomotor plant before sending it on to motor neurons as the command for eye motion. (a) Adapted from Lisberger SG, Morris EJ, and Tychsen L (1987) Visual motion processing and sensory–motor integration for smooth pursuit eye movements. *Annual Review of Neuroscience* 10: 97–129. (b) Adapted from Stone LS, Beutter BR, and Lorenceau J (2000) Visual motion: Integration for perception and pursuit. *Perception* 29: 771–787.

continuous control system that attempts to minimize retinal image velocity through negative feedback. A retinal motion error signal or retinal slip (primarily a retinal velocity signal) is computed in area MT and sent to the brain stem as a command to drive eye acceleration. Meanwhile, ongoing eye velocity is maintained by a positive feedback circuit through the cerebellum which acts as an integrator of the acceleration commands. Although retinal image motion models can do a good job of explaining pursuit responses to a single white spot moving on a dark background (the only situation in which retinal image motion is identical to object motion), they cannot explain human pursuit responses to the wider range of visual conditions (and retinal stimuli) experienced when tracking a realistic object (which generates a set of disparate retinal local-edge motions) across a realistically textured environment.

Early studies revealed problems with the core idea that retinal motion error and eye velocity positive feedback form the command signal ultimately driving pursuit eye movements. The earliest pursuit studies observed zero phase-lag pursuit of sinusoidal motion, demonstrating a predictive component to the pursuit response that cannot be accounted for by eye velocity memory. In 1976, Steinbach showed that humans could pursue the horizontal motion of a rolling wagon wheel when only a few illuminated dots were visible on the rim. The perceived horizontal motion of an invisible rolling wheel is tracked, even though the retinal motions of the visible dots are cycloidal. Any observer who pursues this wagon wheel stimulus becomes immediately aware that pursuit does not simply respond to the motion in the retinal image. An additional red flag was raised in 1988 when Newsome, Wurtz, and Komatsu found signals related to ongoing eye motion in area MST, an area shown by both lesions and microstimulation studies to be causally involved in motion perception as well as generating the motor command for pursuit. Thus, the cortical signal driving smooth pursuit is not simply a retinal error signal but, rather, one more related to object motion in head- or world-centric coordinates. Moreover, that same year, Dursteler and Wurtz found that MST lesions cause direction-specific pursuit deficits, with no effort to make smooth corrections of the large residual retinal motion error during the poor steady-state tracking performance. These findings put into question any model of pursuit that proposes a negative feedback circuit that simply attempts to drive retinal motion to zero.

Numerous studies have shown clear links between pursuit and perceived motion, further distancing pursuit behavior from raw retinal velocity errors. First, perception and pursuit show the same speed and direction discrimination performance and are similarly affected by nonlinear directional anisotropies such as the oblique effect, suggesting that rate-limiting neural speed and direction signals are shared by perception and pursuit. Furthermore, analysis of the trial-by-trial variation in human perceptual and pursuit direction responses shows higher correlation than expected by chance from independent mechanisms (**Figure 2(a)**). Thus, perception and pursuit share a limiting internal direction noise source, thereby undermining the theory that pursuit and perception have separate and independent, but fortuitously equal, underlying direction signals. Second, high-level cognitive expectations affect perception and pursuit equally. For example, in 2001, Krauzlis and Adler showed that when the likely direction of stimulus motion is cued prior to each trial, humans generate similar perceptual and pursuit performance biases toward the likely direction. Third, pursuit and perception appear to be fooled in the same way by visual illusions. For example, in 1996, Ringach, Hawken, and Shapley showed that humans generate a pursuit vergence response to the illusory motion in-depth of the kinetic depth effect. Fourth, the time course of the computation of object motion is similar for perception and pursuit. In particular, a human psychophysical study by Shiffrar and Lorenceau in 1996 and a human pursuit study by Masson and Stone in 2002 showed that the temporal integration of an initial set of local edge motion signals into a bona fide object motion signal is similarly sluggish (on the order of a few hundred milliseconds) for both perception and pursuit. In 2001, Pack and Born found a similarly sluggish temporal evolution of the direction signals encoded in the firing rate of MT neurons and those driving smooth eye movements in monkeys. Fifth, when presented with ambiguous image motion, perception and pursuit choose the same arbitrary interpretation of object motion, influenced by the same static image properties. In particular, when Madelain and Krauzlis asked observers to pursue a motion stimulus whose direction is completely ambiguous such that an observer can select a leftward or rightward percept at will, each perceptual reversal was associated with a pursuit reversal. Furthermore, on average, the perceptual reversal precedes the pursuit reversal by nearly 100 ms, consistent with perception driving pursuit within an object-motion pursuit model (**Figure 3**).

Finally, in 2001, Alais and Lorenceau showed that the spatial configuration or shape of ambiguous line drawings affects their perceived motion. In this regard, humans show similar effects of object shape on pursuit (**Figure 4**). For example, the motion of a diamond occluded by vertical windows appears rigid and is both veridically perceived and accurately

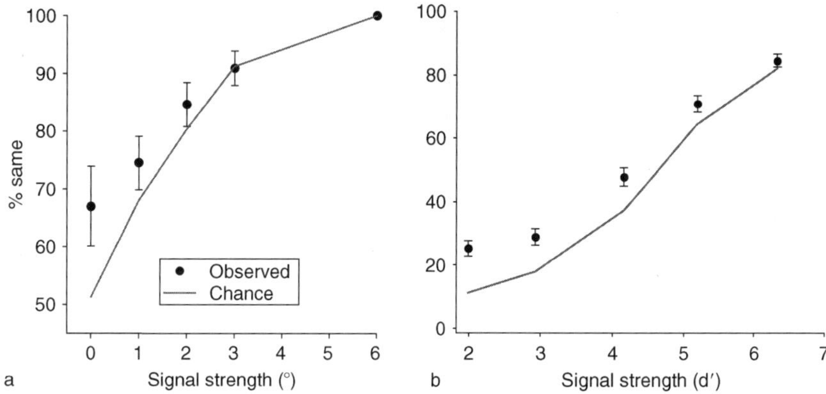

Figure 2 Covariation analysis (also called % same or choice probability). (a) Shared internal direction noise for pursuit and perception. In a simultaneous study of perceptual and pursuit direction signals, the binary psychometric and oculometric decisions were highly correlated across the entire range of signal strengths tested. The correlation expected by chance for two independent mechanisms is 50 % in the no-signal condition and increases monotonically to 100 % in the high-signal condition in which both decisions are always correct and therefore trivially the same. This figure plots the % same (the percentage of trials for which the pursuit and perceptual binary direction decisions were the same) for a single observer as a function of signal strength (direction difference in degrees from a cardinal axis). Note that the observed correlation was significantly higher than expected by chance (error bars show 95% confidence intervals). (b) Shared response to external noise for saccades and perception. In sequential studies of perceptual and saccadic localization with an identical set of noisy search images, the 10-alternative forced choice (10AFC) psychometric and oculometric decisions were correlated across the entire range of signal strengths tested (signal-to-noise levels in d′ units). The correlation expected by chance from two independent mechanisms is 10 % in the zero SNR condition and increases monotonically to 100 % for an extrapolated high SNR condition in which both decisions are always correct and therefore trivially the same. This figure plots the % same (the percentage of image samples for which the perceptual and saccadic 10AFC decisions were the same) for a single observer as a function of signal strength (ratio of peak luminance of the target to the amplitude of the pixel luminance noise). Note that the observed correlation was significantly higher than expected by chance (error bars show standard errors). (a) Adapted from Stone LS and Krauzlis RJ (2003) shared motion signals for human perceptual decisions and oculomotor actions. *Journal of Vision* 3: 725–736. (b) Figure based on data from Beutter BR, Eckstein MP, and Stone LS (2003) Saccadic and perceptual performance in visual search tasks: I. Contrast detection and discrimination. *Journal of the Optical Society of America A* 20: 1341–1355.

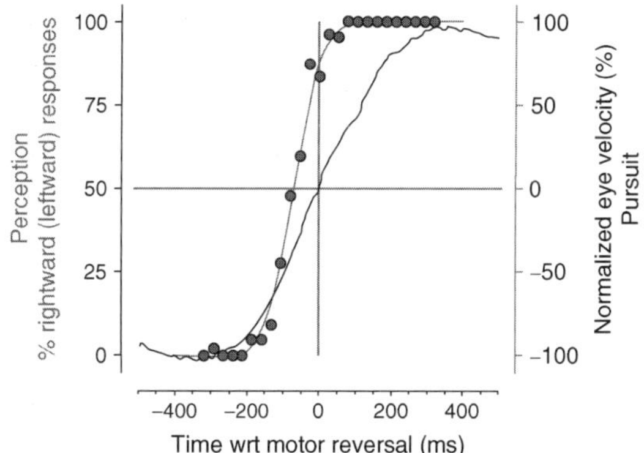

Figure 3 Correlated pursued and perceived direction reversals for completely ambiguous motion. For a stimulus that can be perceived as moving rightward or leftward at will, the data show that the perceptual reversal (plotted as percentage rightward or leftward judgments) preceded the oculomotor direction reversal (plotted as mean eye velocity) by slightly less than 100 ms, consistent with perceived motion driving pursuit. The retinal image motion is constant throughout but pursuit changes from rightward to leftward (or vice versa) synergistically with the reversals in perceived motion, which is inconsistent with all retinal image motion models of pursuit. Adapted from Madelain L and Krauzlis RJ (2003) Pursuit of the ineffable: Perceptual and motor reversals during the tracking of apparent motion. *Journal of Vision* 3: 642–653.

pursued. However, the motion of a similarly occluded cross (defined by the exact same segment image motion but merely spatially rearranged) is perceived as nonrigid; the coherent two-dimensional (2-D) object motion interpretation is presumably interfered with by the distracting vertical motion of the segments. Pursuit of a diamond moving along an isotropic trajectory shows an isotropic response (i.e., vertical and horizontal pursuit gains are equal), consistent with the motion of a rigid object. However, pursuit of the cross shows lower overall gain and a clear vertical bias, consistent with the nonrigid object motion percept and the vertical segment motion inference. This finding suggests that object shape information, presumably from the ventral pathway, is influencing perception and pursuit in parallel. Moreover, even an extended version of the retinal image motion model that attempts to minimize the sum (or vector average) of all the retinal segment motions would predict that pursuit of the cross and pursuit of the diamond would be identical.

The emerging picture is that pursuit is driven by a signal related to perceived object motion and not directly by retinal image motion. An object motion model of pursuit (**Figure 1(b)**) can not only explain

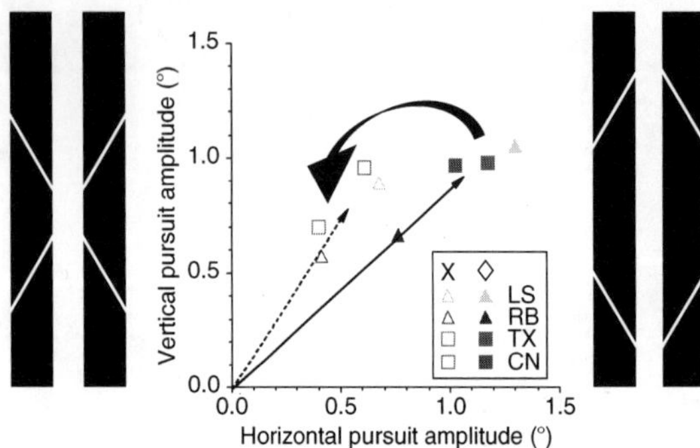

Figure 4 Different pursuit for identical retinal motion related to differences in object shape. Moving occluded line figures with identical object motion trajectories and identical segment motions (but with the segments in different relative retinal locations) can nonetheless be perceived and pursued differently. The data show the horizontal and vertical pursuit amplitudes of four observers in response to a diamond (solid) or a cross (open) configuration representing the same object motion along an isotropic 2-D Lissajous figure. The diamond is perceived to move rigidly and is pursued with an isotropic high-gain response. The cross, however, appears to move nonrigidly and is pursued with a low-gain trajectory biased in the vertical direction of the segment motion. The fact that both of these stimuli generate 2-D trajectories at all is inconsistent with retinal image motion models, which would generate nearly exclusively vertical pursuit in response to the vertical retinal segment motion. More important, the fact that identical physical object motion is pursued differently when different nonmotion information generates different object motion percepts is strong evidence that pursuit is driven by an object motion signal shared with perception. Adapted from Stone LS, Beutter BR, and Lorenceau J (2000) Visual motion: Integration for perception and pursuit. *Perception* 29: 771–787.

the wider range of new phenomena described previously but also takes into consideration the wealth of physiological findings demonstrating an extensive role for both parietal (MST) and frontal (frontal eye field (FEF) pursuit area) cortex in trajectory estimation (including prediction). It also acknowledges that these areas, not just MT, provide a major component of the descending pathway to brain stem and cerebellar structures involved in the generation of the motor output signal driving pursuit. The role of cortex in this new view is not to calculate derivatives of retinal motion but, rather, to compute a best estimate of object motion from the available visual information (both dynamic and static) within a cognitive and attentional context. If an object motion signal is sent down to the brain stem (instead of a retinal error signal), then the role of the cerebellar feedback loop must also be reassessed. If object motion is the descending cortical output signal, then the only processing needed to optimize the oculomotor command to the plant is to high-pass prefilter the eye velocity command to compensate for the low-pass filtering of the oculomotor plant. Indeed, the output signals from the cerebellum supporting pursuit have been shown to be a prefiltered version of the subsequent eye velocity signal. Such prefiltering could be achieved via a positive feedback loop that mimics the plant. Another important virtue of this model, in addition to its ability to reconcile a wide range of behavioral and physiological pursuit observations, is that it is easily generalized to other motor systems, whereby the cerebellum would act as a compensator for other motor plants all driven by the same cortical object motion signal (or another relevant perceptual signal). Thus, the hand and the eye can work synergistically when tracking a moving object.

Saccades and Visual Target Selection

The linear systems theory view of the saccadic system has been dominated by variants of a retinal offset model (**Figure** 5(**a**)). In this view, the saccadic system is essentially a simple, quasi-linear, bang-bang control system that rapidly corrects retinal position offset by driving this offset to zero through negative feedback. A retinal position error signal from primary visual cortex (V1), modulated by inputs from other cortical areas, is sent down to the superior colliculus (SC) of the midbrain as the retinal target position signal. When a particular locus in the SC map reaches a threshold, that location relays a command for desired eye position to brain stem structures that generate the neural pulse and step signals needed to accelerate the eye and then hold it in its new position, respectively. Although this model includes a detailed description of brain stem structures, as with the retinal image motion pursuit model, the entire visual and decision-making process is the trivial calculation of an unambiguous retinal error signal – in this case, position instead of velocity. Again, such a retinal signal is only unambiguous in the degenerate case of a small spot on a dark background. Furthermore, it is has long been known that nonretinal signals can drive voluntary saccades, such as auditory or visual memory signals.

During approximately the past decade, a number of laboratories have turned their attention to understanding the visual processes underlying saccadic target selection in search and search-like tasks using more realistic visual stimuli with targets of variable signal strength, embedded in external image noise, among similarly salient nontarget 'distractors,' and/or with differing *a priori* location probabilities. These studies have revealed a rich complexity of signal processing, requiring broadly distributed interactions between parietal and frontal cortex and the midbrain.

Numerous studies have illustrated clear links between saccades and perception, further distancing saccadic behavior from raw retinal offset signals. First, it

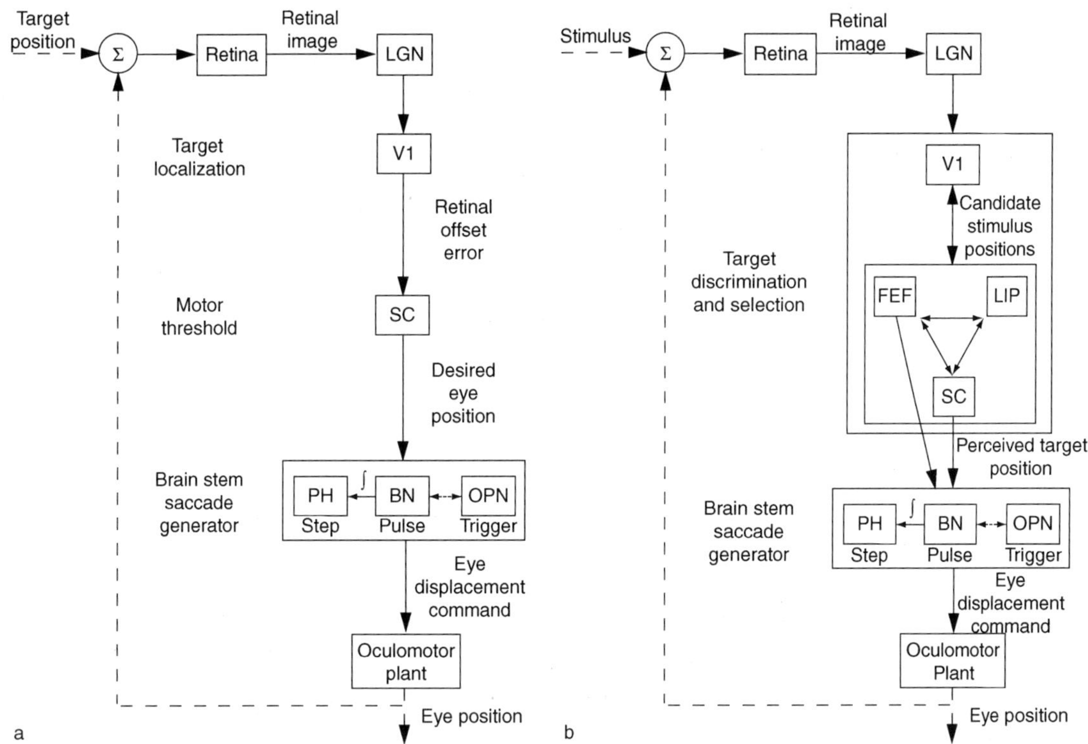

Figure 5 Saccade models. (a) Retinal offset error models. In this framework, a retinal offset signal is computed in primary visual cortex (V1) (with input from parietal and frontal cortical areas) and then send to the superior colliculus (SC) of the midbrain. When that signal reaches threshold, the SC sends a desired eye position signal to brain stem saccadic structures, which generate the command for eye displacement. (b) Target selection models. In this framework, the totality of the retinal image is processed in parallel to identify candidate target locations. A network that includes the lateral–intraparietal area (LIP), the frontal eye fields (FEF), and the SC works to select a single target using the available bottom-up sensory data modulated by top-down cognitive and attentional factors. The resulting perceived target position signal is then sent to brain stem saccadic structures, which generate the command for eye displacement.

has been shown that saccades and perception appear similarly affected by spatial illusions. For example, saccades (and hand pointing as well) show systematic spatial deviations in the same direction as the spatial misperceptions for stimuli that evoke the Muller–Lyer illusion. Although early reports of this effect on saccades were conflicting, when the saccadic task relies on a visual feature that is distorted by the illusion, the motor response reflects the perceptual illusion. Second, contrast detection and discrimination thresholds are equal for perception and saccades. More important, using noisy search stimuli, the correlation between the external image noise-driven responses of saccades and perception is higher than expected by chance from two independent mechanisms (**Figure 2(b)**). Thus, saccades and perception appear equally vulnerable to those random spatial features of a particular noise sample that appear target-like. Third, using classification image analysis (a form of reverse correlation), by combining the hundreds of noise samples (sans target) that generated erroneous responses, one can construct an image of the virtual target that saccades and perception were looking for (i.e., an estimate of the template or overall receptive field used in the decision-making process). Not only are the shapes of the classification images from saccadic and perceptual decisions indistinguishable but also their common shape differs significantly from that of the target (**Figure 6**). Indeed, both images are a high-passed version of the target, which may indeed be optimal if one is searching for the target embedded in the low-pass filtered noise commonly associated with visual neural signals.

The emerging view is that a complicated network between the parietal and frontal cortex, as well as the SC, converges to select a single target using both bottom-up sensory data and top-down cognitive knowledge, expectation, and/or anticipation of reward. Furthermore, ascending feedback from the SC to visual cortical areas appears to play an important role in this process by driving attention-like modulations of visual processing, thereby influencing

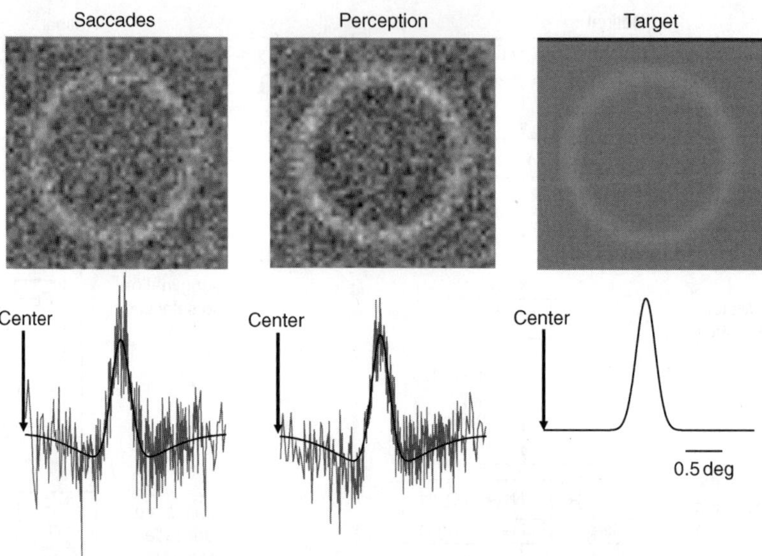

Figure 6 Classification image (CI) analysis reveals the saccadic and perceptual 'receptive field' used to search for the brightest 'O' among dimmer Os. The top row shows the raw CI for saccades and perception, respectively. The bottom row shows the normalized and polar averaged cross-section of the receptive fields. Note that the perceptual and saccades receptive fields are both high-pass filtered versions of the Gaussian stimulus cross-section and are well described by difference of Gaussian functions (solid black lines under the red data traces). Thus, not only is the receptive field shape the same for saccades and perception but also the perceptual and saccades receptive fields are more similar to each other than they are to the actual target, providing strong evidence of a shared target template used by perception and saccades during search.

perception, although the exact nature of these modulations is not well understood. The target selection model of saccades (**Figure 5(b)**) acknowledges the simple fact that the saccadic system is not finding a single target presented in a vacuum but, rather, is selecting the most behaviorally relevant target from among many candidate possibilities. Thus, rather than thinking of visual target localization as a trivial thresholding of a single highly salient spot, studies have reframed saccadic targeting within the context of signal detection theory, addressing the nontrivial question of how to decide where to look next when the target is inconspicuous or is similar to surrounding distractors. Saccadic and perceptual search can be described as a template-matching task in the presence of noise and spatial uncertainty; the template captures essential contrast and shape information about the searched-for target albeit not necessary perfectly matched to the target (**Figure 6**). Indeed, the similarity of the classification images for perception and saccades (and their shared difference with the actual target shape) strongly suggests that the saccadic system has access to the same shape information as perception, presumably from shared ventral pathways supporting both perception and action.

Although the new framework for saccadic targeting embraces a novel view of visual processing, unlike pursuit, the proposed new visual front end for saccades does not require a fundamental reinterpretation of the role of brain stem saccade-generating structures. However, it is becoming increasingly clear that the SC is not merely a feed-forward output relay to brain stem structures but, rather, plays a key role in the target selection process, along with the lateral intraparietal (LIP) area and the FEF. Consistent with this distributed responsibility for target selection, Schiller and colleagues showed that bilateral removal of either the SC or the FEF leaves the ability to make saccades intact, whereas bilateral removal of both areas destroys that ability. Furthermore, studies in both the Wurtz and Newsome laboratories have demonstrated that stimulation of the SC can modulate perceptual performance, justifying the elevation of the SC into the target-selection network, which was formerly considered to be exclusively cortical.

A New Framework for the Visuomotor Control of Pursuit and Saccades

The major paradigm shift that has occurred in the study of pursuit and saccades is the realization that the visual processing part of the sensorimotor problem is more complicated than originally thought.

When humans 'see' by taking the neural signals coming from the approximately 1 million ganglion cells in each eye to create a full-color 3-D model of the world around them, quite a complicated process has occurred. The sensory information available represents two 2-D projections of the world, one from each retina, and is therefore necessarily incomplete. The human visual system must use the available sensory data (bottom-up information) as well as *a priori* knowledge about the world (top-down information) to infer a best guess of what is actually out there. As such, all visual perception is illusion; what we call illusions are merely those rare instances when the brain's best guess is obviously wrong.

Complex interactions between frontal, parietal, inferotemporal, and occipital cortex, along with the midbrain, are used to combine bottom-up and top-down information into a time-varying best estimate of the oculomotor target. For pursuit, the reconstruction of the target object's motion in the world takes time. An early quick estimate of object motion using the vector average of local edge motions appears to drive early perceptual and pursuit responses, with a more accurate estimate emerging with a time constant on the order of 100 ms. The standard linear system control theory approach of considering only the initial 100-ms 'open-loop' pursuit response to characterize the internal visuomotor transfer function therefore misses much of this elegant, yet sluggish, computational process. Object motion estimation of realistic targets takes time because, after the initial sensory transduction, the visual system must first segregate from the background those pieces of the retinal image that represent individual local motion features. The system must then selectively integrate those pieces that properly belong together into a whole object whose global motion can then be computed. This process is inherently ambiguous because the data set is incomplete (although over time the ambiguity of the object trajectory can resolve itself). Thus, the perceptual and pursuit systems must make visual choices. The preponderance of evidence gathered during approximately the past decade argues that perception and pursuit make the same choice using shared visual motion processing mechanisms broadly distributed across parietal and frontal cortex, with likely input from inferotemporal cortex as well.

For saccades, localizing the target object is also a complex, time-consuming visual process involving both parallel and serial components: parallel because all portions of the visual field are being processed simultaneously and serial because, at low target salience, a sequence of discrete fixation steps is traced as one searches for the target. Presumably, during each fixation, a target-like template is being compared with incoming noisy sensory data in order to determine the 'best' next location to foveate, with multiple locations constantly competing for attention. The preponderance of evidence indicates that perception and saccades make the same choices using shared spatial visual processing mechanisms broadly distributed between parietal and frontal cortex, with inputs from the superior colliculus and inferotemporal cortex as well.

Another difference between the traditional oculomotor models (**Figures 1(a)** and 5(**a**)) and the new frameworks (**Figures 1(b)** and 5(**b**)) is the coordinate system of the visual signals driving motor actions. The traditional view of saccades and pursuit assumes that the controlled visual signals are in raw retinal coordinates: retinal position, velocity, or even acceleration error signals to be minimized by negative feedback. Not only do the aforementioned MST studies rule this out for pursuit but also a behavioral study of the direction signals driving perception during fixation and pursuit by Krukowski and colleagues in 2003 showed that the limiting direction noise and even the oblique effect are not in retinal coordinates but, rather, in head- or world-centered coordinates. This finding shows that performance in an apparently simple direction discrimination task is limited by neural signals beyond area MT (the highest area mapped in retinal coordinates) and thus in area MST (an area in which retinal motion signals are combined with eye and head motion signals) or another motion area further along in the dorsal pathway. Indeed, there is even direct physiological evidence that some MST neurons encode object motion in world coordinates.

The cortical signals driving saccades are also not simply in retinal coordinates. LIP and FEF both encode target location in 'oculocentric' coordinates, which comprise a coordinate system in which target location is constantly being updated with respect to the current eye position using anticipatory signals about future eye movements (even in the absence of visual feedback). This updating process, first described by Colby, Duhamel, and Goldberg, effectively keeps the target location stably encoded in head-centered space – yet bouncing around in the retinal map with every saccade – presumably as part of the mechanism keeping the world perceptually stable during saccades. Sommer and Wurtz characterized an oculomotor feedback pathway from SC to FEF, via the mediodorsal thalamus, and have further shown that interruption of the corollary discharge signal from the SC disrupts the proper updating of target location, thereby demonstrating that the SC plays a key role in the coordinate system transformation for target localization performed within the cortex.

Clearly, the frameworks in **Figures 1(b)** and 5(**b**) are mere cartoons that require much fleshing out. Nonetheless, they succinctly represent the concatenation of a number of conceptual advances that are guiding the next generation of oculomotor researchers and cortical physiologists. Regrettably, this short article can mention only a small number of the many important recent findings. Many researchers are actively working to understand the visual processing for saccade target selection and pursuit object motion estimation and the associated neurophysiological underpinnings. Although much progress has been made, the picture of how an extended network of cortical (and even subcortical) areas interact to shape synergistic perception and sensorimotor control remains incomplete.

Conclusion

Because the sensory 'image' of the world is inherently ambiguous, humans must generate a best-estimate solution to this complex puzzle, using noisy incomplete data and cognitive strategies to construct an internal 3-D model of visual space, in order to interact with their environment and ultimately to survive in the real world. Perhaps, our coherent multisensory perception of the world evolved from the need for the brain to provide a single, decisive interpretation of an ambiguous and incomplete set of visual (and other) signals in order to coordinate the actions of multiple motor systems. Indeed, above and beyond the parsimony argument about limited cortical processing resources, it is difficult to imagine an evolutionary advantage of each neural system developing a set of independent, potentially conflicting, private solutions to the visual problems of detection, discrimination, and target selection.

See also: Active Perception; Attention and Eye Movements; Basal Ganglia and Oculomotor Control; Brainstem Control of Eye Movements; Cerebellum and Oculomotor Control; Contextual Interactions in Visual Perception; Cortical Control of Eye Movements; Eye and Head Movements; Eye Movement Disorders; Oculomotor Control: Anatomical Pathways; Optokinetic Eye Movements; Pursuit Eye Movements; Saccade–Pursuit Interactions; Saccades and Visual Search; Saccadic Eye Movements; Target Selection for Pursuit and Saccades; Vision for Action and Perception.

Further Reading

Beutter BR, Eckstein MP, and Stone LS (2003) Saccadic and perceptual performance in visual search tasks: I. Contrast detection and discrimination. *Journal of the Optical Society of America A* 20: 1341–1355

Dassonville P and Bala JK (2004) Perception, action, and Roelofs effect: A mere illusion of dissociation. *Public Library of Science Biology* 2: e364.

DeGrave DDJ, Franz VH, and Gegenfurtner KR (2006) The influence of the Brentano illusion on eye and hand movements. *Journal of Vision* 6: 727–738.

Eckstein MP, Beutter BR, Pham BT, Shimozaki SS, and Stone LS (2007) Similar neural representations of the target for saccades and perception during search. *Journal of Neuroscience* 27: 1266–1270.

Goldberg ME, Bisley JW, Powell KD, and Gottlieb J (2006) Saccades, salience and attention: The role of the lateral intraparietal area in visual behavior. *Progress in Brain Research* 155: 157–175.

Ilg UJ (2002) Commentary: Smooth pursuit eye movements: From low-level to high-level vision. *Progress in Brain Research* 140: 279–298.

Ilg UJ, Schumann S, and Thier P (2004) Posterior parietal cortex neurons encode target motion in world-centered coordinates. *Neuron* 43: 145–151.

Krauzlis RJ (2005) The control of voluntary eye movements: New perspectives. *Neuroscientist* 11: 124–137.

Krauzlis RJ, Liston D, and Carello CD (2004) Target selection and the superior colliculus: Goals, choices, and hypotheses. *Vision Research* 44: 1445–1451.

Krauzlis RJ and Stone LS (1999) Tracking with the mind's eye. *Trends in Neuroscience* 22: 544–550.

Krukowski AE and Stone LS (2005) Expansion of direction space around the cardinal axes revealed by smooth pursuit eye movements. *Neuron* 45: 315–323.

Lisberger SG, Morris EJ, and Tychsen L (1987) Visual motion processing and sensory–motor integration for smooth pursuit eye movements. *Annual Review of Neuroscience* 10: 97–129.

Madelain L and Krauzlis RJ (2003) Pursuit of the ineffable: Perceptual and motor reversals during the tracing of apparent motion. *Journal of Vision* 3: 642–653

Milner AD and Goodale MA (1995) *The Visual Brain in Action.* New York: Oxford University Press.

Stone LS, Beutter BR, and Lorenceau J (2000) Visual motion: Integration for perception and pursuit. *Perception* 29: 771–787.

Schiller PH and Tehovnik EJ (2005) Neural mechanisms underlying target selection with saccadic eye movements. *Progress in Brain Research* 149: 157–171.

Stone LS and Krauzlis RJ (2003) shared motion signals for human perceptual decisions and oculomotor actions. *Journal of Vision* 3: 725–736

Smeets JB and Brenner E (2006) 10 years of illusions. *Journal of Experimental Psychology: Human Perception and Performance* 32: 1501–1504.

Sparks DL (2002) The brainstem control of saccadic eye movements. *Nature Reviews Neuroscience* 3: 952–964.

Thompson KG and Bichot NP (2005) A visual salience map in the primate frontal eye field. *Progress in Brain Research* 147: 251–262.

Prefrontal Cortex

J M Fuster, University of California, Los Angeles, CA, USA

The cortex of the anterior pole of the brain can be subdivided, histologically and physiologically, into three major parts. They have been most clearly identified and extensively investigated in the frontal lobe of the primate: (1) the primary motor cortex, a strip of agranular cortex rostral and adjacent to the central sulcus; (2) the premotor cortex, a conglomerate of cytoarchitectonically transitional areas, including the supplementary motor area (SMA); and (3) the prefrontal cortex, which constitutes the largest and most anterior of the three components and which in the primate has a prominent internal granular layer (IV) and for this reason is designated as the granular frontal cortex. The three components can be well distinguished in the external convexity of the frontal lobe; in the cingulate and inferior (orbital) aspects of the lobe, the first two components are absent and the granular cytoarchitecture of the prefrontal cortex blends more or less gradually into that of limbic cortex behind it.

All three parts of the frontal cortex are functionally involved in behavior. The premotor and motor areas participate in the preparation and execution of specific movements, whereas the prefrontal cortex participates in cognitive aspects of behavior. Although its functions have not been completely elucidated, current knowledge strongly indicates that the prefrontal cortex is essentially engaged in the organization of goal-directed behavioral sequences. Furthermore, the prefrontal cortex seems essential for goal-directed rational thinking. Thus, the functional integrity of this cortex is necessary for the temporal organization of behavioral actions as well as of the 'internal actions' that constitute logical reasoning.

Development

Phylogenetically, the prefrontal cortex is the most rostral portion of the neocortex. It is one of the cortical regions to undergo the latest and most expansive development in the course of evolution (**Figure 1**); this is especially true for the cortex of the external prefrontal convexity, which is the part of frontal cortex most heavily involved in cognitive functions. Such development reaches a maximum in the human brain, where the prefrontal cortex constitutes nearly one-third of the neocortex. Ontogenetically, the prefrontal cortex also develops relatively late. In the human, its myelinization is not complete until the second decade of life.

Connections

The prefrontal cortex is connected with many other cerebral structures. Its extrinsic connectivity has certain peculiarities that distinguish it from other neocortical regions. They are as follows:

1. Reciprocal connections with anterior and dorsal nuclei of the thalamus; the prominent links of the prefrontal cortex with the nucleus medialis dorsalis are conventionally used as the criterion for the definition of this cortex in all species.
2. Reciprocal connections with several sensory processing areas of posterior association cortex; afferent inputs from various sensory systems (somatic, visual, auditory, and olfactory) arrive in the prefrontal cortex, which therefore may be considered cortex of polymodal sensory convergence and association.
3. Reciprocal connections with limbic formations, especially the hypothalamus, the amygdala, and the hippocampus, which are known to be involved in certain aspects of emotion, motivation, and memory.
4. Efferent connections to subcortical structures involved in motor control, such as the basal ganglia; further, through the basal ganglia, the cerebellum, and the thalamus, the prefrontal cortex has indirect connective access to the neighboring motor areas of the frontal lobe.

In addition, the prefrontal cortex, as in other associative regions of the neocortex, is reciprocally connected with diencephalic and mesencephalic nuclei and reticular formations with diffuse cortical projection. As in other regions, some afferent (corticocortical) connections in the prefrontal cortex have been noted to terminate in columnar transcortical patterns of distribution.

Neurotransmitters

All major types of neurotransmitter terminals and receptors are represented in the prefrontal cortex. The principal monoaminergic afferent systems from the brain stem and limbic structures innervate the prefrontal cortex. Conversely, the prefrontal cortex sends descending monoaminergic efferents to the thalamus, hypothalamus, subthalamus, and the core of the lower brain stem. Norepinephrine and dopamine seem to be synthesized and concentrated in

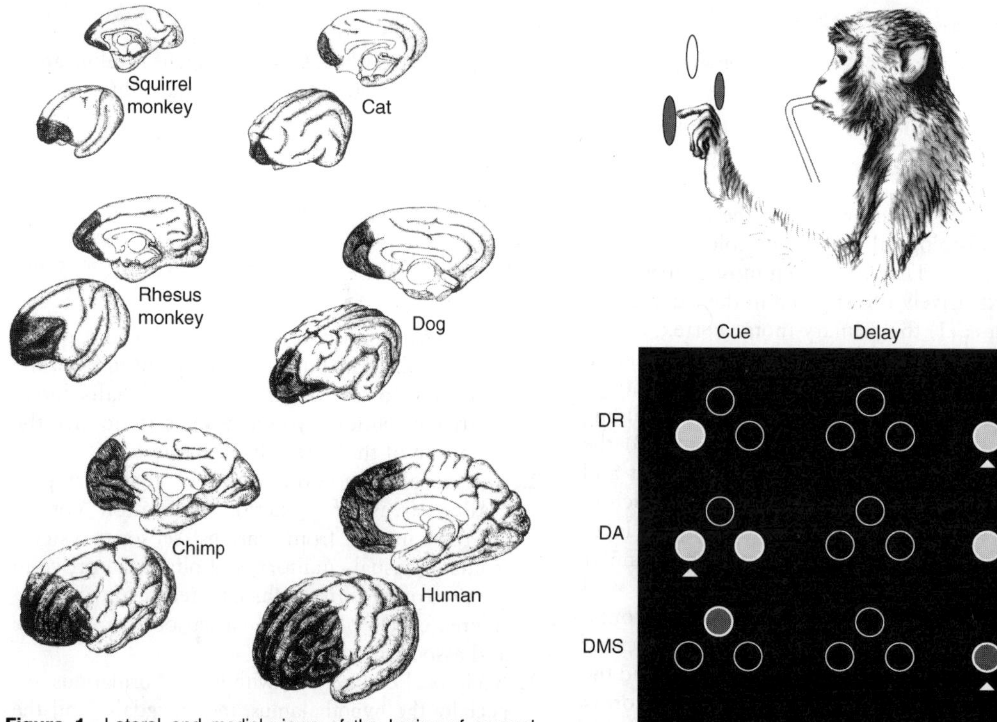

Figure 1 Lateral and medial views of the brains of several species. The prefrontal cortex is indicated by dark shading.

Figure 2 Monkey facing a panel with stimulus–response buttons for performance of delay tasks (mouth spigot for delivery of liquid reward). Below, the sequence of events in three such tasks: delayed response (DR), delayed alternation (DA), and delayed matching-to-sample (DMS). A DR trial begins with brief illumination of a button (right or left, randomly changing); after a delay of a few seconds, two buttons are simultaneously lit, and the animal must press the one lit at the start of the trial. In DA, the animal must alternately press the right and the left of a pair of buttons that are simultaneously lighted between delays. In DMS, the trial begins with brief presentation of a sample color, red or green (upper button); after the delay, both colors appear in the lower buttons, and the animal must press the one matching the sample color; both that color and the positions of the two colors in the lower buttons are changed randomly between trials. (White triangles mark the site of correct response).

higher quantities in the prefrontal cortex than in posterior sensory and associative cortex. The reverse is true for serotonin. The prefrontal region is the recipient of abundant cholinergic fibers from the basal nucleus of Meynert (or its equivalent in the rat and the cat). This nucleus is a relay in a cholinergic system of ascending connections that originates in the brain stem reticular core and diffusely projects to the cerebral cortex. Both catecholamine and acetylcholine systems have been postulated to mediate, in a yet unspecified manner, the participation of the prefrontal cortex in cognitive processes, memory in particular.

Neuropsychology

Lesions of the prefrontal cortex cause changes in various aspects and forms of behavior. The magnitude of the changes depends on the location and extent of the lesion. This has been most systematically studied in primates, but the general characteristics of the behavioral changes observed are the same in all species in which they have been investigated.

The best known alterations resulting from lesions of the dorsolateral prefrontal convexity are deficits in learning and performance of various structured behavioral tasks that have one common feature: the necessity to execute motor acts in accord with sensory information no longer present in the environment. The temporal discontinuity between information and action (cross-temporal contingency) is an essential element of these tasks (**Figure 2**). Thus, the deficit is neither sensory nor motor but has to do with the ability of the animal to integrate, across a span of time, sensory input with appropriate action. However, the degree of deficit depends not only on the length of that time but also on the novelty and complexity of the sensory stimulus or stimuli before it.

It also depends on whether the stimulus–response coupling required for the task is merely one of two or more similar and alternative couplings in the behavioral repertoire of the animal. If only one specific signal calls for one specific act, without the competing possibility of similar signals and acts, no deficit can be seen after prefrontal lesion, however long the time between the signal and the action.

Most typical and documented are the deleterious effects of prefrontal lesions, especially if they involve the lateral convexity, on the performance of delay tasks (e.g., delayed response, delayed alternation, delayed matching to sample) and discrimination reversal tasks. All such tasks impose the need to bridge a cross-temporal contingency between information and action, as well as the need to reject similar alternatives.

Lesions of inferior (orbital) or medial prefrontal cortex may also disrupt to some extent the performance of behavioral tasks, especially if they require the inhibition or suppression of a prepotent and well-established tendency or response alternative. Inferior lesions severely disrupt such tasks as conditioned inhibition and successive discrimination, where that requirement is critical for successful performance but the bridging of cross-temporal contingencies is not.

Summing up, cortical lesion experiments show that the prefrontal cortex, unlike other parts of the cerebral cortex, is essential for the formation of goal-directed structures of behavior that demand cross-temporal integration and the rejection of inappropriate alternatives. The behavioral effects of selective cortical ablations and reversible lesions (by cooling) in the monkey suggest that this is accomplished by the joint action of a temporally retrospective function of short-term memory – also called 'working memory' – and a function of control of internal interference. The former seems mainly based in dorsolateral, the latter in inferior (orbital) prefrontal cortex.

Although clinical observations of the effects of frontal lobe pathology were made long before the relevant animal lesion studies had been carried out, the data from prefrontal lesions in the human have been less systematically investigated and are more difficult to evaluate than those from nonhuman primates. Nevertheless, in recent years, rigorous neuropsychological studies of patients with frontal lobe lesions have shed new light on the nature of symptoms that are commonly encountered in such patients (e.g., difficulties in attention, recent memory, planning). These studies also reveal a remarkable degree of similarity between the prefrontal syndromes of humans and animals. It has now been shown that humans with lesions of the prefrontal convexity, like monkeys with such lesions, exhibit deficits in performance of short-term memory tasks (e.g., delayed matching) and tasks that require the ordering of items in time. In the human, as in the monkey, lesions of orbital prefrontal cortex disrupt the ability to perform tasks demanding the inhibition of strong response tendencies (e.g., discrimination reversal, go/no go). Thus, also in humans, prefrontal lesions result in deficits of short-term memory and control of interference.

As might be expected from these observations, the human subject with a prefrontal lesion is likely to be deficient in the temporal organization of sequential behaviors, such as the spoken language, that rely heavily on cognitive operations. The most dramatic language difficulty resulting from prefrontal pathology is Broca's aphasia, a severe deficit in the construction and articulation of speech resulting from lesions of a small area of the left inferolateral prefrontal cortex. Lesions of more anterior and superior cortex induce more subtle deficits, characterized by a general impoverishment of language and trouble in the construction of elaborate propositions; there is a diminution of spontaneous speech production and of the use of dependent clauses.

In humans, as in animals, extensive bilateral lesions involving most or all areas of the prefrontal cortex result in a generalized blunting of affect and emotions. Apathy and neglect characterize the subject's attitude toward others and the environment. Circumscribed lesions of dorsolateral prefrontal cortex induce cognitive deficits but only rarely changes in emotional behavior. On the other hand, in the monkey, orbital lesions result in fear and loss of normal aggressiveness; in the human, the effects are more variable and frequently include disinhibition, abnormal excitability, irritability, and poor ethical judgment. It is worth noting that the high incidence of emotional abnormalities deriving from ventromedial (in contrast to dorsolateral) prefrontal lesions is probably related to the anatomical and functional relationships between the ventromedial prefrontal cortex and the limbic structures of the hypothalamus and the temporal lobe.

Electrophysiology

Slow electrical potentials and sustained changes of neuronal discharge can be recorded from the prefrontal cortex in the time elapsing between a stimulus and a consequent delayed response to it. A surface-negative potential occurring between these two mutually contingent events is commonly known as the contingent negative variation (CNV) or expectancy wave. It may be observed in both humans and animals. Cellular discharge shows important correlations with this field potential. By microelectrode recording in the monkey, large numbers of prefrontal cells can be seen to undergo altered discharge throughout the delay (seconds or minutes) that separates cue from choice in a delay task. The sustained activation of some prefrontal cells during that delay depends on the behavioral significance and the physical attributes of the cue. That of others depends on the characteristics of the impending motor response. Cells of the first type appear to participate in the short-term memory process; those of the second appear to do it in the preparation for movement. The two types of cells are found interspersed in certain areas of dorsolateral prefrontal cortex.

The posterior fringe of the dorsolateral prefrontal cortex bordering the premotor cortex contains the so-called frontal eye fields. Electrical stimulation of sites in these cortical fields elicits conjugate eye movements. The cells within them show increases of discharge in temporal relation to ocular movements. In an animal conditioned to move its eyes in response to a visual stimulus, some cells are activated right after the stimulus, some right before the movement, and still others through the time that separates the two. Thus, like the neurons in the dorsolateral prefrontal cortex at large, but on a shorter timescale, eye field neurons seem to be involved in the temporal integration of sensory stimuli with their consequent motor responses.

Metabolism and Blood Flow

Modern methods yielding images of the working human brain by the use of computer tomography and radioactive tracers reveal that blood flow and metabolic activity increase in prefrontal areas of the cortex during the ideation and programming of speech and motor sequences. Premotor and motor areas mainly show activation during the performance of speech and skeletal movements. In the past few years, neuroimaging has revealed the activation of the human dorsolateral prefrontal cortex during performance of short-term memory tasks. Increased prefrontal metabolism has been demonstrated during memorization of verbal or visual material. The activation of dorsolateral prefrontal and premotor cortices has also been found related to the preparation of movements that are dependent on the material memorized. Therefore, the metabolic studies in the human confirm the basic inferences from neuropsychological and neurophysiological studies in nonhuman primates, namely, that the neuronal populations of dorsolateral prefrontal cortex are involved in the retention of sensory information for prospective action, as well as in the preparation of motor systems for that action. Both are essential for organizing behavior in the time domain.

General Conclusions

In conclusion, the functions of the prefrontal cortex are not yet fully understood, but the evidence from human and animal studies points to a critical role of this cortex in the temporal organization of behavior. The prefrontal cortex may play that role by the coordinated works of at least three subordinate functions, each with a somewhat different topographic representation within the prefrontal region: (1) short-term memory, (2) short-term set for action, and (3) control of interference. Thus, the various sectors of prefrontal cortex, heterogeneous as to connectivity and apparent behavioral function, may cooperate with one another and with other parts of the brain in providing the cognitive support that the organism needs to bridge cross-temporal contingencies and to form goal-directed and temporally extended structures of behavior.

See also: Aphasia: Sudden and Progressive; Brodmann's Areas; Cerebral Cortex; Neocortex: Origins; Prefrontal Cortex: Structure and Anatomy; Prefrontal Contributions to Reward Encoding; Premotor Cortex in Primates: Dorsal and Ventral; Premotor Areas: Medial; Synaptic Plasticity: Learning and Memory in Normal Aging.

Further Reading

Fuster JM (1995) *Memory in the Cerebral Cortex: An Empirical Approach to Neural Networks in the Human and Nonhuman Primate.* Cambridge, MA: MIT Press.

Fuster JM (1997) *The Prefrontal Cortex: Anatomy, Physiology and Neuropsychology of the Frontal Lobe.* Philadelphia, PA: Lippincott-Raven.

Fuster JM (2001) The prefrontal cortex – an update: Time is of the essence. *Neuron* 2: 319–333.

Goldman-Rakic PS (1984) Modular organization of prefrontal cortex. *Trends in Neuroscience* 7: 419–429.

Swartz BE, Halgren E, Fuster JM, Simpkins F, Gee M, and Mandelkern M (1995) Cortical metabolic activation in humans during a visual memory task. *Cerebral Cortex* 3: 205–214.

Prefrontal Cortex: Structure and Anatomy

H Barbas, Boston University, Boston, MA, USA

Overview

The prefrontal cortex has been associated with central executive functions, involved in selecting relevant information and ignoring irrelevant information for the task at hand. To accomplish these functions the prefrontal cortex must have access to information from structures associated with sensory perception, memory, and emotions. Indeed, the prefrontal cortex receives a wealth of information from a large variety of cortical and subcortical structures. In turn, the prefrontal cortex issues projections to the same structures, targeting both excitatory and inhibitory neurons, a pattern that likely underlies the selection of relevant signals and the suppression of irrelevant signals. Within the prefrontal cortex there is division of labor and specialization, so that distinct areas receive and issue topographically organized projections. The participation of different prefrontal sectors in complex behavioral settings appears to be complementary. A key distinction of prefrontal cortex among high-order association areas is its orientation for action, facilitated by its rich and diverse connections with motor control systems.

The prefrontal areas commonly associated with central executive functions are the lateral areas (**Figure 1(b)**), particularly the areas around the posterior principal sulcus and prearcuate region. These areas have a role in cognitive tasks, requiring the selection, retrieval, and temporary holding of information long enough to accomplish a task at hand. The prefrontal cortex, however, has additional components on the medial and orbitofrontal surfaces, which have a key role in the function of the prefrontal cortex (**Figures 1(a)** and **1(c)**). The posterior parts of medial and orbitofrontal cortices belong to the cortical component of the limbic system by virtue of their architecture and connections (**Figure 1**, dark blue). Damage to prefrontal limbic areas in primates has detrimental consequences on emotional behavior and social interactions. The limbic components of the prefrontal cortex have strong connections with the rest of the prefrontal cortex, providing the anatomic basis for the merging of pathways associated with cognitive and emotional processes.

Location of the Prefrontal Cortex in Primates

The frontal lobe extends from the central sulcus to the frontal pole. This large cortical expanse includes about half of the entire cortex in primates. The prefrontal cortex occupies roughly the anterior half of the frontal lobe in macaque monkeys, and about two-thirds in humans. The primary motor cortex, also known as M1 (or area 4 of Brodmann), marks the posterior extent of the frontal lobe, and the premotor cortex (also known as area 6) is interposed between the primary motor and prefrontal cortices (**Figures 1** and **2**). Species other than primates have a prefrontal cortex, and at least in mammals it is found in front of the premotor cortex. In birds, a region thought to be analogous to the prefrontal cortex, on the basis of physiological properties and connections, occupies the posterior pole of the telencephalon.

The prefrontal cortex is greatly expanded and specialized in primates, and its architectonic organization and connections have been studied most widely in nonhuman primates, and more specifically, in macaque monkeys. In this species, the lateral aspect of the prefrontal cortex extends from the arcuate sulcus to the frontal pole (**Figure 1(b)**, light blue). The medial prefrontal cortex lies in front of the medial parts of the premotor cortex –the supplementary motor area (SMA), or MII – and the cingulate motor areas, and extends from the anterior part of the corpus callosum in the anterior cingulate to the medial part of the frontal pole (**Figure 1(a)**). The orbitofrontal cortex occupies the basal aspect of the brain. In macaque monkeys it is located behind the eye socket, and forms a concave shape around the orbit (**Figure 1(c)**). This large cortical region extends from the olfactory areas and the anterior insula to the basal surface of the frontal pole.

Global and Local Architecture

The prefrontal cortex is composed of 13 principal architectonic areas in the human in the classic map of Brodmann (**Figure 2**), and 12 in the nonhuman primate rhesus monkey, as depicted in the map of Walker (**Figure 3**). These classic maps have been modified by several investigators, and nearly all architectonic areas in the macaque monkey prefrontal cortex have been further subdivided into two or more subdivisions, now numbering over 20 in this species. The

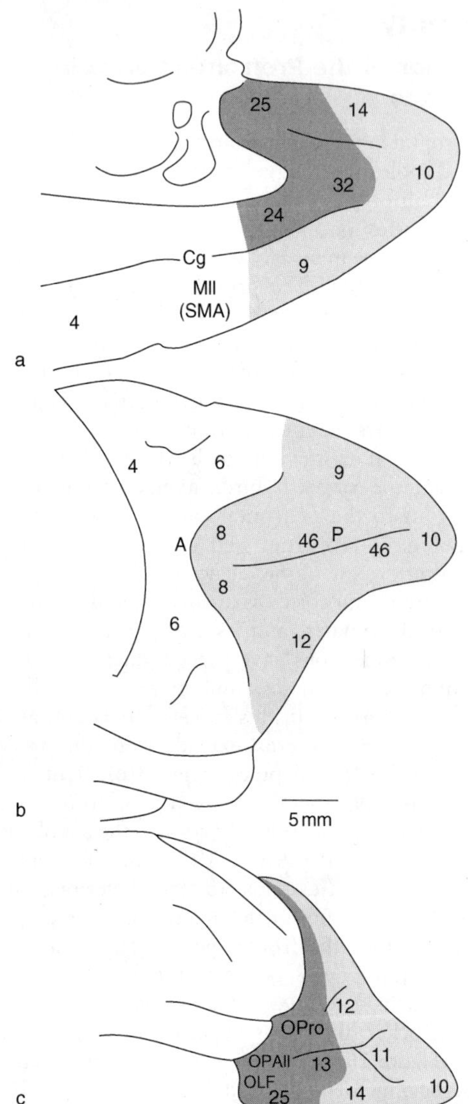

Figure 1 The principal architectonic areas of the prefrontal cortex of the rhesus monkey brain (shaded areas), depicting the (a) medial, (b) lateral, and (c) orbital surfaces. Light blue shading indicates eulaminate areas, with six cortical layers and a distinct granular layer IV. Dark blue shading indicates areas with fewer than six layers (noneulaminate) and which have a poorly developed layer IV (dysgranular) or no granular layer IV (agranular). The prefrontal cortex is bounded posteriorly by the premotor cortices (supplementary motor area MII; SMA) on the medial surface (a), and area 6 on the lateral surface (b). A, arcuate sulcus; Cg, cingulate sulcus; MII SMA, supplementary motor area; OLF, olfactory area; OPAll, orbital periallo cortex; OPro, orbital proisocortex; P, principal sulcus.

classic maps were largely based on brain sections stained for Nissl substance, which labels the cell bodies of neurons and glia. More recent maps have relied on an increasing number of specific neurochemical and molecular markers that aid in delineating architectonic borders by labeling distinct classes of neurons. Nevertheless, the Nissl stain has provided the most reliable information about the organization of the cortex (because architectonic areas vary reliably in overall density) and the relative distribution of neurons in different cortical layers.

The popular name 'frontal granular cortex' is based on the presence of a well-delineated granular layer IV, which is particularly prominent in lateral prefrontal cortex. Most prefrontal areas, including the entire lateral surface, the anterior medial surface, and the anterior orbitofrontal region, have six layers, including a granular layer IV, and thus are called eulaminate (**Figure 1**, light blue). However, the width and density of neurons in layer IV vary widely among prefrontal areas. Layer IV is densest and widest in lateral prefrontal area 8 and posterior area 46 (prearcuate region) of macaque monkeys (**Figure 4**), and least developed in anterior medial and anterior orbitofrontal areas (**Figures 1(a)** and **1(c)**, light blue). But not all prefrontal cortex has a granular layer IV. The most posterior parts of the medial and orbitofrontal cortex have fewer than six layers and are either agranular, meaning that they lack granular layer IV, or dysgranular, meaning that they have a poorly developed layer IV (**Figures 1(a)** and **1(c)**, dark blue). In the posterior orbitofrontal and anterior cingulate areas the deep layers (V and VI) predominate in cell density in comparison with the upper layers (II–III) (**Figure 5**). In contrast, all eulaminate prefrontal areas, and particularly the lateral areas, have a well-developed granular layer IV and a broad layer III, which is densely populated with neurons. The geographically and structurally distinct sectors of the prefrontal cortex have some common connections as well as some specific connections that underlie their specialization.

Common and Specialized Thalamic Connections of Prefrontal Cortices

All prefrontal cortices have bidirectional connections with the mediodorsal (MD) thalamic nucleus. In fact, the prefrontal cortex has often been defined as the cortical region that is connected with the MD thalamic nucleus. This definition is only approximate, because the prefrontal cortex is also connected with thalamic nuclei other than the MD nucleus, and conversely, the MD thalamic nucleus projects to areas outside the classic geographic extent of the prefrontal cortex, albeit more sparsely. Nevertheless, the MD thalamic nucleus is robustly connected with all prefrontal cortices in a topographic manner. Lateral prefrontal cortices are connected with the lateral

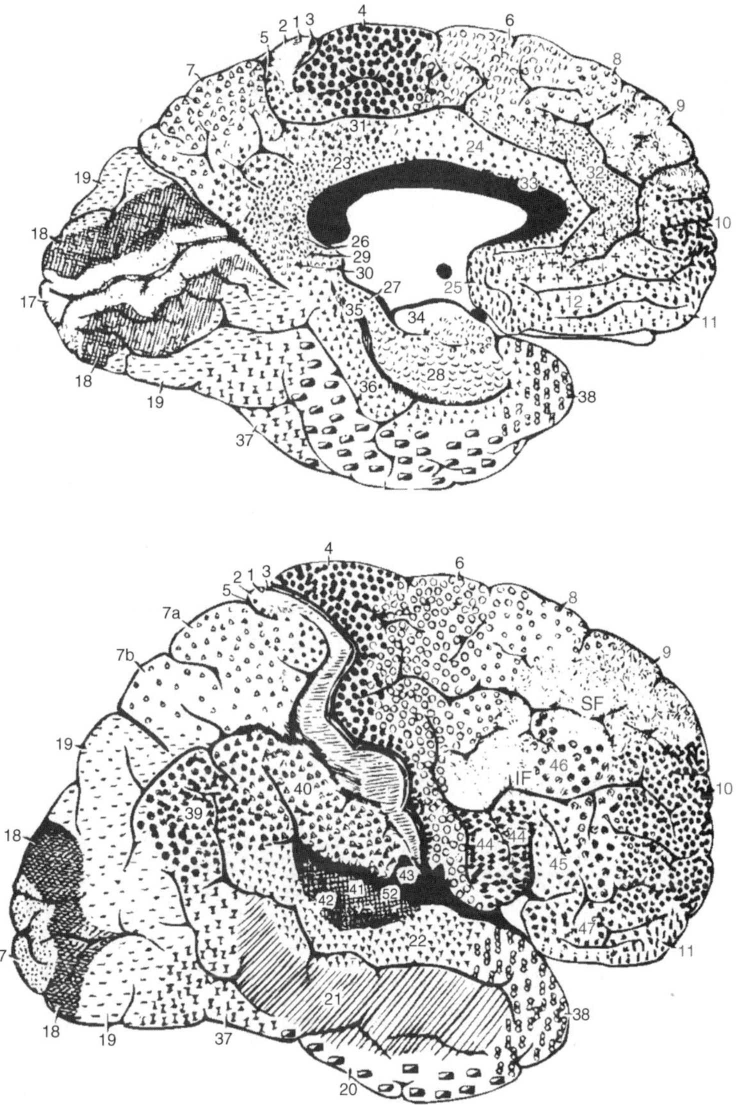

Figure 2 The architectonic map of the human cortex by Brodmann. Prefrontal areas are shown by numbers in red. The medial surface is shown on the top, and the lateral surface is shown on the bottom. IF, inferior frontal sulcus; SF, superior frontal sulcus.

parts of the MD thalamic nucleus, including its most lateral or multiform sector, and with the adjacent parvicellular sector. 'Multiform' refers to the various shapes of neurons, and 'parvicellular' refers to the small size of neurons. Medial and orbitofrontal cortices are connected mainly with the medial, or magnocellular (large cell), sector of the MD thalamic nucleus.

In addition to their connections with the MD thalamic nucleus, the prefrontal cortex is connected with other thalamic nuclei, including the ventral anterior, the medial pulvinar, intralaminar, medial, and anterior nuclei. Lateral prefrontal areas are connected primarily with the MD thalamic nucleus, and have only sparse connections with midline nuclei, but they have connections with some intralaminar nuclei and the medial pulvinar. On the other hand, orbitofrontal and posterior medial prefrontal areas have significant connections with midline and intralaminar nuclei, anterior nuclei, and the medial pulvinar, but still have substantial thalamic connections with the MD thalamic nucleus.

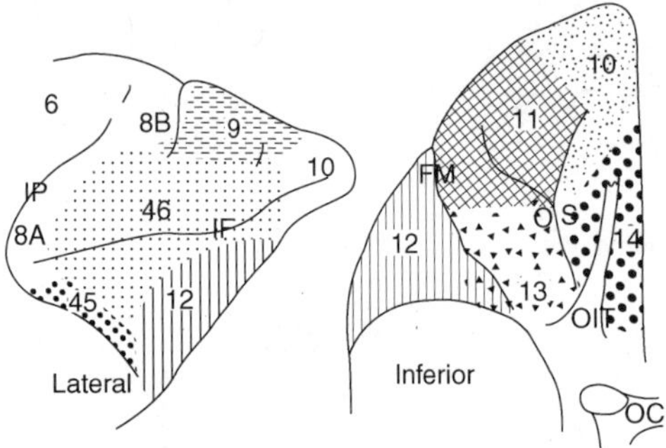

Figure 3 Architectonic areas of the rhesus monkey prefrontal cortex according to the map of Walker. The lateral surface is on the left, the orbital surface (inferior) is on the right; the medial surface is not shown.

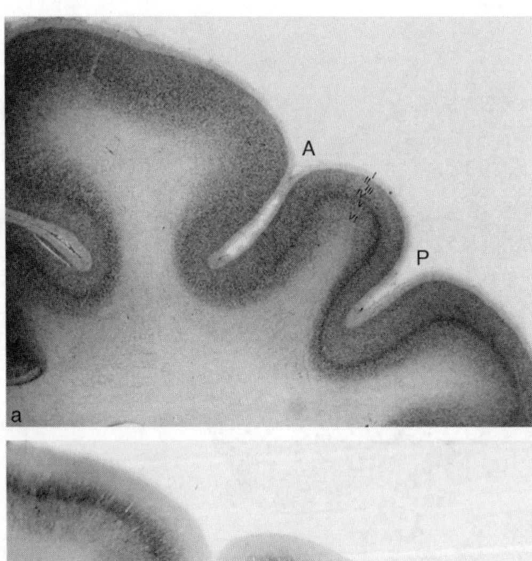

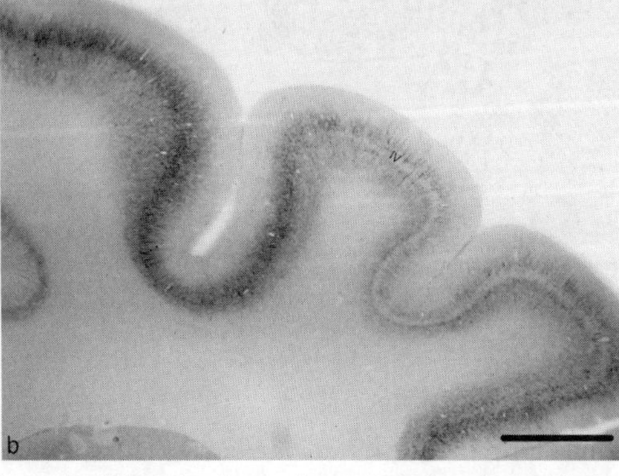

Figure 4 Example of granular prefrontal cortices. (a) Cross section (coronal) through the posterior part of prefrontal cortex of a macaque monkey (*Macaca nemestrina*), showing granular prefrontal cortex within the lateral bank of the arcuate sulcus (A) and adjacent cortex (to the right), and within the banks of the principal sulcus (P). The section was stained with cresyl violet to show the cell bodies and glia. Roman numerals indicate cortical layers. (b) A section at about the same level through the prefrontal cortex of a rhesus monkey brain stained with an antibody to neurofilament protein (SMI-32), which labels neurons in layers II–III and V–VI but not in layer IV. The empty zone in this frame shows clearly the position of granular layer IV. Medial is to the left. Scale bar = 3 mm.

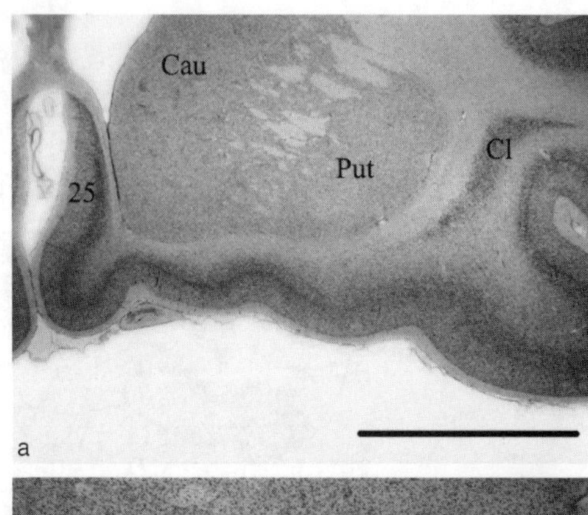

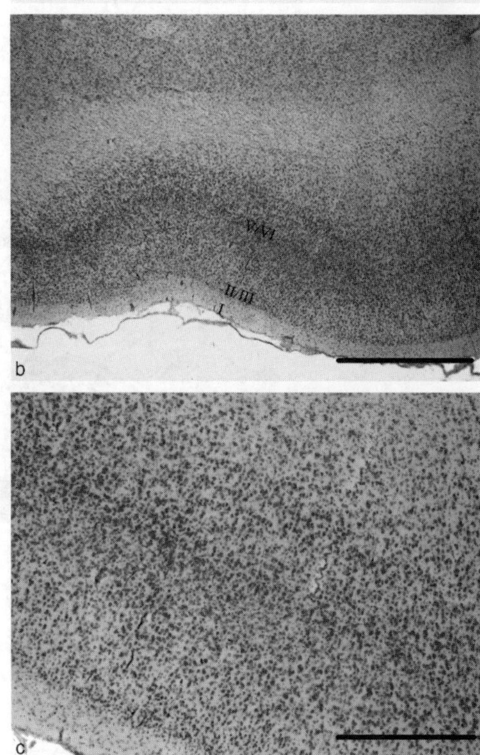

Figure 5 Example of agranular and dysgranular prefrontal cortices. (a) Low-power brightfield photomicrograph showing agranular- and dysgranular-type cortex on a coronal section through the orbitofrontal region of a macaque monkey (*Macaca nemestrina*) stained for Nissl substance. Area 25 on the medial surface is also dysgranular. (b, c) The orbitofrontal cortex at higher magnifications. Medial is to the left. Scale bar = 5 mm (a), 1 mm (b), 400 μm (c). Cau, caudate; Cl, claustrum; Put, putamen.

Specialized Connections of Prefrontal Cortices with Other Cortical Systems

Projections from Sensory Association Areas to Prefrontal Cortices

One of the key sources of information to the prefrontal cortex comes from most cortical sensory and polymodal association areas. The primary koniocortices ('dustlike'), which include visual area V1, somatosensory area 3b, and auditory area A1, do not project directly to the prefrontal cortex. On the lateral surface of the prefrontal cortex, projections from visual association cortices reach several areas in the prearcuate region, targeting robustly area 8, which includes the frontal eye fields, and the posterior extent of the principal sulcus (area 46) and lateral area 12. Auditory association cortices project to several sites within the lateral prefrontal cortex, targeting robustly the frontal polar cortex (area 10), several sites of the dorsal bank of the principal sulcus (area 46), and the anterior tips of the limbs of the arcuate sulcus, including the anterior part of dorsal area 8, and area 9. Projections from somatosensory cortices reach the central portion of the principal sulcus (ventral area 46) and the subadjacent area 12. Cortices which are not unimodal, identified as those with neurons that respond to stimuli from two or more modalities, project to prefrontal cortices as well. On the lateral surface these projections originate mostly from the depths of the upper bank of the superior temporal sulcus, and to a lesser extent from the inferior parietal lobule.

Medial prefrontal areas receive projections from auditory association cortices, from polymodal areas in the depths of the upper bank of the superior temporal sulcus and perirhinal region, and only sparse projections from either visual or somatosensory association cortices. The orbitofrontal cortex, on the other hand, receives projections from all unimodal sensory cortices, including the primary olfactory cortices, and visual, auditory, somatosensory, and gustatory association cortices, as well as from polymodal association areas in the superior temporal and perirhinal regions.

There is a big difference in the topography of sensory projections to prefrontal cortices. The prearcuate cortex receives projections from posterior visual association areas, which represent relatively early stages of visual processing. The frontal eye fields seem to be specialized for processing signals from a large variety of visual association cortices, extending from as far back as V2 in the occipital region, up to the anterior parts of the inferior temporal visual association cortices. In contrast, orbitofrontal cortices receive projections from anterior inferior temporal cortices, where the visual receptive fields are global.

There is a comparable organization in the projections from auditory association areas to prefrontal cortices. The prearcuate cortex (area 8; at the tip of the upper limb of the arcuate sulcus) and posterior area 46 receive projections from posterior auditory association cortices in the superior temporal gyrus; these cortices are comparatively close to the primary auditory cortex. In contrast, orbitofrontal and medial prefrontal areas receive projections from the anterior superior temporal gyrus, from areas that process signals associated with species-specific vocalizations in nonhuman primates. Similarly, projections from other sensory association areas to the posterior orbitofrontal cortex originate in late-processing sensory association cortices. Visual input to orbitofrontal cortex, for example, originates in the anterior inferior temporal cortex, where neurons have large visual receptive fields and have a role in visual memory. The only exception is the input from primary olfactory areas to posterior orbitofrontal cortices.

Interface of Prefrontal Projections with Excitatory and Inhibitory Systems

One of the fundamental functional attributes of the prefrontal cortex is the selection of relevant signals and the suppression of irrelevant signals in behavior. This function can be illustrated by the interaction of prefrontal cortices with temporal auditory association cortices. Damage to the lateral prefrontal cortex after a stroke, or in pathological aging, impairs the ability of humans to ignore irrelevant auditory stimuli and thus to follow a conversation in a noisy environment. This function is likely mediated through robust projections from prefrontal cortices to auditory association cortices. Long-distance prefrontal pathways to sensory cortices are excitatory in nature, but they interface with both excitatory and inhibitory systems in auditory association areas. These pathways may form the anatomic substrate for choosing relevant signals and ignoring irrelevant signals. Similar interactions occur between medial prefrontal areas and auditory association areas. Interestingly, medial prefrontal areas in the anterior cingulate are hypoactive in schizophrenia, which likely affects medial prefrontal to temporal cortical communication. The same types of interactions with both excitatory and inhibitory systems occur between prefrontal and parietal cortices, as well as with other sensory and high-order association cortices.

Pathways Related to Specific Aspects of Memory Processing in the Prefrontal Cortex

Lateral Prefrontal Areas and Working Memory

Posterior lateral prefrontal areas are robustly and bidirectionally connected with lateral intraparietal areas, a region associated with visuomotor functions. Connections with the visuomotor parts of the lateral intraparietal cortex are restricted to the prearcuate region, including the cortex within the anterior bank of the arcuate sulcus and the adjacent cortex (area 8), and to the posterior quarter of the principal sulcus (caudal area 46) in macaque monkeys. The prearcuate and lateral intraparietal cortices have in common a role in selective attention, required in cognitive operations. The strong and bidirectional connections that link these distant cortices suggest that they may function in concert in cognitive operations. The posterior cingulate cortex, which has a role in oculomotor responses and attentional processes, is also connected with the prearcuate cortex.

Posterior Medial and Orbitofrontal Areas and Long-Term Memory

Medial and orbitofrontal cortices are robustly connected with structures associated with long-term memory. These areas include the perirhinal region (areas 35 and 36), the entorhinal cortex (area 28), and the parahippocampal cortex (areas TF and TH). In addition, posterior orbitofrontal areas, and especially medial prefrontal cortices in the anterior cingulate, receive projections from the hippocampal formation, originating from the subiculum, presubiculum, and CA1 fields. Posterior medial prefrontal areas share long-term memory functions with the hippocampus, and their damage in humans results in memory deficits.

Pathways for Emotional Processing

Among prefrontal cortices, the posterior orbitofrontal and posterior medial cortices have the heaviest connections with the amygdala, a group of nuclei in the temporal lobe associated with emotional processing. Most of these connections involve the basal complex of the amygdala, especially the basolateral nucleus, and to a lesser extent the cortical and lateral nuclei. The projections of the posterior orbitofrontal cortex with the amygdala are particularly specialized, as they terminate heavily onto a group of nuclei known as the intercalated masses, which are composed of inhibitory neurons and have a role in the internal processing of the amygdala. The connections of posterior orbitofrontal areas are with the posterior half of the amygdala, which, in turn, receives projections from all sensory association cortices (**Figure 6**). One hypothesis is that the rich direct and indirect sensory inputs to posterior orbitofrontal cortices underlie the process through which events acquire emotional significance.

Posterior medial prefrontal cortices also have substantial connections with the amygdala. Projections from posterior medial prefrontal cortices reach heavily the output nuclei of the amygdala to hypothalamic and brain stem autonomic centers, and also terminate onto hypothalamic autonomic centers (**Figure 7**). In monkeys, posterior medial prefrontal cortices in the

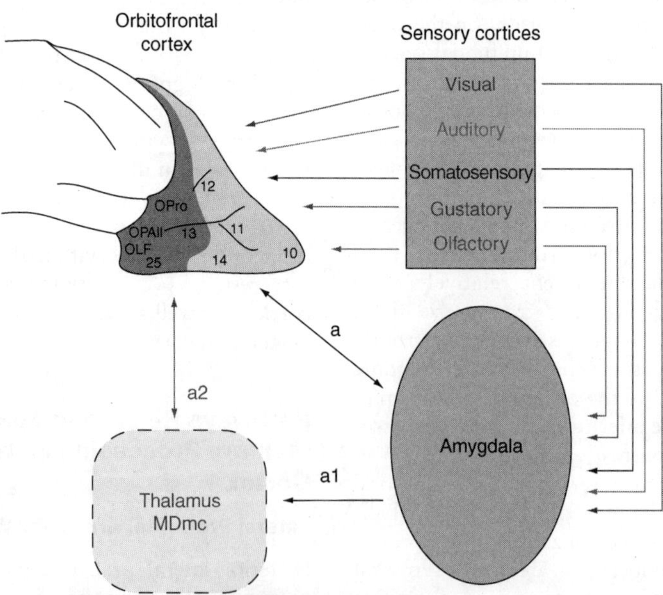

Figure 6 Multiple sources of projections to orbitofrontal cortices. Projections from sensory association cortices reach orbitofrontal cortex as well as the amygdala, which has bidirectional connections with orbitofrontal cortex (pathway a). The amygdala also projects to the medial (magnocellular) part of the mediodorsal thalamic nucleus (MDmc, pathway a1), which has bidirectional connections with the orbitofrontal cortex (pathway a2). Connections of sensory association cortices with orbitofrontal cortex, or with the amygdala, are also bidirectional (not shown). Architectonic areas indicated by letters are: OLF, olfactory area; OPAll, orbital periallo cortex; OPro, orbital prosiocortex.

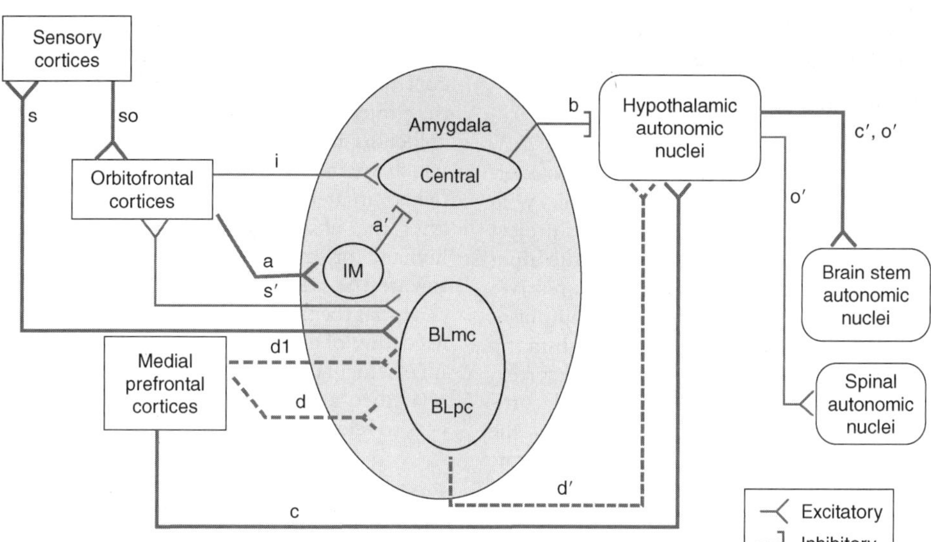

Figure 7 Summary of the connections of orbitofrontal and medial prefrontal cortices associated with perception and expression of emotions. The orbitofrontal cortex and the amygdala receive projections from every sensory modality through the cortex (pathways so, s), and are robustly connected with each other, providing the structural basis for direct (so) and indirect (s′) sensory information to the orbitofrontal cortex. Orbitofrontal axons terminate heavily in the intercalated masses (IMs) of the amygdala (pathway a), which then project to the central nucleus of the amygdala (pathway a′). The central nucleus projects to hypothalamic autonomic nuclei (pathway b). A direct pathway (c) from posterior medial prefrontal cortex reaches hypothalamic autonomic nuclei, which project to brain stem autonomic nuclei (pathway c′) and to spinal autonomic nuclei (pathway o′). Medial prefrontal cortices also project to the parvicellular basolateral nucleus of the amygdala (BLpc, pathway d), and to the magnocellular basolateral nucleus of the amygdala (BLmc, pathway d1), which project to hypothalamic autonomic nuclei (pathway d′), providing sequential pathways through which posterior medial prefrontal areas may influence hypothalamic autonomic nuclei (dotted pathways). A lighter pathway from orbitofrontal cortex terminates directly on the central nucleus of the amygdala (pathway i). Thickness of the lines represents the density of the projections. Red, inhibitory pathways; green, excitatory pathways. Reproduced from Barbas H, Saha S, Rempel-Clower N, and Ghashghaei HT (2003) Serial pathways from primate prefrontal cortex to autonomic areas may influence emotional expression. *BMC Neuroscience* 4:25, copyright 2003 Barbas H et al; licensee BioMed Central Ltd.

anterior cingulate region have a direct role in vocalization associated with emotional communication, emitted in fear or distress, such as at the sight of a predator.

Connections of Prefrontal Cortices with Neurotransmitter-Specific Systems

Like other cortical systems, the prefrontal cortex receives projections from modulatory neurotransmitter systems, including cholinergic projections from the basal forebrain, noradrenergic projections from the locus coeruleus, dopaminergic projections from the substantia nigra/ventral tegmental area, and serotonergic projections from the raphe nuclei. These systems have a role in the attentional and cognitive functions of the prefrontal cortex. In macaque monkeys and rats, the strongest interactions of the basal forebrain are with orbitofrontal and posterior medial prefrontal cortices and are distinct for being bidirectional, in contrast with other prefrontal cortices, which receive, but do not send, projections to the basal forebrain.

In the lateral prefrontal cortex a delicate balance in the availability of dopamine and noradrenaline appears to be crucial in optimal performance on working memory tasks in nonhuman primates. These functions are thought to be mediated through projections from neurotransmitter-specific systems, which target dopamine receptors of the D1 type, and adrenergic receptors of the α-2A type. Disruption of the optimal levels of these neurotransmitters in stress impairs performance on working memory tasks. Imbalance in the neurotransmitter equilibrium in prefrontal cortex may underlie attention-deficit/hyperactivity disorder in humans.

Another system with widespread connections to all sectors of the prefrontal cortex is the hypothalamus, which projects widely to all prefrontal cortices, but has bidirectional connections only with posterior orbitofrontal and posterior medial prefrontal cortices (**Figures 1(a)** and **1(c)**, dark blue). Some of these projections from the hypothalamus to the cortex may be histaminergic, constituting yet another neurochemically distinct pathway.

Common Connections of Prefrontal Cortices with Motor Control Systems

Linkage of Prefrontal Cortices with the Basal Ganglia

The prefrontal cortex is in an ideal position to exercise executive control through its multiple links with motor control systems. All prefrontal cortices project to the neostriatum (caudate and putamen), the input center of the basal ganglia. The neostriatum receives projections from all cortical areas, but the output of the basal ganglia (the globus pallidus and substantia nigra reticulata) reaches selectively the frontal cortex, including the motor/premotor and prefrontal cortices. Information from the basal ganglia reaches the frontal cortex indirectly, through specific thalamic nuclei. The principal nuclei involved in this system, as it pertains to the prefrontal cortex, are the mediodorsal nucleus and the ventral anterior nucleus, and to a lesser extent the anterior medial nucleus, all of which have bidirectional connections with the prefrontal cortex. Distinct prefrontal areas are influenced by the basal ganglia through parallel pathways, suggesting that they have specific roles in behavior. However, the segregation of pathways through the basal ganglia is relative rather than absolute, so that the pathway from lateral prefrontal cortices to the basal ganglia through the thalamus reaches not only lateral prefrontal cortices, but the adjacent premotor cortex as well. These connections suggest that lateral prefrontal cortices have multiple interactions with premotor cortices for action.

The projections of the prefrontal cortex are directed to the anterior part of the neostriatum, terminating mostly in the caudate nucleus. These projections have a certain degree of topographic organization, so that lateral prefrontal areas reach mostly the dorsal part of the caudate nucleus, medial areas project to a more medial position within the caudate, and posterior orbitofrontal cortices project to the ventral striatum. The latter is also known as the limbic striatum, and is also connected with the amygdala and the hippocampus. The limbic striatum projects through a relay in the ventral pallidum to the medial (magnocellular) part of the mediodorsal thalamic nucleus, which has strong bidirectional connections with the posterior orbitofrontal cortex (**Figure** 6) and the anterior cingulate.

Specialized Connections of Prefrontal Areas with Motor Control Systems

Lateral Prefrontal Cortices Are Linked with Brain Stem and Cortical Premotor Systems

Prearcuate prefrontal cortices are connected with neighboring premotor areas, which, in turn, are connected with the motor cortex, suggesting that the prefrontal cortex has close access to cortical motor control systems. Another specialized motor circuit is the projection of the frontal eye fields to the superior colliculus and brain stem oculomotor control systems, which are involved in eye movements. The frontal eye fields, situated within cortical area 8, were so named after the observation that damage to the area in humans or monkeys temporarily shifted the eyes toward the side of the lesion. It subsequently became clear that the frontal eye fields are not necessary for the execution of eye movements. It is now known that the involvement of the frontal eye fields in eye movement is related to attentional processes and to orienting the eyes to relevant stimuli in the environment.

Posterior Parts of Medial and Orbitofrontal Cortices Have Access to Central Efferent Autonomic Structures

The medial and orbitofrontal cortices have a different role in motor control. The posterior orbitofrontal cortex and, especially, the anterior cingulate cortex are connected with hypothalamic and brain stem autonomic structures (**Figure** 7), which innervate peripheral organs, such as the heart, the lungs, and the gut, the activities of which are markedly changed in emotional arousal. These prefrontal areas, therefore, have a role in motor control associated with emotional expression. These circuits are consistent with evidence that damage to orbitofrontal cortex in humans impairs the ability to respond appropriately in emotional situations. Conversely, overactivity of the orbitofrontal cortex is seen in patients with anxiety disorder and obsessive–compulsive disease.

Medial prefrontal cortices have an additional specialization within the motor domain, namely emotional vocalization, effected through a projection to brain stem structures that innervate laryngeal muscles necessary for phonation. This pathway has a role in emotional communication, such as the characteristic cries emitted by monkeys in emotional distress.

There are also other projections from orbitofrontal and, especially, anterior cingulate cortices to central autonomic structures targeting noncholinergic parts of the basal forebrain. One of these basal forebrain regions is the ventral striatopallidum, found in the dorsal half of the basal forebrain, and another is the extended amygdala, which is made up of groups of neurons scattered from the central nucleus of the amygdala through the basal forebrain to the bed nucleus of the stria terminalis. These specialized pathways provide parallel avenues from anterior cingulate and posterior orbitofrontal cortex to central autonomic structures.

Functional Relatedness of Cortical and Subcortical Connections of Prefrontal Cortices

Structures that are anatomically connected collaborate in distinct functions. For example, lateral prefrontal cortices in the posterior part of the principal sulcus and the adjacent prearcuate cortex have a role in working memory, as do the parts of the MD thalamic nucleus with which they are bidirectionally linked. Experimental inactivation of the lateral prefrontal cortex disrupts neuronal responses in the MD thalamic nucleus, observed during working memory tasks, suggesting the interdependence of these structures in behavior. The frontal eye fields have additional thalamic connections with intralaminar neurons, and in both structures neurons have visual and visuomotor properties. The prearcuate and lateral intraparietal regions are also strongly connected bidirectionally, and both have a role in oculomotor responses related to cognitive operations.

Posterior orbitofrontal and anterior cingulate areas are connected with the magnocellular part of the MD thalamic nucleus and with midline and anterior thalamic nuclei, and all of these structures have a common role in long-term memory and emotional memory. Similarly, the polymodal nature of projections to the posterior orbitofrontal region is matched by an equally polymodal input from the same high-order sensory association cortices to the amygdala (**Figure 6**). In turn, the amygdala and the orbitofrontal cortices have strong bidirectional connections, involving the same parts of the amygdala that receive input from sensory and polymodal cortices (**Figure 7**). Finally, medial prefrontal cortices have the strongest connections with central autonomic structures in several distinct brain regions. These pathways include hypothalamic and brain stem autonomic centers, basal forebrain structures, and nuclei of the amygdala that are preferentially connected with central autonomic structures.

Summary

Specialized sectors of the prefrontal cortex have a distinct set of connections and complementary roles in cognition, memory, and emotion. Cortical input to each prefrontal sector is complemented by connections with functionally related subcortical structures. The connections of the prefrontal cortex with the MD thalamic nucleus appear to unify them as one cortical region, though they occur with topographically and functionally distinct sectors of the MD thalamic nucleus, consistent with the specialization of each region in cognitive, mnemonic, and emotional operations.

Notwithstanding the distinctiveness of the set of connections of each prefrontal sector, there are connections between prefrontal sectors, suggesting that they function synergistically in behavior. Moreover, the different sectors of the prefrontal cortex target specific layers of each other, in an intricate but highly ordered communication system. The posterior orbitofrontal and anterior cingulate areas, for example, issue projections through their deep layers, and their axons terminate in the upper layers of eulaminate prefrontal cortices, especially layer I, suggesting 'feedback' communication. Conversely, eulaminate prefrontal areas communicate with anterior cingulate and orbitofrontal cortices through their supragranular layers (layers II–III), and their axons reach the middle–deep layers of noneulaminate cingulate and posterior orbitofrontal cortices. Reciprocity of connections is a common feature in cortical systems and appears to be fundamental to normal function. In their participation in bidirectional circuits, posterior orbitofrontal and the anterior cingulate cortices may function as feedback systems to the neuraxis. The frequent involvement of posterior medial and orbitofrontal cortices in neurologic and psychiatric diseases may be related to disconnection of feedback systems necessary for the synthesis of cognition, memory, and emotions, as these areas are linked with other parts of the prefrontal cortex.

See also: Emotion Systems and the Brain; Frontal Cortex Evolution in Primates; Frontal Eye Fields; Orbitofrontal Cortex: Visual Functions; Prefrontal Cortex; Reward Neurophysiology and Orbitofrontal Cortex.

Further Reading

Alexander GE, Delong MR, and Strick PL (1986) Parallel organization of functionally segregated circuits linking basal ganglia and cortex. *Annual Review of Neuroscience* 9: 357–381.

Arnsten AF and Li BM (2005) Neurobiology of executive functions: Catecholamine influences on prefrontal cortical functions. *Biological Psychiatry* 57: 1377–1384.

Barbas H, Ghashghaei H, Rempel-Clower N, et al. (2002) Anatomic basis of functional specialization in prefrontal cortices in primates. In: Grafman J (ed.) *Handbook of Neuropsychology*, pp. 1–27. Amsterdam: Elsevier Science B.V.

Brodmann K (1909) *Vergleichende Lokalizationslehre der Grosshirnrinde*. Leipzig: Barth.

Chao LL and Knight RT (1997) Prefrontal deficits in attention and inhibitory control with aging. *Cerebral Cortex* 7: 63–69.

Damasio AR (1994) *Descarte's Error: Emotion, Reason, and the Human Brain*. New York: G. P. Putnam's Sons.

DeOlmos JS and Heimer L (1999) The concepts of the ventral striatopallidal system and extended amygdala. *Annals of the New York Academy of Sciences* 877: 1–32.

Foote SL and Morrison JH (1987) Extrathalamic modulation of cortical function. *Annual Review of Neuroscience* 10: 67–95.

Fuster JM (1989) *The Prefrontal Cortex*. New York: Raven Press.

Goldman-Rakic PS (1988) Topography of cognition: Parallel distributed networks in primate association cortex. *Annual Review of Neuroscience* 11: 137–156.

Joel D and Weiner I (1994) The organization of the basal ganglia–thalamocortical circuits: Open interconnected rather than closed segregated. *Neuroscience* 63(2): 363–379.

Lynch JC and Tian JR (2005) Cortico-cortical networks and cortico-subcortical loops for the higher control of eye movements. *Progress in Brain Research* 151: 461–501.

McFarland NR and Haber SN (2002) Thalamic relay nuclei of the basal ganglia form both reciprocal and nonreciprocal cortical connections, linking multiple frontal cortical areas. *Journal of Neuroscience* 22: 8117–8132.

Nauta WJH (1979) Expanding borders of the limbic system concept. In: Rasmussen T and Marino R (eds.) *Functional Neurosurgery*, pp. 7–23. New York: Raven Press.

Neafsey EJ (1990) Prefrontal cortical control of the autonomic nervous system: Anatomical and physiological observations. *Progress in Brain Research* 85: 147–166.

Petrides M (1996) Lateral frontal cortical contribution to memory. *Seminars in the Neurosciences* 8: 57–63.

Rose J and Colombo M (2005) Neural correlates of executive control in the avian brain. *PLoS Biology* 3: e190.

Usher M, Cohen JD, Servan-Schreiber D, et al. (1999) The role of locus coeruleus in the regulation of cognitive performance. *Science* 283: 549–554.

Uylings HB, Groenewegen HJ, and Kolb B (2003) Do rats have a prefrontal cortex? *Behavioral Brain Research* 146: 3–17.

Walker AE (1940) A cytoarchitectural study of the prefrontal area of the macaque monkey. *Journal of Comparative Neurology* 73: 59–86.

Relevant Website

http://brainmaps.org – Interactive high-resolution brain atlas (Regents of the University of California, Davis campus).

Prosopagnosia

D Tranel and N L Denburg, University of Iowa Hospitals and Clinics, Iowa City, IA, USA

Introduction

Prosopagnosia is a neurological term of Greek origin (Greek *prosop*, face, + a + Greek *gnosis*, to know), used to denote a condition in which patients lose the ability to recognize familiar faces. The disorder is confined to the visual realm, and the affected patient cannot arrive at the meaning of some or all previously known faces, despite normal or near-normal visual perception and intact alertness, attention, intelligence, and language. Most patients manifest a comparable defect in the anterograde compartment; that is, they cannot learn new faces despite adequate exposure. Prosopagnosia is usually caused by cerebrovascular disease, head injury, or cerebral tumors. In some instances, it can occur in the setting of a degenerative condition such as Alzheimer's disease, although in these cases it is usually part of more widespread neuropsychological dilapidation. Finally, prosopagnosia can arise during early childhood, with deficits presumably present from birth.

Prosopagnosia (or face agnosia) is the most frequent and well established of the visual agnosias. The phenomenon has been noted since the nineteenth century, and it has been the focus of considerable scientific inquiry. The fascination with prosopagnosia stems from the oddity of the disorder, along with the opportunity it provides to investigate perception, learning, and recall of complex and unique knowledge. From a clinical standpoint, the condition is also important, and given its devastating effect on its victims, accurate diagnosis and management are essential. Investigation of prosopagnosia has been marked by controversy regarding the relative importance of perceptual versus mnestic factors in the development of the condition and a dispute about whether prosopagnosia requires bilateral lesions or can be caused by unilateral damage.

Neuropsychological and Neuroanatomical Correlates of Prosopagnosia

The face recognition defect in prosopagnosia typically covers both the retrograde and anterograde compartments. Patients can no longer recognize the faces of previously known individuals and are unable to learn new ones. They are unable to recognize the faces of family members, close friends, and in the most paradigmatic instances, even their own face in a mirror. On seeing those faces, the patients experience no sense of familiarity, no inkling that those faces are known to them; that is, they fail to conjure up consciously any pertinent information that would trigger recognition. However, the recognition disorder is confined to the visual modality, and recognition via other modalities (e.g., hearing recognizable voices) is unaffected.

As with other forms of agnosia, prosopagnosia must be distinguished from disorders of naming, that is, it is not an inability to name faces of persons who are otherwise recognized as familiar. There are numerous examples of face naming failure, from both brain-injured populations and the realm of normal everyday experience, but in such instances, the unnamed face is invariably detected as familiar, and the precise identity of the possessor of the face is usually apprehended accurately. In prosopagnosia, however, the defect sets in at the level of recognition. Needless to say, the patients will also manifest a face naming impairment (they will not name faces they cannot recognize), but this is artifactual and not a true naming defect. Several major types of prosopagnosia can be distinguished.

Pure Associative Prosopagnosia

In this variety, the recognition impairment is relatively pure in the sense that it is confined to the visual modality and occurs in the setting of normal or near-normal visual perception. Associative prosopagnosia largely conforms to the strict definition of agnosia, that is, "a normal percept stripped of its meaning" (Teuber's classic definition of agnosia; Teuber, 1968: 274–328). The patients perform normally on standard neuropsychological tests of visuoperceptual discrimination and visuospatial judgment. As noted, recognition via other sensory modalities is unaffected, and on hearing the voices of individuals whose faces go unrecognized, the patients will instantly recognize the identities of those individuals. Even within the visual modality, the defect is highly circumscribed. For instance, patients may be able to recognize individuals on the basis of a distinctive feature (e.g., hairstyle) or gait or posture.

Most patients with pure associative prosopagnosia also have achromatopsia, an acquired impairment of color perception. The combination of the defects is due to the contiguity of the neural processing systems for form and color and their sweeping damage by one lesion. The color perception defect *per se*, however, does not account for the face recognition impairment, and normal individuals can easily recognize faces in black-and-white. The ability to read may or may not

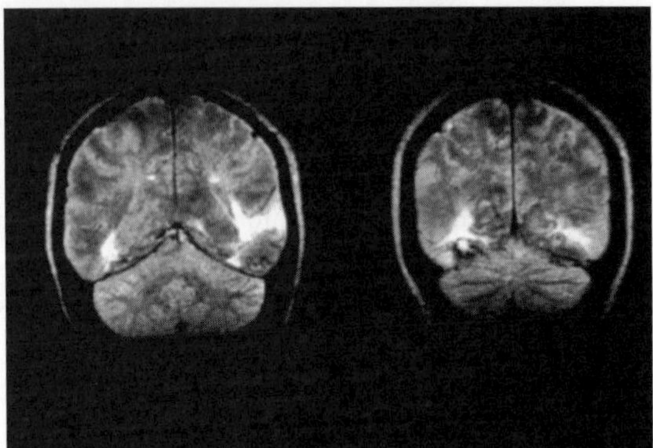

Figure 1 Illustration of the neuroanatomic findings of a patient with pure associative prosopagnosia.

be affected in prosopagnosia patients, depending on the location of the lesion in the left occipital region. When the lesion encompasses both the left occipitotemporal region and the left periventricular region (the white matter beside, beneath, and behind the occipital horn), reading impairment (alexia) coexists with prosopagnosia.

Pure associative prosopagnosia is caused by bilateral damage in inferior occipital and temporal visual association cortices, that is, in the inferior component of cytoarchitectonic areas 18 and 19 and part of the nearby cytoarchitectonic area 37 (see **Figures 1** and **2** for an illustration of the neuroanatomic findings in such a patient). Most cases are due to cerebral infarctions caused by occlusion in posterior cerebral artery branches. Head injury and cerebral tumors, especially gliomas originating in one occipital lobe and traversing into the opposite hemisphere via the splenium of the corpus callosum, can also produce prosopagnosia. Prosopagnosia in connection with lesions (bilateral or unilateral) located exclusively above the calcarine fissure, in superior visual association cortices, has never been reported, although there are cases of face agnosia in which on one or both sides, the inferior lesions extend upward above the calcarine fissure.

Apperceptive Prosopagnosia

Face agnosia in the setting of significant visuoperceptual disturbance has been termed 'apperceptive' prosopagnosia. Apperceptive face agnosics have defects in basic visual perception, demonstrable on neuropsychological testing, which compromise abilities such as matching of unfamiliar faces, judgment of line orientations, and mental manipulation of pictures and picture fragments. It should be noted, however, that such defects are not so severe as to compromise most aspects of basic form vision; thus, the condition conforms in a broad sense to the definition of agnosia. As in other forms of recognition, perceptual processes on the one hand and recognition–recall processes on the other cannot be rigidly compartmentalized. Even in 'pure' cases of associative prosopagnosia, there may be fairly subtle, albeit important, disturbances of high-level integrative perceptual abilities which cannot be detected by available probes. Also, any explanation of face agnosia tied to perceptual factors must reconcile the fact that most patients with visual perceptual defects, even severe ones, do not lose their ability to recognize faces. That is, visuoperceptual disturbance as detected by neuropsychological probes does not necessarily cause face agnosia. For these reasons, it is useful to maintain a distinction between associative and apperceptive prosopagnosia because generally it is possible to determine whether the condition is largely due to memory defects (associative) or to high-level perceptual defects (apperceptive).

Apperceptive face agnosia is most often associated with bilateral damage to 'early' visual association cortices or with damage in right visual association cortices within the occipital and parietal regions. It appears that the damage must involve both the inferior and superior components of posterior visual association cortices (areas 18 and 19), mesially and laterally, for severe and lasting face agnosia to develop. In most cases, parts of areas 39 and 37 on the right will also be damaged. **Figure 3** illustrates the neuroanatomic findings in such a patient.

Developmental Prosopagnosia

Some individuals never develop a normal capacity for learning faces. They have a lifelong deficiency in learning and recognizing faces that ought to have been readily mastered, and since the problem begins in childhood, it is appropriate to call it 'developmental' prosopagnosia. Developmental prosopagnosia has not been widely reported or studied, but it may be far more frequent than suspected, its apparent rarity being because affected persons tend to conceal their disability. It is probably associated with learning disability for other classes of visual stimuli which, like faces, require individual identification and have many similar exemplars. Neural correlates for this condition are in the early stages of being identified, and the findings point to the potentially important role of the midfusiform gyrus and the inferior occipital gyrus. The youngest documented case of developmental prosopagnosia was recently reported. Briefly, patient AT was studied at approximately 5 years of age. AT has both a negative medical history and a negative MRI of the brain. Intellect falls in the very superior range, and he came to medical attention during preschool because of problems recognizing individuals who were well known to him. AT's difficulties are mainly

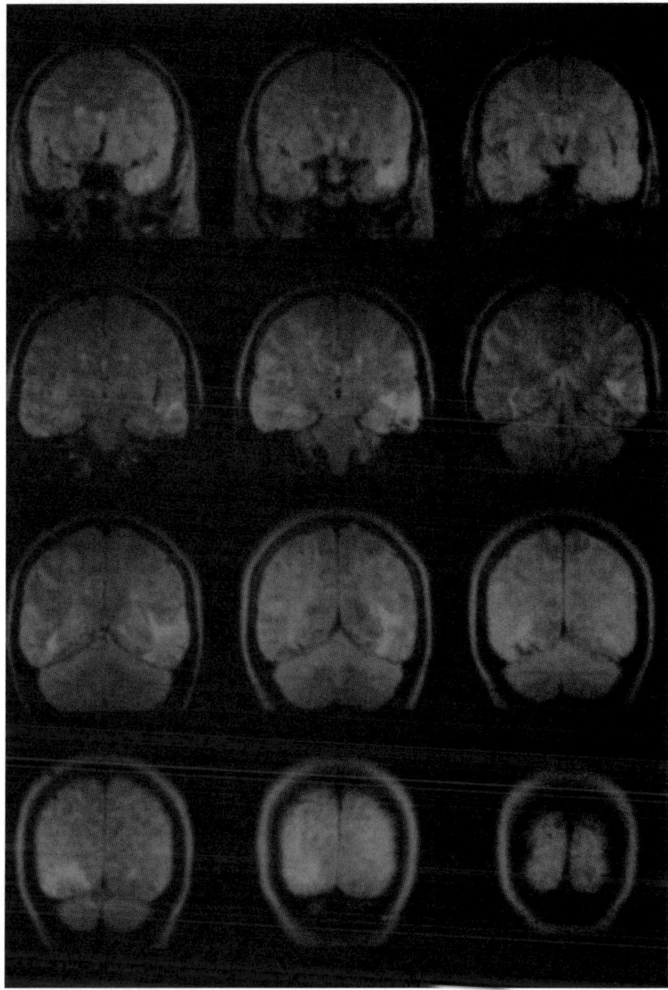

Figure 2 Illustration of the neuroanatomic findings of a patient with pure associative prosopagnosia.

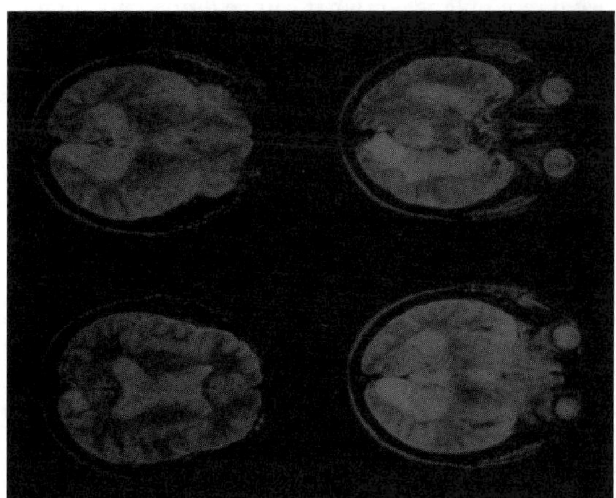

Figure 3 Illustration of the neuroanatomic findings of a patient with apperceptive face agnosia.

associative in nature, although he does manifest aspects of apperceptive prosopagnosia, as demonstrated by defects in certain aspects of visuoperception. Interesting parallels with the experimental research in acquired prosopagnosia in adults are evident in this case and are noted in the section titled 'Nonconscious discrimination of familiar faces.'

A recent study identified a subgroup of patients with Asperger's disorder who manifested prosopagnosic-like defects, suggesting the possibility of occipitotemporal dysfunction in patients with social developmental disorders.

Other Aspects of Face Processing

Nature and Extent of the Defect

In prosopagnosia, the recognition impairment occurs at the most subordinate taxonomic level, that is, at the level of identification of unique faces. Prosopagnosics are fully capable of recognizing faces as faces; that is, performance is normal at the superordinate taxonomic level. Also, most prosopagnosics can recognize facial expressions, and can make accurate determinations of gender and age based on face information. These dissociations highlight the fact that recognizing faces at the level of unique identity is a highly demanding task which requires the brain to distinguish between numerous exemplars that bear a high degree of resemblance to one another.

Although face agnosics recognize any number of visual entities at basic object level, such as cars as cars, buildings as buildings, and dogs as dogs, they often fail to recognize these items at the subordinate level of unique identity. Thus, similar to the problem with faces, they are unable to recognize the specific identity of a particular car or building. These recognition impairments are common in prosopagnosia and underscore the notion that the core defect in face agnosia is the inability to disambiguate fully individual visual stimuli. In fact, cases have been reported in which the most troubling problem for the patient was in classes of visual stimuli other than human faces, such as a farmer who lost his ability to recognize individual dairy (Holstein) cows or a birdwatcher who became unable to tell apart various subtypes of birds.

Prosopagnosic patients can often recognize identity from movement. This means not only that their perception of movement is intact but also that they can evoke appropriate memories from the perception of a unique pattern of movement. Combined with the finding that recovery of identity from motion can be impaired by lesions in superior occipitoparietal regions, these findings underscore the separable functions of the 'dorsal' and 'ventral' visual systems, the dorsal one being specialized for spatial placement, movement, and other 'where' capacities and the ventral one being specialized for form detection, shape recognition, and other 'what' capacities.

Nonconscious Discrimination of Familiar Faces

Some prosopagnosic patients show accurate covert or nonconscious discrimination of familiar faces despite their complete inability to recognize those faces at overt level. For example, it has been shown that prosopagnosics generate large, discriminatory electrodermal responses to familiar faces that are otherwise unrecognized. Preserved covert face discrimination has been demonstrated in other experimental paradigms, such as reaction time tasks and forced choice procedures. In the electrodermal paradigm, covert face discrimination has even been demonstrated for faces from the anterograde compartment, indicating that the brain can continue to learn new visual information even without conscious influence. In the earlier mentioned developmental case, it was found that AT's covert face discrimination based on an autonomic index was normal, suggesting that the brain is capable of acquiring some information about familiar faces, even without conscious recognition.

Recovery

Prosopagnosic patients often become quite adroit at using nonface information to recognize the persons around them. For example, they rely on voice, or gait, or a distinctive visual feature. Regarding the latter, it is often helpful to add a distinctive feature in situations in which recognition is highly demanded but difficult. At a crowded social gathering, for example, the patient's spouse might wear a special hat or other article of clothing, which would facilitate rapid and accurate identification by the patient. There is also evidence to suggest that the prosopagnosic individual may benefit from a local, components-based examination of the face rather than a holistic, configural approach. Generally speaking, though, the earlier in the course of recovery that compensatory strategies such as these can be taught, the better the chances for healthy adaptation to the disability.

Unanswered Questions

An issue which has remained central in the study of prosopagnosia is the mechanism of the defect and in particular, the reason the recognition of faces is affected so much more severely than the recognition of other visual stimuli. It has been proposed that faces, more so than many other types of items, have two important qualities: First, they are highly similar in terms of physical structure, that is, they have high visual resemblance or what can be termed homomorphism. Second, they are numerous, and it is necessary to tell them apart at the unique, individual level. It does not suffice, for example, to recognize a good friend as simply a female person or as a female person who works at the hospital. Rather, recognition must take place at the level of unique identity. Together, these factors make faces a 'visually crowded' category, which may explain the vulnerability of familiar face recognition to acquired brain disease.

Other questions remaining in the study of prosopagnosia concern the reasons some prosopagnosic patients are able to generate covert responses to familiar faces while other patients cannot. A related question concerns the relationship among different indices of covert discrimination – for example, are skin conductance responses, reaction times, and eye movement patterns all tapping into the same discrimination mechanisms?

On another point, much still remains unknown about the neural mechanisms of developmental prosopagnosia. Finally, a recent finding regarding covert discrimination of faces in the setting of 'childhood amnesia' raises many interesting questions. Specifically, it has been shown that when school-age children (e.g., ages 10–15) are shown faces of former classmates who were known only in the early developmental years for which much information is not readily retrievable into declarative memory (especially ages 2–5), the children generate discriminatory skin conductance responses even for faces that are entirely 'forgotten' by overt measures. This finding warrants further investigation.

See also: Agnosia; Recognition Memory; Representation of Color.

Further Reading

Barton JJS, Cherkasova MV, Hefter R, Cox TA, O'Connor M, and Manoach DS (2004) Are patients with social developmental disorders prosopagnosic? Perceptual heterogeneity in the Asperger and socio-emotional processing disorders. *Brain* 127: 1706–1716.

Baudouin J-Y and Humphreys GW (2006) Compensatory strategies in processing facial emotions: Evidence from prosopagnosia. *Neuropsychologia* 44: 1361–1369.

Behrmann M and Avidan G (2006) Congenital prosopagnosia: Face-blind from birth. *Trends in Cognitive Sciences* 9: 180–187.

Benton AL (1990) Facial recognition. *Cortex* 26: 491–499.

Damasio AR, Damasio H, and Van Hoesen GW (1982) Prosopagnosia: Anatomic basis and behavioral mechanisms. *Neurology* 32: 331–341.

Damasio AR, Tranel D, and Damasio H (1990) Face agnosia and the neural substrates of memory. *Annual Review of Neuroscience* 13: 89–109.

De Renzi E (1986) Prosopagnosia in two patients with CT scan evidence of damage confined to the right hemisphere. *Neuropsychologia* 24: 385–389.

Hadjikhani N and de Gelder B (2002) Neural basis of prosopagnosia: An fMRI study. *Human Brain Mapping* 16: 176–182.

Jones RD and Tranel D (2001) Severe developmental prosopagnosia in a child with superior intellect. *Journal of Clinical and Experimental Neuropsychology* 23: 265–273.

Landis T, Cummings JL, Christen L, Bogen JE, and Imhof H-G (1986) Are unilateral right posterior cerebral lesions sufficient to cause prosopagnosia? Clinical and radiological findings in six additional patients. *Cortex* 22: 243–252.

Meadows JC (1974) The anatomical basis of prosopagnosia. *Journal of Neurology, Neurosurgery, and Psychiatry* 37: 489–501.

Sergent J and Villemure J-G (1989) Prosopagnosia in a right hemispherectomized patient. *Brain* 112: 975–995.

Teuber HL (1968) Alteration of perception and memory in man: Reflections on methods. In: Weiskrantz L (ed.) *Annals of Behavior Change*, pp. 274–328. New York: Harper & Row.

Tranel D and Damasio AR (1985) Knowledge without awareness: An autonomic index of facial recognition by prosopagnosics. *Science* 228: 1453–1454.

Tranel D, Damasio AR, and Damasio H (1988) Intact recognition of facial expression, gender, and age in patients with impaired recognition of face identity. *Neurology* 38: 690–696.

Tranel D, Damasio H, and Damasio AR (1995) Double dissociation between overt and covert face recognition. *Journal of Cognitive Neuroscience* 7: 425–432.

Psychophysics of Attention

H E Egeth, Johns Hopkins University, Baltimore, MD, USA

Introduction

The amount of information available to our senses greatly exceeds the information processing capacity of our brains. How we deal with the overload is the topic of this article – attention. More specifically, this article focuses on the study of visual attention. The purpose of the article is not to summarize the neuroscience of attention, but to introduce the basic behavioral findings that have motivated interest in the concept.

Perhaps the most fundamental points about attention are that it is limited, and that it is selective. It allows an organism to select the information that is most relevant to its current goals. With attention we are not simply passive recipients of stimuli; instead, we play an active role in our interactions with the environment.

Before proceeding, it is worth making an important philosophical point. When we say something like "it allows an organism to select..." there is a real danger that we may reify the 'it.' We should remember that there is not a homunculus directing traffic in our heads; referring to attention as an active 'it' is a convenient verbal simplification. In fact, the selectivity of attention may be better thought of as an emergent property of our nervous system. In this brief overview of the field of attention we will touch on (1) evidence of limited capacity and (2) the nature of attentional selectivity.

Attention Is Limited

Enumeration

Some of the earliest experiments in psychology amounted to demonstrations of the limits of attention. For example, Jevons, a nineteenth-century researcher, picked up handfuls of beans and threw them into a box, and after glancing at them briefly, attempted to say how many there were. He found that he was essentially perfect when there were up to four beans, but beyond four made progressively more errors. Many variations of this experiment have been carried out. When reaction time is measured, the time required to respond increases only slightly from one to about four, and increases more steeply thereafter. The ability to enumerate small numbers of items quickly and accurately has been referred to as 'subitizing.' The widely, but not universally, accepted explanation is that a few items (up to about four to six, depending on the methodology) can be apprehended simultaneously; beyond that elements are presumably enumerated one at a time, or, if there is time pressure, their numerosity may be estimated.

Multiple-Item Tracking

Imagine an array of, say, ten gray disks appearing on a computer screen. They are all moving in erratic, random trajectories. One of them is marked as a target by blinking several times, but it then reverts to gray and keeps moving along with the other nine disks. Your task is to follow it for, say, 12 s. At that time the disks stop moving and a probe (a small box) appears around one of the gray disks. Your task is to indicate whether or not the probed item was the one that had been marked by flashing. Could you do it? Yes, indeed. This is a trivial task. Now imagine a trial on which not one but two of the ten disks are marked by flashing, and then after 12 s a single disk is probed and you are asked if this is one of the two that had been marked by flashing. Could you do this? Yes; this is a bit more difficult, but not much. However, as the number of marked disks increases there comes a point at which you simply cannot keep track of additional elements. That point varies across observers, but is approximately three to five disks.

Span of Immediate Memory

In a classic experiment by Sperling, when individuals were shown a 3×4 matrix of letters (four letters in three rows) briefly (say for about 0.1 s) and were asked to report as many as possible, they typically reported only four to five letters. In another condition, individuals were presented with a high-, medium-, or low-frequency tone, the tone indicating which one row (top, middle, or bottom) of the matrix they were to report. In this case they were able to report all four letters in a row when the tone came before or very shortly after the visual display. As the tone was selected randomly on each trial, this means that individuals briefly had access to all twelve letters in the display. However as the tone was delayed, performance declined, until, after as little as a 0.25 s delay, performance reached the same level as the whole report technique (i.e., about four or five letters). Thus, this research provides evidence of a high-capacity short-lived sensory memory (often referred to as iconic memory), followed by a small-capacity short-term memory store.

Psychologists have wondered whether the numerical similarity of the capacity limits (three to four items) shown in the these kinds of studies (enumeration, multiple-item tracking, and immediate-memory span) is evidence of a common limitation, or is just a coincidence. A strong case has been made for a common limit, due ultimately to the ability of attention to hold just three to four items at once. However, the issue is not yet settled. A related point is whether the limitation is properly described in terms of a fixed number of 'slots,' with one 'item' assigned to each slot. This is far from a trivial issue, as the definition of an item is by no means straightforward. For example, is the word 'attention' a single visual object, or are the nine letters composing it the proper units of analysis, or are the line segments composing those letters the proper units?

Visual Search

A popular method of studying perceptual processes is to have an individual look for a designated target item in a display that contains several distractors. Typically, the number of distractors is varied, although the number of targets has also been manipulated. Performance is assessed by measuring reaction time and/or accuracy of performance. Visual search provides a remarkably versatile tool for exploring many aspects of perception and attention with a task that has considerable ecological validity, as it is ubiquitous in everyday life.

One important characteristic of visual search is its efficiency, where by efficiency we refer to the slope relating total search time to the number of stimuli in the display. When search requires a simple discrimination, such as a circle among triangles, a 4 among Cs, or a red item among blue items, the process is highly efficient; the slope of the search function is often near zero. As adding additional items does not incur a cost in search time, such a result implies parallel processing of all elements in the display. Although a search based on a simple feature such as color or line orientation can be done in parallel, when a search target is defined as a conjunction of features (e.g., the target is a red horizontal line segment and distractors are a mixture of black horizontals and red verticals), then search time is often found to increase linearly with the number of stimuli in the display. One interpretation of such results is that efficient 'feature' searches are performed by preattentive mechanisms that can analyze the entire display at once. Searches for conjunctively defined targets, however, require sequential inspection of items, as attention is responsible for conjoining the separate features that constitute a visual object. (Although it is common to take linearly increasing reaction time functions to imply that processing is serial, it has been known for many years that this is not necessarily a safe assumption.)

The feature-integration theory of attention has been very influential. One appealing aspect of this theory is that it is based on known functions of the brain. It seems to suggest that elementary features detectable by early visual processing areas of the brain can be processed over the entire visual field at once, whereas dealing with combinations of elementary features, which presumably requires higher level cortical processing, must be done one item at a time, to avoid a 'combinatorial explosion.' However, over time, some problems with the theory have appeared. One difficulty is that several studies have demonstrated that there are feature combinations that can be processed in parallel. For example, efficient search has been found for brick-shaped objects drawn in such a way that their apparent orientation depended solely on their shading (i.e., which surface looked like it was directly illuminated). That is, a misoriented brick could be found in a background of uniformly oriented distractor bricks independent of the number of those distractors. It is possible to consider such demonstrations as either embarrassments to feature-integration theory or as discoveries of surprising new elementary features (although that claim seems inelegant and unparsimonious, as the number of such new 'features' has become substantial). Worse yet for the theory, there is clear evidence that a feature/shape conjunction can be processed in parallel. There is now even some doubt about the idea that simple features are processed preattentively; this is covered in the next section, in the discussion of the attentional blink. Finally, there are also some interesting effects of familiarity that seem inconsistent with the theory. For example, individuals have been asked to search for a single backward N among several normal Ns or a single normal N among several backward Ns. The latter search was fast and parallel, while the former search was slower and serial. The physical features of the targets and nontargets in these two searches were essentially identical; it is not obvious how the theory can account for the results. Indeed, these data suggest that familiarity itself may be serving as a feature. Could familiarity be detected by early visual areas? There is functional magnetic resonance imaging (fMRI) evidence of widespread reorganization of activity in the visual pathway after extensive training on a perceptual task. Retinotopic cortex is involved, although this is presumably activated in a top-down fashion.

As a result of these problems, several competing interpretations have been proposed. For example, in the 'guided search' model, attention is guided by preattentive processes to the location of likely target items. The ultimate identification of an item as the target or not requires attentive scrutiny of the item. The efficiency of a search depends on the amount of preattentive information available to guide search. This varies from the great efficiency of searching for a red patch in an array of green patches, through conjunction search, to the extremely inefficient search that occurs when the target and distractors share the same features (e.g., looking for a randomly rotated L among several randomly rotated Ts).

Doing Two Things at Once

In the preceding examples individuals may have had to deal with multiple stimuli, but the task in each case was in some sense unitary (count the objects, repeat back all of the letters, etc.) There has also been a great deal of research in which quite different tasks have been combined; what has been at issue is the extent to which tasks can be performed without mutual interference. The general expectation based on everyday experience is that it is difficult to do several things at once (e.g., pay attention to two simultaneous conversations). In contrast, multitasking is possible in some cases (e.g., driving while listening to the radio). Thus the research effort has largely been directed at finding out just which tasks are difficult to combine, and why. One part of this effort has been a search for special conditions in which tasks might be combined without loss, as such conditions might have implications for real-world scenarios, such as using a cell phone while driving.

Some early research with continuous tasks suggested that even fairly complex pairs of tasks that initially interfered with one another – such as typing visually presented text and shadowing (i.e., repeating back) a message played through earphones – could, after sufficient practice, be done as well together as separately. However, with complex continuous tasks it is often possible to interleave components of the tasks so as to minimize or even eliminate the amount of temporal overlap between components of the two tasks. (An extreme example: a centerfielder could probably read a book during the 'slack time' when he is not actively engaged in the game.) Scientists wishing to achieve a more fine-grained analysis of dual-task performance have used simplified tasks to permit a closer analysis of stimulus–response relations. Perhaps the most well-developed analyses come from the psychological refractory period paradigm. In this paradigm two stimuli are presented, S1 and S2, with a variable stimulus-onset asynchrony (SOA). Typically, study participants are instructed to respond as quickly as possible to each stimulus with the appropriate response, R1 and R2, respectively. When the two tasks are widely separated in time there should be no interference between them and we can obtain baseline reaction times (RTs). As the stimuli are presented closer together in time, the reaction time to the second stimulus (RT2) will tend to increase. Most strikingly, in some cases, as the time between stimuli becomes less than about 300 ms, RT2 increases about 1 ms for each millisecond that the SOA is decreased. It is this kind of result, suggesting a clear inability to produce R2 at the same time as R1, that led to the nomenclature of a refractory period, by analogy to the refractory period of neurons.

Another example of the difficulty of responding to two stimuli presented close together in time is known as the attentional blink (AB). In a typical AB task, a rapid series of stimuli (e.g., digits or letters) is presented at fixation, typically at a rate around 10 items per second, and either one or two targets can appear within the stream. The AB refers to a decrement in the detection or identification of the second target (T2) when it occurs soon after the presentation of the first target (T1), to which a response is required. Early models of the attentional blink assumed that T2 processing is impaired because attention is temporarily fully occupied by processing of T1.

In an instructive example, a stream of letters was presented at fixation. There were two targets. The first was a green letter; all of the other letters in the stream were black. The green letter was followed after a variable delay (the lag) by the second target, which was a ring of Gabor patches (a Gabor patch is, essentially, a small patch of parallel stripes) in the periphery surrounding one of the later letters in the stream. Participants had to name the colored letter and also indicate if all of the Gabor patches were oriented in the same direction or if one was misoriented by 90°. In a control condition, individuals could ignore the stream of letters and just indicate if the ring of Gabor patches contained an orientation oddball. Performance in the control condition was about 90% correct and did not vary with the lag between the green letter and the Gabor patches. In the experimental condition, performance was poor (about 60% correct) when the Gabor patches were simultaneous with the green target letter, and improved to nearly 90% correct when the lag between the green letter and the Gabor patches was 700 ms.

What makes these results interesting are the implications they may have for the study of visual processing. The detection of a Gabor patch differing by 90° in orientation from an otherwise uniformly oriented set of patches should be handled preattentively according to feature-integration theory, and, indeed, the reaction time to detect a Gabor patch misoriented by 90° is independent of the number of other patches – which is precisely the diagnostic that has been taken to indicate preattentive processing in discussions of feature-integration theory. Why then should there be a large dual-task decrement? One possible answer is that it takes a really difficult competing task, such as is presumably provided by the attentional blink paradigm, to show that orientation discrimination, while easy, is not completely attention free. However, it is also possible that the deficit is not due to T1 stressing attentional capacity for feature processing; it may be that the attentional blink reflects difficulty with one or more higher level functions, such as maintaining executive control of a task set in the face of a fast-moving sequence of targets and nontargets. The attentional demands of various kinds of perceptual discriminations remain a topic of great interest and the final word has not yet been written.

Attention Is Selective

The preceding evidence points to a variety of limitations on attentional capacity. It is clear that we cannot process everything, at least not at once. What is it that determines just what it is that we do process? William James distinguished between passive and active attention. Today, the corresponding terms for passive attention are usually 'bottom-up,' 'stimulus-driven,' or 'exogenous,' while corresponding terms for active attention are 'top-down,' 'goal-directed,' or 'endogenous.' What we attend to is determined both by properties of the stimulus array (e.g., a sudden loud sound, or a movement in the periphery) and by our goals and intentions. Much research has examined the nature of the interaction between, and relative importance of, stimulus-driven and goal-directed sources of control.

The brute fact of selectivity has been demonstrated many times. In the technique known as shadowing, used in studies of dichotic listening, different messages are played to individuals over left and right earphones. Study participants are instructed to repeat back the message played to one ear. They are able to do this quite well. What is especially interesting is the analysis of what information individuals extract incidentally from the unattended message in such circumstances. They can report a change from speech to a pure tone, or a change from a male to a female voice. However very few persons notice a change from English to German or a change from normal to reversed speech when these changes were in the same voice. Most important is the near-total lack of comprehension of the message in the unattended ear. Related experiments have been performed in vision. Participants were shown two episodes on optically superimposed video screens. One was a ballgame and one was a handgame. Participants counted unpredictable events (e.g., the number of times the ball was passed from one player to another). In some conditions individuals were instructed to attend to just one of the episodes; in some conditions they were asked to attend to both. One finding concerned capacity; participants were reasonably accurate when they had to monitor one episode, but they could not deal with both simultaneously. The other finding concerned selectivity. The episodes occasionally contained distinctly odd events (e.g., a woman carrying an umbrella walking through the ballgame). After seeing the episodes, participants were asked about these odd events; they were often entirely unaware of those that occurred in the unattended episode. This kind of result has since been dubbed inattentional blindness and has been the subject of several more analytic studies.

The interaction of stimulus-driven and goal-directed attention is illustrated in a series of studies concerned with the capture of attention by featural singletons (e.g., the lone red element in a display of green elements) or by sudden onsets of a new stimulus object in a field of persisting objects. In one experiment participants searched for a target letter in an array of three or six other letters. This is a demanding search task in which reaction time increases with the number of letters in the display. Stimuli started out as placeholders (like the figure 8 of a digital clock), and at a certain point in time selected segments were deleted, revealing letters. In some conditions a new object was added to the display at the moment when the letters were being revealed (i.e., a letter was displayed in a location that had not contained a placeholder). Importantly, the location of the sudden onset was in no way predictive of the location of the target. This new object attracted attention; if it was the specified target character, reaction times were fast and independent of display numerosity, but if it was not the target, reaction times increased with display numerosity. Thus the sudden onset of a new object appears to capture attention in a stimulus-driven fashion. A follow-up experiment was conducted to determine if there is something special about sudden onsets. In this case the displays contained a single character that was unique with respect to color or brightness (e.g., a red element when other elements were green). Strikingly, reaction time was the same whether or not the display contained a singleton. In other words, unlike a sudden onset, color and brightness singletons did not automatically attract attention. This study raised at least two questions that have been the subject of further investigation: (1) Is it really the case that feature singletons do not capture attention? (2) Is the sudden onset of a new object really different from other kinds of featural singletons with respect to its ability to capture attention?

Do Feature Singletons Automatically Capture Attention?

In some studies, performance on displays containing an irrelevant singleton is compared to performance when displays contain no irrelevant singleton. For example, in one study participants were presented with displays consisting of colored circles or diamonds arranged around an imaginary circle. A line segment of a variable orientation appeared inside each shape; the task was to determine the orientation of the line segment within a target item. The target item was defined as the unique green diamond among green circles. Search was parallel – that is, independent of display size – but was significantly slower when one of the circles was red than when all elements were green. When the color singleton was made less salient than the shape singleton by changing the colors in the display, the color singleton no longer slowed search for the shape singleton; indeed when the roles of the original color and shape dimensions were reversed (color target and shape distractor), the more salient shape singleton now slowed search for the color target. Note that the color singleton provided no information about the target. This study was interpreted as showing that attention is captured automatically by the most salient element in the display.

An alternative to this analysis is that what an individual first attends to depends not just on the salience of stimuli, but also on the individual's task set. It has been suggested, for example, that salient stimuli may only attract attention when individuals adopt the strategy of searching for a feature discontinuity (singleton-detection mode). When individuals adopt the strategy of searching for a specific, known-to-be-relevant, feature (feature-search mode), bottom-up capture can be overridden. In tasks where both strategies are available to the individual (e.g., where the target is a specific feature and also a singleton, such as a green circle among green triangles), both search strategies are available. Therefore, an irrelevant singleton may or may not cause interference, depending on which strategy the individual adopts. In support of this claim it has been shown that when singleton-detection mode is discouraged, and individuals are forced to resort to feature-search mode, a salient distractor no longer interferes with search.

There has been an ongoing debate about the extent to which the most salient item captures attention automatically, as opposed to capturing attention only when an appropriate strategy has been selected. Be that as it may, the consideration of search strategies has led to new findings. For example, circumstances can be arranged to force individuals to search in time rather than in space. Individuals viewed a central rapid serial visual presentation stream (just as in the attentional blink paradigm) in which a target letter was defined by being a particular color (e.g., red). On critical trials, an irrelevant color stimulus could appear in the periphery during one frame of the stream. Interestingly, the irrelevant stimulus reduced the probability of an individual identifying the target letter, when that irrelevant stimulus preceded the target by 200 ms. That is, even though the peripheral stimulus was irrelevant and did not have to be responded to, it had the same effect as a first target in the attentional blink paradigm. That sounds like automatic capture by the irrelevant stimulus, but there is a critical additional finding: the existence of this interference effect was dependent on whether the individual was in singleton-detection mode or feature-search mode. In one experiment, to induce singleton-detection mode, the letters were all gray except for one that was red. (In fact, half the individuals were tested with red, half with green.) Note that when there is just one colored character in a stream of otherwise all gray characters, either feature search or singleton detection could have been applied. In this experiment, regardless of whether an individual was in the search-for-red or search-for-green group, both red and green peripheral distractors produced substantial, and equal, interference with target detection. In a second experiment, multiple colors were used in constructing the letter stream. Again the target was either red or green (different groups of individuals), but now the individuals had to look for a particular color, whereas in the first experiment they could have searched for 'anything chromatic.' Now, individuals who searched for a red target only suffered interference when the distractor was red, and individuals who searched for a green target only suffered interference when the distractor was green. Follow-up experiments established that the interference was due to a spatial capture of attention.

Are Sudden Onsets Special?

An influential account of how performance in search tasks might be affected by nominally irrelevant singletons is that participants in search experiments always adopt one or another sort of attentional control setting that determines what will be selected. (We have already come across this notion; singleton detection and feature search can be considered specific examples of attentional control settings.) To test this idea, participants searched for a target character that could be either a color or an onset singleton across blocks. Immediately preceding each search display another display appeared that contained a cue that was itself either a color or an onset singleton in one of the (four) potential target locations. It was explained to the participants that the location of the cue was independent of the location of the target. The chief result was that target reaction times were strongly dependent on the cue location, but only when the cue matched the target dimension. For example, if the task was to identify a color singleton, then reaction time was faster when the target was in the same location that the cue had occupied than when it was in another location. However, when participants had to identify a color singleton, the location of an onset cue had no effect on reaction time. This finding is contrary to the notion that the sudden onset of a new object is unique in that it captures attention automatically (i.e., in a stimulus-driven fashion). The possibly special status of sudden onsets is controversial and remains a topic of lively current interest.

Conclusion

The study of attention has been of keen interest to psychologists for over a century. A great deal of progress has been made in understanding the limitations of our perceptual and cognitive processes, and the selectivity these limitations force on us. Most of this research has used psychophysical methods solidly within the behavioral tradition. However over the past 20–30 years the conceptual and methodological armamentarium available to study attention has been expanded in scope by the growth of the neurosciences.

See also: Attention: Models; Attentional Networks; Attentional Networks in the Parietal Cortex; Attentional Functions in Learning and Memory; Human Methods: Psychophysics; Short Term and Working Memory; Visual Attention.

Further Reading

Burnham BR (in press) Displaywide visual features associated with a search display's appearance can mediate attentional capture. *Psychonomic Bulletin & Review.*

Cowan N (2001) The magical number 4 in short-term memory: A reconsideration of mental storage capacity. *Behavioral and Brain Sciences* 24: 87–185.

Enns JT and Rensink RA (1990) Sensitivity to three-dimensional orientation in visual search. *Psychological Science* 1: 323–326.

Folk CL, Remington RW, and Johnston JC (1992) Involuntary covert orienting is contingent on attentional control settings. *Journal of Experimental Psychology: Human Perception & Performance* 18: 1030–1044.

Jonides J and Yantis S (1988) Uniqueness of abrupt visual onset in capturing attention. *Perception and Psychophysics* 43: 346–354.

Joseph JS, Chun MM, and Nakayama K (1997) Attentional requirements in a 'preattentive' feature search task. *Nature* 379: 805–807.

Leber AB and Egeth HE (2006) It's under control: Top down search strategies can override attentional capture. *Psychonomic Bulletin & Review* 13: 132–138.

Lien M-C, Ruthruff E, and Johnston JC (2006) Attentional limitations in doing two tasks at once: The search for exceptions. *Current Directions in Psychological Science* 15: 89–93.

Mandler G and Shebo BJ (1982) Subitizing: An analysis of its component processes. *Journal of Experimental Psychology: General* 11: 1–22.

Neisser U and Becklen R (1975) Selective looking: Attending to visually specified events. *Cognitive Psychology* 7: 480–494.

Olivers CNL, Stigchel S van der, and Hulleman J (2005) Spreading the sparing: Against a limited-capacity account of the attentional blink. *Psychological Research* 8: 1–14.

Pashler H (1998) *The Psychology of Attention.* Cambridge, MA: MIT Press.

Pylyshyn ZW and Storm RW (1988) Tracking multiple independent targets: Evidence for a parallel tracking mechanism. *Spatial Vision* 3: 179–197.

Sperling G (1960) The information available in brief visual presentations. *Psychological Monographs* 74(no. 11): 1–30.

Theeuwes J (2004) Top-down search strategies cannot override attentional capture. *Psychonomic Bulletin & Review* 11: 65–70.

Treisman A and Gormican S (1988) Feature analysis in early vision: Evidence from search asymmetries. *Psychological Review* 95: 15–48.

Wang Q, Cavanagh P, and Green M (1994) Familiarity and pop-out in visual search. *Perception & Psychophysics* 56: 495–500.

Wolfe JM (2003) Moving towards solutions to some enduring controversies in visual search. *Trends in Cognitive Sciences* 7: 70–76.

Referentiality and Concepts in Animal Cognition

K Zuberbühler, University of St. Andrews,
St. Andrews, UK

> No name belongs to a particular thing by nature, but only because of the rules and usage of those who establish the usage and call it by that name. (Plato, *c.* 360 BC)

Introduction

Communication happens when individuals exchange information by means of a common system of behavior, an inherently social event. Human language is a particularly remarkable example, and the quest for its evolutionary origins is a scientific problem of continued interest. One popular approach is to examine the cognitive capacities of nonhuman animals, especially those of primates, during natural acts of communication. The comparative approach is based on the premise that human language is built on a number of cognitive capacities with independent evolutionary histories, some with phylogenetic roots deep in the primate lineage.

Precisely what capacities are required for language? An article by Hockett in 1960 has been particularly influential. He identified 13 different design features that are common to all languages. Some are shared with animal communication systems; others appear to be uniquely human. The distinction between human speech and primate vocal behavior is particularly interesting since the two differ in only four design features (**Table 1**).

Referential Communication and Semanticity

A key property of language is that it allows speakers to use distinct utterances in order to convey information about objects and events in the outside world. This by itself is not a uniquely human trait, however. Honeybees are able to communicate about the location of distant food sources, and many animal species produce acoustically different alarm calls for different predators. For nonhuman primates, the classic example for such referential signals is the vervet monkey alarm calls. These primates produce acoustically distinct vocalizations to some of their predators, such as eagles, leopards, or pythons. When others hear a group member's alarm call to a python, they respond in ways that suggest the call is meaningful to them, for instance, by scanning the surrounding area for the snake they assume is present. Another example is the West African Diana monkeys, which produce acoustically different alarm calls to leopards and crowned eagles. These calls convey the biological class of the predator and are not simple responses to situational circumstances or perceived threat (**Figure 1**).

Eavesdropping is common in alarm situations, both within and across species. For example, yellow-casqued hornbills live sympatrically with Diana monkeys in the Taï Forest, Ivory Coast, and occasionally feed on the same trees. Crowned eagles threaten both species, but only leopards also attack the monkeys. Field playback experiments have shown that the hornbills not only recognize these two predators by their calls but also discriminate between the eagle and leopard alarm calls of the Diana monkeys, despite the fact that acoustic differences are very subtle (**Figure 2**).

Although the relation between monkey alarm calls and their meanings is arbitrary, the ontogenetic processes leading to the link are not. Infant vervet monkeys give eaglelike alarm calls to numerous flying objects, such as storks or falling leaves, and only with experience do they learn to restrict call use to the genuinely dangerous raptor species. The main alarm-call types develop fairly rigidly, as do the underlying psychological states that elicit them. Social learning subsequently leads to fine-tuning of the range of events that warrant call production, within the predetermined categories. Although widely accepted, the empirical basis for this model is not very strong, suggesting that further research could alter our understanding of how primates acquire semantic competence.

What sorts of mental processes do animals experience when responding to predator-specific alarm calls? Are these calls truly meaningful to them, in the sense that they are linked with specific mental representations, or are call production and comprehension possible without complex processing – a kind of cognitive knee-jerk reflex? These are difficult problems and some researchers thus prefer the term 'functional reference' to acknowledge that what superficially resembles human referential communication may be the product of different cognitive processes. For nonhuman primates, at least, there is relatively good evidence that individuals experience some fairly specific mental representations when hearing each other's calls.

In one study, the cognitive processes experienced by primates when listening to their own eagle or leopard alarm calls were investigated. The question was whether monkeys simply responded to the physical

Table 1 Design features in which human speech is thought to differ from primate communication

Design feature	*Human language*	*Primate communication*
Displacement	Information about past, present, and future events	Communication about present events only
Productivity	Generation of novel meanings; familiar pieces are reassembled into new utterances	No semantic creativity; closed call systems
Transmission	Socially learned and culturally transmitted	Genetically hard-wired signals
Duality of patterning	Small stock of meaningless phonemes to build meaningful morphemes	Holistic utterances, no permutations

Adapted from Hockett CF (1960) The origin of speech. *Scientific American* 203: 89–96.

features of the calls or whether they were capable of generating a mental representation of the corresponding predator (i.e., the semantic content of their calls). In the experiment, different groups of Diana monkeys were exposed to one of three different prime stimuli: the shrieks of a crowned eagle, a male's alarm calls to an eagle, or a male's alarm calls to a leopard (**Figure 3**). Five minutes later, the same monkey group heard a second stimulus, the shrieks of a crowned eagle. Hence, depending on the condition, the two playback stimuli did or did not correspond semantically. Results showed that eagle shrieks did not elicit new alarm calls when monkeys were previously primed with eagle shrieks or monkey eagle alarm calls, in contrast to when they were primed with monkey leopard alarm calls (**Figure 3**). Therefore, when responding to each other's vocalizations, nonhuman primates activate mental representations, which are responsible for subsequent behavioral patterns.

The Semiotic Triangle

In humans, the relation between speech utterances and world entities is mediated by mental concepts in the form of a semiotic triangle (**Figure 4**). A number of studies suggest that this model may also be useful in explaining some animal communication systems. For phylogenetic reasons, the focus is on nonhuman primates, although an increasing number of nonprimate species have demonstrated that some of the crucial cognitive capacities are not uniquely primate.

Thoughts

Accessing mental processes in animals is not a trivial task – the 'other mind' problem in philosophy. Although it is possible to systematically study an animal's behavioral responses to a stimulus, the only way to access underlying cognitive processes is by inference. A common custom is to select the most parsimonious mechanisms from a selection offered by human psychology, but this practice habitually causes discomfort and ongoing debate. Nevertheless, much empirical progress has been made in describing how animals mentally represent their worlds – that is, the kinds of conceptual structures they build and maintain to interact with their environment. It is important to know that in humans mental concepts can exist independently of language. Some mental concepts are well established in prelinguistic infants well before language is acquired. In some cases, infants have demonstrated competence in dealing with abstract mental concepts in ways that exceeded that of adults.

One important technique to study concept formation in animals is to train individuals to respond to a number of real-world exemplars, which are members of a particular category. In a subsequent testing phase, subjects are then asked to make choices in response to novel stimuli. In one pioneering study, pigeons learned to distinguish between unfamiliar photographs that did or did not contain trees, suggesting they possessed a natural concept for tree. An intriguing example is honeybees, which have been shown to form concepts of sameness and oddity. Thus, complex abstract concepts are widespread throughout the animal kingdom and are not restricted to primates or even vertebrates.

Human intelligence is thought to have evolved in the social realm, however, and research on social concepts is therefore of particular interest. One study of long-tailed macaques has become somewhat of a classic. Monkeys were trained to select photographs showing pairs of familiar group members, either mother–offspring dyads or other pairings. The study animals successfully mastered novel dyads, demonstrating that they utilized a concept analogous to the human mother–child affiliation. It has also been claimed that chimpanzees are able to match black-and-white photographs with faces of unfamiliar mothers and their sons, providing further support for mother–offspring social concepts in primates but also suggesting that phenotypical markers play a role during categorization. In another study, rhesus monkeys watched video clips showing an agonistic interaction between two unfamiliar conspecifics. Not only was it

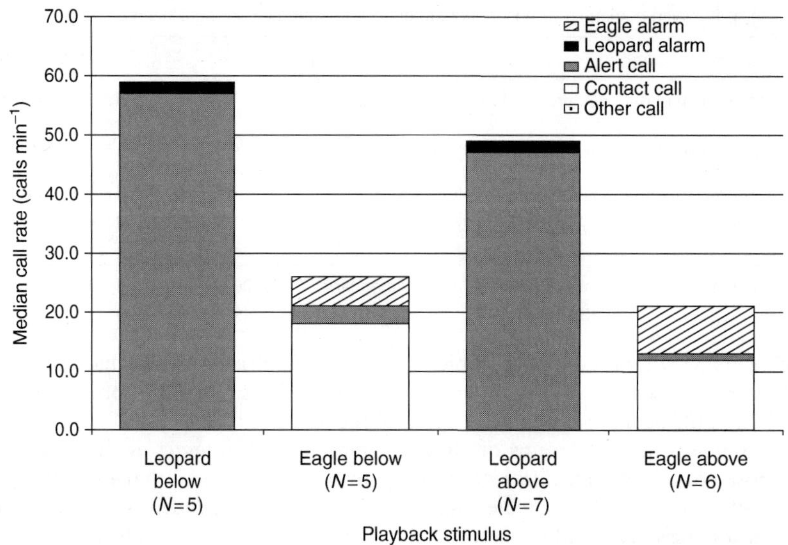

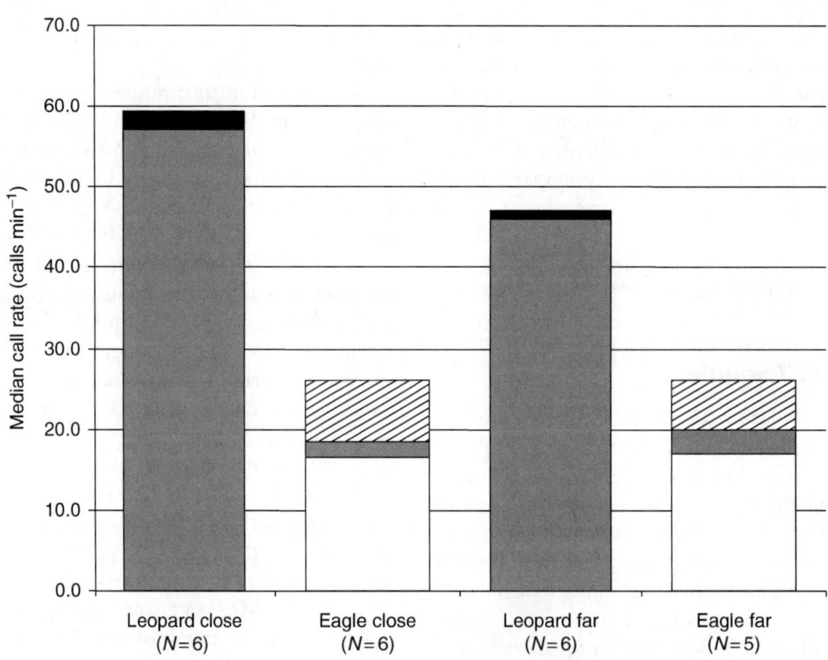

Figure 1 Diana monkey alarm calls convey information about the biological class of the predator, not its distance or direction of attack. Nearby group members respond with the same vocal behavior to the growls of a leopard (or shrieks of a crowned eagle, respectively) regardless of whether or not the calls were broadcast at close distance or from within the canopy above or on the ground. Adapted from Zuberbühler K (2000) Referential labelling in Diana monkeys. *Animal Behaviour* 59: 917–927.

possible to train subjects to select the dominant individual in the interaction but also the subjects continued to do so when watching novel video clips – a demonstration that they possessed a social concept for dominance.

Despite these examples of primate social intelligence, there is a widespread consensus that nonhuman primates are unable to attribute mental states to one another, an activity that humans engage in from early childhood. However, empirical work has led to some

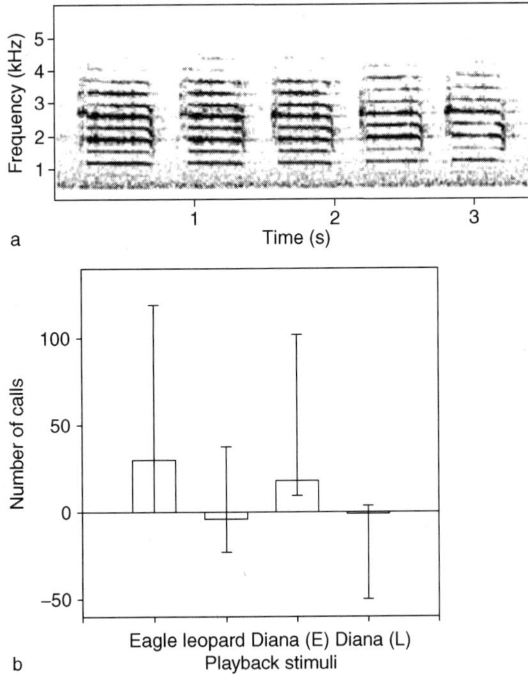

Figure 2 Responses of yellow-casqued hornbills of Tai forest to various predator-related acoustic stimuli. (a) Spectrogram of typical 'long' calls. Rate of production of this call type increased after playback of eagle calls and Diana monkey eagle alarm calls. Five individual calls are presented here. (b) Median and interquartile ranges of differences between the number of hornbill calls before and after playback of different stimulus types. Hornbills increased numbers of calls after playback of eagle shrieks significantly more than after playback of leopard growls. The same differences were found after playback of Diana monkey eagle and leopard alarm calls (Diana E and L). Adapted from Rainey HJ, Zuberbühler K, and Slater PJB (2004) Hornbills can distinguish between primate alarm calls. *Proceedings of the Royal Society of London Series B-Biological Sciences* 271: 755–759.

interesting amendments. Chimpanzees have been found to be capable of predicting the movements of more dominant competitors based on assessing the competitor's visual perspective. Related to this, when chimpanzees and other great apes interact with a human experimenter who is looking behind a barrier, they tend to position themselves such that they can see what the experimenter is looking at, suggesting that they attempt to take the experimenter's visual perspective. A number of non-ape species have shown comparable skills. When given the choice between two experimenters who were capable or incapable of seeing a food item, rhesus monkeys preferentially retrieved the food items from the visually unaware experimenter. In an experiment with ravens, the view of individuals during caching was manipulated, thereby creating competitors that were either knowledgeable or ignorant of the cache location. Results

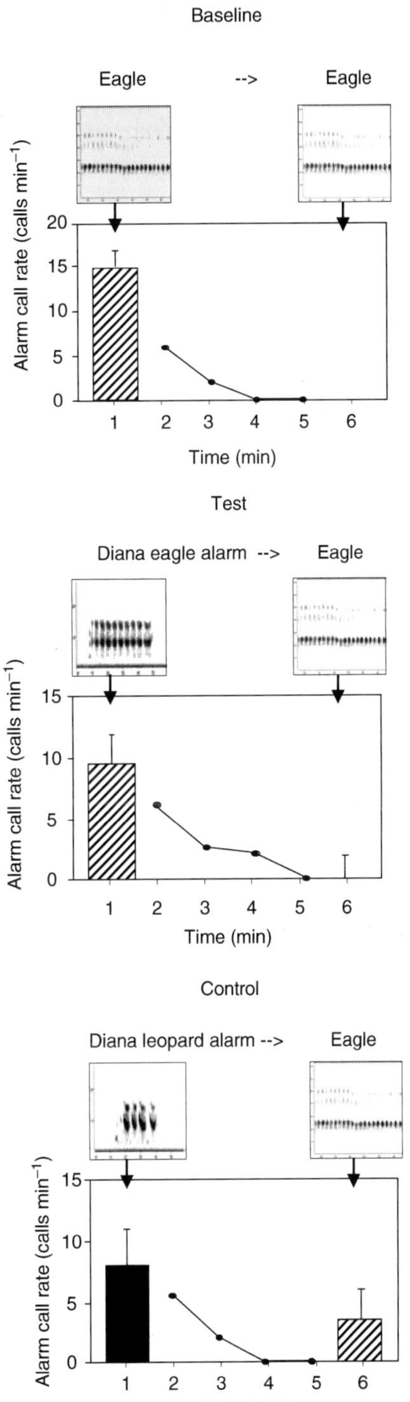

Figure 3 Design and results of a prime probe experiment to investigate the cognitive processes underlying Diana monkey alarm-call production. Analogous results were obtained if leopard growls were used as predator stimuli. Adapted from Zuberbühler K, Cheney DL, and Seyfarth RM (1999) Conceptual semantics in a nonhuman primate. *Journal of comparative Psychology* 113: 33–42.

demonstrated that ravens adjusted their subsequent behavior depending on a competitor's knowledge – that is, whether or not it previously had witnessed the caching event. In addition, ravens can follow gaze around barriers similar to primates, further suggesting that they make judgments of the visual perspective of other individuals.

In summary, although primates and other animals are able to understand what others see or have seen in the past (i.e., that they know), there is currently no evidence that they can reflect on what they know or that they recognize and share each other's intentions, which has potentially significant consequences, particularly for cultural development.

Symbols

Vocal repertoires Primate vocal repertoires, and those of many other species, are often said to be genetically predetermined, suggesting that individuals have little control over vocal production, similar to some nonverbal utterances in humans, such as laughing or crying. Although the main thrust of this argument remains unchallenged, some empirical studies have provided a number of clarifications.

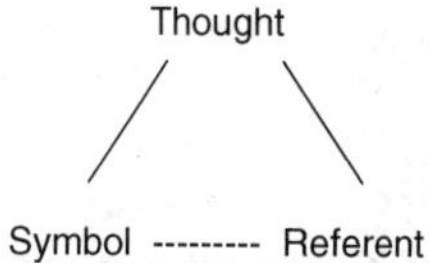

Figure 4 The semiotic triangle of referential communication.

First, several studies have shown that adult primates can change the acoustic structure of some of their calls, usually following significant social events. In Campbell's monkeys, adult females exchange contact calls as part of their daily social interactions. Each individual produces a certain number of acoustic variants, but these patterns collapse after changes in group composition. Playback of females' currently produced call variants reliably triggered vocal responses from other group members, whereas the same female's former, no longer used call variants caused long-term cessation of vocal behavior, indicating that the calls form part of a long-term social memory. Chimpanzee pant hoot vocalizations are a further example of vocal behavior that can undergo acoustic modifications depending on the social circumstances.

Second, the apparatus used by nonhuman primates for vocal production is not fundamentally different from that of humans. Sound is generated by the larynx, from which it radiates into the supralaryngeal vocal tract that acts as an acoustic filter. During speech, the shape of the vocal tract changes rapidly due to the movements of the various articulators, such as the lips, tongue, jaw, or larynx. The same basic processes have been found in Diana monkeys. Males produce alarm calls that contain formants with variable structure. Crowned eagles elicit calls with little or no formant transition, whereas leopards elicit calls with strong transitions (**Figure 5**). These acoustic modifications are the result of constrictions in their vocal tract formed by various articulators, similar to what takes place during speech production.

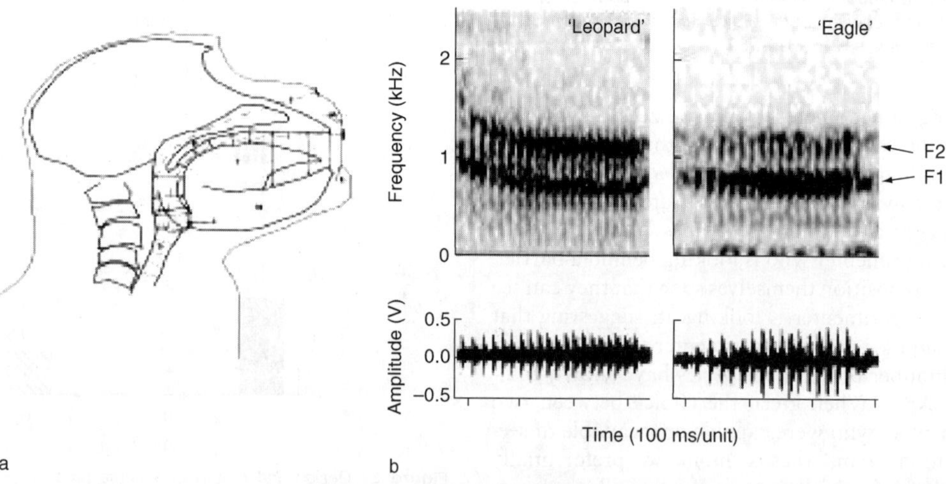

Figure 5 Vocal production mechanisms in a nonhuman primate. (a) Cross section of a Diana monkey vocal tract highlighting locations where acoustic filtering takes place due to constrictions. T, tongue; M, mandible; uL, upper lip; lL, lower lip; P, palate; Tr, Trachea. (b) Formant structure and transitions in Diana monkey eagle and leopard alarm calls. F1, first formant; F2, second formant. Adapted from Riede T, Bronson E, Hatzikirou H, and Zuberbühler K (2005) Vocal production mechanisms in a non-human primate: morphological data and a model. *Journal of Human Evolution* 48: 85–96.

Despite these similarities, there are vast differences between human and nonhuman vocal production. Humans are enormously skillful in producing rapid and precise articulatory movements, particularly with the tongue. As a result, humans are able to create a rich array of sounds, whereas sound production in nonhuman primates seems to be confined to a limited number of call types. For example, whereas modern English operates with approximately 40 different phonemes, male Diana monkeys possess only two (**Figure 5**). It has been suggested that this human specialization may be linked to a particular gene, *FoxP2*, since damage to this gene causes a severe speech disorder due to a lack of orofacial control. The human *FoxP2* is slightly different from those of the other nonhuman primates, suggesting that human–primate difference in orofacial control could be caused by this genetic difference.

Combinations of calls In contrast to speech, animal communication is considered to be holistic and lacking features that mark particular relationships between one call and another – Hockett's notion of duality of patterning. Although some animals combine acoustic units into patterned sequences, this behavior usually only serves to advertise identity, status, or quality, with no evidence of any sort of referential function.

A number of studies have provided empirical evidence that may require revision of current theory. At least two species of nonhuman primates have been found to combine calls into structurally more complex units, thereby modifying the semantic content of the entire utterance. An example is provided by free-ranging Campbell's monkeys. Like the Diana monkeys described previously, male Campbell's monkeys produce acoustically distinct alarm calls to leopards and eagles. However, if males witness other disturbing events that are not directly linked with these predators (e.g., a falling tree or a fleeing forest duiker), they usually produce a pair of low-sounding 'booms' before giving a series of alarm calls. Playback experiments have shown that other monkeys ignore such boom-introduced alarm calls, suggesting that the booms selectively change the meaning of subsequent alarm calls from predator-specific alarm signals to more general sign of disturbance (**Figure 6**).

Second, work on free-ranging putty-nosed monkeys in Nigeria has revealed similar results. In this species, the males produce two basic alarm call types, the 'hacks' and 'pyows.' These calls are not predator specific because males produce them to both eagles and leopards. Instead, callers concatenate the two calls into different sequence types, and these sequences are predator specific. In other words, putty-nosed monkeys encode predator class at the level of the call sequence and not at the level of the individual call. In addition, the males produce a peculiar pyow–hack sequence used to instigate group progression.

In summary, some primates do assemble calls into higher-order sequences and thereby generate information that is unrelated to the meaning conveyed by constituent elements. Although these combinatorial

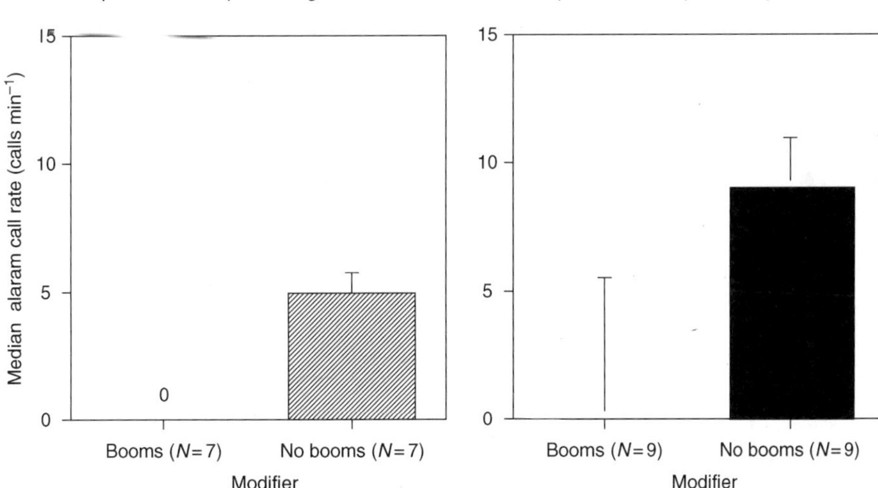

Figure 6 Diana monkey responses to Campbell's monkey eagle or leopard alarm calls in the presence or absence of preceding boom calls. Artificially adding boom calls prior to an alarm-call sequence deletes the predator-specific meaning of these calls. The hatched bar indicates the median number of Diana monkey eagle alarms in the first minute after playback, the solid bar indicates the median number of Diana monkey leopard alarm calls. Adapted from Zuberbühler K (2002) A syntactic rule in forest monkey communication. *Animal Behaviour* 63: 293–299.

systems may lack the generative power of recursion, they provide an efficient means of increasing message repertoire without the need to invent new calls.

Referents

The final element in the semiotic triangle is the referent – that is, the kinds of entities that trigger vocal behavior in nonhuman primates. Most progress has been made in two contexts that are of particular evolutionary relevance: finding food and avoiding predators.

Food discovery Many primates vocalize when finding food. Although the underlying mental processes are not well understood, two factors appear to be particularly relevant: the social setting during call production and the food. Food-associated calls attract nearby listeners, and in some species callers exert some control over this process by adjusting call production. For example, chimpanzees are more likely to produce food-associated calls, the so-called rough grunts, if the food source is divisible and anticipated competition is likely to be low, a pattern also found in bonobos. These processes are not limited to primates. Male chickens produce specific calls upon discovering food, more likely so in the presence of a potential mate. Hens respond to the calls with anticipatory feeding movement, suggesting that the calls contain basic referential information. In ravens, there is a relation between food type encountered by the caller and call rates produced.

In chimpanzees, food quality is unrelated to call rates. In one study, calls from captive individuals were recorded in response to nine different food items, ranked by the individuals as high, medium, or low preference. There was no evidence for food labels with the low and medium preference class; acoustic differences were only significant between the three preference classes. Surprisingly, however, calls given to the high preference foods were acoustically distinct, suggesting that referential labels for food items can emerge in captive conditions. In a related study, it was investigated whether these call variants are meaningful to recipients. Rough grunts, given in response to bread and apples, were played back to recipients, and the subsequent amount of search effort underneath an apple and a bread tree was measured. Results demonstrated that the focal animal spent significantly more time and search effort underneath the correct tree (i.e., the tree corresponding to the call type played before), demonstrating that chimpanzees are able to attend to the subtle acoustic differences inherent in their food calls and that they are meaningful to them (**Figure 7**).

Predator detection Predator-specific alarm calls are a common feature of primate and nonprimate vocal behavior. Monkeys convey the biological category of the predator, but other information is sometimes also encoded. For example, some species, such as white-browed scrubwrens or California ground squirrels, adjust their calling behavior as a function of predator distance. Domestic chickens mainly distinguish between events on the ground or in the air, regardless of predator species. Gunnison's prairie dogs' alarm calls differ depending on the color of

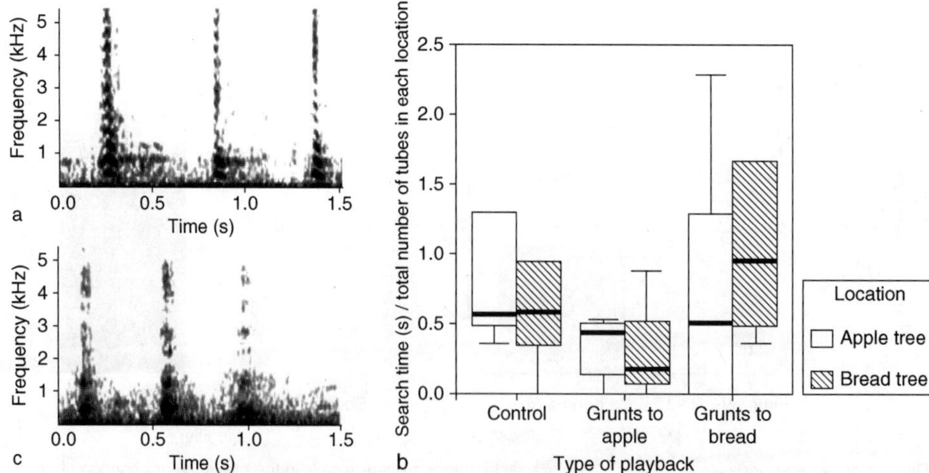

Figure 7 Chimpanzee food grunts are referential signals. (a) Rough grunts given in response to two different food items – bread (top) and apples (bottom). (b) Search behavior of the focal animal in response to playbacks of apple grunts and bread grunts given by different group members. The subject devoted more search effort underneath the food tree, indicated by the food grunts played back earlier. Adapted from Slocombe KE and Zuberbühler K (2005) Functionally referential communication in a chimpanzee. *Current Biology* 15: 1779–1784.

clothes and general shape of human experimenters, and black-capped chickadees' alarm calls convey the size of potential predators with the number of D-notes in the 'chick-a-dee' alarm calls, a relevant source of information for recipients.

Similar to food calls, alarm call production in primates is under significant social control. In vervet monkeys, high-ranking individuals alarm-called at higher rates than low-ranking ones. The presence of offspring also increased alarm call rates in females, whereas males called at higher rates when with an adult female than when with other adult males. Primates may even keep track of the alarm-calling behavior of other group members. A field study reported that male Thomas langur responded with alarm calls to a model tiger and continued to do so until every member in their group had give at least one alarm call, suggesting that males keep track of which group members have and have not yet called.

Social events Primates routinely use vocalizations during social interactions, and in some cases the acoustic structure of calls varies with the social situation. The social calls of baboons have been studied in depth. During social interactions, subordinate animals tend to produce fear barks to approaching dominant group members, whereas dominants give grunts to signal their willingness to interact peacefully. These types of call exchanges have been used to experimentally mimic different types of social interactions to nearby listeners. In one experiment, individuals not only recognized the rank orders of the different group members but also recognized to which matrilineal kin group the individuals belonged.

Similarly, chimpanzees often scream when participating in agonistic interactions. In one study at Budongo Forest, Uganda, the vocal behavior of a large number of different individuals was recorded during agonistic interactions, such that each individual contributed the same number of calls both as a victim and as an aggressor. Results showed that the screams given in the two roles differed in a number of subtle acoustic features, providing reliable cues of the identity of the individuals involved and their social role. The degree to which listeners take advantage of this rich set of acoustic information needs to be explored.

Conclusion

The long-standing notion that the meaning of an utterance is nothing more than its use also has some relevance in animal communication. Nonhuman primates heavily rely on vocal communication, particularly those species whose primary habitat is the forest, where visual contact is limited and unreliable. Primates actively attend to each other's calls, and they are able to extract multifaced levels of information from individual calls and the way in which calls are arranged into different sequences. There is also evidence that primates understand something about the causal structure of the events that were responsible for the production of the various vocal signals produced by conspecifics and other animals. At the same time, primates have only limited control over their articulators and the vocal signals they can produce, but many of the fundamental principles of speech production are already well established.

A neglected area of research relates to the problem of how much primates take their audience into account and whether callers intentionally inform each other about events they have just witnessed rather than responding to the events directly. Anecdotal observations with chimpanzees suggest that individuals utilize vocalizations to affect the behavior of particular group members, although there is no clear evidence that this is for the sake of sharing information only. Chimpanzees are able to make judgments about other's intentions, even without being specifically trained to do so. For example, individuals behave differently depending on whether a human experimenter is unwilling or unable to give them food. Similarly, free-ranging baboons recognize when a call is directed at themselves rather than at other individuals. After hearing a threat grunt of a more dominant female, subjects moved away more quickly after having received aggression than grooming from that female, suggesting that baboons make inferences about the target of the caller's attention – a first crucial step toward the recognition of other individuals' intentions and motives.

One central Hockettian claim that has received comparably little attention throughout the years is that animal communication is thought to take place in the here and now only (**Table 1**). This point is interesting because the past is clearly an important psychological variable for many animal species. For example, there is evidence that scrub jays are able to recall particular food caching events in the past, including where and when they have occurred. Free-ranging gray-cheeked mangabeys of Kibale Forest, Uganda, can take the weather condition over the previous few days into account when searching for figs. The monkeys were more likely to revisit fig trees following several days of warm and sunny weather compared to after cooler, cloudier periods, presumably because they knew that temperature and solar radiation affect the ripening rate of figs. Given that animals are able to process information about past events, particularly in the context of foraging, why is there no evidence that they also communicate about them? Perhaps there are deep reasons for this; perhaps future empirical work will reveal unexpected communication capacities.

Human language is a culturally transmitted behavior. It is maintained by children who try to understand and mimic utterances produced by relevant social figures, a process that starts very early in life. A number of studies have shown that nonhuman animals, including dogs, birds, and apes, can be brought to understand spoken language to some degree. Social processes, particularly the ability to share attention and intention, appear to play a crucial role in language acquisition in humans, an ability that emerges early on during human ontogeny. The degree to which joint attention and joint intention and related social processes play a role in the acquisition of meaning in animal communication is not well understood. The current state of the art is that even human enculturated apes show a total lack of attempts to share attention with others. This peculiar lack of social intelligence is widely regarded as the main reason why humans' common system of behavior to exchange information, spoken language, is so much more complex and powerful than those of any animal species. As usual, however, future work may tell a different story.

See also: Animal Communication: Honesty and Deception; Facial Expression in Primate Communication; Game Theory and the Economics of Animal Communication; Language: Nonhuman Animals; Primate Communication: Evolution; Signal Design Rules in Animal Communication; Social Interaction; Social Interaction Effects on Reward and Cognitive Abilities in Monkeys.

Further Reading

Cheney D and Seyfarth R (1992) How monkeys see the world. *Behavioral and Brain Sciences* 15: 135–182.

Crystal D (1997) *The Cambridge Encyclopedia of Language.* Cambridge, UK: Cambridge University Press.

Emery NJ and Clayton NS (2005) Evolution of the avian brain and intelligence. *Current Biology* 15: R946–R950.

Fitch WT (2000) The evolution of speech: A comparative review. *Trends in Cognitive Sciences* 4: 258–267.

Hockett CF (1960) The origin of speech. *Scientific American* 203: 89–96.

Hurford JR (2007) *The Origins of Meaning.* Oxford, UK: Oxford University Press.

Lieberman P (2002) On the nature and evolution of the neural bases of human language. *Yearbook of Physical Anthropology* 45: 36–62.

Marcus GF and Fisher SE (2003) FOXP2 in focus: What can genes tell us about speech and language? *Trends in Cognitive Sciences* 7: 257–262.

Marler P, Evans C, and Hauser MD (1992) Animal signals: Reference, motivation, or both? In: Papoucek H, Jürgens U, and Papoucek M (eds.) *Nonverbal Vocal Communication: Comparative and Developmental Approaches*, pp. 66–86. Cambridge, UK: Cambridge University Press..

Pepperberg IM (1999) *The Alex Studies.* Cambridge, MA: Harvard University Press.

Segerdahl P, Fields W, and Savage-Rumbaugh S (2005) *Kanzi's Primal Language.* New York: Palgrave.

Seyfarth RM and Cheney DL (2003) Signalers and receivers in animal communication. *Annual Review of Psychology* 54: 145–173.

Tomasello M (1999) *The Cultural Origins of Human Cognition.* Cambridge, MA: Harvard University Press.

Tomasello M and Call J (1997) *Primate Cognition.* New York: Oxford University Press.

Zuberbühler K (2003) Referential signalling in non-human primates: Cognitive precursors and limitations for the evolution of language. *Advances in the Study of Behavior* 33: 265–307.

Zuberbühler K (2006) Alarm calls – Evolutionary and cognitive mechanisms. In: Brown K (ed.) *Encyclopedia of Language and Linguistics.* Oxford: Elsevier.

Relevant Websites

http://www.budongo.org – Budongo Conservation Field Station.

http://www.psychol.cam.ac.uk – Cambridge University, Department of Experimental Psychology.

http://www.gsu.edu – Georgia State University; see Language Research Center.

http://www.wjh.harvard.edu/~mnkylab – Harvard University, Cognitive Evolution Laboratory.

http://www.haskins.yale.edu – Haskins Laboratories (Yale University).

http://www.eva.mpg.de – Max Plank Institute for Evolutionary Anthropology; see Wolfgang Köhler Primate Research Center.

http://psy.st-andrews.ac.uk – School of Psychology, University of St. Andrews; see Research – Origins of Mind.

http://www.csl.sony.fr – Sony Computer Science Lab Paris.

http://nationalzoo.si.edu – Smithsonian National Zoological Park; see Think Tank.

http://www.alexfoundation.org – The Alex Foundation.

Sleep Deprivation and Brain Function

S P A Drummond, University of California at San Diego and Veterans Affairs San Diego Healthcare System, San Diego, CA, USA
B S McKenna, San Diego State University, University of California at San Diego, and Veterans Affairs San Diego Healthcare System, San Diego, CA, USA

Introduction

The behavioral and cognitive consequences of sleep deprivation have been the subject of scientific investigation for over 100 years, since the pioneering work of Patrick and Gilbert in 1896. In general, sleep deprivation produces neurobehavioral deficits in experimental tasks of alertness, attention, memory, cognition, learning, and motor responses, as well as performance deficits in operational settings (e.g., on the highway and in the factory). Despite the wealth of knowledge concerning the behavioral effects of sleep loss, much less work has examined the neurophysiological effects of sleep loss. This article discusses what we have learned about the effects of sleep deprivation on brain function from the perspective of functional neuroimaging studies. First, the definitions of sleep deprivation and brain function are covered. Then we review the literature in which functional neuroimaging is used to study sleep deprivation. Because the widespread application of functional neuroimaging techniques is still relatively new, there are fewer than 20 such studies published. However, rather than providing a detailed review of each one, we highlight the common findings and provide details only when they are illustrative or of particular interest. Finally, we provide a synthesis of the various findings.

Definitions

Sleep deprivation in humans can be broadly classified into three categories: total sleep deprivation (TSD), partial sleep deprivation (PSD), and sleep fragmentation. TSD is the complete lack of sleep for at least one night and often longer. PSD involves restricted sleep for multiple nights, that is, individuals obtaining an inadequate amount of sleep for several consecutive nights. Sleep fragmentation is repeated awakenings from sleep throughout the night. This results in a decreased amount of sleep but a normal time spent in bed. This article focuses on the research on TSD because all published neuroimaging studies in healthy adults to date have used this paradigm.

The term 'brain function' can be used to describe activity ranging from the cellular level (e.g., production of neurotransmitters) to the systems level (e.g., interactions among several brain regions). Functional neuroimaging refers to a set of technologies that allow researchers to examine brain activity with various spatial and temporal resolutions and relate that activity to behavior. Here we focus on two aspects of brain function typically examined in functional neuroimaging studies: (1) that cognitive performance is a behavioral measure often conceptualized as the output of brain function and (2) that functional neuroimaging techniques all provide some measure of brain metabolism. The two functional neuroimaging techniques that have been used most commonly to understand the effects of sleep deprivation are positron emission tomography (PET) and functional magnetic resonance imaging (fMRI). The specific PET technique used measures glucose metabolism over the course of 45 min (although the signal is dominated by activity in the first 20 min). The measure of brain function obtained in the fMRI studies is a complex signal called the blood oxygen-dependent (BOLD) signal. When neurons in a local area increase firing rates (e.g., in response to a cognitive demand), blood flow and blood volume in that area increase. These, in turn, increase oxygen delivery to the area. However, more extra oxygen is delivered than is needed, and the net result is an elevated level of oxyhemoglobin in the local region of activity. It is this elevated level of oxyhemoglobin that produces the BOLD signal. fMRI has a temporal resolution on the order of seconds. Both techniques allow investigators to examine the regions of the brain that are involved in processing a cognitive task being performed by a subject. Brain regions showing positive signal changes when an individual performs the task are said to be activated.

Functional Neuroimaging Studies of Sleep Deprivation

This section reviews the findings from the PET and fMRI studies examining sleep deprivation in healthy young adults. The various reports are categorized by the type of cognitive task examined. Not surprisingly, the type of task has a tremendous influence not only on the brain regions activated when the subject is well rested but also on how brain activation changes with sleep deprivation.

Attention Tasks

There are many types of attention (e.g., sustained, selective, spatial, and divided), but functional neuroimaging studies have examined only sustained attention and short-term visual attention. Sustained attention is the ability to focus on a single task for an extended period of time. Visual attention refers to the need to process a short stream of visual stimuli and respond to a specific target. In well-rested individuals, sustained attention relies on the right middle frontal gyrus and inferior parietal lobe and, to a lesser extent, on the left inferior parietal lobe and bilateral thalamus. Shorter-term visual attention tasks rely more heavily on the extrastriate cortex, as well as the fusiform, lingual, and superior parietal regions, depending on the specific target of attention.

The first study to use neuroimaging to examine TSD was a PET study involving a sustained attention task in which individuals pressed a button every 3 s for 45 min. Along with a decrease in alertness, this study showed decreased whole-brain metabolism of glucose following approximately 32 h of TSD. In addition, the frontal and temporal lobes showed a decrease in absolute metabolic rates, whereas the parietal lobes showed an increase and the occipital lobes showed no change. The largest decreases, however, were seen in the thalamus, basal ganglia, and cerebellum. These findings are consistent with a later PET study of sustained attention in which subjects performed a serial addition task for 45 min. That study showed a significant drop in cerebral metabolic rates in most brain regions after 24 h of TSD, which continued throughout 72 h of TSD. Both these studies used very long tasks and only examined brain function averaged across the entire task.

Two other studies used fMRI to examine attention after TSD on a finer temporal scale. The first measured visual attention over 40 s and found that increased activation in the ventrolateral thalamus supports intact attention after TSD. The final study used an even finer temporal scale to examine performance on the psychomotor vigilance task (PVT), which measures sustained attention and arousal lability. In this task, an individual presses a button as soon as a millisecond counter starts, which begins randomly within a predetermined interval. The task lasts 10 min and requires sustained attention. Within a testing session, performance on the PVT has been thought to reflect state instability (the variability (waxing and waning) in performance produced by the increased sleep drive during TSD). Findings showed that the frontoparietal sustained attention network supported fast reaction times whether the subjects were well rested or sleep deprived. These brain regions did not respond during slow reaction times under normal sleep conditions (which is probably why those reaction times were slow). Interestingly, however, these same regions showed increased responses immediately following slow reaction times after TSD. This was thought to reflect individuals reengaging in the task following a slow response because they received feedback regarding this slow reaction time. In essence, then, a slow reaction time prompts compensatory effort from an individual, and this compensatory response is captured in fMRI as an increase in activation in the frontoparietal sustained attention network following the slowest reaction times. A final noteworthy finding is that the study also suggests that the mechanism underlying poor performance after TSD is either (1) the impaired ability of the brain to appropriately allocate resources to task-specific brain regions or (2) the inability to inhibit activation within brain regions that actively interfere with performance.

Overall, it appears that TSD results in decreased brain responses in regions underlying sustained attention demands, as well as diminished performance on sustained attention tasks. Nonetheless, it appears that sleep-deprived individuals can indeed engage these attention regions for brief periods while sleep deprived, but only when accompanied by compensatory activation within the thalamus. This brief engagement allows for intermittent normal levels of performance, despite the fact that average performance across the entire task is diminished with TSD. This set of findings illustrates the importance of the temporal scale at which brain function is measured during TSD.

Learning Tasks

Learning is an essential task for humans, and there are multiple types of learning and memory that rely on various brain systems. Verbal learning (i.e., memorization of language-based material) is the only type of learning studied with functional neuroimaging techniques in the context of sleep deprivation. Studies of TSD have examined brain function during the encoding of verbal material, but none has directly studied recall or recognition of learning materials. Cortical regions associated with verbal encoding are almost exclusively in the left hemisphere and include the medial temporal structures, inferior frontal gyrus, premotor areas, middle temporal gyrus, and cerebellum.

Unlike sustained attention tasks, in which brain function generally decreases with TSD, verbal encoding tasks elicit increased activation in several brain regions after TSD. The most reliable increases are seen in the left and right inferior frontal gyri, as well as the left-hemisphere inferior and superior parietal lobes. This increased activation is typically associated with intact, or only minimally impacted, performance on the learning tasks. In fact, the increased activation within the parietal lobes is directly related to performance after TSD; individuals showing the greatest activation within the left inferior parietal regions after TSD show the best learning performance after TSD.

In addition, the difficulty level of the verbal learning task also influences brain function with TSD. This was demonstrated in a study comparing learning an easy word list versus learning a hard word list. During the memorization of easy words, brain activation did not differ between well rested and TSD states. Memorization of hard words, however, elicited strong increases in brain activation after TSD, and those increases were directly related to performance. The influence of task difficulty in verbal learning has also been examined by employing a distracter task to interfere with learning. That study showed a similar result, with the learning-plus-distraction condition showing greater cerebral responses after TSD than after a normal night of sleep. Once again, the greater the increase in activation with TSD, the better the subjects performed on the learning task. Interestingly, in all the studies that examined verbal learning, the left parietal lobes showed increased activation following TSD and individuals showing the greatest increases in this region also showed the best performance after TSD. This suggests that the left inferior parietal lobe plays a key role in maintaining verbal learning performance during TSD.

Finally, one recent study examined cerebral responses during a verbal learning task from a network perspective using functional connectivity analyses. This study showed that memorization of easy words and hard words each activated the same brain regions (the left and right inferior frontal gyrus and left inferior and superior parietal lobes) but that the interconnections among those regions differed. Following TSD, this study found that the interactions among brain regions within these networks changes. Specifically, in both cases, the interhemispheric connection within the frontal lobe weakened, whereas the intrahemispheric connection between the inferior and superior parietal lobes increased. Thus, this study suggests that changes, positive or negative, in cerebral activation with TSD may reflect alterations in communication among brain regions rather than simply increased or decreased activation within discrete brain regions.

Working Memory

Working memory, also called executive function, has long been a popular cognitive domain in TSD research. This is because (1) working memory tasks typically rely, at least in part, on brain function within the prefrontal cortex; (2) the prefrontal cortex has traditionally been thought of as the brain region most vulnerable to TSD; and (3) electroencephalography (EEG) studies have consistently demonstrated that changes in the frontal lobes following TSD contribute to cognitive performance deficits. The term 'working memory' refers to a large number of cognitive functions, however. It is likely that the specific aspect of working memory examined in any given study influences the measured effect of TSD on brain function. The types of working memory tasks used in functional neuroimaging studies of TSD include those requiring arithmetic, maintenance of information, and manipulation of information.

Arithmetic working memory relies on activation within the bilateral dorsolateral prefrontal cortex, anterior cingulate gyrus, and bilateral parietal lobes. Two studies examined arithmetic working memory following TSD. One of those is the PET study previously discussed in the section on attention tasks. This study showed widespread decreases in glucose metabolism during task performance starting after 24 h of TSD. However, activation in this study was confounded by the sustained attention demands of the task. The second study was an fMRI study examining serial subtraction after 35 h of TSD. Even though this study measured brain activation over 40 s intervals (thereby reducing the sustained attention demands), it confirmed the decreased responses within task-related brain regions following TSD. In both studies, subjects showed diminished performance with TSD.

Tasks requiring maintenance of information in working memory elicit bilateral activation in the prefrontal, precentral, and inferior parietal regions, as well as in the insula and thalamus. Tasks requiring the manipulation of information in working memory show more extensive activation in those same areas, reflecting the fact that manipulation requires more cognitive resources than simple maintenance. The studies examining brain function after TSD during tasks requiring maintenance and/or manipulation of information in working memory have reported both increased and decreased activation with TSD. Some of that inconsistency can be attributed to the task difficulty, similar to the verbal learning studies. More specifically, tasks requiring only the maintenance of information in working memory are more likely to show deceased activation, whereas those requiring the manipulation of information are more likely to show increased activation with TSD. Furthermore, increasing the difficulty level within either a maintenance or manipulation task also results in greater activation during TSD. This is evident from a study that used a grammatical transformation task to manipulate task difficulty and found a stronger modulation of activation in task-related regions as difficulty increased following TSD, compared to the degree of modulation after normal sleep.

Overall, the effect of TSD on the cerebral response to working memory demands remains unclear. It appears that arithmetic demands (at least those not overlearned) produce decreased activation after TSD. The brain response to other working memory tasks probably depends on the specific nature of the task demands and the specific subregions with the prefrontal cortex underlying performance of those specific demands.

Visuospatial Functioning

Visuospatial functioning refers to those cognitive processes involved in visual perception of spatial relationships among objects. One example of visuospatial functioning involves the recognition of objects, such as circular line configurations, that have no verbal properties. In imaging experiments using recognition of nonverbal objects, visual association areas in the ventral visual stream are commonly activated along with the precuneus, an area associated with the dorsal visual stream. As with working memory tasks, studies using visuospatial tasks have shown both increases and decreases in cerebral activation following TSD. Most commonly, activation in the visual association cortex and precuneus decreases after TSD, and this correlates with decreased behavioral performance. Regions showing increased activation during recognition of nonverbal objects after TSD include the basal ganglia and insula. Interestingly, the one study that attempted to use a more real-world spatial navigation task (a piloting task) found exclusively increased activation after TSD, including in both visuospatial processing regions and dorsolateral executive controls regions.

Summary and Conclusion

Research using functional neuroimaging techniques to better understand the effects of sleep deprivation on brain function is still in the early stages. Most studies have taken a relatively descriptive approach; they administered various tasks to examine the differences in brain function after normal sleep and after TSD. A few studies have used more sophisticated manipulations such as parametrically manipulating task demands or functional connectivity analyses. Despite the fairly small number of studies in this area, some generalizations can be made about the results. There appear to be two distinct brain responses to cognitive challenges during TSD. The first is characterized by decreased activation relative to the well-rested state and diminished performance; this can be thought of as an impaired brain response. The second type of response is characterized by increased activation and relatively intact performance; this has been interpreted as a compensatory recruitment response.

Compensatory Recruitment Hypothesis

The compensatory recruitment hypothesis states that the brain has the ability to recruit additional cognitive resources during task performance following TSD that it typically does not recruit to perform the same task when the subject is well rested. These resources are then engaged in performing the task, and the more an individual engages these cognitive resources following TSD, the better the individual performs the task. It is this correlation between recruitment (measured as activation) and performance that makes the process compensatory. Clearly, however, such recruitment does not always occur because several studies reported decreased activation with TSD. Three broad classes of factors are thought to influence whether, and where in the brain, recruitment occurs following TSD: (1) cognitive task-related factors (What is the subject asking the brain do to?); (2) the length and type of sleep deprivation; and (3) individual difference variables (i.e., some individuals are able to recruit new resources and others are less able).

The studies reviewed here suggest that cognitive task factors certainly play a role in brain function following TSD. For example, sustained attention tasks seem to show impaired brain responses following TSD, whereas verbal learning tasks consistently show increased activation. In addition, each study that systematically manipulated the task difficulty showed that increasing the task difficulty facilitated the compensatory recruitment response. We might think that there is a functional limit to this difficulty-influenced recruitment; however, no study to date has effectively demonstrated such a limit. A similar argument could be made with respect to the length of sleep deprivation. After enough sleep loss, even the verbal learning tasks that consistently show recruitment with TSD should show decreased activation; however, only one published study took functional neuroimaging measurements at multiple time points during TSD. This was the PET study showing decreased glucose metabolism after 24, 48, and 72 h of TSD. Because this study did not even show recruitment at the first time point, it cannot serve as a test of this aspect of the hypothesis. Likewise, no study has examined any length of PSD. The final factor thought to affect recruitment is individual differences, which has only been investigated in a few preliminary studies and, thus, also remains largely untested.

Future Directions

Clearly, much work needs to be done before we will fully understand the impact of sleep deprivation on brain function. All three factors proposed to affect cerebral activation following TSD need more research. Cognitive task-related factors are the most well-studied area. Nonetheless, we need to design cognitive tasks better so as to focus on very specific aspects of cognition rather than on general domains of cognition. For example, instead of examining working memory generically, investigators should employ event-related designs to examine the various components of working memory (e.g., attention, working memory buffer, manipulation, and encoding/retrieval). To the extent this has been done already, the results suggest that some components are more sensitive to TSD than others. Furthermore, future studies should use more real-world tasks when possible. For the second factor, models of PSD need investigation. This is a more realistic model of sleep loss in day-to-day life. Behavioral studies have suggested that a week of 4 or 6 h in bed per night produces cognitive deficits on some tasks similar to 24 or 48 h, respectively, of TSD. However, the time course of the deterioration and whether the brain can show compensatory recruitment during PSD remain unknown. Finally, behavioral data show that some individuals are relatively resilient to the effects of TSD on specific tasks, whereas others are more vulnerable. Understanding the source of those differences could lead to important advances in job selection, safety training, and effective countermeasures to sleep deprivation. Currently, we do not even know if demographic measures such as age, education, IQ, and gender play a role in the brain's response to TSD. Other variables to consider include the subject's mastery of a given task, genomic and gene expression differences, and prior experience with sleep deprivation. Work in this area is growing exponentially. The promise is that a better understanding of the consequences of sleep deprivation, and the factors that protect against the negative consequences, will help us better understand the function of sleep itself.

See also: Autonomic Dysregulation During REM Sleep; Endocrine Function During Sleep and Sleep Deprivation; fMRI: BOLD Contrast; Immune Function During Sleep and Sleep Deprivation; Metabolic Syndrome and Sleep; Positron Emission Tomography (PET); Sleep and Sleep States: PET Activation Patterns; Sleep Deprivation: Neurobehavioral Changes; Sleep-Dependent Memory Processing; Stimulant and Wake-Promoting Substances; Thermoregulation During Sleep and Sleep Deprivation.

Further Reading

Chee MWL and Choo WC (2004) Functional imaging of working memory after 24 hr of total sleep deprivation. *Journal of Neuroscience* 24: 4560–4567.

Chee MWL, Chuah LYM, Venkatraman V, et al. (2006) Functional imaging of working memory following normal sleep and after 24 and 35 h of sleep deprivation: Correlations of fronto-parietal activation with performance. *NeuroImage* 31(1): 419–428.

Choo WC, Lee WW, Venkatraman V, Sheu FS, and Chee MWL (2005) Dissociation of cortical regions modulated by both working memory load and sleep deprivation and by sleep deprivation alone. *NeuroImage* 25: 579–587.

Drummond SPA, Bischoff-Grethe A, Dinges DF, et al. (2005) The neural basis of the psychomotor vigilance task. *Sleep* 28: 1059–1068.

Drummond SPA, Brown GG, Gillin JC, et al. (2000) Altered brain response to verbal learning following sleep deprivation. *Nature* 403: 655–657.

Drummond SPA, Brown GG, Stricker JL, et al. (1999) Sleep deprivation-induced reduction in cortical functional response to serial subtraction. *NeuroReport* 10: 3745–3748.

Drummond SPA, Meloy MJ, Yanagi MA, Orff HJ, and Brown GG (2005) Compensatory recruitment after sleep deprivation and the relationship with performance. *Psychiatry Research: Neuroimaging* 140: 211–223.

Drummond SPA, Smith MT, Chengazi V, and Perlis ML (2004) Functional imaging of the sleeping brain: Review of findings and implications for the study of insomnia. *Sleep Medicine Reviews* 8: 227–242.

Mu Q, Nahas Z, Johnson KA, Yamanaka K, et al. (2005) Decreased cortical response to verbal working memory following sleep deprivation. *Sleep* 28: 55–67.

Portas CM, Rees G, Howseman AM, et al. (1998) A specific role for the thalamus in mediating the interaction of attention and arousal in humans. *Journal of Neuroscience* 18: 8979–8989.

Stricker JL, Brown GG, Wetherell LA, and Drummond SPA (2006) The impact of sleep deprivation and task difficulty on networks of fMRI brain response. *Journal of the International Neuropsychological Society* 12: 591–597.

Thomas ML, Sing HC, Belenky G, et al. (2000) Neural basis of alertness and cognitive performance impairments during sleepiness. I: Effects of 24 h of sleep deprivation on waking human regional brain activity. *Journal of Sleep Research* 9: 335–352.

Wu JC, Gillin JC, Buchsbaum MS, et al. (1991) The effect of sleep deprivation on cerebral glucose metabolic rate in normal humans assessed with positron emission tomography. *Sleep* 14: 155–162.

Social Interaction Effects on Reward and Cognitive Abilities in Monkeys

J R Stevens and M D Hauser, Harvard University, Cambridge, MA, USA

Introduction

When given a choice between receiving $100 in 30 days and $110 in 31 days, most people wait for the larger, more delayed reward. However, when the choice is between $100 today and $110 tomorrow, many people shift their preferences to the smaller, immediate reward despite the same difference of $10 and 1 day. Reward properties – such as time to receipt – play a crucial role in our processing of rewards. However, reward processing does not only occur for individual decisions but also for social interactions; we must decide whether to cooperate or compete with others for rewards. Humans stand out in the animal kingdom as exceptional cooperators, both in terms of the form that cooperation assumes as well as the nature of rewards attained. Regarding form, we are unique in the stability of our reciprocal interactions and in the scale of our cooperative coalitions, entailing multiple nation states in times of war. In terms of rewards, we are of course motivated, like all other animals, by the central survival payoffs such as food and water but also by abstract entities such as money, the promise of future support, and positions of power such as a king, president, or head of an academic department. To maintain these complicated interactions and evaluate the nature of reward, we must possess a number of prerequisite cognitive abilities. Here, we view this problem through the lens of evolutionary biology, asking which aspects of our cognitive machinery, and the social interactions it supports, are uniquely human and which are shared with other primates. Though we focus on lemurs, monkeys, and apes, we acknowledge that many of the processes we document are unlikely to be restricted to the primates, and, in many cases, there is already comparable evidence from other mammals and birds. We begin by reviewing a suite of cognitive mechanisms that are involved in both human and nonhuman primate reward processing. This article is particularly focused on the subset of situations with quantifiable rewards. We then describe the kinds of social interactions that are part and parcel of primate life, especially the highly social monkeys and apes. Finally, we merge these two sections and consider how constraints on primate cognition may limit the complexity of primate social interactions.

Primate Cognition

To set up the problem of reward processing in animals, we can distinguish between asocial, individually based processes and social ones. The primary difference is whether access to rewards entails competitive or cooperative social interactions or instead can be achieved by an individual on its own. Some processes operate across asocial and social contexts. For example, an individual seeking food as a reward must discriminate between food and nonfood objects, quantify the amount of food available and its relative value, recall where food is located in the environment as well as the timing of its seasonal availability, and inhibit the temptation to take a small, immediately available reward over a larger, more valuable but delayed reward. Social interactions add a layer of complexity to these processes, raising questions about the extent to which individuals can generate expectations about what others want and intend, their competitive abilities, and the value of a coalitionary partner.

Primates are an ideal group in which to study the comparative cognition of reward processing because they are phylogenetically closely related to humans and because primate species vary in their life histories, mating systems, and foraging ecologies. Thus, we can not only explore how these different socioecological parameters uniquely shape each species' capacity for reward processing but also explore the extent to which there are more general, derived mechanisms, having evolved before humans diverged from their phylogenetic ancestors.

Properties of Rewards

For folivorous, frugivorous, and omnivorous primates, individuals must distinguish between edible and inedible items, especially given the possibility of ingesting potentially toxic items. For many animals, recognition of edible foods entails using chemical cues, color patterns, textures, and shapes. And in some cases, these cues or features are detected in the context of social interactions. For example, in a study of rhesus macaques (*Macaca mulatta*), an experimenter ate one of two novel food items while a subject watched. The experimenter then placed new copies of each these food items on the ground and allowed the subject to approach and select one. Consistently, subjects picked the food item eaten by the experimenter. To assess which features mediated response selection, a set of follow-up conditions put different features into competition, using artificially created foods. For example, in one condition, the experimenter ate an orange sphere while holding a blue cube and then presented a blue sphere and an orange cube. Subjects consistently picked the orange cube, showing that in the context of a social foraging problem, rhesus macaques use color over shape to identify valuable food.

Number

To reliably process rewards, animals must be able to quantify reward amounts, either using number or some continuous dimension of amount such as volume. There are at least two naturally occurring situations in which number would appear to matter for primates: aggressive competition between groups and foraging for food. In black howler monkeys (*Alouatta pigra*) and chimpanzees (*Pan troglodytes*), individuals attend to the number of competitors. Playback experiments demonstrate that a group of males is more likely to approach foreign males if the numerical odds are in their favor. Additionally, in many primate species, two or three individuals will form coalitions to defeat either a single dominant individual or a smaller coalition. Although these coalitions involve small numbers, they nonetheless require some capacity to quantify the number of competitors to acquire rewards such as mates or foraging areas.

Studies of foraging in animals show that individuals often maximize the rate of energetic returns, choosing patches with more over less food. Since estimates of rates of return depend on quantifying amount of food consumed over time, researchers have asked whether animals count the pieces, estimate the volume, or time the foraging periods in a patch. For instance, when given the choice between two different amounts of apple slices, rhesus macaques consistently picked two apples over one, three apples over two, and four apples over three. But when presented with five versus four apple pieces, some animals picked four and some five. Without training, rhesus monkeys can quantify the number of pieces of food up to about four but thereafter appear to rely on a general estimate of amount.

Based on an overwhelming number of carefully controlled experiments, it is now fair to say that animals have a number sense that likely consists of two naturally available systems. One system allows animals to quantify individuals up to about four with precision; the second allows them to approximate number but without any limits on magnitude. In the precise system, as evidenced by the rhesus macaque example, primates are limited to representing four items simultaneously in short-term memory. Human infants and adults demonstrate a similar limit in a variety of tasks, suggesting continuity across development and across species. In the approximate system, primates can discriminate between approximate quantities using analog magnitudes, in which performance is limited by the ratio between the quantities and is independent of absolute value. Other work on operantly trained rhesus macaques demonstrates that ratio determines numerical discrimination between quantities ranging from 1 to 30 items. Ratio is important because it suggests that primate numerical competence conforms to Weber's law, a psychophysical process in which the accuracy of discriminating different quantities scales with the magnitude of the quantities. Again, human infants and adults also represent large approximate numbers and show similar signature ratio limits.

Timing

Predicting the timing of reward availability is a critical capacity for primates. In many species, crucial elements of the diet are only seasonally available, requiring both timing and planning. For example, when chimpanzees discover a source of ripe palm nuts, they not only invest in the processing of these nuts with stone hammers and anvils, but often leave behind particularly good hammers, retrieving them on future visits. Studies conducted with captive apes reveal that they can recall the kinds of tools needed for certain tasks, and retrieve them in the service of planning for future tasks. Based on their patterns of movement, it is also clear that many primates store information about fruiting cycles, enabling them to time the optimum period of visitation and harvesting.

Like number, the capacity to time events is based on a mechanism that, both behaviorally and neurobiologically, shows the signature of the analog magnitude system that underlies number. Importantly, timing exhibits the scalar property of Weber's law: the variance of timing accuracy scales with interval magnitude and is therefore a function of the ratio between magnitudes. For instance, rhesus macaques showed similar accuracy levels between timing events with a 1:1.5 ratio, regardless of whether the discrimination was 4 versus 6 s, 6 versus 9 s, 8 versus 12 s, or 10 versus 15 s. Unfortunately, little work has explored primate timing abilities beyond a few seconds, with the exception of periodic timing of circadian cycles. Moreover, the work is largely restricted to studies involving operant training, with no work on the relationship between timing and the role of social or ecological contexts.

Impulsivity

Animals must often combine quantity and temporal information to choose between rewards available over different time intervals (intertemporal choice). For example, imagine a monkey encounters a tree full of unripe fruit but with only a few ripe fruit available: should it spend the time and energy to consume the few ripe fruit now or wait for the rest to ripen? Waiting would yield a higher reward amount, but the future is uncertain – another monkey may eat the fruit in the meantime, winds may knock them into a stream below, or a fungus may infest and spoil the perfectly good fruit. This uncertainty may have provided a strong adaptive benefit for impulsivity.

Decision makers can make intertemporal choices by means of at least two mechanisms. The first mechanism simply assumes that the forager maximizes its food intake rate over repeated foraging bouts. This rate maximization account predicts that foragers should maximize the total energy gained from rewards over the total time spent acquiring and processing the rewards. Evidence from operant experiments suggests that cotton-top tamarins (*Saguinus oedipus*) and common marmosets (*Callithrix jacchus*) may use rate maximization strategies when trading off future benefits. Temporal discounting represents the second mechanism and involves the subjective devaluation of future rewards. If animals discount the future (as the example in the introduction implied), delayed rewards are less valuable than immediate rewards, potentially resulting in impulsive choice. In experiments that estimate discounting levels, subjects are presented with two stimuli: one associated with a small, immediate reward and the other with a large, delayed reward. The discounting level is 'titrated' by incrementally increasing the delay-to-large until subjects are indifferent between choosing the large, delayed reward and the small, immediate reward. Therefore, researchers can find indifference points between immediate and delayed rewards over a range of small and large reward amounts. Psychologists have extensively studied discounting in rats and pigeons, but fewer studies have investigated primate discounting. Surprisingly, the handful of primate discounting studies that have been conducted demonstrate that cotton-top tamarins, common marmosets, brown capuchin monkeys (*Cebus apella*), and rhesus macaques show similar impulsivity levels to rats and pigeons.

The high levels of discounting observed for most nonhuman animals suggests that when rewards are distributed over time, individuals place a premium on immediacy, forgoing delayed rewards. This not only puts severe constraints on the foraging strategies of monkeys and apes, but constrains other behaviors such as cooperation, territory defense, and mate selection.

Inhibitory Control

Inhibiting prepotent responses to reward is a difficult task for nonhuman animals. Clearly, natural selection has favored a strong drive to obtain the largest reward available. This is evidenced by the performance of a number of primate species on the reversed-contingency task in which subjects must reach toward the smaller of two visible rewards to receive the larger reward. Brown and black lemurs (*Eulemur fulvus* and *Eulemur macaco*), tamarins, squirrel monkeys (*Saimiri sciureus*), rhesus macaques, orangutans (*Pongo pygmaeus*), gorillas (*Gorilla gorilla*), bonobos, and chimpanzees all invariably choose the large reward, only to receive the small reward – they seem incapable of controlling their desire to reach for the larger reward amount.

The reversed-contingency task has proven difficult for primates to solve but not impossible. A number of techniques can circumvent the inhibitory control problem. First, sheer repetition can allow subjects to choose the smaller and receive the larger food reward. Most subjects do not solve the task after 200 trials, though some are at chance rather than repeatedly choosing the smaller amount. After 400–2500 trials, however, six rhesus macaques received the larger reward in over 90% of trials. Thus, massive exposure to the reversed contingencies can eventually trump the inhibitory problems. Second, imposing costs for 'incorrect' choice can facilitate receiving the larger reward. By withholding all food when subjects pick the larger quantity, macaques and squirrel monkeys eventually learn to pick the smaller quantity; tamarins stick with the losing strategy, picking the larger and getting nothing at all. This suggests that part of the failure to point to the smaller quantity is due to the lack of costs associated with pointing to the larger quantity. Finally, including a mediator between seeing the food and receiving the food can curb the impulse to choose the larger reward amount. This has been most noticeably documented by an experiment testing chimpanzees trained on the Arabic number symbols from 1 to 6. Instead of choosing between one food treat versus four treats, the chimpanzees chose between a card with the numeral 1 written on its face and a card with the numeral 4; each card covered up the corresponding number of food treats. The chimpanzees quickly learned to pick the number 1 card and received four treats, indicating chimpanzees can learn a rule like "Point to the one you don't want to get the one you want." Surprisingly, once they learned this rule with symbols, they were incapable of generalizing to the same problem with food presented on its own. Therefore, it seems as though the difficulty of this task results from the chimpanzees' strong motivation to reach for food rather than an inability to learn the reverse-contingency rule.

Memory

Memory is a multifaceted cognitive ability with clear evolutionary importance. Researchers have delineated several different types of memory that are applied to different types of information. Here we will focus on three types of memory – short-term, spatial, and episodic memory. One of the simplest tasks used to test short-term memory is the delayed-response task. In this task, a reward is placed under one of two (or more) identical but spatially separated stimuli. After a retention interval, subjects are allowed to chose one of the stimuli and receive the rewards if correct. Comparative data show that rhesus macaques are fairly good at remembering the location of the food item. They begin with about 80% accuracy after only a few seconds and drop to about 68% accuracy after a 15 s retention interval. Marmosets, however, though also starting at 80% accuracy, drop to 58% accuracy at 15 s, only slightly better than chance. Though some evidence suggests that the Old World monkeys may retain information better than the New World monkeys, this is by no means a universal, with capuchin monkeys being a notable exception to the rule.

Spatial memory plays an important role in primate reward acquisition. Recalling when and where food rewards are distributed is critical in foraging situations. In fact, some have suggested that foraging problems have posed strong evolutionary pressures on primate cognition, with species that feed on spatially and temporally variable foods showing higher levels of brain encephalization than species that feed on more stable food sources. Numerous studies have demonstrated strong spatial skills in primates, particularly in analogs to the radial arm maze. In this task, feeder stations placed throughout an enclosure are baited before subjects enter. After a subject finds all of the stations, researchers bait only some of the stations and, following a retention interval, record whether the subjects first attempt to feed at the previously baited stations. Most of the experiments on primates show high accuracy over retention intervals as long as 24 h. As predicted by the adaptive specialization hypothesis, species that search over longer distances for food in the wild tend to be more accurate at longer retention intervals (e.g., frugivorous golden lion tamarins (*Leontopithecus rosalia*) are more accurate than gummivorous Wied's marmosets (*Callithrix kulhi*)). Additionally, the contingency between space and reward plays an important role. Common marmosets, for instance, are more accurate in a win-stay paradigm in which previous food locations predict current locations than in a win-shift paradigm in which subjects are not rewarded for visiting previously visited food stations.

Probably one of the most interesting and controversial areas of primate memory is episodic memory. There is a feisty debate in the literature about whether nonhuman animals have the ability to mentally travel in time to recall previous experiences. The benchmark requirements for demonstrating episodic memory include showing that animals know 'what,' 'where,' and 'when' an experience occurred. Though this is difficult to study in nonlinguistic creatures, recent research provides suggestive evidence of episodic-like memory in corvids and primates. For example, up to 24 h after receiving a particular food item from an experimenter, a gorilla correctly identified the food type received and the experimenter from whom it was received.

Theory of Mind

Another highly contentious area of primate cognition is theory of mind. As mentioned earlier, this aspect of primate cognition is not strictly about reward. Yet, the capacity to make inferences about what others know, desire, believe, and intend often leads directly to cooperative and competitive rewards, and most of the experimental studies use food as a motivator to explore these mental states.

Early studies failed to find evidence of theory of mind in primates. One explanation for these failures was that the studies relied on animals making inferences about human mental states in contexts involving cooperation, as opposed to asking animals to make inferences about each other in the context of competition. Though several primate species do cooperate (see below), competition is far more common and may represent the most basic form of social interaction among animals. To test this hypothesis, recent studies of monkeys and apes have used both competitive and cooperative tasks, contrasting conspecific pairings as well as conspecific–heterospecific pairings. There is increasing evidence that monkeys and apes make inferences from seeing to knowing. Chimpanzees, for instance, can take the visual perspective of other individuals to understand whether they can see occluded food rewards: subordinate chimpanzees preferentially approach rewards that are obscured from the view of dominant individuals. Rhesus monkeys show similar abilities, stealing food primarily from experimenters without visual access to the food rather than from those that do have access. Though visual perspective taking is only one component of having a theory of mind, it plays a significant role in the competitive and cooperative interactions of primates. What remains to be explored is whether primates go beyond this elemental capacity, attributing intentions, desires, and beliefs to others.

Primate Social Interactions

In socially living animals, such as some of the lemurs and most monkeys and apes, obtaining rewards is often coupled with socially competitive or cooperative interactions. In some instances, helping another individual yields payoffs for the helper, while in other cases, helping is costly for the helper. The existence of the latter poses a puzzle given the generally accepted Darwinian assumption that behavior evolves via natural selection to provide fitness benefits to the individual. Specifically, what selective pressure has favored individuals who provide benefits to other individuals?

Here, we address the evolution of cooperation by describing four different models (mutualism, kin selection, reciprocity, and punishment), focusing on evidence from monkeys and apes. We operationally define cooperation as social interactions resulting in a net benefit for all participants; here, benefit is measured in terms of increasing reproductive success.

Mutualism

The simplest type of cooperative behavior provides direct benefits to the cooperator, in addition to other individuals. Therefore, benefits to others are by-products of benefits to self. This model of cooperative behavior is termed by-product mutualism. Any individual that defects (does not cooperate) in mutualistic situations will, by definition, do worse than a cooperator; therefore, in the absence of a temptation to defect, cooperation provides the best option. Importantly, mutualism does not depend on the identity of one's partner and thus can occur between any members of the same species and even members of different species.

Mutualism is a common form of cooperation, with cooperative hunting providing a prime example. When multiple individuals cooperate to hunt the same prey, they can both increase the probability of successful prey capture and reduce the individual costs associated with hunting. Cooperative hunting provides mutualistic benefits only when the per capita intake rate increases with group size. Therefore, a pair of hunters would have to capture more than twice as many prey items as a solitary hunter. This typically requires the success rate of solitary hunters to be fairly low, making cooperation particularly successful. Increased success combined with lower hunting costs can lead to direct, immediate, and simultaneous fitness benefits for cooperative hunters, particularly when hunting small or difficult prey. For example, wild chimpanzees often cooperatively hunt arboreal monkeys. Although different populations vary, there is evidence that in some populations the per capita intake rate increases with group size, suggesting that the hunting is cooperative. Cheaters that do not hunt are discouraged by receiving only small amounts of meat in food-sharing bouts following a kill. Thus, it is in an individual's best interest to participate in a hunt to acquire the much-sought-after meat.

In the laboratory, mutualism has been documented in a variety of primates, including marmosets, capuchin monkeys, and chimpanzees. Typically, when joint action is required to receive separate benefits for each player, subjects succeed in cooperating. However, when food is monopolizable instead of divided between players, cooperation breaks down. That is, when immediate rewards are available, primates cooperate. But once competition reduces the probability of reward, there is no guarantee of immediate benefit and no apparent mechanism capable of maintaining cooperation. In a recent study of captive chimpanzees, individuals confronted an opportunity to manipulate an apparatus for a food reward; on some trials, the focal subject had to recruit the help of another individual in order to manipulate the apparatus and on other trials, the focal could operate the apparatus alone. Subjects only recruited help when two individuals were required to obtain the food reward. Moreover, in a second experiment, subjects selectively recruited effective helpers over ineffective helpers, demonstrating a keen knowledge of the role of others in the mutualistic acquisition of rewards.

Kin Selection

Whereas mutualism poses no problem for classic Darwinian theory, altruistic cooperation does as the actor incurs a cost while benefiting another. Kin selection provided the first clear theoretical solution to the paradox of altruism. Individuals may bias cooperation toward their genetic relatives because it helps propagate their own genes shared by common descent. What looks altruistic from an individual's perspective actually serves self-interest from the gene's view. Individuals have a certain probability of sharing a gene (r, the coefficient of relatedness) with relatives due to common descent. If the benefits to kin discounted by this coefficient of relatedness outweigh the costs of helping, altruism toward kin can evolve.

Kin selection may be particularly powerful in primates because of the close-knit family groups found in many species. With a few notable exceptions, including chimpanzees, nonhuman primates follow the general mammalian pattern of philopatry in which males leave their natal groups upon reaching reproductive maturity whereas females stay in their natal groups for life; consequently, most primate groups consist of closely related female kin and genetically unrelated males. Kin selection theory predicts that individuals should preferentially help relatives and should help in proportion to their coefficient of relatedness. These types of quantitative predictions have proven difficult to test in primates, but there are data showing kin-directed helping, particularly in coalition formation and food sharing.

Primates frequently form coalitions in which multiple individuals form an alliance in agonistic interactions with other group members. This is particularly prevalent in primate species with matrilineal dominance hierarchies, such as macaques and baboons. In these species, females often assist relatives in aggressive encounters with other group members. Notably, the probability of coalitionary support tapers off with increasingly distantly related kin – mothers almost always aid offspring but are less likely to aid nieces and nephews. Therefore, as relatedness increases, these primates are more likely to pay costs associated with helping kin. Additionally, individuals are more likely to form coalitions with kin than nonkin against higher-ranking opponents, suggesting that they will pay a higher cost of helping related individuals. Male primates can also form coalitions, often to guard or acquire sexually receptive females. In situations in which few mating opportunities exist for males, these kin-based coalitions are especially relevant because aiding kin helps ensure the propagation of one's genes, even in the absence of direct mating opportunities. This is the case in red howler monkeys (*Alouatta seniculus*), where coalitions of related individuals have longer tenure in a troop (and therefore more mating opportunities) than unrelated individuals. Though many instances of coalitionary support are directed to kin, some are directed to nonkin and may be attributable to other benefits such as mutualism and reciprocity.

One of the most often-reported examples of apparent altruism is food sharing – voluntarily allowing another to consume food that one individual possesses. Food sharing is, of course, very common between mother and offspring for numerous primate species. However, it also occurs between grandparents and grandoffspring, siblings, and even adult relatives, often scaling with relatedness. In captive macaques, for instance, mother–daughter pairs ($r = 0.5$) frequently fed from the same food bin. Both grandmother–granddaughter pairs and sister–sister pairs ($r = 0.25$) co-fed at intermediate rates, and aunt–niece pairs ($r = 0.125$) co-fed at low levels indistinguishable from unrelated pairs. Though it is unclear what proportion of food transfers occurs between relatives, kin-based sharing likely explains the bulk of sharing in numerous species.

Reciprocity

Reciprocity occurs when an individual pays a short-term cost of cooperation for the future benefit of a social partner's reciprocated cooperation. As a form of altruistic cooperation, reciprocity aims to explain cooperative behavior among genetically unrelated individuals (thereby eliminating kin selection as an explanation) often using a unique type of social interaction termed the prisoner's dilemma. The keys aspects of the prisoner's dilemma are (1) cooperation maximizes the total payoff to everyone involved in the interaction (mutual cooperation provides more benefits than mutual defection); however, (2) any individual will receive a higher personal payoff by defecting, so a sizable temptation to cheat exists. Pursuing unilateral cooperation in this game is not a stable strategy.

Theoreticians suggested that reversing roles as donor and recipient of altruism may reduce the temptation to defect because it largely commits individuals to invest in future cooperation. When the fitness payoffs sum over a series of interactions with the same partner, reciprocal strategists can reap the benefits of mutual cooperation. The reciprocal strategy tit-for-tat, in which a player starts out cooperating and copies its opponent's behavior in previous interactions, can successfully dominate simulated populations of social partners engaging in prisoner's dilemma games, winning out over many alternative behavioral strategies. If the probability of interacting again exceeds a critical level, a reciprocal strategy can maintain cooperation.

Many authors have reported examples of reciprocity in animals, including primates, spanning such contexts as food sharing, grooming, and coalitions associated with mating opportunities. Unfortunately, in most cases these purported examples of reciprocity have either never been replicated or have been challenged by alternative explanations for the patterns of interaction, including especially kin selection and mutualism. Another alternative explanation, symmetry-based reciprocity, occurs when the reciprocal pattern can be explained by the symmetrical relationship between individuals. For instance, if individuals A and B interact frequently and cooperate, their behavior will appear to be reciprocal even though it is based on symmetrical interactions rather than contingent cooperation. This contrasts with calculated reciprocity (such as tit-for-tat) in which individuals track debts owed and favors given when deciding whether to cooperate.

A field study of olive baboons (*Papio anubis*) provided one of the first reports of reciprocity. Males formed coalitions in order to drive off rival males and gain access to reproductively active females. Data suggested that males took turns reaping the benefits, implying evidence of reciprocity. The robustness of this finding, however, is unclear, given that a subsequent study of a different population of baboons did not find the same reciprocal patterns, and a study of a closely related species proposed an alternative, mutualistic explanation.

Another example comes from experimental tests of food sharing in captive capuchin monkeys. When pairs of capuchins were placed in adjacent chambers separated by a mesh partition, if individual A allowed individual B to consume dropped scraps of food in one particular trial, then B tended to allow A to gather scraps in the next trial. Because the food transfer is primarily passive and costs may be minimal, these results can be explained by a mutual tolerance between individuals. Therefore, the capuchins do not appear to be assessing the costs and benefits of their actions, making calculated reciprocity an unlikely explanation of capuchin food transfers.

Finally, in a series of experiments with captive cotton-top tamarins, subjects could pull a tool to give food to an unrelated recipient without getting any food for self. Tamarins pulled the tool most often for partners that always pulled and infrequently for partners that never pulled. The frequency of cooperation was, however, less than 50%, and as each game progressed, the amount of food given dropped. Tamarins, therefore, maintained moderate levels of cooperation with other cooperators, but the degradation of cooperation over time suggests an unstable system; in fact, game theoretic modeling of the data suggest that reciprocity crashes if an opponent fails to cooperate on two consecutive opportunities.

In summary, there are few examples of true, calculated reciprocity among monkeys and apes. Most putative examples can be explained by symmetry-based reciprocity, mutualism, or kin selection. Given the simplicity of the preconditions for reciprocity and the apparent ubiquity of reciprocity in humans, its rarity in primates (and other animals) is surprising. We take up this issue in the section on cognitive constraints on reward processing.

Punishment

Punishing individuals that defect can potentially impose enough costs to offset the temptation to cheat, and, like reciprocity, can elicit future cooperation. Punishment involves energetic costs, and, when accomplished by means of aggression, also involves the costs of risked injury. Consequently, as an adaptive behavior, punishment is a selfish strategy, favoring actions that ultimately benefit the punisher by eliciting cooperative behavior from the recipient of punishment. As defined, punishment resembles reciprocity, which should occur when it elicits cooperative behavior directed strictly at the reciprocator. Despite the theoretical interest, punishment is not well documented in animals; in fact, though animals act aggressively toward others in the context of resource defense (e.g., territoriality, dominance interactions), there are few examples in the context of cooperation.

Whereas punishment penalizes past behavior with the hope of future reward, a similar behavior called harassment penalizes present behavior to elicit immediate reward. Harassment occurs when an individual imposes costs such as aggression on another to induce immediate cooperation, thereby providing instant benefits to the harasser. Harassment may also influence future as well as current cooperation, suggesting that it can lead to punishment strategies. For instance, if a defector is in the process of consuming an entire food resource, a harasser could impose costs on the defector aimed at obtaining some portion of the food resource immediately. Whereas punishment appears relatively rare among animals, harassment may be more common. For instance, after capturing prey, chimpanzees frequently allow other individuals to consume part of the meat. Observational work has demonstrated that harassment best accounts for the pattern of food sharing, taking the form of individuals incessantly begging for food with hand gestures, grabbing at the food, and placing their hands over the mouths of the food possessors. In this context, harassment was costly for the food owner (food intake rate decreased as the number of beggars increased), owners shared more often when beggars harassed frequently and intensely, and when sharing occurred harassment levels decreased. Controlled experiments corroborated these findings with captive chimpanzees, as well as squirrel monkeys (*Saimiri boliviensis*), a species that rarely cooperates.

Harassment may, of course, influence future as well as current cooperation, suggesting that it may lead to punishment strategies. One example comes from rhesus macaques. When individuals find food, they often give food calls, an altruistic act that recruits others to the food source, thereby potentially benefiting kin. However, individuals sometimes find food and suppress their calls. If no one detects these silent discoverers, they reap more food rewards than those who announce their discoveries. If, in contrast, they are detected, then they are aggressively attacked, leading to an even larger loss of food to the attacker. Thus, aggression yields an immediate benefit of accessing food for the attacker, clearly qualifying it as a case of harassment. In addition, the aggression may have a punishing effect on silence by eliciting future food calls. That is, aggressive behavior influences both immediate and future benefits.

The Cognitive Psychology of a Cooperator

Many researchers have argued that the frequency of complex social interactions in primates underlies the evolution of their cognitive abilities. Negotiating a complicated network of allies and enemies, dominants and subordinates, and mates and competitors has created selective pressure for cognitive abilities such as transitive inference, theory of mind, and deception. Though this connection between sociality and cognition has been well recognized, the cognitive constraints on social interaction have often been ignored. Put simply, much of the work on primate cognition has focused on how large brains enable rich social interactions instead of how limited cognitive abilities may constrain the range of social interactions. Here, we take up this 'cognitive constraints' perspective.

Mutualism and kin selection are both theoretically well-understood and empirically well-documented models of cooperation. By contrast, reciprocity and punishment, while theoretically feasible, are rare among primates (although harassment may be more widespread). Therefore, despite models purporting the evolutionary stability of all of these types of cooperation, some types occur much more frequently than others. Unfortunately, a strictly adaptive perspective has limited power to explain the frequency of mutualism and kin biased cooperation and the rarity of reciprocity and punishment. A proximate perspective that links with the ultimate problem can, however, reveal how cognitive constraints limit or facilitate particular forms of cooperation.

The proximate approach emphasizes critical aspects of reciprocity and punishment that differ markedly from mutualism and kin-biased cooperation. In both reciprocity and punishment, the fitness benefits associated with cooperation depend on the partner's behavior: cooperation should only occur when the partner responds by reciprocating or punishing. When this contingent response occurs in the future, the temporal delay introduces cognitive challenges that may constrain the emergence and stability of cooperation. Animals can easily implement strategies that yield immediate benefits, such as mutualism and harassment, because individuals do not have to track benefits over time. With a time delay between cooperating and receiving return benefits, however, individuals must invest in an uncertain future. Delayed benefits impede learning the consequences of cooperation, place greater demands on the capacity to recall previous interactions, and trade off short-term fitness gains for long-term gains. Here we highlight how several key cognitive constraints play a role in mutualism, kin-biased cooperation, reciprocity, and punishment, thereby uniting the two sections of this essay.

Cognitive Constraints on Mutualism and Kin-Biased Cooperation

Because no temptation to cheat exists in mutualistic interactions, individuals should always cooperate. As a result, mutualism requires no special cognitive abilities above and beyond the challenges inherent in the cooperative behavior itself. Kin-biased cooperation does, however, require additional cognitive capacities. At a minimum, it requires the capacity to direct cooperative actions to related individuals.

Mechanisms of kin recognition include recognition alleles, phenotype matching, and spatial and familiarity cues. The recognition allele hypothesis predicts that individuals can compare a particular phenotypic cue (auditory, olfactory, visual, etc.) to an innately specified template. Such a model requires few cognitive skills other than discriminating the cue associated with relatedness. The closely related phenomenon of phenotypic matching occurs when an individual compares a conspecific's phenotypic cues to a learned template. This requires specialized perceptual and computational systems that detect cues at an early stage to form a template, then test cues against the template to discriminate kin. Though recognition alleles and phenotypic matching provide the most direct forms of kin recognition and have been observed in some animal species, they do not appear to be common mechanisms of primate kin recognition. Instead, primates seem to use a simple set of rules such as spatial and familiarity cues to discriminate kin. Often primates may use rules such as 'be nice to individuals near your home' or 'help those that you grew up with' to direct the benefits of cooperation toward kin. These familiarity mechanisms require little in the way of cognitive abilities, building on general laws of learning by association, and seem to be widespread throughout the primates.

Cognitive Constraints on Reciprocity and Punishment

The original formulation of reciprocity had three requirements for evolutionary stability: (1) the reciprocated benefit must outweigh the immediate cost, (2) individuals must interact repeatedly, and (3) individuals must recognize each other. These requirements, however, most likely underestimate what is cognitively necessary for both developing and maintaining a system of stable reciprocity. In particular, the delay between the cost of a cooperative act and the benefit of reciprocated cooperation introduces a number of cognitive challenges. Like reciprocity, punishment can involve a delay between a costly act and a beneficial payoff, and in these cases it faces similar constraints. For this reason, we consider the constraints on reciprocity and punishment together, pointing to differences where appropriate.

Individual recognition Like kin selection, reciprocity and punishment require directing cooperation to others. Unlike kin selection, however, where altruistic acts are disseminated simply as a function of coefficients of genetic relatedness, reciprocity and punishment require targeting specific individuals. Therefore, the delayed, contingent response required for both reciprocity and punishment necessitates that individuals can distinguish different partners. Mechanisms for individual recognition appear to be the norm among animals, including lemurs, monkeys, and apes. Consequently, the paucity of evidence for reciprocity and punishment across primates cannot appeal to individual recognition as a constraint.

Number, amount, and time Numerical abilities can play a key role in reciprocity when individuals must precisely quantify the reward amounts being reciprocated. When primates engage in a bout of reciprocity, they will either be limited to small numbers of objects in cases where the exchange must be precise (a banana for a banana), or they will be freed from this constraint where approximate exchanges are tolerated. The same prediction holds for cases where the currency is time, such as the duration of a grooming bout. If one monkey grooms another for 10 min, the groomer will most likely accept as fair exchange a reciprocated grooming bout of 8–12 min. As reward quantity and time magnitudes increase, quantification accuracy decreases, making equitable exchange more difficult and leaving opportunities for cheaters to exploit the judgment errors. This constraint only applies when variance exists in the quantity and time magnitudes. If the exchange is always a banana for a banana, these quantification abilities are superfluous.

Inhibitory control and impulsivity Reciprocity is itself an inhibitory and impulsivity problem: can an individual inhibit the choice of the immediate large benefit to gain the delayed larger benefit? Like the reversed-contingency task, the chooser must first reach for the undesirable over the desirable reward. The first move can be likened to giving away food. By avoiding the temptation of the larger immediate reward, the first move is costly to self. As data on the reversed-contingency task in primates show, the cost often appears too great and the inhibitory system too weak.

The second move, waiting for the reciprocated benefit, is analogous to the intertemporal choices described earlier. Individuals must choose between the immediate reward of defecting and the long-term reward of cooperating. Indeed, a number of researchers have predicted that impulsivity can reduce the value of reciprocated benefits. Experimental data on variation in human impulsivity and cooperation validate the view that a preference for immediate rewards may inhibit reciprocity. Impulsivity correlates with cooperation such that individuals who prefer immediate gains also cooperate less frequently. In parallel, blue jays (*Cyanocitta cristata*) show stable cooperation in a prisoner's dilemma, only following an experimental reduction in their preference for immediacy. Although primates have not been tested in both impulsivity and cooperation tasks, it seems highly probable that a significant constraint on their capacity for reciprocity emerges from their steep discounting functions. Similar abilities are required for punishment: punishers must pay an immediate cost of punishing to achieve a future, discounted reward.

Memory Episodic memory may very well be required to implement reciprocity. Because individuals must track the actions ('what') of previous partners ('who') the last time that they interacted ('when'), fairly sophisticated memory systems may be required for reciprocity. Even if episodic memory itself is not required, limitations in memory decay, interference, and capacity can also constrain the frequency of reciprocity and punishment. Memory decay proceeds rapidly over time; therefore, longer time intervals between cooperative acts may make reciprocity and punishment more difficult. Even with short time delays between cooperative interactions and few distractions, every potential new partner increases the computational load of tracking debts owed, favors given, and costs imposed. Keeping score of reciprocal obligations and punishment with the extensive social network found in many primate species may place a computationally intensive burden on memory systems. Although few studies examine learning and memory constraints in primate cooperation, studies of human cooperation suggest that these constraints can pose challenges for maintaining stable cooperative relationships.

Theory of mind Understanding the knowledge of others is critical to strategic reasoning. 'I know that you know that I know that you know…' is a central assumption of economic decision making required for rational agents in economic games. If, however, natural selection acts as the 'rational agent' by selecting for individuals that make good decisions, this capacity may not be required for individuals if they use simple rules that approximate the outcome of fully rational choice. Therefore, it is possible for primates to implement reciprocity without full theory of mind capacities. At present, only a few studies have attempted to integrate issues concerning mental state attribution with those involved in cooperation. For example, recent demonstrations of visual perspective-taking abilities in primates suggests that they might be able to attend to rewards that others seek, possibly aiding their ability to recognize cooperative situations. However, despite this evidence, recent work shows that chimpanzees do not demonstrate other-regarding preferences; that is, they do not preferentially acquire food rewards in such a way as to give food to others. Instead, they appear to be completely indifferent to how their own reward-based actions can benefit other individuals. In contrast, in the study of tamarins mentioned above, individuals were more likely to cooperate with individuals who intentionally gave food as an altruistic act as opposed to individuals who gave the same amount of food as an accidental by-product of an otherwise selfish act. Further study of what monkeys and apes understand of the goals, beliefs, and intentions of others will elucidate whether limitations in these areas constrain other-regarding preferences.

Conclusions

With increasingly sophisticated and ecologically relevant tasks, we are closing in on those aspects of reward processing and social cognition that have uniquely evolved in humans and those that evolved by common descent with other primates and, possibly, other nonprimate animals. We suggest that reward processing and social cognition are intimately linked, setting up cognitive constraints on the evolution of cooperative behavior. We do not propose that these reward-processing constraints are immutable. If the evolutionary benefit of cooperation is great, selection pressure may circumvent these constraints. This, however, is likely to occur in a domain-specific manner rather than a domain-general manner. For instance, food-caching species such as squirrels may suspend inhibitory and impulsivity problems when hiding nuts away for winter. Yet, this ability has evolved to solve a very specific problem and likely does not apply generally to the species' decision-making strategies. Therefore, domain-general cognitive systems must evolve to allow many of the more complex forms of cooperation. The possibly unique presence of reciprocal cooperation and punishment in humans may be directly attributable to a combination of our keen number sense, patience, inhibitory control, memory capacity, and theory of mind.

See also: Connectivity of Primate Reward Centers; Episodic Memory; Games in Monkeys: Neurophysiology and Motor Decision-Making; Goal-Directed Behavior Theories; Neuropsychology of Primate Reward Processes; Prefrontal Contributions to Reward Encoding; Primate Communication: Evolution; Representation of Reward; Reward and Learning; Reward Neurophysiology and Primate Cerebral Cortex; Social Brain: Evolution.

Further Reading

Axelrod R and Hamilton WD (1981) The evolution of cooperation. *Science* 211: 1390–1396.

Boesch C and Boesch H (1989) Hunting behavior of wild chimpanzees in the Tai National Park. *American Journal of Physical Anthropology* 78: 547–573.

Boysen ST and Berntson GG (1995) Responses to quantity: Perceptual versus cognitive mechanisms in chimpanzees (*Pan troglodytes*). *Journal of Experimental Psychology: Animal Behavior Processes* 21: 82–86.

Chapais B and Berman CM (2004) *Kinship and Behavior in Primates*. Oxford: Oxford University Press.

Hampton RR and Schwartz BL (2004) Episodic memory in nonhumans: What, and where, is when? *Current Opinion in Neurobiology* 14: 192–197.

Hare B, Call J, Agnetta B, and Tomasello M (2000) Chimpanzees know what conspecifics do and do not see. *Animal Behaviour* 59: 771–785.

Hauser MD, Chen MK, Chen F, and Chuang E (2003) Give unto others: Genetically unrelated cotton-top tamarin monkeys preferentially give food to those who altruistically give food back. *Proceedings of the Royal Society of London, Series B* 270: 2363–2370.

Hauser MD and Spelke ES (2004) Evolutionary and developmental foundations of human knowledge: A case study of mathematics. In: Gazzaniga M (ed.) *The Cognitive Neurosciences III*, pp. 853–864. Cambridge, MA: MIT Press.

Kacelnik A (2003) The evolution of patience. In: Loewenstein G, Read D, and Baumeister RF (eds.) *Time and Decision: Economic and Psychological Perspectives on Intertemporal Choice*, pp. 115–138. New York: Russell Sage Foundation.

Meck WH (2003) *Functional and Neural Mechanisms of Interval Timing*. Boca Raton, FL: CRC Press.

Stevens JR (2004) The selfish nature of generosity: Harassment and food sharing in primates. *Proceedings of the Royal Society of London, Series B* 271: 451–456.

Stevens JR, Hallinan EV, and Hauser MD (2005) The ecology and evolution of patience in two New World monkeys. *Biology Letters* 1: 223–226.

Tomasello M and Call J (1997) *Primate Cognition*. Oxford: Oxford University Press.

Trivers RL (1971) The evolution of reciprocal altruism. *Quarterly Review of Biology* 46: 35–57.

Spatial Cognition

C L Colby, University of Pittsburgh, Pittsburgh, PA, USA

Behavioral Studies of Spatial Cognition in Humans

Spatial Abilities

Spatial cognition involves not one but many specific abilities. These include locating points in space, determining the orientation of lines and objects, assessing location in depth, appreciating geometric relations between objects, and processing motion, including motion in depth. These spatial skills can be applied to imagined objects as well as to external stimuli, as in the classic experiments on mental rotation. These experiments showed that observers take longer to determine whether two objects are identical when the degree of mental rotation needed to align them increases. Similar kinds of basic processes contribute to spatial cognition in the auditory and somatosensory domains.

Multiple Frameworks for Spatial Representation

Our subjective experience strongly suggests that we have direct access to a single coherent and overarching representation of space. Whether we locate an object by sight, smell, hearing, or touch, we can respond to it with equal ease and with any motor system at our command. This introspection is misleading. There is no evidence for the existence of a single, explicit, topographic representation of space suitable for incorporating every kind of sensory input and generating every kind of motor output. On the contrary, the evidence points to multiple representations of space, in a variety of coordinate frames, each closely linked to separate output systems designed to guide specific motor effectors.

The particular representation of space in use at any time depends on the task the subject is trying to perform. For example, if you were to draw out a route for a hiking trip on a map, the route would be in the coordinates of the map, the piece of paper. If you were then going to walk along that route, you would have to begin by locating your current position within that coordinate frame and constructing a representation of the route with respect to your starting point. The first, map-based representation is an example of an allocentric representation, in which locations are represented in reference frames extrinsic to the observer. Allocentric representations include those centered on an object of interest (object-centered) and those in environmental (room-centered or world-centered) coordinates. The second representation, the one in the coordinates of the hiker's current position, is an example of an egocentric representation, in which locations are represented relative to the observer. Egocentric representations include those in eye-centered, head-centered, hand-centered, and body-centered coordinates. Experimental work in humans indicates that multiple reference frames can be activated simultaneously.

Neural Basis of Spatial Cognition

Impairments of Spatial Cognition in Humans

Much of our knowledge about the neural basis of spatial cognition comes from observations in patients with spatial deficits following brain damage. These include a wide range of perceptual and motor deficits, such as poor localization of visual, auditory, or tactile stimuli; inability to determine visual or tactile line orientation; impaired performance on mazes; impairment on tests of mental spatial transformations; right–left confusion; poor drawing; impaired eye movements to points in space; misreaching; defective locomotion in space; and amnesia for routes and locations. As can be seen from this partial list, spatial behavior involves many kinds of skills, and not surprisingly, a number of brain regions have been implicated in spatial cognition and performance.

Broadly speaking, the parietal lobe is responsible for spatial perception and representation of immediate extrapersonal space, whereas temporal and parahippocampal cortices are more involved in topographic memory and navigation. The frontal lobe receives input from both parietal and temporal cortex and is responsible for generating actions. An important point about deficits in spatial cognition in humans is that they are far more common after right hemisphere damage than left. Although patients with left hemisphere damage may also exhibit spatial deficits, it is clear that the right hemisphere in humans has a superordinate role in spatial processing and behavior.

Impact of Parietal Lesions in Humans on Spatial Cognition

Two kinds of spatial deficits following parietal lobe damage are particularly illuminating. First, a common sensorimotor deficit is difficulty in using visual information to guide arm movements, referred to as optic ataxia. Patients with optic ataxia have difficulty with everyday tasks that require accurate reaching under visual guidance, such as using a knife and fork. They both misdirect the hand and misorient it with respect to the object, and they are most impaired when using the contralesional hand to reach for an object in the contralesional half of space. A second, classic disorder of spatial cognition in humans is the tendency to ignore one half of space, called hemispatial neglect. The most common form of neglect arises from damage to the right parietal lobe and is manifested as a failure to detect objects in the left half of space. Neglect is more than just a visual deficit, however. It can occur separately or jointly across many sensory modalities. Moreover, neglect occurs with respect to many different spatial reference frames. A patient with right parietal lobe damage typically neglects objects on the left, but left may be defined with respect to the body, or the line of sight, or with respect to an attended object. Furthermore, this neglect is dynamic, changing from moment to moment with changes in body posture and task demands.

Neglect is apparent even in the purely conceptual realm of internal images. Patients exhibit neglect when asked to imagine a familiar scene, such as a city square, and describe the buildings in it. The portion of space that is neglected changes when they are asked to imagine the scene from a different viewpoint. As **Figure 1** illustrates, neglect can occur with respect to an internal image constructed by the individual. Patients with neglect show evidence of using multiple reference frames, just as intact individuals do.

Impact of Parietal Lesions in Monkeys on Spatial Cognition

The role of parietal cortex in spatial cognition has been explicitly tested in animal studies. Monkeys with posterior parietal lobe lesions exhibit many of the same deficits seen in humans, including deficits in the appreciation of spatial relations between objects and impairments in eye movements and reaching. They perform normally on tests of object discrimination but are selectively impaired on a spatial task that requires them to judge which of two identical objects is closer to a visual landmark. In contrast, monkeys with temporal lobe lesions are unimpaired on the spatial task but fail to discriminate between or recognize objects. This double dissociation between the effects of lesions, in combination with the discovery of distinctive cortical inputs to the parietal and temporal lobes, led to the concept of the dorsal and ventral visual-processing streams. The ventral stream processes information about object form and color and is necessary for object recognition. In contrast, the dorsal stream processes information

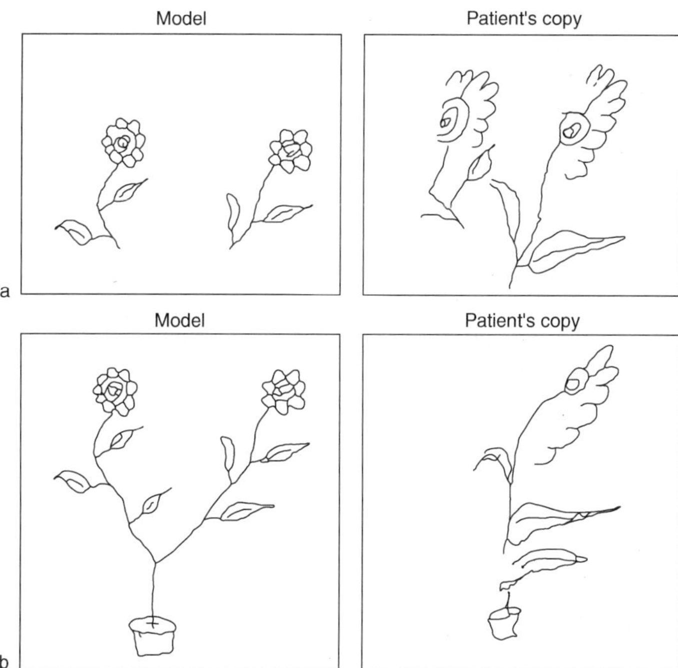

Figure 1 A test for object-centered neglect. When asked to copy the two drawings on the left, a patient made the two copies on the right. Detail is omitted from the left half of each object rather than from the left half of the drawing as a whole. Reproduced from Marshall JC and Halligan PW (1993) Visuo-spatial neglect: A new copying text to assess perceptual parsing. *Journal of Neurology* 240: 37–40, with permission.

about where objects are located and how to acquire or avoid them.

Neurons in the dorsal stream encode several types of visual information important for spatial perception. Neurons in specific dorsal stream areas are selective for orientation, depth, direction and speed of motion, rotation, and many other stimulus qualities appropriate for perceiving spatial information. The dorsal visual-processing stream leads to posterior parietal cortex, where many kinds of visual information converge, including information about stimulus shape. An equivalent set of somatosensory processing areas send tactile information to anterior parietal cortex.

Visual and somatosensory signals converge on single neurons within the intraparietal sulcus, which divides anterior and posterior parietal cortex. Auditory signals have also been demonstrated to contribute to spatial processing in monkey parietal cortex.

Spatial Information Is Encoded in Multiple Reference Frames

The standard approach for investigating the role of parietal neurons in spatial processing is to record electrical activity from individual neurons while the monkey performs a spatial task. Because brain tissue has no sensory receptors, fine microelectrodes can be introduced into the brain without disturbing the animal's performance. By recording neural responses during carefully designed tasks, neural activity can be related directly to the sensory and representational processes that underlie spatial behavior. The general conclusion from these studies is that the function of parietal cortex is to transform spatial information from its original sensory coordinates into the motor coordinates necessary for the guidance of action. The specific kind of coordinate transformation depends on the anatomical area within parietal cortex and the task to be accomplished. Several cortical areas have been defined within the parietal lobe in monkeys. Two examples of parietal areas with distinct forms of spatial representation are described next.

Head-centered spatial representation in the ventral intraparietal area The ventral intraparietal area (VIP) is located in the floor of the intraparietal sulcus, where inputs from high-order visual and somatosensory cortex converge. In the visual domain, VIP neurons are characterized by direction and speed selectivity, and they resemble neurons in other dorsal stream visual areas that process stimulus motion. Surprisingly, these same neurons were discovered to respond to light touch on the head and face. The somatosensory and visual receptive fields of individual neurons exhibit strong spatial correspondence: they match in location, size, and even their preferred direction of motion.

The existence of spatially matched receptive fields raises an interesting question: What happens when the eyes move away from primary position? If the visual receptive fields were simply retinotopic, they would have to move in space when the eyes do and so would no longer match the location of the somatosensory receptive field. Instead, for many VIP neurons, the visual receptive field moves to a new location on the retina when the eyes move away from the straight-ahead position. For example, a neuron that has a somatosensory receptive field near the mouth and responds best to a visual stimulus moving toward the mouth will continue to respond to that trajectory of motion regardless of where the monkey is looking. The conclusion is that these neurons have head-centered receptive fields: they respond to stimulation of a certain portion of the skin surface and to the visual stimulus aligned with it, no matter what part of the retina is activated. Neurons in area VIP send projections to the region of premotor cortex that generates head movements. Area VIP neurons contribute to the visual guidance of head movements and may play a special role in hand, eye, and mouth coordination. They operate in a head-centered reference frame in order to generate appropriate signals for a particular motor effector system, namely that which controls head movements.

Eye-centered spatial representation in the lateral intraparietal area In contrast to area VIP, neurons in the lateral intraparietal area (LIP) construct an eye-centered spatial representation. Individual neurons become active when a salient event occurs at the location of the receptive field. This can be a sensory event, such as the onset of a visual or auditory stimulus; a motor event, such as a saccade toward the receptive field; or even a cognitive event, such as the expectation that a stimulus is about to appear or the memory that one has recently appeared. The level of response reflects the degree to which attention has been allocated to the site of the receptive field.

As discussed for area VIP, the animal's ability to make eye movements raises an interesting question about spatial representation. Neural representations of space are maintained over time, and the brain must solve the problem of how to construct an accurate spatial representation when a receptor surface moves. With each eye movement, every object in our surroundings activates a new set of retinal neurons. Despite this constant change, we perceive the world as stable. Area LIP neurons contribute to this perceptual stability by using information about the metrics of the eye movement to update the spatial representation

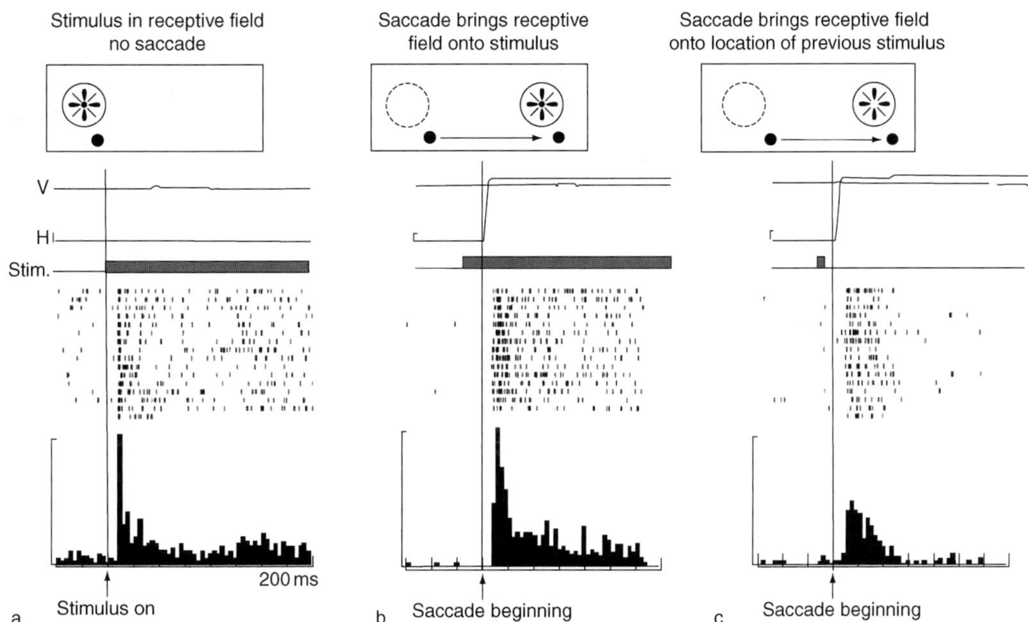

Figure 2 Remapping of visual memory trace activity in area LIP. The activity of a single neuron was recorded under three different conditions. (a) Simple visual response to a constant stimulus in the receptive field, presented while the monkey is fixating. The rasters and histogram are aligned on the time of stimulus onset. (b) Response following a saccade that brings the receptive field onto the location of a constant visual stimulus. (c) Response following a saccade that brings the receptive field onto the location where a stimulus was presented previously. The stimulus is extinguished before the saccade begins so it is never physically present in the receptive field. The neuron responds to the updated memory trace of the stimulus. H, horizontal eye position; V, vertical eye position. Reproduced from Duhamel JR, Colby CL, and Goldberg ME (1992) The updating of the representation of visual space in parietal cortex by intended eye movements. *Science* 255: 90–92, with permission.

of a salient location. In a simple saccade task, LIP neurons are activated when the monkey makes an eye movement that brings a previously illuminated screen location into their receptive field. These neurons respond to the memory trace of the earlier stimulus: no stimulus is ever physically present in the receptive field, either before or after the saccade. The explanation for this striking finding is that the memory trace of the stimulus is updated at the time of the saccade. Before the saccade, while the monkey is looking straight ahead, the onset of the stimulus activates a set of LIP neurons whose receptive fields encompass the stimulated screen location. They continue to respond after the stimulus is extinguished, maintaining a memory trace of the stimulus. At the time of the saccade, a corollary discharge, or copy of the eye movement command, containing information about the metrics of the saccade arrives in parietal cortex. This corollary discharge signal causes the active LIP neurons to transmit their stored representation of the stimulus to the new set of LIP neurons whose receptive fields will encompass the stimulated screen location after the saccade. The representation of the stimulated location is dynamically updated from the coordinates of the initial eye position to the coordinates of the final eye position (**Figure 2**).

The significance of updating lies in what it reveals about spatial representation in area LIP. It demonstrates that the representation is dynamic and is always centered on the current position of the fovea. Instead of creating a spatial representation that is in purely retinotopic (sensory) coordinates, associated exclusively to the specific neurons initially activated by the stimulus, area LIP constructs a representation in eye-centered (motor) coordinates. The distinction is a subtle one but critical for the ability to generate accurate spatial behavior. By representing visual information in eye-centered coordinates, area LIP neurons tell the monkey not just where the stimulus was on the retina when it first appeared but also where it would be now if it were still visible. The result is that the monkey always has accurate spatial information with which to program an eye movement toward a current or remembered target. The transformation from sensory to motor coordinates puts the visual information in its most immediately useful form. Compared to a head-centered or world-centered representation, an eye-centered representation has the significant advantage that it is already in the coordinates of the effector system (oculomotor) that will be used to acquire the target. Humans with unilateral parietal lobe damage fail on an eye movement task that depends on an eye-centered representation of a remembered target position. This failure presumably reflects an impairment of the updating mechanism in parietal cortex.

In summary, posterior parietal cortex plays a critical role in spatial cognition. Physiological studies in monkeys show that parietal neurons represent spatial locations relative to multiple reference frames, including those centered on the head and the eye. Individual neurons combine spatial information across different sensory modalities (in area VIP), and specific spatial reference frames are constructed by combining sensory and motor signals (in area LIP). In accord with the physiology, human neuropsychological studies show that neglect can be expressed with respect to several different reference frames.

Frontal Lobe Mechanisms of Spatial Cognition

The parietal lobe transforms sensory representations of attended objects into the motor coordinate frames most appropriate for action. It does not actually generate those actions. Dorsal stream outputs to frontal cortex provide the sensory basis, in the correct spatial framework, for producing specific motor outputs. The following sections describe different types of spatial representations found in distinct regions of frontal cortex.

Head-centered and hand-centered visual receptive fields in premotor cortex Two different forms of spatially organized visual responsiveness have been described in ventral premotor cortex. First, in a subdivision representing facial movements (area F4), neurons respond to visual stimuli at specific locations relative to the head, much like those described

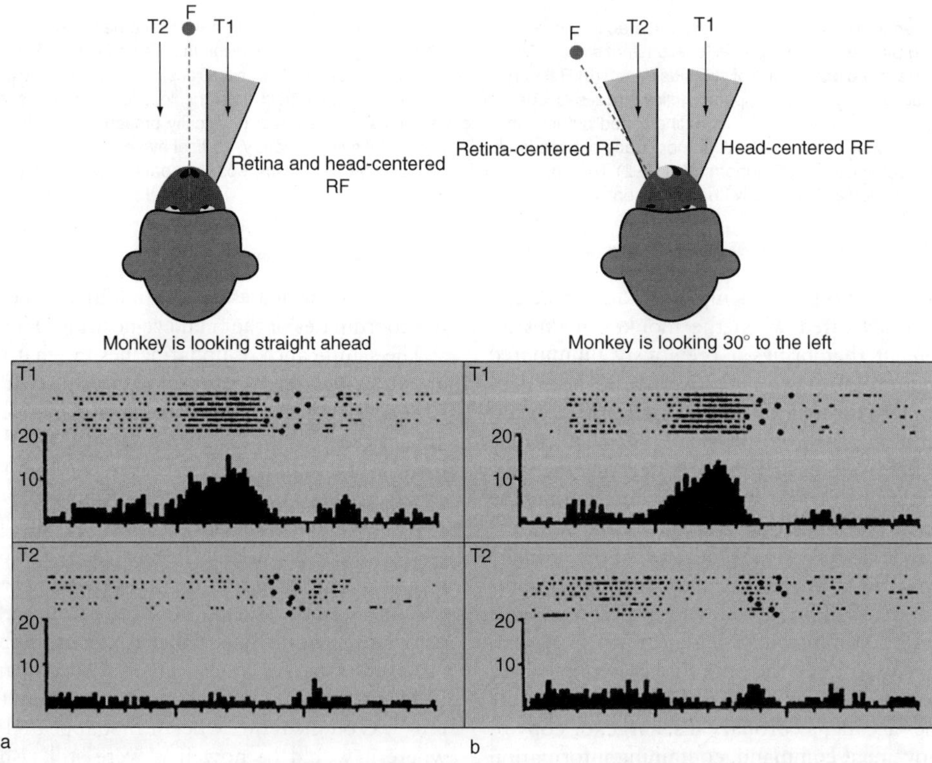

Figure 3 Data from a neuron in the premotor cortex with a head-centered visual receptive field (RF). (a) While the monkey was looking straight ahead at a fixation point (F), an object approached and receded, traveling either along trajectory 1 (T1, to the right of the head) or along trajectory 2 (T2, to the left of the head). The neuron fired strongly only when the object approached along trajectory 1. (b) When the monkey looked at a new fixation point on the far left, the neuron still responded only when the object approached along trajectory 1, indicating that the receptive field is tied to the location of the head and not to the location of the retina. The timelines above each raster and histogram show the horizontal and vertical eye position during one trial. The timeline below shows the position of the visual object as it comes toward and then moves away from the monkey. Adapted from Fogassi L, Gallese V, di Pellegrino G, et al. (1992) Space coding by premotor cortex. *Experimental Brain Research* 89: 686–690, with permission.

previously in area VIP. These neurons have been characterized by recording activity while objects approach the monkey's head along various trajectories. The preferred trajectory is constant with respect to the head, and it is not affected by changes in eye position. This specific zone of premotor cortex receives inputs from area VIP and uses the same form of spatial representation. In both cases, stimuli are represented in the motor coordinate frame that would be most useful for acquiring or avoiding stimuli near the face by means of a head movement (**Figure 3**).

A different kind of spatial representation has been observed in a subdivision of premotor cortex involved in generating arm and hand movements (area F5). Here, neurons respond to visual stimuli presented in the vicinity of the hand. When the hand moves to a new location, the visual receptive field moves with it. Moreover, the visual receptive field remains fixed to the hand regardless of where the monkey is looking, suggesting the existence of a hand-centered representation. A fascinating observation indicates that some neurons in this area are capable of even more abstract forms of representation. Some neurons in premotor cortex are activated both when the monkey grasps an object, such as a raisin, and when the monkey observes the experimenter performing the same action. These mirror neurons encode not just the monkey's own motor actions but also the meaning of actions performed by others.

Object-centered spatial representation in the supplementary eye field Actions are directed toward objects in the environment and toward specific locations on an object. Picking up your coffee cup requires that you locate both the cup in egocentric space and the handle in relation to the cup. The spatial reference frame that guides such movements is not limited to the egocentric representations described previously. Evidence from the supplementary eye field (SEF) demonstrates that single neurons can encode movement direction relative to the object. The SEF is a division of premotor cortex with attentional and oculomotor functions. Neurons here have visual responses and are also active before and during saccades. In monkeys trained to make eye movements to particular locations on an object, SEF neurons exhibit a unique form of spatial selectivity: they encode the direction of the impending eye movement

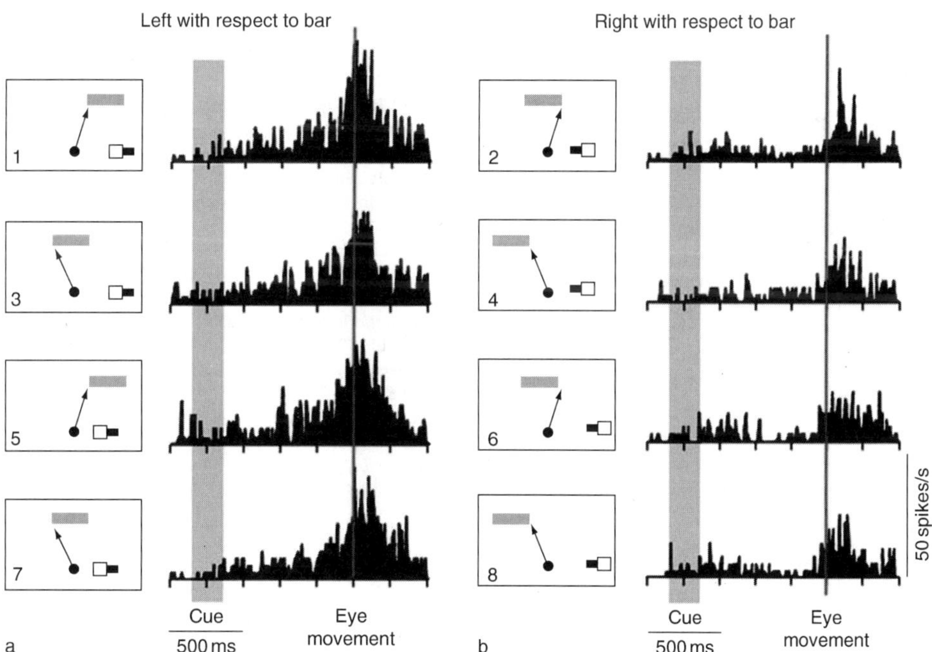

Figure 4 Data from a neuron in the SEF selective for the object-centered direction of eye movements. The monkey was trained to make eye movements to the right or left end of a horizontal bar. A cue appeared on the small sample bar shown in the lower right of each panel (1–8) to tell the monkey which end of the target bar (top in each panel) was relevant on a given trial. The arrow in the panel next to each histogram indicates the direction of the eye movement. The neuron fired strongly when the eye movement was directed to the left end of the target bar (left column) regardless of whether the physical movement of the eye was up and to the right (panels 1 and 5) or up and to the left (panels 3 and 7). Reproduced from Olson CR and Gettner SN (1995) Object-centered direction selectivity in the macaque supplementary eye field. *Science* 269: 985–988, with permission.

as defined relative to an object-centered reference frame. For example, a given neuron may fire when the monkey looks toward the right end of a bar placed at any of several different locations on the screen, regardless of whether the eye movement is a rightward or leftward saccade. Moreover, the same neuron will fail to respond when the monkey makes a physically identical eye movement toward the left end of the bar stimulus (**Figure 4**).

This remarkable result indicates that single neurons can make use of quite abstract spatial reference frames. Object-centered spatial information could potentially guide arm movements as well as eye movements. Moreover, neuropsychological evidence indicates that an object-centered reference frame can be used to direct attention: some patients exhibit object-centered neglect after parietal lobe damage. Parietal lobe lesions in monkeys likewise produce impairments on tasks that require an object-centered spatial representation.

Conclusion

Behavioral and neuropsychological studies indicate that we make use of multiple spatial representations in the perception of extrapersonal space. Neurophysiological studies are beginning to uncover the neural mechanisms underlying the construction of these egocentric and allocentric spatial representations. We can conclude that spatial cognition is the product of many brain areas with distinct representations of space.

See also: Attentional Networks in the Parietal Cortex; Multisensory Convergence and Integration; Neural Coding of Spatial Representations; Parietal Cortex and Spatial Attention; Prefrontal Cortex; Sensorimotor Integration: Attention and the Premotor Theory; Sensorimotor Integration: Barrels, Vibrissae and Topographic Representations; Spatial Orientation: Our Whole-Body Motion and Orientation Sense; Spatial Cognition and Executive Function; Spatial Transformations for Eye–Hand Coordination; Spatial Cognitive Maps; Vision for Action and Perception.

Further Reading

Barbieri C and De Renzi E (1989) Patterns of neglect dissociation. *Behavioural Neurology* 2: 13–24.

Behrmann M (2000) Spatial reference frames and hemispatial neglect. In: Gazzaniga M (ed.) *The Cognitive Neurosciences.* Cambridge, MA: MIT Press.

Bisiach E and Luzzatti C (1978) Unilateral neglect of representational space. *Cortex* 14: 129–133.

Colby CL (1998) Action-oriented spatial reference frames in cortex. *Neuron* 20(1): 15–24.

Colby CL and Goldberg ME (1999) Space and attention in parietal cortex. *Annual Review of Neuroscience* 22: 319–349.

Duhamel JR, Colby CL, and Goldberg ME (1992) The updating of the representation of visual space in parietal cortex by intended eye movements. *Science* 255: 90–92.

Fogassi L, Gallese V, di Pellegrino G, et al. (1992) Space coding by premotor cortex. *Experimental Brain Research* 89: 686–690.

Fuster JM (1997) *The Prefrontal Cortex: Anatomy, Physiology and Neuropsychology of the Frontal Lobe,* 3rd edn. Philadelphia: Lippincott-Raven.

Gallese V, Fadiga L, Fogassi L, and Rizzolatti G (1996) Action recognition in the premotor cortex. *Brain* 119: 593–609.

Graziano MS (2001) Is reaching eye-centered, body-centered, hand-centered, or a combination? *Review of Neuroscience* 12(2): 175–185.

Heilman KM, Watson RT, and Valenstein E (1985) Neglect and related disorders. In: Heilman KM and Valenstein E (eds.) *Clinical Neuropsychology.* New York: Oxford University Press.

Kakei S, Hoffman DS, and Strick PL (2003) Sensorimotor transformations in cortical motor areas. *Neuroscience Research* 46(1): 1–10.

Marshall JC and Halligan PW (1993) Visuo-spatial neglect: A new copying text to assess perceptual parsing. *Journal of Neurology* 240: 37–40.

Olson CR (2003) Brain representation of object-centered space in monkeys and humans. *Annual Review of Neuroscience* 26: 331–354.

Olson CR and Gettner SN (1995) Object-centered direction selectivity in the macaque supplementary eye field. *Science* 269: 985–988.

Rizzolatti G and Craighero L (2004) The mirror-neuron system. *Annual Review of Neuroscience* 27: 169–192.

Shepard R and Cooper L (1986) *Mental Images and Their Transformations.* Cambridge, MA: MIT Press.

Snyder LH (2000) Coordinate transformations for eye and arm movements in the brain. *Current Opinion in Neurobiology* 10(6): 747–754.

Ungerleider L and Mishkin M (1982) Two cortical visual systems. In: Ingle DJ and Mansfield RJW (eds.) *Analysis of Visual Behavior,* pp. 549–586. Cambridge, MA: MIT Press.

Spatial Cognition and Executive Function

M Behrmann, CarnegieMellon University and Center for the Neural Basis of Cognition, Pittsburgh, PA, USA
S Shomstein, George Washington University, Washington, DC, USA

Introduction

Representing and exploring the space around us is fundamental to human cognition. The study of spatial cognition, both at the psychological and neural level, is extensive, encompassing parallel investigations of many different types of spatial knowledge and many different spatial tasks. For example, there is now a large literature concerned with the processes involved in deriving spatial relations between objects or between parts of objects, and with the way these processes differ from other mechanisms involved in object recognition, such as the representation of the parts alone.

A rather different form of spatial processing, which is also the topic of much current investigation, concerns the nature of the spatial representations engaged during the learning of the spatial layout of the environment. Two forms of spatial knowledge, both of which are deemed critical for navigation purposes, have been described in these investigations of spatial cognition: survey knowledge (based on an external perspective or an aerial or maplike view), which allows access to the global spatial layout, and route knowledge, which is the perspective represented by a ground-level observer. Recent functional neuroimaging studies have suggested that these two spatial processes recruit both a common network of cortical regions but also additional, differentiable regions of cortex. Consistent with this, in individuals with unilateral hemispheric lesions, several brain areas appear to be involved in retracing a route from the end to the beginning, including the right hippocampal formation, the right posterior parietal cortex, the right dorsolateral prefrontal cortex, and the right temporal lobe. The hippocampus also plays a particular role in path integration; specifically, individuals with lesions to the right (but not left) hippocampus are inconsistent in their navigation to previously viewed targets, and they also show a systematic underregistration of linear displacement (and/or velocity) during walking. Whereas the hippocampal coding appears to be specific to certain places in the field, parietal neurons code route maps in a more scalable and versatile form, independent of the size and spatial configuration of the navigational field.

A further strand of experimental studies concerned with spatial cognition has explored the psychological and neural mechanisms mediating spatial working memory. Keeping spatial information active online (even for extended periods of time) engages dorsal areas of lateral prefrontal cortex, posterior parietal cortex, and possibly even the hippocampal formation, and damage to these areas significantly impairs working memory. Finally, much research is concerned with delineating the nature of the underlying spatial representations, with specific emphasis on determining the reference frames or spatial coordinates employed for sensory information encoding. In some regions of cortex, the spatial position of the input is defined with respect to an eye-, head-, and/or body-centered frame of reference or sometimes some mixture of these different reference frames. While parietal cortex appears most involved in these egocentric forms of representation, in which the reference frame is centered on the observer, superior parietal cortices represent information allocentrically, independent of the observer, although, of note, these egocentric and allocentric representations appear to be somewhat interdependent. Of great interest, too, are the means whereby spatial information is updated – as the eyes move or as the observer navigates, the spatial positions of items in the environment change. To achieve a stable and robust representation, information must be constantly updated, and studies concerned with spatial updating have been (and continue to be) conducted with humans and nonhuman species, using a variety of methods, including lesion studies, functional magnetic resonance imaging, and single-unit recording.

As is evident from this brief overview, spatial cognition is multifaceted, and spatial representations are derived in the service of many different forms of cognition. Importantly, too, these different spatial representations are not mutually exclusive and much research remains to be done to specify the differences and commonalities among these representations and the spatial tasks in which they are engaged. This article focuses specifically on the spatial representations mediated by parietal cortex, often assumed to be the preeminent area involved in spatial processing. Two major lines of investigation are summarized, with one set of data primarily derived from studies of individuals with parietal lesions and the other set of data acquired from functional brain imaging studies (mostly functional magnetic resonance imaging).

Parietal Lobe and Spatial Representations

Anatomical Delineation of Parietal Cortex

The parietal lobe forms about 20% of the human cerebral cortex and is divided into two major regions, the somatosensory cortex and the posterior parietal cortex (**Figure 1**). Posterior parietal cortex, located at the junction of multiple sensory regions and projecting to several cortical and subcortical areas, is engaged in a number of cognitive operations, many of which involve spatial representations. Parietal cortex is separated from the frontal lobes by the central sulcus and from the occipital lobes by the parieto-occipital fissure. Since the 1940s, hundreds of studies have documented the behavioral consequences of parietal lesions in humans and monkeys, with primary emphasis on the perturbation of perceptual and action space following these lesions.

Parietal Lobe and Spatial Representations: Evidence from Hemispatial Neglect

In humans, the deficit that affects the representation of space following unilateral hemispheric lesion is referred to as hemispatial neglect ('neglect,' for short). Following brain damage, particularly to the right hemisphere (see **Figure 2** for examples of lesions giving rise to neglect), individuals typically exhibit a variety of symptoms, including impaired representation of information appearing on the side of space contralateral to the lesion. These individuals may fail to report or to orient to sensory information on the contralateral side of space. Standard bedside tests, such as having the patients draw a clock from memory or copy a clock, bisect some lines, or cancel lines on a page, are typically used to elicit neglect (see **Figure 2(b)** for examples of patients' performance on such tests). Individuals may also show neglect of information appearing in contralesional personal space, in that they may eat, dress, and/or shave only the ipsilesional side. Furthermore, the eye and hand movements of such individuals may also be somewhat restricted to the ipsilesional side, and there is a perseverative tendency (perhaps induced by the failure to keep track of spatial locations) to revisit the same regions on the ipsilesional side. Interestingly, even in the absence of sensory input, neglect may be evident: the patients report only ipsilesional information in tasks of mental imagery and may show a paucity of contralesional saccades even when moving their eyes in the dark. Note that the neglect disorder does not arise from a primary motor or sensory deficit *per se* and is generally thought to arise from a deficit in attending to and representing the contralateral information.

Neglect also occurs more frequently and with greater severity following right than left hemisphere lesions (see also evidence from functional imaging studies on hemispheric asymmetry of parietal activation), and so we refer to neglect of left-sided information as a convenience throughout the following discussion. The scientific study of hemispatial neglect has been especially captivating over the past few decades and has continued to shed light on the mechanisms supporting spatial representation.

A critical question repeatedly addressed in the neglect literature is whether spatial information from different sensory modalities is processed in similar fashion. Although a majority of the studies have explored visual neglect, the question of interest is whether the underlying spatial map, perturbed by parietal damage, is specifically visual or utilized by other modalities as well. If the latter holds, then one might expect to observe neglect across multiple sensory modalities. Indeed, the consensus is that the representation of and awareness of space involve input from multiple sensory

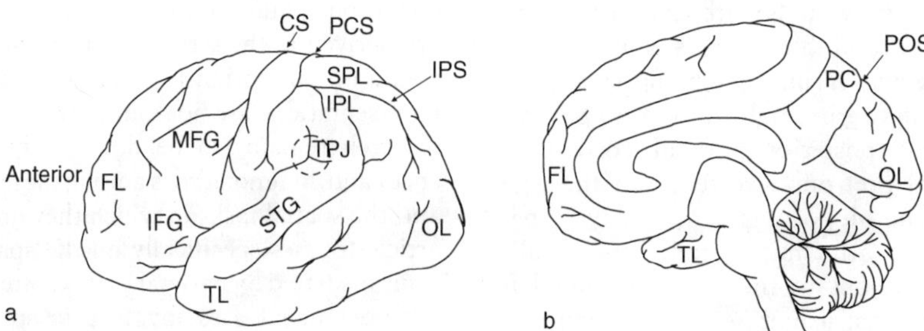

Figure 1 (a) Schematic depiction of relevant anatomical landmarks projected onto the (a) lateral and (b) medial surfaces of the human brain. Parietal cortex (PC) is located posterior to the postcentral sulcus (PCS), which lies posterior to the central sulcus (CS), and superior to the occipital lobe (OL). It is divided by the intraparietal sulcus (IPS) into the superior parietal lobule (SPL) and the inferior parietal lobule (IPL). The continuation of the SPL on the medial side, anterior to the parieto-occipital sulcus (POS), is called the cuneus. The frontal lobe (FL) is divided into the middle frontal gyrus (MFG) and the inferior frontal gyrus (IFG). The superior temporal gyrus (STG) runs along the superior extent of the temporal lobe (TL) and terminates at the temporoparietal junction (TPJ).

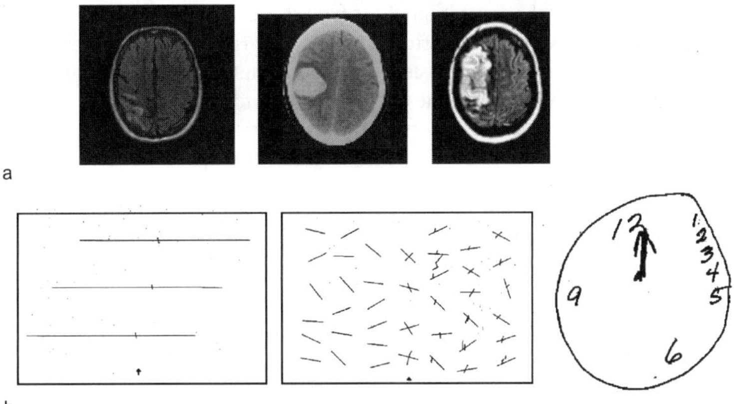

Figure 2 (a) Examples of structural scans from three different individuals, all of whom show hemispatial neglect following right parietal lobe lesions. Note that the right hemisphere is on the left of the image. (b) Examples of performance of three different patients with hemispatial neglect, using bedside tests of line bisection, line cancellation, and clock drawing from memory.

modalities: patients with visual neglect have difficulty localizing sounds and also experience problems in specifying the location of tactile input. Also, prism adaptation (see later for more details) appears to affect visual as well as proprioceptive input, further attesting to the cross-modal nature of spatial representation. Of course, one cautionary note in reaching this conclusion is that the lesions in humans are typically large and may implicate many regions of parietal cortex (in contrast to the lesions in nonhuman primates or the single-unit recording studies wherein the target areas are more circumscribed). With the advent of high-resolution structural imaging, we can start delineating better, in the neglect patient, the exact site of the lesion, the extent to which different parietal regions are affected, and the consequences of these more limited lesions on behavior.

Given that parietal cortex appears to derive a representation of space, one issue that has been under considerable investigation concerns the nature of competitive interactions between information appearing further on the ipsilesional or contralesional side of space. Consistent with ideas emerging from 'biased competition' accounts, there is a view that suggests that information appearing more contralesionally is assumed to compete with more rightward information, perhaps 'extinguishing' it entirely. If the contralesional information appears temporally in advance of the more rightward information or is much more salient than the rightward information, it might not be so readily extinguished and might ultimately be reported. It is also the case that if the contralesional information can be integrated or perceptually grouped with the rightward information, it, too, might survive the competitive interaction and be reportable. Although much of the emphasis has been on a spatial gradient with greater activation as one proceeds from left to right, there is also growing consensus that there is a temporal delay in representing spatial information (enhanced or prolonged 'attentional blink'), even when the information appears in the midline.

One recent domain in which considerable progress has been made concerns the nature of recovery of spatial attention deficits in individuals with hemispatial neglect. An intervention procedure used in some recent studies to ameliorate hemispatial neglect is to adapt the patients to prisms, which serves to induce a rightward displacement of the visual field. Several studies have successfully reported reduction in the severity of hemispatial neglect following prism adaptation and have shown that the eye movements postadaptation (in individuals with right-sided lesions and left-sided neglect) are significantly more rightward deviated than was the case prior to the intervention. Although many questions remain as to the mechanisms that give rise to this lateral-displacement postadaptation (Is it a redistribution of spatial attention? Is it visuomotor in nature?), and even though the consequences of adaptation are not very prolonged, the technique has proved to be remarkably valuable in flexibly altering the behavior of the patients with neglect, and much remains to be done in this domain.

Even without prism adaptation, following standard rehabilitation procedures, individuals with hemispatial neglect do show a decrement in the bias to orient rightward as well as showing a significant improvement in attention reorienting to the contralateral space. Of particular interest in recent investigations, as revealed in functional imaging studies, is that the behavioral improvement even in these standard treatment procedures is correlated with reactivation of multiple cortical areas, which previously evinced weak or no task-related activity (even though some of these areas were anatomically intact). The opportunity to use functional imaging procedures to track recovery and perhaps to identify the optimal procedures for reinstituting cortical activation is promising and offers a new method for developing and assessing rehabilitation procedures.

Parietal Lobe and Spatial Representations: Evidence from Lesion Analyses

The advent of high-resolution imaging (and its relative ease of accessibility) has also enabled investigators to track the lesion site in greater detail than has been possible in the past and to reevaluate the anatomical underpinnings of hemispatial neglect. While neglect has been most commonly associated with the inferior parietal lobule and also the temporoparietal junction (TPJ; see **Figure 1**), the underlying anatomical substrate has come under increased scrutiny. For example, some findings suggest that the superior temporal gyrus (STG) is the critical site of cortical damage associated with neglect and subcortical sites, including the putamen, and, to a lesser extent, the caudate nucleus within the basal ganglia and the pulvinar within the thalamus have also been implicated. Yet others have argued that a disconnection between the frontal and the inferior parietal region, brought about by a lesion of the superior longitudinal fasciculus, gives rise to chronic neglect. A further set of investigations has suggested that parietal cortex has a more dorsal and a more ventral stream and that each may play a slightly different role, with more superior regions engaged in voluntary, goal-directed attention and more inferior regions more engaged in bottom-up detection of salience or novelty. Finally, large-scale studies report that neglect arises after lesions to any one of multiple nodes making up a distributed spatial-attentional network, including temporal, parietal, frontal, and occipital cortices as well as basal ganglia and thalamus (in order of incidence). The continued development of more sophisticated imaging techniques and methods of lesion analysis will be critical in outlining the neural substrate of spatial representation and possibly even in differentiating subtypes of neglect and their cortical signatures.

Parietal Lobe and Spatial Representations: Evidence from Functional Imaging Studies

Thus far, the role of parietal cortex in spatial representation has been considered based on findings from human lesion studies. Converging evidence from functional imaging studies has recently contributed enormously to elucidating the mechanisms underlying spatial representation. For example, one robust finding is that when cues direct an observer to a spatial location in which an upcoming target is likely to appear, activation is noted in superior frontal, inferior parietal, and superior temporal cortices. Spatial attentional selection serves to facilitate perception of stimuli (e.g., objects), as reflected in enhanced speed of processing of attended information. Given the increased access to functional imaging, researchers have spent considerable effort to shed light on the mechanism subserving spatial attentional orienting. A primary focus of such studies has been to determine the anatomical loci within the human cortex that give rise to the attentional biasing signal (i.e., the source or process that directs or shifts attention) that ultimately initiates the sensory enhancement of the selected stimulus (i.e., the effect). In this next section, we summarize findings from these studies, showing the differential involvement in the source versus the effects of attentional manipulations.

Effects of Spatial Selection: Enhancement of Sensory Signals

Studies of the effects of visual attentional selection have revealed behavioral facilitation and enhanced cortical responses to information appearing in attended spatial locations. Neurophysiological studies investigating the effects of top-down attentional bias have demonstrated that when a cell is presented with a stimulus in its receptive field (RF), the neural response to that stimulus is increased when attention is covertly directed to it as compared to when the stimulus is in the RF but attention is either unfocused or is diverted elsewhere. For example, in their seminal study, Moran and Desimone first identified the classical RF of a V4 neuron and its corresponding effective and ineffective stimuli (i.e., stimuli that drive the cell strongly and weakly, respectively). The monkeys were trained to attend to stimuli in a specific location within the visual field while ignoring stimuli at another location. Both effective and ineffective stimuli were presented within the RF and the responses of the V4 neurons were strongly modulated by the spatial attentional locus: the firing rate to the preferred stimulus was only one-third as great when the monkey did not attend to it as compared to when the preferred stimulus was attended. In fact, what was particularly interesting about this study is that when attention was directed to one of two stimuli in the receptive field of a V4 cell, the effect of the unattended stimulus was attenuated, as if the receptive field had contracted to include only the attended stimulus. This type of spatial attentional enhancement was found to increase with task difficulty and was observed throughout early sensory regions within the visual cortex.

Several neuroimaging studies in humans have also documented early sensory enhancement following top-down spatial attentional allocation. In the majority of these experiments, individuals are presented with stimuli appearing to the left or right of fixation and are asked to direct their attention to either side of the fixation point (i.e., shifting their attention either to the left or the right side of space) (**Figure 3**). Directing spatial attention to the left hemifield results in increased stimulus-evoked neural activity of the early visual areas in the right hemisphere, whereas directed spatial attention to the right hemifield is accompanied by increase of activity in the early visual areas of the left hemisphere. Studies employing event-related potentials (ERPs) take advantage of the fact that visual stimuli typically elicit two early waveform components, which are termed P1 (first positive, occurring 100–200 ms after stimulus onset) and N1 (first negative). These effects are robust and are observed even during passive viewing of input. Of relevance, the P1 and N1 components are modulated (i.e., increase in negativity and/or positivity) when visual stimuli are being attended to, as opposed to when spatial attention is diverted elsewhere in the scene. The modulation is manifest by a change in the amplitude of these components, while the component latency remains the same when the stimuli are attended or ignored. In summary, spatial attention serves to modulate sensory signals elicited by the stimuli in the early sensory cortex (i.e., areas V1–V4) and also in higher order areas such as the motion-sensitive region (MT+), fusiform face area (FFA) selective for face processing, and other higher order regions within the human cortex.

Sources of Spatial Orienting Signal

Several regions within monkey and human posterior parietal cortex (PPC) have been identified as coarsely representing spatial topography as it relates to the source or trigger of a spatial attentional orienting signal. For example, neurons in the lateral intraparietal area (LIP) of the monkey cortex fire in response to the location in space to which attention was cued, representing the voluntary allocation of attention to a specific region in space. Several regions within the human parietal and frontal cortices – inferior parietal sulcus (IPS), superior parietal lobule (SPL), and the frontal eye fields (FEFs) – are also identified as playing a critical role in spatial attentional selection. Functional magnetic resonance imaging (fMRI) studies have demonstrated that activity in these frontal and parietal regions is spatially selective, such that stronger activity is noted when attention is directed toward spatial locations in the contralateral field.

Several fMRI studies support the proposal that the top-down attentional signal (the implementation of the cue) arises at least partially from the parietal

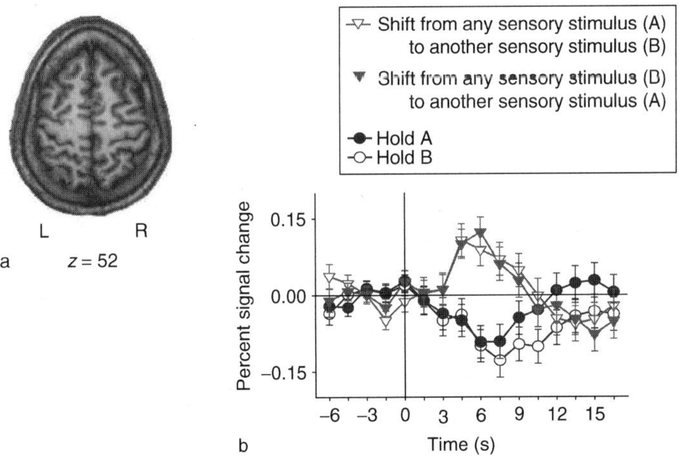

Figure 3 (a) A representative slice through a high-resolution reconstructed brain of an individual performing an attentional shifting task. The activation (shown in red) is obtained by contrasting activity during shifts of attention between the sensory stimuli (could be, for example, from left side of space to right side of space, or from auditory stimuli presented to the left ear and to the right ear) with activity when holding attention within a sensory stimulus. The cluster of activated voxels encompassed within the white circle is in the right superior parietal lobule. (b) Blood oxygen-level-dependent signal extracted from the right superior parietal lobule reflects transient activity elicited within this region following shifts of attention from one sensory stimulus to another. Note that activity within this region remains low for sustained attention (hold trials). From Shomstein S and Yantis S (2006) Parietal cortex mediates voluntary control of spatial and nonspatial auditory attention. *Journal of Neuroscience* 26(2): 435–439.

cortex, with an additional contribution from the frontal cortex – what has been termed the frontoparietal attentional network. For example, when individuals are asked to covertly direct their attention following a cue to a spatial location in the visual display in preparation for a target, areas in the occipital lobe respond transiently to the cue, while areas in the posterior parietal cortex along the inferior parietal sulcus exhibit a more sustained response. The sustained activity in the PPC is assumed to reflect the source of the attentional orienting signal: it could not be linked to either visual stimuli or motor responses *per se* and its activity was time locked to the period during which individuals paid attention to the peripheral future target location.

It is important to understand the precise function of the parietal lobe's involvement in attentional control. At least two possibilities regarding the time course of parietal lobe activity following spatial shifts of attention must be considered. The first possibility is that the PPC provides a continuous signal that maintains the locus of attention at a specific spatial location – the 'sustained hypothesis.' In other words, once the individual has decided to change the locus of spatial attention, the PPC issues a signal that will be sustained until another change in the locus of spatial attention is made (i.e., sustained increase in neural activity). Another possibility is that the PPC issues a transient brief signal to shift the attentional state – the 'transient hypothesis,' such that once the locus of spatial attention needs to be redirected elsewhere, the PPC issues a transient signal that dissipates quickly once the attentional shift has been made. This latter hypothesis also predicts that the locus of attention is maintained by other areas, presumably frontal areas within the frontoparietal network.

Several recent studies examined the exact involvement of the PPC in attentional shifting tasks by adjudicating between these two hypotheses. In a typical task, individuals are shown two streams of input presented peripherally to the left and right of fixation and are initially instructed to monitor one stream for a cue (for example, a digit among the stream of letters). The identity of the cue indicates to the individuals whether they should maintain attention on the current stream or shift attention to the other stream. The critical finding is revealed when one compares cortical activity related to shifting the attentional focus from one spatial location to another with activity related to maintaining the attentional focus on a single stream. When attention was shifted between spatial locations, the time course of the blood oxygen-level-dependent (BOLD) signal in the right SPL and inferior parietal lobule (IPL) exhibited transient activity (see **Figure 3**). The transient nature of the signal elicited by the SPL suggests that this area of the parietal cortex is the source of a brief attentional control signal to shift attentive states to a new spatial position, and is not the source of a continuous signal to actively maintain the new attentive state.

Sources of Nonspatial Orienting Signal

Although the focus thus far has been on spatial representation and attending to spatial regions containing input, the top-down attention-shifting signal is not restricted to spatial shifts alone, and this region is activated when individuals shift their attention between any two dimensions of the input. For example, shifts between superimposed houses and faces, shifts between two different features of an object, or shifts between two different sensory modalities all selectively activate the PPC. Whereas spatial shifts are accompanied by increased activation in the SPL region of the parietal lobe, nonspatial shifts are accompanied by increased activity in the precuneus region, the continuation of the SPL on the medial side of the parietal lobe (see **Figures 1** and **3**). This anatomical distinction between spatial and nonspatial shifts of attention clearly deserves a more thorough investigation. We should note that additional attentional functions could be mediated by some of the same subareas of parietal cortex already described. For example, both an anterior part and an inferior part of the intraparietal sulcus appear to be activated in a visual conjunction task, even in the absence of multiple distractors, and this occurs to a greater extent in the left than in the right hemisphere. By contrast, activation of a more posterior region of the intraparietal sulcus appears to be contingent on the presence of distractors. Much work remains to be done to outline the various attentional functions mediated by the parietal cortex and also, in parallel, to map out the behavioral and neural mechanisms associated with spatial representation.

Conclusion

Spatial cognition is a complex, multifaceted set of processes that are engaged in a large variety of tasks, including, for example, mental rotation, spatial navigation, and spatial working memory. The exact nature of the spatial knowledge implicated in these different tasks remains to be determined. We have focused on behavioral and neural mechanisms involved in representation of spatial locations, with evidence drawn from neuropsychological studies of individuals with hemispatial neglect and neuroimaging studies of spatial attentional selection (and the ensuing sensory enhancement). As is evident, the findings are probably more complicated than we might have thought, given the progress made to date on these topics. In particular, better use of structural and functional imaging has led to fine-grained reconsideration of previous findings. Some of the received wisdoms regarding hemispatial neglect have come under scrutiny, and the fMRI findings have opened new avenues of investigation. Among the outstanding issues are the mechanisms giving rise to the neglect in the first place (for example, a deficit in spatial attention, a problem in spatial updating, or competition between inputs). The neural locus of neglect has also come under reconsideration and many questions remain. Findings from functional imaging studies have also opened new domains of investigation. In particular, the imaging studies have suggested that spatial positions in the world can be selectively attended and that these attentional effects are robust and are present throughout the visual (and auditory) system, and attending to specific stimuli modulates the cortical areas involved in processing the input. The posterior parietal cortex appears to play a dominant role in signaling and implementing the attentional shift from one location (or feature or object) to another, as reflected in the transient activity in posterior parietal cortex.

See also: Attentional Networks in the Parietal Cortex; Cognition: An Overview of Neuroimaging Techniques; Executive Function and Higher-Order Cognition: Neuroimaging; Neglect Syndrome and the Spatial Attention Network; Neural Coding of Spatial Representations; Parietal Cortex and Spatial Attention; Spatial Orientation: Our Whole-Body Motion and Orientation Sense; Spatial Memory: Assessment in Animals; Spatial Transformations for Eye–Hand Coordination; Spatial Cognition; Spatial Cognitive Maps.

Further Reading

Bisley JW and Goldberg ME (2003) Neuronal activity in lateral intraparietal cortex and spatial attention. *Science* 299: 81–86.

Chambers CD and Mattingley JB (2005) Neurodisruption of selective attention: Insights and implications. *Trends in Cognitive Science* 9(11): 542–550.

Corbetta M, Kincade JM, and Shulman GL (2002) Neural systems for visual orienting and their relationships to spatial working memory. *Journal of Cognitive Neuroscience* 14(3): 508–523.

Corbetta M, Kincade MJ, Lewis C, et al. (2005) Neural basis and recovery of spatial attention deficits in spatial neglect. *Nature Neuroscience* 8(11): 1603–1610.

Luck SJ, Girelli M, McDermott MT, et al. (1997) Bridging the gap between monkey neurophysiology and human perception: An ambiguity resolution theory of visual selective attention. *Cognitive Psychology* 33: 64–87.

Malhotra P, Coulthard E, and Husain M (2006) Hemispatial neglect, balance and eye-movement control. *Current Opinion in Neurology* 19(1): 14–20.

Merriam EP, Genovese CR, and Colby CL (2003) Spatial updating in human parietal cortex. *Neuron* 39(2): 361–373.

Moran J and Desimone R (1985) Selective attention gates visual processing in the extrastriate cortex. *Science* 229: 782–784.

O'Craven KM, Rosen BR, Kwong KK, et al. (1997) Voluntary attention modulates fmri activity in human mt-mst. *Neuron* 18(4): 591–598.

Philbeck JW, Behrmann M, Levy L, et al. (2004) Path integration deficits during linear locomotion after human medial temporal lobectomy. *Journal of Cognitive Neuroscience* 16(4): 510–520.

Serences JT, Schwarzbach J, Courtney SM, et al. (2004) Control of object-based attention in human cortex. *Cerebral Cortex* 14(12): 1346–1357.

Shelton AL and Gabrieli JDE (2002) Neural correlates of encoding space from route and survey perspectives. *Journal of Neuroscience* 22(7): 2711–2717.

Shomstein S and Behrmann M (2006) Objects modulate competition in human parietal and extrastriate cortices. *Proceedings of the National Academy of Sciences of the United States of America* 103(30): 11387–11392.

Shomstein S and Yantis S (2006) Parietal cortex mediates voluntary control of spatial and nonspatial auditory attention. *Journal of Neuroscience* 26(2): 435–439.

Treue S and Maunsell JHRM (1999) Effects of attention on the processing of motion in macaque visual cortical areas mt and mst. *Journal of Neuroscience* 19: 7603–7616.

Tversky B (1991) Spatial mental models. In: Bower GH (ed.) *The Psychology of Learning*, pp. 109–145. San Diego: Academic Press.

van Asselen M, Kessels RP, Kappelle LJ, et al. (2006) Neural correlates of human wayfinding in stroke patients. *Brain Research* 1067(1): 229–238.

Vandenberghe R, Gitelman DR, Parrish TB, et al. (2001) Functional specificity of superior parietal mediation of spatial shifting. *NeuroImage* 14(3): 661–673.

Wojciulik E and Kanwisher N (1999) The generality of parietal involvement in visual attention. *Neuron* 23: 747–764.

Yantis S, Schwarzbach J, Serences JT, et al. (2002) Transient neural activity in human parietal cortex during spatial attention shifts. *Nature Neuroscience* 5(10): 995–1002.

Spatial Cognitive Maps

B Poucet and E Save, Université de Provence, Marseille, France

Introduction

Several theories have been developed to account for spatial learning. For S–R theorists, spatial learning consists of chaining together a number of motor responses linking relevant external stimuli (stimulus–response associations). This view was challenged by Tolman in 1948, who argued that rats do not merely base their actions on S–R associations, but internally reorganize acquired spatial information so as to form cognitive representations of the environment. In other words, rats learn the location of a place where they have been rewarded independently of the specific movements necessary to reach it. Tolman explained this ability by introducing the notion of a cognitive map, a mental representation held by the rat in which it encodes the elements of a task and the spatial relationships between these elements. An important property of cognitive maps is that they allow animals to react to stimuli that are not immediately present since the relationship of such stimuli to those actually perceived is maintained in the representation. Thus, the rat can be aware of the properties of the environment beyond their field of perception. The major consequence of such a representation is that it bridges informational gaps about the environment, thus conferring greater flexibility and efficacy to behavior.

Tolman's notion of cognitive map was further developed by O'Keefe and Nadel in 1978, who proposed a theoretical framework to account for spatial behavior and its neural bases. They made a distinction between two main processes used by rats to perform spatial tasks. They proposed that rats can use either a taxon system or a locale system. The taxon system is based on S–R associations, whereas the locale system is based on spatial relationships in the form of a cognitive map (**Figure 1**). They further proposed that the brain regions subserving these forms of spatial navigation are different and at least partially independent.

Spatial Strategies

The number of studies which support the hypothesis that animals form a mental representation of their environment is quite impressive. This does not mean, however, that animals rely exclusively on spatial representations to orient in space. Performing specific responses, approaching particular cues, or even learning conditional associations about the sensory consequences of specific movement sequences may be efficient strategies in a number of situations. Nevertheless, in spite of their efficacy, such strategies do not confer behavior with the degree of flexibility afforded by the use of a cognitive map.

Selection of appropriate navigational strategies is primarily determined by the perception of space, that is, by the nature of the cues that can be used for navigation. There are two main categories of spatial cues: allothetic and idiothetic cues. Allothetic cues are provided by the environment and include visual, olfactory, and auditory information. Idiothetic cues are derived from the animal's own movements, including information provided by the vestibular, proprioceptive, and somatosensory systems, efference copies of motor commands, and external motion-related information such as optic flow. Although this article is about navigation based on cognitive maps, it is useful to briefly describe other strategies useful for moving efficiently in space.

Cue Navigation

The simplest navigational strategy is to move toward or away from a directly perceived cue. The use of such a system requires a radial stimulation gradient field centered on the source. The notion of gradient field refers to the variation of intensity of the source as a function of the distance. In the simplest case, intensity varies monotonically with the distance. The animal can therefore reach the goal, that is, the origin of the gradient, by navigating in the gradient direction or conversely, avoid a place by navigating in the opposite direction. A gradient field may originate from auditory and olfactory cues. Navigation toward a conspicuous visual cue has similar characteristics. The visual cue is considered to be at the center of a radial gradient where the gradient direction corresponds to the direction of the light flux. Then, reducing the distance from the visual cue (that leads to an increase of the apparent cue size) is equivalent to navigating along the axis of greatest intensity. The animal can also use a similar mechanism to reach a hidden goal that is closely associated with a salient landmark (called a beacon). A landmark is therefore considered as an intermediate goal whose spatial contiguity with the real goal has been learned through an associative process.

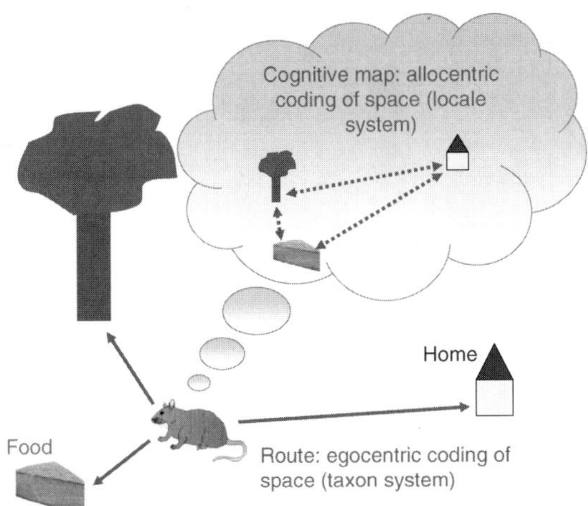

Figure 1 The two systems for encoding spatial information proposed by O'Keefe and Nadel in 1978. Cognitive mapping (locale system) involves building a representation of a part of space that encodes the relationships between environmental landmarks (e.g., the nest, a tree, and a food source), independently of the animal's location (allocentric coding). Using a route (taxon system) involves encoding the location of landmarks relative to the animal's position (egocentric coding).

Guidance

If the goal cannot be directly perceived and if there is no landmark closely associated to the goal, the animal must rely on environmental landmarks to navigate. One strategy is to use landmarks as directional cues. Guidance, therefore, requires that the animal directs its attention to particular landmarks and maintain some egocentric (i.e., relative to the animal) spatial relationships with respect to these landmarks to reach the goal. A place-recognition process is then needed to identify the goal location. Rats may be guided either by individual or configurations of landmarks. For example, they may be able to memorize a view (or snapshot) of the spatial arrangement of landmarks seen from the goal and so adjust movements until a current view matches a memorized view.

Routes

To reach a remote goal, cue navigation and guidance may be elaborated into route learning. In route learning, rats may memorize a sequence of associations coupling specific landmarks and motor responses, for example, "after reaching the rock, turn left." Each landmark is considered as an intermediary goal and the sequence of these goals constitutes a route. Routes allow rapid navigation at the expense of behavioral flexibility, however. Environmental changes altering the sequence of landmarks may be fatal to successful navigation. In addition, retracing the route cannot be achieved by simply inverting the order of the landmarks, but requires active learning of a new sequence.

Path Integration

Path integration, or dead reckoning, relies on an 'egocentric' (self-centered) coding process, which allows an animal to memorize a location (usually the starting point of its journey) in relation to its own position. This form of navigation relies on idiothetic (self-motion) cues, which are used to update a vector that specifies, in egocentric coordinates, the distance and head-referred direction of the goal from the animal's current location. Its major drawback is that the computation of these parameters is subject to cumulative error. If the cumulated error is great enough, the animal may miss its target. Although the egocentric coding process is unreliable, its precision can be improved if information is recalibrated from visual or other sensory information available from the environment. It is not clear, for rats or humans, whether any reliance is placed on path integration except when external sensory information is missing or inadequate.

Allocentric (Place) Navigation

Allocentric navigation refers to the process of determining and maintaining a course or trajectory from one place to another by using environmental cues. It requires formation and use of a map-like representation of the environment (a cognitive map) which encodes the allocentric relationships between landmarks and places, independently of the animal's position. The use of a mapping strategy allows an animal to reach a goal from a variety of points, including over trajectories that it has not previously used. A rat is thus able to infer its location relative to particular places whose position is encoded in the representation and compute optimal trajectories to reach these places. Place navigation is flexible because if a possible path is obstructed, or if a landmark is missing, the animal is still able to generate successful trajectories by performing detours and short-cuts and by adapting its navigational behavior to environmental changes.

One of the most versatile test to study place navigation is the Morris water maze task, in which the animal swims in a circular tank filled with opaque water in order to reach a submerged or visible platform, which is the only place to which it can escape from the water. In the place version of the task, there is no cue closely associated with the platform. Localization of the hidden platform can only be performed

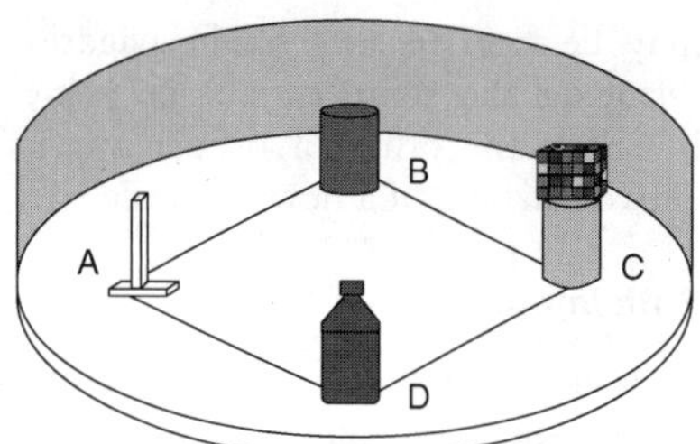

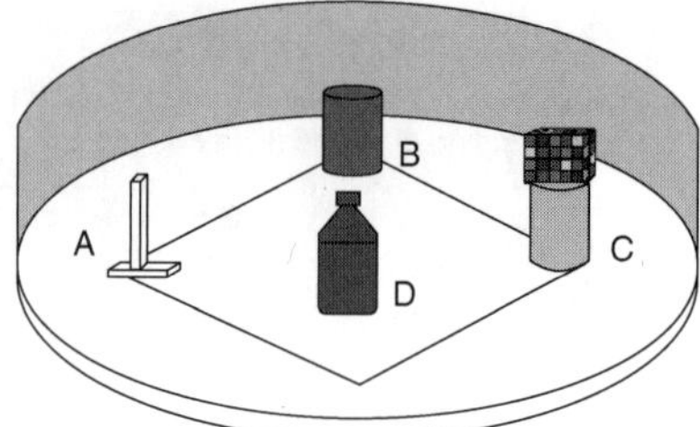

Figure 2 Role of exploration in updating cognitive maps. A typical protocol involves the rat exploring an enclosed apparatus containing a set of objects in stable locations. After the rat is familiar with this object configuration, a change is made in the spatial arrangement of objects (here a single object, D, is slightly moved from its original location). When reintroduced into the apparatus, animals usually display an exploratory reaction toward the moved object, indicating that they detect the change and update their cognitive map accordingly.

and learned by using distal room cues. To prevent the animal from using a local view for guidance, different starting places are used on successive trials. It is therefore assumed that learning results in the elaboration of a cognitive map. Acquisition of the Morris navigation task however also requires procedural memory and working memory. Procedural memory allows the rat to learn that it must swim, find an escape platform, climb on the platform, etc. Working memory results in learning that the platform is at a specific location, which rats can often do in a single trial after mastering the procedural details of the task.

Exploration and Spatial Cognitive Maps

Although an obvious function of cognitive maps is to indicate where potentially important objects are located in space, they can be used for other purposes. As a matter of fact, animals need to be familiar with the surroundings and will not behave according to their primary motivation, such as hunger or thirst, until they recognize and identify where they are in space. This ability to locate oneself in the current environment depends on prior exploration. In fact, navigation and exploration are so intimately related that accurate navigation cannot occur without preliminary exploration of the environment. The major function of exploration is information gathering and storage and so it is necessary for the formation of spatial representations. An advantage of such storage is that it may allow detection of unexpected new information in an otherwise familiar environment. For example, if place recognition is not achieved, exploration occurs again so that the cognitive map comes to match the real environment as closely as possible, therefore providing the animal with spatial invariants. Exploration may lead either to a new representation or to the updating of a former spatial representation.

An illustration of the updating process is provided by studies which show that changing the spatial configuration of objects in a previously explored arena induces a renewal of exploratory activity mostly aimed at the displaced objects (**Figure 2**). The protocol consists of two successive phases: habituation and spatial change. First, repeated exposure to the same configuration of objects results in habituation of exploratory activity, that is, a decrement in the response with increasing familiarity. It is hypothesized that during this phase, rats acquire some knowledge of the spatial characteristics of the environment. Habituation thus reflects the elaboration of a spatial representation. Once habituation is achieved, the animals are exposed to a new configuration of the same familiar objects. A renewal of exploration following this change is assumed to reflect that the animal (1) encodes certain spatial relationships and (2) is able to compare the previous and current situations. Such renewal is thus an adaptive behavior aimed at updating the spatial representation of the environment. It is therefore clear that there is a constant interplay between exploration and the cognitive map, with exploration allowing for initial buildup and subsequent updating of the map, which in turn drives further spatial behavior, including exploration, within the animal's current environment.

What Is the Information Stored in Spatial Cognitive Maps?

That animals are able to use representations of their environment does not mean that they encode all aspects of the spatial surroundings. In fact, evidence suggests that the information content of spatial cognitive maps can be quite selective.

Configurations of Cues and Geometry

In most spatial tasks, performance appears to rely on configural rather than on individual landmarks. Up to a point, removing specific cues in tasks such as the water maze place navigation task (or the radial arm maze tasks) usually does not alter animal's performance to a great extent. In contrast, rearranging these cues can be quite detrimental to task solution. Based on the analysis of exploratory patterns, it can also be demonstrated that changing the spatial configuration of discrete objects in a familiar arena induces a renewal of exploratory activity. Further analyses of exploratory responses confirm that the animal keeps a record of the spatial arrangement of the objects, but that this record is specific to certain classes of spatial relationships. In general, changes that induce the strongest responses are those that affect either the overall geometrical arrangement of the object set, or the topological relationships among the objects. The configuration seems to be privileged over the absolute position of objects. Thus, spatial geometry seems to constitute an important piece of information contained in the map. In other studies, rats were placed in a rectangular chamber and were required to visit the four corners of the chamber. Each corner contained a different amount of food and was associated with a distinctive visual insert. Two opposite corners had the most bait while the remaining two opposite corners had the least bait. After the animals mastered the task (i.e., visited each corner according to a decreasing order from the most baited to the least baited arm), a number of probe tests were conducted based on transformations of the initial distribution of the inserts. The rats' patterns of visits to the food locations were remarkably insensitive to the modifications made in the spatial arrangement of the inserts. Rather, the animals used the rectangular shape of the experimental chamber as a means to locate the various food sources. Thus, rats ignore obvious landmarks and attend to landscape features instead in reorienting themselves in symmetric environments. Although they are aware of the landmarks, they simply do not appear to use them for certain purposes. The rules governing when landmarks or landscapes are used in behavior remain to be fully explicated. Current thinking suggests that local landmarks are not used to determine directions in space, nor to define a spatial framework within which such directions can be nested. Rather, landscape features are seemingly used for these purposes.

Distal versus Local Landmarks

Landscape features are not the sole markers of the spatial arrangement. Distal landmarks provide another major source of information on which spatial navigation can rely. In general, animals will preferentially use such distal information when it is available, to the detriment of local cues. As an example of the greater efficiency of distal cues in guiding spatial behavior, consider the navigation performance of rats trained in the water maze navigation task. In this task, a swimming rat can escape from water by locating a safe platform relative to the array of visual cues located 'outside' the swimming pool. After a few training trials (usually fewer than 30), the rat swims almost directly toward the platform. In contrast, when the task is changed so that rats have to rely on three objects placed directly in the swimming pool (local cues) to locate the platform, many more trials are required before the rat displays direct navigation paths.

Distal information also predominates when it conflicts with movement-related information such as that provided by path-integration mechanisms. While path-integration-based homing behavior in hamsters is barely altered by the manipulation of local cues, it can be easily altered by manipulating distal information. To understand why distal cues are so effective in controlling place navigation, it is necessary to realize that only distal cues maintain their reciprocal relationships with respect to the animal during its motion. Thus the perceived reciprocal relationships between distal cues are minimally affected by an animal's movements. On the contrary, the perceived reciprocal relationships between local cues are subject to strong changes during movements. Since a cognitive map contains absolute topographical information rather than information about egocentric locations relative to the animal, it becomes evident that distal cues provide a more reliable source of information for localization since they retain relatively stable relationships as the animal moves about the environment.

Metrics and Topology

The evidence reviewed above indicates that rats possess a representation of the configural aspects of the distal environment. This representation is not homogeneous, however: animals process certain locations in a more detailed way during exploration. This is not very surprising because space is not homogeneous. It is more surprising, however, that the topological relationships among such locations (e.g., whether they are in the same vicinity) often have stronger control over spatial behavior than do metric relationships (e.g., their absolute distance in Euclidean space). It is therefore possible that spatial representations can be both topological, therefore affording relatively unstructured information about the connectivity within space (e.g., place A is directly connected to place B but not to place C), and metric (e.g., place A is a certain distance and direction from place B), affording more detailed information about specific

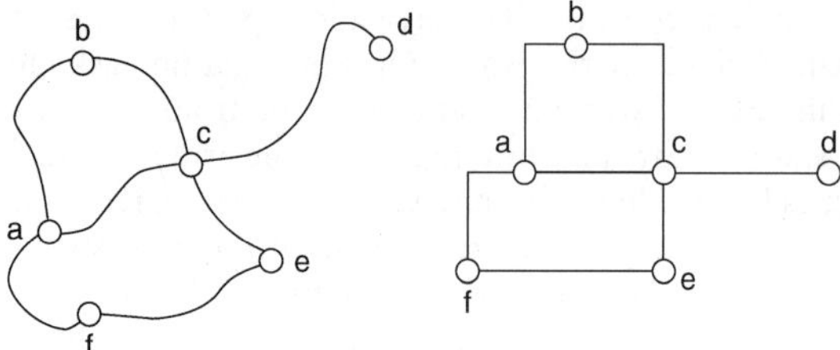

Figure 3 Metric and topological information can be used separately to describe space. The left part of the figure shows a environment in which a set of spatial locations (a–f) are connected to each other by specific paths. An arbitrary topological transform of the spatial network is shown in the right part of the figure. The topologically equivalent network preserves the topological properties of vicinity and connectivity between the locations, but not the metric relationships (i.e., angles and distances between locations).

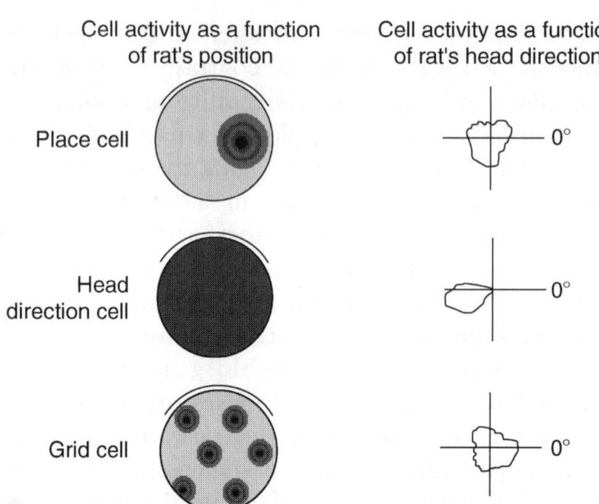

Figure 4 Main properties of place cells, head direction cells, and grid cells. Cells are usually recorded as a rat explores a cylindrical environment in which a single landmark (a cue card) is attached to the apparatus wall (shown as an arc at 12:00 in the figure). The left-hand and right-hand parts of the figure show the typical positional firing rate map and directional polar plot for each type of cell, respectively. Place cells discharge only at a specific location (shown as concentric colored circles at 3:00 in the positional firing rate map) but have no strong directional selectivity (the directional polar plot does not reveal strong direction variability). On the contrary, head direction cell firing depends on the heading of the animal (e.g., at 180°) independently of its location (no specific place is associated with increased firing). Finally, the discharge of grid cells resembles that of place cells but they have multiple, regularly spaced fields. Note that other cells exist that can combine these different properties (e.g., have both location and direction correlates).

relationships among places (**Figure** 3). The advantage of this dual format is that topological information is more rapidly acquired than metric information because metric encoding would largely rely on motion-related signals provided by repeated movements between places. However, direct empirical support for dissociation between topological and metric encoding of spatial information is still awaited.

Neural Bases of Spatial Cognitive Maps

Damage to almost any portion of the brain can result in impairments in spatial navigation. The question, however, is whether the brain is organized so that the two modes of spatial coding, egocentric and allocentric, are dissociated. This question is not trivial because it is not easy to disentangle the contribution of motion-related signals (which provide the basis for egocentric coding) to the allocentric coding of spatial information which likely involves movements in space. In spite of this difficulty, several studies have shown that the two systems may be distinct. Substantial evidence suggests that taxon navigation is subtended by basal forebrain structures such as the dorsal striatum, whereas locale navigation is subtended by temporal lobe structures including the hippocampus. Striatal lesions in rats impair the performance of egocentric localization tasks, while leaving unaffected the performance of equally difficult tasks that did not require egocentric localization. In contrast, hippocampal lesions produce place learning impairment in place navigation tasks, such as the water maze, but generally do not affect performance in egocentric tasks (e.g., cue navigation). Recent evidence for a functional dissociation between the effects of lesions of the striatum and lesions of the hippocampus confirm that these two brain regions are involved in egocentric coding processes (cue, guidance, and route strategies) and allocentric coding processes (place strategy), respectively.

The role of the hippocampus in spatial navigation based on a place strategy is further supported by the existence of cells that carry a spatial signal. Such cells are found in the hippocampus proper and closely related structures, and can roughly be classified as place cells, head direction cells, and the more recently discovered grid cells.

Place cells are hippocampal pyramidal cells whose firing is strongly correlated with the location of a freely moving rat in its environment. Head direction cells are primarily found in the postsubiculum, and the anterior and lateral dorsal thalamus. Their firing depends on the heading of the animal independently of its location. Finally, grid cells are found in the dorsocaudal medial entorhinal cortex. These cells are activated whenever the animal's position coincides with any vertex of a regular grid of equilateral triangles spanning the surface of the environment. Together, grid cells provide a directionally oriented, topographically organized neural map of the spatial environment (**Figure** 4). A common feature of all these cell populations is that their firing is primarily controlled by salient visual cues and motion-related signals although other sensory cues can be used to maintain coherent activity. In addition to these populations of cells, the hippocampal formation contains neurons whose spatial signals are more complex. For example, cells in the subiculum have both location and direction correlates. It appears, therefore, that the hippocampus and related structures form a system where spatial information is processed and coherently organized and lies at the core of a widespread neural network concerned with the processing of spatial information. Although current evidence suggests that normal hippocampal function is required for place navigation, its exact role is still a matter for debate. In addition, it is not clear how the information processed in the hippocampus is passed onto other brain areas involved in spatial processing. A number of other cortical structures (e.g., entorhinal, retrosplenial, prefrontal, or parietal cortex) and subcortical structures such as several thalamic nuclei have been hypothesized to contribute to place navigation. The specific role of these structures in relation to the hippocampus remains to be elucidated. Nevertheless, recent findings suggest that the human hippocampus hosts cells that look very much like hippocampal place cells in the rat, thereby strengthening researchers' interest for a better understanding of the computational properties of these systems.

Conclusion

The hypothesis that the hippocampus is the locus of a cognitive map has resulted in a growing interest into the neural basis of animal spatial cognition. Current evidence suggests that rats are able to build spatial representations of their environment so as to navigate with efficiency. Data on the neural mechanisms potentially associated with the processing of spatial information are accumulating rapidly. We currently know many pieces of the puzzle, but are still far from understanding how they are put together. Nevertheless, neuropsychological studies of spatial cognition in the rat routinely provide new data likely to shed light on how spatial information is handled by the brain, and therefore to help us understand how complex human behaviors are implemented in neural activities.

See also: Magnetic Sense in Animal Navigation; Neural Coding of Spatial Representations; Parietal Cortex and Spatial Attention; Spatial Memory: Assessment in Animals; Spatial Cognition and Executive Function; Spatial Cognition; Synaptic Plasticity and Place Cell Formation.

Further Reading

Gallistel CR (1990) *The Organization of Learning.* Cambridge: MIT Press.

Hafting T, Fyhn M, Molden S, Moser M-B, and Moser EI (2005) Microstructure of a spatial map in the entorhinal cortex. *Nature* 436: 801–806.

Jeffery K (ed.) (2003) *The Neurobiology of Spatial Behaviour.* Oxford: Oxford University Press.

Muller RU (1996) A quarter of century of place cells. *Neuron* 17: 813–822.

O'Keefe J and Nadel L (1978) *Hippocampus as a Cognitive Map.* Oxford: Clarendon.

Poucet B (1993) Spatial cognitive maps in animals: New hypotheses on their structure and neural mechanisms. *Psychological Review* 100: 163–182.

Save E and Poucet B (2000) Involvement of the hippocampus and associative parietal cortex in the use of proximal and distal landmarks for navigation. *Behavioral Brain Research* 109: 195–206.

Taube JS (1998) Head direction cells and the neurophysiological basis for a sense of direction. *Progress in Neurobiology* 55: 225–256.

Thinus-Blanc C, Save E, and Poucet B (1998) Animal spatial cognition and exploration. In: Foreman N and Gillett R (eds.) *A Handbook of Spatial Research Paradigms and Methodologies*, pp. 59–86. Hove, UK: Psychology Press.

Tolman EC (1948) Cognitive maps in rats and men. *Psychological Review* 55: 189–208.

Wiener SI and Taube JS (eds.) (2005) *Head Direction Cells and the Neural Mechanisms of Spatial Orientation.* Cambridge: MIT Press.

Relevant Websites

http://www.bris.ac.uk – Neural Basis of Spatial Memory, Centre for Synaptic Plasticity, University of Bristol.

http://instruct1.cit.cornell.edu – Neuroethology of Rat Spatial Navigation: The Role of Place Cells, Academic Technologies

http://en.wikipedia.org – Place cell, Wikipedia.

Spatial Orientation: Our Whole-Body Motion and Orientation Sense

D Merfeld, Massachusetts Eye & Ear Infirmary, Boston, MA, USA

Introduction

Our sense of body motion and orientation can be divided into two overlapping and interacting systems – one that senses head motion and head orientation with respect to the external world and a second that senses relative motion and orientation of the various body segments. This article focuses on our sense of motion and orientation with respect to the external world. This sense has nine degrees of freedom. It includes our sense of motion – three dimensions of rotational motion and three dimensions of linear motion. It also includes our sense of three-dimensional orientation, which we explicitly define as the combination of heading direction (i.e., which way am I facing? or yaw orientation) as well as tilt of the head with respect to gravity (e.g., pitch and roll with respect to the normal upright posture).

Although somatosensory cues provide a substantial influence on our sense of motion and orientation, the predominant contributors to our sense of motion and orientation are the vestibular and visual systems. This article focuses on the contributions of the vestibular system because this sensory system is often overlooked, compared to the more commonly known sensory systems. The vestibular system is made up of specialized sensory end organs dedicated to measuring head motion and orientation. In brief, the vestibular system in each inner ear consists of three semicircular canals, which sense three dimensions of head rotation, and two otolith organs, which sense three dimensions of head linear acceleration and gravity. The anatomy and physiology of the vestibular end organs are discussed very briefly next.

In addition to perceptual contributions, the vestibular system makes crucial contributions to several reflexive motor responses. These include (1) reflexive eye movements, called vestibuloocular reflexes, that improve visual acuity by helping stabilize images on the retina; (2) reflexive cardiac and respiratory responses, called vestibulo-autonomic reflexes, that help stabilize autonomic tone; and (3) reflexive postural responses, called vestibulo-spinal reflexes, that help stabilize our head and body with respect to gravity, assisting us as we walk and stand upright.

Although the vestibular system makes critical contributions to the forementioned reflexive responses, the vestibular system is also a sensory system that contributes to our perception of motion and orientation. This sense is often neglected relative to the commonly known five classical senses. This may be due to the inconspicuous nature of vestibular function, which almost always operates at an automated level. Patients suffering from rapid-onset vestibular disorders often become acutely aware of the fundamental contributions of the vestibular system to perception only when the vestibular system fails. The importance of the vestibular system is also emphasized by the fact that it appeared very early in evolutionary terms. The fossil record shows the presence of morphologically distinct vertical semicircular canals – not unlike mammalian vertical semicircular canals – dating back 400 million years.

Because the vestibular system is often overlooked as a sensory system, we compare the principal characteristics of the vestibular system to the principal characteristics shared by other sensory systems. First, as defined by Johannes Müller, physical stimuli activate specific nerve fibers that connect to the central nervous system to yield specific sensations – a concept referred to as specific sense energy. As a related concept, detailed in the *Principles of Neuroscience*, all sensory systems share "three common steps: (1) a *physical stimulus*, (2) a *chain of events* transforming the stimulus into nerve impulses, and (3) a response to this signal in the form of a *perception* or conscious experience of the sensation" (p. 412, 4th edn.). The relevant specific sense energy is discussed for the canals in the section titled 'Specific sense energy – semicircular canals' and for the otolith organs in the section titled 'Specific sense energy – otolith organs.' Second, all sensory systems mediate four stimulus characteristics – modality, location, intensity, and timing – that can be quantitatively correlated with perception. The relevant stimulus characteristics of the vestibular system are discussed in the section titled 'Vestibular senses information coding.' Because rotation yields changes in orientation, physical rotation and physical orientation are directly coupled to one another. If any observer knows the orientation of the head at some time point (time A) and also knows the head's complete rotation history between time A and a second time point (time B), we can correctly calculate its orientation at any time between times A and B). On the other hand, our perceptions of motion and orientation can, unlike true physical motion, be inconsistent.

Such inconsistencies are illustrated in the next section, which also provides compelling evidence for the contributions of the visual and vestibular systems to our sense of motion and orientation.

Example

Imagine that a human subject is upright with respect to gravity and looks at the inside of a sphere that is rotating in roll about an Earth-horizontal axis (**Figure 1(a)**). At first, the subject reports that he or she is stationary and that the visual display is rotating; both perceptions are veridical. However, if the subject continues to observe the rotating visual display for just a little longer (~10 s or more), he or she typically begins to perceive a sensation of self-rotation in the direction opposite the rotation of the visual display (**Figure 1(b)**). This illusory perception of self-motion evoked by visual motion is called vection, or more specifically rotational vection, and it demonstrates the visual contributions to our sense of self-rotation. Similarly, if subjects view a visual scene that is translating (e.g., the train next to theirs) while they are stationary, this often induces a perception of linear motion called linear vection, or, if subjects view a stationary display that is tilted (e.g., a tilted room), this can induce an illusion of self-tilt.

Paradoxically, subjects experiencing rotational vection, like that just described, seldom report that they are tumbling head over heals as they would if they truly were rotating to the extent that they perceive. In fact, subjects typically experience a simultaneous illusory sensation of tilt that gradually builds up to some relatively constant level (**Figure 1(c)**). These perceptions are often described as a sensation of motion without getting anywhere. These sensations are contradictory because if the perceived rotational motion were real it would yield continuously varying changes in perceived tilt, not a stable perception of some constant amount of tilt. This demonstrates that our sense of motion and orientation is not limited to perceptions that are consistent with physically possible motions and orientations.

This example can also be used to illustrate the role played by the vestibular system in our sense of motion and orientation. First, patients who have severe and complete damage in the vestibular periphery often report greater vection than normal subjects. Second, astronauts report greater vection when weightless than when on Earth. Third, astronauts experiencing rotational vection in weightlessness report a head-over-heals tumbling sensation, which is absent on Earth. This shows that the body's detection of gravity, which is measured by the otolith organs, inhibits the head-over-heels tumbling sensation here on Earth. Taken together, these findings show that the vestibular system makes a substantial contribution to our sense of motion and orientation. This is not surprising because the vestibular system is specialized to sense head motion and head tilt with respect to gravity.

Specific Sense Energy – Semicircular Canals

Like most sensory receptors, the semicircular canals respond primarily to a single physical stimulus, which for the semicircular canals is rotational motion. More specifically, the physical stimulus is angular acceleration, although the fluid mechanics of the canal yield a mechanical integration such that the neural response

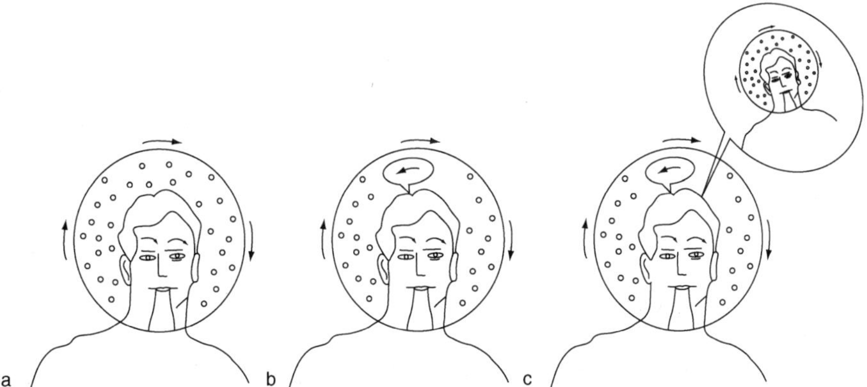

Figure 1 Roll vection: (a) sketch of a subject viewing a visual display rotating in roll; (b) subject beginning to experience vection (a sense of self-rotation in the direction opposite the rotation of the visual display); (c) roll vection is often accompanied by an illusion of roll tilt that is induced by the perceived roll rotation. For demonstration purposes, the visual display is shown as being transparent. Initially, subjects correctly sense that they are stationary and the visual display is rotating. In (c), the direction of the perceived tilt is consistent with the tilt direction that would have occurred if the subject were truly rotating in roll.

in first-order vestibular afferent neurons represents angular velocity over a broad range of physiological frequencies. A brief description of the physiological chain of events leading to peripheral transduction in the semicircular canal follows: (1) angular acceleration of the head yields fluid movement in the canals with respect to the head, which (2) deflects the cupula, which (3) deflects hair cell cilia, which (4) gates mechanically sensitive ion channels, which (5) alters the receptor potentials, which (6) alters the neurotransmitter release rate, which (7) alters the firing rate of afferent neurons innervating the canal.

Finally, there is no question that we perceive rotation. Skeptics can be rotated on a rotating chair (e.g., bar stool) with their eyes closed to show them that they perceive rotation even in the absence of cues providing a visual reference. Although the actual motion thresholds in the dark depend on the frequency content of the motion, at physiological frequencies, many normal subjects perceive angular velocities above 1–2 $^\circ s^{-1}$ and angular accelerations above approximately 0.2–1 $^\circ s^{-2}$. Consistent with Müller's notion of specific sense energy, a similar sense of rotation is evoked when the neurons innervating the canals are activated via electrical stimulation.

The perception of rotation about an Earth-vertical rotation axis has dynamic characteristics that mimic a high-pass filter (**Figure 2**); this is expected because the first-order afferent neurons from the canals are known to have high-pass response dynamics when the afferent response is compared to angular velocity stimuli. More specifically, at frequencies below approximately 0.025 Hz, little or no rotation is perceived. As the stimulation frequency increases, so does the perceived rotation. At moderately high frequencies (between 0.2 and 0.8 Hz), the sensation of rotation appears to plateau at a level that slightly underestimates the rotation.

That the semicircular canals are a predominant contributor to rotational sensation is demonstrated by the fact that patients in the dark with complete bilateral absence of vestibular function do not perceive rotational motion that would be detected easily by normal subjects. These patients do maintain the ability to perceive rotation in the light, when visual cues are available, especially at lower frequencies. In fact, it has been shown that signals from the visual periphery indicating visual motion (as opposed to foveal visual motion cues) converge with the afferent canal neurons in the vestibular nuclei, which is in the brain stem one synapse from the vestibular periphery.

The semicircular canals sense head rotation and evoke a perception of rotation. (Although we can argue that the perceived quantity is angular velocity, whereas the physical stimuli is actually angular acceleration, which is then mechanically integrated

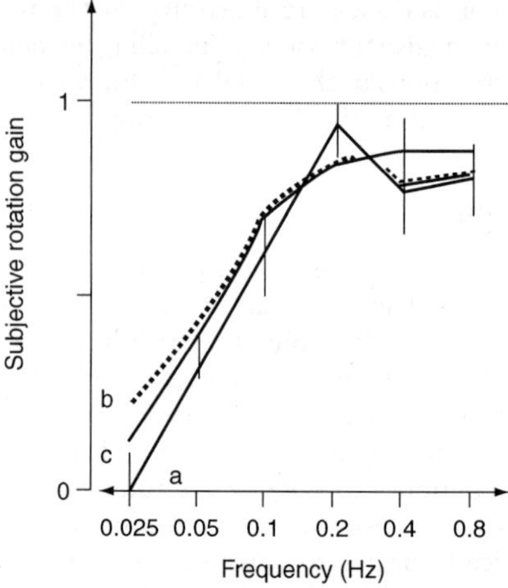

Figure 2 Magnitude of yaw rotation perception as a function of rotation frequency during sinusoidal rotations of the whole body. The three curves represent three different assays of perceived rotation, each of which yields a very similar measure of perceived rotation. Trace a shows perceived rotation in complete darkness; trace b shows perceived rotation when a single head-stationary object was viewed; and trace c shows perceived rotation when a single object rotated at twice the angular velocity of the subject. From Mergner T and Becker W (1990) Perception of horizontal self-rotation: multisensory and cognitive aspects. In: Warren R and Wertheim A (eds.) *Perception & Control of Self-Motion*, pp. 219–263. Hillsdale, NJ: Lawrence Erlbaum.

by the end organ such that the neural response most closely relates to angular velocity, this is not a critical distinction.) Hence, the dimensionality of the physical stimulus and the perceived quantity are the same. This direct relationship between the physical stimuli and the perceived quantity is interesting; no other sensory system has a more direct relationship between the perception and the primary physical stimulus. For example, the dimensionality of the perception evoked by physical stimulation (hearing, sight, smell, taste, and touch) and the actual physical stimulation (pressure waves, photons, chemical, and pressure) is not identical for any of the commonly known sensory systems.

Specific Sense Energy – Otolith Organs

While most sensory receptors respond primarily to a single physical stimulus, the otolith organs, which sense both gravity and linear acceleration, provide an interesting exception. All linear accelerometers, including the otolith organs, respond equivalently both to gravity and linear acceleration, which is consistent with Einstein's equivalence principle which posits that linear acceleration and gravity have equivalent effects.

While probably important only to aficionados, it is interesting to note that one can define the physical stimulus to the otolith organs as the vector difference between gravity and linear acceleration. The corresponding force is called the gravito-inertial force. Under this definition, one could consider gravito-inertial force as the operating stimulus, which would mean that otolith organs, like the majority of sensory systems, respond primarily to a single stimulus. However, gravity and linear acceleration are different physical stimuli from a perceptual viewpoint. Nonetheless, they are indistinguishable in their effects from a physical viewpoint. There is no way, without separate information, to dissect the gravito-inertial force into portions due to each source. This is not an axiom of physics, but an inference from the observation that the gravitational and inertial masses (defined by Newton's law of gravitation and Newton's second law, respectively) have been measured to be equal to a very high degree of precision. Einstein made the assumption of perfect equality explicit in his equivalence principle, and built the theory of general relativity upon this assumption.

The physiological chain of events that yield neural responses in the otolith organs is similar to the cascade previously described for the semicircular canals. A brief description of the chain of events leading to peripheral transduction in the otolith organs follows: (1) linear acceleration of the head and/or the presence of a gravitational field deflects a membranous gel layer that is embedded with calcium carbonate crystals called otoconia, which (2) deflects hair cell cilia, which (3) gates mechanically sensitive ion channels, which (4) alters the receptor potentials, which (5) alters neurotransmitter release rate, which (6) alters the firing rate of afferent neurons innervating the otolith organ.

Because the otolith organs respond equally to two classically distinct forms of stimulation – linear acceleration and gravity – two distinct 'perceptual' responses are evoked by otolith stimulation. The issue of how this sensory ambiguity is resolved by the nervous system is discussed elsewhere.

The otolith organs contribute to tilt perception – the perception of the orientation of the head with respect to gravity. This sensation is both stable and relatively precise. Most young normal subjects can – even in a dark room – correctly estimate when tilted from upright by as little as 1–2° or so. Furthermore, for static tilts, subjective indications of perceived tilt more or less accurately reflect the actual physical tilt for tilts up to 90° (**Figure 3**), although consistent overestimates and underestimates of tilt angle are reported. If the subjects are tilted dynamically using sinusoidal stimuli, the subjective tilt responses remain somewhat constant across the frequency range of 0.005–0.8 Hz, although subjective tilt was accurately reported for high frequencies and somewhat overestimated at low frequencies (**Figure 4**). Because of the equivalence of gravity and linear acceleration, subjects report an illusion of tilt in the dark when they are dynamically accelerated using sinusoidal stimuli, even in the absence of actual physical tilt. This illusion is large at low frequencies (<0.05 Hz) before declining precipitously, such that almost no tilt illusion is experienced at frequencies of 0.2 Hz and higher (**Figure 4**).

The otolith organs also contribute to translation perception. In the absence of vision, normal subjects perceive linear motion having linear accelerations as small as approximately 0.05–0.10 m s^{-2} (510 mG) and linear velocities as small as approximately 0.02 ms^{-1} (<0.05 mph). In addition, when humans are exposed to steps of linear acceleration, the time that it takes to detect the direction of the motion (i.e., Is the motion to the left or right?) decreases as the magnitude of the linear acceleration increases (**Figure 5**).

Vestibular Senses Information Coding

As stated in the *Principles of Neuroscience*, "all sensory systems convey four basic types of information when stimulated – *modality*, *location*, *intensity*, and *timing*. Together these four elementary attributes yield sensation" (p. 412, 4th edn.). We look at vestibular function here as it relates to our sense of motion and orientation from the perspective provided by these four basic sensory system characteristics.

Generally, modality defines the general class of stimulus. As already discussed, the vestibular system has three modalities because it responds to rotational motion, linear acceleration, and gravity – with three dimensions for each of the three modalities. More specifically, the semicircular canals respond to rotation, with the nearly orthogonal canals sensing rotation in each of the three spatial dimensions, whereas the otolith organs respond to gravity in each of three dimensions and respond to linear acceleration in each of three dimensions.

Generally, location refers to the spatial distribution of the energy spectrum for each individual modality. For example, for touch and vision, the spatial distribution of the afferent neurons encodes the spatial location of the object (vision) or point of body contact (touch). For hearing, the spatial distribution of the afferent neurons represents the frequency of the acoustic stimulation. For the vestibular system, the spatial distribution of the afferent neurons represents the direction of motion or the direction of gravity. To use a specific example, neurons innervating the lateral canals respond nearly exclusively to yaw head

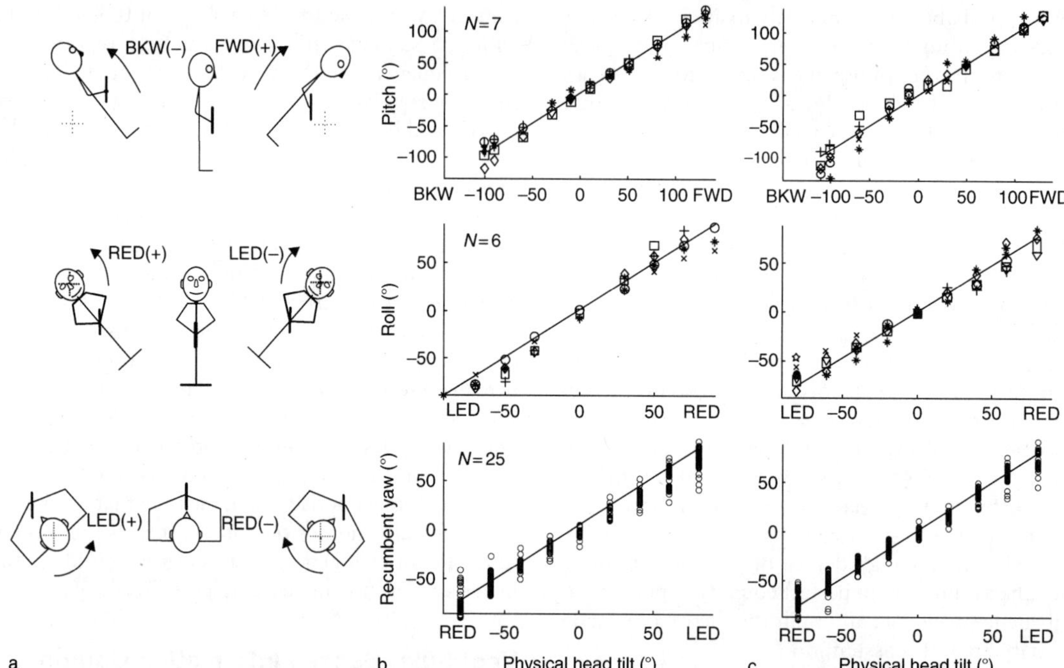

Figure 3 Tilt perception for static pitch (top row), roll (middle row), and yaw (bottom row) tilts: (a) sketches defining pitch, roll, and yaw and associated conventions; (b) tilt perception provided by subjects using a handheld haptic device; (c) tilt perception provided by subjects verbally. To first-order, perceived tilt accurately reflects the actual tilt for all three tilt directions, although roll tilts were slightly overestimated and yaw tilts were slightly underestimated. BKW, backward; FWD, forward; LED, left ear down; RED, right ear down. From Bortolami SB, Pierobon A, Dizio P, and Lackner JR (2006) Localization of the subjective vertical during roll, pitch, and recumbent yaw body tilt. *Experimental Brain Research* 173: 364–373.

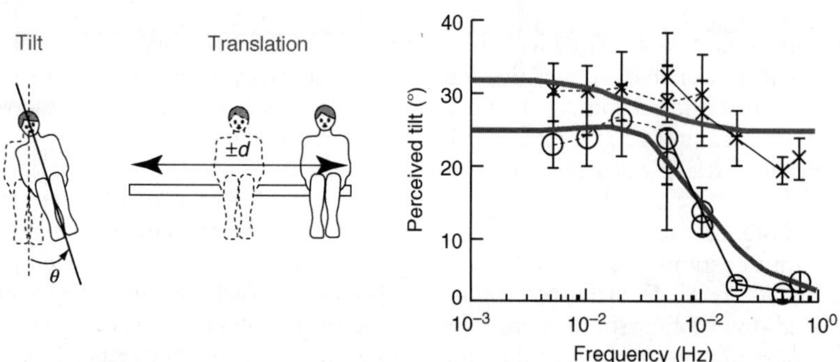

Figure 4 Magnitude of roll tilt perception, which is tilt to the left or right, provided by subjects using a two-handed task as a function of frequency between 0.005 and 0.7 Hz. Tilt stimuli: Roll tilt perception during applied sinusoidal roll tilts are shown (indicated by x) with a modeling prediction overlaid in green. Translation stimuli: Illusory roll tilt perception reported during sinusoidal linear accelerations (indicated by o), with no actual tilt stimuli, are shown with a modeling prediction overlaid in red. Adapted from Park S, Gianna-Poulin C, Black FO, Wood S, and Merfeld DM (2006) Roll rotation cues influence roll tilt perception assayed using a somatosensory technique. *Journal of Neurophysiology* 96: 486–491. Roll tilt modeling prediction from Merfeld DM, Park S, Gianna-Poulin C, Black FO, and Wood S (2005) Vestibular perception and action employ qualitatively different mechanisms I: Frequency response of VOR and perceptual responses during translation and tilt. *Journal of Neurophysiology* 94: 186–198.

rotations, responding minimally to rotations that do not include yaw head rotations. Similarly, the other semicircular canals, the anterior and posterior canals, respond only to rotational motion aligned with the anterior and posterior canal planes, respectively. A similar relationship holds true for the otolith organs. Individual neurons have spatial tuning characteristics that result in the neuron firing when a component of

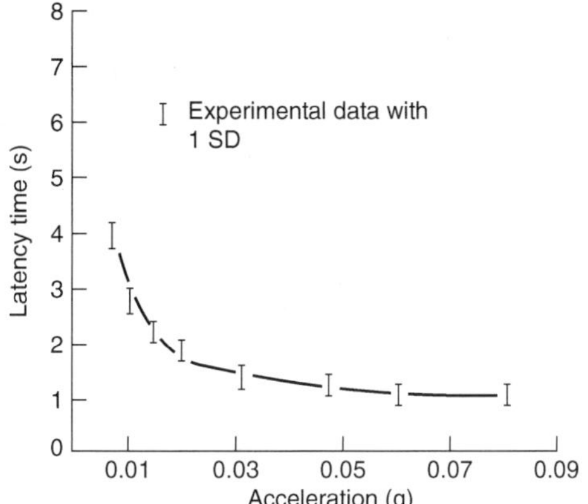

Figure 5 Latency between the start of a linear acceleration step and the subjective indication of the direction of linear motion, shown as a function of the level of linear acceleration; this latency is often called the time-to-detect. The time-to-detect decreases as the magnitude of the acceleration step increases. In this paradigm, the relationship between the time-to-detect and the linear acceleration magnitude covary in a manner consistent with the subjects correctly detecting the direction of motion when they attain a velocity of approximately 0.20 m s^{-1}. SD, standard deviation. From Young L (1984) Perception of the body in space: Mechanisms. In: Darian-Smith I (ed.) *Handbook of Physiology: The Nervous System*, pp. 1023–1066. Bethesda, MD: American Physiological Society.

gravity or linear acceleration aligns with that neuron's axis of maximal sensitivity, which is determined by the polarity of the innervated hair cell(s).

Generally, stimulus intensity is signaled by the firing rate of the afferent neurons. Neurons in the vestibular system of primates have a relatively high tonic baseline activity of approximately 100 action potentials per second. The firing rate of these neurons increases for motion in one direction and decreases for motion in the opposite direction. Within the normal physiological range, the magnitude of the change in the neural firing rate of each individual neuron represents the intensity of the motion. For rotations at physiological frequencies (circa 0.1–5 Hz), the magnitude of the neural firing rate for neurons innervating the semicircular canals scales nearly linearly with angular velocity until the stimulus becomes so large that saturation effects predominate. Similarly, for the otolith organs, the magnitude of the neural firing rate scales roughly linearly with (1) the component of linear acceleration aligned with the sensitive direction of each neuron innervating the otolith organ and/or (2) the gravitational component aligned with the sensitive axis of each otolith neuron. It is interesting to note that, saturation effects aside, the vestibular afferent responses change roughly linearly with stimulus intensity. This differs from most other sensory systems, in which the afferent response varies with the logarithm of the stimulus intensity.

The timing of the physical stimulus is nearly instantaneously indicated by changes in the neural firing rate of vestibular neurons. At physiological frequencies, the firing rate of each neuron innervating a semicircular canal increases and decreases in near synchrony with increases and decreases in the angular velocity. Similarly, the firing rate for neurons innervating the otolith organs increases and decreases in near synchrony with linear acceleration and/or gravitational stimulation.

Summary

The vestibular system is a sensory system that makes crucial contributions to our sense of motion and orientation. The subjective experiences evoked by the vestibular system include perceptions of angular velocity and linear velocity and perceptions of both tilt and heading. These subjective experiences are evoked by objective physical stimuli; the semicircular canals sense angular acceleration, whereas the otolith organs sense both linear acceleration and gravity. These physical stimuli lead to sensory transduction, which cause changes in the neural activation of the vestibular afferents. This neural activation is a first step in the physiological processes that lead to neural representations of the physical stimuli, which are sometimes called internal representations. Such internal representations are the brain's way of storing and processing the external physical stimuli and combining the vestibular information with other information – like information provided by visual cues, somatosensory cues, and/or cognitive cues – to best inform us about our motion and orientation.

See also: Auditory/Somatosensory Interactions; Canal–Otolith Interactions; Hair Cells: Sensory Transduction; Motion Sickness; Neural Coding of Spatial Representations; Spatial Cognition and Executive Function; Vestibular System; Vestibulo-Autonomic Responses; Vestibulo-Ocular Reflex; Vestibulospinal System and Eye–Head/Neck Movement; Vision: Mechanisms of Orientation, Direction and Depth; Visual–Vestibular Interactions.

Further Reading

Benson A (1982) The vestibular sensory system. In: Barlow H and Mollon J (eds.) *The Senses*, pp. 333–368. Cambridge, UK: Cambridge University Press.

Bortolami SB, Pierobon A, Dizio P, and Lackner JR (2006) Localization of the subjective vertical during roll, pitch, and recumbent yaw body tilt. *Experimental Brain Research* 173: 364–373.

Gardner E and Martin J (2000) Coding of sensory information. In: Kandel E, Schwartz J, and Jessel T (eds.) *Principles of Neural Science,* 4th edn., pp. 411–429. New York: McGraw-Hill.

Guedry F (1974) Psychophysics of vestibular sensation. In: Kornhuber HH (ed.) *Handbook of Sensory Physiology*, pp. 1–154. New York: Springer.

Howard I and Templeton W (1966) *Human Spatial Orientation.* New York: Wiley.

Kandel E, Schwartz J, and Jessell T (2000) *Principles of Neural Science,* 4th edn. Upper Saddle River, NJ: Prentice-Hall.

Merfeld DM, Park S, Gianna-Poulin C, Black FO, and Wood S (2005) Vestibular perception and action employ qualitatively different mechanisms I: Frequency response of VOR and perceptual responses during translation and tilt. *Journal of Neurophysiology* 94: 186–198.

Mergner T and Becker W (1990) Perception of horizontal self-rotation: Multisensory and cognitive aspects. In: Warren R and Wertheim A (eds.) *Perception & Control of Self-Motion*, pp. 219–263. Hillsdale, NJ: Lawrence Erlbaum.

Park S, Gianna-Poulin C, Black FO, Wood S, and Merfeld DM (2006) Roll rotation cues influence roll tilt perception assayed using a somatosensory technique. *Journal of Neurophysiology* 96: 486–491.

Young L (1984) Perception of the body in space: Mechanisms. In: Darian-Smith I (ed.) *Handbook of Physiology: The Nervous System*, pp. 1023–1066. Bethesda, MD: American Physiological Society.

Strategic Control of Memory

B A Kuhl and A D Wagner, Stanford University, Stanford, CA, USA

Introduction

Cognitive control mechanisms permit memory to be accessed strategically and so aid in bringing knowledge to mind that is relevant to current decisions and actions. A fundamental component of the strategic control of memory is the resolution of interference from competing, irrelevant representations. This article considers how the ventrolateral prefrontal cortex (VLPFC) regulates mnemonic competition in multiple memory systems. We initially discuss how damage to lateral prefrontal cortex impacts mnemonic function and then consider recent neuroimaging and focal lesion findings that highlight the distinct roles that subregions of the VLPFC play in the control of memory.

Lateral Prefrontal Cortex

The lateral prefrontal cortex (PFC) consists of ventral, dorsal, and frontopolar subregions. In this article, we primarily focus on the function of VLPFC. In the human (**Figure 1(a)**), VLPFC corresponds to the inferior frontal gyrus, which includes (moving caudally to rostrally) the inferior frontal pars opercularis (Brodmann area (BA) 44), inferior frontal pars triangularis (BA 45), and inferior frontal pars orbitalis (an area that Petrides and Pandya term area 47/12, which corresponds to the lateral portion of BA 47). Whereas Petrides and Pandya refer to area 47/12 and BA 45 collectively as the mid-VLPFC, distinguishing these regions from the caudally situated BA 44, in this article we functionally distinguish area 47/12 from BA 45. Thus, we use anterior VLPFC to refer to the inferior frontal pars orbitalis (area 47/12), mid-VLPFC to refer to the pars triangularis (BA 45), and posterior VLPFC to refer to the pars opercularis (BA 44). We note that the caudal portion of area 47/12 actually lies ventral (rather than rostral) to BA 45 (**Figure 1(a)**). The inferior frontal sulcus in humans (and the principal sulcus in monkeys) marks the approximate boundary between the VLPFC and the dorsolateral PFC (DLPFC). In terms of anatomical connectivity, the VLPFC is strongly connected with cortical areas in the lateral temporal lobe and medial temporal lobe (MTL), including (but not limited to) the inferotemporal cortex, superior temporal cortex, and, more medially, perirhinal and parahippocampal cortices.

Mnemonic Deficits Following Lateral Prefrontal Damage

Neuropsychological studies in humans and lesion studies in animals indicate that insult to the lateral PFC can produce memory impairments that are qualitatively distinct from those observed following MTL damage. Whereas MTL damage results in an amnesic condition that reflects the inability to encode and retrieve new declarative memories – long-term memories for events (episodic memory) and facts (semantic memory) – lateral PFC damage impairs the strategic regulation of multiple forms of memory, including declarative memory and working memory. Significantly, impairments in episodic memory, semantic memory, and working memory following lateral PFC damage are often most apparent when performance requires the resolution of interference, which led Moscovitch, Shimamura, and others to propose that lateral PFC subserves cognitive control mechanisms that regulate how we work with or dynamically filter memory.

Episodic Memory Deficits

Patients with lateral PFC damage show modest impairments in their ability to encode and retrieve episodic memories, with these deficits being particularly apparent when memory for target information is required in the face of distraction. Here we illustrate these deficits by highlighting a number of well-documented paradigms in which PFC patients are impaired.

First, PFC patients show disproportionate deficits on tests of free recall compared to item recognition. Theorists have argued that the unconstrained nature of free recall increases the likelihood of mnemonic competition or interference. Second, even within recognition tests, PFC patients show impairments when distracter items at test (foils) are similar to items from the study list. In other words, PFC patients suffer interference from items that are similar to those they studied, as evidenced by false claims of having studied these items. Third, in tests of source memory, in which memories for individual items must be attributed to a particular learning context – a discrimination that presents high interference because irrelevant contexts are often highly salient – PFC patients exhibit disproportionate deficits relative to tests of item recognition. Fourth, the use of AB–AC learning paradigms reveals that learning an AC association is disproportionately impaired in PFC patients (i.e., patients show a heightened sensitivity to proactive interference). In such paradigms, the patient's

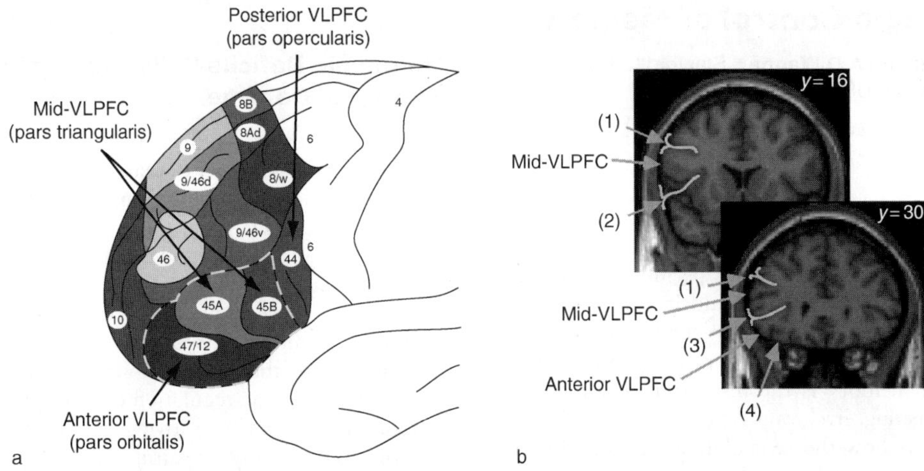

Figure 1 Anatomical divisions of the ventrolateral prefrontal cortex (VLPFC) in the human: (a) representation of the cytoarchitectonic subdivisions of the lateral prefrontal cortex (PFC); (b) coronal slices through the PFC depicting the anatomical boundaries that define the mid-VLPFC and anterior VLPFC. The subregions of the VLPFC include the pars orbitalis, pars triangularis, and pars opercularis, corresponding to the anterior VLPFC (area 47/12), mid-VLPFC (area 45), and posterior VLPFC (area 44), respectively. (Note that we use the term mid-VLPFC to refer to area 45 only, adopting anterior VLPFC to refer to area 47/12.) As shown in (b), both the anterior and mid-VLPFC lie ventral to the inferior frontal sulcus (1). In caudal slices, the mid-VLPFC is bounded ventrally by the insular sulcus (2), and in rostral slices it is bounded by the horizontal ramus of the lateral fissure (3). The anterior VLPFC is bounded ventrally and medially by the orbital gyrus (4). (a) Adapted from Petrides M and Pandya DN (2002) Comparative cytoarchitectonic analysis of the human and the macaque ventrolateral prefrontal cortex and corticocortical connection patterns in the monkey. *European Journal of Neuoscience* 16: 291–310. (b) From Badre D and Wagner AD (2007) Left ventrolateral prefrontal cortex and the cognitive control of memory. *Neuropsychologia* 45(13): 2883–2901.

memory for AC pairs is largely compromised by increased intrusions of the earlier learned AB associations. Moreover, even when sequentially studying two unrelated lists of items (i.e., the lists do not share common associates), PFC patients show disproportionate list 1 interference when trying to learn list 2. Finally, when PFC patients are provided with a subset of items from a previously studied list as retrieval cues (i.e., part-list cueing), the high salience of the provided items results in increased impairment in the patients' ability to recall the remaining (unpresented) items from the list. Collectively, these and other observations indicate that the ability to resolve interference in episodic memory is compromised following lateral PFC damage.

Semantic Memory Deficits

Just as PFC patients show impairments in unconstrained episodic memory tests, they also show deficits in unconstrained tests of semantic retrieval. For example, patients show reduced total output on verbal fluency tasks, which involve freely generating as many unique exemplars as possible in response to a semantic or orthographic cue. This impairment is thought to partially reflect patients' heightened sensitivity to output interference stemming from the initially retrieved exemplars. Significantly, this interference-dependent deficit during semantic or lexical retrieval stands in contrast to the typically unimpaired ability of PFC patients to recognize semantic structure or evaluate semantic relationships. Beyond verbal fluency tasks, patients with damage to the left lateral PFC fail to show normal semantic priming when the meaning of a semantic cue (the prime) is a context-dependent homograph, compared to words with less ambiguous meanings. This impairment may be due to PFC patients failing to retrieve the appropriate stimulus meaning when the prime is ambiguous, thereby preventing priming from occurring. Both these deficits are consistent with the perspective that the lateral PFC is recruited during controlled semantic retrieval, as well as when interference between competing semantic or lexical representations must be resolved.

Working Memory Deficits

In tests of working memory, PFC patients are often unimpaired, as measured by simple tests of verbal span. However, in tests in which maintenance is complicated by interference from irrelevant information, lateral PFC damage tends to result in impairment. For example, in delayed recognition tests, PFC patients are particularly sensitive to the presence of distracters during the delay. When compared to patients with damage to the MTL, PFC patients show impairments at all delay intervals as long as distracters are present, whereas patients with MTL damage show impairments principally at long delays. A similar observation comes from studies of PFC-lesioned monkeys. Whereas it was initially believed that PFC-lesioned monkeys were unable to remember the location of a food item that was hidden for only a short delay, it was later shown that this apparent memory deficit could be eliminated if the delay period was held in total darkness. In other words, the monkey's memory deficit was a function of the interfering effects of visual input during the delay period. Strikingly, not only do PFC patients show impaired working memory performance due to distracters, but PFC patients also show exaggerated electrophysiological responses in cortical areas that process the modality of the distracting information, suggesting that when distraction is present, the PFC is responsible for gating activity in regions that would otherwise process the distracting information. Further evidence that lateral PFC damage results in an inability to filter or gate irrelevant distracting information comes from studies of negative priming. In such studies, healthy controls typically showed increased reaction times when processing a stimulus that was previously a distracter (i.e., these previous distracters showed negative priming). By contrast, frontal patients showed the reverse effect – facilitated processing of stimuli that previously served as distracters – which suggests that the patients had difficulty preventing the processing of the distracters.

Functional Specificity within Lateral Prefrontal Cortex

Although data from frontal patients provide compelling evidence that one contribution of the lateral PFC to the strategic control of memory is to regulate interference, the lack of anatomical specificity that typically accompanies naturally occurring PFC lesions in humans often precludes the determination of the specific functional contributions of particular PFC subregions. In an attempt to specify the mechanistic contributions of the subregions of the VLPFC to the control of memory, we consider in the next section evidence from functional neuroimaging studies and from recent reports of patients with lesions focused on subregions of VLPFC. As we discuss, extant data implicate the mid-VLPFC as a key component of the neural circuitry that resolves mnemonic interference, be it within working memory, semantic memory, or episodic memory.

Memory and the VLPFC

Focal lesion studies with monkeys have shown that damage to the inferior convexity (the monkey homolog of the human inferior frontal gyrus), but not to the DLPFC, causes perseverative tendencies in contexts in which the prior response learning must be reversed. Similar perseverative errors are a classic hallmark of human frontal lobe damage, as is often revealed through errors on the Wisconsin Card Sorting Task, when subjects must override a previously established, but now irrelevant, response set. As already noted, the strategic control of working memory, semantic memory, and episodic memory often requires conceptually similar mechanisms that permit the overriding of interference from irrelevant representations. Functional neuroimaging data in humans, complemented by focal lesion evidence, now indicate that the left mid-VLPFC regulates mnemonic interference by enabling the selection of relevant representations in the face of mnemonic conflict, whereas the left anterior VLPFC controls access to, and guides the retrieval of, long-term semantic knowledge. Response override or inhibition, by contrast, appears to differentially depend on regions in the human right VLPFC.

Left Mid-VLPFC and Interference in Working Memory

Extensive evidence for the role of the left mid-VLPFC (BA 45) in resolving mnemonic interference comes from a variant of the Sternberg working memory paradigm (**Figure 2(a)**). In this task, participants encode a target set of stimuli (e.g., four letters), which they then attempt to maintain in working memory across a brief delay. Following the delay, a probe (e.g., a letter) is presented and participants make a yes/no decision as to whether the probe is in the currently maintained memory set. Critically, some negative probes (i.e., probes to which the subject should respond no) come from the immediately preceding memory set (negative recent probes), whereas other negative probes have not appeared in either the present or the preceding memory sets (negative nonrecent probes) (**Figure 2(a)**). Given this structure, negative recent probes are associated with interference because subjects must attribute the familiarity of the probe to its having been in the preceding memory set to correctly reject the probe as not being a member of the current memory set. Thus, comparisons of negative recent to negative nonrecent trials provide leverage on the neural mechanisms that are engaged in the face of this mnemonic interference.

Jonides and colleagues were the first to demonstrate that functional activation in the left mid-VLPFC is greater during negative recent relative to negative nonrecent trials, a pattern that has been replicated and extended by others (**Figure 2(b)**). Subsequent data indicated that (1) the response in the left mid-VLPFC during negative recent trials is

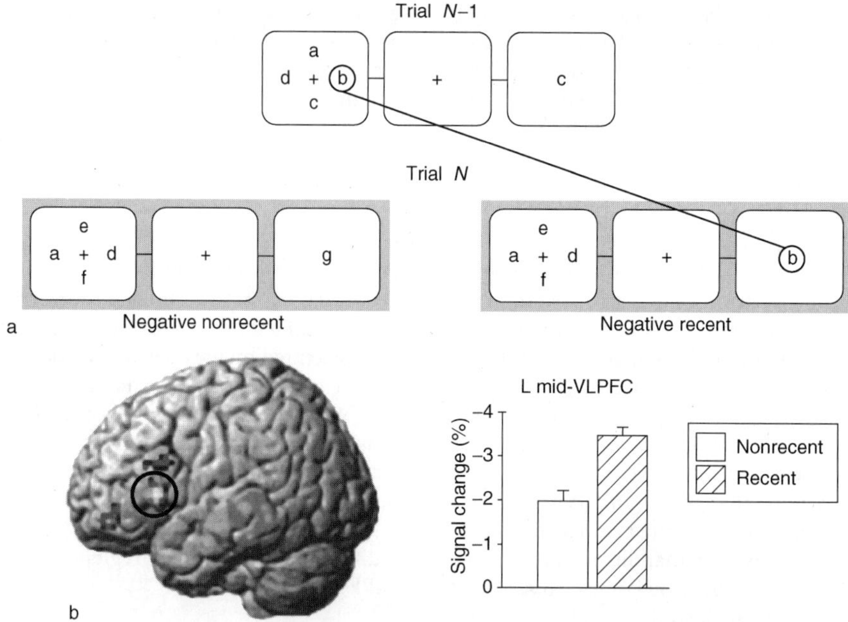

Figure 2 Interference resolution in the Sternberg working memory task: (a) a representative version of the task; (b) representative fMRI data. As shown in (a), during the task subjects maintain a set of four letters in working memory until a probe letter appears, at which point subjects indicate whether the probe is a member of the currently maintained set (positive probe) or is not a member of the current set (negative probe). Interference occurs when a probe is not a member of the current set, but is a member of the immediately preceding set (negative recent probe), relative to situations in which the probe is a member neither of the current set nor of the immediately preceding set (negative nonrecent probe). In (b), the fMRI data reveal greater activation during negative recent vs. negative nonrecent trials in the left mid-VLPFC (circled), reflecting that the presence of interference in working memory is accompanied by greater recruitment of the left mid-VLPFC. fMRI, functional magnetic resonance imaging; L, left; VLPFC, ventrolateral prefrontal cortex. Adapted from Badre D and Wagner AD (2005) Frontal lobe mechanisms that resolve proactive interference. *Cerebral Cortex* 15: 2003–2012.

restricted to the probe period of the trial, which is consistent with the fact that interference is a function of the probe's familiarity, and (2) when directly interrogating the DLPFC, a similar difference between negative recent and nonrecent trials is not typically observed, suggesting a specific role of the left mid-VLPFC in resolving interference in this task. Moreover, in a compelling study motivated by the aforementioned neuroimaging data, Thompson-Schill and colleagues showed that PFC patients with damage that spared the left VLPFC demonstrated interference effects that were comparable in magnitude to those in healthy controls, whereas one patient, R.C., with a focal lesion that damaged almost the entire extent of the left BA 45, exhibited an exacerbated interference effect despite relatively normal working memory performance when interference was minimal. Complementing these data, Postle and colleagues observed that when repetitive transcranial magnetic stimulation (TMS) – which transiently disrupts cortical function – was applied to the left VLPFC during the probe period in healthy humans there was a similar increase in susceptibility to interference to that seen in patient R.C. By contrast, TMS disruption of the primary motor, primary somatosensory, or supplemental motor area did not affect the ability to resolve interference in this task. Collectively, these data demonstrate that the left mid-VLPFC makes necessary contributions to resolving interference from currently irrelevant information in working memory. A leading hypothesis is that this region enables the selection of relevant active information over irrelevant active representations.

Left VLPFC and Declarative Memory Retrieval

Complementing the working memory literature implicating the left mid-VLPFC in resolving interference from recently activated but now irrelevant mnemonic representations are patient and imaging data that suggest that the left mid-VLPFC also supports selection during retrieval from declarative memory (i.e., semantic and episodic memory). For example, as already discussed, demands on interference resolution during semantic retrieval may be greater when available retrieval cues are unconstrained, and it is under these conditions that left PFC patients show impairments in generating semantic knowledge.

Such impairments may reflect an inability to select relevant representations from among competing alternatives.

Functional neuroimaging and focal lesion data converge on the left mid-VLPFC as being central for mediating the selection of relevant semantic representations. For example, in an influential functional magnetic resonance imaging (fMRI) study, Thompson-Schill and colleagues compared semantic processing under conditions that varied the demands placed on selection. Across several tasks, low-selection conditions were constructed such that they involved retrieving dominant, or prepotent, semantic information, whereas high-selection conditions involved retrieving nondominant semantic information from among competing representations. Significantly, the imaging data revealed that the left VLPFC (BAs 44 and 45) was consistently more active during the high-selection (vs. low-selection) conditions, demonstrating that this is a replicable characteristic of left mid-and/or posterior VLPFC function. Subsequent neuropsychological work by Thompson-Schill and colleagues revealed that it is the proportion of damage to this left VLPFC region, but not the gross lesion size, that strongly predicts the magnitude of behavioral impairment on high-selection semantic retrieval tasks.

Related data have increased the precision of our understanding of left mid-VLPFC function and its relation to the functions of the surrounding anterior and posterior VLPFC subregions. In particular, Badre and colleagues demonstrated that selection demands during semantic processing tasks are specifically associated with the same left mid-VLPFC subregion (BA 45; pars triangularis) that resolves interference in working memory tasks (**Figure** 3(**a**)). Moreover, these researchers observed a functional dissociation within the left VLPFC, indicating that the left mid-VLPFC supports selection from among active representations, whereas the more rostrally and ventrally situated left anterior VLPFC subregion (area 47/12; pars orbitalis) controls the retrieval of semantic representations stored in the lateral temporal cortical areas. This functional distinction between the left mid-VLPFC and anterior VLPFC appears replicable and generalizeable; Gold and colleagues reported a similar functional pattern using a lexical decision task – namely that the left anterior VLPFC was associated with controlled semantic retrieval and the left mid-VLPFC was associated with resolving interference from irrelevant active representations.

Evidence for functional segregation within the left VLPFC has also come from studies comparing semantic versus phonological control. For example, neuroimaging studies of phonological rehearsal and phonological analysis of stimuli have implicated the left posterior VLPFC (BA 44; pars opercularis), suggesting that this VLPFC subregion is critical for representing and maintaining phonological codes. On the other hand, neuroimaging studies of semantic retrieval and analysis of stimuli have implicated the left anterior VLPFC. Significantly, these dissociations between the left anterior and posterior VLPFC have been observed in studies that directly contrasted tasks that differentially depend on semantic and phonological control. Moreover, Devlin and colleagues have shown that TMS to the left anterior VLPFC differentially disrupts concurrent semantic processing, whereas TMS to the left posterior VLPFC differentially disrupts concurrent phonological processing, demonstrating that these subregions are necessary for distinct forms of control.

Functional distinctions between the left VLPFC subregions are also apparent during tasks that probe episodic memory. For example, Dobbins and colleagues observed that the left mid-VLPFC is associated with selecting between episodic details in the course of making a source judgment (**Figure 3(b)**), whereas the left anterior VLPFC is associated with semantically elaborating on the cues used to probe episodic memory. Further, during episodic encoding, Dolan, Fletcher, and colleagues demonstrated that left mid-VLPFC activity increases when prior learning interferes with to-be-encoded information (i.e., when the resolution of proactive interference is required). Collectively, these data suggest that the left mid-VLPFC contributes to the resolution of interference during all forms of declarative memory, whereas the left anterior VLPFC controls the retrieval of semantic knowledge that is not retrieved in an automatic (bottom-up) manner. Moreover, when considered along with the evidence that the left mid-VLPFC resolves interference within working memory, extant data favor the hypothesis that the left mid-VLPFC serves a domain-general role of resolving mnemonic interference.

Right VLPFC and the Control of Memory

We have thus far focused on how the left VLPFC contributes to interference resolution and other forms of cognitive control; however, it should be emphasized that the right VLPFC is sometimes coactive with the left VLPFC during tasks that require overcoming mnemonic conflict. Nevertheless, although the right VLPFC may support control functions that are conceptually analogous to those supported by the left VLPFC, it appears that (in the human) the right VLPFC at least partially differs from the left VLPFC in the domain of knowledge on which is operates. For example, Aron and colleagues, among others,

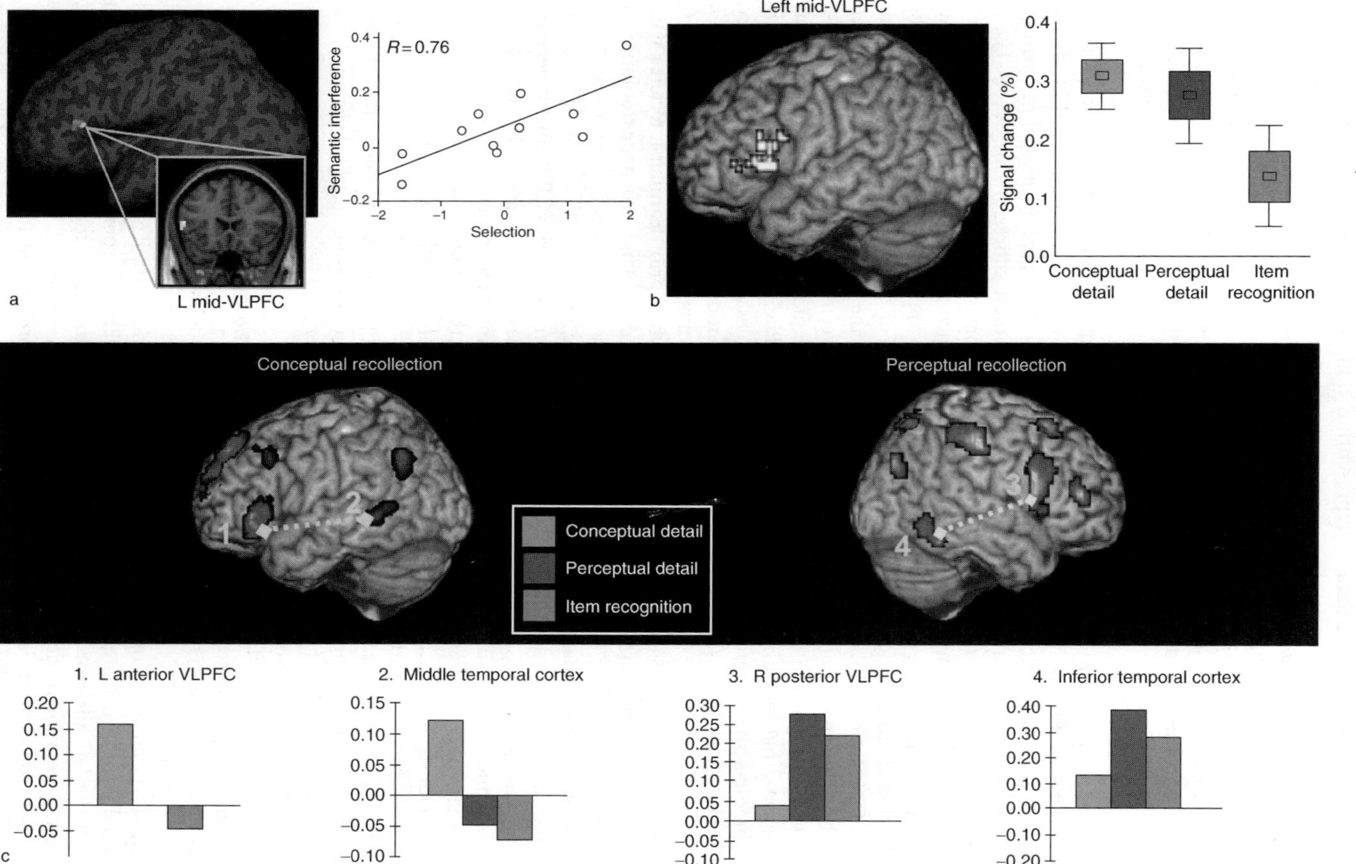

Figure 3 PFC contributions to the control of declarative memory: (a) a behavioral selection measure derived from performance during various semantic retrieval tasks; (b) the left mid-VLPFC during episodic retrieval; (c) the left anterior and right posterior VLPFC during episodic retrieval. In (a), the selection measure was exclusively associated with the magnitude of activation in the left mid-VLPFC (left). For example, this selection measure was tightly correlated with the magnitude of interference-related activation in the left mid-VLPFC during semantic retrieval (right). As shown in (b), during episodic retrieval, the left mid-VLPFC was differentially engaged when source details (conceptual or perceptual) were selectively retrieved, compared to simple item recognition. As shown in (c), during episodic retrieval, the left anterior VLPFC (1) was selectively engaged during recollection of conceptual source details, functionally coupling with the middle temporal cortex (2). By contrast, the right posterior VLPFC (3) was engaged during perceptual recollection and during recognition of familiar vs. novel objects, functionally coupling with the inferior temporal cortex (4). L, left; PFC, prefrontal cortex; VLPFC, ventrolateral prefrontal cortex. (a) Adapted from Badre D and Wagner AD (2005) Frontal lobe mechanisms that resolve proactive interference. *Cerebral Cortex* 15: 2003–2012. (b, c) Adapted from Dobbins IG and Wagner AD (2005) Domain-general and domain-sensitive prefrontal mechanisms for recollecting events and detecting novelty. *Cerebral Cortex* 15: 1768–1778.

reported that functional activation in the posterior aspect of the right VLPFC is consistently implicated in situations in which prepotent motor responses must be inhibited or when well-learned stimulus–response contingencies must be reconfigured. Moreover, these researchers demonstrated that when the right VLPFC is damaged, subjects display increased susceptibility to interference at the response level, highlighting the necessary contribution of this VLPFC subregion to response inhibition.

By contrast, other data indicate that the right VLPFC may contribute to the orienting of visual attention toward task-relevant object representations (and away from distracters). Significantly, with respect to the control of memory, this latter role of the right VLPFC in orienting to visuo-object representations has been observed in a number of mnemonic contexts, including discriminating novel from encountered visual objects, encoding faces and complex visual scenes into episodic memory, recollecting object–object associations, and recollecting perceptual details about previously encountered objects (**Figure** 3(c)). Thus, the extent to which the right VLPFC (as opposed to the left VLPFC) is engaged at least partially depends on the modality of the mnemonic representations attended, with the right VLPFC preferentially engaged during visuospatial processing and the left VLPFC engaged during phonological and semantic processing (**Figure** 3(c)). Significantly, although the right VLPFC has been implicated in visuo-object attention and in resolving competition at the response level, functional understanding of the subregions within the right VLPFC is not as well advanced as that of the homologous structures in the left VLPFC.

Concluding Comments

Interference resolution is a fundamental aspect of efficient mnemonic processing and may represent a principal way in which cognitive control interacts with memory. This interaction is critically enabled by control mechanisms that depend on the lateral PFC for their operation. This article focuses on the delineation of the mechanisms supported by the VLPFC, but it should be noted that the VLPFC must dynamically interact with the posterior neocortical association areas and with the MTL to implement the control of memory. Further, although VLPFC functions are clearly important for the resolution of mnemonic interference, the VLPFC also interacts with the DLPFC and frontopolar cortical areas that subserve other forms of cognitive control. Next we briefly illustrate each of these points.

To regulate memory-relevant processes, PFC control mechanisms must interact with systems that support or store long-term mnemonic representations. One line of evidence for such frontal-posterior interactions comes in the form of coactivations within functional neuroimaging studies. For example, fMRI studies of episodic remembering indicate that the left anterior VLPFC coactivates with the left middle temporal cortical areas that represent conceptual knowledge during controlled attempts to recollect such details about the past (**Figure** 3(c)). Analogously, the right VLPFC coactives with bilateral occipito-temporal areas that represent visuo-object form during attempts to recollect such details (**Figure** 3(c)). Moreover, as previously alluded to, lesions to the lateral PFC result in the failure to regulate processing in such posterior neocortical areas, demonstrating that the lateral PFC is necessary for gating the processing of distracting or interfering stimuli. Collectively, these data illustrate the top-down role of PFC control mechanisms in regulating perception, memory, and action.

With respect to cross-regional interactions within the PFC, it is important to emphasize that other structures in the DLPFC and frontopolar cortex are also often engaged in situations in which control must be implemented to accomplish a mnemonic goal. For example, DLPFC activation is frequently observed during complex working memory tasks, during attempts to remember past events, and during many tasks that require response selection or the resolution of response conflict. Although the specific nature of interactions between the DLPFC and VLPFC have yet to be well characterized, it is hypothesized that the DLPFC may operate at a higher stage in the processing hierarchy relative to the VLPFC, serving to perform operations on the products of VLPFC processing.

Thus, it is clear that the strategic control of memory is multifaceted. Future research promises to further illuminate how cognitive control emerges through lateral PFC function, allowing us to strategically wrest control of our memories, bringing them in line with current goals.

See also: Cognition: An Overview of Neuroimaging Techniques; Event-Related Potentials (ERPs); Inhibitory Control over Action and Memory; Neuroimaging; Prefrontal Cortex: Structure and Anatomy; Prefrontal Cortex; Short Term and Working Memory; Spatial Cognition and Executive Function; Working Memory: Capacity Limitations.

Further Reading

Aron AR, Robbins TW, and Poldrack RA (2004) Inhibition and the right inferior frontal cortex. *Trends in Cognitive Sciences* 8: 170–177.

Badre D, Poldrack RA, Paré-Blagoev EJ, Insler RZ, and Wagner AD (2005) Dissociable controlled retrieval and generalized selection mechanisms in ventrolateral prefrontal cortex. *Neuron* 47: 907–918.

Badre D and Wagner AD (2005) Frontal lobe mechanisms that resolve proactive interference. *Cerebral Cortex* 15: 2003–2012.

Badre D and Wagner AD (2007) Left ventrolateral prefrontal cortex and the cognitive control of memory. *Neuropsychologia* 45(13): 2883–2901.

Dobbins IG and Wagner AD (2005) Domain-general and domain-sensitive prefrontal mechanisms for recollecting events and detecting novelty. *Cerebral Cortex* 15: 1768–1778.

Dolan RJ and Fletcher PC (1997) Dissociating prefrontal and hippocampal function in episodic memory encoding. *Nature* 388: 582–585.

Feredoes E, Tononi G, and Postle BR (2006) Direct evidence for a prefrontal contribution to the control of proactive interference in verbal working memory. *Proceedings of the National Academy of Sciences of the United States of America* 103: 19530–19534.

Gold BT, Balota DA, Jones SJ, Powell DK, Smith CD, and Anderson AH (2006) Dissociation of automatic and strategic lexical-semantics: Functional magnetic resonance imaging evidence for differing roles of multiple frontotemporal regions. *Journal of Neuroscience* 26: 6523–6532.

Gough PM, Nobre AC, and Devlin JT (2005) Dissociating linguistic processes in the left inferior frontal cortex with transcranial magnetic stimulation. *Journal of Neuroscience* 25: 8010–8016.

Henson RN, Shallice T, Josephs O, and Dolan RJ (2002) Functional magnetic resonance imaging of proactive interference during spoken cued recall. *Neuroimage* 17: 543–558.

Iversen SD and Mishkin M (1970) Perseverative interference in monkeys following selective lesions of the inferior prefrontal convexity. *Experimental Brain Research* 11: 376–386.

Jonides J, Smith EE, Marshuetz C, Koeppe RA, and Reuter-Lorenz PA (1998) Inhibition in verbal working memory revealed by brain activation. *Proceedings of the National Academy of Sciences of the United States of America* 95: 8410–8413.

Martin RC and Cheng Y (2006) Selection demands versus association strength in the verb generation task. *Psychonomic Bulletin & Review* 13: 396–401.

Moscovitch M and Melo B (1997) Strategic retrieval and the frontal lobes: Evidence from confabulation and amnesia. *Neuropsychologia* 35: 1017–1034.

Petrides M and Pandya DN (2002) Comparative cytoarchitectonic analysis of the human and the macaque ventrolateral prefrontal cortex and corticocortical connection patterns in the monkey. *European Journal of Neuoscience* 16: 291–310.

Shimamura AP (2000) The role of the prefrontal cortex in dynamic filtering. *Psychobiology* 28: 207–218.

Shimamura AP, Jurica PJ, Mangels JA, Gershberg FB, and Knight RT (1995) Susceptibility to memory interference effects following frontal lobe damage: findings from tests of paired-associate learning. *Journal of Cognitive Neuroscience* 7: 144–152.

Thompson-Schill SL, D'Esposito M, Aguirre GK, and Farah MJ (1997) Role of left inferior prefrontal cortex in retrieval of semantic knowledge: A reevaluation. *Proceedings of the National Academy of Sciences of the United States of America* 94: 14792–14797.

Thompson-Schill SL, Jonides J, Marshuetz C, et al. (2002) Effects of frontal lobe damage on interference effects in working memory. *Cognitive, Affective, & Behavioral Neuroscience* 2: 109–120.

Thompson-Schill SL, Swick D, Farah MJ, D'Esposito M, Kan IP, and Knight RT (1998) Verb generation in patients with focal frontal lesions: A neuropsychological test of neuroimaging findings. *Proceedings of the National Academy of Sciences of the United States of America* 95: 15855–15860.

Task Switching

D W Schneider and G D Logan, Vanderbilt University, Nashville, TN, USA

Introduction

Task switching is widely considered to be at the nexus of executive control in the human cognitive system. The ability to switch tasks is thought to require extensive high-level cognitive processing, ranging from instantiating abstract representations to preparing task-specific processes and monitoring response selection and execution. The behavioral outcome of this processing is a robust switch cost – slower and more error-prone performance when switching tasks than when repeating tasks.

Switch costs are frequently interpreted as reflecting the duration of time-consuming executive control processes that reconfigure the cognitive system when switching tasks, although this idea is debated in the behavioral literature on task switching. Some researchers have questioned whether switch costs are valid indices of executive control processes, whereas others have challenged the very notion that task switching involves executive control. There is abundant evidence indicating that basic psychological processes subserving attention, memory, and perception contribute to switch costs, compromising the interpretation of many behavioral effects as diagnostic evidence of executive control. Given that the cognitive architecture underlying switch costs and related effects is a matter of debate, it is important to exercise caution when interpreting proposed linkages between neural activity and specific cognitive processes putatively involved in task-switching performance.

With or without full appreciation of this point, many researchers have begun to explore the neural correlates of task switching. An increasing focus on identifying the neural substrates of various components of task-switching performance has produced a wealth of knowledge about task representation, selection, preparation, and switching. However, the quest to identify switch-specific neural mechanisms has proven to be challenging, with mounting evidence indicating that a distributed frontoparietal cortical network underlies task-switching performance.

Task Representation

To perform a task, it is necessary to have access to a representation of the associations between relevant stimuli and responses (i.e., task or stimulus–response mapping rules). A task representation can be considered part of a broader configuration of the cognitive system known as a task set, which includes task-specific processes that act on these representations. Many researchers propose that switching tasks requires reconfiguring the existing task set, in part to instantiate different task rules.

A brain area that is strongly implicated in task representation is prefrontal cortex (PFC). It has been proposed that PFC is involved in the acquisition, representation, and maintenance of abstract task rules for goal-directed behavior. These task rules are assumed to be extracted from past experience, in part through myriad connections to and from sensory and motor areas throughout the brain. The strongest evidence that PFC encodes task rules comes from single-cell recordings in monkeys performing different tasks. When monkeys are cued to adopt a specific task rule for responding to a stimulus, a substantial proportion of single neurons in PFC have been found to fire selectively for a given task rule. These neurons were considered rule selective because they fired after cue onset or during the delay period following the cue, regardless of the specific cue used to signal the task rule. Moreover, monkeys were able to generalize the rule to new, unseen stimuli. Such rule-selective neurons have been identified throughout dorsolateral, ventrolateral, and orbital PFC.

Task rule-selective neurons have also been found in parietal cortex. There is evidence that single neurons in the lateral bank of the intraparietal sulcus (IPS) and on the angular gyrus may encode task rules. These neurons had markedly increased firing approximately 400 ms after cue onset and fired regardless of the perceptual cues associated with each rule, suggesting that abstract task information (rather than the sensory features of the cues) had been encoded.

The evidence implicating prefrontal and parietal cortices in task representation suggests that these brain areas should be active when switching tasks, based on the proposal that task switching involves changing the existing task representation or task set. This suggestion is supported by several studies on task selection, preparation, and switching.

Task Selection, Preparation, and Switching

The primary goal in many task-switching situations is the selection and performance of a relevant task in the face of irrelevant, competing tasks. Task selection becomes crucial when stimuli are multivalent (i.e., associated with more than one task), creating ambiguity about which task to perform. Such ambiguity can be resolved by presenting a task cue prior to or in conjunction with the imperative stimulus, enabling researchers to investigate the neural underpinnings of how tasks are selected, prepared, or switched in advance or during task execution.

Much of our knowledge concerning task switching has come from studies involving event-related functional magnetic resonance imaging (fMRI), in which researchers measure changes in the blood oxygen level-dependent (BOLD) signal elicited by different types of trials. The basic analytical strategy has been to contrast task switches with task repetitions (or other baselines) to determine which brain areas are more 'active' (i.e., generate stronger BOLD signals) when switching tasks. Although there are potential problems with this strategy (discussed later), it has yielded a large body of knowledge about the neural basis of task switching.

Neural Correlates of Task Switching

As with task representation, there is evidence that PFC underlies task selection, preparation, and switching. There is a general consensus that PFC is involved in various activities related to executive control, such as selective attention, task management, goal maintenance, and the regulation of on-line processing involving the contents of working memory. Evidence suggesting that PFC is involved in goal maintenance in dual-task and task-switching situations has come from several fMRI studies. For example, dual-task performance that involves keeping a single goal in mind activates dorsolateral PFC (Brodmann area (BA) 9), whereas keeping a primary goal in mind while performing concurrent subgoals tends to activate dorsal frontopolar PFC (BA 10). Some researchers have proposed that goal activation in PFC may bias or configure processing in other brain areas to enable implementation of the relevant task set, implying top-down control over task processing. Direct evidence in support of this proposal comes from single-cell recordings in split-brain monkeys performing a cue–stimulus association task; activity in inferior temporal cortex related to task processing was found to be modulated by activity in PFC.

The notion that PFC is involved in selecting and maintaining goals in preparation for performing or switching tasks is the main conclusion from many studies. Bilateral dorsolateral PFC (BA 9/46) activation has been observed following different types of task cues in task switching, suggesting that cue-based selection of task goals is subserved by PFC. Evidence indicates that a similar type of cue-elicited task preparation may occur in an area at the junction of the inferior frontal sulcus and inferior precentral sulcus – the so-called inferior frontal junction (which includes parts of BA 6, 8, and 44). Activation in the inferior frontal junction is separate from that associated with cue encoding and is thought to reflect task management or the updating of task representations in preparation for task switching. However, activity associated with task-switching performance extends to other regions of PFC, such as frontopolar, ventrolateral, and medial PFC.

Regarding the medial surface of the frontal lobes, researchers have also focused on the role of anterior cingulate cortex (ACC; BA 24/32) in task-switching performance. ACC is thought to play an important role in resolving conflict situations and monitoring for errors; therefore, it is likely involved in task selection when stimuli are multivalent and there is a chance of performing the wrong task. In dual-task performance, ACC activation has been interpreted as reflecting response selection among competing alternatives. In task-switching performance, ACC activation has been observed when switching between Stroop color–word tasks, which are thought to require executive control processes to resolve stimulus-induced conflict (e.g., the word 'green' printed in the color red). Even in non-Stroop task-switching situations, ACC is sometimes active and tends to be accompanied by activity in dorsolateral PFC, especially when tasks occur unpredictably and stimulus onset is uncertain. This latter point has received some attention in studies on the effects of manipulating task predictability, either by contrasting fixed and randomized task orders or by comparing cues that either specify the upcoming task or only indicate whether to switch or repeat tasks. These studies have led to the emerging idea that PFC is organized along an anterior–posterior axis, with activation becoming more anterior as task performance requires more endogenous (i.e., internal) control.

Another anterior–posterior axis figures prominently in neuroimaging research on task switching, although this axis extends across the brain from prefrontal to parietal cortex. Consistent with some of the studies on task representation, there is evidence that areas of parietal cortex are highly active when switching tasks. One such area is the IPS (BA 39/40), which has been found to be more active for task-switching than dual-task performance. The IPS is more active when task order is unpredictable rather than predictable, although there is also evidence of its involvement in cue-elicited task preparation. Moreover, there is emerging evidence for possible functional dissociations in parietal cortex, with posterior areas being more active when switching between task-relevant dimensions, and anterior areas being more active when switching between stimulus–response mapping rules.

These activations in parietal cortex tend to be interpreted in relation to activations in PFC. As mentioned previously, PFC is thought to provide top-down control signals for coordinating neural activity in other brain areas. Some researchers have interpreted activation in PFC as reflecting the selection of task-relevant neural pathways or instantiation of the appropriate task representation, with concurrent activation in parietal cortex reflecting the organization or implementation of task-specific stimulus–response mapping rules. In other words, PFC is viewed as the source of preparatory signals for biasing activation in parietal cortex and other brain areas.

Although much of the neuroimaging literature tends to emphasize the involvement of the frontal and parietal cortices in task-switching performance, many other brain areas have been found to be more active when switching than when repeating tasks, such as the cerebellum and various regions in the temporal and occipital cortices. The consistency of these activations across studies is unclear, and functional interpretations of their roles in task switching are lacking, in part because researchers have been more captivated by the frontal and parietal cortices. An important avenue for future research on task switching will be to delve into these relatively unexplored brain areas to determine if and how they contribute to the broader network of neural activity underlying task-switching performance.

Rule Switching

Given that task switching is often thought to require changing task (or stimulus–response mapping) rules, it is useful to search for neural correlates of rule switching in related experimental paradigms. One such paradigm is the Wisconsin Card Sort Test (WCST), which was a precursor to some of the modern research on task switching. In the WCST, subjects are given a set of cards on which stimuli of varying number, color, and shape are printed. The task is to learn to sort the cards into piles related to a specific stimulus dimension (e.g., color), based on feedback from the experimenter. After many consecutive correct responses (indicating that the sorting rule has been learned), the relevant stimulus dimension is surreptitiously changed, and subjects have to discover the new sorting rule (e.g., shape). The process of adopting a new sorting rule is thought to require changing the existing task set; hence, the neural correlates of WCST performance should be similar to the neural correlates of task-switching performance.

There is abundant evidence implicating PFC in WCST performance. Early neuropsychological studies revealed that patients with lesions of dorsolateral PFC performed worse than control subjects. fMRI studies have examined different components of WCST performance within PFC. Activation of the posterior part of the bilateral inferior frontal sulci (BA 45/44) increases as the number of relevant sorting dimensions increases. The right anterodorsal part (BA 46) and bilateral posteroventral parts (BA 8/44) of PFC tend to be more active when a change in the task rule requires shifting attentional set (e.g., to a different stimulus dimension), but only the latter areas are activated when the task rule is merely reversed. Although these findings of bilateral activation in PFC indicate that both cerebral hemispheres are involved in WCST performance, evidence suggests that there is functional specialization, with regions of right lateral PFC activated in response to negative feedback (when the sorting rule changes) and regions of left lateral PFC activated when updating the existing task set. Collectively, these findings of PFC activation, as well as reports of parietal cortex activation, are consistent with the neuroimaging results of many task-switching studies, suggesting that the brain areas involved in WCST performance may overlap with those involved in task-switching performance. Indeed, this suggestion is supported by a meta-analysis of WCST and task-switching studies that revealed a common pattern of distributed frontoparietal cortex activation across these paradigms.

Task-Set Inhibition

The preceding review may convey the misconception that task switching is only about the activation of task representations or stimulus–response mapping rules, but it is important to consider some of the neuroimaging evidence for inhibition in task-switching performance. When switching between different tasks (denoted A, B, and C) across a series of trials, performance is slower on the third trial of an ABA task sequence than a CBA task sequence. This impairment in performance of a recently abandoned task has been attributed to task-set inhibition – the inhibition of a previously relevant (but now irrelevant) task set when performing a different task.

Studies have found evidence suggesting that task-set inhibition involves right PFC, consistent with findings associated with other types of inhibition. Contrasting ABA and CBA task sequences in fMRI work has revealed activation in right lateral PFC (BA 45, 9/46) as well as left inferior temporal cortex (BA 37) and occipital cortex (BA 19). However, these results have been interpreted as reflecting increased task-set engagement in response to inhibition rather than task-set inhibition *per se*. Further evidence for the involvement of right PFC in task-set inhibition comes from the finding that patients with focal lesions of right PFC exhibit no behavioral manifestation of task-set inhibition, unlike patients with lesions of left PFC and control subjects.

Correlations between Neuroimaging and Behavioral Data

If the various inferences about the roles of different brain areas in task switching are valid, then it should be possible to identify correlations between activations in specific regions and behavioral measures of task-switching performance. A positive correlation has been observed between activation of the left inferior frontal junction (as well as the presupplementary motor area) and the magnitude of a behavioral cuing effect (i.e., the decrease in response time with an increased cue–target interval), which has been interpreted as evidence of cue-elicited task preparation. When switching between Stroop color–word tasks, activation of left dorsolateral PFC is strongest for those subjects who exhibit the weakest behavioral effects related to conflict, suggesting a role for this brain area in task preparation, whereas activation of ACC is strongest for those subjects who exhibit the strongest conflict effects, suggesting a role for ACC in performance monitoring. A finding that is related to the aforementioned results concerns a region encompassing parts of the presupplementary motor area and ACC: as activity in this region increases, switch cost increases. This finding has been interpreted as evidence of neural activity increasing in parallel with the degree of interference at the time of task performance, consistent with the observation of increased switch costs with increased activity in task-irrelevant brain areas. However, there have been some reported failures to observe correlations between switch cost and neural activity, which may reflect the fact that multiple brain areas contribute to task-switching performance, a point discussed later.

Switch Specificity

Research on task representation, selection, preparation, and switching implicates an extensive frontoparietal cortical network and many other brain areas in task-switching performance. This distributed neural basis for task switching raises an important question that has motivated many neuroimaging studies: are there any brain areas that are specific to switching tasks? This multifaceted question can be approached from three angles: analytical, empirical, and conceptual.

The Analytical Angle

Identifying a switch-specific brain area in neuroimaging research usually requires contrasting task switch trials with appropriate baseline trials. A common baseline used in fMRI studies is the pattern of activation on task repetition trials, resulting in a task switch–task repetition contrast. When a specific brain area is reliably more active (i.e., generates a stronger BOLD signal) when switching tasks than when repeating tasks, this contrast will tend to be significant. Although some researchers have used this contrast to identify brain areas involved in task switching, an important point that is sometimes overlooked is that the contrast indexes relative, not absolute, activation across different types of trials. In other words, a specific brain area may be active on both task switch and task repetition trials but exhibit stronger activation on task switch trials, yielding a significant contrast. It is clearly inappropriate in this situation to claim that the brain area associated with the contrast is switch specific (i.e., it is only involved in switching tasks), and this problem extends to region-of-interest analyses that are based on the pattern of activation associated with task repetition trials.

This issue can be partially addressed through the use of multiple baselines. For example, some researchers have supplemented the task switch–task repetition contrast with a task repetition–fixation contrast in an effort to separate out those brain areas that are active on task repetition trials. There are two potential problems with this strategy. First, the processing required for nontask events such as fixation may differ substantially from that required for task repetition trials, obfuscating the interpretation of any brain areas that yield significant task repetition–fixation contrasts. Second, application of this strategy requires making the assumption that task switch trials not only include switch-specific processes but also all of the processes engaged on task repetition trials, which may not necessarily be the case. This second problem also applies to the use of other tasks (e.g., Stroop color–word tasks) and situations (e.g., dual-task performance) as comparison conditions for task switch trials. Although these tasks and situations may be comparable to task switching (in that they are thought to require executive control processing), the differences between complex tasks may complicate any inferences regarding switch-specific brain areas.

The Empirical Angle

Analytical issues aside, there is little empirical evidence of switch-specific brain areas. Through the use of multiple baselines, some researchers have found that the same brain areas are active on both task switch and task repetition trials, suggesting that task-switching performance is not restricted to a single brain area and that there is no brain area specifically involved in task switching. This suggestion is supported by contrasts of task-switching performance with other situations (e.g., dual-task performance), which have revealed activation of a common bilateral prefrontoparietal cortical network. Similar findings have emerged from integrative meta-analyses of Stroop and task-switching performance and different types of attention shifting (which included task switching and rule switching). For example, meta-analyses of attention-shifting studies have revealed substantial activation overlap in areas such as medial PFC, medial, superior, and inferior parietal cortex, and premotor cortex (as well as bilateral dorsolateral PFC and bilateral anterior insula, but to a lesser extent); these results have been interpreted as evidence that different types of attention shifting all depend on a similar set of working memory and executive control processes.

Some researchers have argued against the notion of switch-specific brain areas on the basis of other evidence. For example, the lack of a relationship between switch-related neural activity and behavioral measures of task-switching performance has been interpreted as evidence against a switch-specific neural mechanism. An electrophysiological study of changes in the electrical brain potential over frontal cortex, supplemented with fMRI data, did not yield any clear markers of task-switching performance. On a related note, there is evidence that changes in event-related electrical brain potentials following a single task switch trial can persist over a subsequent run of task repetition trials, suggesting that activity on task repetition trials may not be pure (in the sense of not reflecting task switching). A direct implication for fMRI studies of task switching – which typically involve measuring changes in cerebral blood flow over several seconds – is that task repetition trials may not represent an appropriate baseline for task switch trials in standard contrasts.

The Conceptual Angle

The lack of evidence for switch specificity is not surprising if one considers the broader conceptual issue of what is likely involved in task switching. In the behavioral literature, many component processes have been proposed to account for task-switching performance, and it is unlikely that all of these processes are exclusive to task switching or implemented in the same brain area. The idea that task switching requires the integration of various perceptual, attentional, mnemonic, and motor processes is supported by the abundant evidence implicating an extensive frontoparietal cortical network in task-switching performance and the conjecture that frontal areas integrate and coordinate information that is then transmitted to parietal areas for task-specific processing. For these reasons, it may be difficult to find robust correlations between switch cost and neural activity, and the search for switch-specific brain areas may be in vain. Indeed, some authors have argued that attempts to localize any complex cognitive processes in the brain may be misguided because such processes likely involve a distributed, interacting network of brain areas. If this is the case, then perhaps cognitive neuroscientists should focus their efforts on identifying and understanding the functional linkages between different brain areas involved in task-switching performance rather than seeking evidence of switch-specific neural mechanisms.

Conclusion

Despite the fact that the cognitive neuroscience of task switching is only approximately 7 years old, much progress has been made toward identifying the neural correlates of task-switching performance. Research on task representation, selection, preparation, and switching suggests that myriad brain areas – stretching from prefrontal to posterior parietal cortices – are involved in task switching. Although there has been interest in isolating switch-specific neural mechanisms, careful consideration from analytical, empirical, and conceptual angles suggests that no single brain area underlies performance. As researchers continue to delve into the multifaceted nature of task switching, a clearer picture of the intricate functional connections between brain areas will likely emerge, hopefully providing insight into the cognitive architecture of task switching and a window to the broader realm of executive control in human cognition.

See also: Attentional Networks in the Parietal Cortex; Cognition: An Overview of Neuroimaging Techniques; Executive Function and Higher-Order Cognition: Neuroimaging; Parietal Cortex and Spatial Attention; Prefrontal Cortex: Structure and Anatomy; Prefrontal Cortex.

Further Reading

Brass M and von Cramon DY (2004) Decomposing components of task preparation with functional magnetic resonance imaging. *Journal of Cognitive Neuroscience* 16: 609–620.

Buchsbaum BR, Greer S, Chang W-L, and Berman KF (2005) Meta-analysis of neuroimaging studies of the Wisconsin card-sorting task and component processes. *Human Brain Mapping* 25: 35–45.

Derrfuss J, Brass M, Neumann J, and von Cramon DY (2005) Involvement of the inferior frontal junction in cognitive control:

Meta-analyses of switching and Stroop studies. *Human Brain Mapping* 25: 22–34.

Dove A, Pollmann S, Schubert T, Wiggins CJ, and von Cramon DY (2000) Prefrontal cortex activation in task switching: An event-related fMRI study. *Cognitive Brain Research* 9: 103–109.

Dreher J-C, Koechlin E, Ali SO, and Grafman J (2002) The roles of timing and task order during task switching. *NeuroImage* 17: 95–109.

Kimberg DY, Aguirre GK, and D'Esposito M (2000) Modulation of task-related neural activity in task-switching: An fMRI study. *Cognitive Brain Research* 10: 189–196.

MacDonald AW, Cohen JD, Stenger VA, and Carter CS (2000) Dissociating the role of the dorsolateral prefrontal and anterior cingulate cortex in cognitive control. *Science* 288: 1835–1838.

Miller EK and Cohen JD (2001) An integrative theory of prefrontal cortex function. *Annual Review of Neuroscience* 24: 167–202.

Monsell S (2003) Task switching. *Trends in Cognitive Sciences* 7: 134–140.

Pollmann S, Dove A, von Cramon DY, and Wiggins CJ (2000) Event-related fMRI: Comparison of conditions with varying BOLD overlap. *Human Brain Mapping* 9: 26–37.

Rushworth MFS, Passingham RE, and Nobre AC (2002) Components of switching intentional set. *Journal of Cognitive Neuroscience* 14: 1139–1150.

Sohn M-H, Ursu S, Anderson JR, Stenger VA, and Carter CS (2000) The role of prefrontal cortex and posterior parietal cortex in task switching. *Proceedings of the National Academy of Sciences of the United States of America* 97: 13448–13453.

Stoet G and Snyder LH (2004) Single neurons in posterior parietal cortex of monkeys encode cognitive set. *Neuron* 42: 1003–1012.

Swainson R, Cunnington R, Jackson GM, et al. (2003) Cognitive control mechanisms revealed by ERP and fMRI: Evidence from repeated task-switching. *Journal of Cognitive Neuroscience* 15: 785–799.

Wager TD, Jonides J, and Reading S (2004) Neuroimaging studies of shifting attention: A meta-analysis. *NeuroImage* 22: 1679–1693.

Wallis JD, Anderson KC, and Miller EK (2001) Single neurons in prefrontal cortex encode abstract rules. *Nature* 411: 953–956.

Yeung N, Nystrom LE, Aronson JA, and Cohen JD (2006) Between-task competition and cognitive control in task switching. *Journal of Neuroscience* 26: 1429–1438.

Vestibular Influences on Cognition

F W Mast, University of Lausanne, Lausanne, Switzerland

Vestibular Areas in the Cortex

The vestibular system, long described as a sensory system, elicits reflexive eye movements such as the vestibuloocular reflex (VOR). The VOR helps us to keep our gaze fixed on a target while we move our head. Research interests have focused on the neuronal circuits underlying the VOR and computational models have been developed to describe the underlying neuronal network. The VOR has become a suitable paradigm to study how the brain implements a sensorimotor reflex; however, vestibular afferent pathways not only project to brain stem areas, which then elicit eye movements, but also reach other areas in the brain. These include the hippocampus (either directly or via thalamic nuclei) as well as cortical areas identified in primate studies to receive vestibular input (e.g., the area 2v at the tip of the intraparietal sulcus, area 3av in the central sulcus, area 7 in the inferior parietal lobule, and the parietoinsular cortex). More recently, measures of human brain activation by means of neuroimaging techniques (e.g., functional magnetic resonance imaging or positron emission tomography) during caloric stimulation of the semicircular canals or galvanic stimulation of the vestibular system have widely confirmed the existence of these vestibular-related areas. It is noteworthy that some cortical vestibular areas also project back to the vestibular nuclei.

The cortical vestibular areas are interesting because knowledge about them is a necessary prerequisite to explore the influence vestibular stimulation can have on cognitive functions. The relation between vestibular information and cognitive functions is twofold. First, we can study how vestibular information influences cognitive functions, and second, we can study how cognitive influences modify the perception of vestibular stimuli. Regarding the first point, it is particularly interesting to explore which cognitive tasks are affected by vestibular processing, and in what way. The second point studies how influences of cognitive origin can alter the perception of vestibular stimuli. These types of influences are often referred to as 'top-down' information, which can affect relatively early processes. Top-down processing has been studied intensively in many areas of visual perception, but there still is only scarce evidence for its role in the context of vestibular stimulation.

As already mentioned, neurophysiological evidence suggests that several cortical areas receive vestibular input (relevant for the first point), and there also are corticofugal projections from higher cortical areas to lower areas in the brain stem (relevant for the second point).

Influence of Body Tilt on Cognitive Tasks

It needs to be determined which cognitive functions are influenced by vestibular information, and which are not. It is at least conceivable that concomitant vestibular stimulation acts just like an additional task, which absorbs limited cognitive resources, which are then no longer available for the primary task. In this case, vestibular information would act in a rather unspecific way, and any type of cognitive function would be affected in nearly the same way. However, there is evidence that body tilt information from the otoliths has specific effects on cognitive functions.

Body Tilt Influences on Visual Perception Tasks

We first consider the example of orientation acuity, which illustrates how visual perception is influenced by body tilt. When upright persons have to judge the orientation of test stimuli (e.g., two subsequent sine wave gratings in a two-alternative forced-choice paradigm), the acuity estimates show clear meridional anisotropies; orientation acuity is higher for the principal upright and horizontal axes when compared to oblique axes. It was often tacitly assumed that orientation acuity is determined by the orientation of the test stimuli with respect to retinal coordinates. When the head was tilted sideways, however, the meridional variation interacted with head orientation. This finding contradicts an explanation based solely on retinotopically tuned neurons, which cannot explain the effect of head tilt. Similar influences of head tilt were found for other types of visual tasks ranging from visual illusions to visual search.

With perfectly upright observers, no effect of body tilt can possibly unfold, and only when tilted observers are tested can the retinal and gravitational reference frames be decoupled. Interestingly, single-cell recordings from monkey and cat studies further support the influence of body tilt information on early visual cortex. Even though the empirical evidence is still scarce, the findings demonstrate compellingly that orientation selectivity of neurons in early visual cortex is not defined exclusively in retinal coordinates, but rather follows the gravitational upright orientation.

These neurons are in the service of orientation constancy, which is the ability to perceive our environment as stable and upright despite the fact that head tilts inevitably influence how the world outside projects onto the retina. To compensate the potentially disturbing influence of head tilt, the brain uses the information from the otoliths, which signal the amount of head tilt. The otoliths are the primary sensory source of information about head tilt, even though a possible contribution of another gravity-receptive sensory system located in the trunk cannot be ruled out completely. In any case, retinal image shifts due to head tilts are compensated for, thus ensuring orientation constancy. How internal coordinate transformations of retinal coordinates can influence perception is strikingly illustrated by transient room-tilt illusions following central or peripheral vestibular disorders. Upright patients perceive the orientation of their visual environment as upside down or tilted by 90°. Room-tilt illusions are thus an example of what happens when the otherwise functioning visual–vestibular interaction is impaired.

These findings illustrate how performance in simple visual psychophysical tasks can change when the participants are no longer in a perfectly upright body position. In the following sections we shift the focus from the encoding of visual stimuli to information already stored in memory, and describe how higher cognitive functions can be modified by vestibular information.

Body Tilt Influences on Mental Imagery Tasks

What is the spatial frame of reference used by information already stored in memory? Do changes in body tilt influence how we perform mental operations? One of the most studied functions in cognitive psychology is mental imagery. It draws on the ability to generate, inspect, and transform images in our mind. An example of the latter is mental rotation, which is the ability to rotate images in one's mind. It is used when we see objects in an unusual orientation – for example, upside down. To still recognize the objects we need to match the image from the sensory input with a representation stored previously in memory. The more the objects are tilted away from their natural and upright orientation, the longer it takes for observers to respond (e.g., to name the object). It needs to be defined, however, what 'upright' means. Does upright refer to retinal coordinates (which is an egocentric frame of reference) or to a gravitational frame of reference (which is an allocentric frame of reference and therefore independent of the observer)? Again, in the upright body position it is impossible to decouple the two reference frames because they are fully aligned. Only when the observers are tilted can we draw conclusions about their relative influence.

Studies on mental rotation Empirical results have revealed an influence of body position – for example, with letterlike symbols as stimuli in a mental rotation task. Specifically, an observer's' performance was better when the stimuli were aligned with the gravitational vertical than with the retinal vertical. This implies that at least some representations are stored with respect to the gravitational vertical. More recently, the frame of reference has been studied in the context of face perception. Earlier research on face perception has shown that inversion of facial features such as mouth and eyes within an otherwise right-side-up face looks extremely grotesque (the face of a former British prime minister has been used in a well-known demonstration of this), but this grotesqueness disappears almost completely when the face is viewed upside-down (i.e., when picture is rotated by 180°). This phenomenon has been explained by a mental rotation process, which is simply overtaxed by keeping track of all configural information between facial parts when upside-down faces are rotated mentally. In the current context, it is of interest whether the perception of faces is determined by their orientation with respect to eye coordinates. If this were the only factor, changes in body position would not matter. After testing face perception in a variety of different body positions, it turned out that in a body position of 135° roll tilt (the head is between horizontal and upside down), it was more difficult to detect changes in the faces, whereas no such effect was present in the upside-down body position. This suggests that a gravitational frame of reference is involved in the perception of faces, even though the nature of the underlying mechanism is not resolved.

The subjective visual vertical The effect of head-down body positions has been investigated in other studies. For example, the subjective visual vertical shows largest errors in body tilt positions around 135°. Interestingly, not only the deviation from the physical vertical but also the variance reaches its maximum in positions around 120° and 150° roll tilt (whereas in the upside-down body position, 180°, there is much less variance and the errors are smaller). Therefore, the spatial reference information for the perception of the vertical is less reliable, and as a consequence, observers have difficulties in these positions in unambiguously judging the orientation of visual stimuli. In head-down positions around 135°, the deviation between the retinal up and the perceived gravitational is largest and exceeds more than 90° (this is also true for the upside-down body position but there the reference frames are again aligned, albeit in exactly opposite directions). It is noteworthy that observers sometimes report a paradoxical experience when they are in a head-down body position. Some observers tend to perceive two different but distinct verticals, rather than just an increased range of uncertainty.

It has been assumed that less precise sensory information from the otoliths is related to the lack of confidence about the direction of gravity in exactly these unusual body positions. In analogy to the blind spot on the retina, it has been hypothesized that there also is a body tilt stimulus for which there are many less utricular or saccular hair cells with the corresponding direction specificity. It is, however, not yet certain whether the psychophysical results reported in head-down positions can be explained entirely by the properties of receptor physiology. Nevertheless, situations which lead to ambiguous or insufficient perception make the use of cognitive influences more likely, and they may eventually help in resolving what the actual stimulus was.

Currently, there is compelling empirical evidence for the role of body tilt information on perceptual and cognitive tasks, but no theory has yet been proposed describing how these influences can unfold, and what the underlying neuronal mechanisms are. More experimentation is still needed, since many studies varied two body positions only (e.g., upright and lying on the side in the horizontal position), and this is not sufficient to reveal the function the body tilt influence follows. Also, the stimulus dimensions need to be explored more thoroughly – for example, the effect of gravity on the perception of natural scenes may even exceed the effect on faces, because – unlike faces – natural scenes always appear gravitationally upright.

Studies in microgravity Instead of tilting the observers, exposure to microgravity is yet another way to change vestibular information – in particular, the information from the otoliths about the direction of gravity. Astronauts, during long-term missions, experience microgravity onboard the spaceship during several days. A short-term exposure to microgravity for about 20 s can also be reached on Earth by means of parabolic flight protocols onboard an airplane. During microgravity, the astronauts can move freely inside the cabin and receive no sensory input that directly indicates the direction of the vertical. When the pull of gravity is absent, the resting discharge level becomes the only afferent signal from the otoliths. It has been suggested that perceptual consequences can unfold from asymmetries between the otolith discharge levels from the right and left inner ear, and this still is discussed in the context of space motion sickness, for which no clear predictive measure has yet been found. On Earth, however, the presence of gravity provides a strong enough stimulus to override these possible asymmetries.

Interesting in the context of microgravity are orientation illusions. Astronauts are able to voluntarily assign a spatial frame of reference to their environment. They can choose which wall inside the spaceship becomes the floor. On Earth, this is determined by the presence of gravity, and only in the horizontal plane do we sometimes get confused regarding our orientation within the environment (e.g., when ascending from a subway we often start walking in the wrong direction, not taking into account a turn we just made underground).

Still, much research is needed to better understand the effects of microgravity on cognitive functions, both in terms of short-term and long-term exposure. The latter is important because it also includes the effects of a possible adaptation to the new environment. To date, only few studies on cognitive functions have been carried out in microgravity, and some studies report no change when compared to performance on the ground. This finding is not so surprising because, unlike body tilts on Earth, microgravity does not induce any changes in the direction of gravity. Vestibular and visual cues are not in conflict and the observers rely on visual information, such as upright persons on the ground. It has to be noted that only few cognitive studies have been carried out in microgravity, and it would be premature to rule out a yet unexplored effect on other cognitive functions.

Influence of Whole Body Movement on Cognitive Tasks

The preceding findings were obtained under static conditions. The vestibular influence is thus of otolith origin, since any semicircular effects of prior head or whole-body movements dissipated by the time the measurements began. Measurements during whole-body rotation are much more difficult to obtain. For example, the VOR can interfere with the visual encoding of stimuli used for a cognitive study, and this may confound the interpretation of the results. Yet another difficulty is to define an appropriate control condition, in which the body remains stationary. The absence of any vestibular stimulation is easy to achieve but there are several other factors, which are just not controlled for when comparing the results from the same task during the experimental condition (with vestibular stimulation) and the control condition (body and head are still). Inevitably, body movement entails stimulation of other sensory systems, such as skin receptors during acceleration or deceleration of the body (e.g., when we feel pushed backward into the seat during an airplane's takeoff). Not only is it hard to isolate the vestibular system, but the body movement can be experienced just as generally more distracting or even discomforting and therefore can impair performance in the task. Yet another difficulty is of technical nature. Vestibular stimulation requires acceleration or deceleration as stimulus, and not movement at constant velocity, which is not based on any vestibular stimulation. For example, constant yaw rotation around the body longitudinal axis is no longer perceived when the eyes are closed; the person in this situation feels stationary as long as the head is not moved, which then likely results in cross-coupled acceleration stimulation. To sum up, it is not at all trivial to conduct research with clearly defined vestibular stimuli, and, in addition to this, it requires carefully designed tasks if one wishes to measure at the same time performance in a cognitive task.

Visual–Vestibular Interaction

Caloric and galvanic vestibular stimulations have become widely used techniques in vestibular research, and when combined with neuroimaging they have enabled researchers to explore the human brain areas during vestibular stimulation. They have the advantage that one can isolate the vestibular stimulation, and that they can be used while the body is stationary. They provide ways to produce the percept of body movement even though the body remains perfectly still.

Converging evidence based on several studies using different techniques points to a mutual inhibition between vestibular and visual stimulation. During vestibular stimulation the visual cortex is deactivated, and, likewise, during large-field visual stimulation the vestibular cortical areas are deactivated. Such a mutual inhibition serves the purpose of minimizing sensory conflicts. The deactivation of the visual cortex can help suppress inappropriate visual input during vestibular nystagmus.

Why is this mutually inhibitory interaction between visual and vestibular information relevant in the context of cognitive tasks? Independent research in cognitive neuroscience has provided a wealth of knowledge about the role of early visual cortex in visual mental imagery. When study participants have vividly imagined previously memorized images, several neuroimaging studies found early visual activation, in particular when the task required to picture details in images. During caloric stimulation this part of the brain is deactivated and hence it could be expected that imagery abilities are impaired. This was in fact the case, whereas a control task with knowledge-based questions (designed so that they have low imagery content) showed no change during caloric stimulation. This suggests that the influence caloric stimulation has on cognitive tasks is specific and does not generally distract attention.

The role of attentional demands on vestibular processing has also been studied, and the results show that monitoring of orientation is impaired when the level of disorientation is high enough. It has also been shown that cognitive tasks such as backward counting can impair accuracy in orientation tasks. This suggests that monitoring orientation using vestibular information requires mental effort and is therefore not entirely automatic.

Still, however, there is only scarce evidence about how vestibular information relates to cognitive tasks. To date, there is not yet a systematic approach to study cortical vestibular processes and to what extent these brain areas are shared with cognitive functions.

See also: Balance and Posture Control; Canal–Otolith Interactions; Gravitational Effects on Brain and Behavior; Motion Sickness; Nystagmus; Vestibular System; Vestibulo-Autonomic Responses; Visual–Vestibular Interactions.

Further Reading

Berthoz A (2000) *The Brain's Sense of Movement.* Cambridge, MA: Harvard University Press.

Buchanan-Smith HM and Heeley DW (1993) Anisotropic axes in orientation perception are not retinotopically mapped. *Perception* 22: 1389–1402.

Corballis MC, Nagourney BA, Shetzer LI, et al. (1978) Mental rotation under head tilt: Factors influencing the location of the subjective reference frame. *Perception & Psychophysics* 24: 263–273.

Dieterich M (2007) Functional brain imaging: A window into the visuo-vestibular systems. *Current Opinion in Neurobiology* 20: 12–18.

Gaunet F and Berthoz A (2000) Mental rotation for spatial environment recognition. *Cognitive Brain Research* 9: 91–102.

Kaptein RG and Van Gisbergen JA (2004) Interpretation of a discontinuity in the sense of verticality at large body tilt. *Journal of Neurophysiology* 91: 2205–2214.

Lobmaier JS and Mast FW (2007) The Thatcher illusion: Rotating the viewer instead of the picture. *Perception* 36: 537–546.

Mast F, Kosslyn SM, and Berthoz A (1999) Visual mental imagery interferes with allocentric orientation judgements. *Neuro Report* 10: 3549–3553.

Mast FW, Berthoz A, and Kosslyn SM (2001) Mental imagery of visual motion modifies the perception of roll vection stimulation. *Perception* 30: 945–957.

Mast FW, Ganis G, Christie S, et al. (2003) Four types of visual mental imagery processing in upright and tilted observers. *Cognitive Brain Research* 17: 238–247.

Mast FW, Merfeld DM, and Kosslyn SM (2006) Visual mental imagery during caloric vestibular stimulation. *Neuropsychologia* 44: 101–109.

Merfeld DM, Zupan L, and Peterka RJ (1999) Humans use internal models to estimate gravity and linear acceleration. *Nature* 398: 615–618.

Oman CM, Lichtenberg BK, Money KE, et al. (1986) M.I.T./ Canadian vestibular experiments on the Spacelab-1 mission: 4. Space motion sickness: Symptoms, stimuli, and predictability. *Experimental Brain Research* 64: 316–334.

Sauvan XM and Peterhans E (1999) Orientation constancy in neurons of monkey visual cortex. *Visual Cognition* 6: 43–54.

Vision: Mechanisms of Orientation, Direction and Depth

N J Priebe and D Ferster, Northwestern University, Evanston, IL, USA

Primary Visual Cortex

Primary visual cortex is the site of a remarkable transformation in the neural representation of the visual world. The afferent neurons of the retina and the primary visual thalamus, which relays the retinal signals to the primary visual cortex, have circularly symmetric receptive fields and respond to almost any stimulus, as long as the stimulus falls within a broad range of sizes. In sharp contrast, the neurons of primary visual cortex are exquisitely sensitive to several complex stimulus attributes, including orientation of a contour, direction of motion, size, and binocular disparity. In many cases, selectivity is absolute: cortical neurons will not respond at all unless the stimulus matches the neuron's preferences for each of these attributes.

Primary visual cortex has become a model system for neuronal processing by the circuitry of the cerebral cortex. Ultimately, we would like to understand how the higher cortical areas give rise to our recognition of sensory stimuli, decision making, and language comprehension. But, we barely have a way of defining what tasks are performed in these areas, let alone how they are performed. By comparison, the transformations performed by the primary visual cortex on its thalamic inputs – the extraction of orientation and direction information, for example – are complex enough to be interesting, but simple enough to be tractable. The neuronal mechanisms by which cortical receptive properties emerge have therefore become the subject of intense scrutiny and debate.

Orientation Tuning

The basic phenomenon of orientation selectivity is very simple and striking. As Hubel and Wiesel originally demonstrated in their Nobel Prize-winning work of 1962, when a bar or contrast edge is flashed in or moved across a cortical neuron's receptive field at the neuron's preferred orientation, the neuron responds vigorously with a barrage of action potentials. When the stimulus is presented within the same region of visual space but at the orthogonal orientation, the neuron, in most cases, does not respond at all. In cat visual cortex, a vast majority of neurons are orientation selective. In primate visual cortex, all neurons outside layer 4c (the thalamic recipient zone) are orientation selective. Different neurons have different preferred orientations, so that some subset of cortical neurons will respond to a stimulus of any orientation and position. The selectivity of each neuron is roughly Gaussian in shape. That is, a graph of response against stimulus orientation forms an approximately Gaussian-shaped curve, with a half-width at half-height in the range of 10–30°. For cells that give a nonzero response at the nonpreferred orientation, the Gaussian rides on top of an offset the size of the nonpreferred response.

Hubel and Wiesel also showed that orientation-selective cells can be divided into two distinct groups, labeled simple and complex. The receptive fields of simple cells are identified by the presence of two or three (or occasionally more) distinct subregions (or subfields) of their receptive fields. The subregions are defined on the basis of their response to flashing stimuli. ON subregions are defined by the responses evoked at the onset of a stimulus brighter than the background light, or the offset of a stimulus darker than background. OFF subregions are defined by the responses evoked by the onset of dark stimulus, or the offset of a bright stimulus. The subfields are elongated in the direction parallel to the preferred orientation of the cell and are positioned side by side, in the direction perpendicular to the preferred orientation (**Figure 1(a)**). They are also mutually antagonistic: a bright stimulus in an OFF region will diminish the response to a simultaneously presented bright stimulus in an ON region, and vice versa. Complex cells, by definition, lack these distinct subfields and instead respond to flashed stimuli more or less uniformly throughout the receptive field, either with ON responses, OFF responses, or both (**Figure 1(d)**). Since Hubel and Wiesel's first description of simple and complex cells, it has been shown quantitatively that they form two distinct populations, rather than the tails of a single population, when defined through the spike responses. When measured from their synaptic inputs, however, cortical cells form a continuum in which simple cells with highly segregated receptive field subregions lie at one end, and complex cells lie at the other. The transformation between synaptic input and spike output by spike threshold therefore helps to segregate simple and complex cells into distinct groups. In the cat, simple cells predominate in layers 4 and 6, the layers of the cortex that receive direct input from the visual thalamus (lateral geniculate nucleus, or LGN). Complex cells predominate in layers 2, 3, and 5, which predominantly receive input from other cortical cells instead of the LGN.

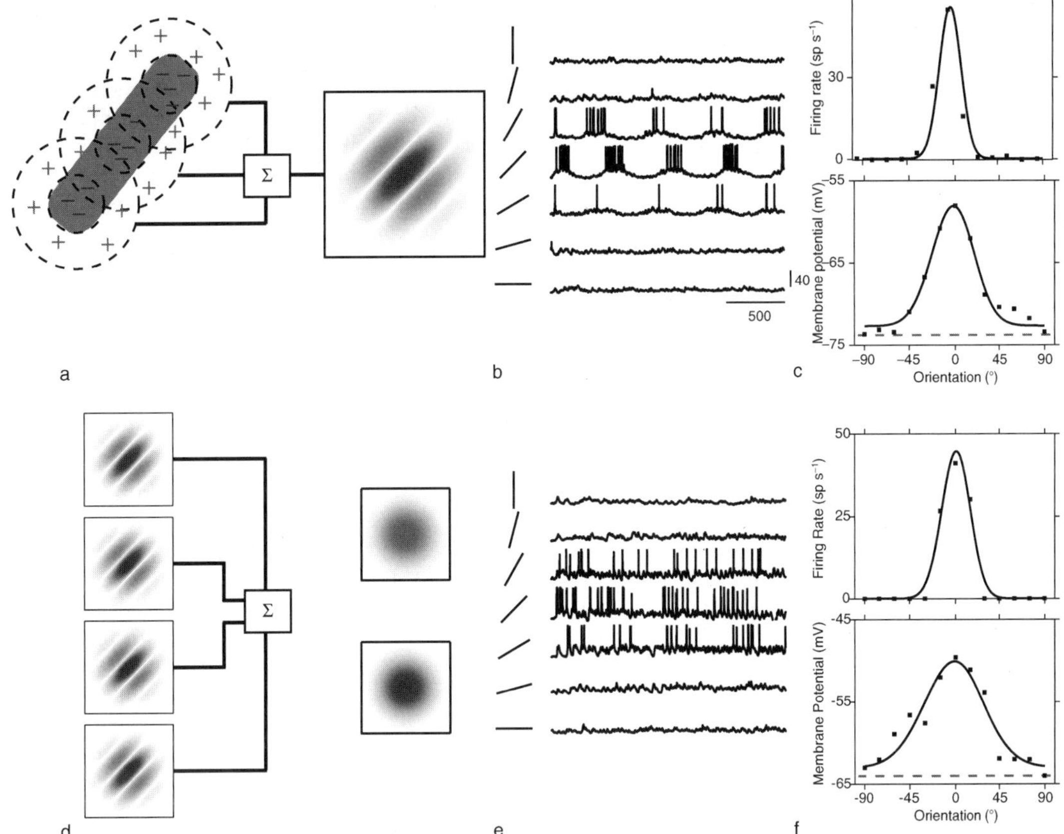

Figure 1 The emergence of orientation selectivity in primary visual cortex. The feed-forward model proposed by Hubel and Wiesel contains two stages, one that creates simple cell responses (top row) and a second that creates complex cell responses (bottom row). (a) In the first stage of the model, thalamic relay cells with circularly symmetric receptive fields converge on a simple cell. The spatial offsets of the relay cell receptive fields create the elongations observed in simple cell receptive fields. Blue indicates locations where a dark stimulus elicits a depolarization; red indicates locations where a light stimulus elicits a depolarization. (b) Elongated receptive fields then give simple cells the orientation selectivity observed in both the membrane potential and the spiking responses to drifting gratings, which elicit a modulated responses. (c) Orientation tuning is narrower for firing rate (top) than for membrane potential (bottom). Values plotted represent the peak (first Fourier component + mean) components of response. (d) In the second stage of the feed-forward model, multiple simple cells with similar orientation tuning but different spatial selectivity converge to create complex cell receptive fields. Complex cells respond to either a dark or a light stimulus placed in the receptive field, as long as the stimulus has the correct orientation. (e) Complex cells respond with a sustained depolarization to a drifting grating, but maintain orientation tuning. (f) Tuning curves for firing rate narrower than those for membrane potential.

Functional Architecture

At the same time that they first demonstrated orientation selectivity, Hubel and Wiesel also laid out what they termed the functional architecture of the cortex, or the way in which neurons with similar receptive field properties are physically arranged within the cortex. Specifically, they showed that all of the neurons in a cortical column – the cells arrayed vertically beneath one point on the cortical surface – have nearly identical preferred orientations. The columns preferring different orientations, in turn, arranged in an orderly fashion. Specifically, Hubel and Wiesel found that an electrode that is advanced in a direction perpendicular to the cortical surface encounters cells with the same preferred orientation. Conversely, as an electrode is advanced in a direction roughly tangential to the cortical surface, each cell encountered has a slightly different orientation from the previous cell. A large sequence of cells shows a smooth progression of orientation, with occasional jumps in orientation or reversals in the direction of the sequence (clockwise to counterclockwise, or vice versa). On average, a full range of orientations is covered by the neurons within a distance of about 1 mm of the cortical surface, which Hubel and Wiesel referred to as an orientation hypercolumn.

Subsequent to these observations from physiological experiments, the exact pattern or map of orientations within a hypercolumn was the subject of considerable theoretical and experimental work. The complete pattern of orientation columns was first revealed in detail by the advent of techniques for imaging neuronal activity *in vivo*. The images are based on almost imperceptible changes in the color of the cortical tissue that occur when active neurons take up oxygen, changing both the color of hemoglobin and the amount of blood flow in the local vasculature. The activity-evoked changes in reflectance of the cortical surface are less than 1/1000th of the total reflectance, but can be detected with an appropriate camera. Alternatively, the cortex can be stained with dyes that dissolve into the neuronal membranes and change their absorption as a function of the local electric field (voltage-sensitive dyes). Here again the optical signals are extremely small, but are much faster than the intrinsic, hemoglobin-based signals. Both types of imaging yield a map of orientations on the cortical surface, showing in both monkey and cat the formation of pinwheel structures, such that neurons lying within the vanes of the pinwheel each have a slightly different orientation preference (**Figure 2**). In a circular track around a single pinwheel, neurons of all preferred orientations would be found, arranged in order of orientation. Pinwheel centers are spaced at roughly 1 mm intervals across the cortical surface, and the vanes of adjacent pinwheels blend into one another. Note that at the centers of the pinwheels the vanes narrow down to essentially zero width, so that cells with very different orientation would lie very close to one another. The optical signals show relatively weak orientation tuning at the pinwheel centers, but because the techniques have spatial resolution somewhat larger than a single cortical cell, there are two possible explanations: the cells at the pinwheel centers could all have weak orientation preference, or the cells at the center could all be well-tuned for orientation but have different orientation preferences. Recent experiments with two-photon Ca^{2+} imaging *in vivo* have achieved single-cell resolution of neuronal activity, and indicate that cells within the pinwheel centers and cells outside the pinwheel are equally selective for orientation. The vanes of the pinwheels narrow, but are sharply defined down to the level of single cells, all the way into the centers.

Cortical Circuitry Underlying Orientation Selectivity

Nearly all discussions about the cortical circuitry underlying orientation selectivity begin with the simple and elegant model that Hubel and Wiesel proposed when they first described orientation selectivity. They noted that the ON and OFF subfields of simple cells are similar to the ON and OFF structures of LGN relay cell centers, which provide the main visual input to the cortex. Simple cell subfields, unlike the centers of relay cell receptive field, are elongated, however, which prompted Hubel and Wiesel to suggest that each simple cell's ON region is constructed from the input from a number of ON-center relay cells that have receptive fields aligned in a row. Similarly, the OFF subfield would be built from input from a set of OFF-center relay cells that have receptive fields overlapping the subregion. According to the model, orientation selectivity in the simple cell arises directly

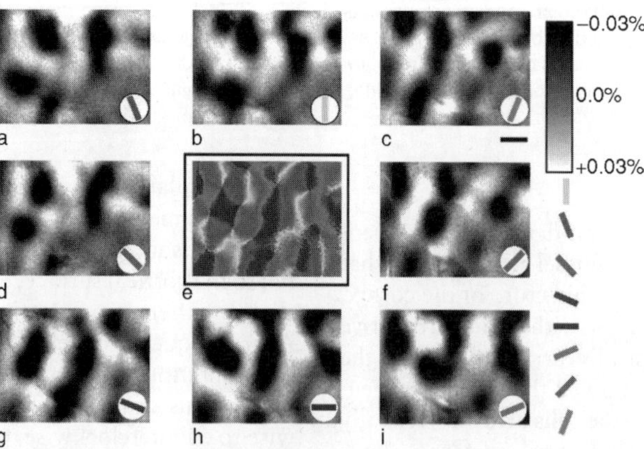

Figure 2 Orientation maps on the surface of primary visual cortex measured with optical imaging of intrinsic signals. Gray-scale images (a–d, f–i) show responses (through both eyes) to stimulation at the orientation indicated by the colored bar inset. Dark regions are areas of strong neuronal response. Angle map (e) shows preferred stimulus orientation (scale at right). Scale bar = 500 μm; medial, up; anterior, to the right. Reproduced from Crair MC, Ruthazer ES, Gillespie DC, and Stryker MP (1997) Ocular dominance peaks at pinwheel center singularities of the orientation map in cat visual cortex. *Journal of Neurophysiology* 77: 3381–3385, used with permission.

from the spatial arrangement of the receptive fields of the presynaptic relay cells (**Figure 1(a)**). When a stimulus is parallel to the subfields, it simultaneously encounters the receptive fields of all of the constituent relay cells. The relay cells therefore synchronously excite the simple cell, bringing it to threshold. Conversely, when a stimulus is perpendicular to the subfield, it can only excite a fraction of the presynaptic relay cells at one time. The stimulus therefore generates some asynchronous excitation in the simple cell, but the excitation is too weak to reach threshold. The spatial organization of the input therefore generates the initial orientation bias in the synaptic input to the simple cell, and spike threshold amplifies the bias into an absolute selectivity in the cell's spike output.

Hubel and Wiesel's model of the relay cell input to simple cells is most likely correct. Recordings from connected pairs of LGN relay cells and simple cells demonstrate that a relay cell makes excitatory contact with a simple cell only if the relay cell receptive field center overlaps the subfeild of the target simple cell with the same response polarity (ON or OFF). In addition, intracellular recordings from simple cells, even with the cortical circuit inactivated so that the only remaining inputs are from relay cells, show strong orientation selectivity. Few would dispute, then, that the spatial organization of the relay cell input generates an initial orientation bias in the input to cortical cells.

There has, however, been dispute over whether the spatial organization of the relay cell input is sufficient to explain all of the simple cell response properties. For example, in several experiments it has been observed that the spatial organization of the receptive field overestimates the width of orientation tuning. From Hubel and Wiesel's model, one would expect that the longer and narrower a cell's receptive field subregions are, the more sensitive the cell will be to orientation. With a long, narrow subfield, a small shift in orientation will create a large mismatch between the stimulus and the receptive field, and therefore strongly reduce the evoked response. In most cells, however, tuning is even narrower than expected.

One proposal for the origin of this narrowing is lateral inhibition in the orientation domain (also called cross-orientation inhibition), in which cells with different preferred orientations inhibit one another. Alternatively, cells with similar preferred orientations and different tuning widths could inhibit one another. Cross-orientation inhibition could also explain two other strongly nonlinear properties of cortical cells: cross-orientation suppression, in which the responses to stimuli of the preferred orientation are antagonized by superimposed stimuli of the orthogonal orientation, and contrast-invariance of orientation tuning, in which the width of orientation tuning does not change with the strength (contrast) of the stimulus. Even more suggestive is the observation that antagonists of γ-aminobutyric acid ($GABA_A$)-mediated inhibition degrades orientation tuning when applied to the cortex.

Despite these strong indications that lateral inhibition among cells with different orientation preference is critical for generating orientation selectivity, direct evidence of lateral inhibition has been hard to find. Many (though not all) intracellular recordings from simple cells show only modest inhibition evoked by stimuli of nonpreferred orientation. Recent work suggests, as an alternative to lateral inhibition, that nonlinear properties of the feed-forward pathway from the LGN to the cortex can account for most of the aforementioned properties of simple cells. Spike threshold, by way of the so-called iceberg effect, for example, can explain why simple cells have such narrow orientation tuning relative to what is predicted by their receptive field maps. In this view, the input from geniculate relay cells determines the aspect ratio of the subfields, and therefore the width of orientation tuning for the synaptic input to the simple cell. Because of the iceberg effect, these inputs are suprathreshold only for a narrow range of orientations near the preferred orientation. Thus, the orientation tuning for the spike output of the cell is much narrower than that predicted by the spatial organization of the receptive field. Similar arguments, based on nonlinearities such as contrast saturation and spike rectification in relay cells, or response variability in cortical cells, can, in turn, can account for cross-orientation suppression and contrast invariance of orientation tuning.

Direction Selectivity

In addition to being selective for orientation, many cortical cells are also selective for the direction of stimulus motion. For a large fraction of both simple and complex cells in primary visual cortex, response strength depends on stimulus direction, with direction being perpendicular to the preferred orientation. Some cells are completely directional and do not respond at all to stimuli of the nonpreferred direction. As with orientation selectivity, direction selectivity is mapped onto the surface of the cortex: within a single orientation column, neurons with different preferred directions are segregated into direction-specific subcolumns. Recent Ca^{2+} imaging of neuronal activity using two-photon laser scanning microscopy has shown that the borders between direction-specific regions of the cortex are extremely precise, with neurons on either side of a sharp border having opposite preferred directions. In primates, direction-selective neurons are also segregated by layers, tending to be located in the lower portion of layer 4 and in layer 6, which then project preferentially to extrastriate cortical areas in the dorsal processing stream.

Cortical Circuitry Underlying Direction Selectivity

As with orientation selectivity, direction selectivity is not represented in the relay cell input to primary visual cortex, and therefore must be computed within the cortex. Because motion in its essence requires a comparison over time and space (Where is the stimulus now? Where was it before?), computing direction requires that the responses of different inputs differ in both time and space. The origin of direction selectivity is still not fully understood, but in simple cells it clearly depends the heterogeneity of response timing within receptive field subregions. Specifically, it has been observed that in direction-selective cells, the latency of the response to a flashed stimulus differs by several tens of milliseconds between one side of the subfield and the other (along the axis perpendicular to the preferred orientation) (**Figure 3(a)**). The cell invariably prefers motion in the direction starting-from the long-latency regions of the receptive field and moving toward the short-latency region (**Figure 3 (b)**). When the stimulus moves in the nonpreferred direction, it encounters the short-latency part of the receptive field first, and the long-latency part later. The inputs from the two parts of the receptive field arrive at the cell at two different times, separated by the sum of the latency difference between the two regions and the time it takes the stimulus to travel from one region to the other. Conversely, when the stimulus moves in the preferred direction, it encounters the long-latency part of the receptive field first and the short-latency part later. If the stimulus travel time is approximately equal to the latency difference, then the inputs from the two parts of the receptive field will sum. The preferred stimulus therefore evokes a larger, though shorter-duration, input, compared to the nonpreferred stimulus.

This mechanism is strongly akin to orientation tuning, but with the orientation in the space–time domain rather than in the purely spatial domain. That is, a two-dimensional (2-D) plot of response latency against stimulus position is tilted for direction-selective cells (those without a gradient of latency across the receptive field), and is vertical for non-direction-selective cells (those with a gradient). Only stimuli with the correct spatiotemporal tilt (which move in the preferred direction) will evoke responses.

Although the preferred direction of motion is well predicted by the tilt of the spatiotemporal receptive field, the degree of selectivity in simple cells is often much greater than that predicted by the spatiotemporal receptive field map, much the same way that the spatial receptive field map underestimates the degree of orientation tuning. And similar to orientation tuning, one proposed explanation is lateral inhibition, in this case in the direction domain, such that direction-selective cells of opposite preferred direction inhibit one another. Once again, however, intracellular recordings from simple cells show little evidence for lateral inhibition. Excitation and inhibition in most cells share the same preferred direction. The apparent mismatch between the predictions of the spatiotemporal maps and recorded direction selectivity can be explained by the nonlinearity inherent in spike threshold. Because spike threshold disproportionately suppresses smaller synaptic inputs relative to larger ones, the direction selectivity of the spike output of cells is much larger than the direction selectivity of their synaptic inputs (**Figure 3(c)**).

The origin of the difference in response latency between different synaptic inputs is not known. Different relay cells could have different visual latencies (e.g., lagged and nonlagged relay cells), or long- and short-latency inputs could originate in different regions (such as the LGN and cortex).

The Aperture Problem

The processing of motion information at the level of primary visual cortex is incomplete. Neurons in primary visual cortex respond to the retinal image through a small aperture, defined by their receptive fields. They are only sensitive to the component of motion perpendicular to their preferred orientation within that restricted area. A cortical cell, then, cannot detect the difference between an optimally oriented stimulus moving in the preferred direction and an indentical stimulus moving at a different angle but higher speed (**Figure 4**). As long as the stimuli are much longer than the receptive field, such that their ends do not cross the receptive field, the stimuli appear identical to the cell and evoke the same response. Disambiguating such stimuli can only occur by integrating information from across the visual field and assembling the small components of the image into larger patterns. For motion, the extrastriate cortical medial temporal (MT) area is thought to be critical to this process.

Disparity Tuning

Information from the right and left eyes converges onto single cells for the first time in primary visual cortex. Throughout the cortex the balance of input from the two eyes (ocular dominance) covers the full

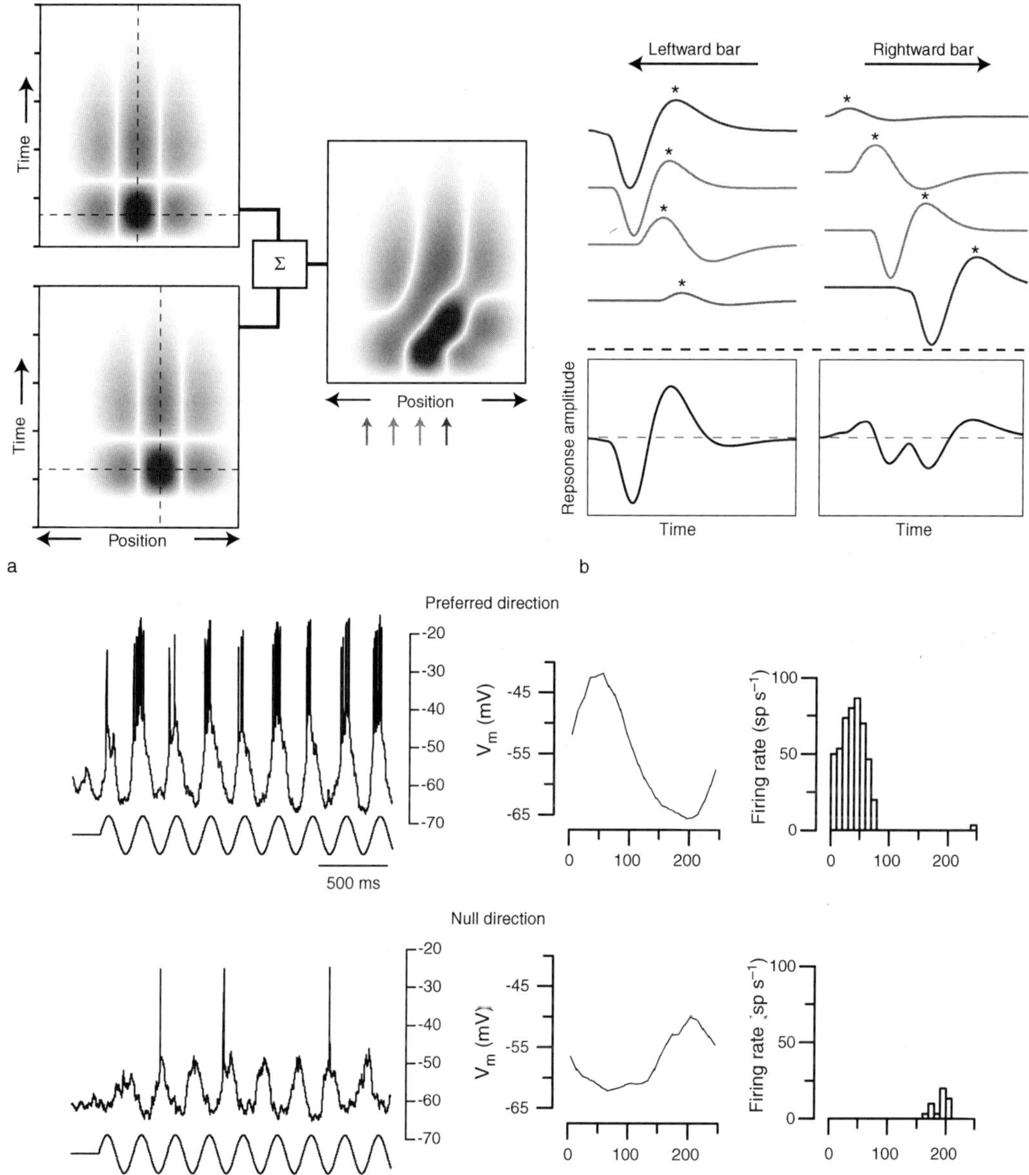

Figure 3 The emergence of direction selectivity in primary visual cortex. (a) Direction selectivity in primary visual cortex emerges due to the convergence of nondirectional responses that differ in both spatial preference and response timing (compare the latency and spatial preference of the two input neurons). The resulting spatiotemporal receptive field is tilted in space and time, a hallmark of direction-selective simple cells. Blue indicates an increase in response to a dark stimulus; red indicates an increase in response to a light stimulus. (b) Tilt in the spatiotemporal receptive field creates direction-selective responses to bars drifting across the receptive field. As a moving bar is sequentially flashed across the receptive field, a response is evoked at location (colored traces, locations indicated by the arrows in (a). For a leftward bar, moving from the purple arrow toward the red arrow, the response peaks at each location synchronously (indicated by the asterisk for each trace). The synchronous responses sum to create a large response to the leftward bar (bottom trace). The peak responses to a rightward bar are asynchronous and the summed response is therefore small. (c) Direction selectivity observed in cortical simple cells is evident both in the membrane potential and in spiking responses. The direction selectivity measured from membrane potential is modest relative to the selectivity observed in firing rate: direction index $= (R_p - R_n)/(R_p + R_n)$, where R_p and R_n are the responses in the preferred and nonpreferred (null) directions; for this example neuron, membrane potential $= 0.36$; firing rate $= 0.80$.

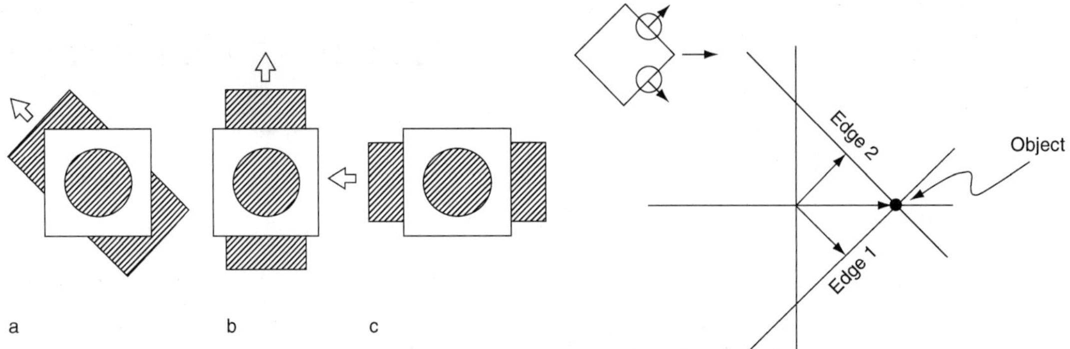

Figure 4 The aperture problem. (a–c) The direction of a drifting grating, moving behind the aperture, is ambiguous. All three conditions have the same apparent motion within the aperture. When information from multiple cells with different orientation preferences is available, the correct direction and speed of a moving diamond can be computed (right panel). By converting the motion components into velocity space (where direction is indicated by angle, and speed is indicated by vector length), each edge gives rise to a family of possible motions (indicated by the line orthogonal to each edge velocity vector). The intersection of these two lines indicates the correct solution to the object's velocity. Reproduced from Adelson EH and Movshon JA (1983) The perception of coherent motion in two-dimensional patterns. *Proceedings of the ACM SIGGRAPH/SIGART Interdisciplinary Workshop on Motion Representation and Perception*, pp. 11–16. © 1983 ACM, Inc. Reprinted by Permission.

range, with some cells receiving excitatory input only from one eye, some receiving predominant but not exclusive input from one eye, and others receiving equal input from the two eyes. Like orientation, ocular dominance is organized into columns, in this case alternating bands of about 0.5 mm thickness, with completely monocular cells near the center of the bands and more binocular cells near the edges.

In most cases, the receptive field of a binocular cortical cell mapped through one eye is identical in all respects to the field mapped through the other eye. Orientation and direction preference are the same, as are receptive field type (simple or complex), size, and position, even if the strength of the responses is different for the two eyes. By position, here, we refer to the relative positions of the receptive fields in the two retinas. That is, the receptive fields are located at the same direction and distance relative to the point of central vision (fovea in primates, area centralis in cats). Thus, the receptive fields are located at correspondent points in the retina, such that images falling on those points would appear to originate from the same point in visual space.

Of course, the images generated by many objects do not fall on correspondent points of the retina, specifically those objects that lie in front of or behind the plane of fixation. As one can easily demonstrate for oneself, for an object in front of the fixation plane the image in the left eye appears to lie to the right of the image in the right eye (and vice versa for objects beyond the fixation plane) (**Figure** 5). This depth-dependent lateral displacement of the two retinal images of an object is called binocular disparity and forms the basis for binocular depth vision.

Many neurons in the primary visual cortex are highly sensitive to binocular disparity. Tuned excitatory cells respond to stimulation in either eye, and tend to respond most strongly to simultaneous stimulation of correspondent points on the retinas – that is retinal disparities at or near 0°. Tuned inhibitory cells respond most weakly at 0 disparity and respond more strongly at disparities on either side of 0. Near cells respond only to crossed disparities, which are generated by objects closer than the fixation plane; far cells respond to uncrossed disparities.

Although their function is still under debate, together, these different types of cells could encode enough information to support depth perception. It has been noted that since the eyes are separated laterally, only horizontal disparities are generated by stimuli out of the fixation plane. If disparity-sensitive cells in the visual cortex feed into the circuitry for depth perception, the reasoning goes, they would be preferentially sensitive to horizontal disparities. Data on this point are equivocal, however.

Much like the aperture problem for direction selectivity, accurately reconstructing the three-dimensional visual world from the signals provided by disparity-sensitive cells presents a formidable computational problem. At the heart of the problem lies the existence of a large number of what are called false stereo matches in the two retinal images, also referred to as the stereo correspondence problem. When looking at a repeating pattern, such as a picket fence, for example, the brain must decide which slats of the fence in the right eye's image match with the slats in the left eye. If the slats lie in the plane of fixation and are spaced at 0.25° intervals, then

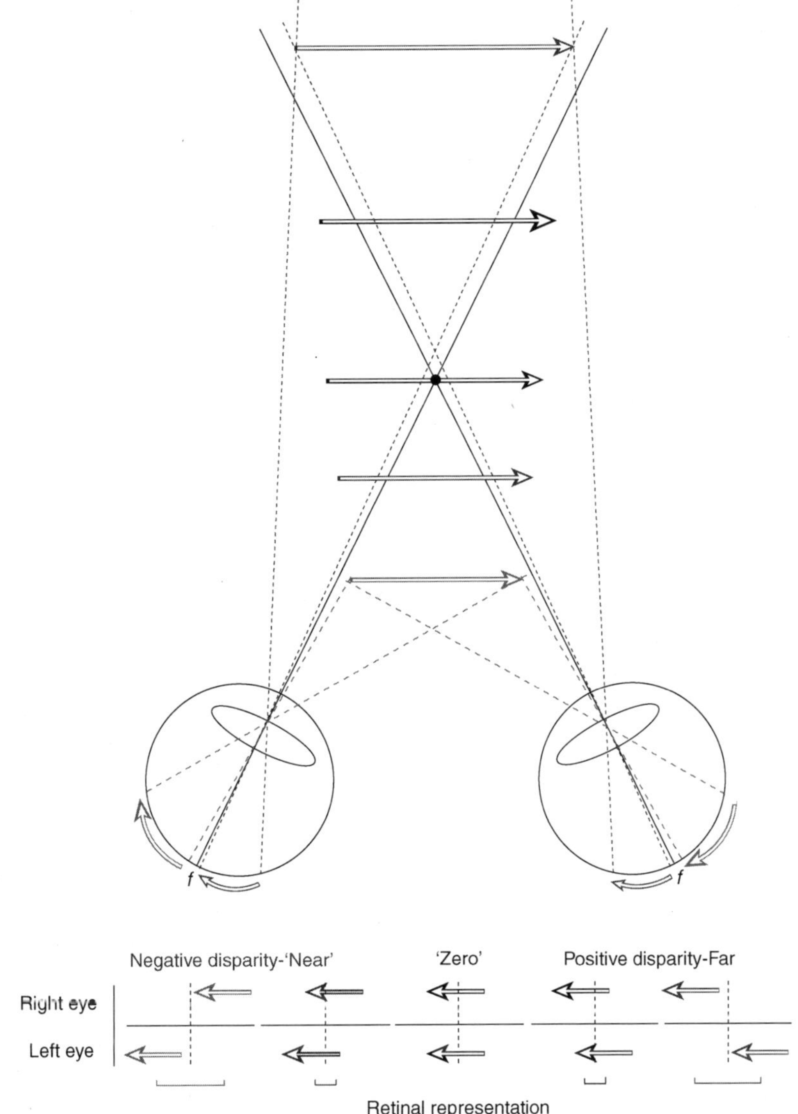

Figure 5 Retinal disparity. The retinal representations of objects at different depths differ in relative position between the right and left eyes. The red and blue arrows are placed at near and far depths, respectively, and their representations occupy different portions of the retinal representations. The retinal images for the red arrow fall on the temporal portion of the retinas, while the blue arrow images lie on the nasal retinas.

disparity-tuned cells that prefer 0°, ±0.25°, ±0.5°, and so forth will all be active. The ±0.25° cells, however, will be falsely matching a slat in one eye, and the adjacent one in the other eye. Only the 0° cells are responding correctly in the sense that a real object exists in the fixation plane. There are number of models as to how the brain suppresses false matches and arrives at a reasonably accurate perception of the three-dimensional stimulus. If the disparity-sensitive cells of primary visual cortex contribute to this process, however, their raw responses to disparity matches are likely further processed in higher cortical areas, such as visual areas V2, MT, and beyond.

Conclusion

The discovery of the response selectivity of cortical neurons by David Hubel and Torsten Wiesel in the early 1960s has raised a variety of questions, all of which have received considerable attention. How does the cortical circuit extract information about orientation, direction, and size from the nonselective signals coming from the retina and thalamus? Why is the visual image parsed into these particular parameters? What advantages do orientation and direction selectivity confer on the animal, and how do they facilitate object detection and recognition at higher cortical levels? How does the circuitry of the cortex develop, and does development require visual experience?

See also: Information Coding; Neural Synchrony and Feature Binding; Perception of Surfaces and Forms; Representation of Movement; Shape Representation in Inferotemporal Cortex; Stereoscopic Vision; Visual Cortex: Mapping of Functional Architecture Using Optical Imaging; Visual System: Multiple Visual Areas in Monkeys; Visual Attention.

Further Reading

Adelson EH and Movshon JA (1983) The perception of coherent motion in two-dimensional patterns. *Proceedings of the ACM SIGGRAPH/SIGART Interdisciplinary Workshop on Motion Representation and Perception*, pp. 11–16.

Anderson JS, Carandini M, and Ferster D (2000) Orientation tuning of input conductance, excitation, and inhibition in cat primary visual cortex. *Journal of Neurophysiology* 84: 909–926.

Anzai A, Ohzawa I, and Freeman RD (1999) Neural mechanisms for encoding binocular disparity: Receptive field position versus phase. *Journal of Neurophysiology* 82: 874–890.

Crair MC, Ruthazer ES, Gillespie DC, and Stryker MP (1997) Ocular dominance peaks at pinwheel center singularities of the orientation map in cat visual cortex. *Journal of Neuroscience* 77: 3381–3385.

Cumming BG and DeAngelis GC (2001) The physiology of stereopsis. *Annual Review of Neuroscience* 24: 203–238.

Finn IM, Priebe NJ, and Ferster D (2007) The emergence of contrast-invariant orientation tuning in simple cells of the cat visual cortex. *Neuron* 54: 137–152.

Gardner JL, Anzai A, Ohzawa I, et al. (1999) Linear and nonlinear contributions to orientation tuning of simple cells in the cat's striate cortex. *Visual Neuroscience* 16: 1115–1121.

Hubel DH and Wiesel TN (1962) Receptive fields, binocular interaction and functional architecture in the cat's visual cortex. *Journal of Physiology (London)* 160: 106–154.

Hubel DH and Wiesel TN (1977) Functional architecture of macaque visual cortex. *Proceedings of the Royal Society of London, Series B* 198: 1–59.

Hubener M, Shoham D, Grinvald A, et al. (1997) Spatial relationships among three columnar systems in cat area 17. *Journal of Neuroscience* 17: 9270–9284.

Marr D (1982) *Vision: A Computational Investigation into the Human Representation and Processing of Visual Information.* San Francisco: W.H. Freeman and Company.

Martinez LM, Wang Q, Reid RC, et al. (2005) Receptive field structure varies with layer in the primary visual cortex. *Nature Neuroscience* 8: 372–379.

Monier C, Chavane F, Baudot P, et al. (2003) Orientation and direction selectivity of synaptic inputs in visual cortical neurons: A diversity of combinations produces spike tuning. *Neuron* 37: 663–680.

Movshon JA, Adelson EH, Gizzi MS, et al. (1986) The analysis of moving visual patterns. *Experimental Brain Research* 11: 117–151.

Movshon JA and Newsome WT (1996) Visual response properties of striate cortical neurons projecting to area MT in macaque monkeys. *Journal of Neuroscience* 16: 7733–7741.

Ohki K, Chung S, Kara P, et al. (2006) Highly ordered arrangement of single neurons in orientation pinwheels. *Nature* 442: 925–928.

Poggio GF and Fischer B (1977) Binocular interaction and depth sensitivity in striate and prestriate cortex of behaving rhesus monkey. *Journal of Neurophysiology* 40: 1392–1405.

Priebe NJ and Ferster D (2005) Direction selectivity of excitation and inhibition in simple cells of the cat primary visual cortex. *Neuron* 45: 133–145.

Priebe NJ and Ferster D (2006) Mechanisms underlying cross-orientation suppression in cat visual cortex. *Nature Neuroscience* 9: 552–561.

Reid RC, Soodak RE, et al. (1991) Directional selectivity and spatiotemporal structure of receptive fields of simple cells in cat striate cortex. *Journal of Neurophysiology* 66: 505–529.

Sillito AM (1975) The contribution of inhibitory mechanisms to the receptive field properties of neurones in the striate cortex of the cat. *Journal of Physiology (London)* 250: 305–329.

Somers DC, Nelson SB, and Shapley RM (1995) An emergent model of orientation selectivity in cat visual cortical simple cells. *Journal of Neuroscience* 15(8): 5448–5465.

Visual Attention

S Treue, German Primate Center, Goettingen, Germany
S Katzner, Smith–Kettlewell Eye Research Institute, San Francisco, CA, USA

The visual system of humans and other primates is an evolutionary success story. It has developed an elaborate peripheral sensor system, the retina, in which the information picked up by more than 100 million receptors is compressed in a highly efficient manner and sent to the central nervous system by 1.5 million axons leaving the eyes. The complexity and level of sophistication of the retina is matched by a dedicated cortical processing hierarchy that encompasses more than 30 anatomically and/or functionally distinct areas covering approximately 50% of cerebral cortex in macaques and 20–30% in humans.

Although such a system picks up a plethora of information, even the highly developed visual cortex of primates would not be sufficient to process it all optimally and equally. Essentially, two interacting systems have evolved to counteract this limitation. A bottom-up system substantially compresses the information picked up by the retinal photoreceptors, and a top-down system dynamically allocates central processing resources for the visual information deemed most relevant in the current situation. The latter system, selective attention, is the focus of this article, but the two systems work hand-in-hand to provide an organism with the information most likely to be of relevance for its survival.

This article concentrates on our understanding of the neural basis of visual attention, emphasizing the most direct methodological approaches, namely single cell recordings from the visual cortex of behaving monkeys and, to a lesser degree, brain imaging measurements in human subjects. The central task for studies aimed at elucidating the neural correlates of attention is to evaluate linking hypotheses – that is, proposals of how the activity of neurons (in visual cortex or elsewhere) could account for the features and perceptual consequences of visual attention. More directly, such studies need to document effects that show the three characteristic features of attention that have been established in psychophysical studies: (1) attention selects relevant information – that is, some sensory signals receive preferential treatment; (2) the processing of selected and unselected information is differentially modulated – that is, attention changes how sensory information is processed; and (3) this selective modulation has perceptual consequences – that is, it changes the weighting or salience of different aspects of the visual environment as a function of their behavioral relevance, creating a representation that enhances some aspects at the expense of others. These three aspects serve as a framework for this article.

Selectivity

Spatial Attention

Directing attention into versus out of the receptive field Early attention research demonstrated that visual attention can be directed to selected locations in the visual field, even covertly (i.e., in the absence of eye movements). Behavioral measurements have shown that stimuli at attended locations are processed faster and more accurate compared to stimuli at unattended locations. Modern imaging studies of attention have measured brain activity during spatial attention tasks and have documented an enhanced activity in retinotopic cortical areas representing the location of the focus of attention.

This spatial allocation of attention has often been likened to a spotlight, suggesting as a neural correlate an enhanced response of a sensory cell and an increased synchrony in the activity of cell populations when spatial attention overlaps a neuron's receptive field. Indeed, studies report modulated responses when attention is directed into the receptive field of neurons from almost every area in visual cortex tested. However, an attentional mechanism that would modulate responses solely depending on whether the 'attentional spotlight' is inside versus outside the receptive field would have very poor spatial resolution beyond striate cortex as receptive fields grow with increasing levels of hierarchy in visual cortex, covering large portions of the visual field in higher areas. Instead, our visual system seems to be able to allocate spatial attention at a finer spatial scale than implied by the large receptive fields in higher areas of visual cortex.

Differential attentional effects inside the receptive field To examine the resolution of the neural mechanisms of spatial attention, several studies have trained monkeys to direct their attention to one of two stimuli inside the receptive field. In most of these studies, one stimulus was matched to the sensory preferences of a cell, whereas the other was not. Responses are generally substantially higher in trials in which the animals are attending to the preferred stimulus. Thus, attention can modulate responses even when it is only switched between two stimuli that are both inside the receptive field, demonstrating that attentional modulation has a better spatial resolution than the size of the receptive fields in these areas (**Figure 1**).

For middle temporal area (MT) neurons the neuronal correlate of the attentional selection of one of two stimuli inside a receptive field has been investigated by carefully mapping the receptive fields while the animal was directing its spatial attention to one of the two stimuli inside the receptive field. Under these conditions, the center of the receptive field shifts toward the attended location with a concomitant slight decrease in receptive field size (**Figure 2**). A similar distortion of receptive field profiles has been observed in area V4 when spatial attention is directed to various positions just outside the receptive field.

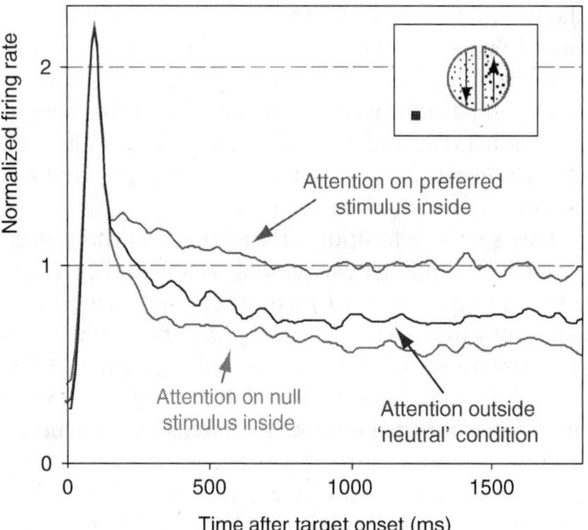

Figure 1 Effect of directing attention to either of two moving stimuli presented inside the receptive field of direction-selective neurons in macaque visual cortex. The inset illustrates the experimental conditions. Two stationary, semicircular apertures containing moving random dots are presented inside the receptive field. One of the dot fields is moving in the preferred direction (red semicircle; upward motion in this example) the other one in the null direction (green semicircle) of the neuron under study. At the beginning of each trial, the animal was instructed to covertly direct attention either to one of the two dot fields or to the fixation point (blue square) while maintaining its gaze on the fixation point. The curves represent firing rates, normalized to the level of sustained activity with attention on the preferred direction semicircle, and averaged across a population of neurons from the middle temporal and the medial superior temporal area. The *x*-axis represents time, with time zero indicating the onset of the visual stimulus. As can be seen, attending to the preferred direction stimulus inside the receptive field increases firing rates (red trace) compared to a condition in which attention is directed to the luminance of the fixation point (blue trace). In contrast, attending to the null-direction stimulus inside the receptive field reduces firing rates (green trace) relative to the fixation point condition. Modified from Treue S (2001) Neural correlates of attention in primate visual cortex. *Trends in Neurosciences* 24(5): 295–300, with permission.

As a consequence of such receptive field shifts, more neuronal processing resources are devoted to attended stimuli. Assuming that neuronal responses provide evidence of the presence of a stimulus at their original receptive field locations, attentional shifts of receptive fields could be the basis of the perceptual overestimation of an attended stimulus' size observed psychophysically.

Although the consequence of the observed shifts in receptive fields is fine-grained changes in visual information processing caused by spatial attention, it should be emphasized that the observed modulation need not be created in the large receptive fields in extrastriate cortex where it has been observed but, rather, could be the consequence of effects on the matrix of small receptive fields in area V1 that together form the large receptive fields in higher areas.

Attention can suppress responses The response modulations that are demonstrated when switching attention from outside to inside the receptive field suggest that directing attention into the receptive field always enhances responses. To investigate this conjecture, a 'neutral' or 'sensory' condition can be used in which attention is directed outside the receptive field, with two (behaviorally irrelevant) stimuli inside the receptive field. Usually, one of the two stimuli is matched to the neuron's preference (e.g., aligned to the preferred orientation), whereas the other is a nonpreferred stimulus. In such a paradigm, the response of the neuron is increased when directing attention toward the preferred stimulus inside the receptive field. However, the response of the neuron will usually drop below the neutral response when attention is directed to the nonpreferred stimulus. Switching attention between two stimuli inside the receptive field combines the suppressive effect of attending to the nonpreferred stimulus with the enhancing effect of attending to the preferred stimulus (**Figure 1**). This push–pull interaction may be one of the reasons why the attentional modulation is typically stronger in experimental paradigms that juxtapose two stimuli inside the receptive field. As a consequence of such attentional effects, the neural representation of attended stimuli is enhanced at the expense of unattended stimuli.

Nonspatial Attention

Feature-based attention The spotlight metaphor suggests a special role for spatial location as the basis for attentional selection, but several studies have demonstrated nonspatial, feature-based attentional modulation as well. Responses in inferior temporal cortex are enhanced, even before the onset of the preferred shape of a neuron, if its appearance was

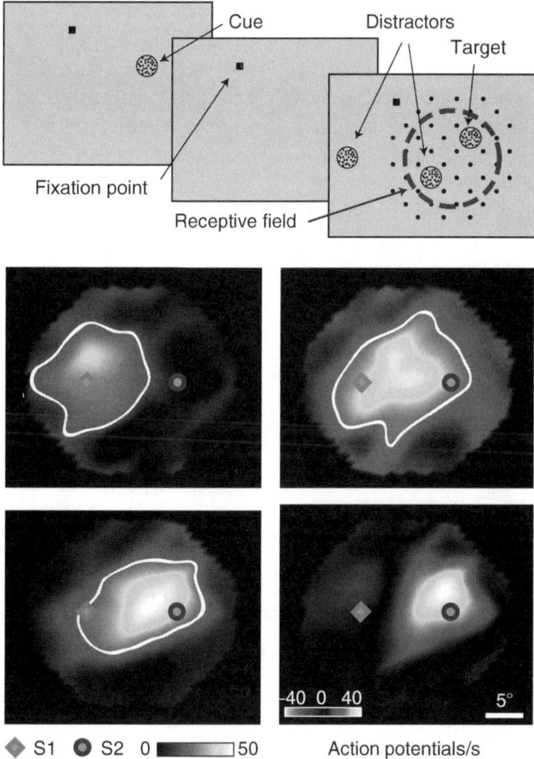

Figure 2 Modulation of receptive field structure by spatial attention. The gray panels at the top represent a computer monitor and illustrate the sequence of events in a single trial of the experiment. After the monkey fixates the small black square, a cue is briefly presented indicating the spatial location of one stimulus (target) that will appear together with two others (distractors). After the cue disappears, three stationary apertures containing moving random dots are presented on the screen, two of which are placed inside the receptive field of the recorded neuron (dashed circle) and the other one is placed outside. While the monkey is attending to the target, trying to detect a subtle change in the direction of motion, an additional small moving pattern is briefly presented at spatially random locations marked with the black dots. Plotting the neuron's response to this pattern as a function of its position describes the spatial structure of the receptive field. The bottom of the figure shows such a receptive field obtained from a single neuron in the middle temporal area. The strength of the response is coded in color, with white indicating the strongest excitation and blue indicating inhibition. The top right panel represents conditions in which attention was directed to the stimulus outside the receptive field. The top left panel and the bottom left panel represent conditions in which attention was directed to the stimulus marked with the green square or to the stimulus marked with the blue circle, respectively. Finally, the bottom right panel represents the difference between the latter two conditions, showing the push–pull effect of spatial attention across the receptive field that underlies the shift of the receptive field center between the conditions. Modified from Treue S, Womelsdorf T, and Martinez-Trujillo JC (2007) Visuelle Aufmerksamkeit: Von Orten, Eigenschaften und Kontrasten. *NeuroForum* 13: 55–60, with permission from NeuroForum.

expected and behaviorally relevant. Similarly, when monkeys are discriminating the orientation of a bar that matches the color of a cue, enhanced responses are observed in area V4 compared to situations in which the color of the bar is different from the color of the cue.

Feature-based attentional modulation that reaches far beyond the confines of the spatial receptive field of a sensory cell has been reported in the dorsal cortical pathway. The activity of MT neurons is higher when the animal is attending to a stimulus moving in their preferred versus nonpreferred direction, even when the attended stimulus is far from the classical receptive field. Thus, attending to a feature, such as a particular direction of motion, enhances the responsiveness of all neurons that prefer this particular stimulus feature, not just those whose receptive field includes the attended stimulus. This global spread of feature-based attention has been confirmed in behavioral and functional brain imaging studies.

Feature-based attentional modulation is comparable in strength to spatial attentional modulation, and the two influences combine additively in appropriate experimental paradigms. The similarity in strength of spatial and nonspatial attention and the additivity of the two modulations have also been observed in the ventral pathway, suggesting a unified system in which the spatial location is just another stimulus feature.

These observations have led to the formulation of the feature similarity gain model of Treue and Martinez-Trujillo. In essence, this model predicts the sign and magnitude of attentional gain modulation based on the similarity between the currently attended feature and the preferences of the neuron under study. Attending to the preferred feature of a given neuron (e.g., its preferred direction) increases neuronal responses, whereas attention to nonpreferred features (e.g., the nonpreferred direction) decreases neuronal responses. Note that the feature similarity gain model also accounts for spatial attentional modulations, interpreting the response reduction when spatial attention is shifted outside the receptive field as a situation of low feature similarity since the attended location is not matched to the preference of the neurons (i.e., its receptive field).

Object-based attention In addition to spatial and feature-based attention, the perceptual grouping of individual stimulus features into visual objects can also strongly influence the allocation of attention. Traditionally, investigations of object-based attention have played a more prominent role in psychophysical and functional magnetic resonance imaging experiments. Typically, two or more visual objects are superimposed such that spatial attention cannot be used to guide the allocation of attention. In such paradigms, features belonging to the same object are generally processed faster and more accurately than features belonging to different objects. Strong evidence for the existence of object-based attentional mechanisms has also been provided by imaging studies comparing activity in functionally defined regions of interest. The visual features of superimposed objects are carefully chosen to differentially activate well-defined cortical regions. Attending to a particular feature can result not only in enhanced activity within the cortical region processing the attended feature but also in enhanced activity within regions processing other, task-irrelevant features of the same object. Therefore, in contrast to feature-based attention, object-based attention is characterized by a transfer of attention from attended to unattended features of the same object. In physiological experiments, it has been difficult to distinguish feature-based attention from object-based attention. A notable exception is a series of experiments in primary visual cortex involving a task in which the animal was trained to mentally trace a curved line while keeping fixation on one of its ending points. Multiunit activity of V1 recording sites overlapping with different segments of the line was simultaneously enhanced if the curve crossing the receptive fields was behaviorally relevant as opposed to when it was not. Such findings indicate that responses of neurons in area V1 depend on whether the stimulus inside their receptive field is part of an attended object.

In summary, different experimental paradigms have revealed apparently distinct forms of attention, depending on whether spatial locations, nonspatial stimulus features, or visual objects are relevant in terms of current behavioral goals. Additional physiological examinations of these phenomena will help to assess the validity of such a strict separation by investigating the basic neuronal mechanisms leading to an enhanced representation of relevant visual information.

Modulation

Multiplicative Modulation of Tuning Curves

The ability of a given neuron in visual cortex to encode a particular stimulus feature is captured by the neuron's tuning curve, the bell-shaped response profile which plots the response of a neuron as a function of some continuous stimulus property, such as orientation or direction of motion. Investigating the neural basis of attentional modulation of information processing therefore requires examining attentional influences on tuning properties. Studies of orientation-tuned cells in area V4 (i.e., the temporal visual pathway) as well as of direction-tuned neurons in MT and medial superior temporal (MST) areas (i.e., the dorsal pathway) have documented that switching spatial attention from outside to inside the receptive field of a given neuron enhances the neuron's responses in a multiplicative manner. Thus, the tuning curves in these two attentional conditions are scaled versions of each other, not differing in their tuning width but only in their amplitude (**Figure 3**). This shows that the allocation of spatial attention into the receptive field of a neuron enhances the neuron's response gain independently of the particular stimulus that drives its response. Moreover, the temporal dynamics of direction tuning in MT neurons show multiplicative modulation by attention in the absence of shifts or changes in shape of the temporal profile. Collectively, these studies show that the highly specific modulation of the response gain of sensory neurons in visual cortex is a central mechanism of attentional influence.

Nonmultiplicative Consequences of Attention

Although both spatial and feature-based attention have been shown to create gain changes (i.e., exert a multiplicative influence on neurons in visual cortex), it is important to note that multiplicative effects can be combined to create nonmultiplicative modulations. One example of such nonmultiplicative modulations is the change in receptive field profiles created

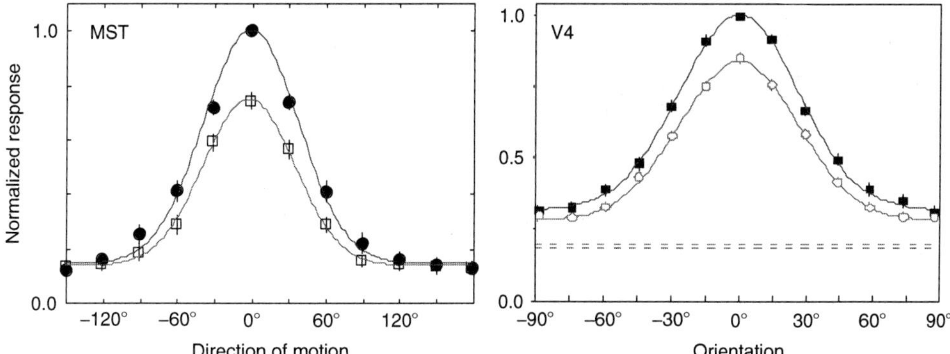

Figure 3 Multiplicative effects of spatial attention on neuronal tuning curves. The red curve in both panels represents the response when attention was directed toward the stimulus inside the receptive field, whereas the green curve gives the response to the same stimulus when attention was directed out of the receptive field. For both pairs, the attentional modulation did not significantly change the width of the tuning curve. The left panel shows firing rates, averaged across a population of neurons from the medial superior temporal area (MST), in response to the direction of a high-contrast moving random dot pattern. The right panel shows the average tuning curve across V4 cells to the orientation of a grating. The dashed lines represent the background firing rates (i.e., the responses of the cells in the absence of a stimulus). Modified from Treue S (2001) Neural correlates of attention in primate visual cortex. *Trends in Neurosciences* 24(5): 295–300, with permission.

when shifting spatial attention within a receptive field or between locations inside and outside the receptive field (**Figure 2**). Nevertheless, this modulation can also be caused by gain changes, if one assumes that spatial attention differentially enhances and reduces the gain of those V1 neurons providing the input to MT neurons and covering the attended and unattended portions, respectively, of the MT receptive field.

Similarly, switching attention from a fixation point to a stimulus moving in various directions inside an MT receptive field creates a systematic but nonmultiplicative change of the direction-tuning curve between the two attentional conditions (**Figure 4**). Note that although even purely multiplicative effects of attention have been shown to improve the signal-to-noise ratio of attended stimuli, this selective modulation is even higher in the case of nonmultiplicative modulations based on gain changes. As such, they usually exert a push–pull influence that cannot be achieved directly through a gain change, suppressing sensory responses to unattended stimuli and enhancing responses to attended stimuli.

Saliency

Comparing Response Modulation by Contrast and Attention

The multiplicative modulation of responses by attention is very reminiscent of the modulatory influence of a number of well-studied stimulus parameters on sensory responses, such as contrast, speed, and motion coherence. This similarity suggests a common neural mechanism that would allow attention to modulate the strength of a stimulus representation by changing its 'effective contrast' or saliency. Alternatively, this similarity in terms of effects might simply reflect the existence of two independent multiplicative systems.

A few studies have addressed this issue by testing whether the effects of stimulus contrast interact with the effects of attention. These studies have measured contrast response functions under different attentional conditions. If the two systems were truly independent, the multiplicative effects of attention should be independent of the level of contrast, and the contrast response function should be scaled by a constant factor along the vertical dimension (**Figure 5(a)**), in the same way as the tuning curves shown in **Figure 2**. If, on the other hand, these two systems share a common mechanism, directing attention should have the same effect as changing contrast and should therefore become evident in a horizontal shift of the contrast response function between attentional conditions. As a consequence, the strongest attentional effects would then be expected for stimuli of intermediate luminance or contrast (**Figure 5(b)**).

Recordings from area V4 have revealed a horizontal shift of the contrast response function, consistent with the notion that contrast modulation and attentional effects share a common mechanism. Studies in MT and MST have also reported such a horizontal shift and have documented the strongest attentional effects for intermediate levels of stimulus luminance (i.e., for levels corresponding to the steepest part of the sigmoidal contrast response function). Altogether, the studies further support the notion of a close coupling between these mechanisms. They could thus underlie the attentional effects on perceived stimulus saliency observed in psychophysical studies (**Figure 5(c)**). Moreover, the

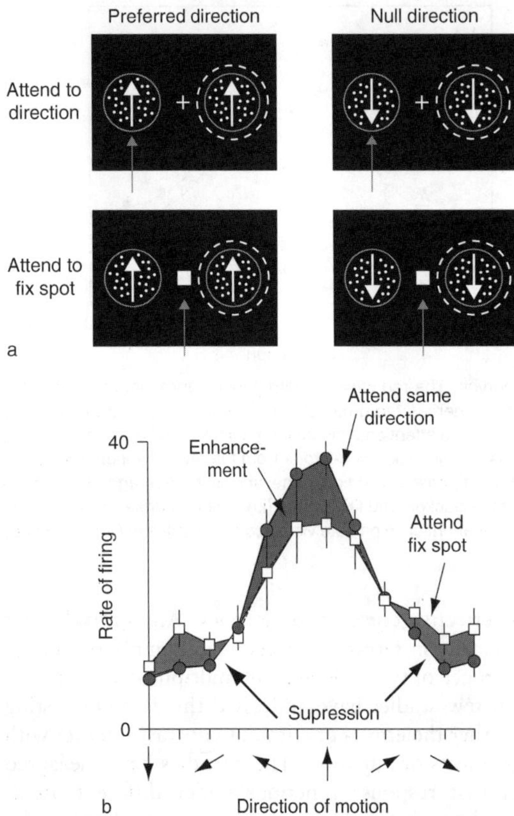

Figure 4 Feature-based attention in the middle temporal area (MT). (a) Schematic representation of tasks used to assess the effects of attention to direction of motion. Two stationary apertures containing moving random dots were presented on the computer monitor. One of them was placed inside the receptive field (dashed white line) of the neuron under study, and the other one was placed outside. The dot patterns always moved in the same direction (white arrows), but different directions of motion were presented on different trials. On some trials (bottom row), the attention of the animal (gray arrows) was directed to the fixation spot to detect a change in luminance. On other trials (top row), a cue at the beginning instructed the animal to pay attention to the motion of the pattern outside the receptive field to detect a subtle change in that motion. (b) Responses of a representative MT neuron to different directions of motion, separately for each attentional condition. Attention to the preferred direction of motion increased the response of the neuron, but attention to the null direction of motion decreased its response. Thus, attention to a particular direction of motion does not increase responses across all neurons. Rather, it has a push–pull effect that increases responses only for neurons that prefer motion close to the attended direction. Modified from Maunsell JHR and Treue S (2006) Feature-based attention in visual cortex. *Trends in Neurosciences* 29(6): 317–322, with permission.

influence of stimulus contrast on the magnitude of the attentional effects might account for the variability in the magnitude of attentional modulation reported in the literature. However, a related study, also recording from area V4, reported a mixture of effects, including multiplicative scaling of the contrast response function by spatial attention, leaving open the possibility of a less direct and more complex relationship between attentional and contrast modulation. Further research is necessary to reconcile these findings.

Forming an Integrated Saliency Map by Spatial and Feature-Based Attention

Our visual environment is represented as the neuronal activity across a population of neurons, with various receptive field positions and preferred feature values. The insights into the neuronal mechanisms of attentional modulation gained from the studies mentioned previously permit inference on the attentional modulation of this population activity, caused by directing attention to a particular feature at a particular location in a complex visual scene. Conceivable could be a scenario in which the visual input creates a fairly homogeneous level of activation across the neuronal population. Spatial attention will increase the gain of all neurons whose receptive field overlaps the current attentional focus, creating an enhanced representation at that location that is akin to a local increase in contrast and that creates a corresponding perceptual effect (**Figure 5(c)**).

Since similarity in terms of features can also be based on spatial location, the feature similarity hypothesis predicts that the attentional modulation within this retinotopic population should vary considerably. Specifically, neurons whose receptive fields only partially overlap the focus of attention will experience less of a gain increase than those centered on the focus – a prediction that has not been tested experimentally.

In addition to this spatially confined modulation of the retinotopic representation, the contribution of the attended nonspatial feature must also be considered. Feature-based attention will cause a differential gain change across the whole retinotopic representation with a particularly strong gain increase for neurons preferring the attended feature and a corresponding gain decrease for those of opposite preference. The total effect will be a population response that is no longer homogeneous but has its highest activity in the group of neurons preferring the attended location and feature, intermediate enhancements at retinotopic locations where the visual input only matches the attended nonspatial feature (i.e., potential targets in a visual search situation), and suppressed responses everywhere else. Combining such modulated population responses across cortical areas could create an integrated saliency map – that is, a topographic representation of relative stimulus strength and behavioral relevance across visual space.

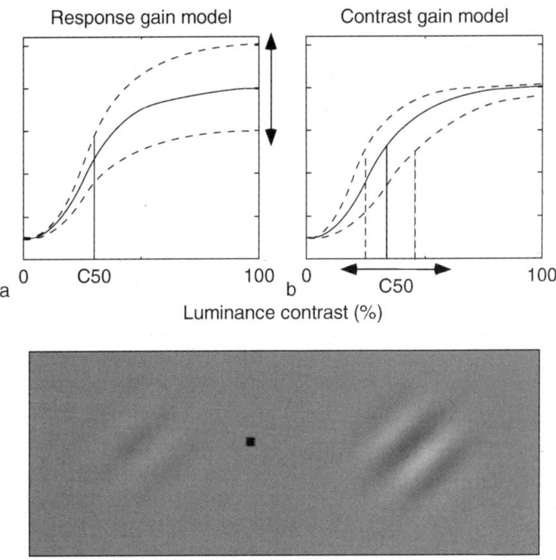

Figure 5 Depiction of the similarity between attentional effects and changes in luminance contrast. (a and b) Possible attentional effects on contrast response functions of visual cortical neurons. According to the response gain model (a), attention modulates the neuronal response to every level of contrast by a constant factor, effectively scaling the contrast response function along the vertical dimension. According to the contrast gain model (b), directing attention is equivalent to changing contrast, resulting in a shift of the contrast response function along the horizontal dimension. A number of studies have provided evidence for the contrast gain model, suggesting that an unattended stimulus of a given contrast will have the same effect as an attended stimulus of lower contrast. An increase in the perceived contrast by attention has been demonstrated in behavioral experiments with human observers and is illustrated in (c). The two stimuli, shown to the left and right of the fixation square, are judged to be equal in contrast if attention is directed to the left stimulus only. Modified from Treue S, Womelsdorf T, and Martinez-Trujillo JC (2007) Visuelle Aufmerksamkeit: Von Orten, Eigenschaften und Kontrasten. *NeuroForum* 13: 55–60, with permission from NeuroForum.

Top-Down and Bottom-Up Response Modulation

The previously outlined attentional modulations of neural activity in visual cortex all result in an enhancement in the activity or the synchrony of cell populations preferring attended stimulus attributes and a simultaneous suppression in the activity of cell populations preferring nonattended attributes. This will create an enhanced representation of attended relative to unattended stimuli, an effect reminiscent of the selective enhancement of particular aspects of the visual input by the hardwired bottom-up coding mechanisms mentioned in the introduction. The similarity of the two systems suggests their combination into the integrated saliency map, in which the visual input is represented not by an individual stimulus' physical strength (e.g., its luminance) but by its saliency (i.e., its difference in features compared to the spatially surrounding visual input). The integrated saliency map combines the bottom-up saliency with the modulatory influence of attention, strengthening or weakening it according to the behavioral relevance of a particular location, feature, or object.

This interaction provides an account for a central function of attention in enhancing the representation of stimuli of intermediate strength while particularly salient stimuli will be well represented even in the absence of attention. This is in good agreement with results from a large body of psychophysical studies demonstrating that highly salient stimuli (known as 'pop-out' stimuli in visual search tasks) need little attentional resource allocation, whereas the same stimuli embedded among similar distractors will only be perceived when attention is directed toward them.

Conclusion

The understanding of attentional influences has advanced considerably beyond the view that attention is a separable influence providing only a late modulation of an otherwise stimulus-driven sensory information processing system. Instead, attention influences the processing of visual information even in the earliest areas of primate visual cortex. This influence seems to shape an integrated saliency map – that is, a representation of the environment that weighs every input by its local feature contrast and its current behavioral relevance. This map enables the visual system to integrate large amounts of bottom-up and top-down information because it provides an efficient coding scheme for the potentially most relevant information in the sensory input. However, by completely integrating bottom-up sensory information and top-down attentional influences, it equates the absence of attention with low stimulus power. This provides a possible explanation for the observation that highly salient stimuli will be processed even in the absence of attention, whereas low inherent salience will often prevent the perceptual representation of unattended parts of complex natural scenes, although exceptions seem to exist for the categorization of the gist of natural scenes.

The brain areas providing the guidance for the top-down attentional effects seem to be tightly linked to those areas responsible for the planning and execution of eye movements in agreement with the frequent need for foveating salient regions of the visual environment for a more detailed analysis.

Although many questions remain, the rapid development of functional imaging techniques and the development of sophisticated paradigms and recording techniques in monkeys trained to perform complex attentional tasks provide the basis for the recent growth in understanding. By bringing together bottom-up stimulus aspects that are often responsible for automatic attentional allocation and top-down influences reflecting voluntary attention, a global map representing stimulus saliency modulated by the current behavioral state of the organism can provide a unified framework for interpreting future findings on attentional effects and their close integration with sensory information processing.

See also: Attention and Eye Movements; Parietal Cortex and Spatial Attention; Thalamic Mechanisms in Vision; Visual Cortex in Humans; Visual Development.

Further Reading

Anton-Erxleben K, Henrich C, and Treue S (2007) Attention changes perceived size of moving visual patterns. *Journal of Vision* 7(11): 1–9.

Boynton GM (2005) Attention and visual perception. *Current Opinion in Neurobiology* 15(4): 465–469.

Carrasco M, Ling S, and Read S (2004) Attention alters appearance. *Nature Neuroscience* 7(3): 308–313.

Desimone R and Duncan J (1995) Neural mechanisms of selective visual attention. *Annual Review of Neuroscience* 18: 193–222.

Downing P, Liu J, and Kanwisher N (2001) Testing cognitive models of visual attention with fMRI and MEG. *Neuropsychologia* 39(12): 1329–1342.

Maunsell JHR and Treue S (2006) Feature-based attention in visual cortex. *Trends in Neurosciences* 29(6): 317–322.

Moore T (2006) The neurobiology of visual attention: Finding sources. *Current Opinion in Neurobiology* 16: 159–165.

O'Craven KM, Downing PE, and Kanwisher N (1999) fMRI evidence for objects as the units of attentional selection. *Nature* 401: 584–587.

Reynolds JH and Chelazzi L (2004) Attentional modulation of visual processing. *Annual Review of Neuroscience* 27: 611–647.

Reynolds JH and Desimone R (2003) Interacting roles of attention and visual salience in V4. *Neuron* 37: 853–863.

Roelfsema PR, Lamme VAF, and Spekreijse H (1998) Object-based attention in the primary visual cortex of the macaque monkey. *Nature* 395: 376–381.

Treue S (2001) Neural correlates of attention in primate visual cortex. *Trends in Neurosciences* 24(5): 295–300.

Treue S (2003) Visual attention: The where, what, how and why of saliency. *Current Opinion in Neurobiology* 13: 428–432.

Treue S, Womelsdorf T, and Martinez-Trujillo JC (2007) Visuelle Aufmerksamkeit: Von Orten, Eigenschaften und Kontrasten. *NeuroForum* 13: 55–60.

Williford T and Maunsell JHR (2006) Effects of spatial attention on contrast response functions in macaque area V4. *Journal of Neurophysiology* 96: 40–54.

Womelsdorf T, Anton-Erxleben K, Pieper F, and Treue S (2006) Dynamic shifts of visual receptive fields in cortical area MT by spatial attention. *Nature Neuroscience* 9(9): 1156–1160.

Working Memory: Capacity Limitations

T Drew and E K Vogel, University of Oregon, Eugene, OR, USA

Working Memory System

Working memory (WM) has been proposed to be a cognitive system that temporarily holds a limited amount of information in an active state so that it may be quickly accessed, integrated with other information, or otherwise manipulated. This type of memory is thought to underlie our ability to perform a wide range of basic tasks such as assigning meanings and syntactic roles to the interdependent words of a complex sentence, understanding the relationships among the ideas within a complex argument, performing mental rotation, and tracking the trajectory of a moving object when the visual input to the brain is continually disrupted by eyeblinks and saccades. Many cognitive processes that require information to be held in an online state are thought to use the WM system as a form of mental workspace to perform their requisite operations. As a result of its central position within cognition, the limited capacity of the WM system reflects one of the more significant processing limitations for human cognition.

Capacity Limits: Central or Modality-Specific?

One of the most notable characteristics of WM is that its storage capacity is highly limited. Most of the early models of short-term memory implicitly or explicitly assumed that it was a unitary memory store, irrespective of modality. In the 1970s, however, Baddeley and his colleagues proposed a multimodal model of WM in which the memories for visual and verbal information are stored separately with independent capacity limits, both controlled by a central executive process. Early support for this model came from dual-task experiments in which little or no interference was found when verbal memory tasks were performed concurrently with visual memory tasks but substantial interference was found for two concurrent verbal tasks or two concurrent visual tasks.

Nelson Cowan, on the other hand, proposed that the capacity limits of WM reflect a more central limit, irrespective of modality. Specifically, his model proposes that WM is not an entirely separate system but is a part of the long-term memory system. Consequently, representations of information in WM are proposed to be the activated portions of long-term memory within two embedded levels. The first level consists of activated long-term memory representations, which are memory representations that have recently been accessed. Although a large number of these representations can be active simultaneously, the highly accurate retrieval of this information is fairly limited as a consequence of interference. By contrast, the second level consists of a small subset of these active long-term memory representations that are held within the focus of attention, which has a capacity limit of approximately four items, irrespective of modality. That is, although there may be independent passive maintenance of information in modality-specific stores, the true capacity limits arise from the central limitation of the focus of attention.

Overview and Approach

At present, the evidence is somewhat mixed with regard to whether WM capacity limits are modality-specific or a single central limitation. Therefore, in the following sections, we consider the capacity limitations of WM separately for the verbal and visual modalities. Where appropriate, however, we also describe how these results can be alternatively accounted for within the Cowan framework. After discussing the common behavioral approaches to measuring WM capacity, we then describe more recent attempts to use neurophysiological methods to measure these capacity limits. In the final section, we summarize work that examines individual differences in WM capacity and how these differences relate to broader cognitive constructs such as intelligence and attentional control.

Verbal Working Memory Capacity – Memory Span Tasks

For over a century, the most common approach to measuring WM capacity has been with variations of the digit span task. In the standard version of this task, subjects are given a randomized list of numbers that they must immediately repeat back in the order of presentation. Subjects are initially presented with lists of two or three digits and if they repeat a list of numbers without making a mistake, the size of the list is increased until they cannot accurately complete the list. On average, most individuals can accurately report approximately seven items, although this number varies substantially across individuals. Similar estimates are typically observed when letters and words are used as the to-be-remembered stimuli.

Although the results of span tasks are often interpreted as reflecting the capacity of WM for verbal material, there are two important constraints that shed light on the nature of storage capacity in this context.

Chunking of Information

Recently, *Psychological Review* named George Miller's 1956 article, "The magical number seven, plus or minus two: Some limits on our capacity for processing information," as its most influential paper. Although many agree that the author intended the title of the paper to be taken as a tongue-in-cheek statement, the meme of short-term memory being limited to "seven plus or minus two" items has permeated the popular literature in psychology for the last 50 years. However, one of the primary ideas expressed in Miller's paper is that the exact number of items that can be held in WM depends heavily on whether the items can be grouped into meaningful units, or chunks. That is, chunking exploits preexisting information about concepts already stored in long-term memory so that new information can be more efficiently held in WM. For example, consider the letter string:

FBICIAFDRJFK

Memory span for this series is generally fairly poor because the 12 letters exceed the typical seven-item limit. However, consider the same items when broken into the following clusters:

FBI CIA FDR JFK

Performance is greatly enhanced under this condition because the units for memory span are four meaningful and familiar concepts rather than 12 independent letters. Thus, the precise number of items that can be held in WM is strongly dependent on what type of information is to be held, whether those items can be clustered into a smaller number of meaningful units, and finally whether the subject attempts to strategically code the incoming information into clusters. Indeed, efficient chunking of information is thought to be a pervasive aspect of daily cognitive life, and it may greatly underlie our ability to perform complex tasks such as reading and playing chess.

Phonological Coding of Verbal Information

The remaining constraint on estimates of verbal WM capacity is derived from studies that have examined the nature of how information is coded in verbal WM. One of the more popular characterizations stems from Baddeley's model of WM. In particular, information maintained in verbal WM is thought to be stored in a phonological loop. Essentially, information is thought to be stored as a phonological or sound-based code within a structure (e.g., a tape loop) that can hold a limited amount of information for a very short period of time. However, this information can be held for much longer durations when the subject subvocally rehearses the phonological information repeatedly to keep it from being lost. There are several pieces of evidence that support the notion of phonological storage in verbal WM. For instance, fewer phonologically similar words (e.g., cap, slap, trap, map) can be held in WM than phonologically dissimilar words. However, memory span is not affected if the words are similar in meaning (e.g, big, tall, huge, wide) or similar looking (e.g., bough, dough, cough, through), which indicates that the phonological properties of the to-be-remembered items are a primary factor for the storage limit. In addition, many studies have shown that memory span is considerably smaller for phonologically longer words (e.g., alimony, Mississippi, testosterone) than for phonologically short words (e.g., hat, boy, up), which indicates that storage capacity is determined by how long it takes to pronounce the information to be remembered. Moreover, an individual's rate of speech also has a direct impact on how many items he or she can hold in a span task, with fast-speaking individuals capable of holding more items than slower-speaking individuals. On the basis of results such as these, many researchers agree that the capacity of verbal WM is determined by how much the individual can say in approximately 2 s. Thus, it appears that the capacity limits of this system are much better understood in terms of time (i.e., 2 s of speech) rather than by numbers of items (e.g., seven plus or minus two). Interestingly, when subjects are prevented from engaging in rehearsal, individuals can accurately report only three or four items accurately. This could be explained by Cowan's central capacity limit theory, in that the phonological loop is a domain-specific storage mechanism and the true capacity limit of attention can be observed when rehearsal is prevented.

Visual Working Memory Capacity: Whole Report

The initial measurement of the capacity of WM for visual information is often credited to George Sperling. In this influential series of experiments, subjects were presented briefly (50 ms) with arrays of 12 random letters and were asked to immediately report as many letters as possible. Across several experiments, subjects could accurately report between four and five items, irrespective of how many total letters were in the array, how they were configured, or how long the array was presented (ranging from 15 to 500 ms). The results of these and other similar experiments suggest that subjects' ability to apprehend information from a brief display is extremely limited and that they are capable of maintaining information about only a relatively few items in memory.

Sperling's estimate of visual WM capacity has two potential limitations as an estimate of visual WM capacity. The first is the possibility of output interference. Subjects were asked to name or write each of the letters they remembered. This may have underestimated WM capacity because the process of transforming the visual input into a reportable form may be too slow to capture the fleeting sensory information before memory capacity is fully exhausted. Furthermore, Sperling used alphanumeric characters as the memoranda, which calls into question whether the items were being held strictly in a visual memory store or whether both verbal WM and visual WM contributed to the capacity estimate. Indeed, because the subjects had to report the identity of the letters at the end of the trial, they must have transformed the visual image into verbal labels. Thus, although suggestive, results from whole report tasks such as these do not provide definitive estimates of the capacity of WM for visual information.

Visual Working Memory Capacity: Features and Objects

In an attempt to measure the capacity of visual WM more directly, we and others developed a variation of Philips' sequential comparison paradigm that is commonly known as the change detection paradigm. In this task, subjects are shown a brief array of simple objects that they must remember (see **Figure 1**). The objects disappear for a short retention period and afterward reappear in the same locations as before. On half the trials, the first and second arrays of objects are identical; on the other trials, one of the objects changes its identity (e.g., shape or color). Subjects make a single button-press response regarding whether the two arrays are the same or different. To examine capacity limitations in this task, the number of items in each array is manipulated to find when performance starts to decline. Luck and Vogel used this task to examine the capacity of visual WM for simple single-featured objects. These objects were bright, suprathreshold colors that were chosen to be highly discriminable from one another so that the task would be limited primarily by memory storage capacity rather than by perceptual and decision factors. Performance was near-perfect for arrays containing one, two, or three items, but declined at higher set sizes. They estimated visual WM capacity to be approximately three to four items, and this was unchanged even when subjects performed a concurrent articulatory suppression task to keep them from verbally labeling the visual items. They also tested whether visual WM capacity is determined by the number of features that must remembered or whether it is determined by the number of objects that must be remembered. To do this, they asked subjects to remember arrays of objects that each possess two features (e.g., color and orientation) to determine whether the additional features consumed more memory capacity. Surprisingly, they found that subjects could remember the same number of multifeatured objects as they could single-featured objects. Indeed, in one experiment, they found that subjects could remember four four-featured objects (i.e., color, orientation, size, and a stripe) just as well as they could remember just four colors. That is, they could retain up to sixteen features as long as they were distributed across four separate objects. Although there are some limitations to the strength of this object advantage, these results have been taken as strong evidence in favor of visual WM capacity being determined by the number of objects to be remembered.

Units of Capacity: Objects or Information Load?

A recent challenge to the object-based visual WM capacity proposal was provided by Alvarez and Cavanagh, who tested whether visual WM capacity was also determined by the information load engendered by various complex object categories. To examine this, they measured visual WM capacity for several object categories of varying complexity (e.g., simple colors, Chinese characters, and three-dimensional shaded cubes) and found that, as the complexity of the remembered objects increased, the memory capacity likewise decreased (see **Figure 2**). That is, subjects could remember approximately 4.5 colored squares (the least complex items), but they could accurately remember only 1.6 shaded cubes (the most complex items). They described these results as indicating a direct trade-off between the required resolution of the items in memory and the number of items that may be maintained in visual WM; complex items that require a high resolution cause a decrease in how many objects can be held in memory.

Recently, Awh, Barton, and Vogel examined whether the lower capacity estimates for complex objects may have been due to an increase in similarity between items in the complex categories. That is, change detection performance depends not only on the number of representations that can be maintained in working memory but also on the observers' ability

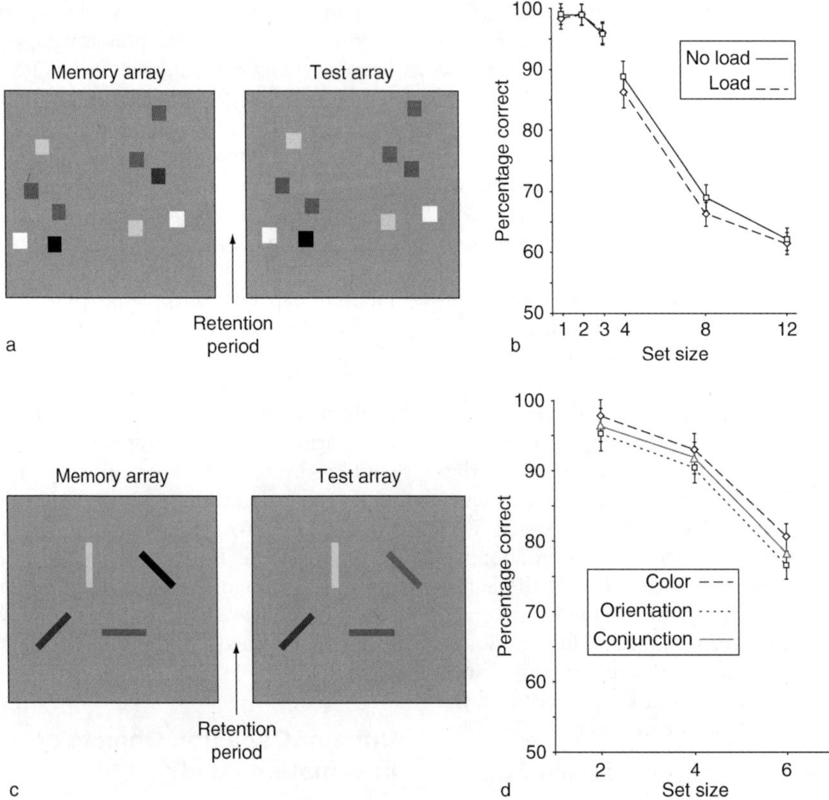

Figure 1 Estimating visual working memory capacity: (a) change detection paradigm using color; (b) memory performance in (a); (c) change detection paradigm using color and orientation; (d) memory performance in (c). In (a), subjects are asked to remember the colors in the memory array across the retention interval. At test, subjects judge the colors to be the same or different as the memory array. As shown in (b), performance in this task is near-perfect for 1, 2, or 3 items and quickly declines at higher set sizes. A concurrent articulatory suppression task has no effect on performance of the visual memory task. In (c), subjects are asked to remember both the color and orientation of the items. As shown in (d), memory performance is equivalent irrespective of the number of features. Adapted from Luck SJ and Vogel EK (1997) The capacity of visual working memory for features and conjunctions. *Nature* 390: 279–281.

to discriminate between these stored representations and the new items that are presented during change trials. If the similarity is high, then changes can be missed in this procedure even though the changed item was stored in memory. Along these lines, Awh and colleagues found that for the object categories used by Alvarez and Cavanagh there was a strong positive correlation between complexity and within-category similarity. Moreover, they found that when within-category similarity was decreased (by using cross-category changes) memory capacity estimates were equivalent for both simple and complex objects (i.e., three to four items). These data suggest that visual WM represents a fixed number of items, regardless of object complexity. These results do not contradict the important observation that change-detection performance is strongly influenced by object complexity. However, it may be that the relationship between object complexity and change detection has more to do with the resolution for making discriminations than with the number of representations that can be maintained in memory.

Neural Measures of Working Memory Capacity

Neuroimaging Since the 1990s, numerous studies using neuroimaging in humans have found increased blood-oxygen level-dependent (BOLD) activation during the retention interval of various WM tasks. This activity is thought to be analogous to delay activity observed in monkey single-unit studies. The sustained BOLD activity is primarily observed in the prefrontal, posterior parietal, and inferotemporal cortices. Although there have been several demonstrations that the magnitude of the activity increases as memory load increases, it is often difficult to

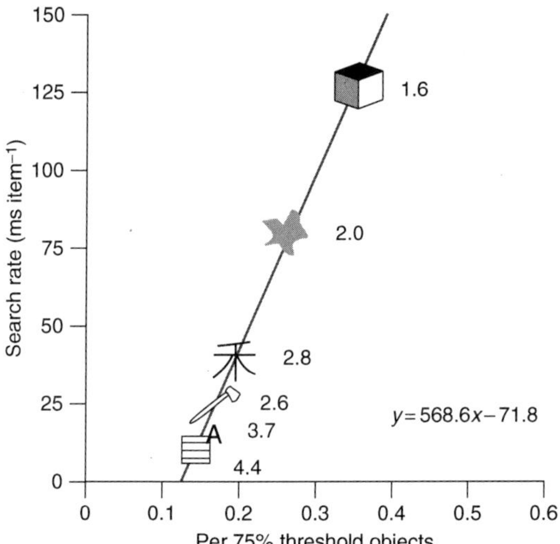

Figure 2 Information load and working memory capacity. As the information load for a type object increases, the estimated number of items that can be accurately remembered decreases from a high of 4.4 objects for color squares to a low of 1.6 for three-dimensional cubes. The search rate for each object type was found by asking subjects to perform a visual search for a specific object among other objects of that type. Search rate is a proxy for the amount of information load for a given object. Adapted from Alvarez GA and Cavanagh P (2004) The capacity of visual short-term memory is set by both the visual information load and by number of objects. *Psychological Science* 15(2): 106–111.

determine whether it necessarily reflects WM storage demands *per se* or whether other, more task-general activity is responsible for the load-related increase in activity. Consequently, it is often difficult to determine whether the increasing activation is due to more memory representations being held in WM or if it is simply the result of the increased difficulty in the high-load conditions.

Within the verbal WM domain, there is one notable functional magnetic resonance imaging (fMRI) study that appeared to distinguish between patterns of neural activity for subcapacity memory loads and supracapacity loads. Specifically, Rypma and colleagues used a letter WM task and found increased activation in the left ventrolateral prefrontal cortex for loads of three items, compared to only one item. This region is in the vicinity of Broca's area, and it is plausible that the increased activity reflects the additional subvocal rehearsal demands for the additional items in verbal WM. Interestingly, when the load was increased from three items to six items, a wide range of prefrontal areas became active. These results suggest that when the verbal WM capacity was exceeded, many additional executive processes are recruited to assist in performing the task.

In the visual WM domain, there are two recent studies that suggested that activity in the posterior parietal cortex is sensitive to WM capacity limits. Todd and Marois used the change detection paradigm for colored items and found that retention period activity in the intraparietal sulcus (IPS) increased as a function of the number of items in memory, but this increasing activity reached asymptote at approximately four items (see **Figure 3**). These results suggest that the activity in the IPS reflects the number of item representations that can be successfully maintained in visual WM because it reaches a ceiling at the known storage-capacity limit of visual WM. Xu and Chun recently replicated and extended this finding by showing evidence that there are three primary areas that show this sensitivity to visual WM capacity limits: the superior IPS, the lateral occipital complex (LOC), and the inferior IPS. Interestingly, they found that the activity in the superior IPS and LOC reached asymptotic levels for smaller array sizes when the memory items were complex than when they were simple. However, the inferior IPS activity reached asymptote at arrays of four items, irrespective of whether the items were simple or complex. Together, these results suggest that a suite of posterior cortical areas underlie visual WM capacity limits and that distinct mechanisms may be sensitive to the necessary resolution and the number of items that can be held in visual WM.

Electrophysiological measures Our laboratory used event-related potentials (ERPs) to observe the storage and maintenance of object representations in visual WM. To do this, we used a modified version of the change detection paradigm in which we presented simple objects in both the left and right hemifields and asked subjects to remember the items in only a single hemifield using an arrow cue (see **Figure 4(a)**). This bilateral stimulus task design allowed us to isolate the ERP activity that is specific to the memory items by dividing electrodes in terms of whether they were contralateral or ipsilateral with respect to the side of the display the subjects were remembering on a given trial. Approximately 250 ms following the onset of the memory array, we observed a large negative wave at posterior electrode sites that were contralateral to the position of the memoranda for a given trial. This activity persisted throughout the retention period until the test array arrived, and we refer to it as the contralateral delay activity (CDA). An important property of the CDA is that its amplitude increases as a function of the number of items that are being held in visual WM. However, like the fMRI studies in the IPS, this amplitude increase reaches asymptote at approximately four items,

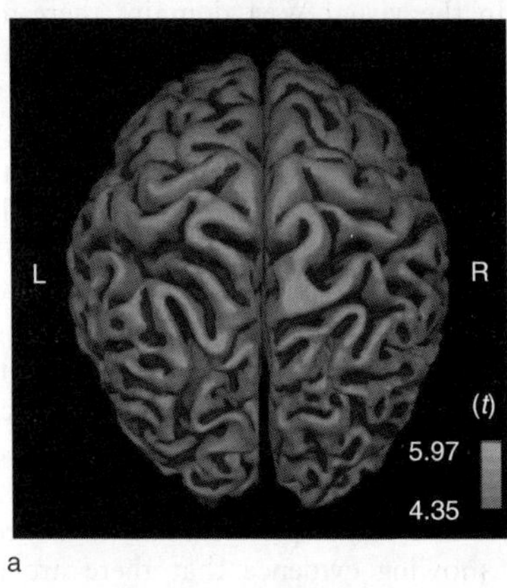

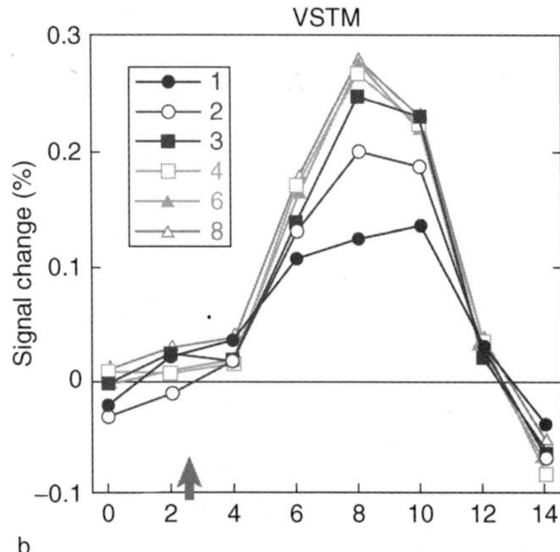

Figure 3 An fMRI measure of visual working memory capacity: (a) a statistical map of activation in the intraparietal sulcus (IPS) during the retention interval overlaid on a structural scan; (b) activation in the IPS as a function of number of memory items. The green arrow represents the time of presentation. Activation in this area increases until there are three items and then asymptotes for four to eight items. fMRI, functional magnetic resonance imaging; L, left; R, right; VSTM, visual short-term memory. Adapted from Todd JJ and Marois R (2004) Capacity limit of visual short-term memory in human posterior parietal cortex. *Nature* 428(6984): 751–754.

indicating that this activity is sensitive to visual WM capacity limits and may reflect the active representations that can be held in memory. Indeed, the precise point at which it reaches asymptote is different for each subject depending on his or her specific memory capacity (see **Figure 4(c)**).

Individual Differences in Working Memory Capacity

Although the capacity of WM is known to be highly limited, these limitations have long been known to vary substantially across individuals. In fact, because WM is thought to play a central role in a wide range of cognitive processes, it is not surprising that an individual's WM capacity is positively correlated with performance on a wide range of cognitive and aptitude measures such as intelligence, reasoning, scholastic performance, math abilities, and ability to acquire a second language. Thus, WM capacity appears to be a core mental construct that underlies an individual's general cognitive ability in a variety of situations. Next, we review two primary correlates of WM capacity: intelligence and attentional control.

Intelligence and Working Memory Capacity

The relationship between WM capacity and intelligence has been well known and studied for over a century. For example, Binet and Simon observed that cognitively impaired children have sharply smaller digit spans than normal children, which prompted the view that WM capacity could provide a window to intelligence. Indeed, to this day, almost all intelligence battery tests include at least some form of memory span component. In the last few decades, researchers began to move away from using digit span as an individual difference measure because it is highly susceptible to strategic performance differences, such as chunking, that often weaken the relationship to intelligence measures. Instead, many use WM measures of processing capacity rather than simple span as a predictor of cognitive performance. For example, Daneman and Carpenter demonstrated strong positive correlations between WM reading span tasks and cognitive aptitude. Their reading span task asked subjects to read sets of random sentences and to remember the last word of each sentence, which they were tested on at the end of the session. Performance on this task was strongly correlated with SAT verbal scores and reading comprehension scores. One currently popular method used to measure WM capacity is operation span (OSPAN). A subject's OSPAN is measured by asking the subject to read a simple mathematical equation, judge the accuracy of the equation, and then read a random word aloud. For example:

$$\text{Is } (3 \times 4) - 6 = 7\text{? Dog}$$

After the task has been repeated several times, the subject is asked to recall as many of the words as possible. Both reading span and OSPAN show strong positive correlations with language comprehension and intelligence measures. However, the relationship between WM capacity and intelligence is not limited to measures of verbal WM, but can also be observed with visual WM measures as well. For example, Cowan and his colleagues recently found

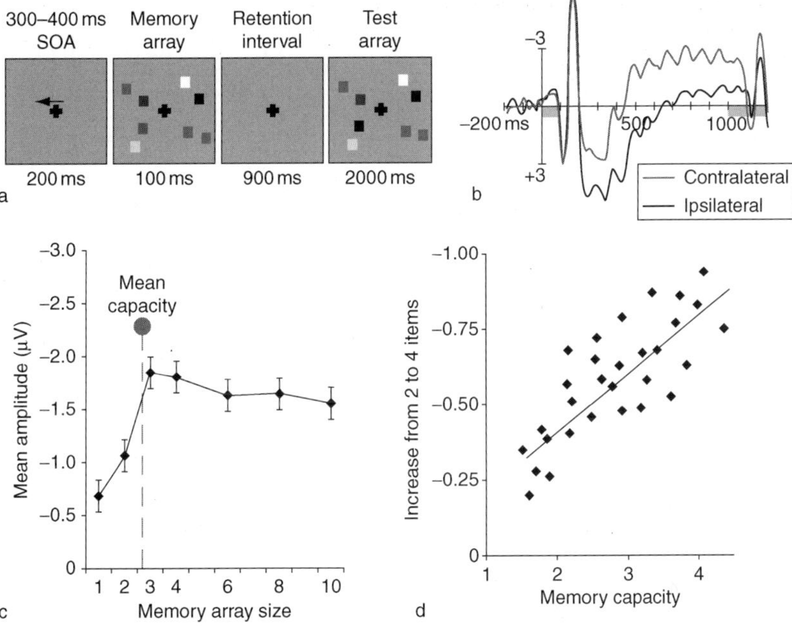

Figure 4 An event-related potential (ERP) measure of visual working memory capacity: (a) a bilateral change detection trial; (b) ERPs time-locked to the memory array; (c) mean amplitude of contralateral delay activity (CDA) during the retention interval; (d) correlation between an individual's memory capacity and the asymptote of the CDA (r=0.78). In (a), subjects are cued to remember the items in one hemifield. After a retention interval, subjects judge whether objects on the cued side of the test array are the same or different than objects in the memory array. In (b), note that negative voltage is plotted upward in the graphs, which show grand-average ERP waveforms time-locked to the memory array and averaged from occipital and posterior parietal electrodes. Ipsilateral and contralateral are defined with respect to the side of the screen that subjects are cued to attend. Gray rectangles represent the time of the memory and test array. As shown in (c), CDA amplitude increases up to approximately three items and then asymptotes at the point when the mean behavioral capacity (approximately three items) is exceeded. In (d), subjects with low memory capacity showed little increase from two to four items compared to high-capacity subjects. Adapted from Vogel EK and Machizawa MG (2004) Neural activity predicts individual differences in visual working memory capacity. *Nature* 428: 748–751.

that individual differences in capacity in change detection paradigms are also strongly predictive of intelligence and scholastic measures, including reading comprehension. This finding is consistent with Cowan's proposal that there is a single central WM capacity because measures that purport to quantify verbal and visual WM capacity are equally predictive of general cognitive ability, suggesting that the same central capacity limit underlies both visual and verbal WM tasks.

Attentional Control and Working Memory Capacity

More recently, researchers have begun to further examine the nature of the relationship between WM capacity and cognitive performance. However, rather than emphasizing the advantages of additional memory storage space, they have proposed that the benefits of a high WM capacity may actually be due to more efficient attentional control, that is, to how the WM system is used to determine the flow of information into WM and reduce the interference from distracting information. To date, there have been many demonstrations of a strong relationship between performance on various attentional control tasks and WM capacity. For example, in the antisaccade task, subjects are asked to look away from the position of a target that abruptly appears on the screen. This task is thought to require attentional control to override the prepotent response to look directly at the new object location. Interestingly, low-capacity individuals are much worse at avoiding eye movements toward distractors than high-capacity subjects. Moreover, WM capacity has also been shown to predict cocktail party effects in which subjects sometimes notice their own names when they are embedded in an unattended auditory channel. Surprisingly, Conway and colleagues found that low-WM-capacity subjects were three times more likely to detect their name than high-capacity subjects. Results such as these question whether the differences between high- and low-capacity individuals are due strictly to storage or processing abilities; it demonstrates that low-capacity subjects may often be processing more information than the high-capacity subjects but that this information may be detrimental to the task at hand. Along these lines, Vogel, McCollough, and Machizawa examined whether there are differences in the ability to voluntarily control what information is stored in visual WM. To do this, they presented subjects with arrays of objects that contained a mixture of relevant and irrelevant objects, and they measured the CDA component to determine how many total objects (including distractors) were stored in visual WM. They found that high-memory-capacity subjects were extremely efficient at keeping the irrelevant distractors from being stored in memory, whereas the low-capacity subjects were highly inefficient at excluding the distractors from being stored and held in memory (see **Figure 5(b)**). Thus, the low-capacity subjects actually held more information in memory than the high-capacity subjects, but this ancillary

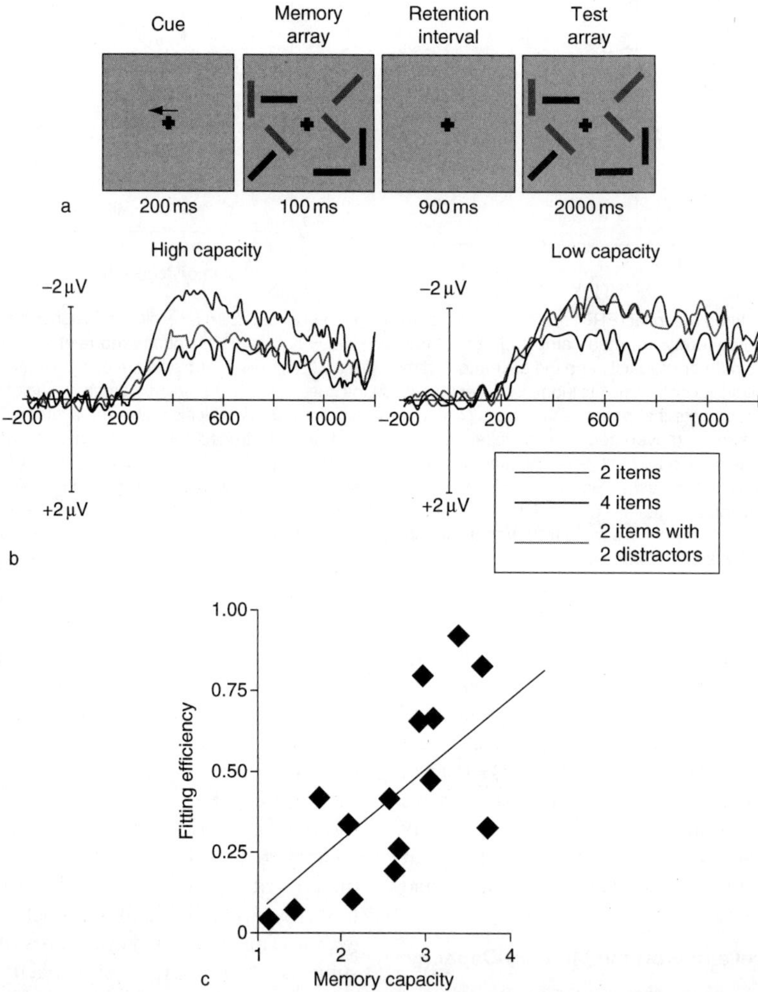

Figure 5 Attentional filtering and working memory: (a) attentional filtering test; (b) mean contralateral delay activity (CDA) amplitude waveforms split between high- and low-memory-capacity subjects; (c) correlation between filtering efficiency and working memory capacity. In (a), subjects were instructed to remember the orientations of only the red items and to ignore the blue items. There were three trial types: two red items alone, four red items alone, and two red items intermixed with two blue distractors. In (b), the CDA amplitude indicates that low-capacity subjects encoded the irrelevant items along with the red items, whereas high-capacity subjects encoded only the red items. In (c), the filtering efficiency measures how similar the CDA amplitude in the distractor condition is to the amplitude in the conditions without distractors. Perfectly efficient attentional filtering would result in equivalent amplitudes for the distractor condition and the two-item condition, resulting in an efficiency score of 1. As memory capacity increases, filtering efficiency also increases ($r = 0.69$). Adapted from Vogel EK, McCollough AW, and Machizawa MG (2005) Neural measures reveal individual differences in controlling access to working memory. *Nature* 438: 500–503.

storage was for irrelevant information. Together, these results suggest that individual differences in WM capacity may actually be the consequence of the attentional control process that determines what information is stored in memory and whether distractions can be resisted rather than the consequence of how much information can be held at one time.

See also: Attentional Functions in Learning and Memory; Cognition: An Overview of Neuroimaging Techniques; Executive Function and Higher-Order Cognition: Neuroimaging; Multiple Memory Systems; Short Term and Working Memory; Spatial Cognition and Executive Function; Strategic Control of Memory; Visual Associative Memory.

Further Reading

Alvarez GA and Cavanagh P (2004) The capacity of visual short-term memory is set by both the visual information load and by number of objects. *Psychological Science* 15(2): 106–111.

Baddeley AD (1986) *Working Memory.* Oxford: Clarendon.

Cowan N (2001) The magical number 4 in short-term memory: A reconsideration of mental storage capacity. *Behavioral and Brain Sciences* 24: 87–185.

Cowan N, Elliott EM, Saults JS, et al. (2005) On the capacity of attention: Its estimation and its role in working memory and cognitive aptitudes. *Cognitive Psychology* 51: 42–100.

Daneman M and Carpenter PA (1980) Individual differences in working memory and reading. *Journal of Verbal Learning and Verbal Behavior* 19: 450–466.

Engle RW (2001) What is working-memory capacity? In: Roediger HL and Nairne JS (eds.) *The Nature of Remembering: Essays in Honor of Robert G. Crowder*, pp. 297–314. Washington, DC: American Psychological Association.

Fuster JM and Alexander GE (1971) Neuron activity related to short-term memory. *Science* 173: 652–654.

Kane MJ, Bleckley MK, Conway AR, and Engle RW (2001) A controlled attention view of working memory capacity. *Journal of Experimental Psychology: General* 130: 169–183.

Luck SJ and Vogel EK (1997) The capacity of visual working memory for features and conjunctions. *Nature* 390: 279–281.

Miller GA (1956) The magical number seven, plus or minus two: Some limits on our capacity for processing information. *Psychological Review* 63: 81–97.

Miyake A and Shah P (eds.) (1999) *Models of Working Memory: Mechanisms of Active Maintenance and Executive Control.* New York: Cambridge University Press.

Rypma B and D'Esposito MD (1999) The roles of prefrontal brain regions in components of working memory. *Proceedings of the National Academy of Sciences of the United States of America* 96: 6558–6563.

Sperling G (1960) The information available in brief visual presentations. *Psychological Monographs* 74(11; whole no. 498): 1–29.

Todd JJ and Marois R (2004) Capacity limit of visual short-term memory in human posterior parietal cortex. *Nature* 428: 751–754.

Vogel EK and Machizawa MG (2004) Neural activity predicts individual differences in visual working memory capacity. *Nature* 428: 748–751.

Vogel EK, McCollough AW, and Machizawa MG (2005) Neural measures reveal individual differences in controlling access to working memory. *Nature* 438: 500–503.

半球特化

Brain Asymmetry: Evolution

A W Toga, K L Narr, P M Thompson, and E Luders, University of California at Los Angeles School of Medicine, Los Angeles, CA, USA

The structural and functional specialization of the two cerebral hemispheres has warranted a tremendous amount of research during the past century. A number of everyday occurrences, whether we are consciously aware of them or not, provide evidence for asymmetrical behavioral traits: the foot preference of the snowboarder, the ear preference of the cell phone user, or the inclination for most people to use their right hands for fine motor activities. Neuroimaging and lesion studies of the brain confirm hemispheric specialization (or lateralization) for specific behavioral functions and show pronounced asymmetries in the structure of some brain regions in the two hemispheres.

Behavioral Traits: Language and Handedness

The most recognized manifestations of functional lateralization are the dominance of the left hemisphere for handedness and language. Approximately 90% of the population is right-handed, with the motor control of the right hand confined to brain regions in the left hemisphere that include the precentral gyrus or primary motor cortices. Observations that language is more severely impaired in response to tumors or strokes in the left hemisphere, as first reported by nineteenth-century anatomists Broca and Wernicke, also confirm that language functions are lateralized to the left hemisphere in most individuals. Specifically, the brain regions supporting language production and some aspects of syntactic processing are localized primarily in anterior left hemisphere regions that include the opercular and triangular sections of the inferior frontal gyrus (Broca's area). Language comprehension, such as understanding spoken words, is processed in the left posterior section of the superior temporal gyrus and around the temporoparietal junction (Wernicke's area). Interestingly, language dominance and handedness are not perfectly correlated. Approximately 97% of right-handers have their speech and language localized in the left hemisphere, whereas 3% demonstrate right hemisphere lateralization or bilateral language representation. These relationships degrade to 70% (right-lateralized) versus 30% (left-lateralized) in left-handed individuals.

Structural Asymmetries

Asymmetric behavioral traits and functional lateralization appear to be accompanied by hemispheric differences in brain structure. Although cursory examination of the human brain fails to expose profound left–right differences, more careful comparisons of the two hemispheres reveal a variety of asymmetric features. Macroscopic asymmetries (e.g., of fissurization) are complemented by microscopic asymmetries (e.g., of dendritic arborization) and by neurochemical asymmetries (e.g., in dopaminergic sensitivity). The first structural hemispheric differences were described in the late 1800s. They were macroscopic and concerned regions surrounding the Sylvian fissure, a deep sulcus on the lateral surface of the brain which separates the temporal lobe from the frontal and parietal lobe. Subsequently, increasingly more features of the brain have been shown as structurally asymmetric. Findings based on simple visual inspections have been confirmed and complemented by observations from manual region-of-interest analyses and from contemporary computational image analysis methods that allow whole-brain measurements. However, the results across laboratories are not always consistent, and the functional significance of structural asymmetries is not always obvious or agreed upon.

Petalias and Related Asymmetries

Among the most prominent observations of brain asymmetry are the right frontal and left occipital protrusions of the surface of one hemisphere relative to the other (**Figure 1**). These protrusions also induce imprints on the inner skull surface, known as petalias. Several studies have shown that these petalias are more prominent in right-handers. A second feature, sometimes regarded as separate from the frontal and occipital protrusions, is that the right frontal region is often wider than the left, whereas the left occipital region is often wider than the right (**Figure 1**). Another related prominent geometric distortion of the hemispheres is known as Yakovlevian anticlockwise torque. This prenatally established pattern encompasses the features described previously and includes the frequent extension of the left occipital lobe across the midline (over the right occipital lobe), bending the interhemispheric fissure toward the right (**Figure 1**). As a consequence, structures surrounding the right Sylvian fissure are also torqued forward relative to their counterparts on the left.

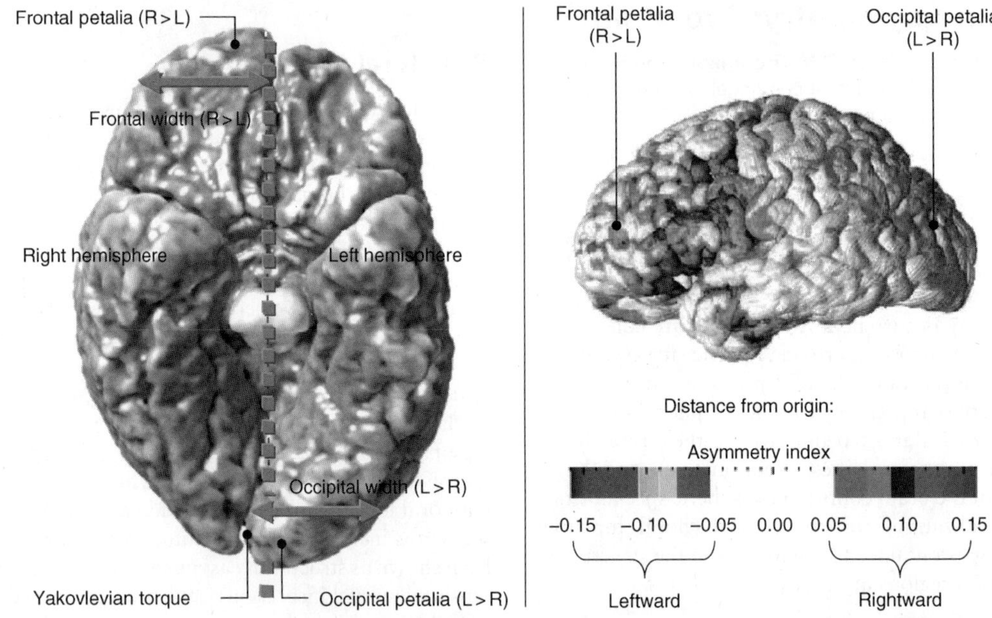

Figure 1 Petalia asymmetry. (Left) A three-dimensional rendering of the inferior surface of the human brain exaggerated to illustrate prominent asymmetries found in the gross anatomy of the two brain hemispheres. Noticeable protrusions of the hemispheres, anteriorly (R > L) and posteriorly (L > R), are observed, as well as differences in the widths of the frontal (R > L) and occipital lobes (L > R). A twisting effect is also observed, known as Yakovlevian torque, in which the left occipital lobe is splayed across midline and skews the interhemispheric fissure in a rightward direction. (Right) The magnitude and direction of hemispheric shape differences, which are estimated by measuring distances from a central point (origin) in the brain to thousands of spatially equivalent cortical surface locations in each hemisphere and by comparing these distances using an asymmetry index. The color scale illustrates anterior protrusions of hemispheric shape in the right hemisphere and posterior protrusions of hemispheric shape in the left hemisphere in one individual.

Sylvian Fissure and Related Asymmetries

At the posterior limit, the right Sylvian fissure curves upward more anteriorly than the left Sylvian fissure in the majority of brains. The Sylvian fissure also typically follows a steeper trajectory in the right hemisphere, whereas it extends further posteriorly and is longer in horizontal length in the left hemisphere (**Figure 2**). In addition to shape asymmetries in the Sylvian fissure, neuroscientists have noted that on the superior surface of the temporal lobe, buried within the Sylvian fissure, there is typically only one transverse gyrus in the left hemisphere, whereas there are two on the right. These transverse gyri (Heschl's gyri) constitute primary auditory cortex. In addition, the extent or area of the cortical surface posterior to the first gyrus of Heschl, a brain region known as the planum temporale (PT), exhibits a hemisphere-specific gross morphology. The PT, a structure involved in the analysis of sound amplitude and frequency, is commonly observed as larger in the left hemisphere. This leftward asymmetry appears to be related to the degree of handedness, with right-handers exhibiting stronger leftward asymmetries than left-handers. Finally, Broca's area (the pars opercularis and pars triangularis of the inferior frontal gyrus, respectively) has been shown to be larger in volume in the left hemisphere than its homolog in the right hemisphere, although opposing results exist.

Notably, the structural asymmetries of Heschl's gyri, the PT, and Broca's area – all brain regions involved in auditory processing or speech perception and production – might constitute the anatomical substrate for language lateralization. In support of this hypothesis, investigators have observed that verbal fluency and the asymmetry of the pars triangularis are correlated in subjects with above average intelligence. In addition, language lateralization appears to follow the direction of the PT asymmetry. Moreover, others have demonstrated a strong leftward PT asymmetry among subjects with left hemisphere speech representation but no consistent PT asymmetry among subjects with right hemisphere speech representation in a sample of left-handers only.

Central Sulcus and Related Asymmetries

The postcentral gyrus is shown to exhibit structural hemispheric asymmetries in the majority of individuals, where the trajectory of the postcentral sulcus

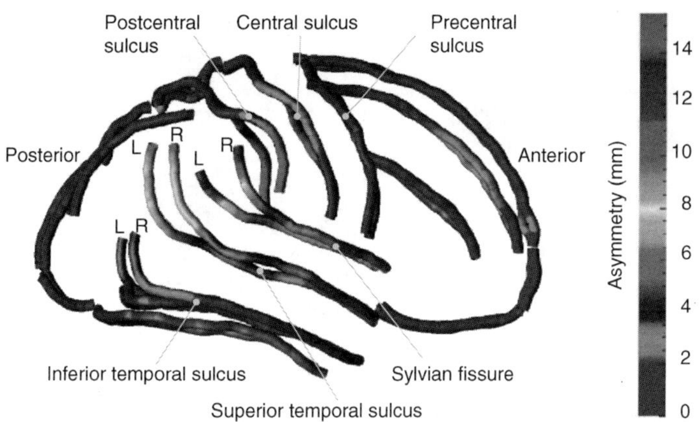

Figure 2 Sulcal asymmetry. From a lateral view, the average shape of the major sulci and fissures for 15 subjects are shown for both the left and the right hemisphere by looking through the brain. The color bar further indexes the magnitude of shape differences between matching sulci in each hemisphere. Note the typical hemispheric differences of the Sylvian fissure (longer in the left (L) and steeper and curving upward more anteriorly in the right (R)), where these asymmetries are largely mirrored in the superior and inferior temporal sulci. Finally, the trajectory of the postcentral sulcus appears to shift more anteriorly in the right hemisphere as opposed to the left hemisphere.

appears to shift more anteriorly in the right hemisphere as opposed to the left (**Figure 2**). This asymmetry may be associated with slope and horizontal length asymmetries of the Sylvian fissure and temporal sulci and may reflect asymmetries in the parietal operculum that complement PT asymmetries in right-handed subjects.

Whereas some neuroscientists have reported that the central sulcus is generally deeper and larger in the right hemisphere, other investigators have observed a rightward asymmetry of the central sulcus in left-handers only, or even a pronounced leftward asymmetry in right-handers. In fact, this latter macrostructural leftward asymmetry was complemented by a microstructural leftward asymmetry in neuropil volume (i.e., tissue compartment containing dendrites, axons, and synapses) in the primary motor cortex located in the precentral gyrus.

Other asymmetries have been detected in subcortical regions that are more proximal to the motor effectors. For example, the right cortical spinal tract is found to be larger than the left in 75% of subjects, and the left pyramid crosses more rostrally and is larger than the right in 82–87% of subjects. Possibly related to asymmetries in regions that supplement motor function, a rightward asymmetry in callosal regions that contain predominantly projections from the motor cortices (e.g., callosal anterior body) has been reported. Finally, anterior cerebellar volumes have been observed as larger in the right hemisphere, whereas posterior cerebellar volumes are reported as larger in the left.

Ventricular Asymmetries

Some hemispheric differences in brain structure may go unnoticed in individual subjects due to the high intersubject variability of anatomy. Population-based brain atlases overcome this problem by averaging three-dimensional models of anatomy across hundreds, or even thousands, of subjects while storing statistics on anatomic variation. Ventricular asymmetry is an example of a statistically significant effect that becomes clear in a group average brain map but is not universally apparent in individual subjects. As demonstrated in **Figure 3**, the left lateral ventricle is typically wider and larger than the right, and the left posterior horn is longer in normal adults. This finding is consistent with volumetric measures and may reflect rapid, asymmetric growth in the overlying language systems; it can occasionally be seen in the embryonic brain, using ultrasound, as early as 29–31 weeks postconception.

Tissue Component Asymmetries

Investigators have also examined the asymmetry of brain tissue compartments; they observed significant hemispheric differences of gray matter (GM) in frontal, temporal, parietal, and occipital regions, that include Heschl's gyrus, the PT, the amygdala, and the hippocampus ($L > R$), as well as in inferior and medial temporal gyrus regions, the lateral thalamus, and the anterior cingulum ($R > L$). Recent analyses have shown hemispheric differences with respect to the thickness of the cortex, where some regions

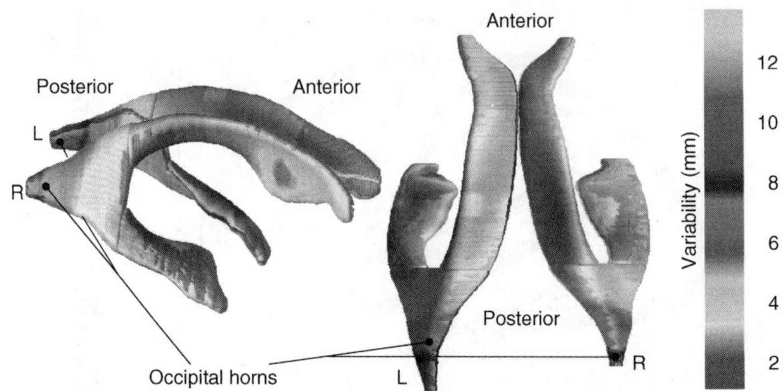

Figure 3 Ventricular asymmetry. The anatomy of the lateral ventricles is shown across subjects ($N = 40$) in three-dimensional view. These maps of average ventricular anatomy show that the left ventricle is larger than the right ventricle. The anatomic asymmetry is clearly localized to the occipital horn, which extends (on average) 5.1 mm more posteriorly on the left than the right. This is consistent with the petalia and torque effects described previously. This asymmetry may go unnoticed in individual subjects due to the high intersubject variability of anatomy.

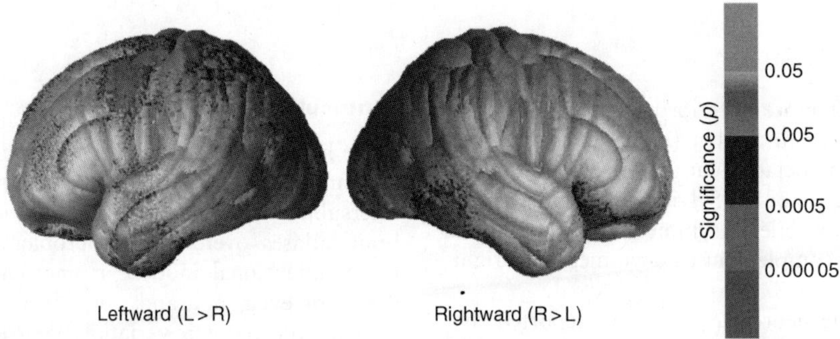

Figure 4 Cortical thickness asymmetry. Statistical maps demonstrating significant hemispheric differences of cortical thickness in a large sample of subjects ($N = 60$). The left brain demonstrates leftward (L > R) asymmetries in the anterior temporal lobe, including the inferior, middle, and superior temporal gyri and the precentral gyrus extending anteriorly to adjacent regions. Two additional larger clusters favoring the left are apparent in the middle frontal gyrus and superior parietal lobe (extending more diffusely inferiorly, covering the inferior parietal lobe and supramarginal gyrus). Smaller clusters of leftward asymmetry are evident in superior frontal regions very close to the midline extending along the longitudinal fissure and in the orbital gyrus. The right brain demonstrates significant rightward asymmetries (R > L) in the posterior inferior temporal lobe and inferior frontal gyrus (comprising the pars orbitalis, triangularis, and opercularis and extending into the extreme anterior tip of the temporal lobe) and near the frontal pole. In general, leftward asymmetries are spread over larger regions than rightward asymmetries.

exhibit pronounced thickness asymmetries that resemble GM asymmetries while other regions reveal distinct asymmetries (**Figure 4**).

Determining Factors of Brain Asymmetries

Heredity versus Environment

Perisylvian asymmetries are already present in children. Their magnitude, however, appears to increase throughout childhood and the teenage years, even after adjusting for developmental increases in brain volume. This suggests that there may be hemispheric differences in white matter maturation, perhaps during the many regional growth spurts in myelination that occur in childhood. It is not certain which factors determine the initiation or amplification of cerebral asymmetries. It appears unlikely that hemispheric differences are solely genetically predetermined. For example, an individual's genotype may not be the only determinant for laterality because many identical twins are discordant for handedness and differ considerably in their expression of PT asymmetry. However, genetic factors appear to influence hemispheric volumes twice as strongly in right-handed twin pairs than in twin pairs with at least one left-hander (non-right-handers). Investigators have hypothesized that the decrement in genetic control of cerebral volumes in non-right-handed twin pairs supports the existence of a 'right-shift' genotype in the majority of the population (expressed as a right hand/left hemisphere bias) that is lost in non-right-handers. Thus, genes appear to be significant contributors to brain and behavioral asymmetries, where the degree of genetic determination also depends on brain structure. For example, GM volumes in perisylvian areas are reported to be under predominantly genetic control, whereas gyral and sulcal patterns have been demonstrated as much less heritable. A number of potential nongenetic contributors to variations in brain asymmetry, including fetal orientation, hormones, and functional adaptations, are discussed later. In addition, gender-specific asymmetries and disturbances in asymmetries as may be associated with some specific diseases are explained.

Fetal Orientation

Asymmetric influences in the prenatal environment may lead to perceptual and motor asymmetries. Two-thirds of fetuses are confined to a leftward fetal position in the third trimester, with their right side facing outward. Lateralization of language perception may result from asymmetries in their auditory experience. For example, the right ear may be better positioned to discriminate high-frequency speech sounds. It has also been argued that asymmetrical vestibular stimulation *in utero* may produce behavioral motor asymmetries later in life. Finally, the exposure to ultrasound in fetal life has been suggested to increase the chances of being left-handed by approximately 30%.

Hormones

In male rats, the right neocortex is thicker than the left. Female rats, on the other hand, display a non-significant trend toward the opposite pattern. Notably, castration at birth, which prevents the flow of androgens from the testis to the brain, blocks the formation of the normal rightward brain asymmetry in male rats. Similarly, neonatal ovariectomy reverses the female pattern to the male pattern. Interestingly, maternal environmental or nutritional stress has been demonstrated to reverse the male-typical asymmetry in fetal male rats to the female pattern by both shifting and depressing a testosterone surge that normally occurs on gestational day 18. These findings suggest that levels of androgenic and ovarian sex steroids, before and after birth, play a role in modulating brain asymmetry, at least in rodents.

In humans, the hormonal determinants for sex-specific symmetries are less understood. In their widely cited theory of cerebral lateralization, Geschwind and Galaburda suggested that elevated testosterone levels might be responsible for deviations from the normal dominance pattern (i.e., right-handedness and leftward language dominance, as well as rightward visuospatial dominance). According to this theory, if testosterone levels are higher than normal *in utero*, consequences include a smaller left hemisphere and even anomalous dominance due to a delay of left-hemispheric growth. This model has been posited to explain the different maturational rates of the sexes (with females generally maturing faster) and also to explain the relative advantage males show for right hemisphere visuospatial tasks and that females show for left hemisphere linguistic tasks. It has also been used to explain the greater incidence of left-handedness in males. Finally, hormonal influences might largely determine gender-specific structural asymmetries, as outlined next.

Gender-Specific Asymmetries

Gender differences in structural asymmetries, with larger interhemispheric differences in males compared to females, have been widely replicated where sex-dependent patterns appear to be complemented by behavioral and neuroactivational scores. To explain greater functional lateralization in men compared to women, it has been suggested that either the functions of the hemispheres are less sharply differentiated in women than in men or, alternatively, that larger commissural systems in women may act to reduce the difference in lateralized response scores between hemispheres. Sex differences in brain organization, both within and between hemispheres, are thought to underlie sex differences in motor and visuospatial skills, linguistic performance, and vulnerability to deficits following stroke and other focal lesions.

With emphasis on structural asymmetries, a larger right hemisphere volume has been identified in male fetuses, but no equivalent pattern has been reported in adults. Other studies have shown a significantly deeper central sulcus in the left hemisphere than in the right, but only in male right-handers; interhemispheric asymmetry was reported absent in female right-handers. Similarly, a larger leftward GM asymmetry in males compared to females has been observed in a region posterior to the central sulcus. Possibly related to these findings, pronounced rightward parasagittal asymmetries have been detected in the anterior callosal body in males but appear to a much lesser degree in females (**Figure 5**). Other

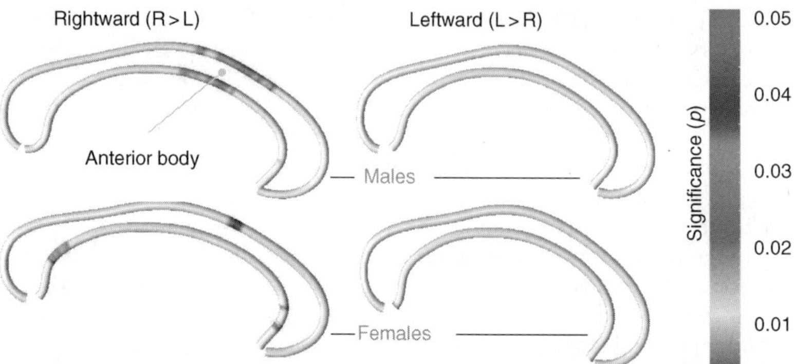

Figure 5 Callosal asymmetry. Statistical maps demonstrating significant gender-specific asymmetries in a large sample of subjects (30 men and 30 women). Differences between callosal thicknesses were measured in the left and right hemispheres several millimeters apart from the midsagittal plane. Rightward asymmetries are largely increased in men, supporting the assumption of a sexually dimorphic organization of male and female brains that involves hemispheric relations and is reflected in the organization and distribution of callosal fibers.

observations of sexually dimorphic cerebral asymmetries include pronounced rightward asymmetries of the planum parietale in right-handed men compared to right-handed women, whereas left-handed subjects demonstrate the opposite pattern. Gender-dependent asymmetries of the inferior parietal lobe and PT, with males having significantly larger leftward asymmetries and females showing reversed, diminished, or no asymmetries, have also been reported. Greater lateralization of right frontal petalias (in right-handers and left-handers) and occipital petalias (in left-handers only) in men compared to women further confirm previous findings of greater frontal and occipital asymmetries in men and reductions of the typical asymmetries in women.

Although the majority of studies suggest diminished asymmetries in female brains, a number of studies also exist that either failed to detect significant gender effects with respect to hemispheric differences or revealed even more pronounced asymmetries in females. A study that analyzed hemispheric differences with respect to the thickness of the cortex observed asymmetry profiles that were similar in both sexes. Notwithstanding, hemispheric differences appeared slightly pronounced in males compared to females, albeit a few regions also indicated greater asymmetry in females compared to males.

Functional Adaptation

Experience-dependent plasticity and asymmetric behaviors may also induce different neuronal changes in the two hemispheres. In rats, the asymmetric use of only one forelimb in the postweaning period induces an asymmetrically larger neuropil volume and lower cell packing density in the motor cortex. In mice with a hereditary asymmetry in their whisker pads, a dominant right whisker pad has been associated with left paw preference. Limb preference may therefore be associated with asymmetries in sensory input, although it is not known whether this relationship is causal.

In humans, professional right-handed keyboard players who had received intensive bimanual training from early childhood are more symmetrical in hand skill tests. Moreover, the absolute length of the central sulcus appears related to the age of commencement of musical training such that those musicians who had started early in life with musical training exhibited the longest sulcus on both sides. These findings suggest that some brain asymmetries are not necessarily genetically determined and may result from lateralized motoric activity and/or sensory stimulation.

Aberrant Asymmetries and Disease

Reduced or even inverted volume asymmetries of the PT have been reported in some subjects with reading disorders or developmental dyslexia, as well as in some people with unusual right-hemispheric dominance for speech. Analogously, functional magnetic resonance imaging studies have shown a pattern of brain activation in stutterers that is shifted toward the right in both motor and auditory language areas. This may suggest an inherent difference in the way in which normal subjects and stutterers process language.

Controversy surrounds reports of altered brain asymmetry in schizophrenia. For example, it has been proposed that altered anatomical and functional asymmetries in schizophrenia constitute a genetic and evolutionary basis for the disease that has developed in concert with hemispheric specialization for language. It has also been suggested that schizophrenia

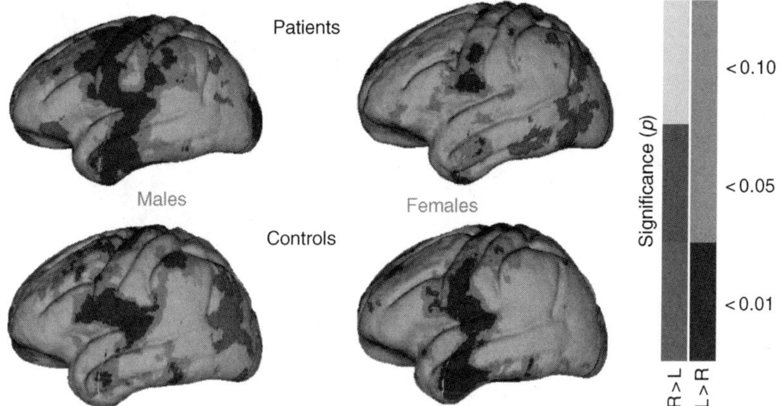

Figure 6 Cortical thickness asymmetry in schizophrenia. Statistical maps show significant hemispheric differences in cortical thickness within groups defined by sex and a diagnosis of schizophrenia ($N = 150$). The patterns of cortical thickness asymmetries appear similar in all groups (leftward asymmetries of thickness in sensorimotor and perisylvian cortices and rightward cortical thickness asymmetries in posterior temporoparietal cortices). Notably, these patterns were not shown to differ statistically in patients with schizophrenia compared to demographically similar healthy comparison subjects.

is due to an anomaly of cerebral dominance, in which an agnosic right shift gene is suggested to be a major contributor toward schizophrenia pathophysiology. Observations of altered structural asymmetries in patients with schizophrenia include the reversal of normal petalias; disproportionately reduced left hemisphere temporal lobe volumes; reduced asymmetries of the PT, the superior temporal gyrus, and the Sylvian fissure; and alterations in hemispheric gyrification indices. Findings indicating intact structural lateralization in schizophrenia, however, are not uncommon. For example, one study failed to detect schizophrenia-related changes in cortical thickness asymmetries in a large sample of schizophrenia patients compared to demographically similar healthy comparison subjects (**Figure 6**). Thickness asymmetries, however, were shown to vary by disease status in non-dextrals.

Some diseases appear to progress asymmetrically. Patients with semantic dementia generally show asymmetric anterolateral temporal atrophy (typically worse on the left side) with relative sparing of the hippocampal formation. In Alzheimer's disease, a spreading wave of GM loss emerges initially in entorhinal and temporal-parietal cortices, sweeping into frontal and ultimately sensorimotor territory as the disease progresses. This sequence occurs in both hemispheres, but left hemisphere regions are affected earlier and more severely. The right hemisphere follows a similar pattern approximately 2 years later (**Figure 7**). Furthermore, cerebrospinal fluid volumes in the Sylvian fissure appear to rise more sharply on the left than the right in patients with dementia compared to normal controls. Additional left-greater-than-right metabolic dysfunctions in a group of patients with early dementia have been observed using positron emission tomography. These disease-related asymmetries suggest either that the left hemisphere is more susceptible than the right to neurodegeneration in Alzheimer's disease or that left hemisphere pathology results in greater structural change and lobar metabolic deficits.

Evolutionary Origins of Anatomical Asymmetries

Brain Size Expansion

Increasing brain size in humans is possibly one of the driving forces in the phylogeny of hemispheric specialization. For example, it has been suggested that the massive evolutionary expansion of the brain may have resulted in a level of complexity where duplication of structures was no longer efficient. Functional incompatibility or the need for simultaneous parallel processing related to increasing cognitive capacities during the course of evolution might also constitute driving forces for the emergence of functionally separated systems. Due to competition for space within the brain, different functions might have been confined to different hemispheres (rather than to different networks within a hemisphere). As a possible consequence, the right hemisphere in humans outperforms the left in the analysis of spatial relations and also shows a tendency for global processes (e.g., with respect to attention and memory storage). The left hemisphere,

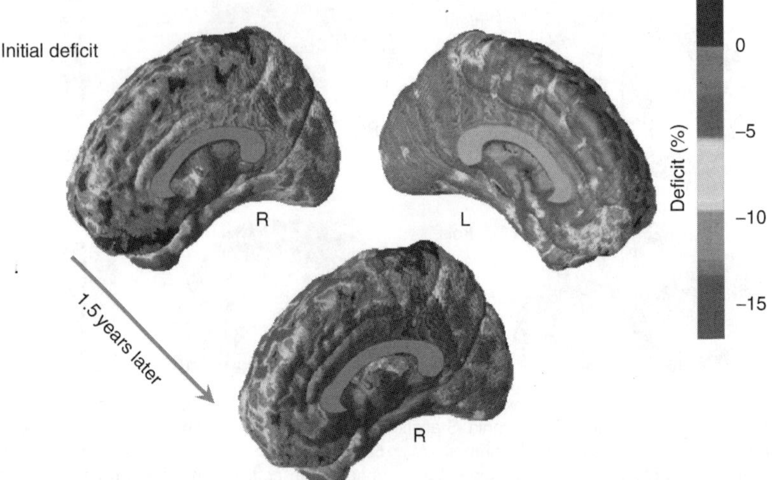

Figure 7 Asymmetrical progression of Alzheimer's disease. These maps show the average profile of GM loss in a group of patients with mild to moderate Alzheimer's disease ($N = 17$) compared to a group of healthy age- and gender-matched controls ($N = 14$). Initially, the right hemisphere (R) is much less severely affected than the left (L), but after 1.5 years the deficit progresses to encompass more of the right hemisphere.

on the other hand, is specialized in language and shows superiority in categorizing (as opposed to global processing).

Time limits associated with the transfer of information across the corpus callosum between the brain hemispheres may also favor development of unilateral networks in larger brains. It has been reported that more asymmetrical brains have a corpus callosum with a reduced midsagittal area relative to more symmetrical ones. In addition, there exists an inverse relationship between forebrain size and relative callosal size accounting for relatively smaller callosal areas in larger brains. Since smaller callosal areas may reflect fewer or thinner fibers connecting the two hemispheres, this suggests the degree of interhemispheric connectedness decreases with increased brain size.

Left-Hemispheric Dominance for Language

The evolutionary development of language in humans may have led to marked volume asymmetries in structures crucial for speech production and perception as well as for motor dominance. For example, in humans, the left PT – an extension of Wernicke's posterior receptive language area – is up to 10 times larger than its right hemisphere counterpart and is perhaps the most functionally significant human brain asymmetry. Language is commonly lateralized to the left hemisphere, and some argue that this is advantageous: (1) it avoids competition between hemispheres for control of the muscles involved in speech, and (2) it may be more efficient to transfer language information between collections of focal areas in a single hemisphere. The main pitfall in arguing that left hemisphere dominance provides an evolutionary advantage is that bilateral language representation, or rightward dominance, is also common. In addition, leftward dominance does not, in general, provide a cognitive advantage.

Left-Hemispheric Dominance for Handedness

A hypothesis first proposed by Condillac in 1746 suggests that the left hemisphere's dominance for language processing evolved from its control of the right hand. The left-hemispheric programming of skilled movement and gesture may have evolved to encompass control of the motor systems involved in speech. Broca's area, in particular, is a premotor module that sequences complex articulations that are not limited to speech. Great apes, including chimpanzees and gorillas, also have an enlarged area 44 (Broca's area). This area controls muscles of the face and vocal tract but is not as well connected with the homolog of Wernicke's area as it is in humans. It has been suggested that nonhuman primates developed a homolog of Broca's area due to a link between primate vocalization and gesture: captive apes usually gesture with the right hand as they vocalize. Research on indigenous gestural languages invented by children in Taiwan and in Nicaragua provides some evidence for the innate relation between gesture and language. Functional neuroimaging studies also suggest that deaf subjects using a gestural sign language activate many of the systems involved in verbal language production. These congruencies in functional anatomy may support the hypothesis that verbal language evolved from gestural language as an outgrowth of the already asymmetric motor control system. It was proposed that language is a relatively recent evolutionary adaptation (not more than 200 000 years old), where the Neanderthal vocal tract was incapable of articulating the range of modern human speech sounds.

Brain Asymmetries in Nonhuman Species

Functional asymmetries in the brain were initially thought to be uniquely human, reflecting unique processing demands required to produce and comprehend language. Nonetheless, functional and structural asymmetries have been identified in nonhuman primates and many other species. For example, Japanese macaques exhibit a right ear advantage for processing auditory stimuli, passerine birds produce song primarily under left hemisphere control, and frogs utilize their left hemisphere to control clasping vocalizations. Moreover, with respect to structural asymmetries, cerebral petalias are seen in phylogenetically older primates (and other species), as evidenced by endocasts from fossilized cranial bones. Similarly, the PT asymmetry also appears in higher nonhuman primates. In most great apes, the Sylvian fissure is longer and straighter on the left side than on the right. It has also been observed that the right hemisphere is generally larger than the left in rats, mice, rabbits, and cats. Although asymmetries in nonhuman species can be strikingly similar to those in humans, asymmetries defined in animal studies may not be easy to extrapolate to humans because the precursors of language-related asymmetries in humans may not be present in other species. The mechanisms that underlie some cerebral asymmetries in humans might differ substantially from those that underpin brain asymmetry in other mammals. Notwithstanding, the existence of hemispheric differences in nonhumans indicates that brain asymmetry is neither unique to humans nor completely dependent on the development of language.

Acknowledgments

This work was supported by NIBIB/NINDS/NIMG grant P01 EB001955 and NIH/NCRR resource grant P41 RR013642. Additional support was provided by the National Institutes of Health through the NIH Roadmap for Medical Research grant U54 RR021813. Additional support was also provided by the National Institute of Mental Health grant K01 MH073990.

See also: Brain Damage: Functional Reorganization; Brain Injury: Functional Recovery After; Brain Connectivity and Brain Size; Brain Development: The Generation of Large Brains; Dichotic Listening Studies of Brain Asymmetry; Hemispheric Specialization and Cognition.

Further Reading

Galaburda AM and Geschwind N (1981) Anatomical asymmetries in the adult and developing brain and their implications for function. *Advances in Pediatrics* 28: 271–292.

Geschwind N and Galaburda AM (1987) *Cerebral Lateralization: Biological Mechanisms, Associations, and Pathology.* Cambridge: MIT Press.

Hellige JB (1990) Hemispheric asymmetry. *Annual Review of Psychology* 41: 55–80.

Hugdahl K and Davidson RJ (2003) *The Asymmetrical Brain.* Cambridge, MA: MIT Press.

Previc FH (1991) A general theory concerning the prenatal origins of cerebral lateralization in humans. *Psychological Review* 98: 299–334.

Toga AW and Thompson PM (2003) Mapping brain asymmetry. *Nature Reviews Neuroscience* 4: 37–48.

Zilles K, Dabringhaus A, Geyer S, et al. (1996) Structural asymmetries in the human forebrain and the forebrain of non-human primates and rats. *Neuroscience and Biobehavioral Reviews* 20: 593–605.

Relevant Websites

http://www.loni.ucla.edu – Laboratory of Neuro Imaging, UCLA.

http://nihroadmap.nih.gov – National Institutes of Health Roadmap for Medical Research.

Dichotic Listening Studies of Brain Asymmetry

K Hugdahl, University of Bergen, Bergen, Norway

Dichotic Stimuli

The stimuli typically used in dichotic listening (DL) studies consist of presentations of pairwise combinations of consonant–vowel (CV) syllables that are made up of the six stop-consonants /b/, /d/, /g/, /p/, /t/, and /k/, and the vowel /a/.Thus, examples of DL stimulus pairs are /ba/–/pa/, /ga/–/pa/, and so on. Another often-used variant of the DL test is the so-called fused rhymed words test. These stimuli are computer synthesized and consist of consonant-vowel-consonant (CVC) pairs. The stimuli are synthesized so that the nondistinctive components of each pair are identical (e.g., /aba/–/aka/). The temporal and auditory spectral overlap between numbers of each pair in this test is so great that they fuse into a single auditory percept.

The Dichotic Test Situation

Preparation of dichotic stimulus materials requires computer editing on each trial of the two CV syllables. The most important aspect of the editing procedure is the synchronization of the onset of the energy release in the two syllables in a pair. The syllables are synchronized on both the consonant and vowel segments, which usually requires access to speech synthesis analysis capability. **Figure 1** shows a computer display of the syllables /ba/ (top) and /pa/ (bottom) that are synchronized on both the consonant and vowel onset.

DL Paradigms

The most commonly used paradigms in DL laterality studies are the free-report paradigm, the forced-attention paradigm, the fused-rhymed paradigm, and the target-monitoring paradigm. In the free-report paradigm, individuals are required to report the items that they heard on each trial as accurately as possible. Only those trials in which a person can identify one item, but not the other, correctly reveal information about brain laterality. Thus, as a general rule, only single-correct trials should be analyzed. An alternative is to instruct the person to answer only for one item on each trial. The experimenter then calculates number of correct reports from the right and left ears, separately. The free-report paradigm requires that the person has intact speech and can give an oral answer. Thus, the free-report paradigm is less well suited for the study of laterality in clinical populations with speech dysfunctions.

In the target-monitoring paradigm, some of the items in the list to be presented are selected as 'targets,' and the person is instructed to indicate (manually or orally) whenever he/she detects a target. Usually CVC syllables or words are used in the target-monitoring paradigm. The target-monitoring paradigm has the advantage that it can be used also with persons who lack expressive speech.

The fused-rhymed paradigm is similar to the free-report paradigm except for the important distinction that the two sounds presented at the ears fuse into a coherent perceptual unit. A characteristic of the fused-rhymed paradigm is that although individuals subjectively report that they hear only one sound, they report this to be the right-ear item.

The forced-attention paradigm allows for the study of attentional influences on brain laterality. The paradigm involves instructing the individual to pay attention only to the right ear, and report only from that ear in half of the trials, and to pay attention to and report only from the left ear in the other half of the trials. Often there is a third condition included whereby the person is not given any specific instructions. In that case, each instructional condition then applies to a third of the trials.

The Right-Ear Advantage

Irrespective of whether nonfused CV syllables or fused CVC syllables are used, the typical outcome in a standard DL test is a greater percentage of correct reports from the right ear, as compared to the left ear. This is called a right-ear advantage (REA) and is a robust empirical finding in both right- and left-handed persons. The REA is most easily seen in response to the consonant, and is difficult to observe in response to the vowel in a CV syllable. It has thus been argued that the REA might reflect hemisphere specialization for rapidly changing auditory stimuli, such as the rapid formant transition seen in the stop consonants. **Figure 2** shows the distributions for correctly reported items from the right-ear (red) and left-ear (blue) stimuli from 694 right-handed adults. Note the apparent shift to the right for the right-ear stimulus distribution.

Attentional Factors

DL also indicates dynamic laterality factors, such as attention, which may modulate a structurally based

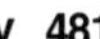

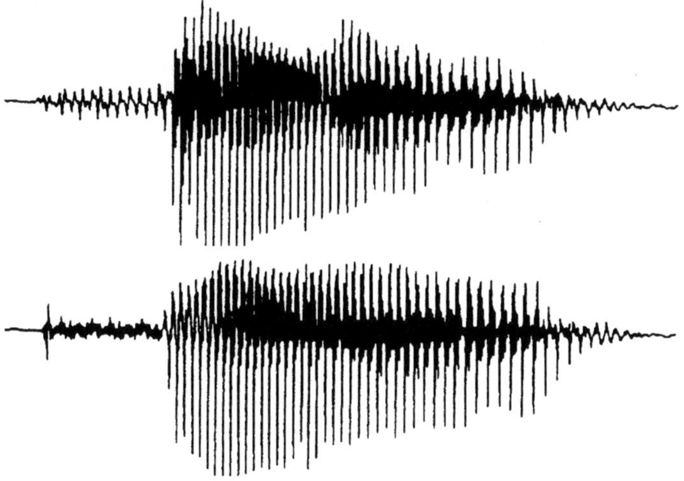

Figure 1 Computer display of the CV syllables /ba/ (top) and /pa/ (bottom) synchronized at the energy release at both consonant and vowel onset segments.

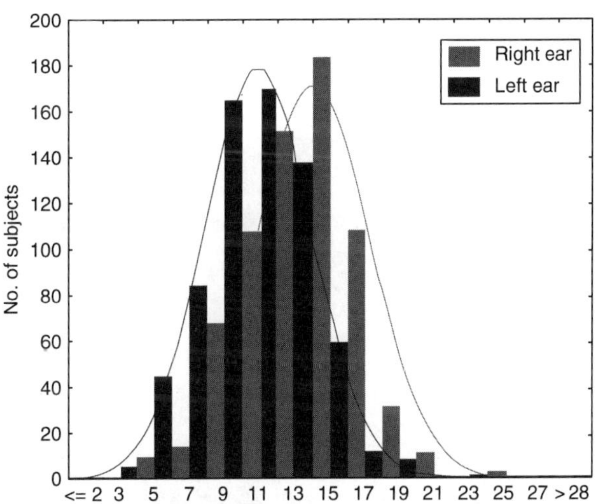

Figure 2 Number of adult study participants ('subjects'; *y*-axis) plotted against correctly reported CV syllables presented in the right ear (red distribution) and left ear (blue distribution), respectively. Data from 694 right-handed adults.

laterality when the individual shifts attention to the right or left side in auditory space. In the typical DL test, one-third of the trials involve a 'nonforced' attentional condition, where individuals are not given any particular instructions regarding deployment of attention. In one-third of the trials the person is instructed to attend to and report from the right ear (forced-right attention), and in one-third of the trials the person is instructed to attend to and report from the left ear (forced-left attention). The REA is increased during the forced-right attention condition, and a left-ear advantage (LEA) is observed during the forced-left attention condition. Thus, attentional factors can sometimes override the basic REA asymmetry, providing evidence for a 'top-down' instruction-driven modulation of a 'bottom-up' stimulus-driven laterality effect. Studies in our laboratory have, however, shown that top-down modulation is reduced in children, particularly before literacy, and in psychiatric patients. The switching of an REA to an LEA during forced-left attention is also dramatically reduced in patients with right-sided brain damage.

Neuroanatomical Basis

The REA is believed to be caused by the fact that although auditory input is transmitted to both auditory cortices in the temporal lobes, the contralateral projections are stronger and more preponderant, interfering with the ipsilateral projections. The advantage for the contralateral auditory projections means that the language-dominant left hemisphere receives a stronger signal from the right ear. The contralateral signal from the left ear to the right hemisphere must first pass the corpus callosum in other to be processed in the left hemisphere. Following the same logic, an LEA indicates the right hemisphere to be language dominant, and a no-ear advantage (NEA) indicates a bilateral language dominance.

In an O^{15}-positron emission tomography (PET) study in our laboratory using a DL target monitoring paradigm, we compared brain activation to CV syllables and musical stimuli that were presented dichotically. The CV syllables and musical stimuli showed opposite activation asymmetries in the temporal lobe. Greater activation was observed in the left superior temporal gyrus to the CV syllable stimuli, while greater activation was observed in corresponding right temporal lobe areas to the musical stimuli. Interestingly, overall activation and the intensity of activation were greater in response to the CV syllable stimuli compared with the musical stimuli. This may indicate specialized cortical networks in the left hemisphere for the processing of linguistic stimuli, also including the planum temporale area. The PET data are shown in **Figure 3**.

Validity and Reliability

The REA to dichotic presentations of CV syllables is usually about 20% in order of magnitude for oral reports, with about 50–70% correct reports from the right ear and 30–50% correct reports from the left ear. The REA is observed in about 85–90% of right-handed persons, and in about 65% of left-handed persons. The magnitude of the REA may, however, vary considerably among individuals within a given ear advantage direction. Scatterplots of DL correct reports from the right and left ears for more than 1000 persons, both children and adults, are seen in **Figure 4**.

The 85% of right-handed subjects to be identified as left-hemisphere-language dominant by the DL technique is about 10% lower than what is obtained

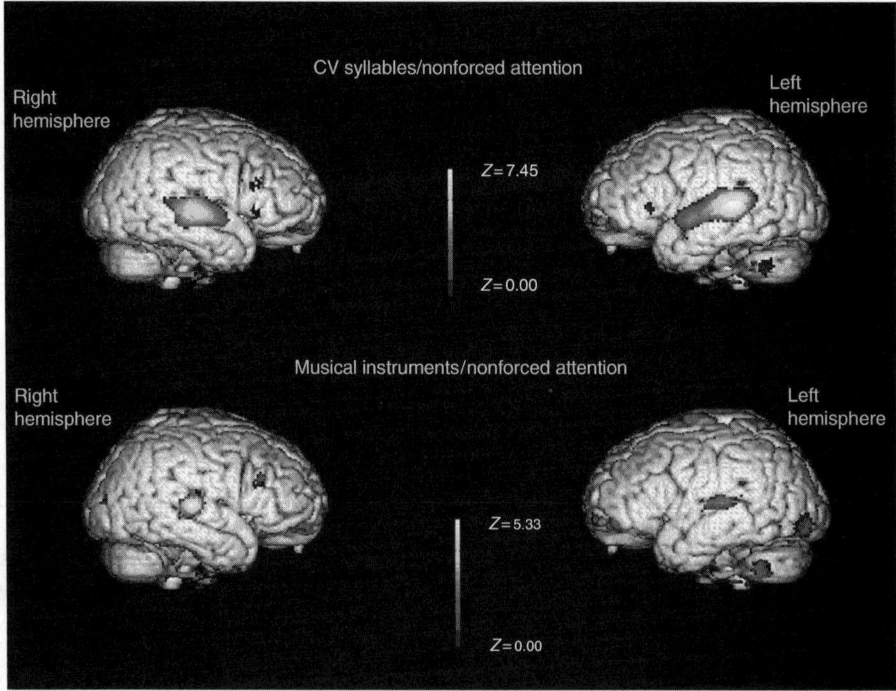

Figure 3 ^{15}O-PET brain activation data in response to CV syllables and musical stimuli. Note the leftward asymmetry for the CV syllable stimuli, and rightward asymmetry for the musical stimuli. Reproduced from Hugdahl K, Brønnick K, Law I, et al. (1999) Brain activation during dichotic presentations of consonant–vowel and musical instruments stimuli: A ^{15}O-PET study. *Neuropsychologia* 37: 431–440, with permission from Elsevier.

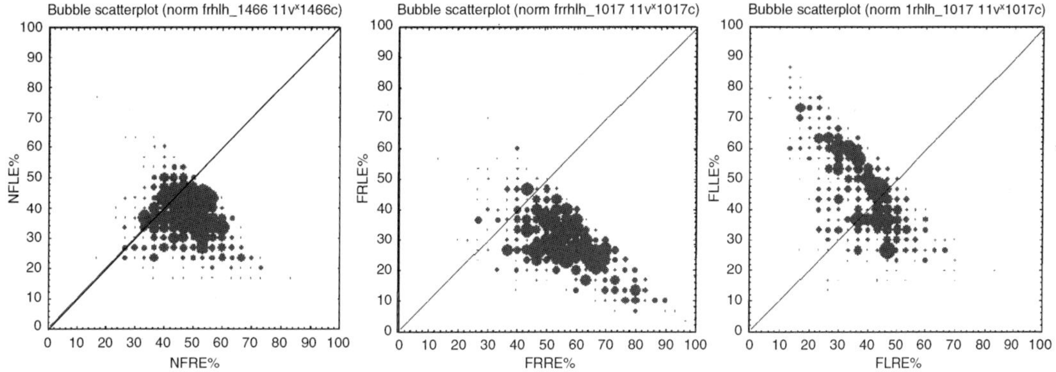

Figure 4 Scatterplots of left- and right-ear correct reports in normal right- and left-handed persons. RE%, % correct right ear reports; LE%, % correct left ear reports, NF, nonforced attention; FR, attention forced to right-ear stimulus; FL, attention forced to left-ear stimulus.

when invasive techniques, like the Wada test, are used. The Wada test involves selective injection of a barbiturate into the right or left hemisphere, 'silencing' the injected hemisphere for about 10 min. The 10% discrepancy between DL and the Wada test probably reflects that DL, in addition to indicating cortical function, also reflects subcortical thalamic influences on language lateralization. DL also picks up perceptual language laterality in addition to expressive speech laterality, whereas the Wada test is an exclusive test of speech laterality. Measures of test–retest reliability vary between 0.70 and 0.90 across different studies. The variation across studies may stem from differences in the reliability index used. However, a study from our laboratory showed that of 17 epileptic patients undergoing both the Wada test for language dominance and DL, 94% of the cases were correctly classified with the DL technique from a stepwise discriminant analysis. The DL results are shown in **Figure 5**, together with an indication of left- (blue dots) or right- (red dots) hemisphere speech according to the Wada test.

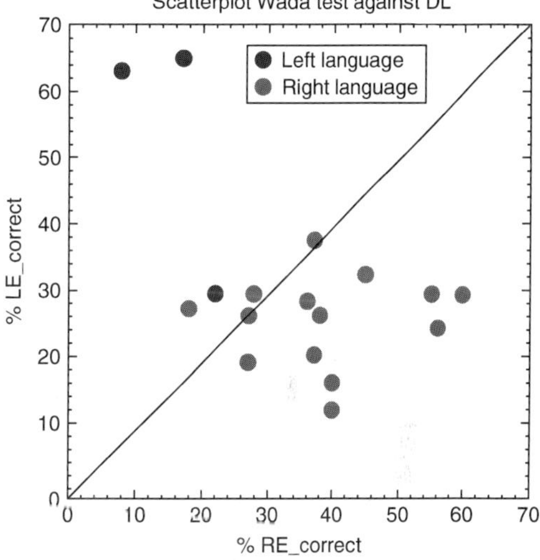

Figure 5 Wada test validation of DL scores from 17 adolescent epileptic patients. Overall, 94% of the group was correctly classified. Data courtesy of Göran Carlsson and Paul Uvebrant, Kiel, Germany, and Göteborg, Sweden.

Calculation of DL Scores

The ear advantage in DL may be calculated in different ways. The most straightforward and simple method is to calculate the number of correct reports from each ear. Since this measure does not compensate for differences in overall performance (i.e., total correct reports) among individuals, some authors favor an index score, where right-ear minus left-ear scores are divided by the sum total of left-ear plus right-ear scores. Still another way of handling DL scores is to display the number of individuals that show a particular ear advantage in scatterplots, as shown in **Figure 4**.

Arousal and Activation

DL scores may be affected by factors other than brain laterality, and it has been shown that individual differences in arousal or activation may attenuate the REA. Specifically, experimental manipulations whereby the persons are made to believe that they will receive an electric shock to their hand whenever they make an error have been shown to drastically attenuate the REA. This is probably caused by an increase in both brain stem reticular and right-hemisphere activation (right hemisphere being particularly sensitive for emotional events), which interferes with left-hemisphere processing of the contralateral right-ear signal.

Studies with the forced-attention paradigm have generally revealed that the REA is not an attentional artifact, with right-handed persons attending to the right side in space, which causes the right-ear signal to be better perceived and reported. Experimental manipulations whereby the person is explicitly instructed to turn his/her head and eyes toward the right or left side in space do not seriously affect the REA.

Developmental Effects

The REA to CV syllables can be observed in children as young as 3 years of age, and is frequently reported in 5-year-old children. The magnitude of the REA does not change with age, but stays rather constant. However, the overall level of performance increases with increasing age. Furthermore, preliterate children also report more items from the right ear during testing following instructions to focus attention to the left ear, as in the forced-attention paradigm. The constancy of the REA across different age levels is taken as an indication that brain laterality is not subject to ontogenetic development, and that it is present already at the infant stage.

Sex Differences and Handedness Effects

Males and females differ regarding several cognitive processes (language, visuospatial skills) that are differentially mediated by the left and right hemispheres. The sexes also differ in disorders related to hemisphere differences in brain function. Various disorders such as dyslexia, hyperactivity, and stuttering occur more frequently among boys than girls. Aphasia is also more commonly seen in males than in females after unilateral left-sided lesions. All this evidence points to the hypothesis that females are either less lateralized than males for certain cognitive functions, or that they have a more diffuse cortical organization for cognitive function.

Similar patterns of responding have been obtained in DL tests, with a greater proportion of males than females showing a REA to CV syllables. Males as a group also show a greater mean REA in the standard free-report DL paradigm. It is known that there are differences in cortical organization between right- and left-handers. Only about 65–70% of left-handers are left-hemisphere dominant for language, compared to 95–99% of right-handers. It then follows that right- and left-handers should also differ in their DL performance to CV syllables. Although not all studies have found significant group-mean differences in ear advantage magnitudes between handedness groups, almost every study has reported a tendency for attenuation of the REA in left-handers compared to right-handers. Usually the difference in the magnitude of the REA between right- and left-handers is in the order of 10–15%. The higher proportion of right-handers showing an REA also seem to be independent of the testing procedure or the kind of paradigm used.

Clinical Populations

Commissurotomized patients with sectioning of the corpus callosum show almost complete suppression of the left-ear signal. This is termed 'paradoxical left-ear extinction' and is explained with reference to Kimura's model of suppression of the ipsilateral auditory pathways under dichotic competition. Thus, in a patient with a split brain, the right-ear signal reaches the left temporal cortex unopposed by the ipsilateral right-ear signal. However, the left-ear signal reaches the right hemisphere, and because of the sectioning of the corpus callosum, it cannot be relayed to the left hemisphere for processing.

DL has been used to assess anomalous brain laterality patterns in, for example, stuttering and dyslexia. Although several studies have reported reduced REA magnitudes in these groups, the evidence is not convincing and more research is needed. The DL technique has also been used in studies of schizophrenia and in affective disorders, under the assumption that these disorders are related to left- and right-hemisphere dysfunctions, respectively. The DL data support a notion that schizophrenia may be associated both with left-hemisphere overactivation and with an interhemispheric transfer deficit, although the findings to some extent are controversial.

Nonverbal Stimuli and Lateralization of Affect

Studies of lateralization of affect have involved both the expression of an emotion, as in facial emotional expressions, and the perception of affect, as in the presentation of an emotional stimulus. To summarize, most studies have revealed a right-hemisphere superiority for both expression and perception of affective, or emotional, events. One question that still arouses controversy in the literature is whether the right-hemisphere superiority for emotional processing is valid for both positive and negative emotions.

DL studies of affect have employed either verbal stimuli differing in prosody (vocal intonation), or nonspeech sounds, such as crying or laughing. DL studies with nonspeech sounds have in general revealed a left-ear advantage in most persons, supporting right-hemisphere processing superiority for these kinds of stimuli. DL studies of differences in prosody to speech sounds have also revealed a larger proportion of persons with an LEA than an REA. However, it is at present unclear whether this is specifically tied to the prosodic component in speech, or whether it is related to an overall right-hemisphere specialization for emotional processing.

See also: Brain Asymmetry: Evolution; Cognitive Neuroscience: An Overview; Hemispheric Specialization and Cognition; Neuropsychological Testing; Psychophysics of Attention; Split-Brain Patients.

Further Reading

Bruder GE (1988) Dichotic listening in psychiatric patients. In: Hugdahl K (ed.) *Handbook of Dichotic Listening: Theory, Methods, and Research*, pp. 527–564. Chichester, UK: Wiley.

Bryden MP (1988) An overview of the dichotic listening procedure and its relation to cerebral organization. In: Hugdahl K (ed.) *Handbook of Dichotic Listening: Theory, Methods, and Research*, pp. 1–44. Chichester, UK: Wiley.

Clark CR, Geffen LB, and Geffen G (1988) Invariant properties of auditory perceptual asymmetry assessed by dichotic listening. In: Hugdahl K (ed.) *Handbook of Dichotic Listening: Theory, Methods, and Research*, pp. 71–83. Chichester, UK: Wiley.

Green MF, Hugdahl K, and Mitchell S (1994) Dichotic listening during auditory hallucinations in schizophrenia. *American Journal of Psychiatry* 151: 357–362.

Hugdahl K (1995) Dichotic listening: Probing temporal lobe functional integrity. In: Davidson RJ and Hugdahl K (eds.) *Brain Asymmetry*, pp. 123–156. Cambridge, MA: MIT Press.

Hugdahl K (ed.) (1988) *Handbook of Dichotic Listening: Theory, Methods, and Research*. Chichester, UK: Wiley.

Hugdahl K and Andersson L (1986) The 'forced-attention paradigm' in dichotic listening to CV-syllables: A comparison between adults and children. *Cortex* 22: 417–432.

Hugdahl K, Brønnick K, Law I, et al. (1999) Brain activation during dichotic presentations of consonant–vowel and musical instruments stimuli: A ^{15}O-PET study. *Neuropsychologia* 37: 431–440.

Hugdahl K, Carlsson G, Uvebrant P, et al. (1997) Dichotic listening performance, intracarotid amobarbital injections in children/adolescent: Comparisons pre- and post-operatively. *Archives of Neurology* 54: 1494–1500.

Hugdahl K, Helland T, Færevåg MK, et al. (1995) Absence of ear advantage on the consonant–vowel dichotic listening test in adolescent and adult dyslexics: Specific auditory–phonetic dysfunction. *Journal of Clinical and Experimental Neuropsychology* 17: 833–840.

Hugdahl K, Nordstrand L, and Engstrand O (1986) A graphic-interactive CAD system for dichotic stimulus alignment (CADDIC). *Psychological Reports, 7, no. 3*. Bergen University of Bergen.

Hugdahl K and Wester K (1992) Dichotic listening studies of brain asymmetry in brain damaged patients. *International Journal of Neuroscience* 63: 17–29.

Wexler BE and Halwes T (1983) Increasing the power of dichotic methods: The fused rhymed words test. *Neuropsychologia* 21: 59–66.

Hemispheric Specialization and Cognition

M T Banich, University of Colorado at Boulder, Boulder, CO, USA

Hemispheric Differences in Cognition

Discovery of Hemispheric Differences in Cognition

Paul Broca, a French neurologist and anthropologist, is generally considered the first person to have clearly illustrated hemispheric differences in cognitive function. As such, he is often said to have discovered the phenomenon. His critical insight derived from his visit with a patient who demonstrated an interesting dissociation in language abilities. Although able to understand what was said to him, the man had an inability to produce speech, being able only to utter the syllable 'tan.' Broca's postmortem analysis of his brain showed that damage was localized to the third convolution of the inferior frontal gyrus in the left hemisphere. Broca then went on to examine other patients who exhibited a similar cognitive profile – an inability to produce speech in the face of a retained ability to comprehend speech. In all cases, the damage was localized to the same region but, most important, always in the left hemisphere – a region now known as Broca's area. As a result of these findings, Broca proposed in 1863 that the left hemisphere is specialized, or dominant, for speech output. Thus, Broca's paper was the first systematic and compelling demonstration of hemispheric specialization of function. In fact, unlike most other aspects of hemispheric specialization, this one is absolute: the right hemisphere has no ability to control speech output in practically all right-handed individuals.

Evidence from Patients with Unilateral Brain Damage

As a result of Broca's discovery, the idea of cerebral dominance was overgeneralized. Probably because language was considered synonymous with thought, his work was interpreted to mean that the left hemisphere was dominant for all aspects of cognitive function. This idea only began to erode gradually over the next century as studies of patients with unilateral brain damage demonstrated different consequences depending on which hemisphere was damaged. As apparent to any neurologist or clinical neuropsychologist, left hemisphere damage usually results in deficits in the domains of verbal, sequential, and analytic processing. For example, aphasia is a common consequence of left hemisphere damage. In contrast, right hemisphere damage typically yields deficits in nonverbal, holistic, and Gestalt processing. For example, deficits in visuospatial processing are more often observed after right hemisphere damage.

Evidence from Split-Brain Patients

In the 1960s, research by Nobel laureate Roger Sperry and colleagues with split-brain patients dramatically demonstrated the relative specialization of the cerebral hemispheres. In these split-brain patients, the main nerve fiber tract connecting the cerebral hemispheres, the corpus callosum, is severed for the treatment of intractable epilepsy. As a result, higher order information, such as that about an item's identity (e.g., a car, the letter 'A,' and the face of Bill Clinton), cannot be transferred from one hemisphere to the other. Thus, information directed to a single hemisphere is functionally isolated to that hemisphere. This situation provides a unique opportunity to examine the relative specialization of the cerebral hemispheres because each hemisphere's capabilities can be examined in isolation from those of its partner. As a result, research with split-brain patients has yielded much important information about hemispheric specialization. Absolute differences have been demonstrated only for a couple of functions, namely speech output and phonological processing, which are under sole control of the left hemisphere. Both hemispheres can perform all other tasks, albeit with differing levels of ability and in different manners. Whereas the left hemisphere has a rich ability to perform most all language tasks, the vocabulary of the right hemisphere is much more limited, as is its ability to process complicated grammatical functions. On the other hand, the right hemisphere is superior at processing most types of spatial relationships, especially those involving three-dimensional relations or complicated geometries.

Perceptual Asymmetries in Neurologically Intact Individuals

The relative specializations of the cerebral hemispheres can also be demonstrated in neurologically intact individuals through the use of methods that essentially pit the hemispheres against one another. These methods, which include tachitoscopic presentation, dichotic listening, and dichaptic presentation, all take advantage of the neuroanatomical wiring of the human brain that transfers information from sensory receptors to the contralateral sensory cortex. In these methods, information is presented laterally so it is received either solely or predominantly by one hemisphere. Then behavioral performance, with regard to either reaction time or accuracy, can be examined depending on which hemisphere initially received the sensory information. These behavioral measures are often referred to as perceptual asymmetries because they reflect the asymmetry in the perception of information depending on the hemisphere to which information was initially directed. Even though the corpus callosum in neurologically intact individuals contains more than 250 million fibers by which the hemispheres can communicate, differences in performance are nonetheless observed. Typically, these effects are in the range of a 10% difference in accuracy in performance or a 20–50 ms difference in reaction time. These studies provide converging evidence with data obtained from patients with unilateral brain damage and from split-brain patients. Myriads of studies have confirmed a left hemisphere superiority for processing verbal information and a right hemisphere superiority for processing nonverbal material, regardless of sensory modality – visual, auditory, or tactile.

Neuroimaging Studies of Hemispheric Specialization

The surge in neuroimaging during the past decade has also served to emphasize that the specializations of the hemispheres are more relative than absolute. These studies have shown that for most all tasks, activation is bilateral, although not necessarily of equal extent nor intensity. Even classic language tasks, such as verbal word reading, activate both hemispheres, although the activation is more left-sided than right-sided. In addition, the complimentarity of the hemispheres is revealed by these studies. For example, single-word processing leads to greater left than right hemisphere activation, but understanding the nonliteral meaning of language, such as analogy or the moral of a story, leads to greater right than left hemisphere activation.

Asymmetries Related to Emotion and Emotional Processing

Hemispheric specialization is not limited to cognitive function; it is found for emotional processes as well. The majority of evidence suggests that the right hemisphere is specialized for the interpretation of emotional information, including information contained in tone of voice and facial expression. Moreover, it is also specialized for the production of emotional cues that serve a communicative function (e.g., a smile that sends a communicative signal to someone else letting him or her know you are happy or pleased).

In contrast, lateralization of mood – that is, the subjective experience of one's internal emotional state – appears to rely on a pattern of brain activation across prefrontal and parietal regions. A large body of research has indicated that asymmetry of activation of frontal regions of the brain is linked to mood states. Greater activation of left than right frontal regions is associated with positive mood and approach behaviors. In contrast, greater activation of the right than left frontal regions is associated with negative mood and avoidance behavior. Moreover, individual differences in these asymmetries have been linked to differences in temperament in infants and to susceptibility to depression in later life. Overlaid on these effects of valence (positive and negative) are differences in activation of right parietal regions, which are linked to arousal. Depressed mood is associated with decreased activity of right parietal regions, whereas the panic associated with heightened anxiety is associated with increased activity of right parietal regions.

Models of Hemispheric Specialization

The broad body of work – from patients with unilateral brain damage, split-brain patients, and studies of perceptual asymmetries with neurologically intact individuals – was originally framed with regard to differences in the type of material that each hemisphere is specialized to process. Initially, the left hemisphere was considered specialized for processing verbal materials, whereas the right hemisphere was considered specialized for processing nonverbal materials. However, in a series of studies in the late 1960s and early 1970s, studies with split-brain patients clearly demonstrated that in many cases both hemispheres were capable of processing a given type of material. What differed, however, was the manner in which they processed that material. This led to a new rubric for understanding hemispheric specialization. The left hemisphere was conceptualized to analyze information in an analytic, piecemeal, and local manner, whereas the right hemisphere was conceptualized to analyze information in a holistic and Gestalt manner. For example, although the right hemisphere of a split-brain patient is superior to the left at identifying a previously viewed face, both can do so. The right hemisphere appears to analyze the overall configuration of the face, such as whether the face is long and narrow or wide and round, and whether the eyes are wide set compared to the width of the face. In contrast, the left hemisphere processes the features or local details, such as the shape of the chin or the eyes. This shift in conceptualizing hemispheric specialization was important because it explained a potential advantage of a specialized brain, namely the ability of simultaneous dual processing. Practically all information can be processed independently and in a distinct manner by each hemisphere at the same time, providing two distinct ways of simultaneously understanding and interpreting the world.

With this conceptual shift, researchers began to explore hemispheric differences from a computational perspective, with the goal of determining the fundamental differences in computations performed by each hemisphere. One early theory suggested that the hemispheres differed in their ability to process low-level sensory information. In particular, the right hemisphere was conceived as being specialized for processing information of low visual spatial frequency – that is, information that does not shift from dark to light within a small degree of visual space. This information generally provides the general contours and outline of visual forms but not the details. In contrast, the left hemisphere was conceived as being specialized for processing information of high spatial frequency – that is, information that shifts quickly, within a given amount of visual space, from dark to light. Such information provides the detail in visual forms. Moreover, asymmetries in higher order cognitive function were posited to emerge from these sensory asymmetries. For example, the overall configuration of a face would be provided by visual information of low spatial frequency, whereas the detailed information would be provided by visual information of high spatial frequency.

This theory was highly influential and has been subsequently modified. Further research demonstrated that the hemispheres appear to be specialized not for the absolute frequency of sensory information but, rather, for the relative frequency, an effect that holds across different sensory modalities. For example, when individuals are presented with information of high auditory frequency, the left hemisphere exhibits a performance advantage for processing the higher half of those high auditory frequencies and the right hemisphere for processing the lower half of those high auditory frequencies. Findings such as these have been expanded to be accounted for by the double-filtering hypothesis, which argues that hemispheric differences arise from an attentional bias in the information that each processes. It is argued that the right hemisphere employs a low pass filter on incoming information, whereas the left hemisphere employs a high pass filter.

Other researchers have focused on why there might be a need to have distinct ways of processing information in each of the cerebral hemispheres. These theories have focused on how the hemispheres might insulate conflicting or independent processes from one another. For example, in the spatial domain it has been argued that the right hemisphere is specialized to coordinate spatial relationships, considered those that provide information about the distance between objects. In contrast, the left hemisphere is specialized for categorical spatial relations that describe the relationship between items (e.g., above, below, to the right of, and to the left of). These two ways of describing information are considered orthogonal to each other because knowing the coordinate information, such as that one item is 3 ft from another, provides no information about categorical information, such as if one item is behind the other. Computational models suggest that these two types of spatial processing are best supported by independent insulated processing systems because the representations required are mutually incompatible and/or create interference. Performance on spatial tasks is superior in a split rather than unitary computational model, suggesting that the hemispheres are specialized to allow for noninterference of processing.

Similar arguments have been made with regard to language processing. Even though the left hemisphere alone has control over speech output and phonological processing, its specialization for language is also relative. Whereas the left hemisphere has been found to be superior to the right hemisphere in aspects of grammar and syntax, the right hemisphere is superior at processing the nonliteral aspects of language, such as discourse, metaphor, and analogy. These differences may arise from incompatible means of semantic access and/or organization. The left hemisphere appears to access words in a very specific, precise, and local manner, whereas the right hemisphere accesses words in a more diffuse manner that allows activation for more far-flung associates. For example, if a paragraph was about gardening, the left hemisphere would quickly hone in on the particular meaning of 'bug' related to insects, whereas the right hemisphere would hold onto a more diffuse set of meanings, including not only the meaning related to insects but also that related to spying devices. As such, the right hemisphere would be better equipped to make connections across sentences and phrases that would allow for discourse and for nonliteral aspects of language comprehension.

Origins of Hemispheric Asymmetry

Although there was once speculation that cerebral asymmetry is a unique feature of the human brain, hemispheric asymmetry is observed in other species, including not only mammals but also fishes, reptiles, and amphibians. The asymmetries observed in behaviors range from those involved in courtship and copulation to escape behavior and limb use (i.e., 'handedness'). These asymmetries are found not only for an individual organism (i.e., a right-sided limb preference in a given animal) but also at the population level. For example, apes tend to use the left hand for stabilizing objects and the right hand for fine motor manipulation. Likewise, 59% of certain species of toad prefer to use their right paw to remove an object affixed to their head.

Because hemispheric asymmetries are observed in many other species, much theorizing has focused on how language processing becomes lateralized. Some theories posit that the association of fine motor coordination of the right hand associated with tool use served as the platform for the fine motor control that is associated with the vocalizations that underlie human language. Other theories posit that a lateralized gestural system, when linked to vocalizations, led to language lateralization. Cross-species support for such an idea is provided by research showing that cells in area F5 of the macaque monkey brain, a region homologous to Broca's area in humans, fire when a monkey sees someone else perform a grasping action similar to one which it has just performed. It has been argued that these 'mirror' neurons underlie the ability to form, through gesture, a common communicative system between individuals. Such a common communicative system would then have evolved to include vocalization. Supporting this idea, gestures linked to speech are produced with much more frequency by the right hand in humans and chimpanzees, whereas gestures that do not have a communicative value (e.g., straightening one's clothes) are not produced asymmetrically.

Developmental Issues and Hemispheric Specialization

Given the evidence for an evolutionary history of lateralization of functioning, it is not surprising that hemispheric asymmetries exist at birth. That is not to say, however, that this pattern cannot be modified by environmental factors. Evidence for an inborn pattern of asymmetry comes from numerous sources. First, gyral and sulcul patterns, which differ between right- and left-handers (who, as discussed later, differ in behavioral asymmetry) are present before birth and not modified thereafter. Second, the effects of hemispherectomy at birth differ depending on whether the left or right hemisphere is removed. Although individuals with only one hemisphere acquire both verbal and nonverbal skills, the degree to which these skills are acquired varies by the hemisphere removed. Individuals with only a right hemisphere perform, on average, better on spatial tasks than those with only a left hemisphere, whereas individuals with only a left hemisphere perform better on verbal tasks than those with only a right hemisphere. Third, asymmetries can be observed in the newborn. These include motoric asymmetries, behavioral asymmetries, and asymmetries in brain responses. For example, a larger evoked response is recorded over the left hemisphere to verbal materials and over the right hemisphere to nonverbal materials.

Thus, it appears that the basic blueprint of hemispheric specialization exists at birth. However, the nature of that blueprint can be altered by environmental factors. For example, it has been well documented that after damage to the left hemisphere during approximately the first 2 years of life, the right hemisphere can acquire the ability to control speech. Somewhat more ambiguous are findings that experience can influence the degree of perceptual asymmetry that is observed. For example, a greater left visual field advantage is observed for holistic processing of faces from a racial group with which one is familiar than for faces of a group with which one is not familiar. Whether this result indicates that the nature of hemispheric specialization is changed by experience, or whether more experience tends to engage more specialized processors in the brain, remains unclear.

The Effect of Handedness

One individual difference, that of handedness, has been clearly linked to patterns of hemispheric specialization for cognitive and emotional function. The relative specializations of the cerebral hemispheres described previously appear to hold only for individuals who are right-handed. In contrast, left-handed individuals, who comprise approximately 10% of individuals worldwide, can have a diverse pattern of lateral organization. This difference is well-known by neurologists and neuropsychologists who have long observed that handedness is an important factor in predicting the types of deficits and the amount of recovery that is likely to be observed after unilateral brain damage. However, there is much variability among left-handers regarding the type of lateralized brain organization they display. In some cases, it is similar to that of right-handers, with the left hemisphere specialized for verbal functions and the right for nonverbal functions. In other cases, it is the opposite, with the right hemisphere specialized for verbal function and the left for nonverbal function. It is estimated that such a brain organization is found in only 1% or 2% of right-handers. Finally, other left-handers exhibit a pattern in which both hemispheres appear to be able to process both verbal and nonverbal information, including speech output. Although much research has attempted to isolate a factor that can predict the type of brain organization a given left-hander will exhibit, for the most part, these efforts have failed. Currently, the leading model of the genetic basis of handedness and its relationship to lateralized brain organization suggests that handedness (and hence brain organization) is randomly distributed, unless one inherits a right-shift allele, which shifts handedness to the right hand and language to the left hemisphere. Such a model assumes that it was evolutionarily advantageous to have motor control of the right hand and control of language co-lateralized to the same hemisphere.

Interhemispheric Integration

After the explosion of research examining hemispheric specialization in the 1970s and 1980s, recent work has examined how the processing of the hemispheres is coordinated and the effects of integration of information between the cerebral hemispheres.

Interhemispheric integration occurs mainly via the massive bundle of nerve fibers connecting the cerebral hemispheres, the corpus callosum. Because information from the peripheral nerves is directed contralaterally, at least for vision, motor, and somatosensory information, integration of information across the hemispheres allows information from each sensory half-field to be bound together. For example, in the visual domain, information is represented contralaterally in V1, V2, and V3a/VP. In fact, there are few, if any callosal connections in BA 17. Representation of information from the ipsilateral visual field first appears at the level of V3a and V4v, which are brain regions whose cells have receptive fields that span the midline. This critical role of the callosum in fusing the sensory worlds is made apparent by split-brain patients who cannot bind information from different sensory fields. For example, if fixated on a central point and shown two items, one on each side visual midline so that they are projected to opposite hemispheres, a split-brain patient cannot determine if they are the same or different.

Although the callosum acts as a mechanism to transfer information between the hemispheres, this transfer involves time costs as well as degradation of information. Transfer of information via the corpus callosum takes approximately 5 ms via the large myelinated fibers that connect sensory and motor areas and 20–50 ms for small unmylineated fibers. The fidelity costs are apparent in old/new memory paradigms. If an item is presented in one visual field, correctly recognizing of that item as previously viewed is poorer if presented to the hemisphere that did not initially view the item as compared to the hemisphere. Such findings are consistent with theorizing that the representations supported by each of the hemispheres are different and are not completely interchangeable.

Integration of information across the cerebral hemispheres plays an additional role above and beyond that of binding together the visual world – that of attentional control. Evidence suggests that the cerebral hemispheres dynamically couple and decouple to meet task demands. When tasks involve relatively low attentional demands, performance is better when all the critical information needed for a decision (e.g., are these two items physically identical?) is directed to a single hemisphere compared to divided between them. It has been proposed that under such conditions, the processing capacity of a single hemisphere is adequate to meet the demands and the cost of interhemispheric communication takes a toll on performance. In contrast, when attentional demands are high, dividing processing between the hemispheres enables more resources to be brought to bear and the advantage provided by these additional resources more than outweighs the cost of callosal transfer. Such an outcome can occur because, as described previously, the specialization of the hemispheres is not absolute but relative, allowing both hemispheres to process almost all types of information. Thus, the additional resources provided by the partner hemisphere, even if not specialized for the task, can nonetheless have a major impact on performance. These findings are consonant with data from individuals in whom the corpus callosum is severed or damaged, such as occurs in multiple sclerosis. A common consequence of callosal damage or insufficiency is problems in attentional control. Although the neural mechanisms that allow the callosum to play such a role remain somewhat obscure, connectionist modeling suggests that the advantage afforded by dividing processing between the hemispheres is an emergent phenomenon of having two somewhat insulated and distinct processors.

Summary

Each of the human cerebral hemispheres has a distinct manner of processing information, with the left hemisphere more adept at attending to and processing more fine-grained information and the right hemisphere more adept at attending to and processing more coarse-grained information. This distinction holds for all types of information, whether verbal or spatial. The complimentarity of these modes of processing means that the human brain contains two processors, each of which provides a unique manner of understanding and interpreting the world.

Moreover, this dichotomy and isolation of processing also provides for a system that can dynamically reconfigure to act in isolation or in tandem depending on attentional demands.

See also: Brain Asymmetry: Evolution; Cognition: An Overview of Neuroimaging Techniques; Dichotic Listening Studies of Brain Asymmetry; Emotional Hormones and Memory Modulation; Memory: Genetic Approaches; Multisensory Convergence and Integration; Split-Brain Patients.

Further Reading

Annett M (2002) *Handedness and Brain Asymmetry: The Right Shift Theory.* New York: Psychology Press.

Banich MT (1998) The missing link: The role of interhemispheric interaction in attentional processing. *Brain and Cognition* 36: 128–157.

Beeman MJ and Chiarello C (1998) Complementary right- and left-hemisphere language comprehension. *Current Directions in Psychological Science* 7: 2–8.

Corballis MC (2003) From mouth to hand: Gesture, speech, and the evolution of right-handedness. *Behavioral and Brain Sciences* 26: 199–260.

Davidson RJ (1992) Anterior cerebral asymmetry and the nature of emotion. *Brain & Cognition* 20: 125–151.

Hellige JB (2001) *Hemispheric Asymmetry: What's Right and What's Left.* Cambridge, MA: Harvard University Press.

Hugdahl K and Davidson RJ (eds.) (2003) *The Asymmetrical Brain.* Cambridge: MIT Press.

Ivry RB and Robertson LC (1998) *The Two Sides of Perception.* Cambridge: MIT Press.

Keller J, Nitschke JB, Bhargava T, et al. (2000) Neuropsychological differentiation of depression and anxiety. *Journal of Abnormal Psychology* 109: 3–10.

Kosslyn SM (1987) Seeing and imagining in the cerebral hemispheres: A computational approach. *Psychological Review* 94: 148–175.

Levy J, Trevarthen C, and Sperry RW (1972) Perception of bilateral chimeric figures following hemispheric deconnexion. *Brain* 95: 61–78.

Monaghan P and Pollmann S (2003) Division of labor between the hemispheres for complex but not simple tasks: An implemented connectionist model. *Journal of Experimental Psychology: General* 132: 379–399.

Sergent J (1985) Influence of task and input factors on hemispheric involvement in face processing. *Journal of Experimental Psychology: Human Perception and Performance* 11: 846–861.

Trevarthen C (1996) Lateral asymmetries in infancy: Implications for the development of the hemispheres. *Neuroscience & Biobehavioral Reviews* 20: 571–586.

Zaidel E and Iacoboni M (eds.) (2003) *The Parallel Brain: The Cognitive Neuroscience of the Corpus Callosum.* Cambridge: MIT Press.

Split-Brain Patients

M E Roser, University of Plymouth, Plymouth, UK
M S Gazzaniga, University of California at Santa Barbara, Santa Barbara, CA, USA

Terminology

The term split brain is used to denote a patient in whom the cortical commissures have been severed, for the relief of epilepsy that cannot be controlled by medication, in an operation known as either a commissurotomy or a callosotomy. A commissurotomy involves severing the corpus callosum, the anterior commissure, and the hippocampal commissure. The massa intermedia, if present, is also severed. A callosotomy involves sectioning of the corpus callosum alone, either completely or partially. In a partial callosotomy, either the anterior or the posterior callosum may be cut. Complete callosal disconnection may result from a staged callosotomy in which the anterior and the posterior parts of the callosum are severed in two separate operations.

History

The split-brain operation in humans was first reported in the early 1940s by the neurosurgeons Van Waganen and Herren, who carried out more than 30 such operations as a treatment for intractable epilepsy. Severing the commissures between the hemispheres prevented the interhemispheric propagation of seizures. These patients were later tested by Akelaitis, who reported that the patients showed no marked effects on behavior beyond the reduction in their epileptic symptoms. This negative finding was congruent with earlier studies of callosal infarcts which suggested that the cortical commissures had little functional role, a state of affairs which prompted Karl Lashley to facetiously remark that the purpose of the corpus callosum was to "keep the hemispheres from sagging."

It was not until the systematic experiments carried out on commissurotomized cats and monkeys by Ronald Myers and Roger Sperry that the importance of the cortical commissures for the transmission of information between the hemispheres became strikingly apparent. Cutting the commissures disrupted the transfer of visual and tactile information, and learned associations, from one hemisphere to the other. The animal studies also suggested that division of the hemispheres would have no catastrophic consequences for human patients because the animals displayed normal behavior outside of the testing situation.

Following the publication of these studies, the commissurotomy operation was carried out on a number of human patients in the early 1960s by the neurosurgeons Philip Vogel and Joseph Bogen. These patients are commonly referred to as the California series and include patients W.J., N.G., and A.A. Other extensively tested patients, including P.S. and J.W., were operated on in the 1970s by Donald Wilson and David W Roberts at Dartmouth Medical School. Many of these patients have participated in a large number of experiments over decades.

The divided human brain offered a unique opportunity for each hemisphere to be studied in relative isolation. The initial investigations of hemispheric communication and asymmetry in humans were carried out by Michael Gazzaniga, working in the laboratory of Roger Sperry. These studies demonstrated the striking disconnection syndrome in which each hemisphere remains unaware of the sensory and gnostic properties of stimuli presented to its opposite number.

Testing Split-Brain Patients

In everyday situations, the split-brain patients appear normal. This is due to the freedom with which they can direct their gaze and movements around in the environment, allowing both hemispheres knowledge of their surroundings. Only when patients are tested in strictly controlled circumstances does the disconnection syndrome become apparent. To test each hemisphere individually, stimuli must be presented to only one hemisphere. Tactile shapes, for example, may be palpated by one hand but hidden from view.

Testing with visual stimuli usually involves the presentation of stimuli to each of the visual hemifields for a duration less than 200 ms, brief enough to preclude a saccade toward the stimulus while it is displayed. Each hemifield projects to the contralateral visual cortex, and thus a stimulus in the left hemifield will be seen by the right hemisphere. In order to achieve lateralized presentation of stimuli, patients are required to fixate on a central point on the display. Stimuli are displayed at locations eccentric to the foveated point by several degrees of visual angle. A chin rest is often used to minimize head movements and infrared eye tracking can ensure that the patient's gaze remains on the fixation point. Using the brief-presentation technique, simple pictures, words, shapes, and colors can be lateralized.

For presentations longer than a few hundred milliseconds, necessary for extended viewing of complex stimuli, steps must be taken to ensure the stimulus remains in one visual hemifield. One method is to prevent foveation by employing a stimulus deflector, which tracks eye movements and adjusts the view of the display accordingly so as to ensure that any saccade toward the stimulus is accompanied by a corresponding movement of the stimulus away from fixation. Another method allows for extended viewing in free, monocular, vision but restricts visual input to one hemisphere through the use of a contact lens that occludes one-half of the visual field. Finally, visual information may be presented in full view of the patient, and thus to both hemispheres, with a response required from only one hemisphere.

Responses are typically collected from the hemisphere to which the stimulus was presented, often by using the hand on the same side as the stimulus. Control of the distal effectors, such as fingers, is thought to be predominantly contralateral. Thus, button presses, as a measure of either simple reaction time or of categorical choice, are often used. In some experiments, a hemisphere may be required to respond by reaching for a picture representing the correct choice.

Care must be taken when testing patients that one hemisphere is not able to cross-cue, or tip off, its opposite number as to the nature of a stimulus or the correct response. Patients are seated with their hands and feet apart. Objects are placed on a soft surface so that they do not make identifying noises when moved.

Neuropsychological Profile

Most patients who have participated in multiple studies over several decades have been assessed as showing verbal, memory, and attentional capacities within normal limits, although scores are often below average. Memory, particularly free recall, shows the greatest deficit, and may result from section of both the corpus callosum and the hippocampal commissure.

Drawing conclusions about function in the brain on the basis of results from split-brain patients is complicated by their history of epilepsy and invasive surgery. Because split-brain patients have diverse medical histories, it is desirable to test as many patients as possible. Often, a multiple case study approach is taken because patients cannot be grouped for comparison with a control group. This heterogeneity does, however, increase the impressiveness of obtaining the same result in two or more patients because consistent patterns of asymmetry are unlikely to have resulted from common neurological history.

Although the brains of callosotomy patients differ greatly from intact brains, evidence from both behavioral testing and functional imaging studies suggests that the patterns of functional lateralization observed in the split brain are congruent with those found in neurologically intact participants in many different cognitive domains. It must be remembered, however, that the divided brain is an unusual situation and that cognitive processes may not operate in the same fashion in each isolated hemisphere as they do in the intact brain. Thus, comparison with a control sample is desirable.

The Disconnection Syndrome

One of the earliest findings from split-brain research was the importance of the corpus callosum for the transmission of information between the hemispheres. The relative isolation of each hemisphere is referred to as the disconnection syndrome and is manifested as poor performance at cross-comparisons of stimuli presented to different hemispheres and, for most patients, an inability to verbally name stimuli presented to the right hemisphere.

Split-brained patients often perform at chance level on tests in which they must decide whether patterns or objects in the two visual fields are the same or different. This includes letters, digits, words, colors, shapes, and luminances. The importance of the corpus callosum for the transfer of information between the visual cortices is also apparent using electrophysiological measures. Sensory evoked potentials are not seen over the hemisphere ipsilateral to a visual stimulus in patients in whom the posterior corpus callosum has been severed. Some patients, however, can judge whether lines on each side are aligned or not. These preserved abilities presumably rely on intact subcortical pathways between the hemispheres.

An inability to name stimuli presented to the right hemisphere can be demonstrated by having the split-brain patient fixate on a central point and flashing stimuli to the left visual field. If the patient is asked to verbally name the stimulus presented to his or her left visual field, he or she is unable to do so because the right hemisphere, in most patients, is not able to produce speech and is separated from the linguistically able left hemisphere. The right hemisphere can, however, control the left hand to find a covered object that corresponds to the stimulus presented. The patient is not able to verbally name the object until it is moved into the right visual field or the right hand.

Other evidence for perceptual disconnection comes from presenting, to each visual field, words that can be combined to form the names of emergent objects. Patients are then asked to draw what they saw. One callosotomy patient, V.P., who has some residual fibers left in her corpus callosum, is able to integrate words presented in the two visual fields (e.g., the words 'head' and 'stone') and draw the emergent object, in this case a headstone. Another subject, J.W., whose corpus callosum was fully cut, did not draw emergent objects when tested but instead drew each object separately. Thus, the perception of complex visual information is divided between the hemispheres of the split brain.

Evidence for the division of attention between the hemispheres is more equivocal. Visual search of an array of objects can be carried out independently by each hemisphere. This was suggested by the observation that the addition of items to the stimulus array impacts to a lesser degree on performance when the objects to be searched are distributed between the two visual hemifields than when the items are all contained within one hemifield. The ability to carry out two independent search processes also leads to a rare advantage in performance for split-brain patients over callosally intact participants.

The ability to divide some attentional processes between the hemispheres does not, however, endow split-brain patients with twice the attentional resources available to neurologically normal individuals. Performance of a demanding task by one hemisphere has been shown to negatively impact upon performance by the other hemisphere, suggesting a finite, shared, pool of attentional resources.

Learned bimanual tasks are not adversely affected by callosotomy, although the acquisition of new skills involving complex bimanual coordination is impaired. Conversely, callosotomy patients can perform some coordination patterns which callosally intact subjects find difficult, such as drawing two different shapes simultaneously, one with each hand. This independence of action following callosotomy suggests that the corpus callosum contributes to the interhemispheric integration of bimanual movement. Some studies suggested that callosal integration is confined to information about movement direction and not timing because temporal coupling of the hands was preserved in callosotomy patients, although recent results have suggested that this only occurs for movements with discrete events.

The divided brain presents an opportunity to study each hemisphere in relative isolation. It can also allow the researcher to obtain double dissociations of cognitive processes if the two processes rely critically on different hemispheres. In one case, seemingly indivisible cognitive processes, such as spoken and written language output, can be separated into lateralized components.

Partial Callosotomy and Callosal Channels

Callosotomy is typically performed in a staged manner, with either the anterior callosum, the genu, or the posterior callosum, the splenium, sectioned first, followed by the remaining fibers if the first operation fails to sufficiently reduce the patient's epilepsy. Because the corpus callosum is organized in a roughly topographic fashion, tests of patients after partial callosotomy can reveal the functional specificity of regions of the corpus callosum. Section of the splenium and midbody disrupts the transmission of visual and somatosensory information between the hemispheres, resulting in poor performance on cross-comparison tasks. Intact anterior pathways are able to support the transfer of semantic information between the hemispheres, allowing patients to perform above chance on tests of naming left visual field stimuli, although performance is often slow and imprecise. Anterior section produces less evidence of disconnection, although the disruption to anterior midbody tracts can affect bimanual coordination for complex motions.

Subcortical Transfer

Each hemisphere of the split brain shows awareness of the presentation of a stimulus to the opposite hemisphere. Simple responses, such as button presses, can be made to stimuli presented in the visual field opposite the response hand. These are known as crossed responses and are subject to a delay, ranging from 30 to 70 ms, relative to uncrossed responses. This delay is thought to index the time taken for transmission of a signal from the hemisphere receiving the stimulus to that making the response, via subcortical channels, and contrasts with 5–15 ms delay for interhemispheric transfer in callosally intact subjects.

The affective content of a stimulus may also be transferred between the hemispheres, as shown by an experiment in which emotive pictorial stimuli were presented to the right hemisphere and were found to affect the judgment of emotionally neutral stimuli, and the patient's current environment, by the left hemisphere.

The complexity of subcortical visual transfer in the split brain is limited to basic spatial information that can support interhemispheric comparisons of stimulus location and alignment. Some experiments suggested that higher order information, such as category or numerical value, could be transferred subcortically and support comparative judgments such as whether a stimulus in one visual field was bigger than a stimulus in the opposite field or whether two stimuli were both of the same categories. The deterioration in performance of stimulus cross-comparisons with increasing set size suggested, however, that this apparent ability was due not to the transfer of complex information but to the responding hemisphere adopting a response strategy based only on the information presented to it. Thus, care must be taken, when testing subcortical transmission in split-brain patients, to ensure that experimental situations truly require transmission for above-chance performance. The transfer of binary information, such as whether a number is odd or even, coupled with response strategies, seems sufficient to explain most instances of apparent higher order transfer.

Hemispheric Specialization

Testing the split brain can reveal whether each isolated hemisphere is competent at a particular task and the degree to which a process can be supported by a single hemisphere. The term specialization, when applied to one of the hemispheres in the split brain, is sometimes used to imply that one hemisphere bears primary responsibility for a particular perceptual, cognitive, or motor process, usually on the basis of a performance difference between the hemispheres. Asymmetries in behavior are often more stark in the divided brain than in lateralized responses from normal controls. Double dissociations between the performances of the two hemispheres on two tasks are sometimes observed, and most fully justify the interpretation that the different processes are predominantly handled by different hemispheres. This is especially true if each hemisphere performs at chance level on one task. Often, hemispheric differences in performance are relative because both hemispheres are capable of above-chance performance. This result is often interpreted as suggesting that the two hemispheres contribute to performance to different degrees. Findings suggesting different levels of competence in each hemisphere are congruent with studies in neurologically normal subjects that suggest that many hemispheric asymmetries are relative, rather than absolute, and can change as task demands change.

Language

Early testing of the split-brain patients revealed their inability to name stimuli in the left visual hemifield and confirmed the primacy of the left hemisphere for the understanding and production of language. In most patients, only the isolated left hemisphere is able to process complex grammar, although in some patients the right hemisphere is capable of making simple grammaticality judgments. The right hemisphere of most patients can understand simple verbal instructions, although these are often accompanied by visual examples presented in central vision. It can also understand simple phrases which, although they contain several words organized grammatically, may be best characterized as single items in a lexicon.

The right hemisphere is able to understand the meaning of words and can choose a picture that represents the item represented by an auditory or visual word stimulus, but in most patients it is unable to match rhyming words and pictures. This suggests that the right hemisphere does not generate the corresponding phonology for the item represented in the picture. However, several patients have demonstrated the development of the ability to verbally name stimuli presented in the left visual hemifield, in one case approximately 10 years after surgery.

Visual Perception

Both hemispheres in the split brain are capable of a range of visual processes, including object recognition, but the right hemisphere displays superiority for visual processes that include a spatial component. The spatial ability of the isolated right hemisphere was demonstrated early in the history of split-brain testing by requiring patients to replicate a pattern by arranging blocks with each hand. This task was performed better, by most patients tested, when using the left hand and patients were frequently unsuccessful when using their right hand. Similarly, tactile patterns are better recognized by the right hemisphere. In the visual domain, the difference in spatial ability between the hemispheres is apparent on a test of mental rotation, which requires the patient to decide whether two objects are mirror images or identical, but rotated, objects. Additional studies have found right hemisphere superiority for judging spatial relations, such as orientation and alignment, between objects. Comparisons of visual stimuli on nonspatial dimensions, such as luminance, can be performed equally well by the two hemispheres.

Based on observations of visual field differences in normal subjects, several dichotomies have been proposed for how visual processes differ between the two hemispheres. These include specializations for processing high- and low-spatial frequencies, the global and local arrangement of arrays, and categorical and coordinate representations of space. Testing in the split brain has not lent strong support to these hypotheses, with several studies failing to show the predicted hemispheric differences. The most common finding was that both hemispheres were capable of performing both modes of processing included within each of the dichotomies, with occasional instances of superior performance by one hemisphere, in line with predictions. This finding is congruent with the view that hemispheric specialization is relative, and fluid, rather than absolute.

The right hemisphere has shown superiority over the left hemisphere for some types of perceptual grouping. Both hemispheres, in two callosotomy patients, were able to group visual stimuli and perceive illusory contours, but only the right was able to group stimuli and perceive an amodally completed object, in which the object's illusory boundaries were partly occluded. This finding suggests that simple perceptual grouping processes are supported by each hemisphere, but complex grouping processes are lateralized.

Differences between the hemispheres are also apparent in the processing of the timing of visual events. The left hemisphere of commissurotomy patient L.B. performed better than the right hemisphere at discriminating between simultaneous and successive lights when delays were very short. In contrast, L.B., and two callosotomy patients, showed a right hemispheric advantage for temporal discrimination of delays between the onsets of two visual stimuli when delays were in the range necessary to produce apparent movement. The two callosotomy patients also showed right hemisphere superiority for determining if the motion of a stimulus was caused by the impact of another stimulus. Thus, the right hemisphere seems superior to the left for the perception of interactions between objects in space and time.

Face Processing

Both hemispheres in the divided brain are able to recognize the self from pictures of the patient's face which are morphed with pictures of the faces of others, although different studies have found opposite hemispheric asymmetries in biases toward identifying faces as either self or other. The right hemisphere in several callosotomy patients has shown greater ability than the left hemisphere in matching pictures of similar faces to a sample, although tests of other patients have failed to find a right hemispheric advantage on tests of face perception. The left hemisphere is better able to voluntarily produce facial expressions of different emotions.

Memory

Some commissurotomy and callosotomy patients have shown lowered performance on tests of general memory ability, although others show little deficit. In affected patients, this deficit is greater than that seen in other domains investigated by standard neuropsychological assessment. Poor memory for new information, such as word associations, contrasts with the intactness of previously learned information and memories of events prior to the surgery. This deficit may result from interruption to both the corpus callosum and the hippocampal commissure and fornix. The involvement of the hippocampal commissure is suggested by the lack of memory deficits exhibited by some anterior callosotomy patients, in whom the hippocampal commissure is spared. Evidence from several patients also suggests that recognition memory may not be affected to the same degree as recall.

Relative hemispheric advantage on memory tests can depend on both the nature of the task and the stimuli. For instance, it was found that in several patients the right hemisphere outperformed the left hemisphere in a test of memory for tactile shapes, but the left hemisphere performed better when patients were required to remember sequences of tactile shapes. Material-specific depth-of-processing effects, in the two hemispheres of two callosotomy patients, and the lack of a catastrophic memory deficit suggest that both hemispheres are capable of memory encoding. The finding also suggests that different material, such as faces and words, are encoded preferentially by one of the two hemispheres.

A tendency for the left hemisphere to elaborate on information it receives may underlie its poor performance on tasks that involve distinguishing between previously seen and novel items with semantic content, such as words or pictorial representations of common scenes. The left hemisphere was found to falsely recognize previously unseen items that were semantically congruent with items shown during the encoding phase. The right hemisphere made no such systematic error.

Higher Cognition

Debate on whether the isolated hemispheres each possess consciousness, either complete or impoverished, has persisted since the publication of early observations from split-brain patients. Both hemispheres display a range of positive competencies, but the mounting evidence for, sometimes subtle, hemispheric differences suggests that consciousness is not identical in the two hemispheres.

The isolated right hemisphere performs poorly on many problem-solving tasks, whereas the left hemisphere remains capable of a level of abstract reasoning comparable to the patient's preoperative performance. The right hemisphere in two callosotomy patients was found to be unable to perform a task involving reasoning about causes, despite this task being solvable by young infants, although the left hemispheres in the same patients performed well.

The left hemispheres of several callosotomy patients have shown a propensity for providing elaborative accounts of their experience and their own behavior, including those initiated by the right hemisphere. If the left hemisphere is challenged to provide an explanation for the behavior of the right hemisphere, patients often reply with interpretation that is consistent with the information presented to the patient's verbally able left hemisphere. The tendency for the left hemisphere to form generalizations about its environment has also been shown in a nonlinguistic test involving the prediction of the location of a forthcoming stimulus. Thus, the interpretive and linguistic processes that allow individuals to make sense of their conscious experience seem to be most fully actualized in the left hemisphere of the split brain.

See also: Attentional Functions in Learning and Memory; Brain Asymmetry: Evolution; Consciousness: Neurophysiology and Visual Awareness in; Consciousness: Neural Basis of Conscious Experience; Dichotic Listening Studies of Brain Asymmetry; Epilepsy; Hemispheric Specialization and Cognition; Memory Representation.

Further Reading

Bogen JE (1993) The callosal syndromes. In: Heilman KM and Valenstein E (eds.) *Clinical Neuropsychology*, 3rd edn., pp. 337–407. New York: Oxford University Press.

Corballis MC (1994) Split decisions: Problems in the interpretation of results from commissurotomized subjects. *Behavioural Brain Research* 64: 163–172.

Gazzaniga MS (2000) Cerebral specialization and interhemispheric communication: Does the corpus callosum enable the human condition? *Brain* 123: 1293–1326.

Gazzaniga MS (2006) Forty-five years of split-brain research and still going strong. *Nature Reviews Neuroscience* 6: 653–659.

Gazzaniga MS, Bogen JE, and Sperry RW (1962) Some functional effects of sectioning the cerebral commissures in man. *Proceedings of the National Academy of Sciences of the United States of America* 48: 1765–1769.

Geschwind N (1965) Disconnexion syndromes in animals and man: I. *Brain* 88: 237–294.

Geschwind N (1965) Disconnexion syndromes in animals and man: II. *Brain* 88: 585–644.

Hugdahl K and Davidson RJ (eds.) (2003) *The Asymmetrical Brain.* Cambridge: MIT Press.

Sperry R (1982) Some effects of disconnecting the cerebral hemispheres. *Science* 217: 1223–1226.

Trevarthen C (ed.) (1990) *Brain Circuits and Functions of the Mind: Essays in Honor of Roger W. Sperry.* Cambridge, UK: Cambridge University Press.

Zaidel E and Iacoboni M (eds.) (2003) *The Parallel Brain: The Cognitive Neuroscience of the Corpus Callosum.* Cambridge: MIT Press.

智　　能

Animal Intelligence: The Search for Animal Intelligence

A A Wright, University of Texas Health Science Center, Medical School at Houston, Houston, TX, USA

Introduction

Discoveries of obvious intelligent behavior by animals are appearing at an accelerated rate. Although examples of ape and monkey intelligence have been known for some time, even avians are casting off their 'bird brain' label. Pigeons, for example, can navigate by landmarks, sun compass, magnetic compass, infrasound sources, and possibly by cues from polarized and ultraviolet light. They can compute a navigational fix to determine their location (if unknown) to find 'home' which would be impossible with a compass alone. Galapagos finches and New Caledonian crows (**Figure 1**) select and fashion tools (e.g., cactus spines, twigs, and leaves) to 'fish' out insects and grubs in tree-limb holes/cracks or under leaf detritus and carry their favorite tools around with them. Clark's nutcracker birds store thousands of pine seeds in hundreds of cache sites (**Figure 2**), with sites varying yearly and often covered with snow during retrieved (**Figure 3**). Alex, a parrot, judges pairs of objects in the laboratory that differ in color, material, and/or shape and answers (in English) to the verbal query 'what's different' or 'what's same.'

Despite such astonishing demonstrations of animal intelligence, there is no answer to the question, What is animal intelligence? Theorists have proposed hierarchies of animal intelligence based on learning rates, learning phenomena (e.g., latent inhibition and tool use), discrimination learning (e.g., two-choice 'learning set' and serial discrimination reversals), abstract concept learning, and self-awareness, but none have withstood the test of time. Consequently, most researchers have turned to the study of specific cognitive phenomena (in laboratory settings, natural settings, social settings, etc.). Nevertheless, comparative cognition invariably gravitates to 'who can do what better.' Inevitably, the focus is on species differences and speculation returns to hierarchies, if but limited hierarchies (e.g., a branch of the evolutionary tree such as corvid or paridae birds). Even single-species studies are often (implicitly) compared to humans (e.g., "... the first demonstration in a nonhuman animal"). By contrast, if the behavioral and neurological mechanisms/processes were known, then similarities and differences should be apparent without resorting to a hierarchy ('better than'). In terms of mechanisms, similarities are as important as differences. Similar mechanisms can have somewhat different outcomes or vice versa. For example, a single test of some cognitive ability (e.g., abstract concept learning) might lead to a premature conclusion that some species (e.g., pigeon) does not possess this cognitive ability (or cognitive module). By contrast, if the study had manipulated critical parameters of concept learning, then it might have been revealed that this difference was only a quantitative difference, not the qualitative absence as concluded. These are among the issues that have guided our selection and discussion of animal cognitive phenomena. Some areas of research that have been considered relevant to animal intelligence are mentioned only in passing (encephalization quotient, consciousness, insight, associative learning, self-recognition in mirrors, animal communication, and animal language) because neither theory nor experiments have proven decisive and the field has moved on, and in other cases it is still too early to assess the reliability/validity and relevance to the field (e.g., theory of mind: seeing–begging, knower–guesser, and deception, social theory of intellect: dominance and imitation).

Stimulus-Bound Concepts

The movie '2001: A Space Odyssey' opens with the allegorical scene of primates discovering tool use and the 'touch stone' of intelligence. Tool use has long been considered a behavior whereby humans exploited their (greater) intelligence, passed down tool use over generations, eventually resulting in tools such as the wheel. Some animals in the wild, such as chimpanzees, use twigs to fish for termites and anvil and hammers to break open hard-shelled fruits/nuts. In laboratories, chimpanzees move stools and swing sticks to get hanging fruit or use rakes to pull food within reach, but this behavior does not seem to be learned by imitation. Interpretation of the tube-trap and stick problem (trap hole on one side of the food) is even less clear. Apes (chimpanzees, bonobos, and orangutans) and capuchin monkeys show successful use of the stick solving this problem, but capuchins, at least, apparently learn by trial and error without understanding which direction of stick poke will avoid the trap. With humans and apes atop the hierarchy of tool use, this seemed to be a promising index of intelligence until birds were also shown to use tools. Tool use by Galapagos finches and New Caledonian crows occurs in the laboratory and New Caledonian crows even construct tools, a feat

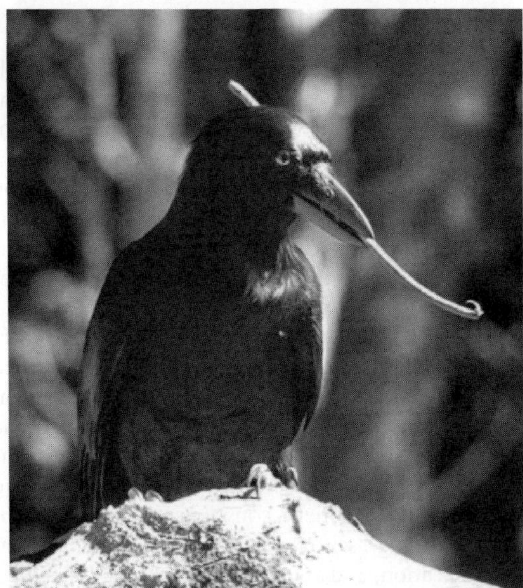

Figure 1 A New Caledonian crow with hooked tool for coaxing food items out of holes and cracks in tree limbs.

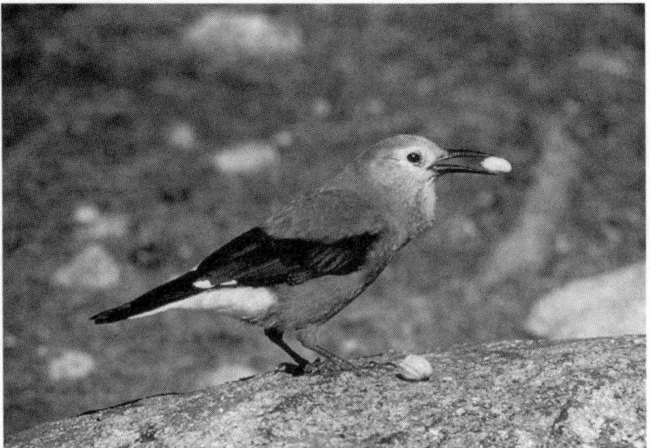

Figure 2 A Clark's nutcracker preparing to cache pinyon nuts. Courtesy of A Kamil.

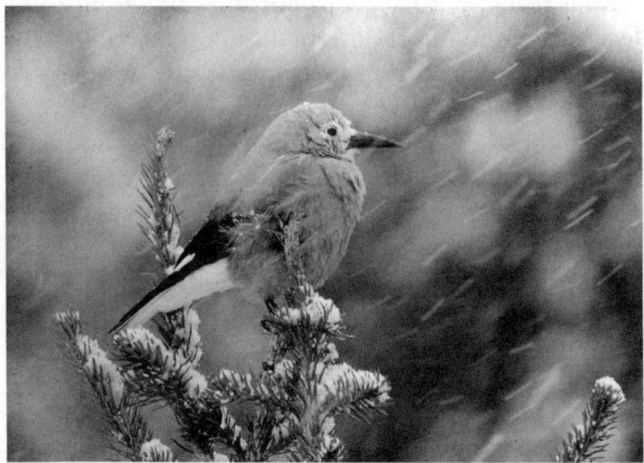

Figure 3 A Clark's nutcracker in winter. Courtesy of A Kamil.

not shown for apes. But here too, captive finches do not seem to learn this tool use by imitation. If these species do not learn tool use by imitation, then the issue becomes how they learn it (i.e., learning mechanisms/processes). The same can be said for other remarkable animal behaviors that, contrary to early speculation, are apparently not learned by imitation (e.g., pilfering cream from milk bottles by English blue tits, pilfering food from backpacks by New Zealand keas, and washing potatoes by Japanese snow monkeys).

Navigation is typically based on relationships among landmarks and/or vector sources (magnetic, sun, and infrasound compasses). The nutcracker's cache retrieval is thought to be dependent on differential weightings of landmarks by a specialized cognitive module. Similar arguments have been made for rats and their spatial abilities. Some of the most remarkable feats of navigation, however, are by insects – animal species that would not stand very high on anybody's intellectual hierarchy. Honey bees, for example, receiving 'dance' communications about a food source strategically evaluate this information according to their knowledge. If the communicated location is an impossible location (e.g., middle of a lake), then they do not fly. If it is adjacent to an island in the middle of the lake, then they will alter the 'flight plan' and fly to the island. At issue is, do honey bees, or any animals, have cognitive maps (i.e., a mental representation of spatial relationships for flexible use)? Navigation in most instances (ants, wasps, bees, and rats) can often be explained by landmarks joined together by movements and local cues resulting in path integration and vector sums – a none too shabby intellectual feat in itself.

Animals (apes, monkeys, and parrots) can learn about number relationships. Monkeys learn to match similar numbers of objects in pictures independent of object size or cumulative area of the objects. They generalize this relational learning to new objects, new sizes, and new numbers and, in some instances, outside the range of numbers used to train the accurate behavior. A gray parrot vocally responds (in English) to the query "how many" and can accurately identify the number of one object type (e.g., keys) mixed with other objects (e.g., rocks). Apes accurately point to Arabic numerals (4, 5, 6, etc.) corresponding to the number of objects even if the objects (e.g., oranges) are hidden in several places. Monkeys too have been shown to identify correct addition (e.g., lemons) by looking longer at incorrect additions. These latter looking-time procedures have the advantage that they require little training, but it is not always clear what cognitive process accounts for such looking-time differences.

Transitive inference has been considered unique to some of the most intelligent species (e.g., humans, apes, and dolphins). Animals discriminate between successive pairs of stimuli taken from a hierarchical sequence of arbitrary stimuli designated by the following letters: A, B, C, D, E. For each successive pair, the choice of the stimulus highest on the hierarchy is rewarded (+) (e.g., A+ vs. B−, B+ vs. C−, and C+ vs. D−). At issue is whether performance will be accurate on a test of B versus D following training. That is, have they learned the hierarchy and can infer that B should be chosen over D without ever been trained on this pair? Although extensive training and a single test example can make for sometimes tricky interpretations, the evidence does indicate that monkeys, rats, jays, and pigeons in addition to humans and nonhuman primates seem to have this ability. Such information adds to the growing list of animal cognitive skills but it hardly lends itself to ranking animals on anything remotely approaching intelligence, and it is not clear whether this task is particularly well suited to investigating the underlying processes.

Animals can learn stimulus relationships and classify/categorize stimuli bound by a category, prototype, or equivalence class. Even pigeons can learn categories (go/no-go tasks) such as person, water, trees, fish, oak leaves, alphabetical letters, and impressionist paintings and as many as four categories (e.g., person, flower, car, and chair) simultaneously. They can accurately transfer to novel category examples. They learn the go/no-go discriminations more rapidly and more accurately if the pictures are grouped by category than when the same pictures are arbitrarily assigned, but they can learn (i.e., memorize) as many as 830 arbitrarily assigned pictures. Pigeons also learn artificial categories (e.g., artificial 'seeds' and geometrical colored shapes and backgrounds). Artificial categories are more amenable to feature analysis (i.e., controlling mechanisms/processes), but these results have often been at odds with feature theory (from human categorization).

Abstract Concept Learning

Abstract concepts are rules about stimulus relationships (e.g., identity). Animals are tested in the laboratory for abstract concept learning in matching-to-sample (MTS) tasks (e.g., sample plus two comparison/choice stimuli) and same–different (S/D) tasks (pairs of stimuli). Rhesus monkeys and apes tested with either junk objects or slide-picture stimuli have for decades shown complete/full concept learning (equivalent training and transfer performance) when tested with novel stimuli. Chimpanzees allowed to play with six different tin cups and six different metal locks showed immediately excellent performance with other stimuli in an MTS task, interpreted as spontaneous abstract concept learning. Although there is little doubt about primates' (apes, baboons, rhesus monkeys, and capuchin monkeys) abstract concept learning ability, other species have been considerably more problematical. Theories of animal cognitive ability and intelligence have been based on which species can (e.g., apes), cannot (e.g., avians), or partially (e.g., dolphins have this ability with auditory stimuli and monkeys with visual stimuli, but not vice versa) learn abstract concepts. Recently, however, this has changed. Dolphins and monkeys have been shown to learn abstract concepts with both visual and auditory stimuli. Even more damning to the hierarchical theories of abstract concept learning is that parrots, crows, rooks, nutcrackers, jays, and pigeons have all showed good (sometimes full) abstract concept learning. Indeed, the amazing feats of intelligent behavior by avians discussed here and elsewhere in this article are even more significant because of the different neural architecture for avians. For example, hemispheric lateralization of function in avians is at least as strong as it is in humans, yet avians have neither a neocortex nor a corpus callosum (and apparently little interhemispheric communication) and these two structures have been in the past thought to be highly correlated with intelligence. Since intelligence is thought to have evolved just like other bodily traits, if intelligence were related to brain size or certain neural structures, then the size of these brain structures should not be modifiable by experience. However, there is abundant evidence (mostly from rats) that size of the hippocampus, corpus callosum, and overall brain size can be altered by experience.

Regarding abstract concept learning, the pigeon is by far the species of greatest focus as well as the most controversial species. In MTS tasks, pigeons have shown full concept learning with cartoon stimuli; they can learn MTS in any of three different (strategic) ways: configural learning, if–then rule learning, or relational learning. Only relational learning leads to abstract concept learning, whereas the other two strategies produce stimulus-specific learning. Moreover, rats learning MTS with different odors (e.g., cinnamon) apparently learn the task relationally (the strategic process necessary for abstract concept learning), exhibit some characteristics of declarative/episodic memory, and require an intact hippocampus to do so.

Pigeons have shown evidence of S/D concept learning with computer-icon arrays, colored geometrical-shape arrays, and travel-slide pictures. In the first case, the degree of concept learning varied with array entropy, but when the array elements were reduced, concept learning diminished and all but disappeared with the minimum of two elements. Work in my laboratory has shown that pigeons tested with travel-slide stimuli are capable of learning the S/D abstract concept with pairs of pictures. No concept learning was found with an 8-item training set. However, successive doublings of the training set improved concept learning to the point where concept learning (i.e., novel stimulus transfer) became equivalent to baseline performance with 256 or more training pictures (**Figure 4**). Similar experiments with capuchin and rhesus monkeys showed more rapid concept learning, and they achieved full concept learning with 128 pictures. These three species showed qualitative similarity in their ability to achieve full S/D abstract concept learning, but they also showed quantitative differences in their rate of concept learning. Pigeons required more exemplars to learn the rule (i.e., larger training set) than monkeys. Further analyses from successive cycles of training set expansion, learning, and transfer testing ruled out generalization (from the training stimulus pairs to the novel transfer pairs) as the mechanism responsible for transfer and concept learning, adding further evidence that these species have learned the higher order concept of S/D.

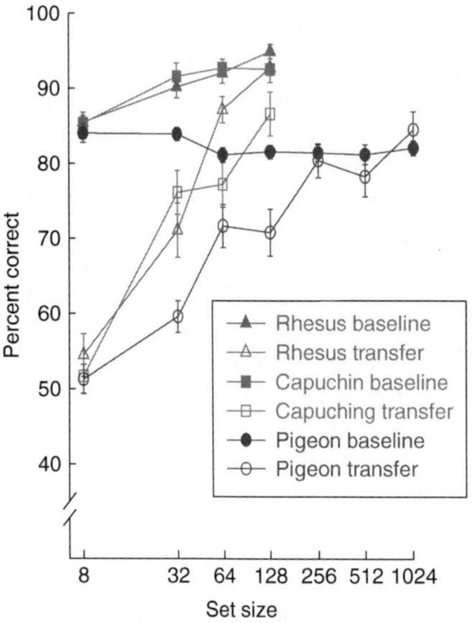

Figure 4 Mean percentage correct performance and standard errors of the mean for baseline performance (solid symbols) and transfer performance (open symbols) at each training set size for rhesus monkeys (triangles), capuchin monkeys (squares), and pigeons (circles). On each trial, a pair of vertically aligned pictures was presented simultaneously along with a white rectangle to the right of the lower picture. If the pair was the same picture, then a response to the lower picture was correct and rewarded. If the pair was two different pictures, then a response to the white rectangle was correct and rewarded. Incorrect choices were unrewarded. All subjects were trained with the same set of eight pictures (100 trials daily) until they were accurate at better than 80% correct and then tested with novel picture pairs (10 novel trials plus 90 training trials) for six sessions. The training set size was then doubled and transfer was tested with novel stimulus pairs after 85% correct performance. This sequence of training-set doubling, retraining, and retesting was repeated several times until transfer was equivalent to baseline (training) performance for each species.

'Higher order' is the watchword for species hierarchies of learning and concept learning in particular. Despite little agreement on most issues, most would probably agree that relations among relations (analogical reasoning) is the highest (most abstract, most difficult) form of abstract concept learning. Supporting the claim of exclusivity would be early evidence that the only animal species capable of this relational feat are chimpanzees because they alone have the ability to recode (tokens and artificial language) abstract relations. However, like previous claims of exclusivity of abstract concept learning, here too failures of other species in analogical reasoning may be the result of training and task failures not cognitive capacity failures. Indeed, baboons have shown similar results using icon arrays, and rhesus monkeys were able to accurately match musical tunes transposed one or two octaves with the first relation being the tunes (a relation among notes) and the second relation being that between the original and transposed tune.

Memory

There is no doubt that many animals have good memory, even by human standards. In addition to the amazing memory ability of nutcrackers to retrieve cached seeds in the natural alpine setting, laboratory studies of monkey memory have shown >70% correct accuracy for sample pictures in a delayed MTS task for 24 h. This good monkey memory occurred with trial-unique pictures so that the animals would not be confused (i.e., proactive interference) from seeing these pictures on previous trials. Although demonstrations of excellent animal memory capture our imagination, research on animal memory has shifted to studies of the memory processes (e.g., rehearsal, decay, consolidation, and interference), different types of memory (episodic, recollection, and familiarity), and brain mechanisms responsible for these different aspects and/or types of memory.

Related to how monkeys in the 24-h memory test might be confused by repeated pictures is what/how animals remember. Do they remember the actual presentation (episode) of the item at the time of test (i.e., episodic memory), or are they just capable of (a vague sense of) familiarity? Familiarity is considered to be a more primitive memory process (hierarchically simpler), associated with less intelligent species, than is episodic memory. Episodic memory and familiarity may be different kinds of memory possibly mediated by different cognitive modules involving different specialized brain areas and neural circuits. Most research on different memory brain areas has been conducted with monkeys and rats and has focused on the medial temporal lobe structures (hippocampus and perirhinal and parahippocampal cortices) for processing of information, the amygdala for emotional significance, and the prefrontal cortex for awareness and planning based on one's own memory (metacognition) and how the memory information will be used. Despite the vast amount of work, only tentative glimpses of a coordinated picture are beginning to emerge. Perhaps the perirhinal cortex might be most critical for object memory, whereas the parahippocampal cortex might be most critical for spatial memory. The hippocampus and prefrontal cortex may be critical for episodic memory through their role in integrating and abstracting information from many other brain areas, including the perirhinal and parahippocampal cortices, thereby associating context information (e.g., 'when and where' information) with the primary memory events ('what' information) and producing evidence of recollection/episodic memory as opposed to item familiarity.

Although human participants can report "I remember" versus "I just know" to indicate episodic versus familiarity memory, respectively, more objective and clever procedures are required for testing animals for these different types of memory. Although it would seem logical for animal research on episodic/familiarity memory to have been done with (nonhuman) primates due to their relative evolutionary proximity to humans, the best and most clever work is actually being done with avians. An additional advantage of working with avians on this issue is that success will have more profound implications because most hierarchical theorists would have apes and/or monkeys being capable of episodic memory – not the proverbial bird brain. Scrub jays have been shown to cache and recover perishable wax worms and nonperishable peanuts in distinctive halves of sand-filled ice cube trays (**Figure 5**). After 4-h delays, the jays first recovered the more desirable wax worms, but after 124-h delays they first recovered peanuts because they had learned that wax worms would deteriorate in 124 h. Thus, they remembered what (peanuts vs. wax worms), when (4 vs. 124 h), and where (which tray side) the foods were stored – requirements of episodic memory. Many

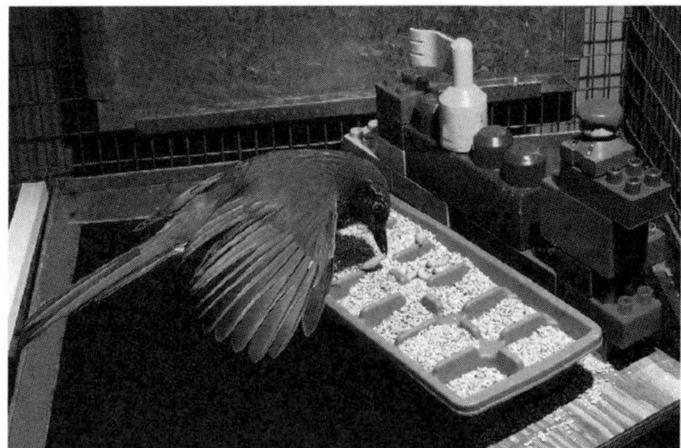

Figure 5 A scrub jay retrieving previously cached wax worms, a food preferred over peanuts at short cache-retrieval times before they deteriorate. Courtesy of NS Clayton.

supporting experiments have replicated these remarkable findings and further explored the processes responsible for this episodic-like memory. Nevertheless, some experts are skeptical that these amazing memory feats by scrub jays may be merely the result of stimulus–response associative learning. However, vast numbers of associative learning studies have shown that associative learning is much more than a collection of stimulus–response reflexes or habits. Rats and other animals in classical conditioning experiments anticipate the future and can even add and subtract anticipated time through complex combinations of forward and backward primary and secondary conditioning. They learn expectations of certain outcomes (what), at certain times (when), and in certain places (where). In these situations, expectations develop over multiple trials (i.e., conditioning) and become reference or generic memory. By contrast, the jays cache a particular item, in a particular place, at a particular time – hence a single episode. Part of the single-episode success may be the act of caching. Caching would be expected to enhance memory for a particular episode, much like the generation effect in human memory. However, the same can be said for taste-aversion memory, which can be a single associative event, a particular stimulus (food taste), and a particular time (as much as several hours or more) before getting sick. Moreover, it has been shown that taste aversion is cognitively flexible (not an automatic stimulus–response association) by manipulations of which of several foodstuffs become associated with sickness. Few would question whether taste aversion is episodic memory because of numerous reports of humans, sometimes decades later, recalling exactly when and under what conditions some previously liked food was inadvertently associated with illness. These so-called 'autonoetic' (self-knowing) reports are considered by some to be the hallmark of episodic memory which, by design or theory, would seem to secure humans as the only animal that definitively possesses episodic memory.

Nevertheless, a delayed-MTS experiment showed that rhesus monkeys, at least, can be consciously aware (metacognition) of their own memories. During retention delays monkeys opted for a memory test and a chance for highly desired reward (peanuts) or else a less desired but certain pellet. Surprise tests showed that they were more accurate when they opted for the test, with the interpretation that they knew when their own memory was good. The key to this interpretation was having the monkeys monitor their memory before the test was presented and thereby avoid confounds of recognition familiarity.

The issues of whether animals have episodic memory, metacognition, or autonoetic experiences aside, animals most certainly have working memory. Indeed, how could any animal learn anything without working memory? Working memory is what is remembered on a particular trial; reference memory is the rules of the task. Good memory observed in natural settings has been tested in laboratory analogues. Nutcrackers have been tested in large arenas where they made as many as 25 caches and accurately recovered these cached seeds 6 months later from 180 possible sites (sand-filled cups). Other caching birds (e.g., tits and chickadees) have been tested in arenas filled with artificial tree limbs where the birds cached seeds in several cloth-covered tree limb holes and later remembered these cache sites from as many as 97 available sites. Many caching birds (scrub jays and nutcrackers) will re-cache if they are observed by another bird or alter their retrieval order (e.g., ravens) to beat the would-be pilferer to the cache site. In at least one case (scrub jays), they re-cache only if they themselves have a history of pilfering from others. Thus, they impute to the observing bird (typically a conspecific) their own pilfering intentions – a prototypical example of so-called 'theory of mind.'

Laboratory tests (e.g., radial arm maze analogues and MTS video monitor images) of single-item memory of some of these caching birds have not always found such remarkably good memory compared to other related species that do not cache. As previously noted, perhaps the act of caching is critical to the good memory. Moreover, the size of the hippocampus does not seem to be highly correlated with the degree of caching or performance on laboratory memory tasks. Current work seems to be more focused on how memory works for these bird species (i.e., processes/mechanisms of landmark navigation) rather than which one has the best memory.

Memory is seldom limited to single items. Certainly in the real world there are collections or streams of things to remember. The study of (human) memory began with memory lists. The hallmark of list memory studies is serial position function (SPF) and its primacy and recency effects (good memory for beginning and ending items, respectively), often revealing a U-shaped SPF. Although animals are notoriously difficult to train in list memory studies, U-shaped SPFs with visual stimuli have been shown for apes, rhesus monkeys, squirrel monkeys, capuchin monkeys, rats, and pigeons. Research on some of the mechanisms/processes responsible for the SPFs has shown that with short four-item lists there is a strong recency effect (last items) at very short retention intervals and little or no primacy effect. As the retention interval is lengthened, the primacy effect develops and the recency effect wanes. Research in my laboratory has shown that these same changes occur for rhesus monkeys, capuchin monkeys, pigeons, and humans (**Figure 6**). The qualitative similarity in these SPFs is complemented by a quantitative difference where the time course of changes takes place in approximately 10 s for pigeons, 30 s for monkeys, and 100 s for humans. The developing primacy effect is counterintuitive because it is an (absolute) increase in memory performance with increasing retention delay. SPFs for auditory stimuli have been shown for dolphins and rhesus monkeys. Rhesus monkeys were tested with short natural/environmental sounds at the same retention delays and list lengths as other rhesus monkeys with visual memory. The auditory SPFs were opposite to the visual SPFs, showing initial strong primacy effects and no recency effects. The recency effects grew with retention delay and the primacy effects waned. Other tests revealed that interference among the list items produced retrieval inhibition and that this inhibition dynamically changed with retention interval. These animal SPFs show some of the mechanisms/processes involved in visual and auditory list memory of these species. They also show that memory is not a unitary system, memory does not decay with time, and rehearsal does not produce the primacy effect – all long-standing tenets of the so-called modal model of memory.

The two examples of work from my laboratory have shown qualitative similarity in abstract concept learning and visual memory processing across such diverse species as humans, New and Old World monkeys, and pigeons. Single tests of these cognitive abilities would likely have shown differences that might have been taken as evidence for a species' differences in

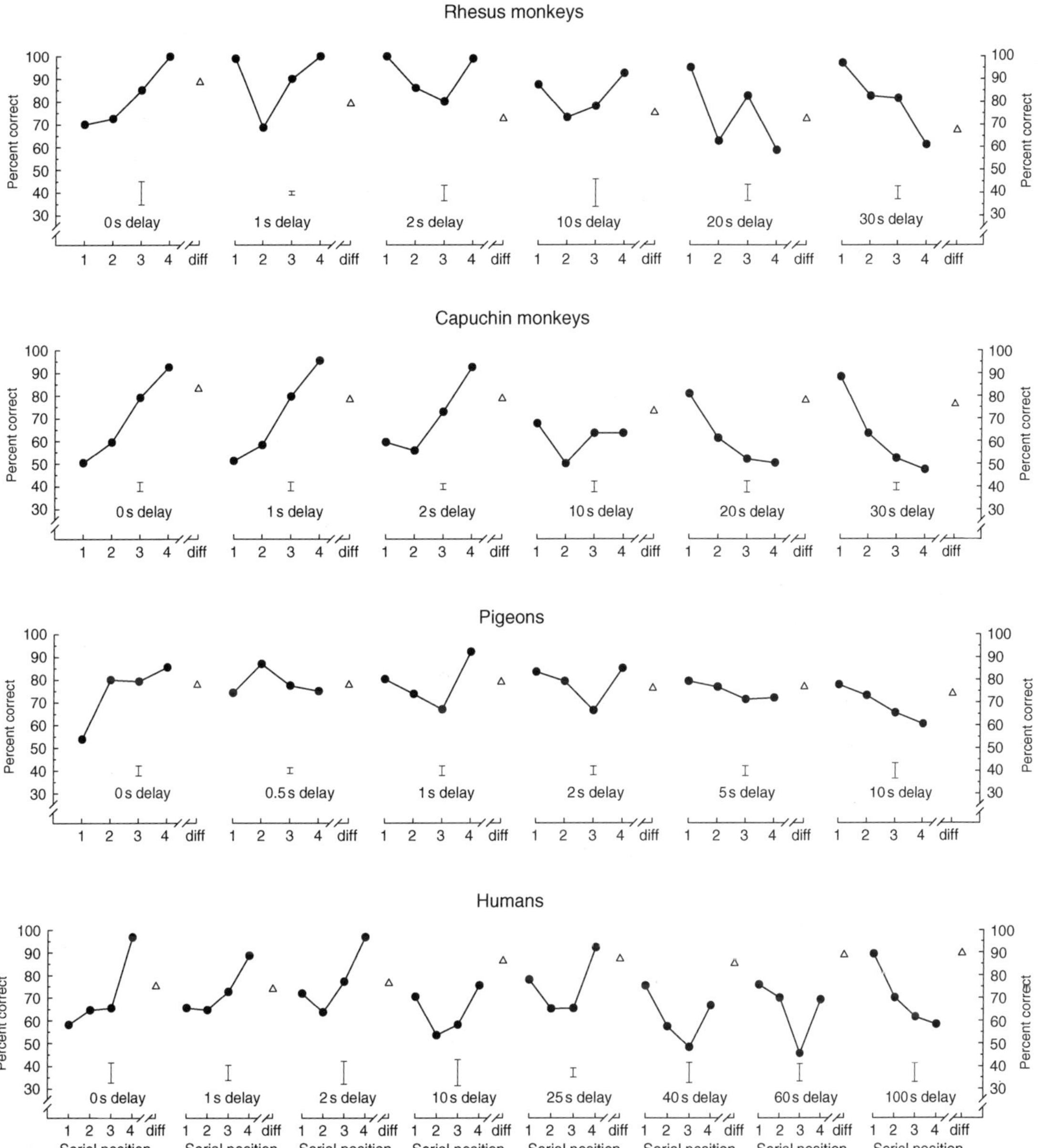

Figure 6 Serial-position memory functions for capuchin monkeys, rhesus monkeys, pigeons, and humans. On each trial, four pictures were briefly presented followed by a retention delay which is indicated in the lower portion of each panel. Subjects responded to indicate their memory of whether a single test picture was or was not in the list. The serial position functions show the results for trials in which the test matched one of the list pictures. (Serial position 4 was the last list item presented.) On half the trials, the test matched no list picture and that performance is shown as 'diff' (different). Test items for monkeys and pigeons were travel slides selected from more than 3000 items; test items for humans were kaleidoscope pictures selected from more than 550 items. The items for all subjects were unique on each daily test session. The error bars are the average standard errors for the four serial positions.

cognitive capability, evolved cognitive modules, and perhaps intelligence. There are differences among species to be sure, but in these cases the differences were quantitative differences. Some of the species (e.g., pigeons) required more exemplars of the rule to learn the abstract concept than monkeys, and in terms of memory, some species had differences in the time course changes of their serial position functions.

See also: Episodic Memory: Assessment in Animals; Executive Function and Higher-Order Cognition: Assessment in Animals; Numerical Intelligence: Neural Substrates; Procedural Learning in Animals; Reasoning and Problem Solving: Models; Referentiality and Concepts in Animal Cognition; Spatial Memory: Assessment in Animals.

Further Reading

Clayton NS, Bussey TJ, and Dickinson A (2003) Can animals recall the past and plan for the future? *Nature Reviews Neuroscience* 4: 685–691.

Emery NJ (2006) Cognitive ornithology: The evolution of avian intelligence. *Philosophical Transactions of the Royal Society B* 361: 23–43.

Olson DJ, Kamil AC, Balda RP, and Nims PJ (1995) Performance of four seed-caching corvid species in operant tests of nonspatial and spatial memory. *Journal of Comparative Psychology* 109: 173–181.

Rogers LJ and Kaplan G (eds.) (2004) *Comparative Vertebrate Cognition*. New York: Kluwer Academic/Plenum.

Shettleworth SJ (1998) *Cognition, Evolution, and Behavior*. New York: Oxford University Press.

Wasserman EA and Zentall TR (eds.) (2006) *Comparative Cognition*. New York: Oxford University Press.

Wright AA (1997) Concept learning and learning strategies. *Psychological Science* 8: 119–123.

Wright AA (1998) Auditory and visual serial position functions obey different laws. *Psychonomic Bulletin and Review* 5: 564–584.

Wright AA and Katz JS (2006) Mechanisms of *same/different* concept learning in primates and avians. *Behavioural Processes* 72: 234–254.

Artificial Intelligence

J Feldman

This article is reproduced from 'Artificial Intelligence in Cognitive Science' in the *International Encyclopedia of the Social & Behavioral Sciences*, Vol 2, pp. 792–796, © 2001, Elsevier Science Ltd.

Overview

Artificial intelligence (AI) and cognitive science are two distinct disciplines, with overlapping methodologies but with rather different goals. AI is a branch of computer science and is concerned with construction and deployment of intelligent agents as computer programs, and also with understanding the behavior of these artifacts. The core scientific goal of AI is to understand the basic principles of intelligent behavior that apply equally to animal and artificial systems. Almost all of the work is mathematical or computational in character and much of the literature is technique oriented.

Cognitive science is an explicitly interdisciplinary field that has participation not only from AI, but also from linguistics, philosophy, psychology, and subfields of other social and biological sciences. The unifying goal of cognitive science is to understand and model human intelligence, using the full range of findings and methodologies of the complementary disciplines. As one would expect, a wide range of techniques from the mathematical, behavioral, social, and biological sciences are employed. Cognitive science, in contrast with AI, is defined more by phenomena than by methodology. There are research groups that are active in both AI and cognitive science, but they tend to produce different types of reports for journals and conferences in the two areas.

Shared Origins in the Postwar Cognitive Revolution

Both AI and cognitive science evolved after 1950, and in their early development were more tightly integrated than at present. For much of the first half of the twentieth century, the Anglo-American study of cognition was dominated by the behaviorist paradigm, which rejected any investigation of internal mechanisms of mind. The emergence of both AI and cognitive science was part of a general postwar movement beyond behaviorist theories, which also included new approaches in linguistics and the social sciences. The idea of computational models of mind was a central theme of what is sometimes called the 'postwar cognitive revolution.' One of the leading early AI groups, under the leadership of Allen Newell and Herbert Simon at Carnegie Mellon, was explicitly concerned with cognitive modeling using the symbolic processes of AI. The current version of this continuing effort is the symbolic cognitive architecture known as Soar (the term derived originally from the concept 'state, operator, and result,' but those currently involved in Soar development prefer not to represent the term as an acronym). Another traditional symbolic approach to modeling intelligence is known as ACT (an acronym for 'adaptive control of thought'). However, there is very little work in contemporary AI that is explicitly focused on modeling human behavior as opposed to intelligent systems in general. There is some continuing work on human and machine game playing, but it is not integrated into the fields of AI and cognitive science.

The central idea of AI is computational modeling of intelligent behavior – its main contribution to cognitive science. The basic notion of a computational model is now commonplace in all scientific fields and many other aspects of contemporary life. One builds a detailed software model of some phenomenon and studies the behavior of the model, hoping to gain understanding of the original system. Much of the work in AI has the engineering goal of producing practical systems, and there is no sharp boundary between AI and other applied fields of computer science and engineering. AI techniques are now commonplace in the full range of business, scientific, and public applications. While all fields use computational models, researchers, in computer science in general and AI in particular, invent and study computational techniques for constructing models, presenting the results of simulations, and understanding the limitations of the simulation. AI has traditionally studied the modeling of the most complex phenomena – those relating to intelligence. Because of the technical challenges arising in the construction of these complex simulations, many innovations in computing have arisen in AI and then have been more widely applied.

Domain-Focused Research That Cuts Across AI and Cognitive Science

The relationship between AI and cognitive science is further complicated by the fact that there are currently several distinct research fields that cut across both disciplines, but have separate journals, meetings, etc. The most prominent of these research areas are speech, language, vision, and neural networks. Each of these fields has thousands of practitioners, many of whom are interested in AI, cognitive science, or both. Appropriately, each of these areas is represented by a vast body of literature. As AI and cognitive science have grown, specialized areas such as language and vision modeling have become largely independent, but they do continue to share the development of underlying methodologies. The main areas that have remained as core AI include knowledge representation and reasoning, planning, and problem solving. The study of learning has evolved somewhat differently (see later). There are some common scientific paradigms that cut across all of these fields, and these are discussed in the following sections as they relate to the social and behavioral sciences. The common thread linking AI to cognitive science is reliance on computational models of different kinds.

Role of Formal Logic in AI and Cognitive Science

To a great extent, the early development of AI was based on symbolic, as opposed to numerical, modeling. This led to the introduction of some novel representations such as those of Soar, but the main effect of this was to align AI with formal logic for much of its early history. In fact, much of the driving force for the creation of the field called cognitive science came from people who saw mathematical logic as its unifying theme. This remains a fruitful approach to AI and constitutes one major area of overlap with cognitive science. Mathematical logic is elegant and well developed and can be shown to be, in some sense, general enough to represent anything that can be described formally. There remains a significant community of linguists, philosophers, and computer scientists for whom logic is the only scientific way to study intelligence.

However, the twentieth century was not kind to categorical, deterministic theories in any field, and cognitive science was no exception. A central issue in the study of cognition has been how to describe the meaning of words and concepts. In formal logic, a concept is defined by a set of necessary and sufficient conditions. For example, a bachelor might be defined as a male who never married. The limitations of classical, all-or-none, categories were already recognized by Wittgenstein, who famously showed that concepts such as 'game' could not be characterized by necessary and sufficient conditions, and were better described as family resemblances. Even the definition of 'bachelor' becomes graded when we consider cohabitation, or how old a male needs to be before being considered a bachelor.

Starting in the 1960s, a wide range of cognitive science studies by Rosch and others showed the depth and complexity of human conceptual systems and their relation to language. This helped give rise to the subfield called cognitive linguistics, which overlaps with cognitive science, but has its own paradigms, journals and conferences. The graded and relational nature of human categories undermined the attempt to create a unified science of mind based on formal logic. Another attack on the formalist program arose from the growing understanding of the neural basis of intelligence. A crucial insight was that basic human concepts are grounded in direct experience and that more abstract concepts are mapped metaphorically to more embodied ones. This undercuts the formalist program, and also leads to a separation of AI, which studies intelligence in the abstract, from cognitive science, which is explicitly concerned with human minds. While much excellent work continues to be done using logic, it is now generally recognized that there are a wide range of phenomena that are better handled by biologically based models and/or some form of numerical, often probabilistic, modeling. For a variety of reasons, the movement to quantitative numerical models followed somewhat different paths in AI and cognitive science, but there are some recent signs of reconvergence.

Learning and the Connectionist Approach to Cognitive Science

As it happens, while the formalists were trying to establish a cognitive science based on formal logic, an antithetical neural network movement was also developing, and this approach has become a major force in cognitive science. The two contrasting approaches to cognitive modeling, neural modeling and logic, were mirrored in the two different methods by which early computer scientists sought to achieve AI. From the time of the first electronic computers around 1950, people dreamed of making them 'intelligent' by two quite distinct routes. The first, 'conventional' AI, is to build standard computer programs as models of intelligence. This remains the dominant paradigm in AI and has had considerable success. The other approach is to try to build hardware that is as brainlike as possible and have it learn the required behavior. The history of this 'neural modeling' approach has been well described. After some promising early mathematical results on learning in simple networks, the neural learning approach to modeling intelligence fared much less well for three decades and had little scientific or applied success. Around 1980, a variety of ideas from biology, physics, psychology, and computer science and engineering coalesced to yield a 'new connectionist' approach to modeling intelligence that has become a core field of cognitive science, and also the basis for a wide range of practical applications. Among the key advances was a mathematical technique (back-propagation) that extended the early results on learning to a much richer set of network structures.

Connectionist computational models are almost always computer programs, but programs of a different kind than those used in, for example, word processing or symbolic AI. Connectionist models are specified as a network of simple computing units, which are abstract models of neurons. Typically, a model unit calculates the weighted sum of its inputs from upstream units and sends to its downstream neighbors an output signal that is a nonlinear function of its inputs. Learning in such systems is modeled by experience-based changes in the weights of the connections between units. The basic connectionist style of modeling is now being used in three quite different ways – in neurobiology, in applications, and in cognitive science. Neurobiologists who study networks of neurons employ a wide range of computational models, from very detailed descriptions of the internal chemistry of the neuron to the abstract units just described. The use of connectionist neural models in practical applications is part of the reconvergence with AI and is discussed in the final section of this article.

In cognitive science, connectionist techniques have been used for modeling all aspects of language, perception, motor control, memory, and reasoning. This universal coverage represents a potential breakthrough; previously, the computational models of, for example, early vision and problem solving used entirely different mathematical and computational techniques. Since the brain is known to use the same neural computation throughout, it is not surprising that neurally inspired models can be applied to all behavior. Unfortunately, the existing models are neither broad nor deep enough to ensure that the current set of mechanisms will suffice to bridge the gap between structure and behavior, but the work remains productive.

Connectionist models in cognitive science fall into two general categories, often called structured and layered networks (also called parallel distributed processor, or PDP, networks). Most modelers are primarily interested in learning, which is modeled as experience-driven change in connection weights. There is a great deal of research studying different models of learning with and without supervision, different rules for changing weights, etc. Because of the focus on what the network can learn, any prewired structure will weaken the results of the experiment. The standard approach is to use networks with unidirectional connections arranged in completely connected layers, sometimes with a very restricted additional set of feedback links. This kind of network contains a minimum of presupposed structure and is also amenable to efficient learning techniques, such as the aforementioned back-propagation method. Most researchers using totally connected layered models do not believe that the brain shares this architecture, but there is an ongoing controversy about the implications of PDP learning models for theories of mind (see the section titled 'Nature and nurture: rules versus connections').

Structured connectionist models are usually less focused on learning than on the representation and processing of information. Essentially all the modeling done by neurobiologists involves specific architectures, which are known from experiment. For structured connectionist models of cognitive phenomena, the underlying brain architecture is rarely known in detail and sometimes not at all at the level of neurons and connections. The methodology employed is to experiment with computational models of the behavior under study that are consistent with the known biological and psychological data and are also plausible in the resources (neurons, computing time, etc.) required. This methodology is very similar to what are called 'spreading activation' models, widely used in psycholinguistics. Some studies combine structured and layered networks, or investigate learning in networks with an initial structure that is tuned to the problem area or the known neural architecture.

Nature and Nurture: Rules versus Connections

Perhaps the most visible contribution to date of connectionist computational models in cognitive science has been to provide a new jousting ground for contesting some age-old issues on the nature of intelligence. Much of the debate has been published in *Science* magazine, which suggests that it is considered to be of major importance by the US scientific establishment. The nature versus nurture question concerns how much of some trait, usually intelligence, can be accounted for by genetic factors, and how much depends on postnatal environment and training. Some PDP connectionists have taken very strong positions, suggesting that learning can account for everything interesting. In the particular case of grammar, an important group of linguists and other cognitive scientists take an equally extreme nativist position, suggesting that humans only need to choose a few parameters to learn grammar. A related issue is whether human grammatical knowledge is represented as general rules or just appears as the rulelike consequences of PDP learning in the neural network of the brain. There is ample evidence against both extreme positions, but the debate continues to motivate a great deal of thought and experiment.

Current and Future Trends

Although the fundamental split between the AI focus on general methods and the cognitive science emphasis on human intelligence remains, there are a growing number of areas of overlapping interest. As already discussed, quantitative neural models are playing a major role in cognitive science. It turns out that the mathematical and computational ideas underlying learning in neural networks have found application in a wide range of practical problems, from speech recognition to financial prediction. The basic idea is that, given current computing power, back-propagation and similar techniques allow large systems of nonlinear units to learn quite complex probabilistic relationships using labeled data. This general methodology overlaps not only with AI but also with mathematical statistics, and is part of a unifying area called computational learning theory. There is also a large community of scientists and engineers who identify themselves as working on neural networks and related statistical techniques for various scientific and applied tasks, along with conferences and journals to support this effort.

While probability was entering cognitive science from the bottom-up through neural models, AI experienced the introduction of probabilistic methods from general theoretical considerations, which only later led to practical application. As discussed earlier, the limitations of formal logic became well recognized in the 1960s. Over the subsequent decades, AI researchers, led by Judea Pearl, at the University of California (Los Angeles), developed methods for specifying and solving large systems of conditional probabilities. These belief networks are now widely used in applications ranging from medical diagnosis to business planning. A growing field that involves both symbolic and statistical techniques is 'data mining,' processing large historical databases to search for relationships of commercial or social importance. Recent efforts to learn or refine belief networks from labeled data are another area of convergence of AI and cognitive science in computational learning theory. Of course, the explosion of Internet activity is affecting AI along with the rest of the computing field. Two AI application areas that seem particularly important to cognitive science are intelligent Web agents and spoken-language interaction.

As the range of users and activities on the Internet continues to expand, there is increasing demand for systems that are both more powerful and easier to use. This is leading to increasing efforts on the human–computer interface, including the modeling of user plans and intentions – clearly overlapping with traditional concerns of cognitive science. One particularly active area is interaction with systems using ordinary language. Whereas machine recognition of individual words is relatively successful, dealing with the full richness of language is one of the most exciting challenges at the interface between AI and cognitive science, and a problem of great commercial and social importance.

Looking ahead, we can be confident that the increasing emphasis on intelligent systems will continue. From the scientific perspective, it is very likely that most of the interdisciplinary research in cognitive science will remain focused on specialized domains such as language, speech, and vision. General issues including representation, inference, and learning will continue to be of interest and will constitute the core of the direct interaction between AI and cognitive science. With the rapid advances in neurobiology, both fields will increasingly articulate with the life sciences, with great mutual benefits.

See also: Animal Intelligence: The Search for Animal Intelligence; Cognitive Neuroscience: An Overview; Cognitive Control and Development; Connectionist Models; Connectionist Models of Language Processing; Executive Function and Higher-Order Cognition: Computational Models; Hippocampus: Computational Models; Memory: Computational Models; Numerical Intelligence: Neural Substrates.

Further Reading

Elman J, Bates E, and Johnson M (1996) *Rethinking Innateness: A Connectionist Perspective on Development (Neural Network Modeling and Connectionism)*. Cambridge, MA: MIT Press.

Lakoff G (1987) *Women, Fire, and Dangerous Things: What Categories Reveal About the Mind*. Chicago, IL: University of Chicago Press.

McClelland JL and Rumelhart DE (1986) *Parallel Distributed Processing*. Cambridge, MA: MIT Press.

Newell A (1990) *Unified Theories of Cognition*. Cambridge, MA: Harvard University Press.

Pearl J (1988) *Probabilistic Reasoning in Intelligent Systems*. San Mateo, CA: Morgan Kaufmann.

Posner MI (ed.) (1985) *Foundations of Cognitive Science*. Cambridge, MA: MIT Press.

Regier T (1996) *The Human Semantic Potential*. Cambridge, MA: MIT Press.

Russell SJ and Norvig P (2000) *Artificial Intelligence*. Upper Saddle River, NJ: Prentice-Hall.

Numerical Intelligence: Neural Substrates

A Nieder, University of Tübingen, Tübingen, Germany

Numbers can be used most flexibly to quantify, rank, and identify virtually everything that is imaginable. Although true counting and mathematics are cultural achievements that are bound to language, it has become evident during the past few decades that basic numerical skills are independent from language. Human adults, infants, and animals are able to nonverbally and approximately grasp the numerical properties of objects or events. Such nonverbal numerical systems are the precursors on which verbal numerical representations build up, and their neural foundation can be studied in animal models.

This article reviews the progress that has been made in our understanding of the neural underpinnings of numerical competence in human and nonhuman primates. It is structured according to the basic concepts numerical quantity, which refers to the empirical property cardinality (the size of a set, also termed 'numerosity'), and numerical rank, which refers to the property serial order.

Numerical Quantity (Cardinality)

Behavior

Animals can discriminate the cardinality of sets. During the past six decades, roughly half a dozen bird and mammal species have successfully been trained to perform several numerical tasks in different modalities. Importantly, animals can transfer their numerical knowledge to numerosities they have not been trained on, which indicates a true understanding of the concept of cardinalities and their sequential arrangement. Moreover, numerical intelligence is not induced by extensive training in the laboratory but can be demonstrated spontaneously in the wild. The data collected for different species indicate that quantity information is indeed exploited by animals in their natural habitat to draw informed choices, for example, in foraging situations or social interactions.

Also, preverbal human infants of several months of age have the capacity to represent cardinality, both in the visual and in the auditory domain. Infants can also engage in rudimentary arithmetic, which was first shown in experiments in which 5-month-old infants were shown basic addition and subtraction operations on small sets of objects.

Human adults can reliably compare the cardinality of sets under conditions that prevent or discourage verbal counting. In contrast to precise verbal counting, however, nonverbal discrimination performance is only inaccurate, or approximate. Some indigenous human cultures that lack number words or have a very restricted concept of verbal counting rely completely on nonverbal cardinality assessment (so-called 'one–two–many' system of 'counting'). Thus, humans without a linguistic number concept can only estimate the number of items by means of a nonverbal quantification system. Together, these studies provide evidence for an evolutionary ancient quantification system which operates independent from language and can thus be studied in animal models.

Numerosity-Selective Neurons

Recordings in monkeys demonstrated the capacity of single neurons to encode numerical quantity. In monkeys performing a visual delayed match-to-numerosity task (**Figure 1(a)**), the highest proportion of numerosity-selective neurons (**Figure 1(c)**) was found in the lateral prefrontal cortex (PFC), irrespective of co-varying nonnumerical parameters. In the posterior parietal cortex (PPC), numerosity-selective neurons were most abundant in the fundus of the intraparietal sulcus (IPS); they were few in other PPC areas or the anterior inferior temporal cortex (aITC) (**Figure 1(b)**). Neurons in a somatosensory-responsive region of the superior parietal lobule (part of area 5) have been reported to keep track of the number of movements, but in a movement-type-dependent manner (i.e., the neurons responded differently whether the monkey's movement was 'push' or 'turn'). Area 5 neurons were not encoding numerosity in visual displays.

Numerosity-selective neurons in the PFC and IPS were tuned for the number of items on a visual display; that is, they showed maximum activity to one of the five presented quantities – a neuron's 'preferred numerosity' (**Figure 1(c)**). All numerosity-selective neurons together formed a bank of overlapping numerosity filters (**Figure 1(e)**), thus mirroring the animals' behavioral performance (**Figure 1(d)**). Interestingly, the neurons' sequentially arranged overlapping tuning curves preserved an inherent order of cardinalities. This is important because numerosities are not isolated categories but, rather, exist in relation to one another (e.g., '3' is greater than '2' and less than '4'); they need to be sequentially ordered to allow meaningful quantity assignments.

The fact that IPS neurons require shorter latencies to become numerosity selective than PFC neurons suggests that the IPS might be the first cortical stage that extracts visual numerical information. Because PPC and PFC are functionally interconnected, that

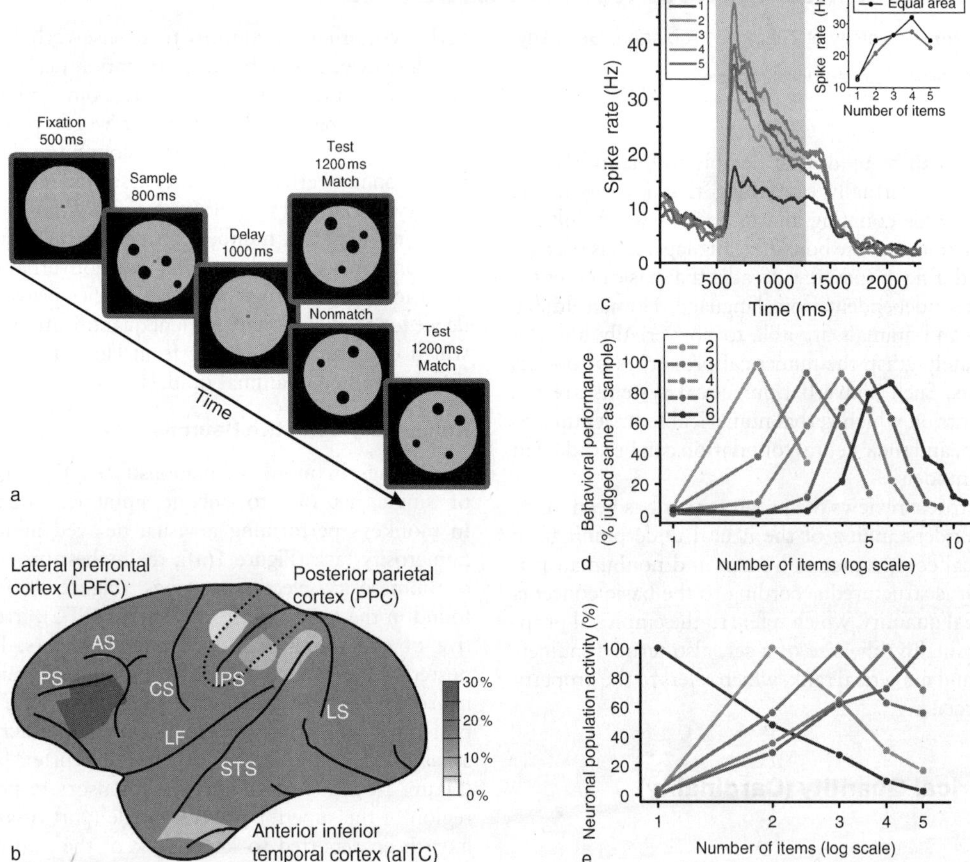

Figure 1 Representation of visual cardinality in rhesus monkeys. (a) Behavioral task. Monkeys performed a delayed match-to-numerosity task. They were required to extract the numerosity in a visual array, memorize it briefly, and match it to the one of two alternative test displays that showed the same numerosity (but with a different visual pattern). (b) Lateral view of the brain of a monkey shows the recording sites in lateral prefrontal cortex (LPFC), posterior parietal cortex (PPC), and anterior inferior temporal cortex (aITC). The proportions of numerosity-selective neurons in each area are color coded according to the color scale. As, arcuate sulcus; Cs, central sulcus; IPS, intraparietal sulcus; LF, lateral fissure; LS, lunate sulcus; PS, principal sulcus; STS, superior temporal sulcus. (c) Responses of a single neuron recorded from the PFC. The neuron showed graded discharge during sample presentation (interval shaded in gray, 500–1300 ms) as a function of numerosities 1 to 5 (color coded average discharge functions). The inset shows the tuning of the neuron and its response to different control stimuli. The preferred numerosity was '4' for this PFC neuron. (d) Behavioral numerosity discrimination functions of two monkeys. The curves indicate whether they judged the first test stimulus (after the delay) as containing the same number of items as the sample display. The function peaks (and the color legend) indicate the sample numerosity at which each curve was derived. Behavioral filter functions are skewed on a linear scale (not shown) but symmetric on a logarithmic scale. (e) The averaged single-cell numerosity tuning functions (from PFC) are also asymmetric on a linear scale (not shown) but symmetric after logarithmic transformation.

information might be conveyed directly or indirectly to the PFC, where it is amplified and maintained to gain control over behavior.

The response properties of numerosity-selective cortical cells can explain basic psychophysical phenomena in monkeys, such as the numerical distance and size effect (**Figure 1(d)**). The numerical distance effect states that it is easier to discriminate quantities that are numerically remote from each other (e.g., 2 vs. 6 is easier than 5 vs. 6), whereas the numerical size effect captures the finding that pairs of numerosities of a constant numerical distance are easier to discriminate if the quantities are small (e.g., 2 vs. 3 is easier than 5 vs. 6). The numerical distance effect results from the fact that the neural filter functions that are engaged in the discrimination of adjacent numerosities heavily overlap. As a result, the signal-to-noise ratio of the neural signal detection process is low, and the monkeys would make many errors. On the other hand, the filter functions of neurons that are tuned to remote numerosities barely overlap, which results in a high signal-to-noise ratio and, therefore, good performance in cases in which the animal has to discriminate sets by a larger numerical distance.

The numerical size effect is based on the finding that neuronal tuning obeys Weber's law: the widths of the tuning curves (or neuronal numerical representations) increase linearly with preferred numerosities (i.e., on average, neurons become less precisely tuned as the preferred quantity increases). Hence, selective neural filters that do not overlap much are engaged if a monkey has to discriminate small numerosities (e.g., 1 and 2), which results in high signal-to-noise ratios and few errors for the discrimination. Conversely, if a monkey has to discriminate large numerosities (e.g., 4 and 5), the filter functions would overlap considerably. Therefore, the discrimination would show a low signal-to-noise ratio, which leads to poor performance.

The Scaling of Numerical Representations

As mentioned previously, the neurons' overlapping tuning curves are orderly arranged along a 'number line' (**Figure 1(e)**). However, what is the scaling scheme of such a number line and are neuronal numerical representations best described on a linear, or a nonlinear, possibly logarithmically compressed scale? The latter would be predicted if Fechner's law holds. Fechner's law states that the perceived magnitude (S) is a logarithmic function of stimulus intensity (I) multiplied by a modality- and dimension-specific constant (k). Since the behavioral discrimination and single-unit tuning functions might be regarded as the monkeys' behavioral and neural numerical representations (**Figures 1(d)** and **1(e)**), the crucial question then concerns which scaling scheme would provide symmetric (i.e., Gaussian) probability density distributions. Both the performance and the single-unit data for numerosity judgments are better described by a compressed scale (**Figures 1(d)** and **1(e)**) as opposed to a linear scale. Therefore, single-neuron representations of numerical quantity in monkeys obey Fechner's law.

Functional Imaging in Humans

In humans, the PFC and the parietal lobe, in particular the IPS, have long been regarded as the prime source for numerical competence. This view, however, was almost exclusively based on verbal and symbolic number tasks, which are only vaguely comparable to numerical magnitude estimation. If anatomical and functional similarities between the brains of monkeys and humans do exist, nonverbal cardinality should be processed in the human brain in equivalent areas as seen in monkeys. Indeed, such a corresponding blood oxygenation level-dependent (BOLD) activation in the IPS of humans has been found using functional magnetic resonance imaging (fMRI) adaptation with numerosities (**Figure 2**). Subjects were repeatedly presented with several visual displays of a fixed numerosity (e.g., 16 dots), without the requirement to discriminate them. The rationale of this protocol is the following: if any region of the brain contains a population of numerosity-selective neurons that are tuned to a specific number of dots and automatically detect numerical information, such a population of detectors should habituate (i.e., decrease its discharge) to numerosities that are repeatedly presented, whereas neurons tuned to other numerosities should not be affected. Such a habituation effect was then 'read out' by recording the event-related fMRI activation to a single deviating numerosity (e.g., 32 dots) that was presented at the end of a display sequence. In fact, the only region in the brain that was significantly habituated to numerosity was the horizontal segment of the IPS (**Figure 2(a)**). With this fMRI adaptation protocol, the average numerosity tuning curve of the underlying neural population could be traced indirectly in humans (**Figure 2(b)**). Similar to single neuron responses in monkeys, fMRI tuning curves in humans seem to be well described on a logarithmic scale, which suggests that the nonverbal number line in all primates is nonlinearly compressed.

Language allows humans to use symbolic representations, and numbers are the symbols that are employed when dealing with numerical information. Interestingly, numerical values that are cued by number symbols and set size have been shown to activate corresponding structures in the brain in humans. The IPS, which has been suggested to play a central role in basic quantity representations, is sometimes the only area specifically activated in simple number detection or comparison tasks. Eger et al. performed fMRI measurements on subjects who were asked to merely detect numerals, letters, or colors which were presented visually (written words and symbols) or acoustically (spoken words). To avoid confounds by response selection and associated cognitive states (e.g., attention), the authors analyzed the presentation of nontarget numerals (numerals that were not required to be detected) and compared it to nontarget letters or colors. The IPS was the only region that exhibited higher activation for numerals, both visually and acoustically (**Figure 3(a)**). Therefore, numerical activation in the IPS seems to be automatic (task independent), supramodal (visual and auditory), and notation independent (irrespective of whether numerals are spoken or written, presented in Arabic notation or spelled-out form). The IPS, however, is

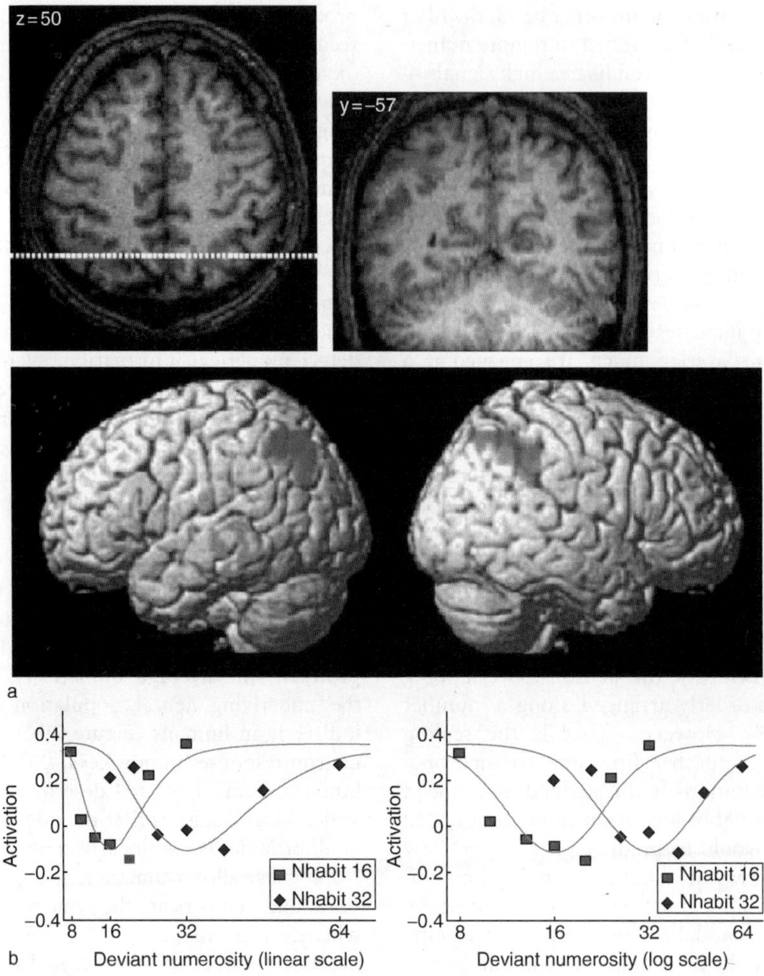

Figure 2 Functional MRI adaptation with numerosities in humans. (a) Regions in the human brain that responded to numerosity changes (i.e., exhibited numerosity selectivity). Colored areas in the axial (top left) and coronal (top right) sections and on the surface image indicate the IPS. (b) Activation difference between the habituation and deviant numerosities resulted in (inverted) numerosity tuning curves that were more symmetrically fitted on a logarithmic (right) than on a linear (left) scale. Adapted from Piazza M, Izard V, Pinel P, Le Bihan D, and Dehaene S (2004) Tuning curves for approximate numerosity in the human intraparietal sulcus. *Neuron* 44: 547–555.

also engaged in more general magnitude judgments. Pinel et al. scanned subjects with fMRI while they compared Arabic numerals for luminance, font size, and numerical value. The authors observed strong overlap in the neural substrates in the three tasks. Number and size, but not luminance, activated a common parietal region, indicating toward an intimate relationship between spatial and numerical representations. This might mean that number-coding neurons are intermingled with other magnitude-coding neurons along the IPS.

Beyond mere encoding of quantity information *per se*, verbal numerical competence requires additional cognitive components. Dehaene and co-workers suggested that verbal counting and calculation engages two more parietal regions: a posterior dorsal parietal area, which is activated by shifts in spatial attention whenever subjects count, and a left angular gyrus area, which is related to linguistic processing. Moreover, simple calculation tasks (e.g., subtraction) typically activate a distributed network that involves parietal, prefrontal, and premotor cortices (**Figure 3(b)**).

Developmental studies confirm that impairments of arithmetical abilities correlate with abnormalities in the organization of parietofrontal networks, and the IPS in particular. Using voxel-based morphometry, Isaacs et al. compared the density of gray matter in adolescents who were born at equally severe grades of prematurity. Half of these subjects (with otherwise normal IQ) suffered from dyscalculia, and the

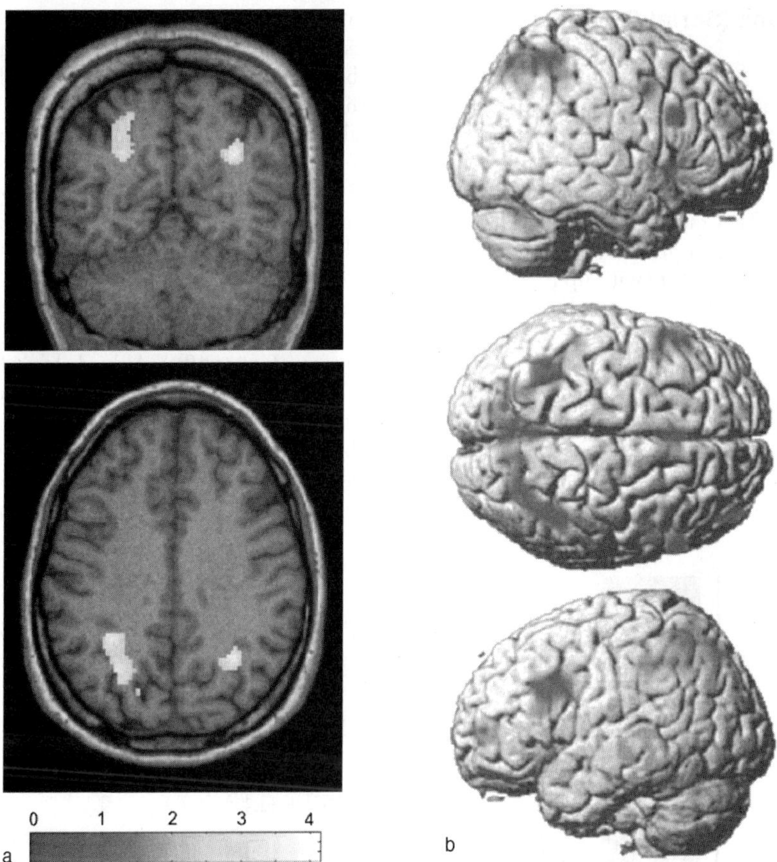

Figure 3 BOLD activation in humans to number symbols and arithmetics. (a) Cortical localization of supramodal responses to numbers (e.g., to both Arabic numerals and spoken number words). Compared to letters and colors, significant bilateral activation was only found deep in the horizontal IPS. (b) Activation pattern observed during subtraction. A covert subtraction task was contrasted with covert naming of the next number in the number line. It resulted in a distributed response pattern involving parietal, premotor, and prefrontal cortices. Adapted from Eger E, Sterzer P, Russ MO, Giraud AL, and Kleinschmidt A (2003) A supramodal number representation in human intraparietal cortex. *Neuron* 37: 719–725.

only region in the brain that showed reduced gray matter associated with arithmetical deficits was the left IPS. Therefore, dyscalculia in children might be the result of specific disabilities in basic numerical processing rather than the consequence of deficits in other cognitive abilities. Arithmetic deficits are also found in certain genetic conditions, such as the Turner syndrome (X monosomy), fragile X syndrome, and velocardiofacial syndrome. In these conditions, fMRI hypoactivation (decreased BOLD activation) was found in the IPS and wider parietofrontal networks.

Neuropsychological Studies

Brain damages in humans can cause relatively selective impairments in dealing with numbers, called acalculia. The most frequent lesions yielding acalculia involve the left inferior parietal area or the left parieto-occipito-temporal junction. In cases of left inferior parietal lesion, acalculia is frequently associated with agraphia, finger agnosia, and left–right confusion in a tetrad of deficits called Gerstmann's syndrome. In addition, calculation deficits have also been observed following left medial frontal, left and right frontal, and temporo-occipital lesions. A major issue in neuropsychological studies is the dissociation between deficits in language and numerical functions, particularly when the left hemisphere is affected. One study has indicated that syntactical mathematical operations (e.g., calculation rules such as solving equations according to brackets) are largely independently represented from linguistic syntax, at least in an adult brain.

Numerical Rank (Serial Order)

Behavior

Numerical rank is the second major numerical concept that shows biological precursors. List learning – the ability to encode and then retrieve an arbitrary list of items in their correct order – opened a window to study how the ordinal rank of objects is learned and stored by animals. Rhesus monkeys learned the serial order of items in several lists with up to seven items. Controlled manipulations of such learned lists showed that the monkeys acquired knowledge of each item's ordinal position.

Single-Unit Studies of Serial Order

Ordinal categorization of visual items requires both information about the rank of an item (e.g., based on temporal order) and its identity. The single-neuron correlate of temporal rank order information in visual lists has been studied in monkeys trained to observe and remember the order in which three visual objects appeared so that the animals could plan a subsequent triple-reaching movement in the same order (**Figure 4(a)**). Neurons in the ventrolateral PFC were selective for visual object properties, whereas neurons in the dorsolateral PFC were selectively tuned to the rank order of the objects irrespective of the visual properties of objects; for example, a rank-order selective neuron would be active whenever the second item of the shuffled lists appears (**Figure 4(b)**). A third class of neurons, found in the ventrolateral PFC, showed the most complex response that was characterized by integrating the objects' sensory and order information; such a neuron would only discharge whenever a certain object appeared at a given position in the sequence.

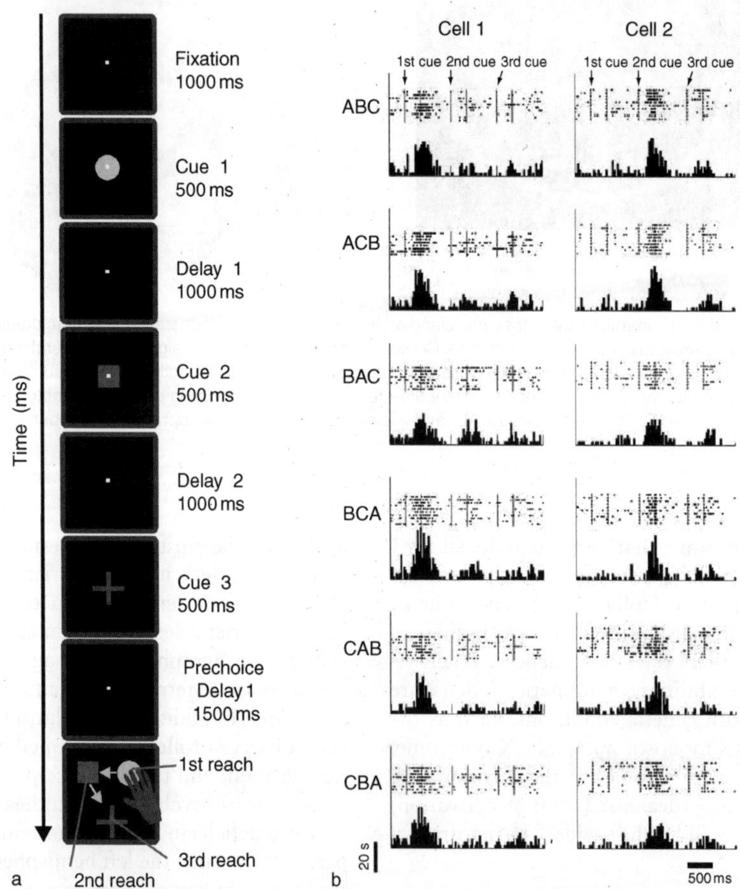

Figure 4 Temporal ordering task and single cell responses from the PFC. (a) Monkeys were required to observe and remember the order in which three visual objects appeared so that the animals could plan a subsequent triple-reaching movement in the same order. (b) Two single neurons encoding the first (cell 1) and the second rank (cell 2), irrespective of the order in which the three items (symbolized by letters ABC) appeared. Neural responses are shown in a dot-raster histogram (top; each dot represents an action potential) and averaged as peri-stimulus time histograms (bottom). Adapted from Ninokura Y, Mushiake H, and Tanji J (2004) Integration of temporal order and object information in the monkey lateral prefrontal cortex. *Journal of Neurophysiology* 91: 555–560.

The lateral PFC is an ideal region in the brain to encode both sensory object properties and rank-order information because it receives massive sensory input from the temporal and parietal lobes, and it projects to premotor and motor areas of the frontal lobe. As a result, neurons that encode the ordinal position of task-related hand or eye movements have been found frequently in prefrontal and a variety of motor-related cortical areas in trained monkeys, such as the frontal eye field (FEF), the presupplementary motor areas (pre-SMAs), the supplementary motor area (SMA), the caudate nucleus, the anterior cingulate cortex (CGa), and even the primary motor cortex (M1). Motor-related areas such as M1, SMA, pre-SMA, and FEF may receive numerical information that has been computed on earlier stages of the cortical hierarchy to perform appropriate serial-order actions.

Human Studies

Based on patient studies, the lateral PFC has been implicated in maintaining temporal order information, which is an integral aspect of episodic memory. It is well-known that damage to the human frontal cortex causes impairment in tasks that require recall of the temporal order of stimuli. A similar ordering impairment has resulted from lesioning the dorsolateral frontal cortex in monkeys, which supports the view that the dorsolateral PFC in primates is important in maintaining information about the order of events. Functional MRI studies of humans show that prefrontal and parietal cortices are more strongly activated for order information (e.g., the order of words in a list) than for item information (the presence of words in a list). In addition, the lateral frontoparietal areas, the basal ganglia, and the cerebellum are preferentially involved in ordinal control of hand movements.

See also: Animal Intelligence: The Search for Animal Intelligence; Cognition: An Overview of Neuroimaging Techniques; Executive Function and Higher-Order Cognition: Neuroimaging; Neuroimaging; Parietal Cortex and Spatial Attention; Prefrontal Cortex: Structure and Anatomy; Prefrontal Cortex; Reasoning and Problem Solving: Models.

Further Reading

Brannon EM and Terrace HS (1998) Ordering of the numerosities 1 to 9 by monkeys. *Science* 282: 746–749.

Dehaene S (1997) *The Number Sense.* Oxford: Oxford University Press.

Dehaene S, Molko N, Cohen L, and Wilson AJ (2004) Arithmetic and the brain. *Current Opinion in Neurobiology* 14: 218–224.

Eger E, Sterzer P, Russ MO, Giraud AL, and Kleinschmidt A (2003) A supramodal number representation in human intraparietal cortex. *Neuron* 37: 719–725.

Gordon P (2004) Numerical cognition without words: Evidence from Amazonia. *Science* 306: 496–499.

Hauser MD, MacNeilage P, and Ware M (1996) Numerical representations in primates. *Proceedings of the National Academy of Sciences of the United States of America* 93: 1514–1517.

Nieder A, Diester I, and Tudusciuc O (2006) Temporal and spatial enumeration processes in the primate parietal cortex. *Science* 313: 1431–1435.

Nieder A, Freedman DJ, and Miller EK (2002) Representation of the quantity of visual items in the primate prefrontal cortex. *Science* 297: 1708–1711.

Nieder A and Miller EK (2004) A parieto-frontal network for visual numerical information in the monkey. *Proceedings of the National Academy of Sciences of the United States of America* 101: 7457–7462.

Ninokura Y, Mushiake H, and Tanji J (2004) Integration of temporal order and object information in the monkey lateral prefrontal cortex. *Journal of Neurophysiology* 91: 555–560.

Piazza M, Izard V, Pinel P, Le Bihan D, and Dehaene S (2004) Tuning curves for approximate numerosity in the human intraparietal sulcus. *Neuron* 44: 547–555.

Pica P, Lemer C, Izard V, and Dehaene S (2004) Exact and approximate arithmetic in an Amazonian indigene group. *Science* 306: 499–503.

Wiese H (2003) *Numbers, Language, and the Human Mind.* Cambridge, UK: Cambridge University Press.

Wynn K (1992) Addition and subtraction by human infants. *Nature* 358: 749–750.

振荡神经活性

Central Pattern Generators

D Bucher, Whitney Laboratory, University of Florida, St. Augustine, FL, USA

Introduction

Repetitive (cyclic) movements underlie crucial behaviors like locomotion (walking, swimming, crawling, and flying), as well as essential vegetative functions like respiration, heartbeat in some invertebrates, chewing, and gut movements. Although both sensory feedback and neuromuscular dynamics play an important role in shaping rhythmic motor output, the basic rhythmic activity patterns are generated by central circuits called central pattern generators (CPGs). These CPGs can, when properly activated, produce rhythmic network activity in the absence of external timing cues, that is, without rhythmic sensory feedback or rhythmic activation by descending neurons.

The most unambiguous demonstration of this principle comes from experiments with isolated parts of the nervous system that produce rhythmic activity *in vitro*, either spontaneously or in response to pharmacological activation. The overall patterning and phasing of such activity very often is surprisingly similar to the basic intact motor behavior and is therefore referred to as a fictive motor pattern or a fictive behavior (e.g., fictive locomotion). Among the first successful demonstrations of the existence of CPGs were experiments with locusts. Those experiments showed that the rhythmic motor output to flight muscles can be generated in the deafferented thoracic nerve cord in an immobilized animal (**Figure 1(a)**). Possibly the most robust mammalian fictive motor pattern is the respiratory rhythm that can be recorded from slice preparations of the brain stem. This activity occurs spontaneously, without electrical stimulation or pharmacological activation (**Figure 1(b)**).

Much effort has gone into understanding the basic cellular and network mechanisms of rhythm generation, with the ultimate goal of linking circuit operation to basic behaviors. Invertebrate CPGs have been invaluable in this endeavor, predominantly because many invertebrate circuits consist of a limited number of individually identifiable neurons with large cell bodies. This makes them tractable systems for establishing circuit connectivity and allows repeated measurements of intrinsic membrane and synaptic properties in unambiguously identified neurons across many different preparations.

In vertebrates, identifying neuron types and characterizing their properties and connections on the basis of electrophysiological and anatomical criteria have been more difficult but have been somewhat successful in the spinal cord of lamprey, amphibians, and cat. Recently, progress has been made in applying new, sophisticated molecular techniques to the study of motor pattern generation, particularly in mice and zebra fish. Such approaches may allow the use of markers for transcription factors to identify groups of neurons and establish the circuit architecture underlying motor pattern generation.

In the following discussion, general principles are introduced that have emerged from the study of a wide range of invertebrate and vertebrate preparations. Mechanisms governing the function of CPGs, the dynamics of their cellular components and their network operations, as well as context-dependent activation and coordination are discussed.

Cellular and Network Mechanisms of Rhythm Generation

Rhythmic motor patterns almost always consist of sequential or alternating activation of antagonistic groups of muscles, and this sequence is seen in the timing of bursts of action potentials between groups of neurons in the underlying CPG. How this rhythmic activity is generated and how bursting and specific relative timing between different neurons is achieved depend on the circuit architecture, the properties of synaptic connections, and the intrinsic membrane properties of CPG neurons.

Synaptic Properties

Even though a wide variety of synapse types may be found in any given CPG, synchronization of neurons that fire in the same phase of the pattern is often achieved or aided by electrical coupling through gap junctions between these neurons, whereas alternating activity is often based on reciprocal inhibitory connections.

Many chemical synaptic interactions in CPGs are based on spike-mediated mechanisms; that is, transmitter is released in response to presynaptic action potentials. However, local interneurons often also rely on graded synaptic transmission; that is, they release transmitter as a graded function of presynaptic membrane potential. In general, it is not clear what the functional significance of graded versus spike-mediated transmission is in the specific context of rhythm generation. However, in a given circuit, the dynamics of these two types of transmission and their interaction with intrinsic neuronal membrane

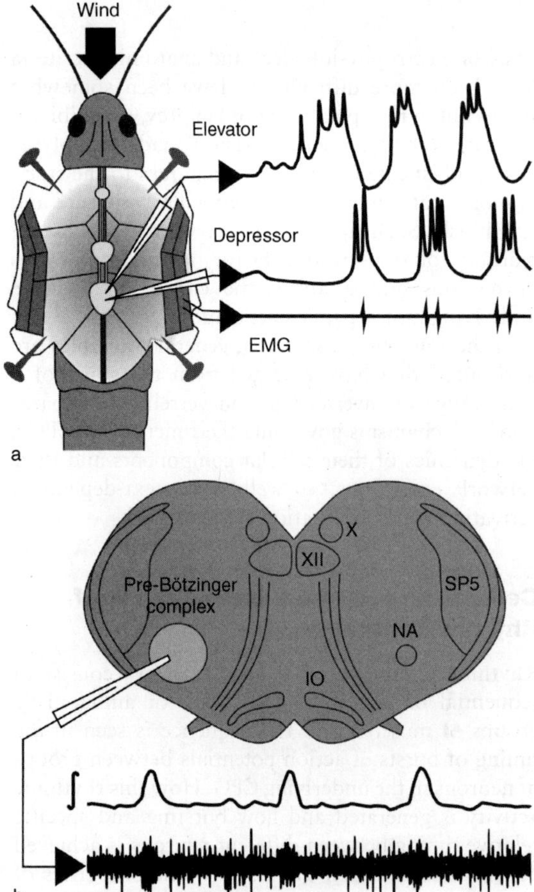

Figure 1 Generation of motor patterns in the absence of sensory feedback. (a) In the locust, rhythmic motor output to flight muscles can be generated in the deafferented thoracic nerve cord in an immobilized animal with wind stimulation to the head. Alternating activity between elevator and depressor motor neurons is generated even though no movement is produced and no sensory feedback reaches the central nervous system. (b) Transverse brain stem slice containing the central pattern generating neurons for respiration in the pre-Bötzinger complex. Population activity is recorded extracellularly (lower trace), and integrated (upper trace) to show rhythmic activity that corresponds to inspiration. XII, hypoglossal nucleus; X, dorsal motor nucleus of vagus; NA, nucleus ambiguus; SP5, spinal trigeminal nucleus; IO, inferior olive. (a) Adapted from Robertson RM and Pearson KG (1982) A preparation for the intracellular analysis of neuronal activity during flight in the locust. *Journal of Comparative Physiology* A 146: 311–320. (b) Adapted from Lieske SP, Thoby-Brisson M, Telqkamp P, and Ramirez JM (2000) Reconfiguration of the neural network controlling multiple breathing patterns: Eupnea, sighs and gasps. *Nature Neuroscience* 3: 600–607.

properties can be quite different, and CPGs exploit the possibilities of both for dynamic circuit operation.

Many synapses show considerable short-term plasticity such as depression, facilitation, or mixtures of both. In CPGs, synaptic dynamics can strongly influence the frequency of rhythmic network activity and the relative timing between different groups of neurons. This is because in rhythmic systems, depression and facilitation cause the strength of a synaptic connection to be dependent on rhythm frequency and on the duty cycle, the number of spikes, or the spike frequency of the presynaptic neuron. In the leech heartbeat CPG, the synaptic strength of connections from a single presynaptic neuron onto several postsynaptic neurons peaks at different times during a single presynaptic burst, as a result of different synaptic dynamics at these connections. Because of synaptic depression, some synaptic connections in the crustacean stomatogastric ganglion become weaker and peak later the faster the rhythm is, and this can help maintain stable relative timing between neurons at different rhythm frequencies.

Intrinsic Neuronal Properties

As in all neural networks, activity does not depend only on synaptic connections but also on a potentially rich complement of voltage-gated ion channels that determine a neuron's intrinsic membrane properties and therefore how it behaves in isolation and in response to synaptic input. A number of intrinsic properties are commonly found in CPG neurons (**Figure 2**). Among them are endogenous bursting properties, postinhibitory rebound, plateau properties, spike frequency adaptation, and restorative sag potentials.

Endogenous bursting means that a neuron can generate membrane oscillations in the absence of synaptic inputs (**Figure 2(a)**). This is an important mechanism of rhythm generation in a number of systems (see the section titled 'Pacemaker and network-based mechanisms').

In other neurons, bursting can be generated on rebound from inhibitory synaptic input (**Figure 2(b)**). This is an important mechanism for the production of alternating activity, and the time course of this rebound is an important determinant of relative timing between alternating rhythmic neurons.

The term plateau potential, or bistable membrane behavior, describes the ability of neurons to generate sustained firing in response to brief and relatively weak depolarizing input (**Figure 2(c)**). If an input crosses a certain threshold, firing activity outlasts the stimulus significantly and can either self-terminate eventually or be shut off by (again, relatively weak) hyperpolarizing input. Plateau properties can therefore uncouple neuronal firing from the duration and strength of excitatory input.

Many CPG neurons show spike frequency adaptation; that is, their firing slows down or ceases during sustained depolarization (**Figure 2(d)**). This can be an important mechanism to ensure that network activity

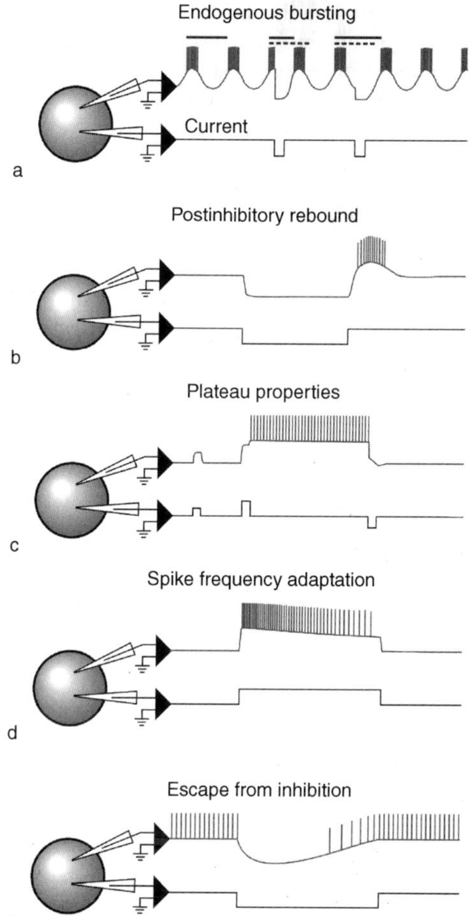

Figure 2 Intrinsic nouronal membrane properties in central pattern generators. Neuronal activity is critically dependent on intrinsic membrane properties that determine how a cell responds to synaptic input. In the absence of synaptic input, some commonly found membrane properties can be demonstrated by assessing the voltage responses to current injection. (a) Endogenous oscillators produce rhythmic activity in the absence of synaptic drive. Rhythmic activity in such neurons can be reset by current injection. Solid lines above the recording trace indicate the cycle duration, and broken lines indicate the unperturbed cycle duration. Whether the following cycle of bursting is advanced or delayed depends on both the sign and the phase of the current injection. The dependency on phase is an important characteristic of oscillators because it determines how synaptic input affects rhythmic activity. (b) Postinhibitory rebound is an overshooting response following hyperpolarizing input that can trigger a burst of action potentials. (c) Plateau potentials are persistent depolarizing responses to brief depolarizing input of sufficient amplitude. The depolarizing response either eventually self-terminates or can be terminated by brief and relatively weak hyperpolarizing input. (d) Spike frequency adaptation is a waning response to continuous depolarization of constant amplitude. Spiking activity can cease before the depolarizing input is shut off. (e) Escape from inhibition is a depolarizing response to hyperpolarizing input and can enable the neuron to eventually start firing action potentials again, despite continuing hyperpolarizing input.

does not get locked into the firing phase of neurons that inhibit functional antagonists.

Neurons that have hyperpolarization-activated inward currents can produce restorative sag potentials in response to inhibitory input; that is, they slowly start to depolarize during sustained hyperpolarization (**Figure 2(e)**). This is an important mechanism for neurons to escape from inhibition.

The ionic basis and the dynamics of the voltage-activated ion channels that are responsible for these properties are relatively well understood in a number of systems, at least to the point that most of the complement of ionic conductances have been identified, characterized, and attributed to certain functions. Some properties are mediated by similar conductances across many cell types and systems, whereas others can be based on a variety of different ionic mechanisms. Even though it is a reasonable approach to attribute certain aspects of a neuron's behavior to specific ionic conductances, especially if pharmacological block of this conductance abolishes this behavior, some caution is advisable. The influence that a specific ionic conductance has on a cell's behavior also depends on the overall complement of other conductances and the relative densities between them. In realistic computer models of neurons, changing the balance between the same set of conductances can change the activity patterns and responses to synaptic input radically.

Pacemaker and Network-Based Mechanisms

Where does the actual rhythmic activity originate? In principle, rhythm generation can be based on intrinsic oscillatory cellular properties or can emerge from synaptic interactions of neurons that are not intrinsically capable of generating rhythmic activity (**Figure 3**). In the first case, rhythmic network activity is based on the endogenous bursting properties of a core group of neurons that drive bursting in other cells (**Figure 3(a)**). Such neurons are referred to as endogenous bursters, oscillators, or pacemaker cells. These neurons synapse onto follower cells that burst as a consequence of rhythmic synaptic input but are tonically active or silent when synaptic input is removed experimentally. Follower neurons can have feedback synapses onto the pacemaker cells and can have rich synaptic interactions with other follower neurons (**Figure 3(b)**). Feedback synapses onto the pacemaker can play an important role in setting both frequency and the phasing of the pattern.

In other networks, rhythmic activity is generated in the absence of any cell-autonomous burst mechanisms and is the result of network connectivity. What may be the simplest form of network-based

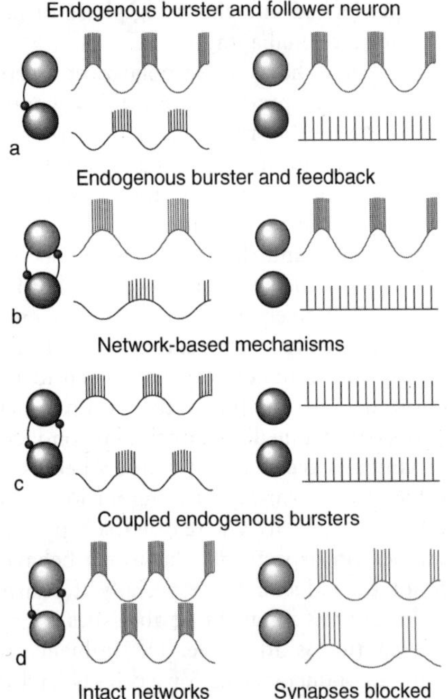

Figure 3 Network mechanisms of rhythm generation. The core mechanism of rhythm generation in a central pattern generator can be based either on endogenous bursting properties or on synaptic interactions of neurons that are not intrinsically capable of generating rhythmic activity. (a) Endogenous oscillators provide synaptic input to follower cells that allows the latter to burst rhythmically, in this case in rebound from inhibition. When synaptic interactions are blocked, the endogenous oscillator continues to cycle, whereas the follower neuron is either silent or fires tonically. (b) Feedback synapses from follower neurons to endogenous bursters can have significant influence on the pattern frequency and phasing. (c) A commonly found network-based mechanism of rhythm generation is reciprocal inhibition. This mechanism is often referred to as half-center oscillation. When synapses are blocked, both neurons are silent or fire tonically. (d) Endogenous bursters can be synaptically coupled to coordinate their bursting and/or stabilize regular rhythmic activity.

mechanisms of rhythm generation is the so-called half-center oscillation (**Figure 3(c)**). Here, reciprocal inhibition leads to alternating patterns of activity between neurons. The transitions from firing in one neuron to firing of the other neuron can be due to such things as release from inhibition when the active neuron shows spike frequency adaptation. Alternatively, the inactive neuron's intrinsic membrane properties can allow it to escape from inhibition, reach threshold, and in turn inhibit the other neuron.

It is not always straightforward to distinguish between cell-autonomous and network-based mechanisms. Some neurons have conditional oscillatory properties; their ability to generate rhythmic activity in synaptic isolation depends on the presence of neuromodulators and, in the intact system, can be dependent on the way the CPG is activated. In addition, pairs of neurons may have strong reciprocal synaptic connections that are essential for establishing robust and regular bursting with specific frequencies and relative timing but may also show endogenous bursting in synaptic isolation, even if this bursting is less robust (**Figure 3(d)**). In fact, a number of circuits show characteristics of both pacemaker-driven and network-based bursting. The circuit motif of reciprocal inhibition, often thought to be a hallmark of network-based rhythm generation, is also widespread in systems that are dominated by pacemaker neurons. In general, which mechanisms dominate may depend on context and how the circuit is activated. That being said, pacemaker-driven rhythmic networks control the mammalian respiratory rhythm and the pyloric rhythm of the crustacean foregut, two motor patterns that are continuously active. In contrast, network-based mechanisms appear to play the most important role in a range of circuits regulating locomotion, a behavior that is executed only in specific contexts.

Activation and Neuromodulation of CPGs

Most rhythmic motor behaviors can occur over a wide range of frequencies and with different durations and relative timing of activity between the muscles involved. For example, movement of a joint can be fast or slow, occur over different angles, and require different relative muscle activation for flexion and extension, dependent on the specific behavioral context. This flexibility is at least partly due to neuromodulators that potentially shape CPG activity into many different forms. The presence of neuromodulators in some cases is required even for the basic operation of a CPG, but in all cases it provides fine-tuning of rhythmic activity. Understanding CPG operation, therefore, requires understanding of not only circuit architecture and the intrinsic dynamics of neurons and synapses; in addition, it requires knowledge of the complement of neuromodulatory substances that affect a given circuit and the consequences that the presence of these substances has for circuit operation. This includes identifying which neurons in a CPG each substance targets and which receptors and ion channels in each cell type are affected. In addition, it is crucial to identify the source of modulatory substances and to know when and how they are released.

Complement and Source of Neuromodulators

The substances that act as neuromodulators can be very diverse and include classical transmitters such as γ-aminobutyric acid and glutamate, biogenic amines such as dopamine and serotonin, a wide variety of peptides, and even gases such as nitric oxide. It is tempting to attribute certain global functions to a single modulator, but the idea that in a specific behavioral context, one modulator is released that changes the motor pattern in the desired way is unlikely to be true. In all systems where the effort has been made, a multitude of substances have been found, and it is more likely that in any given context, different combinations of these substances control CPG operation.

One of the most extensively studied systems in that respect is the stomatogastric ganglion (STG) of crustaceans, which contains CPGs that control the movement of different parts of the stomach. Here, almost 30 different substances have been identified that affect circuit operation (**Figure 4(a)**). These substances reach the STG through the circulatory system as neurohormones or are released into the neuropil by descending modulatory neurons or sensory afferents. Some of the substances are present in both delivery systems, presumably with different consequences because of differences in concentration and spatial distribution. In general, neurohormones affect circuits globally because they have access to the entire nervous system. In contrast, release from neuromodulatory terminals is locally restricted. That being said, paracrine release can lead to a fairly extensive diffusion of these substances, and many modulator actions are likely to be mediated through extrasynaptic receptors.

In some systems, even the CPG neurons themselves can have modulatory cotransmitters. This intrinsic modulation means that the properties of the circuit can be changed as a function of its own activity. In general, cotransmission is a widely found strategy in the modulation of CPGs. In the STG, different identified projection neurons that release the neuropeptide proctolin can elicit different forms of CPG activity. This is partly because they have different complements of cotransmitters that are released at the same time as proctolin.

Divergence and Convergence of Neuromodulator Action

Each modulator has a specific effect on circuit operation because it targets a specific subset of cells in the circuit. It may have different subcellular actions in each cell. In addition, different cells have different combinations of receptors to neuromodulators. Modulators can have a variety of effects in a single neuron (divergence), and different modulators can act on the same subcellular target in a given cell (convergence). In the pyloric circuit of the STG, all these mechanisms have been described.

Dopamine changes the activity of pyloric neurons, particularly the phase relationships, that is, the relative timing between them (**Figure 4(b)**). These effects are based on a wide variety of actions on synaptic and intrinsic neuronal properties (**Figures 4(c)** and **4(d)**). Dopamine enhances the strengths of some chemical synapses and reduces the strength of others. In extreme cases, it can unmask synaptic connections that are not measurable in the absence of dopamine, and it can completely abolish others. In addition, it can alter the strength of electrical coupling between neurons.

Dopamine also affects a number of different voltage-dependent ion channels in pyloric neurons. It has several targets in each neuron, and these sets of targets differ across neurons. In addition, it can have a different effect on the same type of current in different neurons and either enhance or reduce it. In contrast to this divergence of dopamine actions, other substances converge onto the same target. Receptors for many different neuromodulatory substances are found in each pyloric neuron. A large portion of these, particularly the neuropeptides, act on the same voltage-dependent, nonselective, cation channel. In this case, the specificity of neuromodulator action results from different neurons in the circuit having different subsets of receptors.

Descending Commands and the Activation of Specific Patterns

What are the mechanisms of the decision-making process necessary to determine whether a specific motor pattern is elicited or not? This is particularly important in motor behaviors that are elicited only in specific behavioral contexts, but it is also true for specific different forms of continuously active motor output. In some cases, activating a single neuron, or a network of a few, can be sufficient to elicit an entire motor program.

The CPG for swimming in *Tritonia* can be activated by a pair of interneurons called dorsal ramp interneurons (DRI). A swim pattern is maintained as long as DRI is active. DRI is necessary and sufficient to elicit the swim pattern and therefore satisfies the rigorous definition of what is commonly called a command neuron. It receives rhythmic feedback from the CPG and therefore fires rhythmically during fictive swimming. However, it is not part of the CPG, as hyperpolarizing it during a swim pattern that is elicited by electrical stimulation of the CPG does not disrupt CPG activity. It receives excitatory input from sensory neurons and a trigger neuron, Tr1 (**Figure 5(a)**). A brief stimulation of this trigger neuron is sufficient to elicit a swim pattern that outlasts the stimulus substantially. However, DRI can also elicit the swim pattern when Tr1 is hyperpolarized, so Tr1 is sufficient but not necessary in triggering swimming.

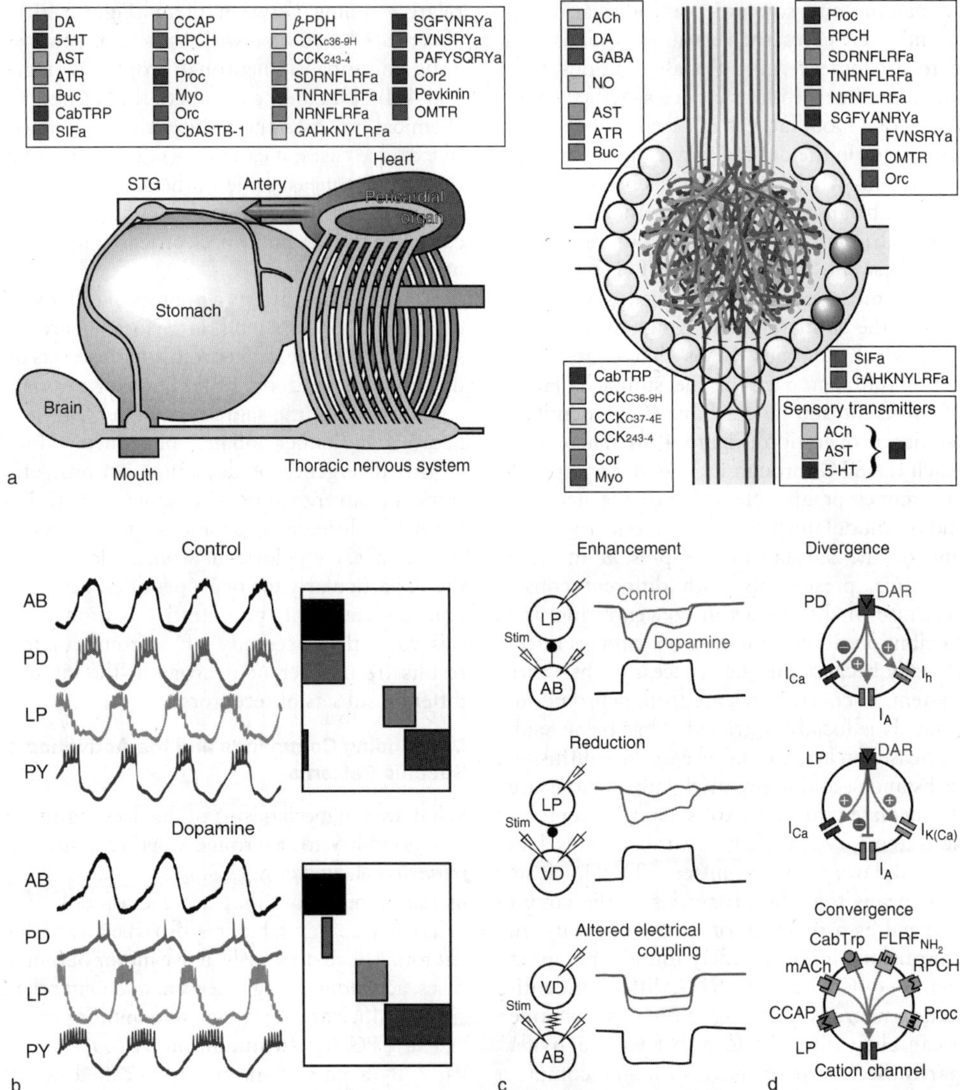

Figure 4 Neuromodulation of central pattern generators (CPGs). (a) The stomatogastric ganglion is modulated by many substances. These substances are either released into the circulatory system (mostly by the pericardial organs) and reach the stomatogastric ganglion (STG) as neurohormones or are released into the neuropil by descending modulatory neurons. (b) Dopamine changes the activity and the phase relationships (relative timing) of CPG neurons in the pyloric circuit of the stomatogastric ganglion. Intracellular recordings show the activity of neurons representative for different phases in the triphasic pyloric rhythm. The bar plots show the activity phases of these neurons in one normalized cycle. (c) Dopamine enhances or reduces chemical synaptic connections and also alters electrical coupling between pyloric neurons. The presynaptic neuron was electrically stimulated and the voltage response in pre- and postsynaptic neuron recorded. Note that chemical synapses are graded. (d) Convergence and divergence of neuromodulator action. Dopamine acts on various voltage-gated ion channels in pyloric neurons. It can act on different subsets of these channels in different neurons and affect the same channel type in different ways in different neurons. In contrast, many modulators, predominantly neuropeptides, activate the same voltage-dependent nonselective cation channel in pyloric neurons. AB, anterior burster neuron; ACh, acetylcholine; AST, allatostatin; ATR, allatotropin; Buc, buccalin; CabTRP, cancer borealis tachykinin-related peptide; CbASTB-1, cancer borealis allatostatin B-1; CCAP, crustacean cardioactive peptide; CCK, cholecystokinin; CCK, cholecystokinin; DA, dopamine; DAR, dopamine receptor; 5-HT, serotonin; GABA, gamma-aminobutyric acid; IA, A-type potassium current; ICa, calcium current; Ih, hyperpolarization-activated inward current; ICa, calcium current; LP, lateral pyloric neuron; Myo, myomodulin; OMTR, orcomyotropin; Orc, orcokinin; NO, nitric oxide; PD, pyloric dilator neuron; PDH, pigment-dispersing hormone; PY, pyloric neuron; VD, ventral dilator neuron; xProc, proctolin; xRPCH, red pigment concentrating hormone; XXa, [peptide sequence]amid. (a) Adapted from Marder E, Bucher D, Schulz DJ, and Taylor AL (2005) Invertebrate central pattern generation moves along. *Current Biology* 15: R685–R699. (b) Adapted from Harris-Warrick RM, Coniglio LM, Levini RM, Gueron S, and Guckenheimer J (1995) Dopamine modulation of two subthreshold currents produces phase shifts in activity of an identified motoneuron. *Journal of*

Such a clear role for descending neurons as in the case of DRI has been found in a number of systems, but it is most likely more common that CPGs are controlled by networks of higher-order neurons and modulatory projections. In that case, different forms of network output can be generated dependent on the relative contribution of different higher-order neurons. In *Aplysia*, the feeding CPG can generate output that is coordinated in two essentially different ways (**Figure 5(b)**). One pattern corresponds to a motor pattern that is used during the ingestion of food. Here, the radula, the mouth part apparatus of mollusks, is protracted while it is open and retracted after a bite, while it is closed. The other pattern corresponds to the rejection of food, when the radula is protracted while it is closed, and retracted while it is open. The choice between these patterns is biased by the relative activity of descending neurons. In the example shown in **Figure 5(b)**, an ingestive pattern is generated when two interneurons, CBI-2 and CBI-3, are activated simultaneously. An egestive (rejection) pattern is generated when CBI-2 is activated while CBI-3 is silent.

In vertebrates, spinal CPGs are subject to modulation by a variety of substances that activate and shape the output patterns they produce. These inputs stem from descending neurons and intraspinal systems. In addition, activation of spinal CPGs is strongly controlled by inhibition from higher centers. An important role in this is played by the pallidum, the output layer of the basal ganglia. The pallidum in turn receives inhibition from the striatum, which is activated by cortical and thalamic inputs. Removal of inhibition in general is an important mechanism of motor program selection. However, to what extent this is a direct influence on the CPGs or rather affects the command circuits that activate CPGs is not clear in most cases.

Coordination of CPGs

Modular Organization of Rhythmic Motor Behaviors

How many CPGs are there? Rather than having one dedicated network for a relatively complex motor behavior like swimming or walking, central pattern generation is inherently modular. 'Unit oscillators' control antagonistic muscle activation for the movement of a single segment or a single joint in an appendage. These rhythm-generating networks need to be coordinated in specific ways to produce specific types of behaviors. For example, swimming movements in lamprey and leech are based on right-left alternation of activity at the segmental level, and this activity can be elicited in reduced preparations with only one or a few segments of the isolated nervous system intact. However, the undulatory movement of the whole body depends on coordination of these segmental patterns along the body axis, in these cases a fixed anterior–posterior phase lag that ensures a sine wave-like movement with a wavelength that matches the body length (**Figure 6(a)**). In the lamprey, this coordination is largely due to central interneuronal coupling so that even the isolated spinal cord displays an intersegmental phase lag similar to that found in the intact animal.

Coordination through Central Coupling or Sensory Feedback

In principle, several mechanisms can be involved in coordinating unit CPGs (**Figure 6(b)**). Apart from central interneuronal coordination, movement generated in response to motor commands in turn produces sensory (e.g., proprioceptive) feedback that can aid in coordinating adjacent oscillators in several ways. In some cases, sensory feedback from one part of the body has access to CPGs controlling adjacent parts of the body. In other cases, movement of one part of the body is transferred via mechanical coupling to other parts of the body, which in turn provide sensory feedback to the local oscillators. In the leech, the intersegmental phase lag during fictive swimming in the isolated nerve cord is reduced in comparison with intact animals. In the intact leech, sensory feedback has been shown to play an additional role in coordinating segmental oscillators. Coordination is even found across segments between which the nervous system had been severed, so that no direct neuronal communication was possible. Therefore, this interaction must have been provided through mechanical coupling.

Sensory feedback plays a particularly important role in shaping motor output and coordinating unit CPGs in behaviors that are heavily dependent on cycle-by-cycle corrections. Terrestrial locomotion takes place in a considerably less-constant medium than do swimming or flying. Therefore, it is no

Neurophysiology 74: 1404–1420. (c) Adapted from Johnson BR, Peck JH, and Harris-Warrick RM (1995) Distributed amine modulation of graded chemical transmission in the pyloric network of the lobster stomatogastric ganglion. *Journal of Neurophysiology* 74: 437–452; and Johnson BR, Peck JH, and Harris-Warrick RM (1993) Amine modulation of electrical coupling in the pyloric network of the lobster stomatogastric ganglion. *Journal of comparative Physiology* 172: 715–732. (d) Adapted from Marder E and Bucher D (2007) Understanding circuit dynamics using the stomatogastric nervous system of lobsters and crabs. *Annual Review of Physiology* 69: 291–316.

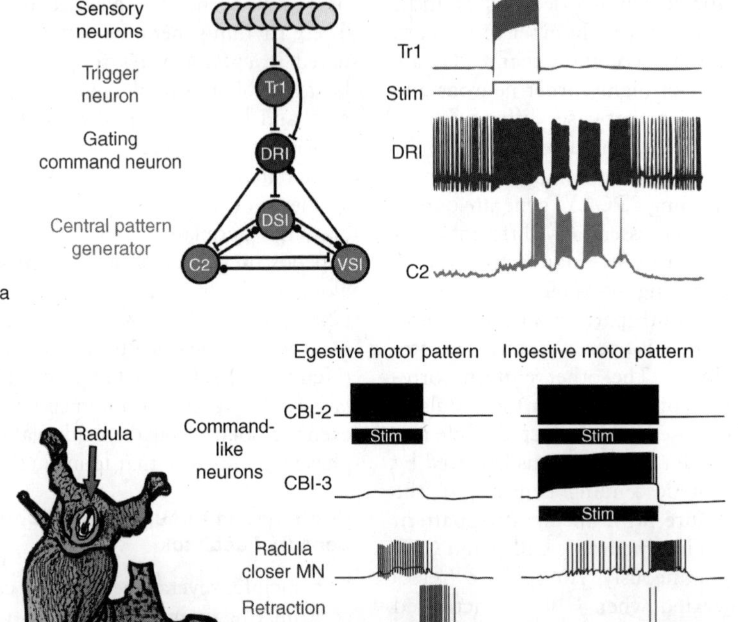

Figure 5 Motor pattern selection. (a) In the *Tritonia* swim system, activation of dorsal ramp interneurons (DRI) is necessary and sufficient to elicit a swim motor pattern. DRI receives excitatory input from sensory neurons and the trigger neuron Tr1. Transient stimulation of Tr1 elicits a swim pattern that outlasts Tr1 activity. (b) In the *Aplysia* feeding system, different relative firing activity of commandlike neurons biases the central pattern generator to express either an egestive or an ingestive motor pattern. These motor patterns correspond to the rejection of food, when the radula is closed during protraction and open during retraction, and to the ingestion of food, when the radula is open during protraction and closed during retraction. When the interneurons CBI-2 and CBI-3 are activated simultaneously, an ingestive motor pattern is elicited. When only CBI-2 is active, an egestive pattern is elicited. (a) Adapted from Frost WN, Hoppe TA, Wang J, and Tain L-M (2001) Swim initiation neurons in *Tritonia diomedea*. *American Zoologist* 41: 952–961. (b) Adapted from Morgan PT, Jing J, Vilim FS, and Weiss KR (2002) Interneuronal and peptidergic control of motor pattern switching in *Aplysia*. *Journal of Neurophysiology* 87: 49–61.

coincidence that much effort has gone into understanding the sensory control of walking. In addition, walking requires a rather complex set of coordinating mechanisms (**Figure 6(c)**). In a single leg joint, antagonistic muscles need to be coordinated to produce alternating contractions. This alternating activity has to be coordinated across several joints to produce alternating stance and swing, that is, a phase in which the leg is on the ground and propels the body, and a phase in which it is off the ground and moves forward to initiate the next stance. Each step sequence has to be coordinated with the step sequences of the contralateral leg and legs in other segments to produce a specific gait. In the stick insect, CPGs controlling different leg joints are operating largely independently in the absence of sensory feedback. Proprioceptors that measure movement in one joint, and mechanoreceptors that measure load or cuticle strain, can entrain and reset CPGs controlling adjacent joints. In contrast, the motor output of the deafferented lumbar spinal cord of the cat resembles stepping movements of the hindleg, with the correct sequence of activation of motor pools controlling hip, knee, ankle, and foot. However, this motor pattern is drastically modified by sensory feedback from predominantly muscular sense organs measuring movement and force.

In addition to modular CPGs that are coordinated for a specific behavioral task, many behaviors involve movements of different body parts that are not part of the same cyclic repetition of sequential muscle activations and run at different speeds. Such coordination

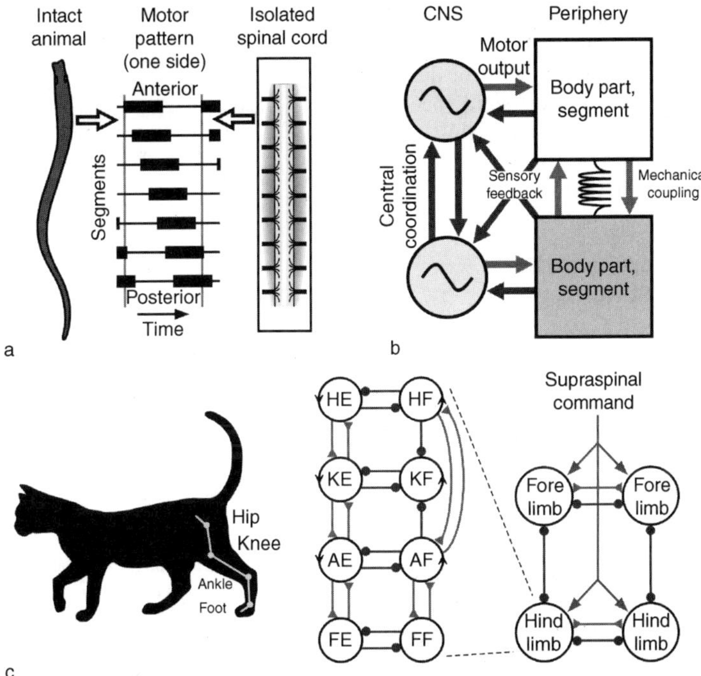

Figure 6 Coordination of motor patterns in different parts of the body. (a) Lamprey swimming consists of a mechanical wave that is transmitted along the anterior–posterior body axis. Alternating right–left activity is expressed with a fixed phase lag between adjacent segments. This pattern of coordination is also seen in the isolated spinal cord during fictive swimming. (b) Schematic of possible coordinating influences between local oscillators. CNS, central nervous system. (c) Coordination of joints and limbs during walking. Alternating extensor (E) and flexor (F) activity is produced at each leg joint (H, hip; K, knee; A, ankle; F, foot), and all joints are coordinated to produce stance and swing phase of the single leg. All limbs are coordinated to produce different gates when activated by supraspinal commands. For example, walking involves mutual inhibitory interaction between right and left, whereas excitatory interaction underlies galloping. (a, c) Adapted from Grillner S (2006) Biological pattern generation: The cellular and computational logic of networks in motion. *Neuron* 52: 751–766.

may be important to avoid mechanical interference between different parts of the body or to tie related behaviors into the same context of operation. For example, the mammalian respiratory rhythm can be coupled to the locomotor pattern during walking or running so that the duration of a respiratory cycle is an integer multiple of the locomotor cycle.

Flexibility of Motor Pattern Coordination

What is the advantage of a distributed, modular arrangement of CPGs? The absence of a dedicated circuitry for a complete behavior means that unit pattern generators can be coordinated in different ways to produce different motor output. We can walk, run, jump, and dance, behaviors that all require alternating activity of antagonistic muscles controlling our leg joints, but with different temporal relationships between different joints and legs. Mammals can walk or gallop, the former requiring alternating activity between left and right and the latter requiring synchronous activation. In the lamprey, the intersegmental phase lag shown in **Figure 6(a)** represents the appropriate coordination for forward swimming. This pattern can be reversed to allow backward swimming. It is interesting that this reversal can also be observed in the isolated spinal cord when the more posterior segments are stimulated appropriately.

Multifunctional Neurons and Circuits

The concept of pattern-generating modules seems to imply that the circuitry that is responsible for controlling local movements is exclusively dedicated to this one specific task. However, there is evidence from a number of systems that shows that this is not true. In the leech nervous system, almost all neurons that are active rhythmically during fictive swimming are also activated during fictive crawling. These motor patterns are mutually exclusive, and the activity phase of particular neurons in the locomotor cycle can be very different between both motor patterns. In the brain stem, pattern generation for breathing, gasping, and possibly other related behaviors like swallowing and coughing share some of the neuronal elements. In the crustacean stomatogastric ganglion, CPG neurons can simultaneously express frequency components of different rhythms that control different parts of the stomach and run at different speeds. Some of these neurons can even completely shift coalitions and, dependent on conditions, can be integral parts of different CPGs at different times.

CPGs as Test Beds for General Principles of Circuit Function and Dynamics

Obviously, analysis of CPG function plays an important role in understanding the neural basis of many motor behaviors and has important implications for the understanding of motor function-related disorders and central nervous system injuries. In addition, studies of CPGs have also elucidated important general principles of network function. Rhythmic firing is a common, if not the prevalent, form of network activity in the brain, spanning systems functioning in a wide range of contexts, from sensory processing to cognitive tasks. Many of the principles that govern these brain functions may be shared with those found to underlie rhythmic motor pattern generation. Furthermore, much of our understanding of circuit dynamics comes from studies of CPGs. This includes both general principles of neuromodulation and important concepts of long-term homeostatic regulation of neuron and network properties. One reason for the successful use of CPGs in studies of network dynamics is that regular rhythmic motor output is relatively easy to measure and quantify. Therefore, CPGs are tractable systems for analyzing the consequences of pharmacological, genetic, or other experimental manipulations on network function.

See also: Autonomic Nervous System: Respiratory Control; Autonomic Nervous System: Central Respiratory Control; Behavioral Hierarchies; Brainstem Respiratory Circuits; Central Pattern Generators: Sensory Feedback; Command Systems; Hormones and Behavior; Neuromodulation; Pattern Generation; Respiration; Walking in Invertebrates.

Further Reading

Büschges A (2005) Sensory control and organization of neural networks mediating coordination of multisegmental organs for locomotion. *Journal of Neurophysiology* 93: 1127–1135.

Dickinson PS (2006) Neuromodulation of central pattern generators in invertebrates and vertebrates. *Current Opinion in Neurobiology* 16: 604–614.

Feldman JM and Del Negro CA (2006) Looking for inspiration: New perspectives on respiratory rhythm. *Nature Reviews Neuroscience* 7: 232–242.

Frost WN, Hoppe TA, Wang J, and Tian L-M (2001) Swin initiation neurons in. *Tritonia diomedea. American Zoologist* 41: 952–961.

Grillner S (2003) The motor infrastructure: From ion channels to neuronal networks. *Nature Reviews Neuroscience* 4: 573–586.

Grillner S (2006) Biological pattern generation: The cellular and computational logic of networks in motion. *Neuron* 52: 751–766.

Harris-Warrick RM, Coniglio LM, Levini RM, Gueron S, and Guckenheimer JE (1995) Dopamine modulation of two subthreshold currents produces phase shifts in activity of an identified motoneuron. *Journal of Neurophysiology* 74: 1404–1420.

Johnson BR, Peck JM, and Harris-Warrick RM (1993) Amine modulation of electrical coupling in the pyloric network of the lobster stomatogastric ganglion. *Journal of Comparative Physiology A* 172: 715–732.

Johnson BR, Peck JH, and Harris-Warrick RM (1995) Distributed amine modulation of graded chemical transmission in the pyloric network of the lobster stomatogastric ganglion. *Journal of Neurophysiology* 74: 437–452.

Kiehn O (2006) Locomotor circuits in the mammalian spinal cord. *Annual Review of Neuroscience* 29: 279–306.

Kristan WB Jr., Calabrese RL, and Friesen WO (2005) Neuronal control of leech behavior. *Progress in Neurobiology* 76: 279–327.

Kupfermann I and Weiss KR (2001) Motor program selection in simple model systems. *Current Opinion in Neurobiology* 11: 673–677.

Lieske SP, Thoby-Brisson M, Telqkamp P, and Raminez JM (2000) Reconfiguration of the neural network controlling multiple breathing patterns: Eupnea, sights and gasps. *Nature Neuroscience* 3: 600–607.

Marder E and Bucher D (2001) Central pattern generators and the control of rhythmic movements. *Current Biology* 11: R986–R996.

Marder E and Bucher D (2007) Understanding circuit dynamics using the stomatogastric nervous system of lobsters and crabs. *Annual Review of Physiology* 69: 291–316.

Marder E, Bucher D, Schulz DJ, and Taylor AL (2005) Invertebrate central pattern generation moves along. *Current Biology* 15: R685–R699.

Morgan PT, Jing J, Vilim FS, and Weiss KR (2002) Interneuronal and peptidergic control of motor pattern switching in *Aplysia. Journal of Neurophysiology* 87: 49–61.

Nusbaum MP and Beenhakker MP (2002) A small-systems approach to motor pattern generation. *Nature* 417: 343–350.

Pearson KG (2004) Generating the walking gait: Role of sensory feedback. *Progress in Brain Research* 143: 123–129.

Ramirez JM and Viemari JC (2005) Determinants of inspiratory activity. *Respiratory Physiology & Neurobiology* 147: 145–157.

Robertson RH and Pearson KG (1982) A preparation for the intracellular analysis of neuronal activity during flight in the locust. *Journal of Comparative Physiology A* 146: 311–320.

Central Pattern Generators: Sensory Feedback

W O Friesen, University of Virginia, Charlottesville, VA, USA

Introduction

Originating near the beginning of the twentieth century, two seemingly incompatible theories informed much of the debate concerning the neural origins of rhythmic movements in animals. One theory, put forth most clearly by Charles Sherrington, held that locomotory patterns, although coordinated by the central nervous system (CNS), arise from sensory feedback and reflexes. Although counterexamples were offered by several investigators, this theory was widely accepted before the 1960s. The second theory, ably proposed by T Graham Brown, held that central pattern generators (CPGs) formed by inhibitory neuronal circuits within the CNS are the source of rhythmic movement patterns. The latter theory gained renewed support from the work of Donald Wilson on locust flight in 1961 and finally became dogma during subsequent decades as more and more CPG circuits were identified in both vertebrates and invertebrates. Near the end of the twentieth century, the importance of sensory feedback for the expression of efficient locomotion received new recognition, leading to a convergence of the two theories. The consensus is that the neuronal circuits underlying locomotion comprise a distributed system that includes both central oscillators and sensory feedback components.

The reemerging recognition that sensory feedback plays an essential role in animal locomotion (and other rhythmic movements) includes the realization that sensory neurons exhibit many of the characteristics that define elements of a CPG. Thus it has now been demonstrated that sensory neurons (1) express rhythmic activity during locomotion, (2) make synaptic contacts with CPG interneurons, and (3) can entrain the CPG when they are stimulated rhythmically. Systems that provide examples of these characteristics include locust flight, swimming in leeches and lamprey, crayfish swimmeret beating, and walking in stick insects and crayfish.

What Is Sensory Feedback?

The neuronal activity patterns that underlie rhythmic movements in a wide variety of animal species are generated by complex neuronal circuits, the CPGs, located within the CNS. In addition, a multitude of sensory receptors, found in the joints, muscles, and other structures of the periphery, detect internal joint positions and movements as well as environmental factors. The overt movements that constitute animal behavior arise from the interplay between the CPGs and sensory feedback from these body structures. Because animals live in environments that are characterized by both temporal change and spatial unpredictability, the instinctive, inherited CPG control circuits cannot be expected to, and do not in fact, generate movement patterns that ensure adaptive behavior. Consequently, CPGs underlying all animal movements are subject to inputs via receptors that monitor the execution of motor commands in relationship to the environment and then provide inputs to motor neurons and to the central neuronal circuits that form the essential core of CPGs. Such inputs modify the neuronal activity patterns arising from the CPG with critical effects on movement amplitude, phase relationships, and the cycle period (or, equivalently, the frequency) of movements. The focus here is on the relationship of CPGs and sensory feedback in a few well-studied invertebrates and a primitive fish, the lamprey. A schematic overview of one such system, which controls the swimming movement in the medicinal leech, illustrates the general properties of the interactions between CPGs, motor output, and sensory feedback (**Figure 1**).

Why CPGs Are Subject to Sensory Feedback

In many animal preparations, the output of the CPG can be observed in greatly reduced preparations, which often include only parts of the CNS. Comparisons of CPG neuronal motor output with activity patterns observed in intact, behaving animals provide the basis for the concept of a CPG, and, more germane here, the comparisons have revealed deficits in motor patterns that arise when sensory feedback is absent. Most prominent, and most important, among such deficits are that neuronal activity patterns generated by CPGs in isolation have increased cycle periods, reduced activity amplitudes and suboptimal phase relationships. Moreover, in the absence of sensory cues, or internal changes in state, motor output tends to represent rather simple movements, such as straight-ahead locomotion, rather than the more complex movements observed in the intact animal.

Unpredictable development There are numerous factors that mandate sensory feedback if animals are to behave adaptively, including body growth during development and maturation. Amplitude and frequency of movements alter with growth; hence, one major consideration is the matching of CPG output to

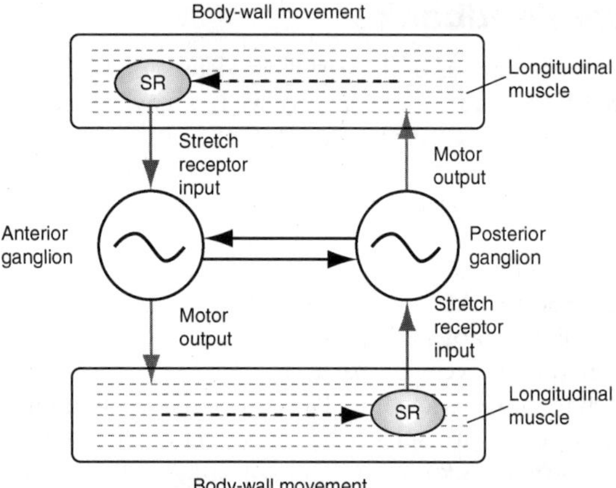

Figure 1 Schematic model for the neuronal control of swimming in the leech. Two segmental central pattern generators (CPGs) within ventral nerve cord ganglia are represented by unit oscillators (∼). These unit oscillators are interconnected and mutually entrained by intersegmental axons that run through nerve cord connectives. The cycle period of the CPG is greater than in the intact animal, whereas intersegmental phase lags are smaller. Segmental motor neurons driven by the CPGs control muscle contraction in their individual segments (red arrows from CPG). When swimming movements are generated by the intact animal, tensions in the body wall, arising from local motor neuron output, mechanical coupling between body wall segments (dashed arrows), and the environment provide sensory feedback (blue arrows) to the CPG. This rhythmic input acts to decrease cycle period and to increase intersegmental phase lags in the intact leech. Symbols: SR, stretch receptor; ∼, CPG. Reprinted from Yu X and Friesen WO (2004) Entrainment of leech swimming activity by the ventral stretch receptor. *Journal of Comparative Physiology* 190: 939–949, figure 6, © 2004 Springer-Verlag, with kind permission of Springer Science and Business Media.

the natural, resonant frequency of limb or body. Although development changes in the CPG and the body structure may be coordinately regulated by genetics, maturation processes depend also on the environment. With the latter not fully predictable, sensory feedback that modifies CPG frequency, phase, and amplitude provides a means of ensuring that body movements are efficient at all stages of growth.

Unpredictable environment Animals live in a wide variety of habitats. Some, like fish or flying insects and birds, move in nearly homogeneous media; nevertheless, obstacles, turbulence, or temperature clines are unpredictable, setting up the essential requirement for sensory input to the CPG, even for swimming and flight. Terrestrial environments exhibit a very high degree of unpredictability; hence it is not surprising that CPGs underlying walking and stepping are even more strongly controlled by sensory inputs.

Compensation for morphological alterations Further requirements for sensory feedback arise from alterations in an animal's form through feeding, accident, or predation. A particularly telling example comes from walking locomotion in insects, which modify their gait immediately when a leg is experimentally amputated. Other examples include seasonal size and weight alterations that require a reprogramming of the motor system but cannot be expected to alter the CPG. Although hormones can reprogram the nervous system to match an animal's activity to its overall condition, only sensory feedback can provide cycle-by-cycle feedback from the environment.

Components of Motor Systems

Motor systems, whether generating the neuronal substrates of locomotion or other rhythmic movements, comprise several elements. Central to these systems are one or more oscillator circuits that generate the rudiments, in period and phase, of the expressed motor activity. Excitatory inputs from higher centers, from sensory input, or from within the circuits themselves stimulate CPG output to pass from a 'resting' stable state, that is, without oscillations, to one that is unstable and hence oscillates with a frequency that may or may not match that observed in the intact animal. Most CPGs are formed entirely, or nearly so, of interneurons. However, motor neurons may constitute most of the CPG, as in the stomatogastric system of crustacea; they may be weakly involved in pattern generation, as in the leech swim CPG; or they may merely serve as followers to drive muscle contractions, as in the lamprey swim circuits. Sensory feedback arises from stretch receptors in muscles, proprioceptors, sensory hairs as in crustacean swimmerets, cuticle receptors that signal load in insects, and stretch receptors in the CNS itself, as in lamprey. These receptors may be spiking or nonspiking, but their function is to provide position, load, velocity, and angle information to the CPG – afferent information that informs the CPG whether the movement commanded is appropriately executed. Alternatively, sensory input modifies CPG function more drastically, as during animal walking, in which sensory processes control phase relationships among limbs and the intensity of motor neuron output and may advance, retard, initiate, or prevent phase transitions.

Experimental Approaches: Techniques and Animal Preparations

Experiments to determine the nature of the sensory receptors and their role in CPG modulation have encompassed a wide range of animal preparations and experimental approaches.

Experimental Approaches and Techniques

Comparison of CPG output and movements of intact animals One methodology employed nearly universally to assess the relative importance of CPG circuits and sensory feedback in the control of animal movements is to compare the neuronal activity patterns expressed in reduced preparations with those of intact, behaving animals. Such comparisons reveal four major aspects of rhythmic activity that are modified by sensory feedback: cycle period, activity amplitude, phase relationships among local outputs, and intersegmental phase relationship. There is a wide range in the relative strength of sensory feedback effects, as illustrated in **Figure 2**, which shows that cycle periods of fictive (isolated CNS) swimming activity in both leech and lamprey are significantly greater than in the intact animal. However, phase relationships remain unchanged by removal of the periphery in the lamprey whereas intersegmental phase lags are reduced by nearly 50% when sensory feedback is eliminated in leeches.

Sensory entrainment A second widely used technique for determining the nature and strength of sensory feedback is to perform entrainment experiments. With this approach, either the body itself (in semi-intact preparations) or sensory receptor membrane potential is modulated rhythmically by the experimenter while the CPG is generating rhythmic output. For many systems, movements or direct current injection into sensory neurons can force the CPG to generate cycle periods that are up to $\pm 50\%$ of the unperturbed values. **Figure 3** illustrates the entrainment technique as it is applied to the swimming rhythm in lamprey. Here physical movements of the rostral or caudal ends of a spinal cord/notochord preparation entrain the CPGs as the movement frequency is set to values both below and above those detected when movements are absent. Such experiments demonstrate that sensory structures, in this case edge cells, have access to the CPG and can modify its properties. Related, alternative approaches are to impede limb or body movements; place a limb into a particular, fixed position; or assess the effects of brief current injection into sensory neurons. Like the entrainment procedure, these alternative methods provide useful information about both the nature and the strength of sensory input in the expression of rhythmic movements.

Animal Preparations

Six preparations and behaviors are described here to illustrate current procedures of, and results from, studies on the relationships between CPG-generated rhythms and sensory inputs during the expression of rhythmic movements. These behaviors are flying in locusts, swimming in leeches and lamprey, swimmeret beating in crayfish, and walking in stick insects and crustacea.

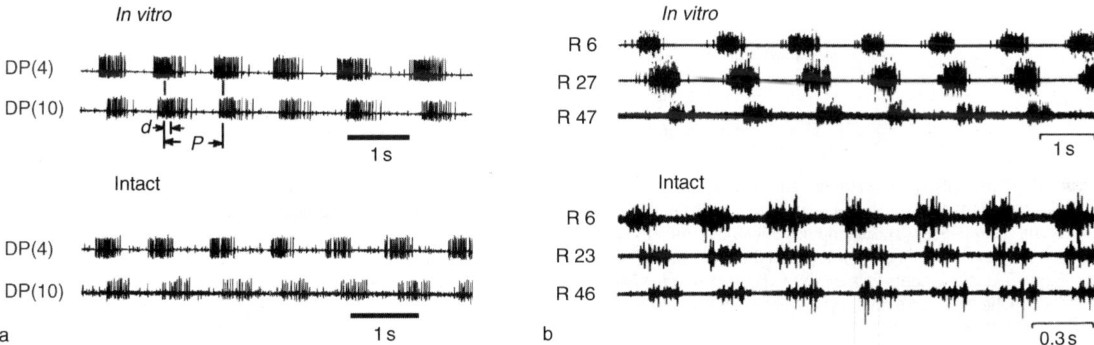

Figure 2 Activity patterns during swimming locomotion: patterns generated by CPGs compared with those expressed by nearly intact animals. (a) Leech swimming. The upper traces (*in vitro*) were obtained from a preparation consisting of the isolated leech ventral nerve cord with electrodes attached to the dorsal posterior (DP) nerves of segments 4 and 10. The lower traces (intact) were obtained from electrodes implanted onto the DP nerves of segments 4 and 10 during swimming in a nearly intact leech. The bursts in these records are axon impulses of cell DE-3, a motor neuron that innervates dorsal longitudinal muscles. P is the cycle period, and d is the intersegmental delay. (b) Lamprey swimming. The upper traces (*in vitro*) depict ventral root activity during fictive swimming. The lower traces (intact) show electromyograph records obtained from an intact swimming lamprey. Letters R and numerals indicate that recordings are from the right side at the segments indicated. Fictive swimming was elicited by bath application of 0.5 mmol l^{-1} D-glutamate. Note the different time calibrations. (a) Reproduced from Pearce RA and Friesen WO (1984) Intersegmental coordination of leech swimming: Comparison of *in situ* and isolated nerve cord activity with body wall movement. *Brain Research* 299: 363–366, with permission from Elsevier. (b) Reprinted from Wallén P and Williams TL (1984) Fictive locomotion in the lamprey spinal cord *in vitro* compared with swimming in the intact and spinal animal. *Journal of Physiology* 347: 225–239, with permission from Blackwell Publishing.

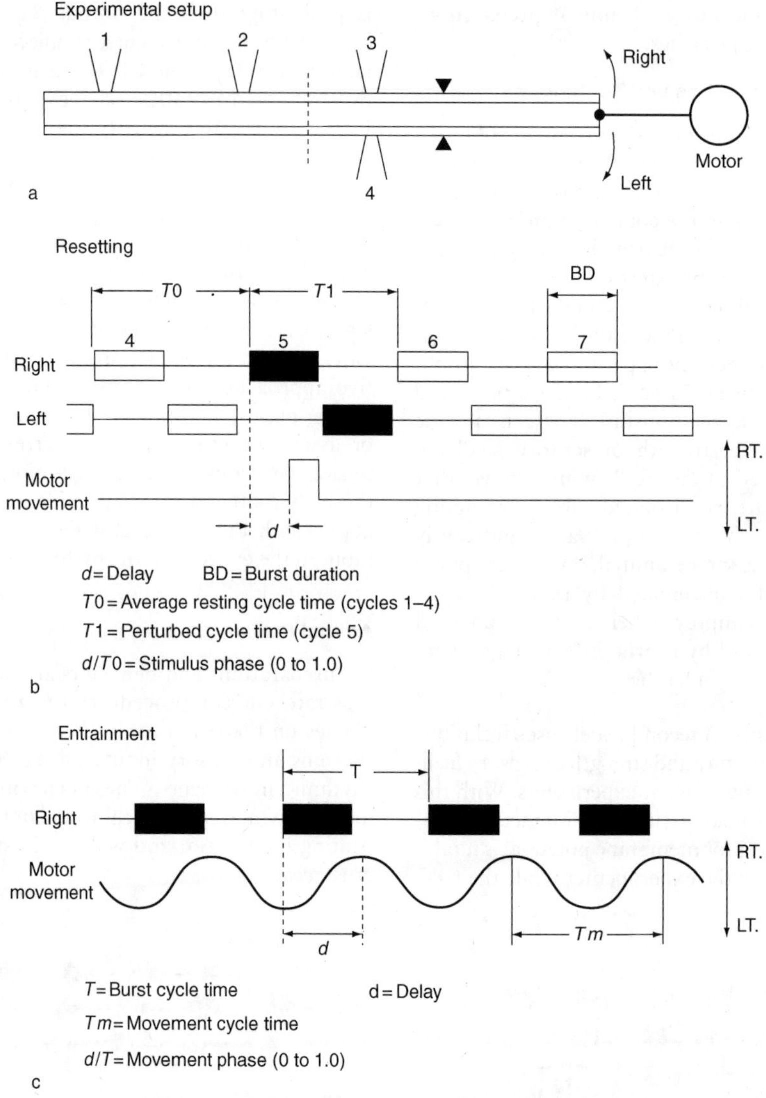

Figure 3 Schematic diagram for entrainment experiments in lamprey. (a) Diagram of the *in vitro* notochord/spinal cord preparation. The caudal (right (RT.)) end of the preparation was rhythmically deflected with a pen motor while the preparation was immobilized to the left (LT.) of the arrowheads. (b) Step inputs. Brief movements (300 ms) of the caudal end at selected phases in the swim cycle were used to determine phase changes (as a fraction of the cycle period) to generate phase response curves (not shown). (c) Entrainment methodology. Sinusoidal movements with a range of cycle periods (*T*) were applied to the preparation; cycle period and the phase relationship (*d*/*T*) between the imposed signal and the fictive motor output were measured. Reprinted from McClellan AD and Jang W (1993) Mechanosensory inputs to the central pattern generators for locomotion in the lamprey spinal cord: Resetting, entrainment, and computer modeling. *Journal of Neurophysiology* 70: 2442–2454; used with permission.

Locust flight Locust flight was the first behavior for which the central role of a CPG was widely accepted. Ironically, locust flight is also among the first clear examples of sensory feedback coordinating animal movements in a well-defined system. Comparisons of flying in nearly intact but tethered animals with the output of the flight CPG in the absence of sensory input reveal the following differences. Wingbeat frequency in tethered flying locust is approximately 15–20 Hz, whereas deafferented preparations exhibit frequencies about half of those values. Moreover, nearly intact tethered locusts stimulated with air currents in a wind tunnel fly continuously, whereas reduced preparations lacking sensory feedback soon terminate the CPG-generated pattern. Stimulation of forewing stretch receptors alters the expressed rhythm in several ways. First, repeated stimulation phase-locked to the flight pattern increases wingbeat frequency. Second, such stimulation prolongs the expression of the motor pattern. These effects are phase-dependent, indicating that they function on a cycle-by-cycle basis rather than through general excitation. Third, stimulation of both forewing stretch receptors at frequencies near the wingbeat frequency entrains the flight rhythm, provided that the frequency of the entraining signal is within 20% of the natural frequency. Single stimuli applied to the stretch receptors can, if appropriately timed, reset the phase of the flight rhythm. The rhythm can also be entrained by sinusoidal depression and elevation of a forewing while the locust is flying in a wind tunnel. The entrainment range for this more natural stimulation is somewhat smaller, with stable entrainment only when the entraining frequency is within 15% of control.

More than modifying the CPG rhythm, forewing stretch receptors appear to be important components of the flight oscillator in locusts. Intracellular recordings from flight CPG interneurons reveal short-latency excitatory input from forewing stretch receptors. Because these receptors are phasically active during flight, can entrain and reset the flight rhythm, and appear to have monosynaptic inputs to CPG interneurons, they are considered to be important elements in the system generating the normal flight rhythm during wing elevation (**Figure 4**). Effects of these receptors and of the tegulae also increase the precision of coordination among the wings. The conclusion is that the forewing stretch receptors and the tegulae (activated by wing depression) are peripheral elements of a complex oscillator system that comprises the CPG and peripheral sensory feedback loops.

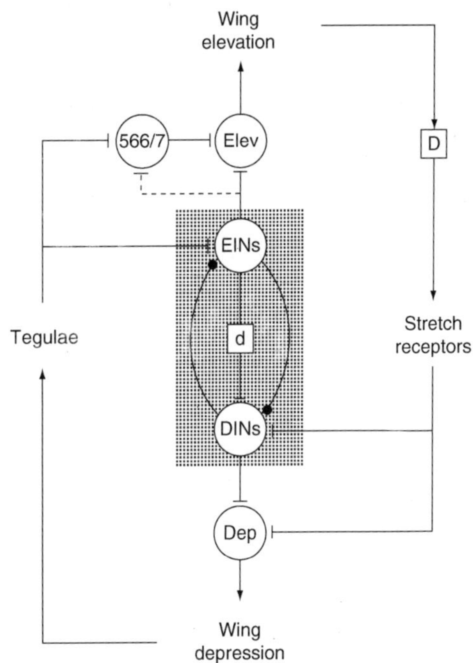

Figure 4 Diagram illustrating identified interactions between sensory afferents and the locust flight central pattern generator (CPG). EIN, elevator interneurons; DIN, depressor interneurons; 566 identified interneurons that participate in the generation of the flight rhythm only when they receive phasic input from tegulae during flight. Elev, elevator motor neurons; Dep, depressor motor neurons; d, delayed excitation; D, long delay, with input arriving at the depressor neurons one cycle subsequent to one that generated the sensory signal. With permission from Pearson KG and Ramirez J-M (1997) Sensory modulation of pattern-generating circuits. In: Stein PSG, Griller S, Selverston AI, and Stuart DG (eds.) *Neurons, Networks, and Motor Behavior*, pp. 225–235. Cambridge, MA: The MIT Press. © 1997 Massachusetts Institute of Technology.

Leech swimming Medicinal leeches are elongated, segmental worms 5–15 cm in length when fully extended. During the prologue to swimming, the leech body flattens and extends in length and width, providing a nearly uniform, flattened profile that is efficient for swimming locomotion. Leeches swim by whole-body undulations that are seen in side-view as a traveling rostrocaudal sinusoidal wave with a cycle period range of 0.3–1 s. The most efficient waveform for this whole-body mode of swimming is a quasi-sinusoidal body wave comprising one wavelength. Commensurate with this theoretical expectation, at any instant, about a single wave length is expressed by swimming leeches. The rhythmic movements of the body are generated by locally antiphasic shortening–lengthening cycles in dorsal and ventral longitudinal muscles. These contraction rhythms, which act against the elevated internal body pressure generated by activity of the flattener muscles, exhibit rostrocaudal phase delays and thereby generate the observed traveling body wave. With some 18–20 body segments actively participating in generating the swim undulations, the intersegmental phase lags in swimming animals are about 20° per segment.

Like other rhythmic movements, the activity cycles, cycle period, and intersegmental phase lags expressed by swimming leeches find a rudimentary origin in a set of interneurons that constitute the CPG. The unit elements of the CPG are found in each midbody ganglion of the leech ventral cord. Although single ganglia are capable of brief, weak swim oscillations when exposed to 50 μmol l^{-1} serotonin, at least two segments are required to generate strong oscillations and intersegmental phase delays. The leech swim CPG comprises more than 13 interneurons per segment, with some participation by sets of dorsal and ventral inhibitory motor neurons. The central oscillator network does not, however, generate the full rhythm expressed in the intact animal. The cycle period generated by the CPG ranges from 0.6 to 2 s, barely overlapping the period range observed in intact animal (0.3–1 s), and intersegmental phase lags expressed by the CPG (about 10° per segment) are only 50% of these of intact animals (**Figure 2(a)**). Thus the isolated CPG does not produce neuronal activity patterns for fast, efficient locomotion.

The sensory inputs that, together with CPG circuits, generate neuronal activity patterns appropriate for efficient swimming arise, at least in part, from segmental stretch receptors, whose somata are associated with dorsal and ventral longitudinal muscles. Stretching the leech body wall induces a hyperpolarization in these receptors, which have peripherally located somata and dendrites and whose giant axons conduct this signal to the CNS electronically.

The importance of sensory mechanisms in leech swimming locomotion was recognized from the beginning of systematic studies of this behavior. For example, leeches were found to swim at a lower frequency in high viscosity media. Moreover, leeches whose movement was restricted mechanically so that they were unable to execute the normal swim undulation altered their movements or aborted ongoing traveling waves. More recently, several types of experiments demonstrated that the stretch receptors can modify the basic activity patterns generated by the CPG. First, in nerve cord–body wall preparations, these receptors encode muscle tension information via membrane potential oscillations, with amplitudes up to 10 mV recorded as the axons enter the ganglia. Second, rhythmic current injection into these receptors can alter intersegmental phase lags by ±5° in a phase-dependent manner. Third, experimentally induced stretch receptor membrane potential oscillations entrain the CPG rhythm if the imposed rhythm is within about 50% of the free-running CPG rhythm. Fourth, brief (several seconds long) current pulses injected into a stretch receptor shift the phase of the ventral nerve cord swim oscillations. Finally, there is direct electrical coupling between at least one of the stretch receptors and a CPG interneuron (**Figure 5**). Hence, as for locust flight, the circuits that generate the swimming rhythm in the leech comprise both the CPG and the peripheral stretch.

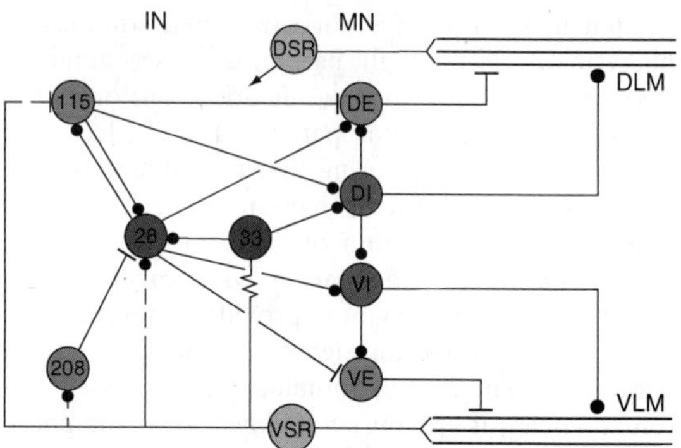

Figure 5 Interactions between stretch receptors and swim-related neurons in leeches. Only a subset of central pattern generator (CPG) neurons (cells 115, 208, 28, and 33) and the phasically active motor neurons are depicted. The ventral stretch receptor (VSR) conveys tension information from the ventral longitudinal muscle (VLM) directly to at least one CPG interneuron, cell 33. IN, interneurons. Motor neuron (MN) designations: DE, dorsal excitor; DI, dorsal inhibitor; VI, ventral inhibitor; VE, ventral excitor; interaction symbols: filled circle, chemical inhibition; 'T,' excitation; resistor, nonrectifying electrical interaction. Dashed interactions appear to be indirect. Interactions between the DSR and the CPG remain unexplored. Reprinted from Cang J, Yu X, and Friesen WO (2001) Sensory modification of leech swimming: Interactions between ventral stretch receptors and swim-related neurons. *Journal of Comparative Physiology* 187: 569–579, figure 1(b), © 2001 Springer-Verlag, publisher. With kind permission of Springer Science and Business Media.

Lamprey swimming Lampreys are primitive fish that swim via anguilliform (eellike) undulations, that, as in leeches, comprise about one wavelength at any moment. The traveling wave results from antiphasic contraction of segmental muscles and from rostra-caudal delays of 1% of the cycle period per segment for a 100-segment animal. Intact lampreys swim with cycle periods ranging from about 0.13 s to more than 0.6 s. The spinal cord of lampreys includes a series of local CPGs. Comparisons of swimming movements in intact animals and motor neuron activity patterns generated within the stationary spinal cord (fictive swimming) show similar patterns (**Figure 2(b)**). Although the range of cycle periods obtained by altering the concentration of the swim-inducing excitatory amino acids (0.7–2 s) in fictive swimming overlaps that observed in the intact animal, the CPG-generated period is normally about twice that of the intact animal. Unlike results from leeches, the intersegmental phase lags in lampreys do not differ markedly in isolated preparations compared with those of intact animals (**Figure 2(b)**). Thus sensory feedback appears to be essential for setting the cycle period but not for phase control during undisturbed swimming in the lamprey.

Sensory feedback during the side-to-side undulations of the swimming lamprey arises, in part, from segmental 'edge cells' within the spinal cord. These cells make synaptic contacts with CPG neurons and with motor neurons. Interactions between the CPG and the edge receptors in the intact animal may, like the CPG itself, comprise a functional oscillator. Experiments on spinal cord–notochord preparations demonstrated that the CPG rhythm can be entrained by mechanical movement of either the rostral or the caudal ends. That is, sensory input arising from these movements could alter the 0.7 Hz 'natural' frequency by a maximum of 50% above and no more than 25% below this control frequency. The range of entrainment depended on the length of the preparation. Short preparations (25 segments) yielded an entrainment range that was nearly twice the range for longer preparations (50 segments). Relative entrainment was also observed with input-to-expressed frequency ratios of 1:2 and 2:1.

Brief movement pulses applied to the spinal cord, as well as current injection into edge cells, can reset the phase of the swimming rhythm of lampreys. Movement pulses, used to generate phase response curves for the spinal cord–notochord preparations, showed phase advances during two-thirds of the cycle, with the largest phase shifts near mid-cycle. Again, it seems likely that, as for locusts and leeches, normal locomotion in lamprey arises both from segmental CPGs and from sensory feedback circuits (**Figure 6**).

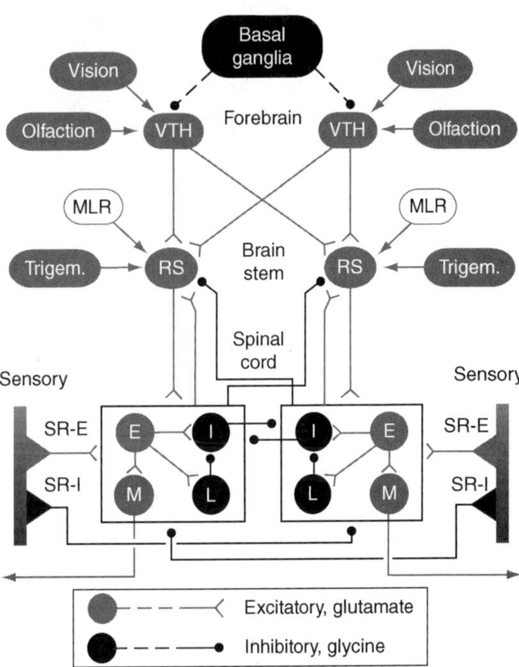

Figure 6 Circuits underlying swimming movements in lampreys. A population of reticulospinal neurons (RS) excites the spinal interneurons and motor neurons. Excitatory interneurons (E), in turn, excite other spinal neurons, including inhibitory interneurons (I) that cross the midline to inhibit neurons on the contralateral side, and lateral interneurons (L) that inhibit ipsilateral interneurons and the motor neurons (M). Spinal stretch receptor neurons (edge cells) include two types; excitatory neurons (SR-E) that excite ipsilateral neurons and inhibitory neurons (SR-I) that inhibit contralateral neurons. Symbols denote populations of cells, not single neurons. Additional control of this system appears to arise from the ventral thalamus (VTH), the trigeminal nuclei (Trigem.), and the mesencephalic locomotor region (MLR). Reproduced from Grillner S and Wallén P (2002) Cellular bases of a vertebrate locomotor system: Steering, intersegmental and segmental co-ordination and sensory control. *Brain Research Reviews* 40: 92–106, with permission from Elsevier.

Crustacean swimmeret beating Crayfish, lobsters, and other decapod crustaceans have abdominal appendages, swimmerets, that beat with metachronal rhythms. The paired segmental CPGs in this system, unlike those described above, provide a basic rhythm that is nearly identical in both cycle period and intersegmental phase lag, about a quarter of the cycle period, to those observed in the intact animal. Although the need for sensory feedback in undisturbed beating is not obvious, execution of swimmeret movements is nonetheless monitored via a set of sensory receptors, including proprioceptors that provide phasic feedback. When, for example, the movement of a swimmeret is experimentally impeded, by fixing the limb at either the retracted or protracted phase in its movement cycle, the central rhythm sometimes stops, sometimes decelerates. In addition to the proprioceptors, lobsters have hairs whose deflection in response to water movements engendered by swimmeret beating can provide rhythmic afferent information. Also, there are two types of hypodermal mechanoreceptors that are likely to be activated when swimmerets beat rhythmically. It appears that swimmeret mechanoreceptor activity, although not required for generating an appropriate activity pattern for swimmeret movement, contributes to the movement of these appendages when normal movement is somehow impeded.

Insect and crayfish walking The neuronal activity patterns that underlie animal walking movements are considerably more complex than the neuronal patterns that underlie flying, swimming, or swimmeret beating. Most animals that utilize walking locomotion have multiple limbs, with each limb comprising multiple segments. Added to those factors is the daunting task of generating effective limb placement on a highly unpredictable substrate. It is therefore not surprising that sensory receptors are closely tied to CPG elements associated with this form of locomotion.

Many forms of animal locomotion can be viewed as the rhythmic alteration of two phases, a power stroke, in which the animal exerts forces on its environment that propel it forward, and a return stroke that returns the limb to the original position for the next power stroke. A major focus for studies of sensory input to the CPG circuits that underlie the walking cycle is the control of transitions between two phases in walking locomotion, the stance and the swing phases. Two additional foci are the control of intra- and interjoint phase angles.

One of the best-studied walking behaviors is that of the stick insect. Each leg in the stick insect has three main joints that are responsible for movements in the horizontal and vertical planes. Muscles associated with the thoracocoxal (TC-) joint drive the leg back and forth, whereas the coxatrochanteral (CTr-) and femur–tibia (FTi-) joints (**Figure 7(a)**) are involved in placing the tarsal segment firmly onto the substrate (during the stance phase) or raising it into the air (during the swing phase). With appropriate stimulation, deafferented thoracic ganglia can be induced to generate the antagonistic motor neuron activity patterns that cause rhythmic joint movements. Because there is little or no coordination among groups of motor neurons associated with different joints in such a preparation, it appears that a unit CPG drives muscles at each joint. The specific neuronal circuits constituting these CPGs remain largely unidentified; however, it is clear that activity in these CPGs is closely coordinated by sensory signals arising from leg proprioceptors and cuticular strain receptors. Coordination of the movements of individual joints occurs by a cascade of sensory information whereby signals from one joint in a leg reset the phase of the CPG that drives a second joint in that leg. These signals include two temporally related sensory modalities: leg weight load and joint position. The effects of such sensory signals are weighted within the CNS to generate locomotory movements.

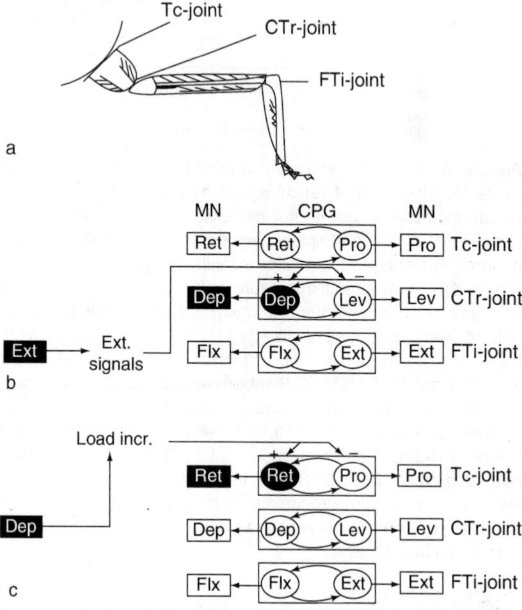

Figure 7 Schematic of sensory influences on the movements of the middle leg of the stick insect. (a) Cartoon of the stick insect leg showing the three main leg joints. (b) Extension position signals (ext. signals) from the FTi-joint switch the phase of the central pattern generator (CPG; Lev to Dep) in the adjacent joint (CTr-joint). The CPGs are denoted by boxes with two interacting neurons, with the active phase indicated by a filled circle. Arrows indicate interactions, but not specific synapses, between hypothesized CPG elements and the antagonistic sets of motor neurons (MNs; rectangles; filled elements are active) they control. (c) Load signals (load increase (incr.)) from the CTr-joint switch the state of the TC-joint CPG (Pro to Ret). TC-joint, –thoracocoxal joint; CTr-joint, –coxatrochanteral joint; FTi-joint, femur–tibia joint; Ret, retraction/retractor; Pro, protraction/protractor; Dep, depression/depressor; Lev, levation/levator; Flx, flexion/flexor; Ext, extension/extensor. Reprinted from Büschges A (2005) Sensory control and organization of neural networks mediating coordination of multisegmental organs for locomotion. *Journal of Neurophysiology* 93: 1127–1135, used with permission.

The specific roles of sensory influences on the CPGs that control the main joints in the stick insect are now known for the phase transitions that occur during step cycles. Two such transitions are illustrated in **Figures 7(b)** and **7(c)**. In **Figures 7(b)**, movement-induced signals from FTi-joint receptors (extension signals, lower left) cause a transition from swing to stance phase. This occurs because this sensory input switches the CPG of the CTr-joint leg to the depressor phase, activating the depressor motor neuron, thereby lowering the leg to begin the stance phase. Next, in **Figure 7(c)**, load receptor activation in the CTr-joint (load increase, left) induced by initiation of the stance phase forces a phase transition from protraction to retraction onto the TC-joint CPG, thereby activating retractor motor neurons that act at the TC-joint and begin the forward propulsion phase of the leg step cycle. Sensory receptor input often has two effects, such as when an increased load increases the activity in flexor motor neurons and hence to muscles that support the animal's weight while simultaneously inhibiting the antagonistic extensors. There appear to be two general coordinating systems: one that initiates transitions between phases of the walking cycle, and one that determines its direction. Computer simulations have demonstrated that the known sensory inputs to control limb motions can, when implemented in a simulated neuronal controller, generate leg stepping movements. Here again, rhythmic locomotory movements arise from combined CPG and sensory interactions. For the stick insect, the role of sensory input influences not only period and phase but the very transitions of the CPG between phases of the activity cycle.

As in stick insects, walking locomotion in the crayfish also arises from CPGs strongly influenced by sensory input. However, unlike the nearly independent joint CPGs of the stick insect, walking CPGs express a coordinated walking rhythm in deafferented preparations. That is, the crayfish CPGs include effective interactions within the CNS while still requiring sensory input to ensure appropriate cycle periods and stable phase relationships. Although the CPGs associated with the eight walking legs in crayfish remain unidentified, at least one sensory structure, the thoracocoxal muscle receptor organ (TCMRO), is known to interact with the CPGs. Rhythmic stretching and releasing of the TCMRO can entrain the CPG, not only locally, but across other legs. The data show that the interactions between sensory input and the CPGs are strong, for the phase relationship between an imposed stimulus rhythm, and the entrained walking cycles is nearly constant. The suggestion is that the walking rhythm is not entrained but actually driven by sensory input. Relative coordination also occurs, with stimulus–response periods of 2:1 or 1:2 when the stimulus frequency lies outside the entrainment range. Direct current injection into the TCMRO afferents also was effective. Overall, sensory input, as in the stick insect, appears to trigger transitions between phases of the movement cycle, and hence sensory input provides essential information to the locomotory CPG in crayfish.

Conclusion: Beyond Sensory Modulation

Just as motor neurons sometimes are integral members of CPGs, even if they are not strictly limited to the CNS, so sensory neurons and muscles may be essential components of circuits that generate rhythmic movements. Sensory input varies in importance among the highly diverse circuits that generate wing movements in locust flight, swimming undulations in the medicinal leech and lampreys, and swimmeret beating and walking locomotion in insects and crayfish. For understanding the physiological bases of rhythmic movements, it appears to be unhelpful to construct artificial divisions between CPGs, motor neurons, muscles, and sensory feedback. A more useful approach is to identify oscillatory subcircuits wherever they occur, whether within the CNS or not; and whether comprising interneurons, motor neurons, effector structures, or sensory receptors. Such subcircuits, together with their mutual interconnections, generate the highly variable and adaptive oscillating patterns that underlie rhythmic animal movement.

See also: Behavioral Hierarchies; Central Pattern Generators; Command Systems; Hormones and Behavior; Neuromodulation; Pattern Generation; Swim Oscillator Networks; Swimming: Neural Mechanisms; Walking in Invertebrates.

Further Reading

Büschges A (2005) Sensory control and organization of neural networks mediating coordination of multisegmental organs for locomotion. *Journal of Neurophysiology* 93: 1127–1135.

Cang J, Yu X, and Friesen WO (2001) Sensory modification of leech swimming: Interactions between ventral stretch receptors and swim-related neurons. *Journal of Comparative Physiology* 187: 569–579.

Delcomyn F (1980) Neural basis of rhythmic behavior in animals. *Science* 210: 492–498.

Elson RC, Sillar KT, and Bush BMH (1992) Identified proprioceptive afferents and motor rhythm entrainment in the crayfish walking system. *Journal of Neurophysiology* 67: 530–546.

Friesen WO and Cang J (2001) Sensory and central mechanisms control intersegmental coordination. *Current Opinion in Neurobiology* 11: 678–683.

Grillner S and Wallén P (2002) Cellular bases of a vertebrate locomotor system: Steering, intersegmental, and segmental co-ordination and sensory control. *Brain Research Reviews* 40: 92–106.

Hooper SL and DiCaprio RA (2004) Crustacean motor pattern generator networks. *Neurosignals* 13: 50–69.

Kristan WB Jr, Calabrese RL, and Friesen WO (2005) Neuronal control of leech behavior. *Progress in Neurobiology* 76: 279–327.

McClellan AD and Jang W (1993) Mechanosensory inputs to the central pattern generators for locomotion in the lamprey spinal cord: Resetting, entrainment, and computer modeling. *Journal of Neurophysiology* 70: 2442–2454.

Pearce RA and Friesen WO (1984) Intersegmental coordination of leech swimming: Comparison of *in situ* and isolated nerve cord activity with body wall movement. *Brain Research* 299: 363–366.

Pearson KG and Ramirez J-M (1997) Sensory modulation of pattern-generating circuits. In: Stein PSG, Griller S, Selverston AI, and Stuart DG (eds.) *Neurons, Networks, and Motor Behavior,* pp. 225–235. Cambridge, MA: MIT Press.

Rossignol S, Dubuc R, and Gossard J-P (2006) Dynamic sensorimotor interactions in locomotion. *Physiological Reviews* 86: 89–154.

Sherrington CS (1947) *The Integrative Action of the Nervous System*, 2nd edn. New Haven, CT: Yale University Press.

Wallén P and Williams TL (1984) Fictive locomotion in the lamprey spinal cord *in vitro* compared with swimming in the intact and spinal animal. *Journal of Physiology* 347: 225–239.

Wilson DM (1961) The central nervous control of flight in a locust. *Journal of Experimental Biology* 38: 471–490.

Yu X and Friesen WO (2004) Entrainment of leech swimming activity by the ventral stretch receptor. *Journal of Comparative Physiology* 190: 939–949.

Gap Junctions and Neuronal Oscillations

M O Cunningham and F E N LeBeau, Newcastle University, Newcastle upon Tyne, UK

Introduction

In addition to neuronal chemical neurotransmission, electrical transmission via gap junctions, which are protein channels that directly link the cytoplasm of adjacent cells, is now known to constitute an important type of cell-to-cell communication. Although initially thought to be important mainly in development, it is now clear that electrical signaling via gap junctions plays an important role in the adult central nervous system (CNS).

Considerable advances have been made in understanding the contribution of electrical signaling, via gap junctions, to neuronal signaling, most notably the role of synchronizing oscillatory or rhythmic activity. Oscillatory neuronal activity underlies the production of the signals recorded with an electroencephalogram (EEG) and reflects the coordinated activity of large populations of neurons. An EEG of the brain reveals rhythmic oscillatory activity in distinct frequency bands that occur during different behavioral states, and can be altered in a number of neurological and psychological diseases. Work from many research groups over the past decade has highlighted the role of electrical signaling via gap junctions in the generation, and/or spread, of synchronous oscillatory network activity. Electrical coupling via gap junctions can occur in both neurons and glial cells throughout the CNS. However, in this article, we focus on electrical coupling in excitatory principal cells and inhibitory interneurons, mainly in the neocortex and hippocampus. We provide an overview of the role of electrical signaling via gap junctions in the generation of oscillatory network activity and discuss briefly the importance of gap junction function in neurological conditions such as epilepsy.

Historical Background

The idea that neurons can form an interconnected network via direct cell-to-cell connections is not a novel concept. Proposed by Camillo Golgi in the late nineteenth century, the 'reticular theory' postulated that the nervous system could form a syncytium consisting of nerve fibers forming an intricate connected network and that the nerve impulse could propagate along such a diffuse network. However, at the same time, Ramón y Cajal's 'neuron doctrine' hypothesized that the nervous system was composed of anatomically and functionally independent units (neurons) with chemical synapses connecting them. Today we understand that in the adult mammalian brain, each of these theories reflects an important aspect of the communication in neuronal networks.

Structure and Properties of Gap Junctions in the CNS

Gap junctions form a continuous link between two separate neuronal structures (**Figure 1**) that allows the direct transmission of electrical signals between neurons. Neurons can be coupled together via gap junctions connecting soma-to-soma, dendrite-to-dendrite, or soma-to-dendrite. More recently, evidence has appeared of gap junctions linking neurons via axon-to-axon connections. The major proteins that form gap junctions are termed connexins (Cxs). Different Cx subtypes are defined by their molecular mass (in kilodaltons). A number of different Cx subtypes have now been identified in the vertebrate CNS, including Cx26, Cx32, Cx36, Cx43, and Cx45, but of these only Cx36 forms have been shown to be specific for neurons. A functional channel connecting two different neurons is formed by the apposition of two connexons, one in the plasma membrane of each neuron. Each connexon contains six Cx proteins. A functional gap junction is thus composed of 12 Cx subunits. Diversity in the composition of connexons in a gap junction can arise, as hemichannels can either consist of the same Cx subtype (homomeric) or different Cx subtypes (heteromeric).

Recently, a new family of gap junction proteins, the pannexins, has been identified in the CNS. Related to innexins, an invertebrate family of gap junction proteins, the so-called pannexins (Px) have been demonstrated to form functional gap junctions in recordings from paired *Xenopus* oocytes. Three Px subtypes have been described in the rat and human genome, with Px1 and Px2 expressed solely in the CNS. There are strong expression patterns for Px1 and Px2 in the cortex and hippocampus, but their functional role in network activity is unknown.

Gap junctions are not simply inert pores between neurons, as they can be dynamically modulated in a number of ways. Evidence suggests that the number of gap junctions, the pattern of expression of Cx proteins, and conductance properties of the individual channels can all be modified by neurotransmitters, second messengers, calcium ion concentrations, intra- and extracellular pH, and transmembrane voltage. This sort of modification occurs during development

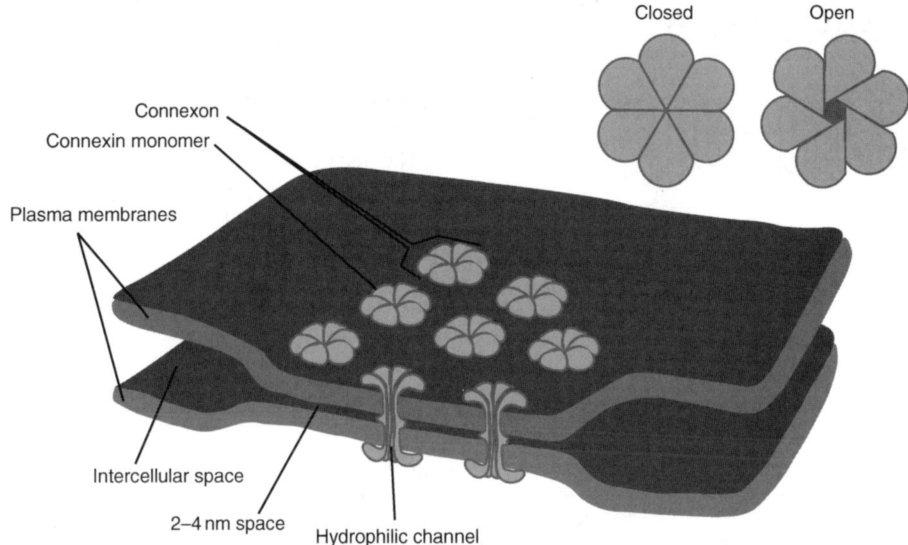

Figure 1 Structure of a gap junction, showing a cluster of gap junctions (yellow) spanning two opposing plasma membranes (blue sheets). The intercellular space narrows at the point of the gap junction, bringing the two membranes into close contact. A gap junction consists of two hemichannels (one in each plasma membrane) that form a continuous channel between the two cells. Each hemichannel contains six connexin proteins, which, as a unit, are called a connexon. Insets show that a conformational change in the connexin proteins allows the gap junctions to open and close in response to modulators such as pH, calcium, and cAMP.

and in response to a variety of factors in the adult. Modulation allows for the complex, connexin-specific regulation of electrical signaling via gap junctions, although to date little is known about the mechanism.

Approaches to Studying Gap Junctions

Evidence for electrical coupling mediated via gap junctions in the CNS comes from using a multidisciplinary approach. The CNS consists of excitatory principal cells and inhibitory interneurons, and there is evidence for electrical signaling in both neuronal populations. Electron microscopy and freeze-fracture studies have anatomically demonstrated gap junctions between both interneurons and pyramidal cells in the cortex.

Early electrophysiological evidence for electrical signaling via gap junctions was obtained by recording from principal cells in the cortex and hippocampus. These studies also showed that certain dyes (e.g., Lucifer yellow) could pass from one principal neuron to another via gap junctions. In dye coupling experiments a specific dye is injected into one cell, and if that cell is coupled to other cells, dye transfer may be detected in the connected cells. However, dye coupling studies are complicated because different connexins may have different permeabilities to dyes, and dye transfer depends on the time for filling and the locations of the gap junctions. For this reason a lack of dye coupling does not completely exclude the presence of functional gap junctions.

Interneurons represent only 10–20% of the neuronal population and are thus difficult to record 'blind' with intracellular sharp electrode techniques. In order to surmount this issue experimentalists have utilized infrared differential interface contrast (IR-DIC) microscopy and whole-cell patch recording techniques. This has made it possible to identify interneurons visually from their basic morphology and thus conduct simultaneous whole-cell patch recordings from two or more interneurons. Using this technique electrical coupling between pairs of interneurons has been demonstrated. When current is injected into one cell to change the membrane potential, a potential change is also seen in the coupled cell (**Figure 2**). The ratio of the potential change in cell 1/cell 2 is termed the coupling coefficient or coupling ratio. As with the dye transfer studies, the absence of electrical coupling potentials cannot totally exclude the possibility that gap junctions may be present at sites too distant for current transfer to be detected with somatic recordings.

Electrically coupled interneurons have now been shown to be widespread in many areas of the vertebrate CNS, including the hippocampus and neocortex. However, elucidating the functional significance of electrical signaling via gap junctions has been made difficult by the lack of specific agents to block gap

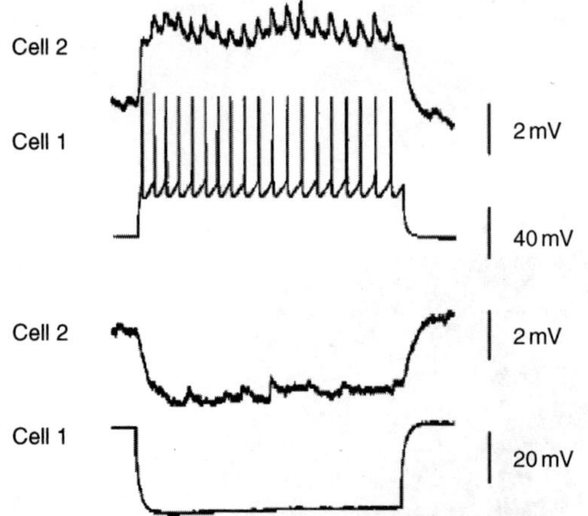

Figure 2 Electrical coupling potentials, showing electrical coupling between fast-spiking interneurons. Paired whole-cell recordings of two fast-spiking interneurons from the hippocampal dentate gyrus region in the mouse are depicted. Traces show the voltage responses in cell 1 following depolarizing (upper) and hyperpolarizing (lower) current injections; voltage responses were also reflected in cell 2 but were smaller in amplitude.

junctions. Uncoupling agents that are currently used include heptanol, octanol, halothane, carbenoxolone, and 18α-glycyrretinic acid. However, these agents will block all gap junctions (including glial gap junctions), making it impossible to clearly identify the importance of any specific gap junctions. Recently, blockers for Cx36 have been described, including quinine and the more specific mefloquine. However, all of these compounds have been reported to have a range of nonspecific effects that could also affect neuronal activity. New strategies have been developed to study the role of electrical signaling via gap junctions using genetically engineered mice that lack specific connexin proteins (see later).

Evidence for Gap Junctions between Principal Neurons

Dye coupling studies show that when one principal cell is injected with dye, often one or two other cells also fill with dye, suggesting direct coupling between the cells. Procedures that increase gap junction conductance (e.g., reduced extracellular calcium) tend to increase the number of dye-coupled neurons. Conversely, the degree of dye coupling is diminished when gap junction conductance is reduced by the application of gap junction blockers. In these and earlier studies, potentials resembling small action potentials (<10 mV) were observed in recordings from the soma of principal cells. Termed fast prepotentials (FPPs), and first observed *in vivo*, these events were initially believed to arise from electrogenesis in dendrites. Subsequent experimental studies, however, suggested that FPPs or spikelets (presently the more commonly used term) represent action potentials in electrically coupled neurons.

The location of the gap junctions that mediate coupling between principal cells has yet to be conclusively demonstrated. Paired whole-cell patch recording techniques have failed to demonstrate significant electrical coupling between the somas of principal cells. However, recent intracellular recordings with sharp electrodes show high levels of coupling between pyramidal cells in the hippocampus. There is evidence to suggest that electrical signaling via gap junctions could be axo-axonic in principal cells. Computational studies first proposed that the fast kinetics of the spikelets seen in pyramidal cells could only be explained if the gap junctions were located between axonal compartments. If the gap junctions were located at remote sites on the dendrites of pyramidal cells, then the electrical-filtering properties of the dendrites would result in slower kinetic properties of the spikelets. Experimental evidence was subsequently provided when one study, using paired recordings from the soma and axon hillock/axon initial segment of the same cell, showed that following antidromic stimulation of the relevant fiber tract, the evoked spikelet appeared first in the axon hillock/initial segment and then in the soma. Subsequent visualization experiments revealed that the path taken by dye loaded into one cell could be followed in real time, as it was observed first filling in the axon and then subsequently in the soma of a second neuron. One recent electron microscopy study has found ultrastructural evidence for gap junctions between pairs of mossy fiber axons in the CA3 region of the hippocampus. However, the identities of the proteins that compose the putative axo-axonic gap junctions are not fully known, although the pannexins and Cx36 have both been proposed as possible candidates.

Evidence for Gap Junctions between Interneurons

Perhaps the greatest advance in our understanding of the role of electrical signaling via gap junctions has come from studies of interneurons. Interneurons in the hippocampus and neocortex consist of a number of distinct subtypes that can be identified on the basis of their morphology, physiological properties, and their expression of specific chemical markers such as peptides or calcium-binding proteins. Early anatomical studies clearly demonstrated evidence for the existence of dendrodendritic or dendrosomatic gap junctions between interneurons in the cortex.

Recent physiological studies have also shown that interneurons can be electrically connected. Electrical coupling between interneuron pairs has been shown to be bidirectional, with current usually flowing equally in both directions. In addition, gap junctions function as low-pass filters in that they preferentially transmit low-frequency signals. Fast signals, such as action potentials, are not transmitted as well and appear in the coupled cell as a truncated spikelet. Nonetheless, spikelets can still facilitate the generation of action potentials in the coupled cell and so enhance the spread of activity. The traditional view of electrical signaling via gap junctions as important for mediating fast excitation is an oversimplification. Gap junctions can transmit depolarizing and hyperpolarizing current equally well. For example, the afterhyperpolarization that follows an action potential is also transmitted to the coupled cell, so a spikelet can be followed by a significant hyperpolarization. Thus electrical signaling can be both excitatory and inhibitory.

A key feature of gap junction coupling observed between cortical interneurons is that it is mainly between interneurons of the same class (e.g., fast-spiking basket cells, multipolar bursting cells, neurogliaform cells, and low-threshold spiking cells). As it has long been postulated that different classes of interneurons are involved in different functions, this specificity of connectivity leads to the formation of distinct networks of electrically coupled interneurons, each of which could be involved in a separate function. In the neocortex, at least five different interneuron networks of electrically coupled cells have now been identified (**Figure 3**). Interneurons belonging to the same morphological class exhibit gap junction coupling, often with a high incidence (e.g., 50% of basket cells coupled). However, only a few cases of electrical coupling between different interneuron classes have been reported. Paired whole-cell patch recordings reveal that electrical coupling between all inhibitory interneurons so far studied is mediated by the same connexin (Cx36). In mice (though not in rats), Cx36 is expressed only in interneurons, and mice that lack Cx36 exhibit no functional electrical coupling between pairs of interneurons. As yet we know nothing about the mechanisms that regulate the specificity of interneuron coupling so as to ensure that connections only form between interneurons of the same type. This remains an important issue to address in the future.

There is strong evidence for the developmental refinement of the cell-specific distribution of gap junctions. The degree of electrical coupling in both rodent and human brain declines with maturation. This decline in the extent of electrical coupling was one reason that electrical signaling via gap junctions

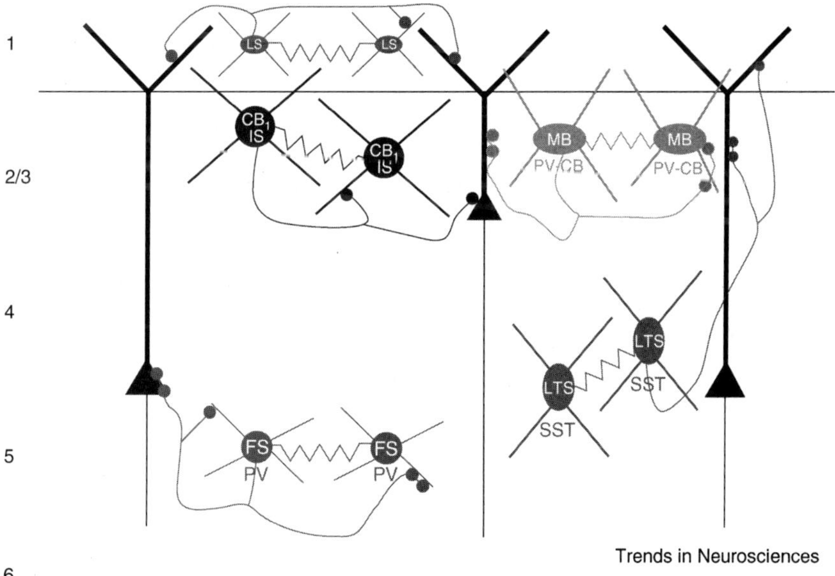

Figure 3 Five networks of distinct electrically coupled γ-aminobutyric acid (GABAergic) interneurons in the cerebral cortex. Numbers indicate cortical laminae. Pyramidal cells are shown in black. Different colored circles represent different interneuron classes that are electrically coupled (jagged lines). Some interneuron classes are also chemically synaptically coupled, and all form synapses onto the pyramidal cells. CB, calbindin; CB_1 IS, cannabinoid receptor-1-expressing irregular-spiking cell; FS, fast-spiking cell; LS, late-spiking cell; LTS, low-threshold spiking cell; MB, multipolar bursting cell; PV, parvalbumin; SST, somatostatin.

was thought to be important mainly in development. However, a number of studies have demonstrated that electrical coupling persists in the adult brain, and computational studies predict that low levels of coupling (e.g., one to two gap junctions per cell) are in fact sufficient to enhance network synchronization.

Gap Junctions and Oscillations of Cognitive Relevance

Oscillatory, or synchronized, network activity occurs in the EEG in different frequency bands during specific behavioral states in mammals, including humans. Oscillations can occur at from less than 1 Hz to several hundred hertz. This broad range of activity is tightly linked to higher cognitive function such as memory formation, sensory perception, and integration. Two types of oscillatory activity in which the role of electrical signaling via gap junctions has been particularly well studied are the gamma frequency (20–80 Hz) and ultrafast (>80 Hz) or very fast oscillations (VFOs). Gamma frequency activity can be recorded in many brain areas but is particularly prominent in the neocortex and hippocampus. It is associated with a number of functions such as sensory perception, attention, learning, and memory. Ultrafast oscillations in the hippocampus are also associated with memory functions, particularly the consolidation of declarative memories.

Role of Electrical Signaling via Gap Junctions in Generating Fast Network Oscillations

A major methodological advance in the study of gamma frequency oscillations has been the ability to study this activity *in vitro*. Persistent gamma oscillations can be induced and sustained in brain slices of hippocampus and cortex by the bath application of drugs that can depolarize both pyramidal cells and interneurons such as kainate, muscarinic, or glutamate metabotropic receptor agonists. Gamma frequency activity cannot be generated in the absence of inhibitory neurotransmission, and several studies have identified specific interneuron classes, particularly fast-spiking basket cells, that fire at gamma frequency during the oscillation and so contribute to the generation of this activity. However, in addition to its role in GABAergic inhibition, electrical signaling via gap junctions also appears to be important for the generation of gamma frequency oscillations. Recent work suggests that electrical coupling between both interneurons and pyramidal cells is important for the generation of gamma frequency activity.

It had been known for some time that application of gap junction blockers (halothane, octanol, and carbenoxolone) can abolish gamma frequency oscillations, but these studies could not distinguish the contribution of electrical signaling via gap junctions in interneurons versus pyramidal cells. However, it is possible *in vitro* to generate a gamma frequency oscillation in which pyramidal cell activity has been blocked – the so-called interneuronal network gamma (ING). Computational modeling studies initially suggested that, along with chemical inhibitory transmission, electrical signaling via dendritic gap junctions between interneurons was important for synchronizing gamma frequency activity. Using the *in vitro* ING model it was found that blockade of gap junctions markedly reduced the synchrony of the oscillations, although some gamma frequency activity still remained.

The contribution of electrical coupling between interneurons to fast network oscillations was tested further using Cx36 knockout mice that specifically lack functional electrical coupling between interneurons. Using the Cx36 mice, in which excitation is intact, it was found that the ability of hippocampal neuronal networks to generate gamma frequency activity was significantly reduced. Reductions in gamma frequency activity were seen both *in vitro* and *in vivo*. At a cellular level, recordings from principal cells and interneurons *in vitro* showed a disruption in the amplitude, rhythmicity, and coherence of inhibitory inputs. Under normal conditions, spikelets in interneurons increase the likelihood of full action potentials being generated in the coupled cells, thus enabling a network of interneurons to fire synchronously. These synchronous inhibitory outputs impinge on the postsynaptic principal cells and control the timing of the spike output, as the principal cells can only fire once the inhibition has decayed. The inability of interneurons in the Cx36 knockout mice to synchronize properly their firing via gap junctions leads to a reduction in the precision of their action potential timing and thus their rhythmic inhibitory output. Behavioral studies have shown that mice lacking Cx36 exhibit learning and memory impairments, an observation consistent with the idea that normal gamma frequency activity is important for these cognitive tasks.

Importantly, the loss of Cx36 did not lead to the complete abolition of gamma frequency activity. A residual gamma oscillation was still present both *in vivo* and *in vitro*. *In vitro* it was shown that this remaining gamma frequency oscillation was blocked by the putative gap junction blocking agent, carbenoxolone. This suggested that some other form of gap junction-mediated signaling is also required for the generation of the gamma frequency activity, and this is now thought to arise from the pyramidal cell population.

Electrical signaling via gap junctions between pyramidal cells was initially proposed to underlie the generation of certain types of ultrafast or 'ripple' activity. Using an *in vitro* brain slice model, high-frequency oscillatory activity, or 'ripples,' occurring at ~80–150 Hz can be generated in the hippocampus in the absence of chemical synaptic transmission when using a nominally calcium-free bath medium. The lack of chemical synaptic transmission in these experiments supports the hypothesis that this activity is dependent on direct electrical connections between neurons. The 'ripple' activity is abolished in the presence of pharmacological blockers of gap junctions, such as halothane or carbenoxolone. At the level of individual neurons, intracellular recording from principal cells revealed that, concomitant with the extracellular field potential 'ripple,' the cells discharged either a full-action potential or a spikelet. The kinetic properties of these spikelets (as discussed earlier) were too fast to be due to dendrodendritic gap junctions, and so axo-axonal connections were proposed. In addition, in the Cx36 knockout mice, this ultrafast oscillatory activity was normal both *in vivo* and *in vitro*, suggesting that interneuronal electrical coupling did not underlie this activity.

More recent work has now demonstrated that the ultrafast oscillations coexist with the gamma frequency activity. Ultrafast oscillations can be generated in the axon plexus of pyramidal cells in the hippocampus. It is currently thought that these high-frequency oscillations occur as a result of random ectopic action potentials (action potentials arising from regions other than the axon hillock) in the axon plexus. This random activity spreads throughout the axon plexus, via axo-axonic gap junctions, resulting in a barrage of fast excitatory synaptic potentials that can be recorded in the interneurons, and provides the necessary excitatory drive for the interneurons. The combination of chemical and electrical connections between the interneurons then allows a synchronized output back to the pyramidal cells at gamma frequency. Gap junctions are therefore required between the pyramidal cells to generate the drive to the interneurons, and the gap junctions between the interneurons are needed to temporally coordinate their activity.

Gap Junctions and Epilepsy

The EEG is an important test in the diagnostic process of treating epilepsy. Traditionally, this approach has been noninvasive, using small, metal electrodes attached to the scalp. This approach is satisfactory for the medical evaluation of the seizure activity. However, there are limitations to this approach. The advent of digital recordings and invasive human studies using depth electrode recordings or subdural electrode mats now allows the measurement of electrical signals with frequencies greater than those recordable with conventional EEG equipment. Using these techniques, ultrafast oscillatory activity has been observed in close proximity to seizure onset zones in both animal models and humans. Indeed, it has been suggested that this type of activity is a reliable electrophysiological marker of epileptogenicity. A common feature of focal epileptic seizure activity, in both humans and experimental models, is the presence of ultrafast oscillations. Thus fast ripples associated with interictal spikes currently provide information on localization and epileptogenicity of the tissue involved in their generation. Evidence from developmental studies further supports a role of gap junctions in epilepsy. Thus genetic linkage mapping demonstrates that Cx36 is a high-ranking positional and functional candidate gene for juvenile myoclonic epilepsy.

A number of molecular biology studies have demonstrated that in neuronal tissue obtained from animal models and human cases of epilepsy there are obvious alterations in the abundance of connexins. Most of this work concerns the expression of connexins, which is limited to astrocytes. Several studies have examined protein and or mRNA expression, but the results from these studies yield conflicting results, with some reporting increases in connexin expression and others reporting decreases. Differences in a number of the experimental parameters applied could account for these discrepancies. It is obvious that more work is required to determine whether Cxs are modified in epileptic tissue, and if so in what directions. Moreover, if putative axo-axonic gap junctions are composed of pannexins, then attempts should be made to examine the expression and localization of such proteins in both human epileptic tissue and tissue from animal experimental models of epilepsy.

Conclusions

Recent advances over the past decade have demonstrated that both chemical signaling and electrical signaling play a central role in cortical communication. It is generally widely accepted that chemical signaling allows for highly complex, specific, and modifiable neuronal communication. However, it is now apparent that electrical signaling mediated via gap junctions can also demonstrate a high degree of functional specificity. Thus, the combination of multiple coexistent synaptic and electrical networks serves to greatly enrich the processing capabilities on neuronal networks.

See also: Epilepsy; Epilepsy: Channelopathies; Gap Junctions and Electrical Synapses; Gap Junction Abnormalities and Disorders of the Nervous System; Neural Synchrony and Feature Binding; Neural Oscillators and Dynamical Systems Models; Neurotransmitter Release: Synchronous and Asynchronous; Presynaptic Receptor Signaling.

Further Reading

Bennet MLV and Zukin RS (2004) Electrical coupling and neuronal synchronization in the mammalian brain. *Neuron* 41: 495–511.

Buzsaki G and Draguhn A (2004) Neuronal oscillations in cortical networks. *Science* 304: 1926–1929.

Connors BW and Long MA (2004) Electrical synapses in the mammalian brain. *Annual Review of Neuroscience* 27: 393–418.

Galarreta M and Hestrin S (2001) Electrical synapses between GABA-releasing interneurons. *Nature Reviews Neuroscience* 2: 425–433.

Hestrin S and Galerreta M (2005) Electrical synapses define networks of neocortical GABAergic neurons. *Trends in Neuroscience* 28: 304–309.

Schmitz D, Schuchmann S, Fisahn A, et al. (2001) Axo-axonal coupling: A novel mechanism for ultrafast neuronal communication. *Neuron* 31: 831–840.

Whittington MA and Traub RD (2003) Interneuron diversity series: Inhibitory interneurons and network oscillations *in vitro*. *Trends in Neuroscience* 26: 676–682.

Information Coding

B J Richmond, National Institute of Mental Health, Bethesda, MD, USA

Published by Elsevier Ltd.

Neuronal Codes

Neural coding describes the study of information processing by neurons. Such studies seek to learn what information is used, and how information is transformed as it passes from one processing stage to another. The field of neural coding seeks to synthesize information arising from many levels of analysis and to explain how integrated behavior arises from the cooperative activity of the neurons in the brain.

Much is known about the biophysics of neuronal responses – that is, how a spike is generated, how the spike acts on the axonal terminal to cause transmitter release, and how transmitters act on the target neuronal receptors. However, the impact of series of spikes is not well known, and it is even less clear what information has been encoded and how that information will be utilized in subsequent processing stages.

It is natural to consider the brain as an information processing machine. It takes in information from physical changes in the environment, including light, touch, and sound, integrates this information with remembered or genetically coded information and then produces organized behavior. In any information processing system, issues to be considered are what is being encoded, what is the code used to transmit the information, how reliable (noisy or not) is the code, and how the information is utilized or decoded.

At the base of this cascade of information processing is the information transformed and transmitted by single neurons. The signal on dendrites and cell body is reflected in fluctuations in the potential difference across the membrane. The signal that is transmitted down the axon is quite different; it is the action potential. This action potential propagates rapidly down the axon. At the axon terminal the arrival of the action potential generally causes the release of a transmitter that affects the membrane of the target neuron. The action potentials mark times at which the cell membrane at the neuronal cell body reaches the firing threshold. Thus, there is a sequence of action potentials containing information about the membrane potential at the neuronal cell body, and it is the information carried by the train of action potentials that provides information at the projection targets for the neurons. This train of action potentials (the spike train) can be considered as elements of a neural code.

Average Rate Codes

The number of action potentials, or 'spikes,' is the critical feature of the neural code. For example, for primary visual cortex, the number of spikes provides information about the orientation of a bar, as shown in **Figure 1**, or, for primary motor cortex, the direction of reaching. For the two examples, the tuning curve can be parameterized by some simple function (e.g., as has been done for reaching direction in primary motor cortex with a cosine or some other similar smooth, unimodal function). This 'tuning curve' then provides a means to estimate the direction of the bar (or movement) from the neural response (**Figure 2**). In higher brain regions (e.g., inferior temporal cortex of the monkey), the neurons respond most strongly to a particular complex object, sometimes a single face or a hand, and a tuning curve for this 'spike count code' can be determined empirically. So far it is generally not possible to parameterize the tuning curve as simply as is done with the aforementioned directional tuning examples. However, for considering the principles underlying neural codes, parameterizing the tuning curve is not critical. Decoding can be studied in any brain region for which the equivalent of this 'tuning curve' is available. The results of experiments using measured tuning curves only become easier to interpret as the knowledge about the tuning function improves. Hence, over the history of single neuronal recording, there has been appropriate emphasis on measuring such 'tuning curves.'

If every presentation of a stimulus elicited the same response, decoding the response would be straightforward; it would only be necessary to measure the response and look up which condition or conditions elicit that response. However, as can be seen in **Figures 1** and **2**, the responses are variable. Many of the possible responses emitted by the primary visual cortical neuron could have been elicited by any of the orientations of the bar (here measured in spike count). In the face of such variability, it is not possible to know unequivocally which stimulus elicited the response. It is possible, however, to determine how likely or probable any particular stimulus might be. In the case shown in **Figures 1** and **2**, one can pick the stimulus that is most likely to have elicited the particular response, and it then becomes possible to estimate how many neurons would be needed to decode the orientation of the stimulus. Thus, even though variability limits the information that a single neuron can encode, a probabilistic estimate of the orientation can be developed. Then, based on these probabilities, some rule for choosing a stimulus can be identified.

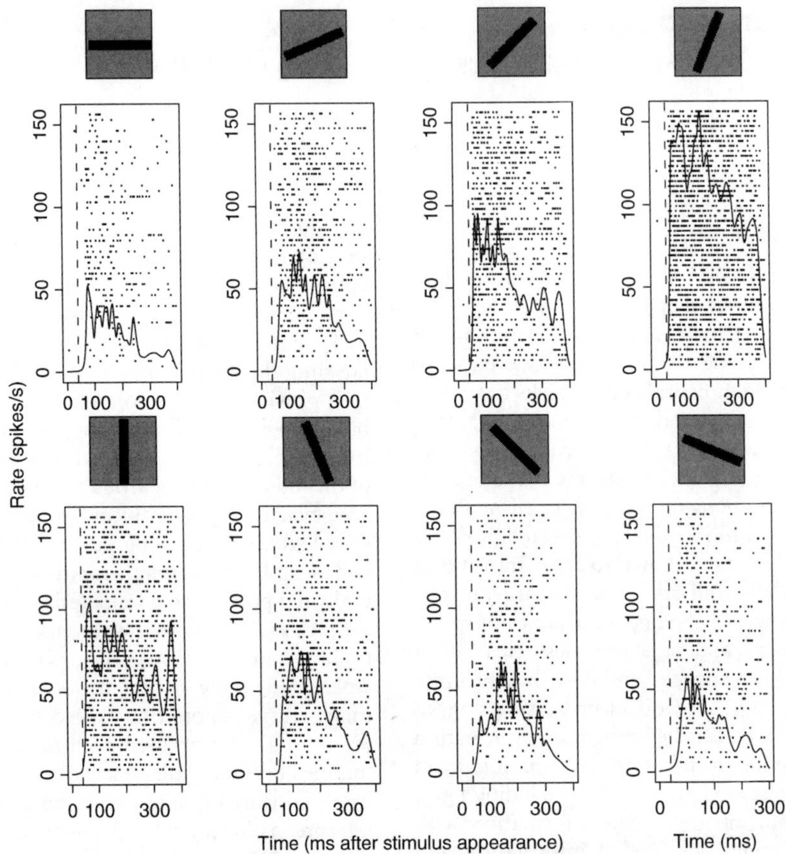

Figure 1 Example of orientation sensitivity of a neuron in primary visual cortex. The black bar at the top of each panel was flashed onto the receptive field (i.e., the position in the visual field that, for that neuron, is sensitive to visual stimulation) of the neuron for 600 ms. The dots in each horizontal row in the panels represent the times that the neuron emitted an action potential. Each row shows a different presentation of the stimulus. Time on the *x*-axis is relative to the stimulus appearance. The third black bar from the left (top and bottom) elicited the most intense response (the largest activity) from this neuron. The large variation in responsiveness from one stimulus presentation to the next can be seen in that successive rows of dots have different numbers of dots, and the dots are in different places for all of these black bars. The smooth black line in each panel is a smoothed average of the spikes across all of the stimulus presentations. This is taken as an estimate of the overall driving of this neuron by its inputs. Modified from Doya K, Ishii S, Pouget A, and Rao RPN (eds.) (2007) *Bayesian Brain: Probabilistic Approaches to Neural Coding*. Cambridge, MA: MIT Press.

The usual rule, and the easiest to implement, is to choose the stimulus that is most likely to have elicited the response; this is the maximum likelihood estimate.

It is because of the response variability that tools from signal processing, statistical pattern recognition, and information theory have become important for studying neural coding. Even though it is obvious that the pattern of spikes can carry additional information, it is easiest to start with the assumption that the spikes are distributed randomly through time, and that only the spike count changes. It then becomes straightforward to add information from the time sequence of the spikes after developing the principles by which to assess the code.

As a first approximation, assume that there is no information in the pattern of spikes. Then measure the information using the spike count alone as a neural code. The only process for which the spikes are equally likely at all times – that is, there is no correlation over time – and hence for which there can be no information in the timing is a Poisson process. A Poisson process is a special case of point process – that is, a process in which there are discrete events that can all be considered identical occurring over time. The only number needed to characterize a Poisson process is the average rate of the events. The variability is proportional to the mean firing rate (**Figure 3**), with the variability being higher when the firing rate is higher, although the mean is not equal to the variance, as would be the case for a pure Poisson process. The source of this variability is not really known, although if a

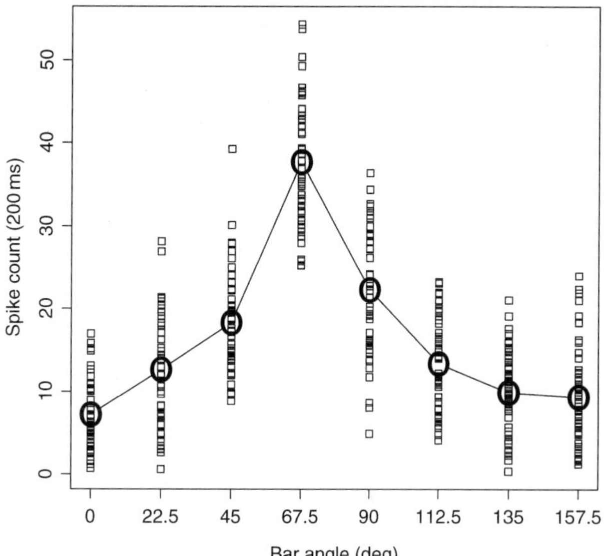

Figure 2 Orientation tuning for the neuron in **Figure 1**. The plot shows the bar angle on the *x*-axis and number of spikes on the *y*-axis. Each small square is the number of spikes emitted in response to one stimulus presentation. The large circles show the average, and the line connects the averages for each viewing. This illustrates the wide variation in the number of spikes emitted even for the same bar on different presentations (the squares in each column). Nonetheless, there is a clear and reliable tendency across trials. Trial-by-trial estimation of the bar orientation can only be done in a probabilistic way, making it necessary to consider how the responses of populations of neurons might be read and decoded. Modified from Doya K, Ishii S, Pouget A, and Rao RPN (eds.) (2007) *Bayesian Brain: Probabilistic Approaches to Neural Coding.* Cambridge, MA: MIT Press.

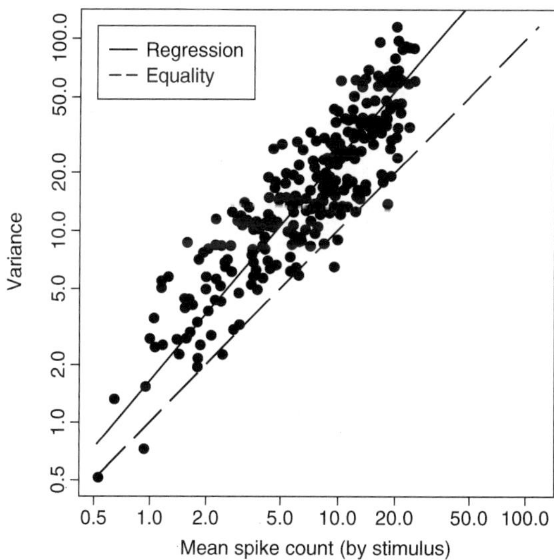

Figure 3 Scatter plot of means vs. variances. Each black dot represents the mean (*x*-axis) and variance (*y*-axis) elicited across many presentations of a single black and white stimulus on the receptive field of a V1 neuron. The solid line is the regression line, and the dashed line is the equality line where the points would lie if the responses arose from a Poisson process. The regression line is parallel to and above the line expected for a Poisson process. From this it can be concluded that the responses have some internal timing structure. From experience it is known that this type of overdispersion is related to point processes in which the points have a tendency to be in groups or 'bursts.'

visual stimulus changes very rapidly, responses can be considerably less variable. It is obvious that the pattern of the spikes over time might be carrying information, and simple considerations of the biophysics of information across synapses make it clear that this temporal 'coding' could easily influence the target neuron.

Two methods commonly used to quantify the effect of this variability are classical analysis of variance (ANOVA), with each stimulus being one level in the stimulus factor (or if a continuous parameter is used to characterize the signal, linear regression), and information theory, which estimates how much the uncertainty about the stimulus being shown is reduced by seeing the response. In ANOVA, in addition to the *p*-value (the probability that all of the levels are the same), the amount of variance explained by each factor (in our example, the orientation) is calculated, and the amount of variance that is left unexplained in this 'model' of the data is also given. Thus, ANOVA (or linear regression) allows the calculation of the signal-to-noise ratio (the explained variance divided by the residual variance). This is a powerful and straightforward approach to quantifying the relation between a set of experimental conditions and the discriminability among conditions that can be achieved using the neural responses. Thus, for the example in **Figures 1** and 2, 70% of the variance can be accounted for, by orientation, and rest is unexplained (for, the purpose here, noise).

Temporal Codes

If it were certain that the responses could be characterized by the spike count or rate alone, tools from linear statistical modeling, such as regression or ANOVA (with possibly some generalization to other types of statistical linear modeling), would be adequate to quantify the relations between stimuli or experimental conditions and responses. However, the responses occur over time, and, as can be seen in **Figure 4**, the rate varies as a function of time. It is natural to ask how much better the stimulus can be determined by using the time course of response, as compared to using the response strength alone. In the example shown in **Figure 4**, the total number of spikes and the variances of these two sets of responses are the same when counted during the whole period of stimulus presentation. It is evident that the variability in both the number and timing of spikes will limit the information carried by the responses. However, it is also clear that the envelope of the firing rate (the low-pass filtered version of the spikes) is different across the two stimuli. Thus, even though these two sets of responses have the same number of spikes over the whole counting interval, the time course of when the spikes occur appears to be different.

There is an ongoing debate about how precisely the timing of spikes needs to be measured to capture all of the information in spike trains. The way for an analysis to become sensitive to the time course of the response is to break the response into epochs of different lengths, and ask whether the information increases as the epochs become smaller. This makes the measurement of the time course more and more precise – that is, as the measurement of the time course becomes more precise. As the epochs become shorter (and there are more of them), the variations in the response that is represented become finer: the response has more 'wiggles.' The difficulty with this approach is that as the epochs become shorter, there are more of them, and the estimate of the firing in each epoch becomes less certain.

One straightforward way to study the temporal pattern of the responses is to use the principal components of the set of responses. The principal components are the eigenvectors of the data domain covariance matrix, and form an orthogonal set of, in this case, temporal waveforms derived from the data. Each response can be represented as a weighted sum of principal components. Information theory is a valuable tool for assessing these types of multidimensional codes, or codes with more than one element. To use information theory, the basic definition of transmitted or mutual information is required. The mutual or transmitted information, $H(r, s)$, is the difference between the entropy of the spike train (or stimulus),

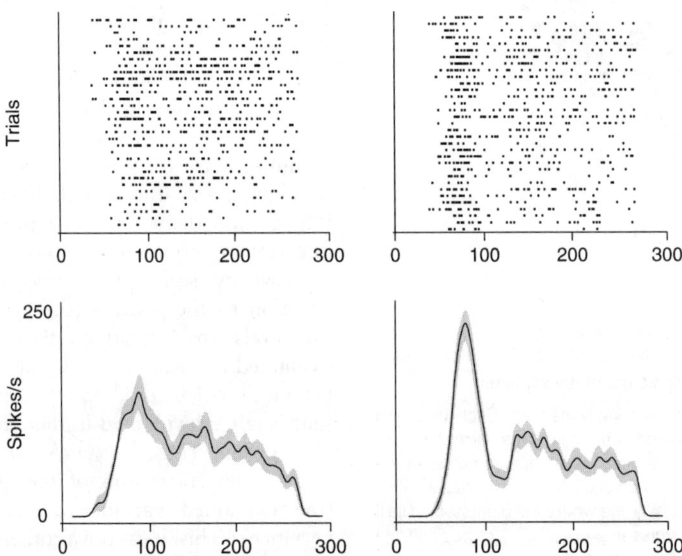

Figure 4 Raster dot diagrams and average spike densities for two stimuli eliciting responses with the same number of spikes. It is clear from this diagram that the pattern of spikes over time, or the pattern of the driving force over time, is different, and ought to be useful for using the spike trains to distinguish the stimuli.

$H(r)$, and the entropy of the response when a stimulus is presented, $H(r|s)$; $H(s, r) = H(s) - H(r|s)$. The entropy is

$$\sum_s p(s)\log(p(s))$$

and the entropy of the stimulus given the response is

$$\sum_s p(s,r)\log(p(s|r))$$

The r and s can be interchanged because mutual information is symmetrical with regard to the sender and receiver of a message, even if the physical channel might not actually be symmetrical (or bidirectional). Information has the strength that the representation of the stimulus and/or the response can be multivariate. With this approach it is possible to compare transmitted or mutual information from different codes. This, then, provides measurements to assess whether one assumed code carries more information than another assumed code.

The responses in **Figure 4** are decomposed using their first few principal components; in **Figure 5**, it can be seen that the value of the first principal component is similar for the two responses, as the spike counts are. The coefficients of the second principal components, however, here have opposite signs. This is because the second principal component has a shape that readily represents the dip (**Figure 4**, left) or lack of it (**Figure 4**, right) seen in these two responses. The weights then become the code elements. The information from one, two, or more principal components can be used as candidate neural codes. Using more than the first two principal components adds little, if any, additional information in this example. For the cases where the principal

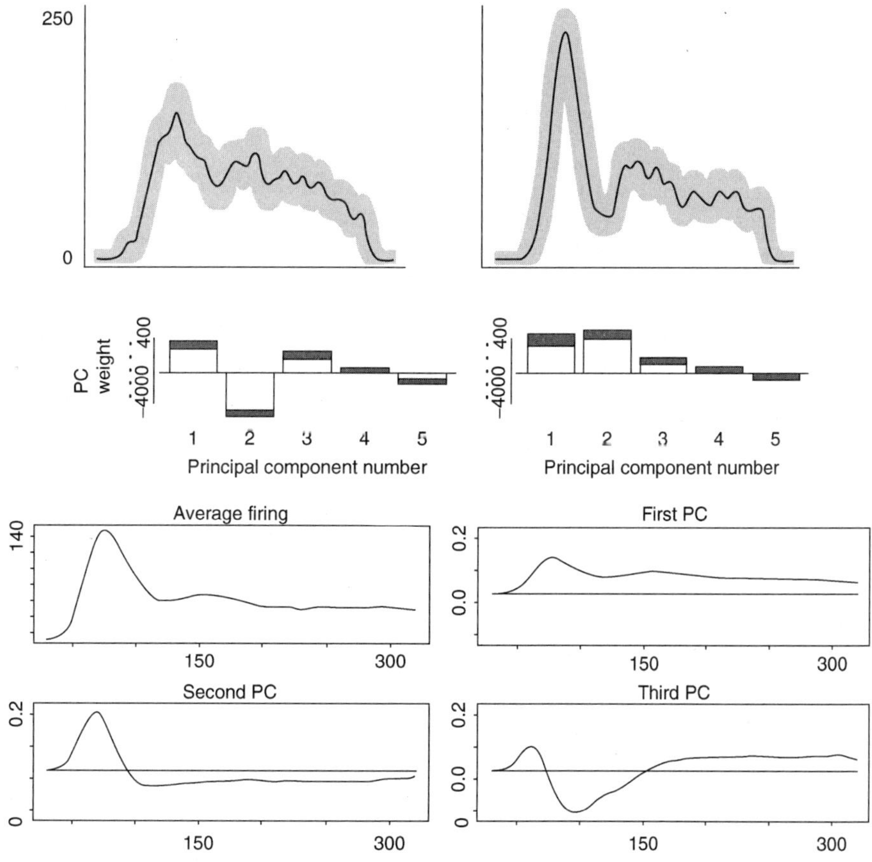

Figure 5 Principal decomposition of the two responses shown in **Figure 3**. The principal components were derived from the covariance matrix calculated from all of the responses to all of the patterns. The average spike densities are shown at the top. The middle panels show the weightings of the first five principal components (PC). The bottom panels show the shapes of the principal components (the eigenvectors of the covariance matrix), as modulations over time. The time-dependent mean (shown as the first waveform, labeled 'Average firing') was subtracted from each response before the covariance matrix was built. The second principal component (labeled 'Second PC') has a shape that, when added to the average, will accentuate the peak or blunt it (by subtracting or inverting this waveform).

components have been used to distinguish responses, the number of them that carry independent information over the preceding ones has been small, between 2 and 5.

In general, slow changes in the neuronal firing are represented by the lower numbered principal components, and as the principal component number goes up, the precision of the timing patterns increases. The need for this small number of principal components suggests that the spikes do not generally need to be represented very exactly in time – that is, blurring them out in time does not hurt the potential decodability of the responses. In the visual system, several experiments have shown that the precision of the spike timing is on the order of 10–20 ms, or longer in these experiments using stimuli that appear and remain on. In contrast to these measurements, if the stimulus is rapidly changing (i.e., if we repeatedly hit the system hard), the responses have spikes tightly time-locked to some temporal feature of the stimulus time series.

The need for more than one principal component suggests that more than one feature of the stimulus (or experimental condition) is encoded (i.e., information is multiplexed). One question is whether different parts of the neuronal responses can be identified with different stimulus characteristics. There are two types of response structures in primary visual cortex that have been given such identifications. These structures are single versus doublet spikes (i.e., whether spikes tend to be grouped into pairs or whether they occur singly). It has been shown that, for complex cells, the amount of clustering is related (tuned) for spatial frequency, and the single spikes are tuned for contrast. It has also been shown for complex cells that the response strength is closely tuned for orientation across a wide range of contrasts, whereas the latency changes substantially with contrast and response strength changes substantially less.

An alternative explanation for the variability is that it arises from encoding sources within the nervous system that do not covary with the stimulus (e.g., arousal or focal attention). These factors might then give rise to unaccounted for variability that is not true noise. At a minimum, the variability will have to be described and its influence on the organization of neuronal responses must be taken in account. The variability is seen both in the number and timing of spikes. Although it was for a long time not completely appreciated, it is now clear that the variability in the number of spikes influences our estimates of relating the number of spikes to their timing.

It is known that the variance becomes greater as the spike count increases. If we plot the coefficients of the variance of the second principal component against its mean for each stimulus, there is only a weak linear relation. The variance of the second principal component, however, is related to the spike count. This can be understood in stochastic terms. Consider stochastic sampling of a uniform point process. If the spikes are placed stochastically, the number of combinations of spikes that arise by chance is

$$\frac{n!}{k!(n-k)!}$$

or, n choose k, where n is the number of bins for the time period (usually taken to be 1 ms) and k is the number of spikes to be placed in the bins. If the number of spikes changes, the number of patterns that occur by chance necessarily also changes; n, the number of bins, is constant, and, k, the number of spikes, changes stochastically across stimulus presentations. For example, 200 choose 2 yields 19 900 combinations of spikes by chance, and 200 choose 3 yields 1 313 400 combinations. Since a small change in spike count can dramatically change the number of spike patterns expected by chance, any effort to describe what happens must first and carefully account for the variability in spike count. This then leads to a line of work to evaluate the impact of this necessary relation between spike count and numbers of spike patterns.

Finally, there is one more indication of this relation between the number of spikes and the number of spike patterns. If the coefficients of the first and second principal components from one neuron are placed on a scatter plot, they fill a cone, with the apex at the lowest spike count. This shows that the number of response types grows with the spike count (and would continue to grow until half the bins could be filled). Thus, when there are only a few spikes, there are only a relatively few spike patterns available for coding.

For a random process, even if not strictly Poisson, the null hypothesis that the spikes are randomly placed so that the overall rate is duplicated can be constructed using order statistics. Order statistics give the unconditional probability distributions for the kth event out of n events. For example, we can calculate the probability distribution for the third event or spike out 10. Order statistics explicitly needs the counts, the density of events (peristimulus time histogram, or PSTH), and the cumulative distribution, all of which we can estimate from data. However, we do not just want this unconditional distribution. Rather if the conditional distribution is available, a decoder or an accurate simulator can be constructed.

The basic equation of order statistics is as follows:

$$h(t) = \binom{n}{k} kF^{k-1}(t)f(t)[1 - F^{n-k}(t)]$$

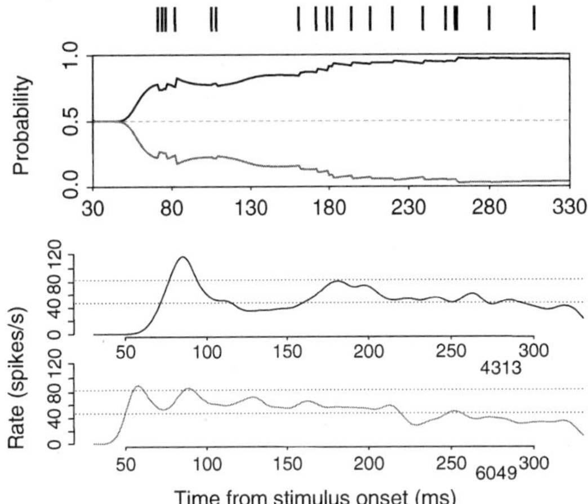

Figure 6 Decoding the spike train at the top for the two responses shown in **Figure 4**. The spike densities are shown again at the bottom in red and black. The *x*-axis on all three panels is time (in milliseconds) after stimulus appearance. The vertical axis on the top panel is the probability of guessing stimulus 1 (black) or stimulus 2 (red). For this spike train, shown by the black vertical tick marks above the top panel, the guessing probability rises quickly (and is correct). Note that the confidence of the guess can decrease at times. It turns out that the latency difference is a key feature for correct decoding in this example. Having a delay in the appearance of the first spike makes the likelihood of stimulus 1 very high.

where $h_1(t)$ is the probability of the spike k at time t; n choose k times k is a normalizing factor, and $F(t)$ is the cumulative distribution from $f(t)$, the rate function over time (estimated as the spike density or peristimulus time histogram). By working recursively, the conditional estimate, based on the time or spikes that have already gone by, can be constructed. This is simplified to be the probability of the first spike over time, $h_1(t)$.

With this recursive relation each successive spike can be considered the next first spike. Next, to construct the probability of the stimulus, regardless of the spike count, the order statistics are weighted by the probability of that spike count occurring, and these are summed. Then the probability of a stimulus s, at time t, through Bayes' theorem, can be estimated, and from this, the probability of the stimulus $p(s, t)$, at time t, can be calculated. Using these new probabilities as the new $p(s|t)$ for $p(s)$, decoding the spike train can be carried out spike by spike. Stepping through the spike train, $p(s)$ is updated. Using a maximum-likelihood rule, for example, a guess is made as to what stimulus is eliciting the spike train (**Figure 6**).

Population Coding

It is certain that activity must be coordinated among large ensembles of neurons, but it is not yet known how information is handled in ensembles. The simplest hypothesis is that the responses of neurons are summed or averaged, with the weight being the experimental condition that is weighted by the tuning in the tuning curve. This vector coding approach is the most influential model of population coding. It is relatively easy to compute. The experimenter can even measure the activity of neurons at different times. It is also straightforward to calculate how many neurons with independent noise are needed to decode from the responses in any condition. This approach is very important, also, for understanding the assumptions underlying mass population measurement approaches such as functional imaging (which actually measures blood flow changes in most cases) and field potentials. These are popular surrogates for having measurements of neural activity, spike trains, membrane potentials, and/or synaptic activity. These approaches assume that the average (presumably some sort of vector average, as in the vector coding approach) reveals functional properties.

The vector averaging code is powerful and is very convenient for computing the results from measuring the tuning curves of lots of neurons. However, it seems likely that the patterns of activity that occur simultaneously, or at least in a coordinated manner, might play an important role. The issue is whether spikes arriving from different inputs to a target neuron have different effects on the target, depending on their relative arrival times. The biophysics of neurons suggests that this should be the case. Before going forward, it is important to point out that the precision with which the coordinated activity must occur is not settled, so there are many investigators trying to make the needed measurements.

Another consideration is whether it matters which neuron carries the spikes. Can the spikes from different neurons be mixed without any loss of information? In the measurements made to this time, the information is greater when the spikes from two neurons are kept separate – that is, it helps to know which neuron carried the spike. This measurement has only been made a couple of times, and must be repeated because it suggests that population measures that only make use of the ensemble average activity will underestimate the information-carrying capacity of the tissue being considered.

A great deal of work has been carried out to look at coordination or synchronization of spikes. The question remains about how precisely the spikes must be represented to account for the information they carry. It is especially important but difficult to determine whether there is information that depends on codes across neuron (e.g., imagine a code based on the difference between the responses of two or more neurons). An intriguing hypothesis about cortical processing is that there are patterns of spikes hidden within the apparently noisy responses of the aforementioned sort. This hypothesis, the synfire chain hypothesis, arises from strong theoretical considerations, in turn arising from straightforward, elegant considerations about cortical connectivity and neuronal biophysical properties. There is some evidence supporting this type of coding, but the number of these hidden patterns is small even in the best examples, so, although this is an elegant idea, the support is not yet very strong.

Another intriguing code that has been suggested is the order of neuronal recruitment. This code gets theoretical consideration, and there is a small amount of evidence that it could be used, at least in the peripheral somatosensory system. It is elegant and simple, but in the face of neurons with ongoing background activity it might be difficult to implement in practice, but it is mentioned here because it emphasizes that latency to onset of firing might (almost certainly does) play an important role in coordination of responses across neurons.

Finally, it seems plausible, and some would say even likely, that there might be dynamically changing neuronal ensembles, especially during learning, and under those circumstances there might be patterns of spikes within and across neurons that are strongly related to cognitive events. A lot of new work is being carried out to collect data from several neurons, even tens of neurons. The evidence about how signals are combined is not at all conclusive. With the advent of new tools from molecular genetics, it is becoming possible to visualize individual members of simple ensembles and make optical recordings of them. Now will come the exciting work of learning how the neural codes from different members of an ensemble are related.

See also: Decoding Neuron Transcriptome by SAGE; Natural Images: Coding Efficiency; Neural Synchrony and Feature Binding; Neural Coding of Spatial Representations; Neural Coding in Primary Motor Cortex; Neural Oscillators and Dynamical Systems Models; Olfactory Coding; Perception of Surfaces and Forms; Perceptual Learning: Neural Mechanisms; Perceptual Learning and Sensory Plasticity; Prefrontal Contributions to Reward Encoding; Spiking Neuron Models; Vision: Mechanisms of Orientation, Direction and Depth; Visual Cortex: Mapping of Functional Architecture Using Optical Imaging; Visual Attention; Visual Motion Models.

Further Reading

Abeles M (1991) *Corticonics.* Cambridge, UK: Cambridge University Press.

Optican LM and Richmond BJ (1987) Temporal encoding of two-dimensional patterns by single units in primate inferior temporal cortex. III. Information theoretic analysis. *Journal of Neurophysiology* 57: 162–178.

Reich DS, Mechler F, and Victor JD (2001) Independent and redundant information in nearby cortical neurons. *Science* 294: 2566–2568.

Reich DS, Victor JD, Knight BW, et al. (1997) Response variability and timing precision of neuronal spike trains *in vivo*. *Journal of Neurophysiology* 77: 2836–2841.

Richmond BJ, Optican LM, Podell M, et al. (1987) Temporal encoding of two-dimensional patterns by single units in primate inferior temporal cortex. I. Response characteristics. *Journal of Neurophysiology* 57: 132–146.

Rieke F, Warland D, de RuytervanSteveninck R, et al. (1996) *Spikes: Exploring the Neural Code.* Cambridge, MA: MIT Press.

Victor JD (2005) Spike train metrics. *Current Opinion in Neurobiology* 15: 585–592.

Wiener MC and Richmond BJ (2003) Decoding spike trains instant by instant using order statistics and the mixture-of-Poissons model. *Journal of Neuroscience* 23: 2394–2406.

Neural Oscillators and Dynamical Systems Models

G B Ermentrout, University of Pittsburgh, Pittsburgh, PA, USA

Introduction

Suppose that a synaptically isolated neuron is injected with a constant current. As the amount of current increases, the neuron might begin to fire action potentials. Or perhaps it will fire a burst of action potentials and then stop firing. Or, if it was already firing, maybe the spikes will stop. On the other hand, consider what happens as a walking horse speeds up: he switches first to a trot and then to a gallop. In both of these cases, some qualitative change in behavior has occurred as some parameter (current in the first case, frequency in the second) changes. How can we put these wildly different phenomena at wildly different spatial and temporal scales on a common footing? Nonlinear dynamics or dynamical systems theory is an area of mathematics which attempts to classify the qualitative differences between systems as their initial states or their parameters change.

Most modeling of neurons, circuits, and systems depends on the simulation of large systems of coupled differential equations: rates of change for voltages, synaptic strengths, etc., are given in terms of the variables themselves. Thus, in this article, we focus on how nonlinear dynamics can help us understand the behavior of the kinds of differential equations that occur in computational neuroscience.

To gain an intuitive feel for the concepts that are introduced in this article, it helps to think of some simple physical systems. A familiar example is a damped pendulum, that is, a solid rod with a weight at the end and with friction. If you move the pendulum, it will rock back and forth several times, eventually returning to the downward position. This position is called an attractor, since perturbations of the pendulum end up back in the downward state. Let us consider a more complicated example. Place a flexible plastic ruler narrow edge down, and place your finger along the top edge. As long as you do not apply too much pressure, the ruler will remain completely straight. If you transiently bend the ruler from the side, keeping the same pressure on it, it will return to a the straight position. Now, apply more pressure on the top of the ruler. Once the pressure becomes too great, the ruler will buckle (bend) to one side or the other. The physical system has gone to a new attractor as the parameter (the applied pressure) changes. The plastic ruler and the pendulum are governed by sets of nonlinear equations, and the goal of dynamical systems theory is to understand their behavior both qualitatively and quantitatively.

Equilibria

We start with a very simple example, a model for a passive membrane:

$$\frac{\mathrm{d}V}{\mathrm{d}t} = (-g_L(V - E_L) + I)/C \qquad [1]$$

Here, $1/g_L$ is the input resistance, E_L is the resting potential, I is the applied current, and C is the capacitance. We divided by the capacitance because it is traditional to put just the derivatives of variables on the left-hand side of the equation. This is a linear differential equation, and we can find a closed form solution, or, even easier, we could pop this onto a computer and solve it. However, to do this, we need one more piece of information: the voltage at a particular point in time, for example, $t = 0$. Thus, we specify $V(0) = V_0$, which is called the initial condition. Rather than solve the equation exactly, we will, instead, introduce the concept of state space and use this to deduce what solutions look like.

In **Figure 1** is a graph showing $\mathrm{d}V/\mathrm{d}t$ on the y-axis and V on the x-axis. The x-axis represents all possible voltages and is called the state space for this system. The y-axis tells us how fast and, more importantly, which direction the voltage goes – to the left means it is decreasing and to the right, increasing. For example, if the initial voltage is to the left of the solid black circle, then $\mathrm{d}V/\mathrm{d}t > 0$ and the voltage increases. Note that as it approaches the filled circle, its rate, $\mathrm{d}V/\mathrm{d}t$, gets smaller so that it decelerates as it gets closer to the filled circle. Initial conditions to the right will decrease until the filled circle is reached. An initial condition starting exactly on the filled circle will stay there forever. For this reason, we call this particular voltage an equilibrium point for eqn [1]. Other terms which are commonly used are steady state and fixed point. Note that all initial conditions move to this unique equilibrium. Thus, we say that it is globally asymptotically stable or that it is a global attractor. No matter what the current injected, there will always be one and only one equilibrium point and it is always stable. In fact, we can write it down explicitly:

$$V_{\mathrm{eq}} = \frac{I + g_L E_L}{g_L}$$

Thus, for this simple linear model, if we call $V(t) = \phi(t;\, V_0)$ the solution to eqn [1] given the initial condition, $V(0) = V_0$, we see that $V(t) \to V_{\mathrm{eq}}$ as $t \to \infty$

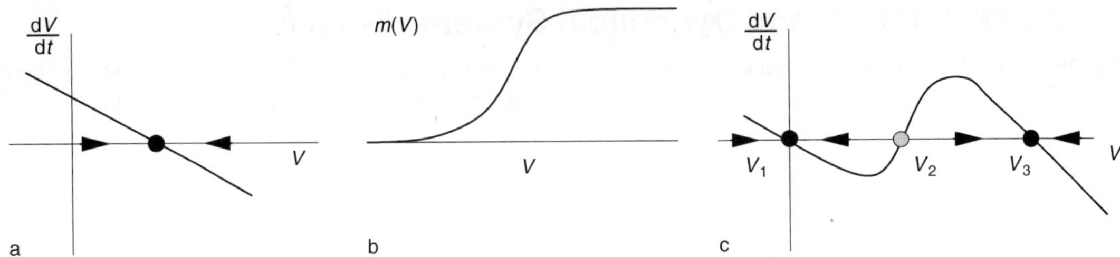

Figure 1 One-dimensional dynamical system showing stable (black) and unstable (gray) equilibria.

for any initial condition. (Note that the function ϕ is introduced to make explicit that the solution depends on the initial value.)

This graphical method may at first seem to be of little use since we can write an explicit solution to the differential equation. However, suppose that in addition to a leak conductance, our membrane has an instantaneous inward current:

$$\frac{dV}{dt} = (-g_L(V - E_L) - g_{Na}m(V)(V - E_{Na}) + I)/C \equiv f(V, I) \qquad [2]$$

where

$$m(V) = 1/(1 + \exp[-(V - V_1)/V_2])$$

(see **Figure 1(b)**). If the inward conductance is large enough, then dV/dt has the form shown in **Figure 1(c)**. It is no longer possible to write down a solution to the differential equation! However, we can use the graphical method to completely understand it. Unlike the left-hand figure, there are now three equilibria. Looking at the arrows on the x-axis, it is clear that initial conditions starting near V_1, V_3 will be driven to respectively, V_1, V_3 while initial conditions near V_2 will be pushed away from V_2. Thus, there are two asymptotically stable equilibria and there is one unstable equilibrium point. Physically, we would never be able to reach the unstable equilibrium, but we would be able to sense it in an experiment. For any initial condition $V(0) > V_2$ will tend to V_3 as time increases, and any initial condition $V(0) < V_2$ will go to V_1. Thus, eqn [2] is bistable; it has two asymptotically stable states and V_2 serves as a separatrix or threshold between the two stable equilibria. Suppose the neuron is resting at V_1 and a brief current stimulus is applied. If the stimulus is small, $V(t)$ will not cross V_2 and will relax back to V_1. If the stimulus is large enough to cause $V(t)$ to cross V_2, then the neuron will tend to the depolarized state, $V = V_3$. All we need now is some sort of delayed outward current and we will have an action potential. Nonlinear dynamics provides a geometric description for the threshold for an active neuron.

More generally, consider a set of n differential equations in n variables:

$$\frac{dx_j}{dt} = f_j(x_1, \ldots, x_n) \quad j = 1, \ldots, n \qquad [3]$$

with initial conditions $x_j(0) = x_{j,0}$. Under fairly general conditions on the functions f_j there is a solution to this which we write in vector form as $X(t) = \Phi(t; X_0)$. In this case the state space is R^n, the set of all n-dimensional vectors, and eqn [3] defines an n-dimensional dynamical system which we can write concisely as

$$\frac{dX}{dt} = F(X) \qquad [4]$$

We call X_{eq} and equilibrium solution to eqn [4] if $F(X_{eq}) = 0$. In our simple example, above, $n = 1$. The familiar space-clamped Hodgkin–Huxley equation consists of four variables, V, m, h, n, and forms a four-dimensional dynamical system. In absence of an applied current, the nerve membrane sits at rest, which is an equilibrium point. We say that an equilibrium point, X_{eq}, is asymptotically stable if all the solutions to eqn [4] with initial conditions that are close to the equilibrium point decay back to the equilibrium point as t increases. The nice geometric picture in **Figure 1(c)** does not help us for higher dimensional systems.

Suppose that A is an $n \times n$-dimensional matrix and that $F(X) = AX$. Then we call this a linear dynamical system. The study of linear dynamical systems is insightful, for, except in special cases (see below), the behavior of any nonlinear system in eqn [4] near an equilibrium point is the same as that of an associated linear system. Consider the following linear dynamical system:

$$\frac{dX}{dt} = AX \qquad [5]$$

Clearly $X = 0$ is an equilibrium point. The general solution to a linear differential equation is a sum of terms of the form:

$$Y(t) = Ve^{at}t^m(\cos bt - c) \qquad [6]$$

where m is a nonnegative integer, a, b, c are real numbers, and V is a constant vector. If $a < 0$, then

$Y(t)$ decays to zero as $t \to \infty$; if $a > 0$, then $Y(t)$ grows exponentially; and if $a = 0$, then the $Y(t)$ grows when $m > 0$ and oscillates when $m = 0$ and $b > 0$. The numbers $\lambda = a \pm ib$ are the eigenvalues of the matrix, A, that is, there is a constant vector, V, such that

$$AV = \lambda V$$

For an $n \times n$ matrix, there are n eigenvalues, roots of the nth order characteristic polynomial

$$pA(\lambda) \equiv \det(\lambda I - A)$$

Combining this fact with eqn [6], we see that all solutions to eqn [5] will decay to the equilibrium point at 0 if $a < 0$ for every eigenvalue of A and that if 'any' $a > 0$, then at least some solutions to eqn [5] will exponentially grow. In the former case, when all the a's are negative, we say that system in eqn [5] is linearly asymptotically stable, and in the latter case when at least one $a > 0$, the system is unstable. The special case $a = 0$ will play an important role later in this article.

Let X_{eq} be an equilibrium solution of eqn [3] or equivalently eqn [4]. Form the following $n \times n$ matrix:

$$B = \begin{pmatrix} \frac{\partial f_1(x_1,\ldots,x_n)}{\partial x_1} & \cdots & \frac{\partial f_1(x_1,\ldots,x_n)}{\partial x_n} \\ \vdots & \ddots & \vdots \\ \frac{\partial f_n(x_1,\ldots,x_n)}{\partial x_1} & \cdots & \frac{\partial f_n(x_1,\ldots,x_n)}{\partial x_n} \end{pmatrix} \qquad [7]$$

and evaluate it at the equilibrium point, X_{eq}. This matrix is called the Jacobi matrix for eqn [4] about the equilibrium point (also often called the Jacobian), and the system $Y' = BY$ is called the 'linearization.' One of the most important results in dynamical systems states that if the linear system defined by the matrix $B(X_{eq})$ is linearly asymptotically stable (all eigenvalues have negative real parts), then the equilibrium point X_{eq} is asymptotically stable as a solution to eqn [4]. This theorem provides a simple way to test the stability of any equilibrium point: form the matrix B and look at its eigenvalues. If all have negative real parts, then the equilibrium is stable; if any have positive real parts, then it is unstable.

Returning to **Figure 1**, the Jacobian is just the slope of dV/dt at the equilibrium point. Thus, if dV/dt has a positive slope through the equilibrium, it is unstable, and if it has a negative slope, the equilibrium is stable. Let us continue to analyze eqn [2] and **Figure 1(c)**, but now we will change the applied current, I. Changing the current just lifts the curve in **Figure 1(c)** up or down. This is shown in **Figure 2** on the left. For large positive or negative currents, there is only one equilibrium point. However, if we start at $I = 0$ where there are three equilibria and hyperpolarize the membrane (decrease I), then the right-most pair of equilibria will move closer to each other (compare blue with black line). As we continue to decrease the current, there is a current value, $I = I_*$, in which both equilibria come together (cyan curve, green circle), and for $I < I_*$, they no longer exist. Unlike the situation when $I = 0$, when $I < I_*$, there is only one equilibrium point (magenta curve, magenta circle). This is qualitatively different from three equilibria. A similar phenomenon occurs when we raise the current; the left-most equilibria merge when $I = I^*$ (red curve, gold circle). In dynamical systems, any time that a qualitative change in behavior occurs as a parameter varies, we say that a bifurcation has occurred. Specifically, when two equilibria merge and disappear, we say that there is a saddle-node bifurcation. This is often called a limit point or turning point bifurcation. Clearly the left-hand picture is useful for a one-dimensional equation, but obviously, if the function $f(V,I)$ is more complicated, we will run out of space and have to draw many different curves for many different values of I. A concise summary of the behavior of this nonlinear system as a parameter varies is shown in the right side of **Figure 2**. A plot is made of the equilibrium values of one of the variables on the y-axis, and the parameter is shown on the x-axis. This curve is called a bifurcation diagram. Traditionally, stable equilibria and unstable equilibria are distinguished by changing the color or line type of the curve. In our figure, stable equilibria are solid and unstable are dashed. The diagram should be read as follows. Pick a value of I and mentally draw a vertical

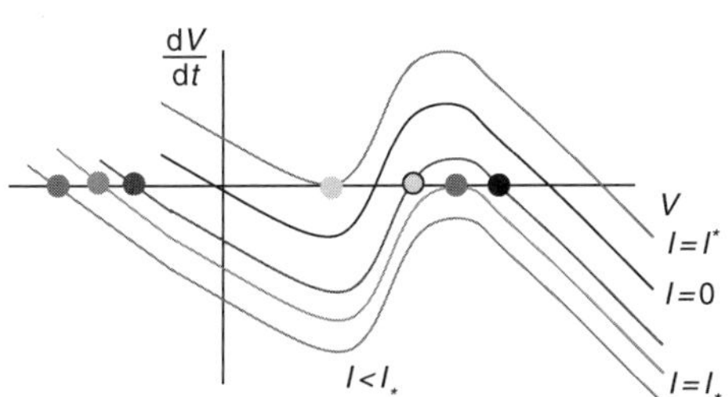

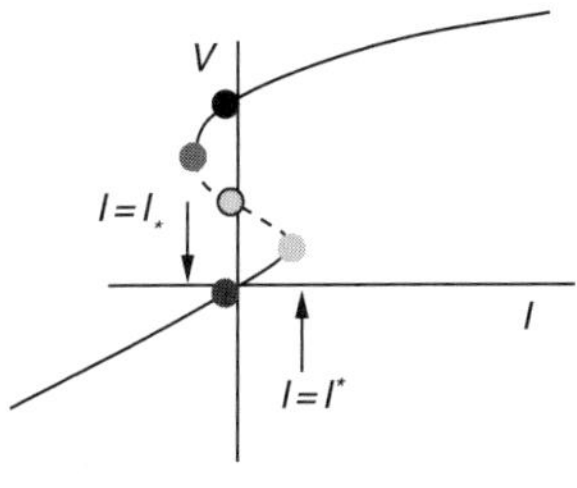

Figure 2 Behavior of nonlinear membrane as the current changes. (Left) Phase space picture. (Right) Bifurcation diagram. Special points are colored green and gold.

line through this value of I. Intersections with the bifurcation diagram correspond to equilibria. Saddle nodes are points where the diagram turns around (hence the name turning point); here, they are at I_* and I^*. **Figure 2**, right, shows that there will be bistability for all currents between I_* and I^*. Suppose that we do the following experiment. Starting at $I = 0$, we gradually increase the current. As soon as it exceeds I^*, the voltage will jump up to the top part of the diagram. Now, we reduce the current. The voltage stays at the upper part of the diagram until the current falls below I_*. Thus, it jumps down at a different current than it jumped up. This phenomenon is called hysteresis, and our neuron has now been endowed with 'memory.' Once in the 'up' state, it will remain there even when the current is brought to zero. Bistability between states (here, equilibria) plays a central role in almost every aspect of the dynamics of single cells and networks of coupled cells.

Before turning to more complex dynamical systems, we close this discussion with an important point. Looking again to **Figure 2**, left, observe that when $I = 0$, the slope through the gray circle is positive while that through the black circle is negative. The linearized system for our model is

$$y' = f'(\bar{V})y$$

where $\bar{V}$ is an equilibrium. If the slope (f') is negative, the equilibrium is stable, and if it is positive it is unstable. At $I = I_*$, the slope at the equilibrium is zero and the linearized system is

$$y' = 0$$

which tells us nothing about stability of the nonlinear system. However, whenever a linearized system has a zero eigenvalue, this is the signature for a possible bifurcation for the nonlinear system. This is true no matter what the dimension of the system.

The methods for finding equilibria and their stability, as well as looking for bifurcations, are not confined to one-dimensional models. Nor are they restricted to single neuron models. As an example of a bifurcation with symmetry, let us consider a mutually inhibitory neural network (**Figure 3**, left):

$$\frac{du_1}{dt} = -u_1 + F(I - gu_2)$$
$$\frac{du_2}{dt} = -u_2 + F(I - gu_1)$$

u_1, u_2 represent the firing rates of two different populations of neurons which are receiving equal inputs, I. The strength of the inhibition is g, and the function $F(u)$ increases with increasing values of u. The reader can imagine this as representing two objects competing for the attention of the network. Since the two populations are identical, there is a symmetric equilibrium point in which $u_1 = u_2 = \bar{u}$. The stability is determined by looking at the linearized system:

$$\frac{dy_1}{dt} = -y_1 - \alpha g y_2$$
$$\frac{dy_2}{dt} = -y_2 - \alpha g y_1$$

where $\alpha = F'(I - g\bar{u})$. Notice that $\alpha > 0$. The Jacobian matrix for this linear system is

$$A = \begin{pmatrix} -1 & -\alpha g \\ -\alpha g & -1 \end{pmatrix}$$

Two-variable systems (also called planar systems) are easy to analyze for stability. Let T be the sum of the diagonal entries of A (called the trace of a matrix) and let Δ be the determinant of the matrix. Then the linear system (and therefore the nonlinear system) will be stable provided that $T < 0$ and $\Delta > 0$. For this example, $T = -2 < 0$ and $\Delta = 1 - g^2\alpha^2$. If the mutual inhibition g is small, or the inputs are small (so that α is

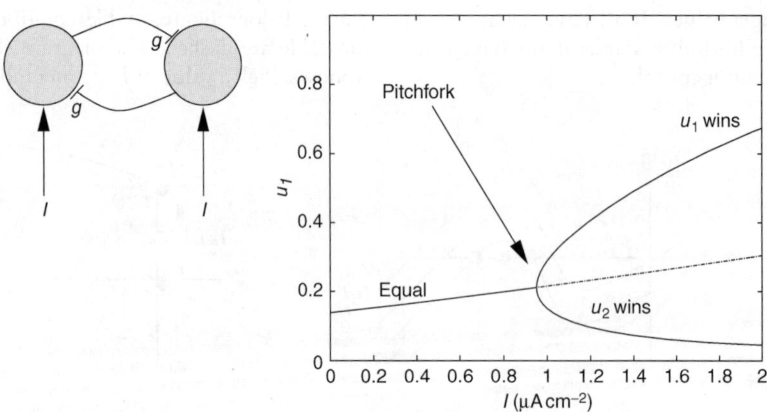

Figure 3 Mutually inhibitory network. (Right) Bifurcation diagram as the input, I, increases.

small), then $\Delta > 0$. If the inputs increase, then Δ could become negative. The equilibrium point is no longer stable. In fact, when the determinant is negative for a planar system, it means that there is one positive eigenvalue and one negative eigenvalue and the equilibrium is called a saddle point. Because of the symmetry of our example, the eigenvalues and corresponding eigenvectors of A are easy to write down:

$$\{\lambda_1 = -1 - g\alpha, \mathbf{v}_1 = [1, 1]^T\}$$

$$\{\lambda_2 = -1 + g\alpha, \mathbf{v}_2 = [1, -1]^T\}$$

λ_1 is always negative, but λ_2 becomes positive when αg exceeds 1. This means that there will be growth along the vector $\mathbf{v}_2$ and decay along the vector $\mathbf{v}_1$. For this reason, $\mathbf{v}_1$ is called the stable set or the stable manifold for the saddle point and $\mathbf{v}_2$ is called the unstable set or unstable manifold. Amazingly, if the linearized system has a saddle point and stable and unstable sets, then the nonlinear system does as well. However, they will not be straight lines.

When the input reaches a critical value so that $\alpha g = 1$, then the determinant is zero and we see that $\lambda_2 = 0$. From the previous discussion, this means that we can expect a bifurcation. **Figure 3** shows the bifurcation diagram for this system. This is very different from the diagram shown in **Figure 2**. Rather than losing solutions as the parameter changes, a solution becomes unstable and two new 'stable' solutions appear. Because of its shape, this is known as a pitchfork bifurcation. It occurs only in systems which have some kind of intrinsic symmetry, but, as this is very common in many physical and biological problems, the pitchfork is a familiar bifurcation. The central line corresponds to the equilibrium point $u_1 = u_2$. As the input increases, when it reaches approximately 1, the symmetric equilibrium point becomes unstable – symmetry is broken. The new equilibria have the form $u_1 = a$, $u_2 = b$ and $u_1 = b$, $u_2 = a$ where $a > b$. A network like this is called winner-take-all since one of the two objects dominates the other. Notice that when $I = 2$, the value a is about ten times larger than the value b.

Planar systems have another advantage over high-dimensional models. Like the one-dimensional models in **Figure 1**, it is possible to sketch the complete behavior of the differential equation. Instead of plotting u_1 or u_2 versus time, plot one against the other. The resulting diagram is called a phase-plane. **Figure 4** shows the phase-plane for the network. Representative solutions (called trajectories; black) appear as curves moving toward the stable equilibrium points, which are filled circles. The advantage of the phase-plane is that it is possible to infer qualitative behavior without actually solving the equations. At each point in the (u_1, u_2) plane, the equations tell us the derivatives, du_1/dt and du_2/dt. These derivatives are tangent to the solutions, so that they show the direction of trajectories. Magenta arrows are drawn at various points in the plane to show the direction. These arrows are called direction fields. Often only a crude approximation of the direction fields is enough: just the eight points on a compass. For example, northeast corresponds to both u_1 and u_2 increasing in time. To determine where u_1 is increasing or decreasing, we only need to determine where u_1 is not changing at all. The graph $du_1/dt = 0$ is called the u_1-nullcline. For our network, $du_1/dt = 0$ when $u_1 = F(I - gu_2)$. This curve is plotted as in red in the phase-plane. The u_2-nullcline, $du_2/dt = 0$ is plotted in green. The nullclines break the phase-plane into regions where the direction fields are similar and their intersections are the equilibria. Thus, much can be gained without ever solving the differential equations. In the right phase-plane, there are two stable equilibrium points separated by an unstable

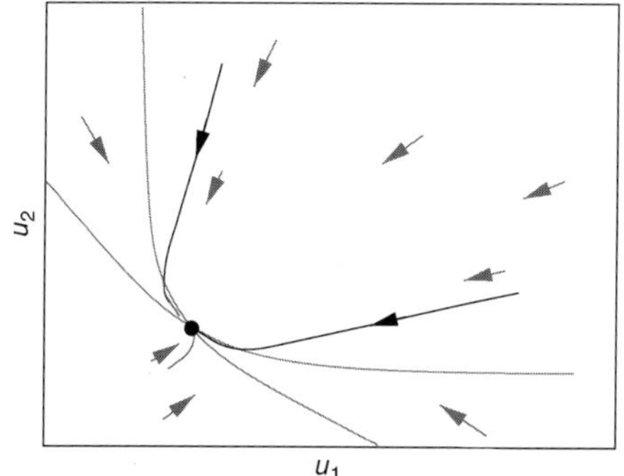

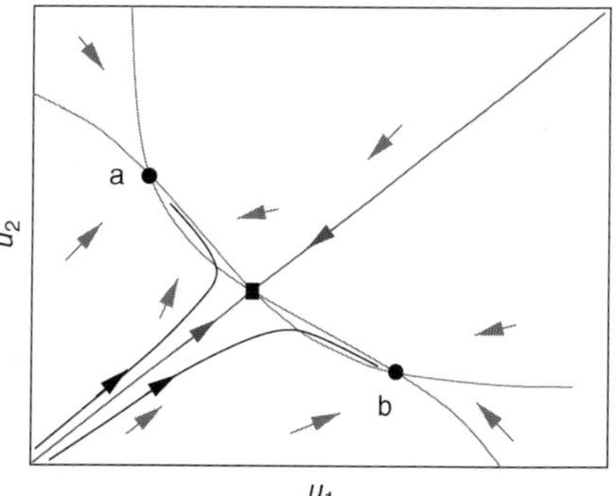

Figure 4 Phase-plane for mutual inhibitory network. Direction fields (magenta arrows) and trajectories (black) are shown. The u_1 nullcline is in red and the u_2 nullcline is in green. For stronger inputs, there are three equilibria. Two (black circles) are stable. Stable (blue) sets for the saddle point (black square) are shown.

saddle point. The stable set of the saddle point (drawn in blue) divides the plane in two. All initial values of (u_1, u_2) above the stable set will end up at the equilibrium point where u_2 wins and u_1 loses, labeled *a*. The opposite occurs when below the line. The upper triangular region of the plane is called the 'basin of attraction' for the equilibrium point *a*.

Limit Cycles

When a neuron is injected with current, it begins to fire repetitively. If the interspike interval is constant, then this pattern of firing is periodic and, in dynamical systems language, is called a limit cycle. A limit cycle is an isolated periodic solution to eqn [4]. All autonomous rhythmic phenomena seen in biology are limit cycles ranging in scales from the 24 h circadian oscillation in the suprachiasmatic nucleus to the 200 Hz ripple in hippocampus. There are several ways in which limit cycles can appear in nonlinear systems. To illustrate these, we will use the simple membrane model of Morris and Lecar:

$$C\frac{dV}{dt} = I - g_L(V - E_L) - g_k n(V - E_k) - gcam_\infty(V)(V - E_{Ca})$$

$$\frac{dn}{dt} = a_n(V)(1 - n) - b_n(V)n$$

Depending on the parameters of the model, as the current increases, rhythmic firing appears in three different ways: (1) Hopf, (2) SNIC, and (3) homoclinic. These three possibilities have been found in almost all published simulations, and there is strong evidence that they are also observed in real neurons.

The best-known mechanism by which a neuron begins to fire periodically is via the Hopf or Andronov bifurcation. Recall that an equilibrium point is stable as long as the real parts of the eigenvalues of the linearized system are all negative. There are two ways in which the real part can switch to positive: (1) a real negative eigenvalue becomes a positive eigenvalue through a zero eigenvalue and (2) the real part of a complex eigenvalue changes sign, leading to an imaginary eigenvalue, $\pm i w_0$. In the former case, saddle node and pitchfork bifurcations occur – the number of equilibria changes. In the latter, there is no change in the number of equilibria, but instead, limit cycles appear. **Figure 5** shows the bifurcation diagram for the Morris–Lecar model as the applied current increases. There is a single equilibrium point, and it changes from stable to unstable as the current increases past about 95. The magenta and green curves plotted in this figure correspond to limit cycles. They depict the maximum and minimum amplitude of the voltage. Like equilibria, the notion of stability can be defined for limit cycles. The magenta curves correspond to unstable and the green to stable limit cycles. The point HB denotes the point of the Hopf bifurcation. Models which undergo Hopf bifurcations have a limited frequency band and a nonzero minimum frequency (often close to w_0). For this model, the frequency ranges from 8 to 14 Hz. The small figures labeled a, b, and c are the phase-planes corresponding to points along the bifurcation diagram. At point (a) there is only a stable equilibrium and the neuron always returns to rest. In point (b), taken between the currents I_1 and I_2, there are two stable states: a stable

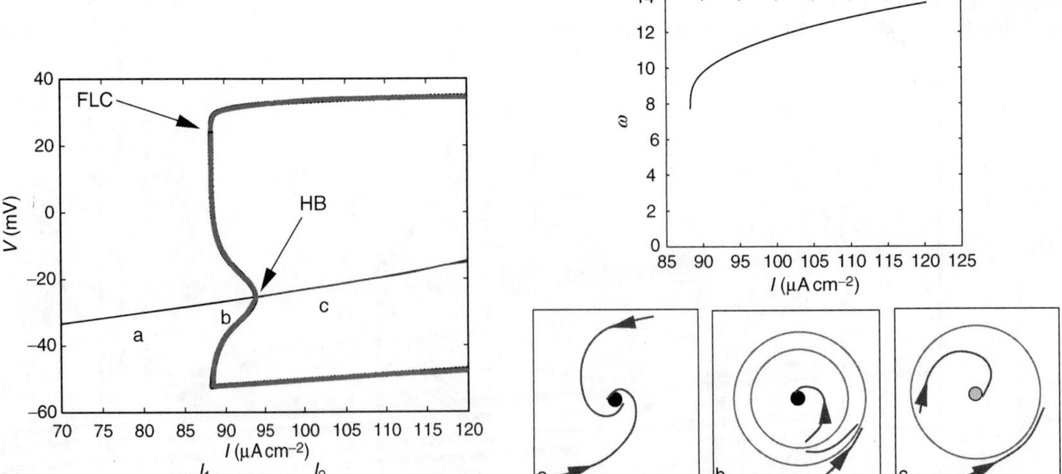

Figure 5 Hopf bifurcation formation of limit cycle. HB, Hopf bifurcation; FLC, fold of limit cycles.

equilibrium and a stable limit cycle. The unstable limit cycle (magenta) separates the plane into two regions. Everything outside of the unstable cycle ends up on the stable cycle and everything inside ends up at the equilibrium. The well-known Hodgkin–Huxley model behaves exactly like this. As the current approaches the value I_1 from the right, the magenta limit cycle and the green limit cycle collide and annihilate. This is called a fold of limit cycles (FLC) and is very much like the saddle-node bifurcation for equilibria: instead of losing two equilibria, two limit cycles are lost. In the transition from (b) to (c), the unstable magenta limit cycle shrinks to the equilibrium and renders it unstable, leaving only the stable limit cycle. There is compelling evidence that fast-spike interneurons in the cortex have this type of bifurcation.

A less well-known, but very important bifurcation to limit cycles is called the saddle-node invariant cycle (SNIC) bifurcation. Most computational models for cortical neurons make the transition from rest to repetitive firing via this bifurcation. An example is shown in **Figure 6**. Unlike the Hopf case, there is never bistability. Rather, there is a smooth transition from rest to rhythmicity. At the point of bifurcation, the frequency of the oscillation goes to zero. Note the huge dynamic range: 0–25 Hz for the simple model. For subthreshold currents, there are three equilibria; two are unstable and one, the rest state, is stable. Phase-plane (a) shows the big picture. The turquoise equilibrium serves as a threshold. If the potential crosses this, then a spike will be emitted before the cell returns to rest. As the current increases, the threshold and the rest state merge (phase-plane (b)) and at larger currents, these two equilibria disappear, leaving just the stable limit cycle and the unstable equilibrium. Comparing phase-plane (c) in the Hopf and SNIC shows that for large enough currents, they cannot be distinguished. However, most neurons (at least in cortex) operate near rest so that the bifurcation matters. We note that near the critical current, I^*, the frequency grows like:

$$\omega = K\sqrt{I - I^*}$$

A key difference between the SNIC and the Hopf is that the Hopf has a much more restricted frequency range and thus is very sensitive to the frequency of the inputs, while the SNIC has a very broad frequency range and no preferred input frequencies. These differences could have important computational consequences: SNIC neurons respond to the total number of inputs (integrators), while Hopf neurons are more sensitive to timing.

The third way in which a limit cycle can appear also involves an arbitrarily low frequency but with a different scaling from the SNIC. The bifurcation diagram is shown in **Figure 7**, and it is more complex than the other two. The frequency also has a large dynamic range, between 0 and 50 Hz. At point (a), there are three equilibria, one stable and two unstable. In phase-plane (a) the unstable set (gold) from the saddle point (turquoise) lies on the outside of the stable set (magenta). As the current approaches the value denoted (b) in the bifurcation diagram, the stable and unstable sets merge to form the red loop in phase-plane (b). This is called a 'homoclinic' solution. Just past the bifurcation point, the homoclinic becomes a stable limit cycle, at point (c) and depicted by the green cycle in phase-plane (c). Note that there is both a stable

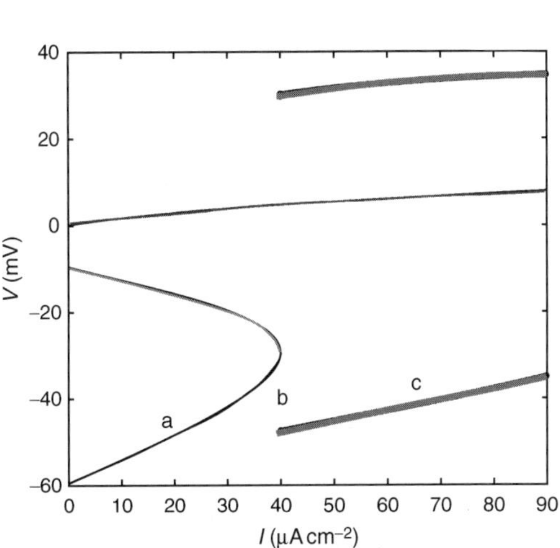

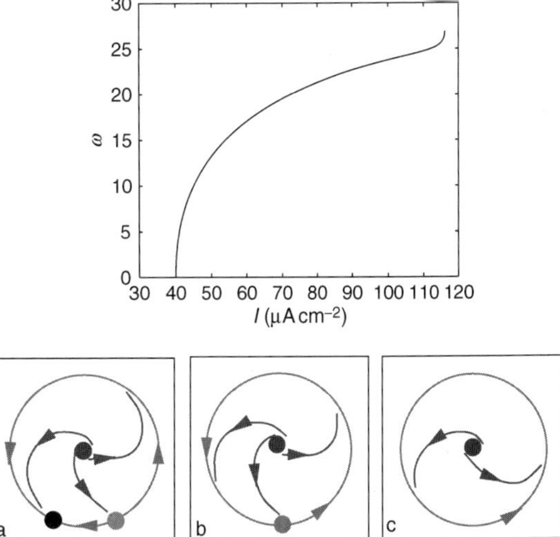

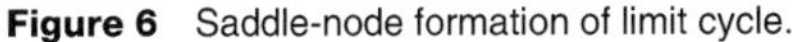

Figure 6 Saddle-node formation of limit cycle.

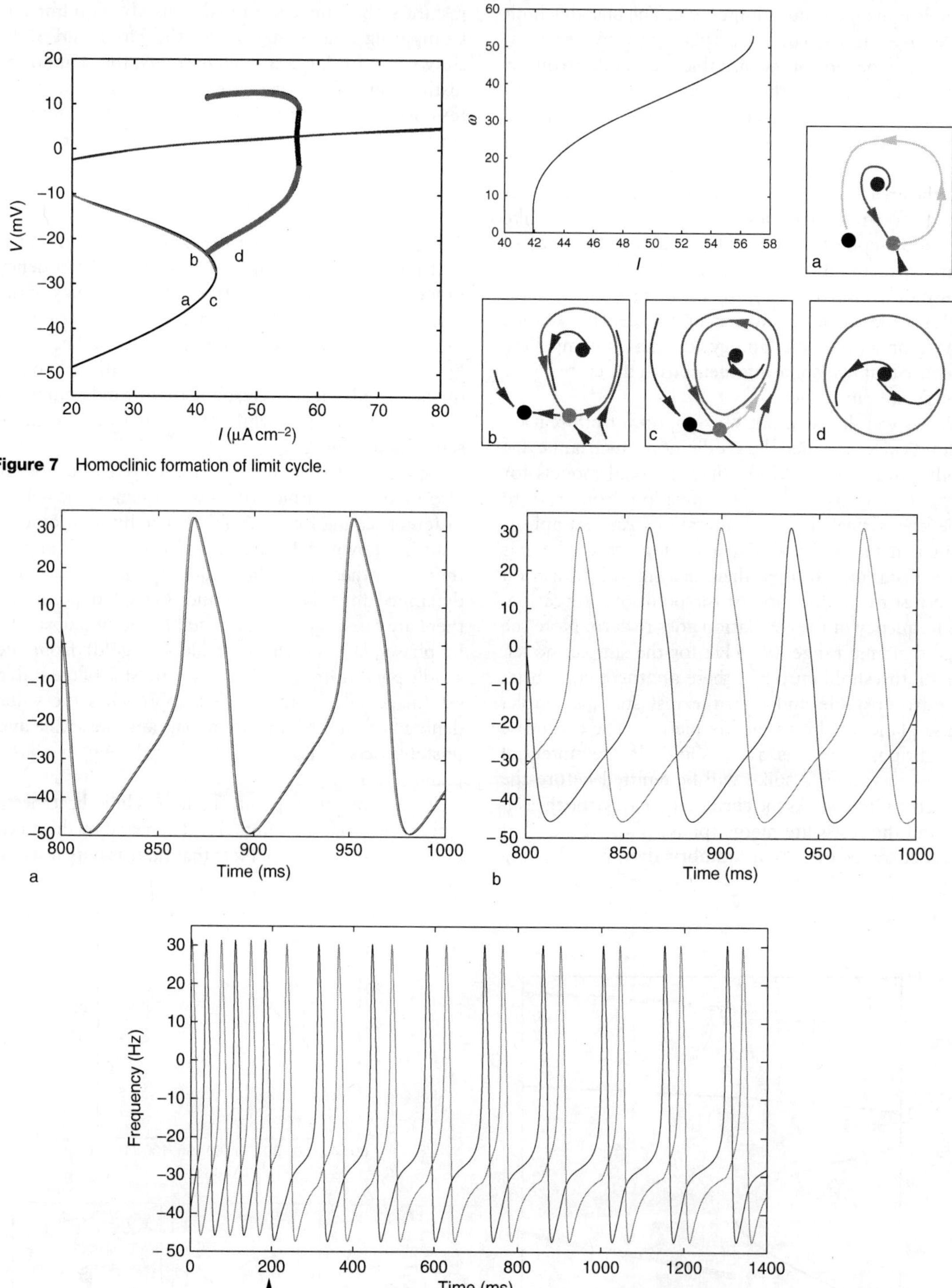

Figure 7 Homoclinic formation of limit cycle.

Figure 8 Bifurcation type determines synchronization properties. (a) Two Hopf neurons synchronize with excitatory coupling; (b) SNIC neurons fire in antiphase. (c) Frequency matters as well – if the frequency is halved, a pair of SNIC neurons switch from antiphase to a nonsymmetric rhythm.

limit cycle and a stable equilibrium (black circle). The stable set of the saddle point (magenta) separates the phase-plane into regions which tend to either the limit cycle or the equilibrium. Finally, as the current increases, the stable equilibrium and the saddle point merge (a saddle-node bifurcation), leaving only the limit cycle and the unstable equilibrium.

The reader may well wonder if these differences matter. Indeed, there seems to be little difference in the shapes of the spikes between the SNIC and the Hopf cases when the neuron is driven to fire at, say, 12 Hz. However, the mechanism by which a neuron makes the transition from rest to firing makes a large difference in how it responds to inputs. This fact is illustrated when two neurons are synaptically coupled into a network. Networks of coupled neural oscillators play a central role in many motor pattern circuits and may be important in sensory perception as well. **Figure 8** demonstrates that the type of bifurcation matters. In (a), the neurons use parameters like those in **Figure 5** and are driven to 12 Hz. Two identical cells are coupled via a synaptic current and, no matter what the initial state, will eventually synchronize. In (b), the parameters are as in **Figure 6**, driven also to 12 Hz. However, no matter what is the initial state, the two neurons will fire alternately in 'antiphase,' a half-cycle apart. Not only does the type of bifurcation matter, but also the frequency Panel (c) shows what happens to a pair as the frequency is halved from 12 to 6 Hz. Instead of firing in a perfect antiphase pattern, there is a switch so that the neurons fire with a short time between respective spikes followed by a long silent period. In the context of the questions posed at the beginning of this article, one can view the frequency-dependent switch shown in **Figure 8(c)** as analogous to a gait switch as an animal speeds up or slows down.

Summary

Nonlinear dynamics provides a means of characterizing the temporal behavior of neurons and networks of neurons. Transitions between different qualitative behaviors as parameters change occur in only a few different ways. Despite differences in timescales and dimensions of the problem, these bifurcations share common features which provide insight into how neurons react to stimuli and the number and variety of states that networks can achieve.

See also: Attractor Network Models; Hodgkin–Huxley Models; Spiking Neuron Models.

Further Reading

Guckenheimer J and Holmes P (1986) *Applied Mathematical Sciences, Vol. 42: Nonlinear Oscillations, Dynamical Systems, and Bifurcations of Vector Fields.* New York: Springer.

Izhikevich E (2006) *Dynamical Systems in Neuroscience: The Geometry of Excitability and Bursting (Computational Neuroscience).* Cambridge, MA: MIT Press.

Koch C and Segev I (1998) *Methods in Neuronal Modeling, 2nd edn.: From Ions to Networks (Computational Neuroscience).* Cambridge, MA: MIT Press.

Strogatz SH (1994) *Nonlinear Dynamics and Chaos: With Applications to Physics, Biology, Chemistry and Engineering.* Cambridge, MA: Perseus.

Neuronal Pacemaking

B P Bean, Harvard Medical School, Boston, MA, USA

Introduction

Neuronal pacemaking refers to the ability of some neurons to generate spontaneous electrical activity by firing action potentials without being stimulated by synaptic input or by input from sensory receptors (**Figure 1**). When spontaneous firing of single neurons is rhythmic and regular, it is often called 'pacemaking,' by analogy to the regular pacemaking of action potentials in the sinoatrial node of the heart. However, firing of a pacemaking neuron need not necessarily trigger firing of downstream cells in a manner analogous to the pacemaker region of the heart. In fact, many neurons with pacemaking electrical activity are inhibitory neurons that release GABA.

Types of Pacemaking Neurons

Many different types of neurons in the mammalian brain have intrinsic pacemaking activity. One broad class of pacemaking neurons comprises neurons that release a variety of modulatory neurotransmitters, including acetylcholine, norepinephrine, dopamine, serotonin, and histamine. Spontaneous activity of such neurons is not surprising, since it appears that many such transmitters are often continuously released so as to produce tonic effects at low levels in a manner that is not cell-specific. Neurons releasing modulatory transmitters are often found to be spontaneously active at typical frequencies of 0.5–10 Hz (action potentials per second) if all synaptic input is removed. In a few cases, such as serotonergic neurons in the dorsal raphe nucleus, the neurons are silent in the absence of all synaptic input but fire rhythmically in a pacemaker-like fashion when there is steady excitation by norepinephrine acting on α-adrenergic receptors.

Many neurons involved in controlling sleep and wakefulness are spontaneously active. Neurons in the suprachiasmatic nucleus of the hypothalamus fire spontaneously at frequencies that show circadian rhythmicity, with faster firing daytime than during nighttime. Hypothalamic neurons that release the neuropeptide orexin, which promotes both wakefulness and feeding behavior, also show pacemaking activity, as do neurons in the tuberomammillary nucleus of the hypothalamus, which release histamine, associated with general stimulatory or activating effects throughout the brain.

A subset of interneurons in the cortex and hippocampus show pacemaking activity. Firing of groups of interneurons is often synchronized, with synchrony mediated both by electrical synapses (gap junctions) and by phase-lock of firing by means of chemical γ-aminobutyric acid (GABA)ergic synapses. It is believed that synchronous firing of networks of interneurons is centrally involved in controlling overall oscillatory activity of the cortex, especially at higher frequencies.

Several neuronal types in the thalamus are spontaneously active. Thalamic relay neurons, which receive sensory input and make glutamatergic projections to the cortex, are spontaneously active during sleep, when their spontaneous activity and synaptic input to the cortex (along with thalamocortical loops of synaptically connected neurons) may serve to underlie slow wave oscillations.

Many neurons throughout the motor system show pacemaking activity. Examples include neurons of the inferior olive; cerebellar Purkinje neurons; neurons in the deep cerebellar nuclei; and a number of neuronal types in the basal ganglia, including GABAergic neurons in the globus pallidus and substantia nigra pars reticulata, glutamatergic neurons in the subthalamic nucleus, giant cholinergic interneurons in the striatum, and dopaminergic neurons in the substantia nigra pars compacta.

Mechanisms of Pacemaking

Changes in the voltage across the membrane of excitable cells are produced by ionic currents flowing through ion channels, transmembrane proteins that form pores through the membrane. Neurons contain dozens of different types of ion channels with differing selectivity to various ions. In most cases, ion channels are normally closed but can be opened ('activated') by changes in membrane voltage. Activation is usually transient, either because the membrane voltage returns to a level that causes closing ('deactivation') of the channels or because of a property called 'inactivation,' whereby channels close even though a change in voltage is maintained. Pacemaking depends on opening of ion channels that pass electrical current flowing from outside to inside the cell. Such current produces depolarization of the cell membrane. In most cases, this current is carried by sodium ions, calcium ions, or both. A variety of different ion channels are involved in different types of pacemaking neurons.

Hyperpolarization-Activated Current

The best-known mechanism of pacemaking involves activation of a voltage-dependent current known as hyperpolarization-activated current (I_h). This current is carried by a family of ion channels called hyperpolarization-activated cyclic nucleotide-sensitive (HCN) channels. I_h is a voltage-gated current with an unusual voltage dependence: it is closed at normal resting potentials and is activated by hyperpolarization, the opposite of the voltage dependence of almost all other voltage-dependent channels, which are opened by depolarization. The HCN channels carrying I_h are permeable to both potassium and sodium, with P_K:P_{Na} ~ 3:1. This gives a reversal potential near −30 mV. The channels begin to be activated by hyperpolarization below −60 to −70 mV, and at these potentials the inward current is carried by sodium ions. The flow of sodium ions into the cells produces depolarization toward threshold for action potential formation.

I_h is present in many neurons. However, many of its properties and a role in spontaneous firing of action potentials were first described in cardiac muscle cells in the sinoatrial node of the heart, where the electrical pacemaking of the heart originates. Because of this association, the channels underlying I_h have sometimes been called 'pacemaker' channels. (It is interesting, however, that although I_h is clearly involved in pacemaking in the heart, blocking the channels generally only slows but does not stop the heartbeat, showing that other channels are also involved.) In mammalian central neurons, I_h appears to play a major role in pacemaking in a subset of pacemaking neurons. These include thalamic relay neurons, large cholinergic interneurons in the striatum, globus pallidus neurons, some interneurons, and a subset of dopaminergic neurons in the midbrain. The role of I_h is often assayed by applying a reasonably selective channel blocker called ZD 7288 (**Figure 2**).

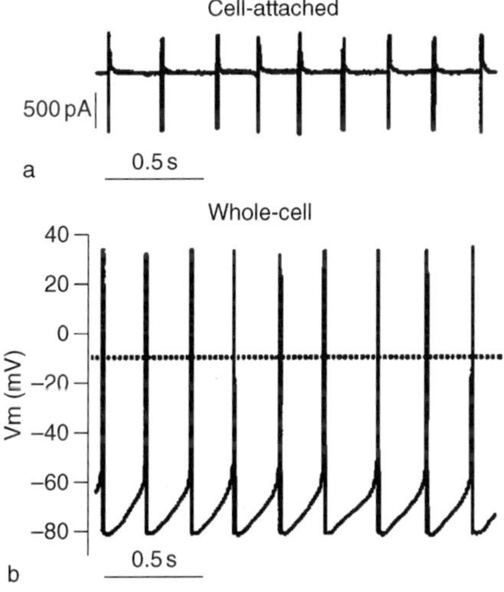

Figure 1 Electrical pacemaking in a suprachiasmatic nucleus neuron. Spontaneous firing of action potentials was recorded first in cell-attached patch mode and then in whole-cell current-clamp mode from an acutely isolated neuron from the suprachiasmatic nucleus of a rat hypothalamus. (a) Action currents from spontaneous firing recorded in cell-attached mode. In this recording configuration, the interior of the cell is undisturbed. (b) Spontaneous firing recorded in whole-cell mode 7 min after breaking through into whole-cell mode. The pipette solution consisted of 123 mmol^{-1} K-methanesulfonate, 9 mmol^{-1} NaCl, 1.8 mmol^{-1} $MgCl_2$, 0.9 mmol^{-1} EGTA, 9 mmol^{-1} HEPES, 14 mmol^{-1} creatine phosphate, 4 mmol^{-1} Mg–adenosine triphosphate, and 0.3 mmol^{-1} guanosine triphosphate, pH 7.3. The external solution included 1.2 mmol^{-1} $CaCl_2$, 3.5 mmol^{-1} KCl, 150 mmol^{-1} NaCl, 1 mmol^{-1} $MgCl_2$, 10 mmol^{-1} glucose, and 10 mmol^{-1} HEPES, pH 7.4. Reproduced from Jackson AC, Yao GL, and Bean BP (2004) Mechanism of spontaneous firing in dorsomedial suprachiasmatic nucleus neurons. *Journal of Neuroscience* 24: 7985–7998.

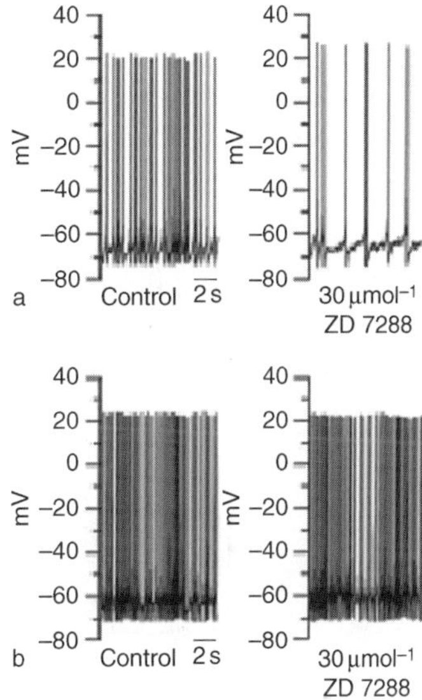

Figure 2 Effect of the hyperpolarization-activated current (I_h) blocker ZD 7288 on pacemaking in two dissociated substantia nigra pars compacta dopaminergic neurons. (a) Left, pacemaking in an acutely dissociated dopaminergic neuron from the substantia nigra par compacta (mouse). To identify dopaminergic neurons, a transgenic mouse line was used in which catecholaminergic neurons in the central nervous system express human placental alkaline phosphatase (PLAP) on the outer surface of the cell membrane. The line was obtained by introducing into the mouse genome PLAP complementary DNA linked to a promoter sequence of the gene for tyrosine hydroxylase. Living dopaminergic neurons were identified before recording by labeling of their membrane with a monoclonal antibody to PLAP directly conjugated to the fluorochrome Cy3 (E6-Cy3). Right, spontaneous firing in the same cell after application of 30 mmol^{-1} ZD 7288 to block I_h. (b) Lack of effect on pacemaking of ZD 7288 applied in a different acutely dissociated neuron (also identified as dopaminergic neuron by antibody to PLAP). Although I_h contributes to pacemaking in the cell in (a), it is not absolutely necessary, and it plays little or no role in the cell in (b). Reproduced from Puopolo M, Raviola E, and Bean BP (2007) Roles of subthreshold calcium current and sodium current in spontaneous firing of mouse midbrain dopamine neurons. *Journal of Neuroscience* 27: 645–656.

Persistent Sodium Current

In many pacemaking neurons, blocking I_h with ZD 7288 has little or no effect on spontaneous electrical activity. In most of these, the spontaneous depolarization activity appears to be due to current through voltage-activated sodium channels that produce steady state, noninactivating sodium current at subthreshold voltages (**Figure 3**). In such neurons, application of tetrodotoxin (TTX), an alkaloid toxin from puffer fish that selectively blocks voltage-dependent sodium channels, silences the firing and produces a stable resting potential (**Figure 3(b)**). Current through voltage-dependent sodium channels can be characterized most clearly in voltage-clamp experiments, in which the voltage of the membrane is controlled (using electronic circuitry) and ionic currents are measured. Current through voltage-dependent sodium channels is usually most obvious as a large transient current that activates rapidly (<1 ms) and inactivates (during several milliseconds) when the membrane is suddenly depolarized from rest. However, voltage-dependent sodium channels can also carry smaller, steady, noninactivating currents. This steady-state current is often called 'persistent' sodium current. It activates with a steep voltage dependence, with activation first evident near −70 or −65 mV and with maximal activation near −40 mV. **Figures 3(c)** and **3(d)** show an example, in which TTX inhibited a steady inward current at −60 mV, as well as a bigger noninactivating current that was activated when the voltage was stepped from −60 to −52.5 mV. **Figure 3(e)** shows current as a function of voltage in the absence and presence of TTX, illustrating a TTX-sensitive inward current (shown subtracted in **Figure 3(f)**) that increases steeply from −65 to −50 mV. This steep voltage dependence produces regenerative depolarization, so if the membrane voltage is depolarized to −65 mV, inward sodium current flows, which produces further depolarization, which activates more channels, which pass larger inward currents, depolarizing the cell further.

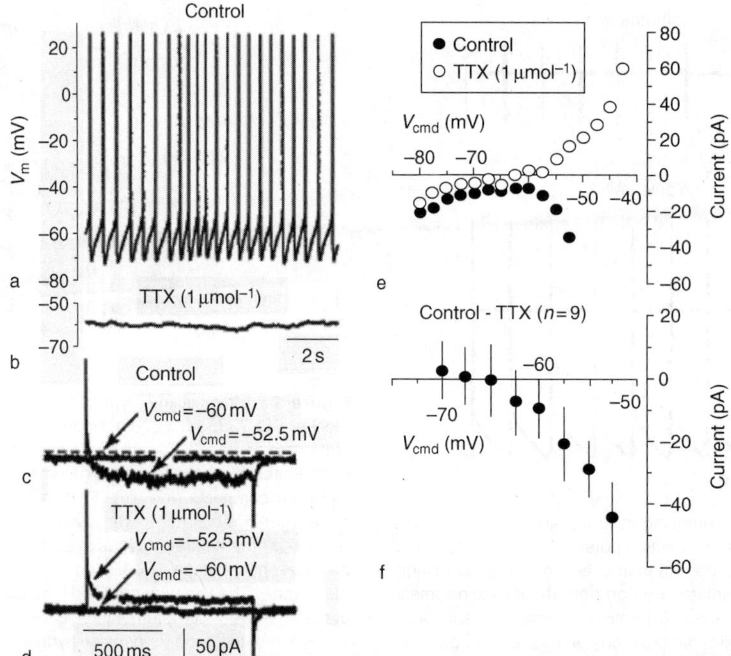

Figure 3 Role of subthreshold sodium current in driving pacemaking in a cholinergic interneuron in the striatum. (a) Spontaneous firing in a striatal cholinergic interneuron. (b) Application of tetrodotoxin (TTX) (1 μmol^{-1}) prevented action potential generation and established a stable subthreshold membrane potential (approximately −60 mV). (c) In voltage clamp, stepping the membrane from a holding potential of −60 to −52.5 mV elicited a slowly developing inward current that persisted throughout the pulse. The dashed line indicates the zero current level. (d) After TTX (1 μmol^{-1}) treatment, the inward current produced by the depolarizing voltage step was absent, and a small outward current was observed. In addition, the zero current level was shifted to −60 mV. (e) The current–voltage plot for a range of voltage steps (V_{cmd}) shows that, under control conditions, there is a region of negative slope conductance at potentials positive to −60 mV and no zero current point in the subthreshold voltage range. The inward current generated by depolarizing steps was blocked by TTX. (f) Voltage dependence of the TTX-sensitive current that was obtained by subtraction for nine neurons and pooled (mean ± standard deviation). V_{cmd}, voltage command. Reproduced from Bennett BD, Callaway JC, and Wilson CJ (2000) Intrinsic membrane properties underlying spontaneous tonic firing in neostriatal cholinergic interneurons. *Journal of Neuroscience* 20: 8493–8503.

This regenerative process continues until the threshold for action potential formation (typically in the range near −55 to −40 mV) is reached.

Evidence suggests that persistent sodium current active at subthreshold voltages is carried by the same population of channels that underlie the transient, inactivating sodium current that underlies action potentials. Models of gating of conventional inactivating sodium channels suggest that with strong depolarization, inactivation of transient sodium channels is ~99.5% complete and that the incomplete nature of inactivation results in steady-state sodium current that activates steeply at voltages between −65 and −40 mV. Virtually all neurons have large transient sodium currents, reaching typical magnitudes of 5–20 nA. Thus, steady-state current at the level of 0.5% would be in the range of 25–100 pA, typical of steady-state persistent sodium currents that are measured. Some neurons, such as pyramidal neurons in the entorhinal cortex, also have specialized sodium channels with more incomplete inactivation that can produce particularly large persistent sodium currents.

The ability of a single population of sodium channels to make both persistent sodium current at subthreshold voltages and transient sodium current at more-depolarized voltage constitutes an intrinsic system of rhythmic pacemaking generated by a single type of ion channel. The presence of a large density of voltage-dependent sodium channels in virtually all neurons implies that virtually all neurons have an intrinsic drive to spontaneous firing. Clearly, many neurons do not fire spontaneously, and pacemaking by this mechanism can be prevented if there is a resting potassium conductance large enough to produce a resting potential negative to −70 mV or so, at which persistent current is first activated. However, the association of persistent sodium current with transient sodium current suggests that pacemaking behavior is an intrinsic propensity of all neurons that use sodium channels for spike formation, requiring the presence of resting potassium channels to prevent or modulate this inherent tendency.

Neurons in which pacemaking appears to be mainly due to persistent sodium current at subthreshold voltages include neurons of the suprachiasmatic nucleus, pedunculopontine nucleus neurons, subthalamic neurons, Purkinje neurons, tuberomammillary nucleus neurons, and neurons of the deep cerebellar nuclei. Even in neurons in which blocking I_h stops pacemaking, it is possible that persistent sodium current plays the major role in generating spontaneous depolarization in the range from −70 mV to threshold, with I_h serving to ensure that the membrane voltage does not fall below −70 mV for very long.

Resurgent Sodium Current

Some pacemaking neurons have an unusual component of TTX-sensitive voltage-dependent sodium current called 'resurgent' sodium current, which activates when the membrane is repolarized to resting potentials following strong depolarizing pulses that have produced maximal inactivation of the sodium channels. Resurgent sodium current appears to arise from an unusual mechanism of inactivation in which channels are plugged by a positively charged intracellular blocking particle after they open. On repolarization, the block is relieved, and the channels carry an inward sodium current transiently before deactivating. This is unlike recovery from the most common mechanism of inactivation in sodium channels, which occurs without any current passing through the channels. Resurgent sodium current gives rise to a component of TTX-sensitive sodium current immediately after a spike. This produces a depolarizing influence and promotes a more rapid approach to threshold than would otherwise occur. Recovery from the mechanism of inactivation associated with resurgent current is faster than recovery from normal inactivation, so as sodium channels pass resurgent sodium current after a spike, they are also recovering from inactivation and able to give transient sodium current on depolarization. This effect also promotes faster firing of a second spike. Resurgent current has been found in several types of neurons that have pacemaking activity at rapid frequencies, notably cerebellar Purkinje neurons (which often fire spontaneously at ~40 Hz), subthalamic nucleus neurons (which often fire at ~20 Hz), and motor neurons of the trigeminal mesencephalic nucleus.

Voltage-Activated Calcium Current

In a few types of neurons, voltage-dependent calcium currents seem to be important for pacemaking. For example, in dopamine neurons in the pars compacta of the substantia nigra, blocking entry of calcium though calcium channels by replacing calcium with cobalt (which is impermeant in most calcium channels) stops spontaneous firing (**Figure 4**), and cessation of firing is accompanied by hyperpolarization, as if a depolarizing inward current carried by calcium has been blocked. This effect of blocking calcium entry is relatively unusual: in many other pacemaking neurons, such as cerebellar Purkinje neurons, subthalamic nucleus neurons, and suprachiasmatic nucleus neurons, blocking calcium entry has little effect on firing frequency (or may speed it) and often produces depolarization rather than hyperpolarization. These effects likely occur because calcium entry is often strongly coupled to activation of calcium-dependent

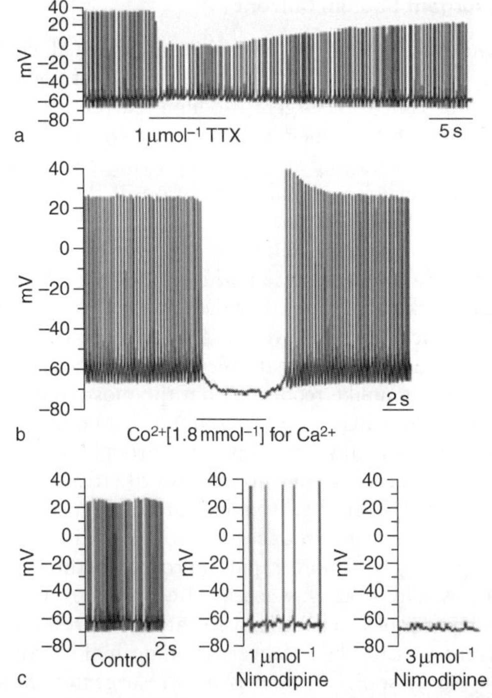

Figure 4 Role of calcium current in pacemaking of dopaminergic neurons from the substantia nigra pars compacta. (a) Effect of tetrodotoxin (TTX) on spontaneous activity in an acutely dissociated dopaminergic neuron from the substantia nigra pars compacta. Spontaneous activity continued, with smaller and broader spikes from a more depolarized potential. (b) Effect of blocking calcium entry (cobalt substitution for extracellular calcium) on spontaneous activity in another dissociated dopaminergic neuron. Immediate hyperpolarization and cessation of pacemaking suggest a role for calcium current. (c) Effect of the L-type calcium channel blocker nimodipine on spontaneous firing in an acutely dissociated dopaminergic neuron from the substantia nigra pars compacta. From Puopolo M, Raviola E, and Bean BP (2007) Roles of subthreshold calcium current and sodium current in spontaneous firing of mouse midbrain dopamine neurons. *Journal of Neuroscience* 27: 645–656.

potassium channels, and the net effect of blocking calcium entry is to inhibit an outward current.

Pacemaking dopaminergic neurons in the pars compacta of the substantia nigra will continue firing action potentials in the presence of TTX (**Figure 4**). This firing appears to be caused by calcium action potentials since it can be inhibited by removal of Ca or by cobalt, which blocks voltage-dependent calcium channels. The calcium current involved in pacemaking of midbrain dopaminergic neurons appears to be at least partly 'L-type' calcium current, since pacemaking is slowed or stopped by L-type channel blockers such as nifedipine and nimodipine (**Figure 4**). Although the dominant type of L-type calcium channels in most neurons (Cav1.2 channels) requires suprathreshold depolarizations for activation (positive to ~−40 mV), L-type current carried by Cav1.3 channels can activate at much more negative voltages, as negative as −70 mV. Evidence suggests that current through Cav1.3 channels may play a major role in pacemaking of dopaminergic neurons in the substantia nigra. It is interesting that Cav1.3 channels are also strongly expressed in the sinoatrial node of the heart and probably contribute significantly to cardiac pacemaking.

Another class of calcium channels that can open at subthreshold voltages and likely contribute to pacemaking in some neurons includes low-threshold, T-type calcium channels (also called low-voltage-activated channels) formed by channels in the Cav3 family. These channels can activate at voltages as negative as −75 mV, but they also inactivate strongly, so that at steady voltages near −60 mV, they are almost completely inactivated. They are likely to contribute to pacemaking primarily when the action potential is followed by a deep afterhyperpolarization lasting long enough to remove inactivation. A significant role for current through T-type channels has been proposed for pacemaking in thalamic relay neurons. However, as there are no blockers that are highly selective for T-type channels, this theory has been difficult to test directly in these or other neurons.

Importance of Resting Potential

A key element regulating the occurrence and frequency of spontaneous firing is the resting potential of a cell. The mixture of conductances that are not voltage-dependent and that determine resting potential of neurons is not well understood. Obviously, a neuron that is continually active does not have a true resting potential. For spontaneously active neurons, the resting potential must be determined when firing is stopped, for example by application of TTX. TTX application usually, but not always, results in a stable resting potential (dopaminergic substantia nigra neurons being one of the exceptions). In general, neurons have resting potentials is the range between −75 and −55 mV, considerably depolarized to the potassium equilibrium potential (near −90 mV for mammalian solutions). Pacemaking neurons frequently have somewhat more depolarized resting potentials than neurons in general, from −60 to −45 mV. The resting potassium conductance of neurons (and all cells) appears to result primarily from expression of 'two-pore domain' family (KCNK) potassium channels, which are not voltage-dependent channels. These channels are highly potassium-selective. In cells with resting potentials considerably positive to E_K, it is unclear whether there is relatively moderate expression of KCNK channels or whether there is additional conductance with permeability to other ions. Some cells with depolarized resting potentials have very high input resistances (i.e., very low resting conductance), and in these, there may simply be relatively little expression of KCNK channels. In lower-resistance cells, there may be substantial expression of KCNK channels but additional expression of background sodium conductances. Evidence for the latter is that in some neurons, replacement of external sodium by the larger cation *N*-methyl-D-glucamine causes hyperpolarization of the resting potential. In some neurons there may also be background calcium conductances that are not voltage-dependent, but these have not been characterized in any detail.

A very simple mechanism of pacemaking is provided by a cell in which there is expression of a reasonably high density of voltage-dependent sodium channels (which provide both persistent steady-state sodium current positive to −65 mV and also transient sodium current to form spikes) along with background conductances that by themselves would produce a stable resting potential positive to −65 mV. Such a cell is likely to fire spontaneously in a pacemaker-like manner as long as the action potential activates potassium conductances that can repolarize the membrane during the falling phase of the action potential sufficiently to provide recovery from inactivation of the transient sodium channels.

Voltage-Dependent and Calcium-Dependent Potassium Conductances as Regulators of Firing Rate

Most neurons have at least a half-dozen to a dozen distinct types of voltage-dependent or calcium-activated potassium channels, and the frequency of pacemaking can be strongly influenced by these conductances. A particular potassium current strongly implicated in control of pacemaking frequency is a current known as 'A-type' current (I_A), generally carried by channels in the Kv4 family, which both activates and inactivates at subthreshold voltages. I_A enables repetitive firing at low frequencies. During the period of relative hyperpolarization after a spike, some inactivation of I_A is removed. Then, as the membrane depolarizes at potentials in the range of −70 to −55 mV (still below threshold for an action potential), I_A increasingly activates and thereby slows the approach to threshold. In the steady state, I_A inactivates nearly completely at voltages positive to about −65 mV, so it eventually inactivates, allowing depolarization to threshold. Expression of a large density of I_A appears common in pacemaking neurons that fire rhythmically at relatively slow frequencies (0.5–5 Hz), such as midbrain dopaminergic neurons. There are other potassium currents that can be activated at subthreshold voltages, notably a current called 'I_D,' which is activated by subthreshold depolarizations, inactivates slowly (more slowly than I_A), and can similarly prolong approach to threshold. However, subthreshold I_D has been characterized mainly in nonpacemaking neurons such as cortical and hippocampal pyramidal neurons, and it is unclear whether there is prominent expression of I_D in pacemaking neurons.

Most voltage-dependent potassium channels require suprathreshold depolarizations to be activated significantly and are not activated in the lead-up to the action potential but rather during the spike itself. Potassium currents through these channels can still influence the frequency of pacemaking if they deactivate slowly enough after the spike repolarizes, pushing the membrane voltage toward E_K as long as they are activated. Of purely voltage-activated potassium channels, channels in the Kv1 family generally have the slowest deactivation kinetics and might influence pacemaking frequency by producing a period of relative hyperpolarization following the action potential.

Calcium-activated potassium currents may also play a major role in regulating firing frequency. During the action potential, there is generally activation of voltage-dependent calcium channels, especially during the falling phase of the action potential, producing a large increase in intracellular calcium, which activates calcium-activated potassium currents. There are two major types of calcium-activated potassium channels: KCa1 channels (also known as 'BK' channels), which are activated both by intracellular calcium and by depolarization, and KCa2 channels (also known as 'SK' channels), which are activated purely by increases in intracellular calcium. Both KCa1 and KCa2 channels are strongly expressed in most neurons. KCa1 channels respond to relatively large increases in intracellular calcium, and they are activated very quickly during the falling phase of the action potential. KCa2 calcium-activated channels respond to lower levels of calcium than do KCa1 channels but have intrinsically slower activation kinetics. Current through KCa2 channels contributes little to the fast repolarization phase of the action potential but helps shape the afterhyperpolarization that follows the action potential. After a spike, KCa2-mediated conductance can last for many hundreds of milliseconds before decaying, probably reflecting the relatively slow decay of intracellular free calcium. In contrast, KCa1 channels generally deactivate far more quickly. The longer-lasting conductance from KCa2 channels gives them a larger role in controlling pacemaking frequency. In several types of pacemaking neurons, block of KCa2 channels (or block of the

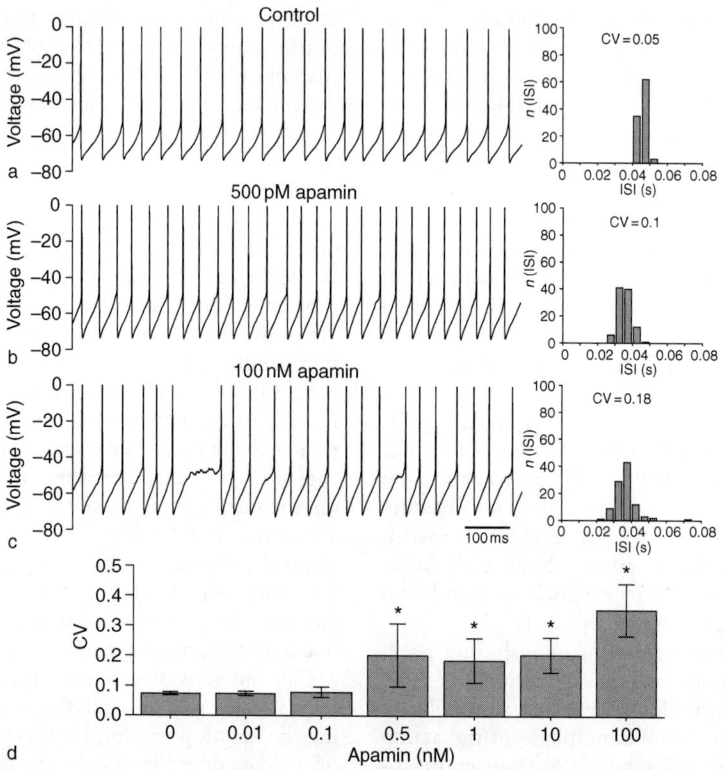

Figure 5 SK(KCa2) calcium-activated potassium channels are critical for the rhythmicity of pacemaking activity in rat subthalamic nucleus neurons. (a) Pacemaking was extremely regular in control conditions. Right, interspike interval histogram generated from 100 interspike intervals. Coefficient of variation (CV) = 0.05; frequency = 21.8 Hz. (b) Partial inhibition of SK channels by 0.5 nmol^{-1} apamin. Firing was less regular (CV = 0.1), and frequency was somewhat faster (28.1 Hz). (c) Complete inhibition of SK channels by 100 nmol^{-1} apamin. Firing was much less regular (CV = 0.18), frequency (27.5 Hz) not much changed from 0.5 nmol^{-1} apamin. Calibration in (c) also applies to (a) and (b). From Hallworth NE, Wilson CJ, and Bevan M (2003) Apamin-sensitive small conductance calcium-activated potassium channels, through their selective coupling to voltage-gated calcium channels, are critical determinants of the precision, pace, and pattern of action potential generation in rat subthalamic nucleus neurons *in vitro*. *Journal of Neuroscience* 23: 7525–7542.

calcium current that activates them) has the striking effect of producing substantially less-regular firing (**Figure 5**). The reasons for this are not clear.

Plasticity of Pacemaking

A number of cases are known in which the frequency of firing of pacemaking neurons can be altered in a relatively long-lasting manner (many minutes to hours). For example, in spontaneously firing neurons in the medial vestibular nucleus, silencing the neurons for relatively brief periods (~5 min) by sustained inhibitory synaptic input can result in increases in the frequency of pacemaking that can last more than 2 h. These neurons serve to transform information about head movement into eye movements and are central to the vestibulo-ocular reflex that keeps appropriate eye position when the head moves. The plasticity of the pacemaking frequency (which is accompanied by an increase in the excitability of the neurons when responding to excitatory stimulation) is believed to constitute a form of motor learning that can recalibrate the gain of the vestibulo-ocular reflex. The mechanism of plasticity of vestibular neurons is thought to involve, during the period of inhibition, a decrease in intracellular calcium that leads to a decrease in basal Cam-kinase II enzymatic activity and a reduction in BK calcium-activated potassium current.

A remarkable example of plasticity is seen in principal neurons in the entorhinal cortex of the parahippocampal region, a key brain area for acquisition and consolidation of working memory. When the conductances in these neurons are modulated by steady activation of muscarinic acetylcholine receptors (known to be important in memory), the neurons acquire the ability to fire in a pacemaker-like fashion at frequencies that can be stepped up or down in a remarkably stable manner (**Figure 6**). Specifically, stimulation with a short (4 s) injection of current (which transiently produces high-frequency firing)

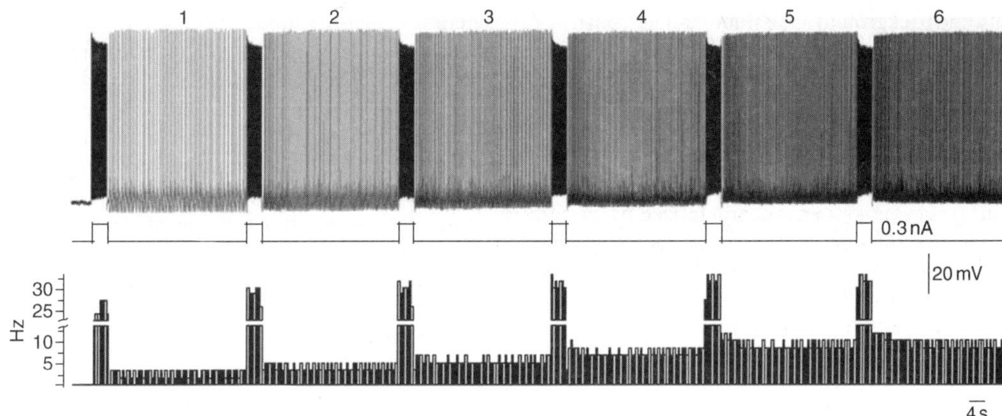

Figure 6 Plasticity of firing frequency in entorhinal cortical neuron exposed to an agonist of muscarinic acetylcholine receptors (10 μmol^{-1} carbamylcholine). Stimulation with a 4 s depolarizing step first induces persistent spontaneous firing (cell was initially quiescent at a stable resting potential of −64 mV). Five more episodes of stimulation each give rise to a further increase in firing frequency, in each case stably expressed until the next stimulation. Top trace shows membrane voltage, middle trace shows injected current, and bottom trace shows frequency of firing. Reproduced from Egorov AV, Hamam BN, Fransen E, Hasselmo ME, and Alonso AA (2002) Graded persistent activity in entorhinal cortex neurons. *Nature* 420: 173–178.

can produce a sustained increase in pacemaking frequency that can last for many minutes. Moreover, this process can be repeated with multiple stimuli, with pacemaking frequency increasing step-wise over a wide range. The increase in frequency can be reversed in a step-wise manner by application of 6 s hyperpolarizing steps that temporarily silence the cell. (Note that the increase in firing frequency following periods of stimulation and the decreases following inhibition are opposite to the plasticity in medial vestibular neurons.) This plasticity constitutes a mechanism of short-term analog memory at a single-cell level. The mechanism is not completely understood but appears to involve increased calcium entry during the period of stimulation that may activate calcium-activated nonselective cation conductances.

Another prominent instance of plasticity of pacemaking behavior occurs in the neurons controlling electric organ discharge of the weakly electric fish *Apteronotus leptorhynchus*. These fish generate an oscillating electric field around their bodies, used for detecting objects and other organisms in muddy water. The oscillatory discharge of electric organ is controlled by pacemaker neurons that fire action potentials at up to 1 kHz, the highest frequency of electrical pacemaking that is known. Because the cells in the pacemaker nucleus are electronically coupled, they have been difficult to study under voltage clamp, and so the ionic conductances underlying pacemaking are not well-characterized. Most likely, pacemaking is generated by TTX-sensitive sodium currents with unusually rapid kinetics, together with rapidly activating and rapidly deactivating potassium channels that keep the spikes short. Pacemaking is extremely regular. However, when two fish using similar frequencies of electric organ discharge share the same area, the one using the higher frequency shifts its frequency higher to avoid jamming of the two signals. This change in pacemaker frequency is normally temporary, lasting only as long as the other signal is present. However, if the exogenous signal is maintained for >30 min, the increase in pacemaking frequency can last for many hours after the other signal is terminated. The mechanism of this plasticity is not understood.

Neurons in the suprachiasmatic nucleus of mammals are the 'master pacemaker' neurons for circadian rhythms in behavior. They fire spontaneously (although sometimes with less regularity than seen in other types of electrical pacemakers), and if the firing of individual neurons is followed, the frequency of spontaneous firing shows a circadian rhythm, higher in the daytime and slower at nighttime (even in nocturnal animals like rats and mice that are less active in the day than in the night). Intensive work over the last decade has identified a molecular clock based on feedback loops of transcription factors and enzymes, involving regulation of translation, dimerization, nuclear translocation, and degradation of multiple elements. However, how the molecular clock is linked to the circadian regulation of electrical pacemaking frequency has been very difficult to determine. Day–night differences in a number of different conductances have been described, including voltage-dependent L-type calcium channels, Kv3-family voltage-dependent potassium channels, BK calcium-activated potassium channels, and background potassium channels, but it has been difficult to definitively ascribe differences in firing frequency to any of the changes in conductance that have been described.

Significance of Pacemaking

The central nervous system is characterized by overall oscillatory electrical activity, as is evident from the oscillatory signals at many different frequencies present in the electroencephalogram. Oscillatory electrical activity occurs at many different levels, including the pacemaking activity of single neurons, oscillations in local networks, and oscillations involving larger-scale connections between brain regions. Oscillatory activity does not require sensory input but rather appears to occur spontaneously (although it can certainly be modified and influenced by sensory input). Presumably neuronal pacemaking at the single-cell level is central in generating the overall spontaneous activity of the brain, amplified and modified by circuits and networks.

Pathophysiology of Pacemaking

It is striking that so many neurons in the motor system are characterized by rhythmic spontaneous firing. Pacemaking activity seems counterintuitive for a system which must often be inactive and in which very rapid events and processing must occur in almost an all-or-none manner. It seems likely that the underlying pacemaking activity of elements of the motor system plays a major role in the generation of oscillatory tremors that characterize diseases such as Parkinson's disease and Huntington's disease. It is not yet clear whether the pathophysiology of tremors involves changes in the pacemaking activity of single neurons, changes in control and circuit connections, or both. It is interesting that a current treatment for Parkinson's disease involves deep brain stimulation of neurons in the subthalamic nucleus, which show prominent pacemaking activity, but the exact mechanism by which deep brain stimulation works is not yet known.

Altered pacemaking mechanisms may also be involved in some other diseases of the nervous system involving hyperexcitability of neurons, including neuropathic pain (some forms of which might involve spontaneous firing of primary pain-sensing neurons, which normally would require input from sensory receptors to be active) and epilepsy.

Summary

In some neurons, electrical pacemaking activity produces spontaneous activity in the absence of any synaptic or sensory input. Such pacemaking activity at the cellular level probably underlies spontaneous oscillatory activity at the level of networks and brain regions, which appears to be a crucial characteristic of the operation of the mammalian brain. There are several different ionic mechanisms of pacemaking in different types of pacemaking neurons, most commonly depending on activation of ion channels that allow entry of either sodium ions or calcium ions into the cell, thus carrying an electrical current that depolarizes the cell membrane to the threshold for firing an action potential.

See also: Calcium and Signal Transduction; Calcium Channels; Calcium Channel Subtypes Involved in Neurotransmitter Release; Calcium Channel and Calcium-Activated Potassium Channel Coupling; Gamma-Amino-butyric Acid (GABA); Large Conductance Calcium-Activated Potassium Channels; Neuromodulation of Sodium Channels; Neuromodulation; Potassium Channel Regulation; Sodium Channels.

Further Reading

Bennett BD, Callaway JC, and Wilson CJ (2000) Intrinsic membrane properties underlying spontaneous tonic firing in neostriatal cholinergic interneurons. *Journal of Neuroscience* 20: 8493–8503.

Chaplan SR, Guo HQ, Lee DH, et al. (2003) Neuronal hyperpolarization-activated pacemaker channels drive neuropathic pain. *Journal of Neuroscience* 23: 1169–1178.

Do MT and Bean BP (2003) Subthreshold sodium currents and pacemaking of subthalamic neurons: modulation by slow inactivation. *Neuron* 39: 109–120.

Egorov AV, Hamam BN, Fransen E, Hasselmo ME, and Alonso AA (2002) Graded persistent activity in entorhinal cortex neurons. *Nature* 420: 173–178.

Forti L, Cesana E, Mapelli J, and D'Angelo E (2006) Ionic mechanisms of autorhythmic firing in rat cerebellar Golgi cells. *Journal of Physiology* 574: 711–729.

Hallworth NE, Wilson CJ, and Bevan M (2003) Apamin-sensitive small conductance calcium-activated potassium channels, through their selective coupling to voltage-gated calcium channels, are critical determinants of the precision, pace, and pattern of action potential generation in rat subthalamic nucleus neurons *in vitro*. *Journal of Neuroscience* 23: 7525–7542.

Hille B (2001) *Ion Channels of Excitable Membranes*. Sunderland, MA: Sinauer.

Jackson AC, Yao GL, and Bean BP (2004) Mechanism of spontaneous firing in dorsomedial suprachiasmatic nucleus neurons. *Journal of Neuroscience* 24: 7985–7998.

Liss B, Franz O, Sewing S, Bruns R, Neuhoff H, and Roeper J (2001) Tuning pacemaker frequency of individual dopaminergic neurons by Kv4.3L and KChip3.1 transcription. *EMBO Journal* 20: 5715–5724.

Maccaferri G and McBain CJ (1996) The hyperpolarization-activated current (Ih) and its contribution to pacemaker activity in rat CA1 hippocampal stratum oriens-alveus interneurones. *Journal of Physiology* 497(Pt. 1): 119–130.

Meredith AL, Wiler SW, Miller BH, et al. (2006) BK calcium-activated potassium channels regulate circadian behavioral rhythms and pacemaker output. *Nature Neuroscience* 9: 1041–1049.

Neuhoff H, Neu A, Liss B, and Roeper J (2002) *I*(h) channels contribute to the different functional properties of identified dopaminergic subpopulations in the midbrain. *Journal of Neuroscience* 22: 1290–1302.

Poolos NP (2004) The yin and yang of the H-channel and its role in epilepsy. *Epilepsy Currents* 4: 3–6.

Puopolo M, Raviola E, and Bean BP (2007) Roles of subthreshold calcium current and sodium current in spontaneous firing of mouse midbrain dopamine neurons. *Journal of Neuroscience* 27: 645–656.

Robinson RB and Siegelbaum SA (2003) Hyperpolarization-activated cation currents: From molecules to physiological function. *Annual Review of Physiology* 65: 453–480.

Smith GT and Zakon HH (2000) Pharmacological characterization of ionic currents that regulate the pacemaker rhythm in a weakly electric fish. *Journal of Neurobiology* 42: 270–286.

Surmeier DJ, Mercer JN, and Chan CS (2005) Autonomous pacemakers in the basal ganglia: Who needs excitatory synapses anyway? *Current Opinion in Neurobiology* 15: 312–318.

Taddese A and Bean BP (2002) Subthreshold sodium current from rapidly inactivating sodium channels drives spontaneous firing of tuberomammillary neurons. *Neuron* 33: 587–600.

Wilson CJ and Callaway JC (2000) Coupled oscillator model of the dopaminergic neuron of the substantia nigra. *Journal of Neurophysiology* 83: 3084–3100.

Wolfart J, Neuhoff H, Franz O, and Roeper J (2001) Differential expression of the small-conductance, calcium-activated potassium channel SK3 is critical for pacemaker control in dopaminergic midbrain neurons. *Journal of Neuroscience* 21: 3443–3456.

Pulsatility in Neuroendocrine Systems

G Leng, N Sabatier, and C Caquineau,
The University of Edinburgh College of Medicine and Veterinary Sciences, Edinburgh, UK

Introduction

A major role of the neuroendocrine hypothalamus is to generate pulsatile patterns of activity that are appropriate for the secretion of each of the pituitary hormones and to regulate these patterns according to specific physiological requirements. How the hypothalamus generates the various patterns varies from system to system; there is no common 'pulse generator' into which different systems can tap to generate their individual rhythms. However, what has been learned of the three best studied systems – oxytocin, the gonadotrophins, and growth hormone (GH) – indicates that there are commonalities as well as differences in the underlying mechanisms.

Oxytocin and vasopressin are secreted from the posterior pituitary as a direct result of the electrical activity of the hypothalamic magnocellular neurons that produce these hormones; thus, pulsatile secretion of oxytocin reflects synchronized burst activation of the oxytocin neurons. However, the process is more complex for the hormones secreted from the anterior pituitary gland. GH, prolactin, thyroid-stimulating hormone, ACTH, follicle-stimulating hormone (FSH), and leutinizing hormone (LH) are all secreted in a markedly pulsatile manner, in at least some physiological circumstances. For the most part, their secretion is regulated by releasing factors and release-inhibiting factors. These factors are released into the hypothalamo-hypophysial portal circulation from the nerve terminals of hypothalamic neuroendocrine neurons that project to the median eminence. In general, the secretion of a pulse of a hormone from the anterior pituitary gland follows release of a pulse of a releasing factor into the portal circulation, and it can be inferred that the pulse of releasing factor release in turn reflects synchronized pulsatile activation of the neurons that make the releasing factor. However, this inference has not been demonstrated directly; the only identified neuroendocrine neurons in which synchronized electrical activation has been directly observed during reflex hormone secretion are the magnocellular oxytocin neurons. These play a key role in forming the paradigm by which we understand the origins and significance of pulsatile hormone secretion.

Oxytocin

In a lactating rat, oxytocin is secreted into the blood in short-lived pulses while the mother is being suckled by the young. These pulses are the result of a brief, synchronized burst discharge of all the magnocellular neurosecretory oxytocin neurons in the supraoptic and paraventricular nucleus of the hypothalamus. Each burst lasts 1–3 s, and during a burst the firing rate of the neurons can exceed 100 action potential/s. The normal spontaneous firing rate of these neurons between bursts is just 1–3 action potential/s. These 'milk ejection' bursts occur at intervals of typically 3–5 min while the young are suckling. The fact that the milk ejection reflex involves intermittent pulsatile response to a continuous suckling stimulus appears to be a general feature in mammals, including humans (**Figure 1**).

In the rat, each milk ejection burst releases approximately 1 mU of oxytocin into the blood from the neurosecretory nerve terminals in the posterior pituitary gland. The released hormone initially travels as a bolus in the blood, and it disperses quickly as it is mixed with the total blood volume. The disappearance rate of the bolus is just a few seconds, much less than the half-life of oxytocin in the blood. This fast disappearance rate makes it very difficult to 'catch' the pulses for measurement by radioimmunoassay of blood samples, but the pulses can readily be detected by online bioassay – measurement of intramammary pressure changes by cannulation of the mammary gland.

The burst discharge of oxytocin cells is still not fully understood. Between bursts, the neurons show little, if any, sign of coordination in their spontaneous activity. However, oxytocin, acting within the hypothalamus, plays a key role in the burst behavior. Oxytocin that is secreted into the blood does not reenter the brain in significant amounts because of the blood–brain barrier, and oxytocin injected peripherally has no effect on the activity of oxytocin neurons, but very large amounts of oxytocin are released from the dendrites of the oxytocin neurons. This dendritic release is regulated semi-independently of peripheral, axonal secretion; dendritic release can be triggered, for instance, by peptides that act on oxytocin neurons to mobilize intracellular calcium stores. Oxytocin injected in small amounts into the brain facilitates the suckling-induced reflex, whereas oxytocin antagonists injected into the brain block it.

Oxytocin is released from the dendrites in response to suckling before any burst discharge is seen. The oxytocin neurons have oxytocin receptors, and activation of these induces calcium mobilization and

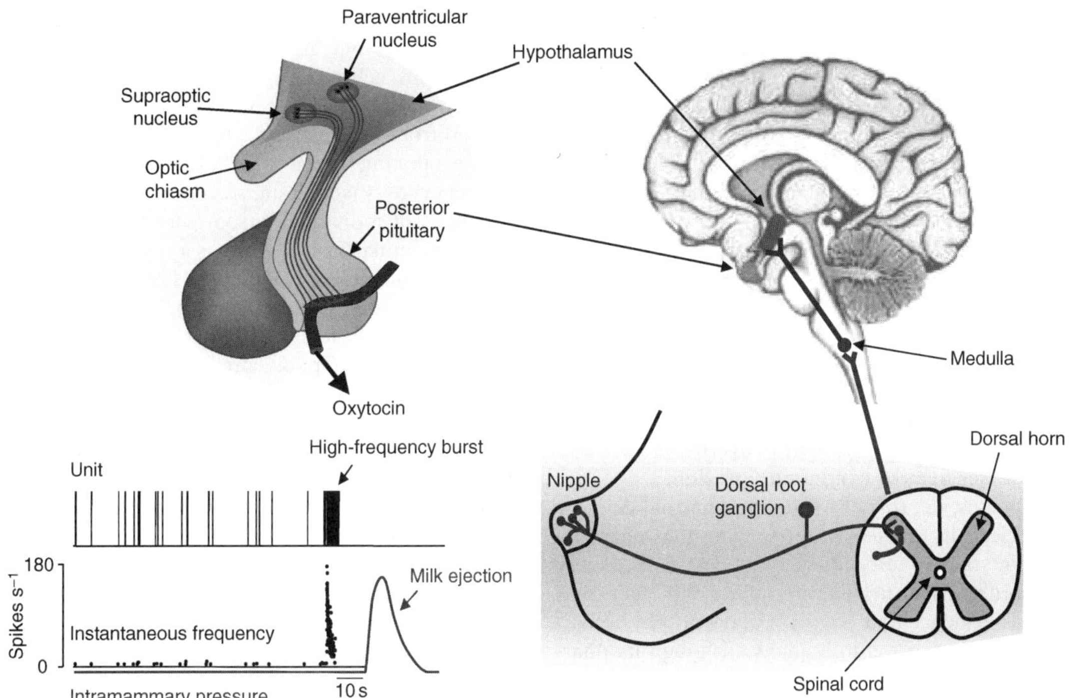

Figure 1 The milk ejection reflex. At the posterior pituitary gland, oxytocin is released from the neurosecretory nerve terminals of magnocellular neurosecretory neurons whose cell bodies are in the supraoptic and paraventricular nuclei of the hypothalamus. When young suckle at the nipples of a lactating mother, the sensory signals travel via the spinal cord and brain stem, resulting in synchronized bursting of the oxytocin neurons. This behavior, first observed by Jonathan Wakerley and Dennis Lincoln in the 1970s, leads to a brief pulse of oxytocin which triggers milk let-down and a transient increase in intramammary pressure. The inset shows the burst from one oxytocin cell preceding an intramammary pressure rise. See Lincoln DW, and Wakerley JB (1974) Electrophysiological evidences for the activation of supraoptic neurones during the release of oxytocin. *Journal of Physiology* 242: 533–554; Wakerley JB and Lincoln DW (1973) The milk-ejection reflex the rat: A 20- to 40-fold acceleration in the firing of paraventricular neurones during oxytocin release. *Journal of Endocrinology* 51: 477–493.

further oxytocin release; thus, there is a positive feedback loop. Oxytocin affects the electrical activity of oxytocin neurons in several ways: It suppresses afferent input to the oxytocin neurons, tending to reduce their spontaneous activity, but it also has a slight direct depolarizing action. In addition, oxytocin can 'prime' dendritic stores of oxytocin, making them more available for subsequent activity-dependent release. The consequence of these factors appears to be that during suckling, oxytocin cells become less responsive to external inputs but increasingly capable of mutual excitation.

The amount of oxytocin secreted as a result of a burst is very large even considering the high rate of spike activity. This is because the nerve terminals in the posterior pituitary show a marked 'frequency facilitation' of stimulus-secretion coupling. An action potential within a burst triggers approximately 100 times as much oxytocin secretion as an action potential that arises spontaneously between bursts. The frequency facilitation is a result in part of the nonlinear effects on exocytosis of the summation of calcium entry through voltage-dependent calcium channels opened by the depolarizing effects of action potentials at nerve terminals. In addition, action potential propagation in the axonal fields in the neural lobe is more efficient in axons that are partly depolarized as a result of potassium efflux from neighboring depolarized axons; thus, action potentials within a burst are less likely to 'fail' at branch points, and they therefore invade more of the neurosecretory terminals.

Synchronized bursting is thus a very efficient way of secreting a large bolus in a brief time. The resulting pulsatile hormone signal is also very efficient for stimulating milk let-down at the mammary gland. When exposed to continuous high concentrations of oxytocin, the myoepithelial cells of the mammary gland on which oxytocin acts desensitize rapidly and become refractory. Accordingly, pulsatile secretion is necessary for the biological efficacy of oxytocin at this site.

Oxytocin is also secreted in pulses during parturition in the rat and other mammals, including humans. Oxytocin is not essential for normal delivery in rodents because transgenic mice without oxytocin can deliver young normally. However, in the rat, the progress of parturition can be interrupted by giving oxytocin antagonists or by pharmacologically blocking oxytocin secretion. In the rat, pulsatile secretion is important for the efficient progress of delivery of the young; when endogenous oxytocin secretion is blocked, parturition is interrupted, but it can be restored by giving exogenous oxytocin. This is achieved much more efficiently by delivering oxytocin in pulses rather than by continuous infusion.

In humans, the role of oxytocin in normal delivery is less clear. In pregnancy, an enzyme that degrades oxytocin, human pregnancy oxytocinase, is highly expressed. When first appreciated, this fact was taken as evidence that oxytocin plays no physiological role in parturition in humans, although its pharmacological potency in inducing uterine contractions has long been known. However, this view has undergone some reappraisal as the importance of pulsatile patterning of secretion has become recognized; the presence of oxytocinase effectively reduces the half-life of a secreted bolus with little effect on its amplitude, and thus oxytocinase might enhance pulsatile patterning of oxytocin rather than eliminate oxytocin completely.

Although pulsatile secretion of oxytocin appears to be very important in lactation and during parturition, there are other circumstances in which oxytocin is secreted continuously. In the rat, oxytocin is secreted continuously when the plasma concentration sodium is high, and the significance of this appears to be that in the rat (but not in all mammals) oxytocin promotes sodium excretion both by a direct action at the kidney and indirectly by activating the secretion of atrial natriuretic factor from the heart. Interestingly, pulsatile oxytocin secretion is an ineffective trigger for natriuresis, apparently because this reflex requires sustained activation of the receptors. Accordingly, continuous secretion of oxytocin and pulsatile secretion of oxytocin can fulfill independent physiological roles – roles that can be combined without conflict.

Vasopressin

Vasopressin neurons, although similar in many respects to oxytocin neurons, do not generate pulsatile vasopressin release in the rat. However, they do generate bursts of activity. These 'phasic bursts' are longer, slower, and more frequent than the bursts of oxytocin cells but are not synchronized among the vasopressin cells and so give rise to continuous secretion rather than intermittent secretion of vasopressin from the posterior pituitary. The significance of the bursting appears to be that it optimizes the efficiency of vasopressin secretion from the nerve terminals of individual vasopressin neurons. Generally, in mammals, vasopressin is a cofactor regulating the secretion of ACTH (acting synergistically with corticotropin-releasing factor), but in most species this regulation is achieved by parvocellular vasopressin neurons of the paraventricular nucleus that project to the median eminence. These parvocellular neurosecretory neurons are functionally independent of the magnocellular vasopressin neurons that project to the posterior pituitary gland, and in most species the concentration of vasopressin secreted from the pituitary is too low for significant action at corticotrophs. However, in some species, notably the horse, vasopressin can be released in large pulses from the posterior pituitary, and these large pulses have an important role in regulating ACTH secretion.

Gonadotrophic Hormones

LH and FSH, coproduced in pituitary gonadotrophs, are secreted in a prominent pulsatile manner in both males and females in response to stimulation by luteinizing hormone-releasing hormone (LHRH), which is released from neurosecretory neurons that project to the median eminence. Whereas magnocellular oxytocin cells are compactly localized in the supraoptic and paraventricular nuclei, the LHRH neurons, of which there are only approximately 1000, are widely dispersed through the preopic/septal area. Nevertheless, these dispersed LHRH neurons are in direct contact with each other via contacts between their dendrites, which in the rat can extend for more than 1 mm. Just as the oxytocin cell dendrites are packed with neurosecretory vesicles, so are those of LHRH neurons, which also express LHRH receptors. Thus, it seems that, as for the oxytocin cells, the pulsatile release of LHRH is a result in part of mutual excitatory interactions between LHRH cells mediated by dendritic release of LHRH.

Again, as for the oxytocin cells, although a basic mechanism for synchronization and pulse generation resides within the LHRH network, afferent inputs to the LHRH cells determine the amplitude and frequency of the LHRH pulses. The gonadal steroids – estrogen and progesterone in the female and testosterone in the male – are powerful modulators of the patterning. The varying steroid environment of the cycling female means that the pattern of

LHRH secretion and hence LH and FSH secretion is different at different stages of the ovarian cycle. The ovarian steroids mediate negative feedback as a result of the gonadotrophic effects of LH and FSH. These negative feedback actions are exerted in the brain but apparently not on the LHRH cells; the LHRH cells express estrogen receptor-β but not estrogen receptor-α (at least not in abundance), but the inhibitory effects of estrogen appear to be mediated mainly by local GABA interneurons and by adrenergic inputs from the brain stem. These two inputs are strongly modulated by direct actions of steroids and are critically important in pulse generation (**Figure 2**).

The LHRH pulses are not transformed 'passively' into LH and FSH pulses by the pituitary gonadotrophs. First, the response of the pituitary gonadotrophs to LHRH is nonlinear: below a critical amplitude, fluctuations in LHRH release will thus be filtered out, whereas above that threshold the dose–response relationship is steep, so the pituitary will thus tend to 'digitize' the LHRH signal. Second, the synthesis of LH and FSH is regulated differentially by the pattern

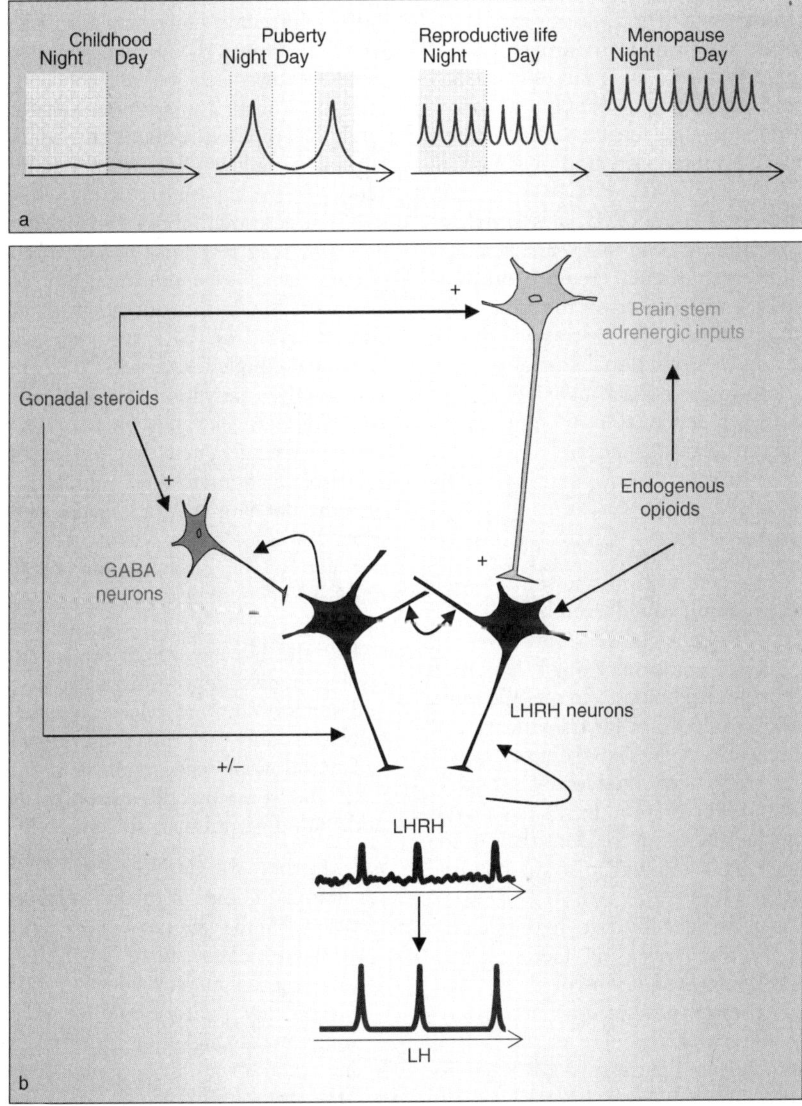

Figure 2 Pulsatile gonadotrophin secretion. (a) The pattern of LH and FSH secretion in mammals varies at different developmental stages, and in women it also varies during the ovarian cycle. (b) LHRH neurons are interconnected via their dendrites and are directly regulated by local GABA neurons, which are targets for estrogen actions. This hypothalamic mini-network is modulated by adrenergic inputs from the brain stem (among others). The resulting LHRH output is filtered and amplified by the pituitary gonadotrophs.

of stimulation by LHRH, so the relative proportions in which these two hormones are secreted will depend on the pattern of LHRH stimulation. Third, estrogen, for example, also has effects at the pituitary; it both stimulates the synthesis of LH and alters how the gonadotrophs respond to a pulsatile LHRH signal. After prolonged exposure to high concentrations of estrogen, the effects of LHRH on LH secretion display 'self-priming'; this has close parallels to the priming of oxytocin cells by oxytocin, which potentiates activity-dependent oxytocin release from the dendrites of oxytocin cells. In both cases, this priming involves a delayed and long-lasting recruitment of neurosecretory vesicles into sites from which their release by exocytosis can be readily evoked. Self-priming in estrogen-primed gonadotrophs means that successive pulses of LHRH can lead to progressively larger pulses of LH secretion, culminating in a dramatic surge release of LH at proestrous. This surge is a prerequisite for ovulation in mammals.

Pulsatile secretion of LH and FSH is essential for normal gonadal function in both males and females. The actions of LH in particular require pulsatile delivery to avoid desensitization of the peripheral targets. Thus, continuous administration of an LHRH agonist results in a functional castration, and this is exploited both for prolonged male contraception and for androgen-deprivation therapy as an adjunct to treatment of prostate cancer.

Growth Hormone

In the male rat, GH secretion from the somatotroph cells of the pituitary gland is dominated by large, 3 h pulses separated by 'troughs' of very low levels of secretion. GH is secreted in a similar pulsatile pattern in most mammals, including humans. In rats and mice, this pulsatile pattern is important for the efficiency of its growth-promoting effects; the sexual dimorphism in body size in rats is largely accounted for by a sexually dimorphic pattern of GH secretion. In the female rat, GH pulses are smaller and more frequent than in the male and the trough levels are higher, so the pulsatile pattern is less marked (**Figure 3**).

GH secretion is controlled by two hypothalamic peptides: growth hormone-releasing factor (GRF), produced by neurosecretory neurons of the arcuate nucleus, and somatostatin, produced by neurosecretory neurons of the periventricular nucleus. It is thought that the underlying pattern of GRF activity is similar in males and females, with the sexually differentiated patterns being produced by different patterns of somatostatin release. Estrogen influences somatostatin neurons, although probably not directly because somatostatin neurons do not express estrogen receptor-α.

Our understanding of pulsatile GH secretion has been limited by the paucity of information about the electrophysiological properties of these hypothalamic neurons and especially about their behavior *in vivo*. In part this is because pulsatile GH secretion does not persist under general anesthesia, which might allow the underlying processes to be observed more directly. However, it is possible to measure GRF and somatostatin release into portal blood and correlate this with GH secretion. These are invasive procedures with limited time resolution, but information from such studies, especially in sheep, has been important in supporting our understanding of GH secretion. However, our understanding mostly comes from measurements of GH concentrations in blood after experimental interventions that affect the release or actions of GRF, somatostatin, and other regulatory factors, including GH, which has negative feedback actions on the hypothalamus.

Much is known about the pituitary somatotrophs and how they respond to somatostatin, GHRH, and ghrelin, which plays an important role in regulating GH secretion by actions at both the hypothalamus and the pituitary. GRF stimulates GH secretion via G-protein-coupled receptors; the transduction pathway involves activation of adenylate cyclase and protein kinase A, elevated levels of cAMP, Ca^{2+} entry through voltage-gated channels, and Ca^{2+}-dependent exocytosis. Somatostatin inhibits GH secretion directly, but it is also a functional GRF antagonist; when somatostatin is present, GRF is less potent at stimulating GH secretion. Somatostatin acts (at separate G-protein-coupled receptors) to oppose the actions of GRF; it reduces the intracellular concentration of cAMP and hyperpolarizes the somatotrophs by increasing potassium conductance. In male rats, GRF and somatostatin are released cyclically and reciprocally to produce the peaks and troughs of GH secretion.

The following features of the pituitary response to GRF and somatostatin are particularly relevant to understanding pulsatile secretion of GH:

- GRF stimulates dose-dependent GH secretion. The sigmoidal nature of this dose–response relationship means that the pituitary acts as a 'band pass filter' for the hypothalamic signal. Small fluctuations of GRF around a low average concentration will be filtered out as below the threshold for activating GH secretion, whereas high concentrations will tend to produce an all-or-nothing secretory response.
- GH secretion in response to GRF desensitizes in a dose-dependent manner. This means that sustained high concentrations of GRF will tend to produce a transient GH response.

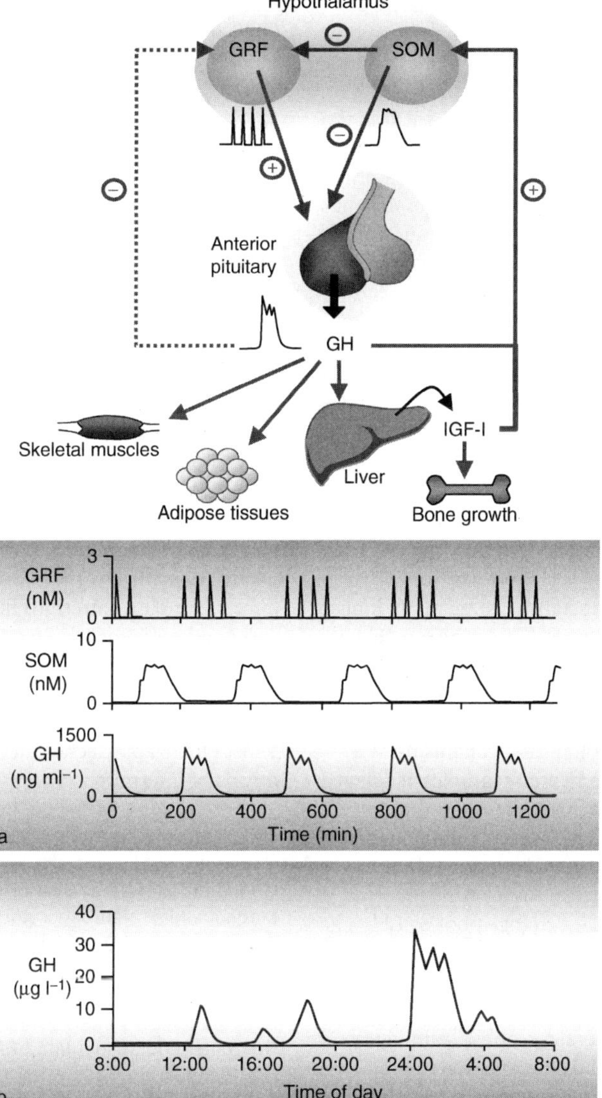

Figure 3 Pulsatile GH secretion. In humans, large pulses of GH are secreted at 3 h intervals. The magnitude of these pulses is maximal at puberty and declines slowly but progressively with age, often leading in old age to increased adiposity, bone frailty, and muscle weakening. The pulsatile pattern of GH secretion is important for its biological efficacy, and it arises as a result of a reciprocal interaction between neurosecretory somatostatin and GRF neurons, regulated by negative feedback from GH and somatomedins (particularly insulin-like growth factor 1 (IGF-I)). (a) The behavior of a computational model of the GH system. Adapted from Macgregor DJ and Leng G (2005) Modelling the hypothalamic control of growth hormone secretion. *Journal of Neuroendocrinology* 17: 788–803. (b) The typical GH profile of an adult man with 3 h pulses and a conspicuously large nocturnal pulse.

- Somatostatin inhibits GH secretion in a dose-dependent manner and can prevent desensitization to GRF; rapid removal of somatostatin causes a GRF-dependent rebound secretion of GH. This means secretion of somotostatin will tend to eliminate low levels of GH secretion and prepare the pituitary to respond to a subsequent GRF pulse.

Thus, GH secretion *in vivo* reflects the activity of hypothalamic neuroendocrine systems, acting via the pituitary, which integrates and filters these signals. These two hypothalamic systems interact; exogenous somatostatin inhibits GRF mRNA expression, and somatostatin has a fast inhibitory effect on GRF neuronal activity and release. Therefore, it seems that

GRF neurons are inhibited following increased activity in somatostatin neurons, and there might also be a complementary influence of GRF on somatostatin neurons.

In addition, GH and somatomedins feed back on the hypothalamus to inhibit the GRF neurons. Administration of GH *in vivo* inhibits GH secretion; this effect develops over approximately 1 h, and it takes another 1 or 2 h for normal secretion to recover. GH suppresses GH secretion in both male and female rats, but females continue to respond to GRF after GH injection, whereas males are unresponsive. This suggests that GH induces a prolonged, delayed release of somatostatin in the male rat but suppresses GH secretion through a different mechanism in the female. Males normally show a more variable response to GRF injections than females that is apparently related to more variable somatostatin release generally.

There is evidence that these negative feedback actions of GH are mediated by effects of GH on the somatostatin neurons; GH appears to trigger a prolonged release of somatostatin, lasting much longer than the original GH challenge. This is also a delayed effect; up to 1 h is required before GH stimulates an increase in somatostatin release. This delay seems too short to reflect changes in synthesis but too long to reflect classic electrophysiological mechanisms.

There are two other documented examples of delayed activation in peptide systems. The first is the self-priming action of LHRH at pituitary gonadotrophs, whereby LHRH potentiates its subsequent effectiveness in estrogen-primed pituitaries, and this involves a delayed mobilization of the secretory pool of LH. The second example is the priming effect of oxytocin on dendritic oxytocin release. There is no direct evidence for priming in somatostatin neurons. However, for both oxytocin neurons and gonadotrophs, priming is a delayed, long-lasting effect that is apparently mediated by mobilization of releasable pools of one peptide in response to the actions of another. A similar effect might underlie the delayed, long-lasting potentiation of somatostatin release by GH.

Synthetic GH secretagogues (GHS), like GH-releasing peptide, also promote GH secretion as GRF does but via different receptors. There are GHS receptors both on somatotrophs and in the hypothalamus, where their actions include activation of the GRF neurons. *In vivo*, GRF and GHS act synergistically; GH secretion is greater when GRF and GHS are applied together than when applied separately. The endogenous ligand for the GHS receptor, ghrelin, is secreted mainly from the stomach and is present in the circulation at high concentrations. Ghrelin is also expressed in a subpopulation of arcuate neurons. The physiological role of ghrelin in regulating GH secretion is unclear, but the potential value of GHS in promoting pulsatile GH secretion has been noted.

Conclusions

Although neuronal networks in the hypothalamus can function as pattern generators, the anterior pituitary gland also plays a major role in filtering, amplifying, and modulating the resulting pattern of hormone secretion. It is increasingly recognized that pulsatile patterns of hormone secretion are near ubiquitous, and even hormones once considered classic endocrine hormones with little neural regulation also display biologically significant pulsatile secretion. Also, underlying the generation of these patterns are mechanisms that appear to be very similar to those which govern pituitary hormone release. The biological importance of pulsatile hormone signals has many implications, including for therapeutic interventions in conditions of hormonal insufficiency. It is difficult, if not impossible, to reproduce a complex pattern of hormonal delivery by exogenous administration. In some cases, drugs that act in the central nervous system show promise for their ability to boost the function of hypothalamic pulse generator systems to 'rejuvenate' dysfunctional systems. Other approaches include developing controlled means of intermittent drug release.

See also: Gonadal Steroid Actions on Brain; Gonadotropin, Neural and Hormonal Control; Gonadotropin-Releasing Hormone: GnRH-1 System; Magnocellular Neurosecretory System: Organization, Plasticity, Model Peptidergic Neurons; Neuroendocrine Aging: Pituitary Metabolism; Neuroendocrine Aging: Pituitary–Gonadal Axis in Males; Neuroendocrine Aging: Hypothalamic–Pituitary–Gonadal Axis in Women; Neurosecretion (Regulated Exocytosis in Neuroendocrine Cells); Oxytocin (Peripheral/Central Actions and their Regulation); Vasopressin/Oxytocin and Receptors.

Further Reading

Alexander SL, Irvine CH, and Donald RA (1996) Dynamics of the regulation of the hypothalamo-pituitary-adrenal (HPA) axis determined using a nonsurgical method for collecting pituitary venous blood from horses. *Frontiers in Neuroendocrinology* 17: 1–50.

Clarke IJ (2002) Two decades of measuring GnRH secretion. *Reproduction Supplement* 59: 1–13.

Clarke IJ and Cummins JT (1987) Pulsatility of reproductive hormones: Physiological basis and clinical implications. *Baillieres Clinical Endocrinology and Metabolism* 1(1): 1–21.

Goldbeter A and Claude D (2002) Time-patterned drug administration: Insights from a modeling approach. *Chronobiology International* 19: 157–175.

Hauffa BP (2001) Clinical implications of pulsatile hormone signals. *Growth Hormone and IGF Research* 11(supplement A): S1–S8.

Kikuchi A and Okano T (2002) Pulsatile drug release control using hydrogels. *Advanced Drug Delivery Reviews* 54: 53–77.

Leng G, Caquineau C, and Sabatier N (2005) Regulation of oxytocin secretion. *Vitamins & Hormones* 71: 27–58.

Leng G and Ludwig M (2006) Jacques Benoit Lecture. Information processing in the hypothalamus: Peptides and analogue computation. *Journal of Neuroendocrinology* 18: 379–392.

Ludwig M and Leng G (2006) Dendritic peptide release and peptide-dependent behaviours. *Nature Reviews Neuroscience* 7: 126–136.

Macgregor DJ and Leng G (2005) Modelling the hypothalamic control of growth hormone secretion. *Journal of Neuroendocrinology* 17: 788–803.

McNeilly AS, Crawford JL, Taragnat C, Nicol L, and McNeilly JR (2003) The differential secretion of FSH and LH: Regulation through genes, feedback and packaging. *Reproduction Supplement* 61: 463–476.

Porksen N (2002) The *in vivo* regulation of pulsatile insulin secretion. *Diabetologia* 45: 3–20.

Robinson IC, Gevers EF, and Bennett PA (1998) Sex differences in growth hormone secretion and action in the rat. *Growth Hormone & IGF Research* 8(supplement B): 39–47.

Russell JA, Leng G, and Douglas AJ (2003) The magnocellular oxytocin system, the fount of maternity: Adaptations in pregnancy. *Frontiers in Neuroendocrinology* 24: 27–61.

Terasawa E (2001) Luteinizing hormone-releasing hormone (LHRH) neurons: Mechanism of pulsatile LHRH release. *Vitamins & Hormones* 63: 91–129.

Veldhuis JD (1998) Neuroendocrine control of pulsatile growth hormone release in the human: Relationship with gender. *Growth Hormone & IGF Research* 8(supplement B): 49–59.

Young EA, Abelson J, and Lightman SL (2004) Cortisol pulsatility and its role in stress regulation and health. *Frontiers in Neuroendocrinology* 25: 69–76.

Sleep Oscillations

A Destexhe, Centre National de la Recherche Scientifique, Gif-sur-Yvette, France

Introduction

The discovery that the brain oscillates during sleep is almost as old as the discovery of the electroencephalogram (EEG). The first human EEG recordings reported oscillations, the type, frequency, and amplitude of which highly depend on behavioral state. In an alert, awake subject, the EEG is dominated by low-amplitude fast activity ('desynchronized EEG') with high-frequency oscillations (beta, gamma), whereas during slow-wave sleep, the EEG shifts to large-amplitude, slow oscillations. The early stage of slow-wave sleep is associated with EEG spindle waves, which occur at a frequency of 7–14 Hz. As sleep deepens, waves with slower frequencies (0.3–4 Hz), including delta waves and slow oscillations, appear and progressively dominate the EEG. During paradoxical sleep, also called rapid eye movement sleep, EEG activities resemble those of wakefulness.

The cellular bases of slow-wave sleep oscillations have been investigated since the first extracellular and intracellular recordings in mammals. The major brain regions identified are the thalamus and cerebral cortex, which are intimately linked by means of reciprocal projections. The activities of thalamic and cortical neurons during sleep have been largely documented by electrophysiological studies. The cellular mechanisms underlying these oscillations depend on many factors, such as the connectivity and intrinsic properties of the different types of thalamic and cortical neurons. To determine these cellular mechanisms, it is necessary to use computational models, which are based on experimental data, and to suggest mechanisms and, if possible, predictions to test them. This type of interaction has been quite successful in the (still ongoing) exploration of the mechanisms of sleep oscillations, which this article attempts to summarize.

Sleep Spindle Oscillations

Sleep spindles are found during the early stages of sleep (sleep stage 2 in humans) and constitute an electrographic landmark for the transition from waking to sleep. Spindle oscillations consist of 7–14 Hz waxing and waning potentials, grouped in sequences lasting 1–3 s and recurring every 3–10 s. Spindle oscillations constitute an interesting and well-constrained problem to investigate by computational models for several reasons. First, these oscillations are generated in the thalamus, which is a well-known structure anatomically, with well-defined connectivity between the different cell types (see circuit in **Figure 1(a)**). Second, spindles are remarkably well documented experimentally and have been extensively characterized both *in vivo* and *in vitro*. Third, this oscillation is generated by an interplay of complex cellular properties (schematized in **Figure 1(b)**, left), such as burst firing, and synaptic interactions via multiple types of postsynaptic receptors (see **Figure 1(b)**, right). Computational models are needed to understand this complex interplay.

The typical electrophysiological features of spindle oscillations are shown in **Figure 1(c)**. The two cell types involved, thalamocortical (TC) and thalamic reticular (RE) neurons, oscillate synchronously and display burst discharges according to a mirror image: RE cells display bursts following excitatory postsynaptic potentials while TC cells burst following inhibitory postsynaptic potentials. While RE cells tend to burst at every cycle of the oscillation, TC cells produce bursts only once every few cycles. These features are typical of spindles recorded in thalamic neurons in different mammals.

Several hypotheses for the genesis of oscillations by thalamic circuits have been proposed. These involve reciprocal synaptic interactions between TC neurons and local inhibitory interneurons, loops between TC and RE neurons, or loops within the RE nucleus. The involvement of the RE nucleus was firmly demonstrated in a series of experiments by Steriade's group. In particular, the deafferented RE nucleus *in vivo* can exhibit spindle rhythmicity in extracellular recordings. In contrast, the RE nucleus does not display autonomous oscillations *in vitro*, but spindles have been observed in thalamic slices based on TC–RE interactions. These *in vitro* spindles display the same intracellular features as *in vivo* (**Figure 1(c)**).

To attempt clarifying these contrasting results, the genesis of spindle oscillations was investigated with computational models. First, models investigated whether the RE nucleus is capable of displaying oscillations consistent with experiments. Models found that RE neurons interacting through γ-aminobutyricacidergic (GABAergic) synapses can generate spindle rhythmicity and suggested different mechanisms. GABAergic interactions between RE neurons can make them oscillate synchronously through mutual inhibitory rebound interactions, either with slow GABAergic synapses or with fast ($GABA_A$ receptor-mediated) GABAergic synapses with extended connectivity. Synchronized oscillations can also be generated

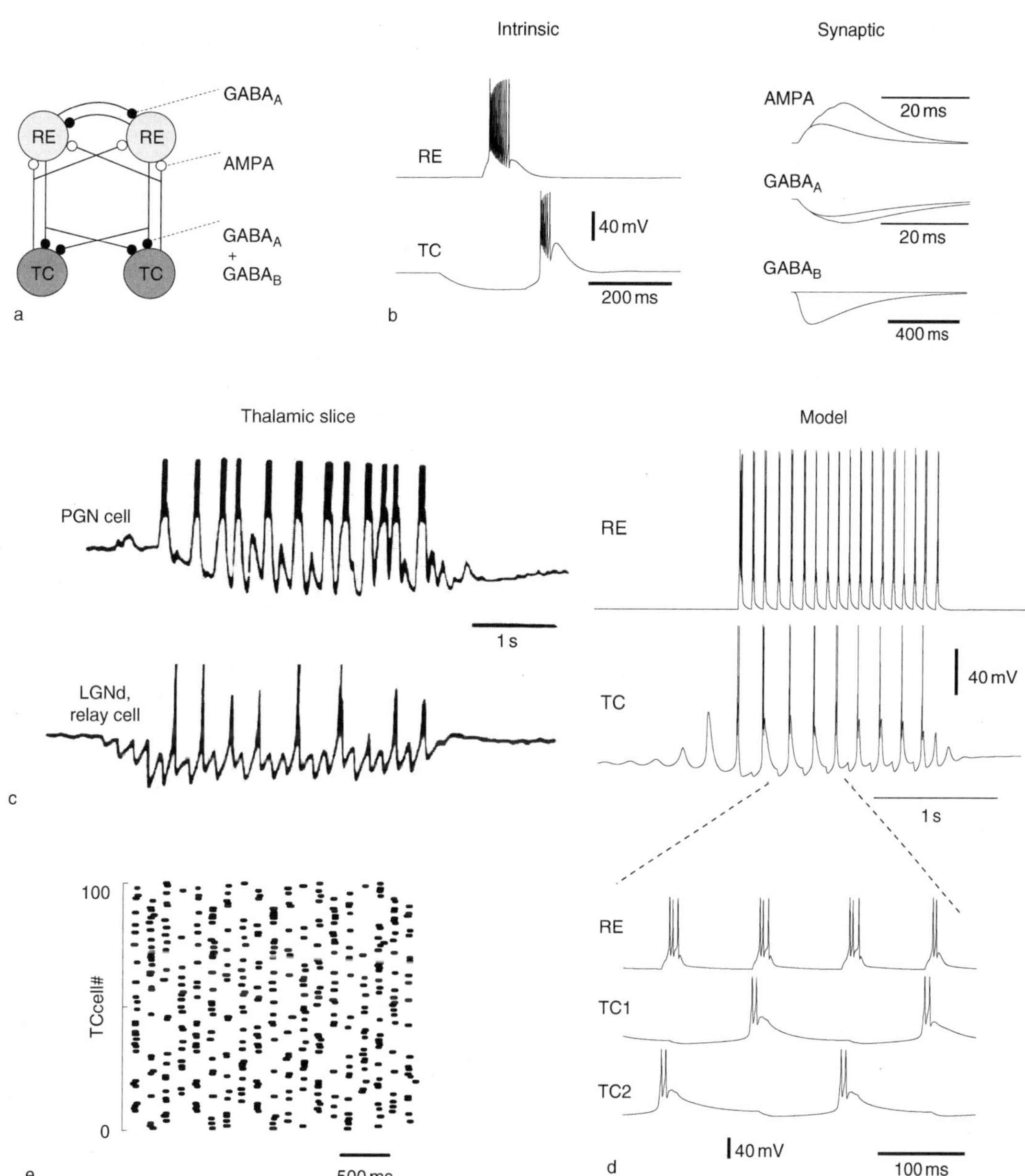

Figure 1 Modeling the interactions between intrinsic and synaptic properties to generate spindle oscillations. (a) Circuit of interconnected thalamocortical (TC) and thalamic reticular (RE) neurons with different receptor types. (b) Models of the intrinsic properties of thalamic neurons (left) and of the synaptic receptor types (right) mediating their interactions. (c) *In vitro* recordings of TC (LGNd) and RE (PGN) neurons from the visual thalamus during spindle oscillations. (d) Computational model of spindle oscillations in circuits of interconnected TC and RE cells. The expanded trace below shows the phase relations of the two cell types. (e) Phase relations of TC cells during spindle oscillations in a different computational model. AMPA, α-amino-3-hydroxy-5-methyl-4-isoxazole propionic acid; GABA$_A$, γ-aminobutyric acid class A receptor; LGN, lateral geniculate nucleus; LGNd, dorsal lateral geniculate nucleus; PGN, perigeniculate nucleus. (a, b, d) From Destexhe A, Bal T, McCormick DA, and Sejnowski TJ (1996) Ionic mechanisms underlying synchronized oscillations and propagating waves in a model of ferret thalamic slices. *Journal of Neurophysiology* 76: 2049–2070. (c) From von Krosigk M, Bal T, and McCormick DA (1993) Cellular mechanisms of a synchronized oscillation in the thalamus. *Science* 261: 361–364. (e) From Wang XJ, Golomb D, and Rinzel J (1995) Emergent spindle oscillations and intermittent burst firing in a thalamic model: Specific neuronal mechanisms. *Proceedings of the National Academy of Sciences of the United States of America* 92: 5577–5581.

from RE neurons connected with depolarizing GABAergic synapses. The presence of gap junctions in the reticular nucleus was also incorporated in models and also reinforced its propensity to oscillate in the spindle frequency range. Thus, models suggest that the intrinsic properties of thalamic RE neurons, combined with their synaptic or electrical interactions, support the RE pacemaker hypothesis.

Second, models including TC and RE cells showed that spindle oscillations can also be obtained from TC–RE loops. This TC–RE loop model is shown in **Figure 1(d)**. Neurons were modeled using Hodgkin–Huxley type representations of Na^+, K^+, and Ca^{2+} voltage-dependent currents, which were based on voltage-clamp data on thalamic neurons. These models reproduced the most salient intrinsic properties of thalamic neurons, such as the production of bursts of action potentials (**Figure 1(b)**). Synaptic interactions were modeled with conductance-based kinetic models, which were used to simulate the main receptor types (α-amino-3-hydroxy-5-methyl-4-isoxazole propionic acid (AMPA), $GABA_A$, and $GABA_B$) identified in thalamic circuits (**Figure 1(b)**, right). Under these conditions, the circuit generated 7–14 Hz spindle oscillations with the typical features identified intracellularly in the different thalamic neuron types. The model reproduced the typical mirror image between TC and RE cells during spindles, as well as the phase relations between cells (see **Figure 1(d)**). In particular, TC cells produced bursts once every two or three cycles, a feature consistently observed experimentally (compare with **Figure 1(c)**). More-irregular behavior, similar to the experiments, was obtained in larger networks (**Figure 1(e)**) or in the presence of the cortex (see the section titled 'Propagation or large-scale synchrony'). The oscillations also showed the typical waxing-and-waning envelope of spindles; this property was due in the model to Ca^{2+}-mediated slow regulation of the hyperpolarization-activated current, a prediction that was verified experimentally.

Thus, models show that the complex bursting properties of thalamic neurons, combined with their interactions through well-defined types of synaptic receptors, account for both RE pacemaker oscillations and spindle oscillations arising from TC–RE loops without assuming pacemaker activity in the RE nucleus. How may such an apparent inconsistency be resolved? This question was addressed by a computational model of the RE nucleus which took into account the action of neuromodulators (such as noradrenaline) in depolarizing RE cells. This model produced oscillations only when a sufficient level of neuromodulator was present. The difference between *in vivo* and *in vitro* preparations may therefore be explained by the limited connectivity between the RE neurons in the slice and/or by the fact that slices lack the necessary level of neuromodulation to maintain isolated RE oscillations. The main prediction from this model is that applying neuromodulators to slices of the RE nucleus should induce oscillations similar to those observed *in vivo*. This prediction still awaits testing.

Propagation or Large-Scale Synchrony?

How spindle oscillations are initiated and distributed in large circuits was investigated with multiple recordings *in vivo* and *in vitro*. Spindle oscillations *in vitro* showed traveling wave patterns, with the oscillation typically starting on one side of the slice and propagating to the other side, at a constant propagation velocity. Traveling spindle waves were simulated by computational models of networks of interconnected TC and RE cells (one-dimensional extensions of the circuit shown in **Figure 1**), in two independent modeling studies. These models were similar in spirit to the circuit shown in **Figure 1(a)** but assumed that there was a topographic connectivity between TC and RE layers, consistent with anatomical data. Under these conditions, the models generated traveling waves consistent with *in vitro* data.

However, in contrast to thalamic slices, the intact TC system *in vivo* does not display clear-cut propagation, but spindle oscillations are synchronized over extended thalamic regions and show little signs for traveling wave activity (**Figure 2(a)**). This large-scale synchrony was lost when the cortex was removed, suggesting that although the oscillation is generated by the thalamus, its synchrony depends on the cortex. To investigate the mechanism underlying large-scale synchrony, a TC network model was developed by combining the previous model of thalamic slices with a model of deep cortical layers. The principal prediction of this model was that, in order to generate large-scale coherent oscillations, the powerful action of cortex on thalamus (via corticothalamic fibers) must be included, and most important, the cortex had to recruit the thalamus primarily through the RE nucleus. Because of the powerful inhibitory action of RE cells, the action of corticothalamic input is 'inhibitory dominant' on TC cells, a property essential to maintain large-scale synchrony by synchronizing the rebound bursts of TC cells. This property of inhibitory dominance is generally observed intracellularly in thalamic neurons when the cortex is stimulated. In these conditions, the same model was capable of generating large-scale synchrony in the presence of the cortex, as well as traveling wave activity in the isolated thalamus (**Figure 2(b)**). Consistent with these models, propagating activity has indeed been observed in the thalamus of decorticated cats *in vivo*.

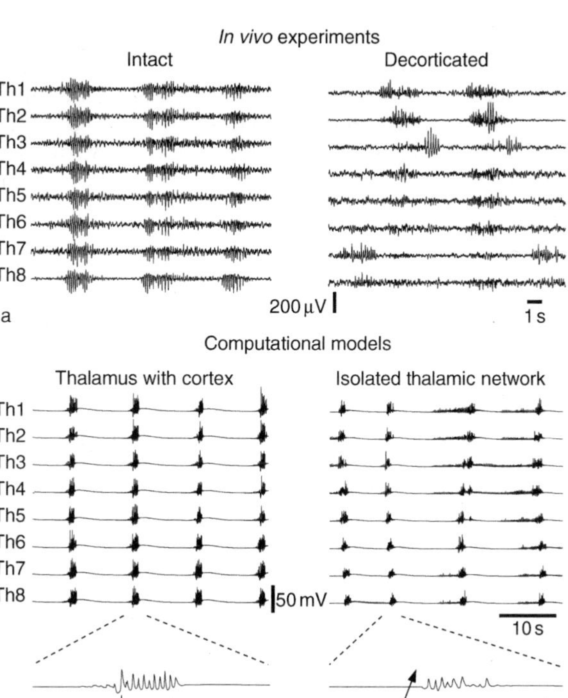

Figure 2 Modeling the large-scale synchrony of spindle oscillations. (a) Multiple extracellular field potential recordings (Th1 ... Th8) in the thalamus of cats *in vivo*. In the intact thalamocortical system (Intact), the oscillations were synchronized over large distances (7 mm between Th1 and Th8). After removal of the cortex (Decorticated), the large-scale synchrony was largely abolished. (b) Computational models of thalamocortical networks displaying large-scale synchrony when cortex was present (left) and local synchrony with traveling-wave activity in the isolated thalamus (right). (a) Adapted from Contreras D, Destexhe A, Sejnowski TJ, and Steriade M (1996) Control of spatiotemporal coherence of a thalamic oscillation by corticothalamic feedback. *Science* 274. 771–774. (b) Adapted from Destexhe A, Contreras D, and Steriade M (1998) Mechanisms underlying the synchronizing action of corticothalamic feedback through inhibition of thalamic relay cells. *Journal of Neurophysiology* 79: 999–1016.

The cortical control of thalamic relay cells through dominant inhibitory mechanisms has important consequences, not only for explaining large-scale synchrony, but also for explaining pathological situations such as absence epileptic seizures. As a result of inhibitory dominance, a too strong corticothalamic feedback can overactivate thalamic $GABA_B$ receptors and entrain the physiologically intact thalamus into hypersynchronous rhythms at ~3 Hz. This scheme may explain the genesis of absence seizures, which are hypersynchronous ~3 Hz rhythms that appear suddenly in the TC system. These seizures can be provoked experimentally by increasing cortical excitability in a physiologically intact thalamus. The TC model accounts for those experiments and can simulate seizures based on inhibitory-dominant corticothalamic feedback. This model directly predicted that manipulating corticothalamic feedback should entrain intact thalamic circuits to generate hypersynchronous rhythms at ~3 Hz, a prediction verified by two independent studies. A similar mechanism, with a different balance between $GABA_A$ and $GABA_B$ receptors, can also generate faster hypersynchronous rhythms (around 5–10 Hz), as observed in rat or mouse experimental models of absence seizures.

Slow-Wave Oscillations

During the deepest phases of sleep (stages 3 and 4 in humans), as well as for some anesthetized states, cortical activity is dominated by delta and slow oscillations, in a frequency range of 0.3–4 Hz. The intracellular correlate of these slow waves is the alternation between depolarized states (up states) and hyperpolarized states (down states), which occurs in perfect synchrony with the EEG (**Figure** 3(**c**)). Thus, entire cortical regions are simultaneously switching between up and down states, as also shown by multiple extracellular studies. The origin of these oscillations seems to be cortical because they survive extensive thalamic lesions, and they are also observed in cortical slices.

One of the interesting features of up states is that this activity is very similar to that during the awake state. This is supported by several observations. First, during the up state, the EEG is of low amplitude, and fast activity is similar to desynchronized EEG. Second, extracellular recordings have shown that the up states obey the same dynamics of firing, have similar local correlations, and display similar relations between EEG and unit firing as wakefulness does. Third, simulating nuclei participating in the ascending arousal system induces periods of desynchronized EEG corresponding intracellularly to prolonged up states. Fourth, conductance measurements from intracellular recordings in anesthetized or EEG-activated states show similar conductance patterns during both states. The absolute conductance is lower in activated states than in up states, but both states are characterized by similar ratios between excitatory and inhibitory conductances. Fifth, computational models of up/down states and of activated states in cortical circuits suggest that both can be generated by similar mechanisms.

Computational models have investigated the genesis of slow-wave oscillations and the associated up- or down-state patterns. These models were based on recurrent circuits of excitatory and inhibitory cortical neurons (**Figure** 3(**a**)). The two main electrophysiological types of cortical neurons were considered, as well as their synaptic interactions through glutamate (AMPA) and GABAergic ($GABA_A$) receptors (**Figure** 3(**b**)). These models showed that up states can be generated by recurrent excitatory and inhibitory connections, which self-sustain the activity (**Figure** 3(**d**)). Different exact mechanisms by which up states begin and terminate have been proposed. Up states can start either by the interaction between subthreshold Na currents (persistent Na current) and miniature excitatory synaptic potentials. Another possible mechanism is spontaneously active cells that would initiate the wave of activity in the network. In either case, none of the mechanisms has been verified experimentally. The termination of the up state is apparently due to a progressive run down of synaptic activity, as indicated by conductance measurements. What causes this run down could be either an intrinsic property, such as the progressive buildup of a slow potassium conductance, or simply depression of excitatory synapses. Both hypotheses are supported by experimental data and are also consistent with the refractoriness of the up states found in slices (this refractoriness could be due to the potassium conductance, or recovery from synaptic depression).

Another property of up/down states is that the duration of the down state is proportional to network size. Down states are typically short *in vivo* (a few hundred milliseconds) whereas they can last up to 20 s in slices. Cutting cortical slabs of different sizes *in vivo* confirmed that the down-state duration varies inversely in proportion to slab size. Here again, this property is consistent with the two mechanisms of initiation outlined above as they both depend on coincident activation of either miniature or spontaneously active cells, both of which will occur more often in large networks.

Models were also used to simulate the transition to the sustained and irregular firing activity during wakefulness. Self-sustained irregular states similar to activated states have been simulated by various models. Only a few models, however, provided the transition from up/down states to activated states. For all such models, up states and activated states are very similar and differ only by the level of excitability of the neurons (mostly by downregulating potassium conductances). Some of these models were confronted to input resistance or conductance measurements and reproduced qualitatively the values measured experimentally. The fact that up states and activated states can be simulated with few differences by the same models is another indication that those two states stem from similar network activity.

A final property of slow waves is that the up states clearly show propagating properties *in vitro*. This propagation can be reproduced by computational models (**Figure** 3(**e**)), assuming that synaptic connections are made locally in the cortical network. In contrast, there is evidence that up states are highly synchronized *in vivo*, because the local EEG is always phase locked with intracellular activity (**Figure** 3(**a**)). Multiple extracellular recordings in natural sleep also demonstrated that the up states of slow waves are highly synchronized across distances up to 7 mm in cortex. A detailed investigation of this synchrony, and the conditions under which up states can propagate *in vivo*, as well as the modeling of such phenomena, still await.

What Is the Role of Slow-Wave Sleep Oscillations?

As mentioned above, the up states during slow waves share many different features of the sustained activity during wakefulness, and thus, up states can be viewed

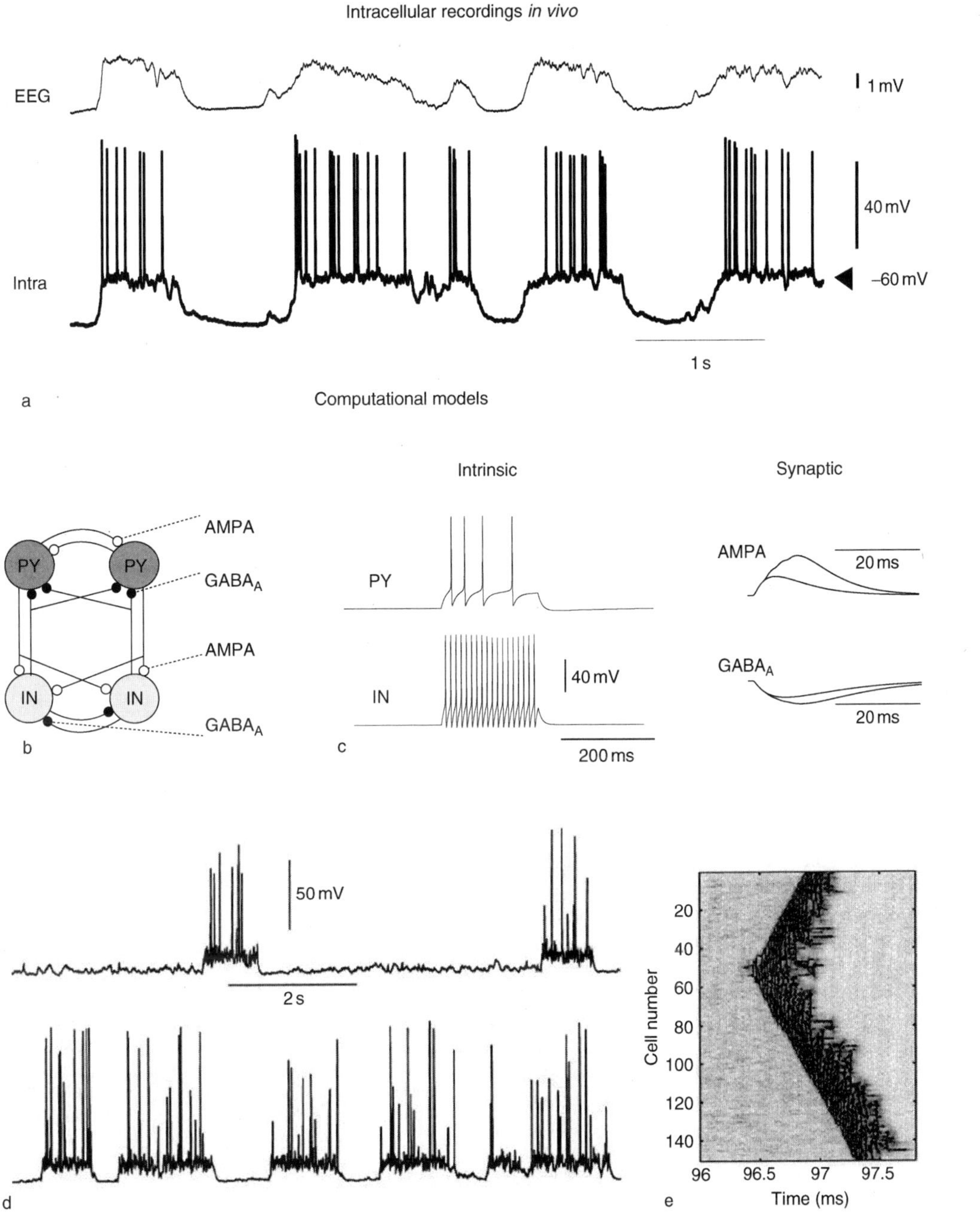

Figure 3 Computational models of slow-wave oscillations in cerebral cortex. (a) *In vivo* recordings of a morphologically identified pyramidal neuron during slow waves. (b) Schematic circuit showing the two main types of cortical neurons, pyramidal cells (PY) and inhibitory interneurons (IN). Those neurons are connected via different types of synaptic receptors, with the two main types illustrated here. (c) Models of the intrinsic properties of cortical neurons (left) and of the synaptic receptor types (right) mediating their interactions. (d) Computational model of slow-wave oscillations arising from reverberation of activity through recurrent connections in networks of cortical circuits. The network displays up and down states with different frequency of occurrence, depending on the level of spontaneous activity. (e) Snapshot of activity in the network, showing the initiation and propagation of the up state. AMPA, α-amino-3-hydroxy-5-methyl-4-isoxazole propionic acid; GABA$_A$, γ-aminobutyric acid class A receptor. (a) Adapted from Rudolph M, Pelletier J-G, Paré D, and Destexhe A (2005) Characterization of synaptic conductances and integrative properties during electrically-induced EEG-activated states in neocortical neurons *in vivo*. *Journal of Neurophysiology* 94: 2805–2821. (d, e) Adapted from Timofeev I, Grenier F, Bazhenov M, Sejnowski TJ, and Steriade M (2000) Origin of slow cortical oscillations in deafferented cortical slabs. *Cerebral Cortex* 10: 1185–1199.

as brief periods of activity in which network dynamics are very similar to the dynamics during wakefulness. This is consistent with the fact that up states would represent 'replayed' events that have occurred previously during the wake state. There is abundant experimental evidence, from birds to higher mammals, for such a replay during sleep.

Why would such a replay occur during sleep and not during wakefulness? There is presently no clear answer to this question, but it was proposed that another type of sleep oscillation, sleep spindles, may be implicated in gating of long-term plasticity mechanisms (for example, permanent changes that require protein synthesis). Computational models of reconstructed pyramidal neurons, combined with intracellular measurements of thalamic inputs during spindles, have shown that the pattern of synaptic bombardment during spindles in the cortex is a strong excitatory-driven depolarization in dendrites, with an equally strong inhibition around the soma, preventing the cell from excessive firing. This pattern is likely to induce massive calcium entry at around 10 Hz in the dendrites, which is an ideal signal to activate molecular gates, such as protein kinase A. Sleep spindles would therefore provide a physiological signal similar to the repeated tetanus used to induce long-term synaptic changes in slices. However, instead of inducing potentiation directly, spindles may in fact provide a 'priming' signal, opening a gate that allows permanent changes to subsequent inputs ('replayed' events mentioned earlier) following the sleep spindles.

Taking those two observations together leads to the following scenario for how these different mechanisms may contribute to memory consolidation during sleep. During conscious experience, latent memories are formed throughout the cortex, together with links to the hippocampal formation that allow top-down retrieval to occur. During the early stages of sleep, spindle oscillations would mobilize the molecular machinery needed for memory consolidation in cortex. In the deeper phases of slow-wave sleep, during the brief periods of wakelike activities (up states), the hippocampal formation would activate latent memories stored in the neocortex ('replay') and induce permanent changes in intrinsic or synaptic conductances. This hypothetical mechanism of memory consolidation during sleep is consistent with all electrophysiological characteristics of sleep oscillations, and it predicts that special correlations between hippocampal and cortical activities should occur during the up states of slow waves. Such correlations have been found recently between cortical slow waves (up states) and hippocampal sharp waves. No computational model has been proposed to date to explain these observations, and certainly they constitute one of the most exciting directions to pursue toward exploring the role of sleep oscillations.

See also: Electroencephalography (EEG); Electrophysiology: EEG and ERP Analysis; Epilepsy; Executive Function and Higher-Order Cognition: EEG Studies; Gap Junctions and Neuronal Oscillations; Sleep and Sleep States: Thalamic Regulation; Sleep Oscillations and PGO Waves; Sleep-Dependent Memory Processing.

Further Reading

Bal T, Debay D, and Destexhe A (2000) Cortical feedback controls the frequency and synchrony of oscillations in the visual thalamus. *Journal of Neuroscience* 20: 7478–7488.

Battaglia FP, Sutherland GR, and McNaughton BL (2004) Hippocampal sharp wave bursts coincide with neocortical "up-state" transitions. *Learning & Memory* 11: 697–704.

Bazhenov M, Timofeev I, Steriade M, and Sejnowski TJ (2002) Model of thalamocortical slowwave sleep oscillations and transitions to activated states. *Journal of Neuroscience* 22: 8691–8704.

Blumenfeld H and McCormick DA (2000) Corticothalamic inputs control the pattern of activity generated in thalamocortical networks. *Journal of Neuroscience* 20: 5153–5162.

Compte A, Sanchez-Vives MV, McCormick DA, and Wang XJ (2003) Cellular and network mechanisms of slow oscillatory activity (<1 Hz) and wave propagations in a cortical network model. *Journal of Neurophysiology* 89: 2707–2725.

Contreras D, Destexhe A, Sejnowski TJ, and Steriade M (1996) Control of spatiotemporal coherence of a thalamic oscillation by corticothalamic feedback. *Science* 274: 771–774.

Contreras D, Timofeev I, and Steriade M (1996) Mechanisms of long lasting hyperpolarizations underlying slow sleep oscillations in cat corticothalamic networks. *Journal of Physiology* 494: 251–264.

Destexhe A (1998) Spike-and-wave oscillations based on the properties of $GABA_B$ receptors. *Journal of Neuroscience* 18: 9099–9111.

Destexhe A, Bal T, McCormick DA, and Sejnowski TJ (1996) Ionic mechanisms underlying synchronized oscillations and propagating waves in a model of ferret thalamic slices. *Journal of Neurophysiology* 76: 2049–2070.

Destexhe A, Contreras D, Sejnowski TJ, and Steriade M (1994) A model of spindle rhythmicity in the isolated thalamic reticular nucleus. *Journal of Neurophysiology* 72: 803–818.

Destexhe A, Contreras D, Sejnowski TJ, and Steriade M (1994) Modeling the control of reticular thalamic oscillations by neuromodulators. *NeuroReport* 5: 2217–2220.

Destexhe A, Contreras D, and Steriade M (1998) Mechanisms underlying the synchronizing action of corticothalamic feedback through inhibition of thalamic relay cells. *Journal of Neurophysiology* 79: 999–1016.

Destexhe A, Contreras D, and Steriade M (1999) Spatiotemporal analysis of local field potentials and unit discharges in cat cerebral cortex during natural wake and sleep states. *Journal of Neuroscience* 19: 4595–4608.

Destexhe A and Sejnowski TJ (2001) *Thalamocortical Assemblies.* Oxford, UK: Oxford University Press.

Destexhe A and Sejnowski TJ (2003) Interactions between membrane conductances underlying thalamocortical slow-wave oscillations. *Physiological Reviews* 83: 1401–1453.

Gloor P and Fariello RG (1988) Generalized epilepsy: Some of its cellular mechanisms differ from those of focal epilepsy. *Trends in Neurosciences* 11: 63–68.

Hodgkin AL and Huxley AF (1952) A quantitative description of membrane current and its application to conduction and excitation in nerve. *Journal of Physiology* 117: 500–544.

Kim U, Bal T, and McCormick DA (1995) Spindle waves are propagating synchronized oscillations in the ferret LGNd *in vitro*. *Journal of Neurophysiology* 74: 1301–1323.

Landisman CE, Long MA, Beierlein M, Deans MR, Paul DL, and Connors BW (2002) Electrical synapses in the thalamic reticular nucleus. *Journal of Neuroscience* 22: 1002–1009.

Ribeiro S, Gervasoni D, Soares ES, et al. (2004) Long-lasting novelty-induced neuronal reverberation during slow-wave sleep in multiple forebrain areas. *PLoS Biology* 2: 126–137.

Rudolph M, Pelletier J-G, Paré D, and Destexhe A (2005) Characterization of synaptic conductances and integrative properties during electrically-induced EEG-activated states in neocortical neurons in vivo. *Journal of Neurophysiology* 94: 2805–2821.

Sanchez-Vives MV and McCormick DA (2000) Cellular and network mechanisms of rhythmic recurrent activity in neocortex. *Nature Neuroscience* 3: 1027–1034.

Sirota A, Csicsvari J, Buhl D, and Buzsaki G (2003) Communication between neocortex and hippocampus during sleep in rodents. *Proceedings of the National Academy of Sciences of the United States of America* 100: 2065–2069.

Steriade M (2003) *Neuronal Substrates of Sleep and Epilepsy.* Cambridge, UK: Cambridge University Press.

Steriade M, McCormick DA, and Sejnowski TJ (1993) Thalamocortical oscillations in the sleeping and aroused brain. *Science* 262: 679–685.

Timofeev I, Grenier F, Bazhenov M, Sejnowski TJ, and Steriade M (2000) Origin of slow cortical oscillations in deafferented cortical slabs. *Cerebral Cortex* 10: 1185–1199.

von Krosigk M, Bal T, and McCormick DA (1993) Cellular mechanisms of a synchronized oscillation in the thalamus. *Science* 261: 361–364.

Wang XJ, Golomb D, and Rinzel J (1995) Emergent spindle oscillations and intermittent burst firing in a thalamic model: Specific neuronal mechanisms. *Proceedings of the National Academy of Sciences of the United States of America* 92: 5577–5581.

Wang XJ and Rinzel J (1993) Spindle rhythmicity in the reticularis thalami nucleus: Synchronization among inhibitory neurons. *Neuroscience* 53: 899–904.

Relevant Website

http://senselab.med.yale.edu – ModelDB, database of freely available model codes, some of which simulate sleep oscillations.

Sleep Oscillations and PGO Waves

M Steriade, Université Laval, Laval, QC, Canada

Behavioral and Electrographic Signs of Sleep Stages

Sleep Onset

The popular view that behavioral quiescence is the sign that heralds sleep may be valid for the full-blown state of sleep but not for the preparatory period during which many animal species display complex motor behaviors directed to find a safe home for sleep. The defining signs of the period when one falls asleep are changes in brain electrical activity (electroencephalogram (EEG)) that are associated with long periods of inhibition in neurons located in the thalamus, a deep structure in the brain and a gateway for most sensory signals in their route to the cerebral cortex. The consequence is that the incoming messages are blocked in the thalamus and the cerebral cortex is deprived of information from the outside world.

In contrast with the rapid awakening from sleep, the period of falling asleep is quite long. Thus, sleep onset may not be exclusively attributable to neuronal mechanisms, which operate on short timescales. It is conceivable that the mechanisms of falling sleep will only be revealed with concerted studies on sleep humoral factors (acting on longer timescale) and on their actions on neurons in critical brain areas. Currently, little is known about the effects of sleep-promoting chemical substances on neurons. The list of putative sleep humoral factors is quite long. Some of them are (1) adenosine, which exerts a tonic inhibitory control on both upper brain stem and basal forebrain cholinergic activating (awakening) neurons; (2) muramyl peptides, which have a chemical structure that is similar to that of serotonin, a neurotransmitter that was implicated in the generation of early sleep stages; and (3) prostaglandin D_2, whose receptors are found in the anterior hypothalamus, thought to be a critical zone for promoting sleep.

The concepts postulating that sleep is a passive phenomenon due to closure of cerebral gates leading to brain deafferentation or, alternatively, an active phenomenon promoted by inhibitory mechanisms arising in some cerebral areas have long been considered as opposing views. However, neurons with inhibitory influences (located in the anterior hypothalamus) act on neurons that exert excitatory influences on the brain (located in the posterior hypothalamus and upper brain stem reticular core), and the final outcome of these relations is the disconnection of the forebrain. Therefore, the two mechanisms (active and passive) of sleep onset are probably successive steps within a chain of events, and they are complementary rather than opposed.

Slow-Wave and Rapid Eye Movement Sleep

Sleep consists of an alternation between two distinct stages. The early stage is characterized by large-scale synchronization of low-frequency EEG activity (0.5–15 Hz), which is generated by the cerebral cortex and thalamus. Synchronization is a state in which two or more oscillators display the same frequency because of mutual influences. The notion of synchronization supposes the coactivation as well as concerted inhibitory processes in a large number of neurons. The summation of neuronal activities is sufficiently large to be recorded with gross electrodes, such as scalp electrodes when recording the human EEG. Because of the prevalent low-frequency waves, this stage is termed slow-wave sleep. This electrophysiological feature is associated with behavioral quiescence and suspension of conscious processes related to the external world because the transmission of signals is inhibited in the thalamus, even before these signals reach the cerebral cortex, the highest site of consciousness. However, not all mental processes are obliterated during slow-wave sleep because the brain oscillations that occur during this stage give rise to synaptic plasticity that underlies processes through which information is stored, such as consolidation of memory traces acquired during the state of wakefulness. Also, a peculiar form of dreaming mentation is present during slow-wave sleep.

The second stage of sleep is associated with rapid eye movements (REMs) and the sign that distinguishes it from the other two states of vigilance (slow-wave sleep and waking) is the largely suppressed motor output (muscular atonia) due to inhibition of spinal motor neurons. In addition, spiky potentials (ponto-geniculo-occipital (PGO) waves), related to ocular saccades, can be recorded from the thalamus and cortex and are regarded as the physiological correlate of dreaming. This state was also termed active because the level of brain alertness is similar to, or even higher than, the state of wakefulness. (This should not imply, however, that slow-wave sleep is inactive from the standpoint of brain functions since neuronal recordings have shown that cortical neurons fire during this stage at almost the same level as during waking.) Thus, REM sleep is a brain-active state associated with paralysis of limbs' muscles. In other words, motor commands from a highly excitable cerebral cortex cannot be executed because of the inhibition of motor neurons in the spinal cord. Although REM sleep seems very similar to wakefulness because of intense brain activity, some differences also exist between these two states, mainly due to more effective inhibitory processes in waking and the virtual silence of monoaminergic neurons. This might explain the psychological differences between the logical thought in waking and the bizarre, illogical, and emotional content of dreaming in REM sleep.

Sleep Oscillations: Sites of Generation and Cellular Mechanisms

Three Major Oscillations Define Slow-Wave Sleep

The brain rhythms that characterize slow-wave sleep are the slow oscillation (0.5–1 Hz) that appears from the onset of full-blown sleep; spindles (7–15 Hz), whose amplitudes are highest during stage 2 of slow-wave sleep; and delta waves (1–4 Hz), which appear in stages 3 and 4, when their great amplitudes may obscure spindles.

The slow oscillation was first described using intracellular recordings from different neuronal types in anesthetized animals and, in the same article, was also detected in EEG recordings during natural slow-wave sleep in humans in which cyclic groups of delta waves at 1–4 Hz recurred with a slow periodicity of 0.4 or 0.5 Hz. The distinctness between delta and slow oscillations also came from human studies showing that the typical decline in delta activity (1–4 Hz) from the first to the second sleep episode was not present at frequencies characteristic for the slow oscillation (range, 0.55–0.95 Hz). The cortical nature of the slow oscillation was demonstrated by its survival in the cerebral cortex after large thalamic lesions and its absence in the thalamus of decorticated animals. This rhythm was recorded in all major types of neocortical neurons, including pyramidal-shaped and local circuit inhibitory neurons. The slow oscillation is composed of a prolonged depolarizing ('up') phase followed by a long-lasting hyperpolarizing ('down') phase. The hyperpolarizations of cortical neurons occur from the onset of sleep and distinguish sleep from the steady depolarization seen during waking (**Figure 1**). The depolarizing phase consists of excitatory postsynaptic potentials (EPSPs), some intrinsic excitatory currents, and also inhibitory postsynaptic potentials (IPSPs) that reflect the action of synaptically coupled local

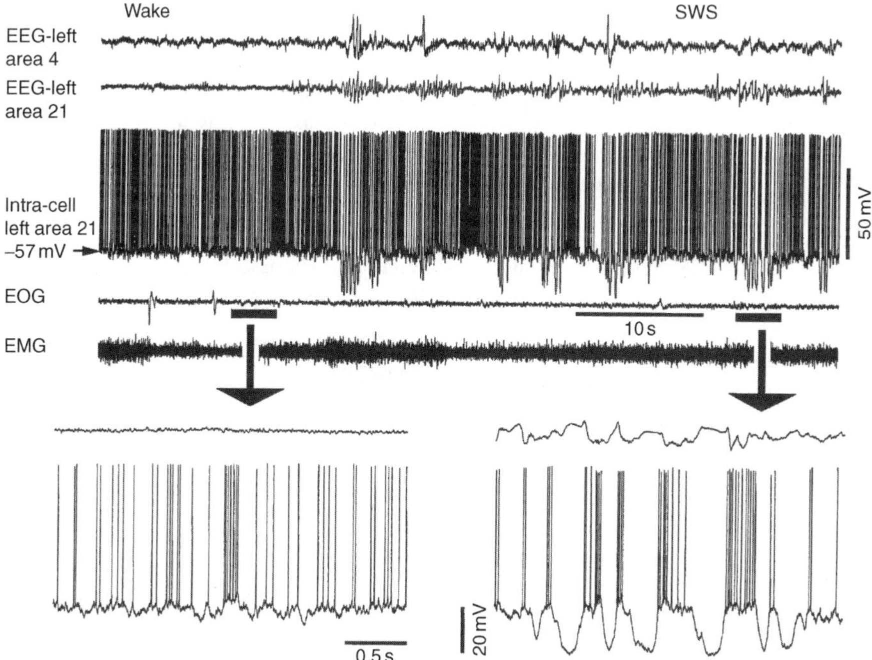

Figure 1 The slow oscillation marks the difference between waking and slow-wave sleep (SWS). Intracellular recording of regular-spiking neuron from left cortical area 21 of chronically implanted cat, together with depth EEG from left areas 4 and 21, electrooculogram (EOG), and electromyogram (EMG). Transition from waking to SWS. Two epochs, one in waking and the other in SWS, are marked by horizontal traces (below EOG) and expanded below (arrows). Note the occurrence of episodic cyclic hyperpolarizations of the slow oscillation since the very onset of SWS, as indicated by EEG.

circuit GABAergic neurons. The hyperpolarizing (silent) phase is not produced by inhibitory interneurons but is due to disfacilitation (removal of synaptic, mainly excitatory, inputs) in intracortical and thalamocortical networks and also to some K^+ currents.

Sleep spindles are waxing-and-waning waves, grouped in sequences that recur every 2–5 s. They are generated in the thalamus, even in the absence of the cerebral cortex, but corticothalamic neurons have a decisive role in the near simultaneity of spindles over widespread thalamic and cortical territories. The pacemaker of spindles is the thalamic reticular nucleus, which consists exclusively of inhibitory (GABAergic) neurons. In the absence of this nucleus, spindles are not seen in the remaining thalamus and cortex, but this oscillation is present in the deafferented reticular nucleus. The cellular mechanisms underlying spindles are as follows. At each spindle wave, thalamic reticular neurons fire spike bursts that impose IPSPs on their targets, thalamocortical neurons. Following IPSPs, thalamocortical neurons discharge postinhibitory rebound spike bursts that are transmitted to cortex, where they rhythmically excite cortical neurons and thus give rise to spindles. The rebound is an intrinsic property of thalamic neurons and depends on a Ca^{2+}-mediated conductance, which is inactive during waking and REM sleep when neurons are depolarized and is de-inactivated (uncovered) during slow-wave sleep when thalamocortical neurons are hyperpolarized.

Some delta waves arise in the cortex without thalamic participation. Another type of delta potentials is generated in thalamocortical neurons through interplay between two of their intrinsic properties.

Coalescence of low-frequency corticothalamic rhythms by the slow oscillation Unlike rhythms that appear within distinct frequency bands and are generated in restricted neuronal circuits of simplified experimental preparations (e.g., isolated thalamic or cortical slices maintained *in vitro* and decorticated or thalamectomized animals *in vivo*), the normal brain does not generally display separate oscillations during slow-wave sleep. Rather, it displays a coalescence of the slow oscillation with other sleep rhythms (spindles and delta) as well as with faster (beta and gamma) rhythms that are superimposed on the depolarizing phase of the slow oscillation (**Figure 2**). The circuitry and neuronal mechanisms that account for the grouping of low-frequency and fast-frequency rhythms by the slow oscillation are discussed later.

During the depolarizing phase of the slow oscillation, the synchronous firing of neocortical neurons impinges upon thalamic reticular pacemaking neurons, thus creating conditions for formation of spindles, which are transferred to thalamocortical neurons and up to cortex, at which level spindles shape the tail of the slowly oscillatory cycle (**Figure 2**, middle panel in 'slow + spindle'). This connectivity explains why a cycle of the slow oscillation is followed by a brief sequence of spindles in thalamocortical neurons and in the cortical EEG (**Figure 2**, left panel in 'slow + spindle'), as seen with intracellular recordings in animal studies as well as with EEG recordings in human slow-wave sleep. The sequence of grapho-elements consisting of an ample surface-positive transient, corresponding to the excitation in deeply lying cortical neurons, followed by a slower, surface-negative component and eventually a few spindle waves, represents the combination between the slow and spindle oscillations. It is termed the K-complex and is a reliable sign for stage 2 of human sleep, but it is apparent in all stages of slow-wave sleep. These investigations indicate that K-complexes are the expression of the spontaneously occurring, cortically generated slow oscillation, although K-complexes can also be evoked by sensory stimuli during sleep.

Why fast rhythms are also observed during slow-wave sleep The unexpected association between a slow sleep rhythm and fast oscillations that are conventionally regarded as defining the electrical activity of waking and REM sleep is explained by the voltage dependency of fast oscillations. Indeed, cortical and thalamic neurons generate beta and gamma oscillations at relatively depolarized values of the membrane potential. Thus, fast rhythms are sustained during the steady depolarization of cortical neurons during waking and REM sleep, selectively appear over the depolarizing phase of the slow sleep oscillation, and are absent during the hyperpolarizing phase of the slow oscillation (**Figure 2**). The association between slow oscillation and fast rhythms has also been reported in human sleep.

Fast Oscillations during REM Sleep and Wakefulness

Beta and gamma waves (20–80 Hz) occur spontaneously during REM sleep and waking and are evoked by intense attention, conditioned responses, tasks requiring fine movements, or sensory stimuli. Beta and gamma rhythms can interchangeably be termed fast because neurons may pass from beta to gamma oscillation in very short periods of time (0.5–1 s), with slight depolarization of cortical neurons. Studies in humans have also shown that there is no precise cutoff between the beta and gamma bands since these activities may fluctuate simultaneously, as indicated by increased activities within both beta and gamma frequency bands (20–40 Hz) during cognitive processes implicating memory. The synchronized fast

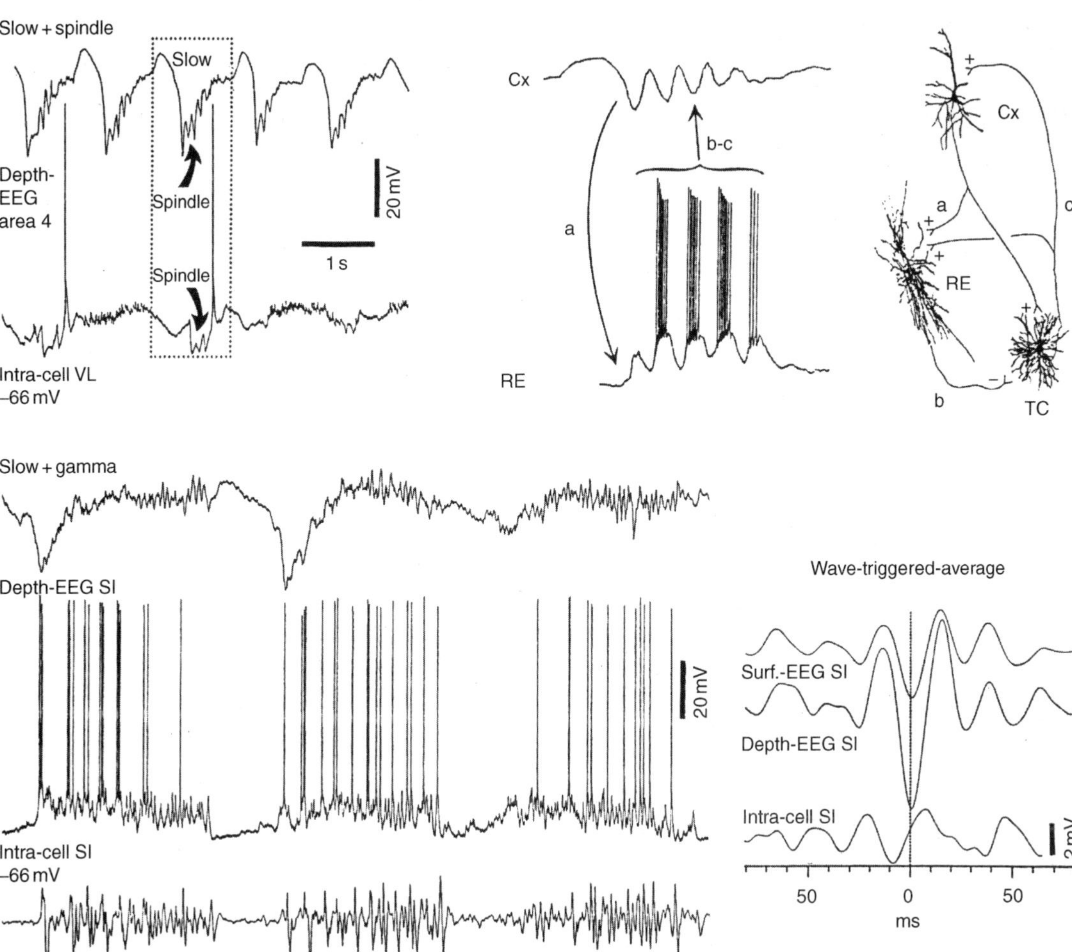

Figure 2 Coalescence of slow oscillation with spindle and gamma rhythms. Intracellular recordings from cortical and thalamic neurons in cats. Slow + spindle, combined slow oscillation and spindle. (Left) Depth EEG from cortical area 4 and intracellular recording of thalamocortical neuron from ventrolateral (VL) nucleus. The excitatory component (negative depth EEG wave, downward deflection) of the slow cortical oscillation (0.9 Hz) is followed by a sequence of spindle waves at 10 Hz (arrows). One typical cycle of these two combined rhythms is indicated by the dotted box; note the inhibitory postsynaptic potentials in the VL neuron leading to a postinhibitory rebound. (Right) Top and bottom traces represent field potential from the depth of association cortical area 5 and intracellular recording from thalamic reticular (RE) neuron. In neuronal circuits (far right), synaptic projections are indicated with small letters, corresponding to the arrows at left, which indicate the time sequence of the events. The depolarizing phase of the field slow oscillation (depth-negative, downward deflection) in the cortex (Cx) travels through the corticothalamic pathway (a) and triggers in the thalamic reticular nucleus (RE) a spindle sequence that is transferred to thalamocortical cells (TC) of the dorsal thalamus (b) and thereafter back to the cortex (c), where it shapes the tail of the slow oscillatory cycle (middle panel). Slow + gamma, fast activity (40 Hz) crowns the depolarizing phase of the slow oscillation. Three traces depict depth EEG waves from primary somatosensory cortex (S1), intracellular recording from S1 neuron, and filtered intracellular trace (between 10 and 100 Hz). Note the fast waves (40 Hz) during the depolarizing phase of the slow sleeplike oscillation and the absence of such fast waves during hyperpolarization.

rhythmic activity led to hypotheses postulating that linkages between spatially distributed oscillatory elements in the visual cortex may be the bases for pattern recognition function. However, beta and gamma activities are also present in the spontaneous activity of neurons and EEG, and these oscillations have been recorded under deep anesthesia when cognitive processes are suspended.

The best candidates for generation and synchronization of fast activities are fast rhythmic-bursting neurons. These neurons are both corticothalamic excitatory and local circuit inhibitory neurons, which may serve synchronization of fast activities within corticothalamic circuits and also be part of the role played by cortical inhibitory neurons in these oscillations. The thalamus and neocortex display coherent beta and gamma rhythms. At variance with the long-range synchrony of the slow sleep oscillation, fast rhythms are synchronized over restricted cortical territories and within specific circuits between thalamocortical and neocortical areas.

Synaptic Plasticity Induced by Sleep Oscillations

Far from being epiphenomena of intrinsic properties and synaptic operations in cortical and thalamic neuronal networks, with little or no functional significance, sleep oscillations lead to synaptic plasticity and are implicated in memory consolidation. Earlier views that considered sleep to be associated with widespread inhibition throughout the cortex and subcortical structures, which would lead to abolition of cognitive and conscious events, have been challenged by intracellular recordings during natural slow-wave sleep demonstrating rich spontaneous firing of neocortical neurons. These data refute the assumption that cortical neurons are inactive in this state. Although external signals are blocked at the thalamic level during slow-wave sleep, mainly because thalamocortical neurons are inhibited during spindle oscillations, the intracortical dialog is maintained and the responsiveness of cortical neurons to cortical volleys is even increased during slow-wave sleep. In humans too, this cortically evoked response is stronger in slow-wave sleep than in waking. That the neocortex is active during slow-wave sleep suggests a reorganization/specification of neuronal circuits. This view is supported by studies using indicators of neuronal activities during slow-wave sleep in humans, revealing more marked changes in those neocortical areas that are implicated in memory tasks and decision making during wakefulness.

Then, spontaneously occurring brain rhythms may lead during sleep to increased responsiveness and plastic changes in the strength of connections among neurons, a mechanism through which information is stored. Next, the results of animal experiments and human studies on synaptic plasticity are briefly presented.

The experimental model of sleep spindles is the sequence of augmenting responses, defined as thalamically evoked cortical potentials that grow in size during the first stimuli at a frequency of approximately 10 Hz, which mimics the initially waxing pattern of spindle waves. In the intact brain, augmenting responses evoked by rhythmic thalamic stimulation are characterized in cortical neurons by an increase in the secondary depolarization, at the expense of the primary EPSP. Synaptic plasticity is not only seen by progressively enhanced amplitudes of responses during the pulse train but also by persistence of self-sustained potentials, with the same pattern and frequency as those of responses during the prior stimulation period (**Figure 3(a)**). Stimulation of the corticothalamic projection with pulse trains at 10 Hz results in evoked responses and also, after protracted stimulation, in 'spontaneously' occurring spike bursts whose form and rhythmicity are similar to those of evoked responses, as if the repetition of volleys was imprinted in the 'memory' of the corticothalamic network (**Figure 3(c)**). Short- and medium-term (5–30 min) neuronal plasticity can occur inside cortical circuitry, even in the absence of the thalamus (**Figure 3(b)**).

Thus, besides their role in cortical disconnection through inhibition of incoming messages in the thalamus, sleep spindles are also operational in important cerebral functions. During spindles, rhythmic and synchronized spike bursts of thalamic neurons depolarize the dendrites of neocortical neurons, which is associated with massive Ca^{2+} entry that may provide an effective signal to efficiently activate Ca^{2+}/calmodulin-dependent protein kinase II, implicated in synaptic plasticity of excitatory synapses.

Similar phenomena, with Ca^{2+} entry in dendrites and somata of cortical neurons, occur with rhythmic spike trains associated with oscillations in the slow (0.5–1 Hz) or delta (1–4 Hz) frequency bands, during later stages of slow-wave sleep. The hypothesis that the slow oscillation is responsible for the consolidation of memory traces acquired during the state of wakefulness is supported by data showing that slow and delta oscillations are implicated in the cortical plasticity of the developing cortex.

These experimental data are congruent with human studies demonstrating that the overnight improvement of discrimination tasks requires some steps, including those in early slow-wave sleep stages. Also, procedural memory formation may be associated with oscillations during early sleep stages. The early part of night sleep favors retention of declarative memories, whereas the late part of sleep favors retention of nondeclarative memories.

At variance with the commonly used notion of global brain processes in slow-wave sleep are two major findings reported in humans subjects: slow-wave sleep activity increases 2 h after a motor learning task, and the enhancement is expressed locally in parietal association areas that receive converging visual and proprioceptive inputs relevant to spatial attention and skilled actions.

The increased cortical activity that accounts for consolidation of memory traces during slow-wave sleep also explains the presence of dreaming mentation during this state. In slow-wave sleep, dreaming is rational and repetitive, in contrast with the vivid, illogical, and emotional perceptions during REM

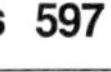

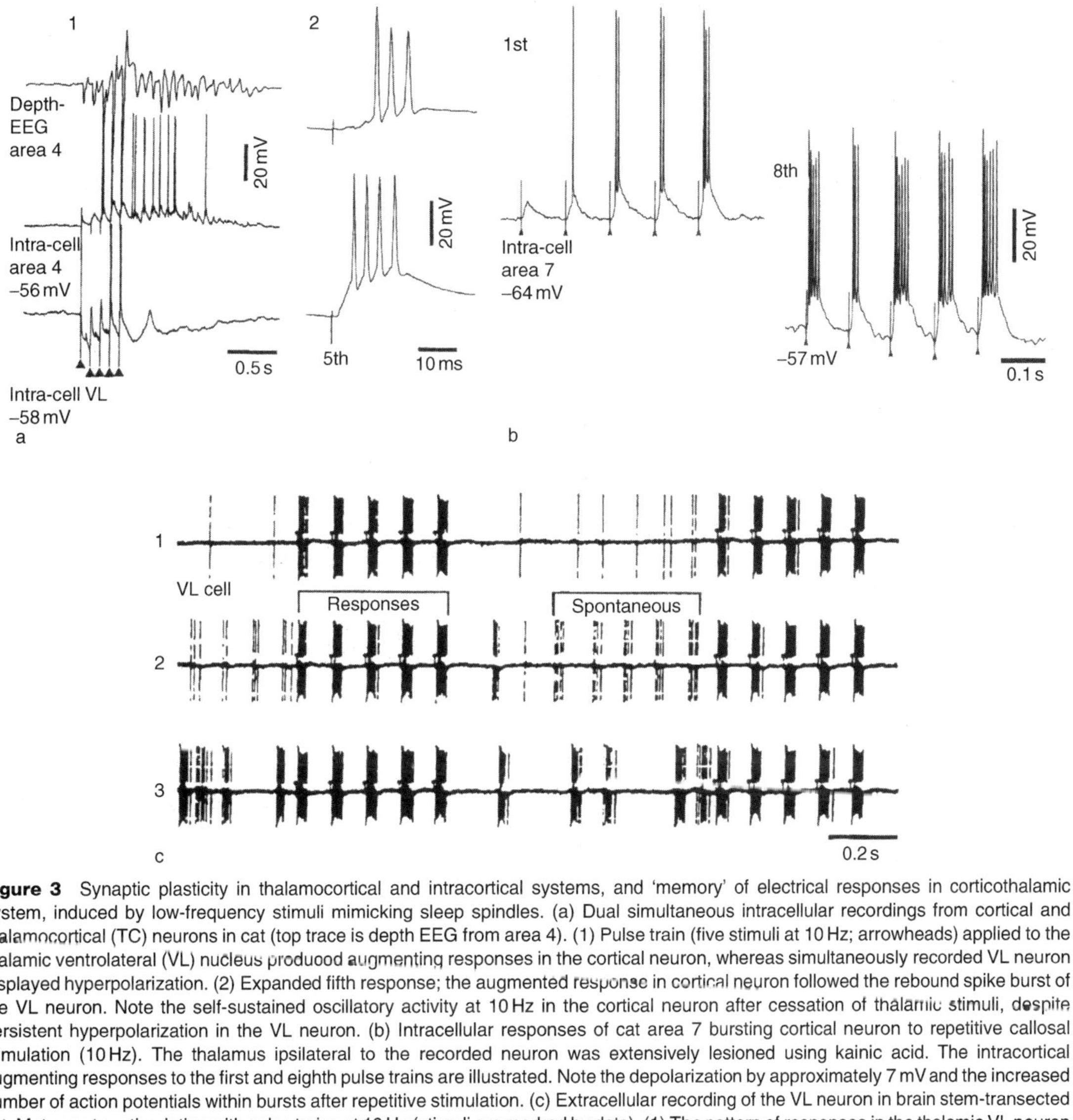

Figure 3 Synaptic plasticity in thalamocortical and intracortical systems, and 'memory' of electrical responses in corticothalamic system, induced by low-frequency stimuli mimicking sleep spindles. (a) Dual simultaneous intracellular recordings from cortical and thalamocortical (TC) neurons in cat (top trace is depth EEG from area 4). (1) Pulse train (five stimuli at 10 Hz; arrowheads) applied to the thalamic ventrolateral (VL) nucleus produced augmenting responses in the cortical neuron, whereas simultaneously recorded VL neuron displayed hyperpolarization. (2) Expanded fifth response; the augmented response in cortical neuron followed the rebound spike burst of the VL neuron. Note the self-sustained oscillatory activity at 10 Hz in the cortical neuron after cessation of thalamic stimuli, despite persistent hyperpolarization in the VL neuron. (b) Intracellular responses of cat area 7 bursting cortical neuron to repetitive callosal stimulation (10 Hz). The thalamus ipsilateral to the recorded neuron was extensively lesioned using kainic acid. The intracortical augmenting responses to the first and eighth pulse trains are illustrated. Note the depolarization by approximately 7 mV and the increased number of action potentials within bursts after repetitive stimulation. (c) Extracellular recording of the VL neuron in brain stem-transected cat. Motor cortex stimulation with pulse trains at 10 Hz (stimuli are marked by dots). (1) The pattern of responses in the thalamic VL neuron in early stages of rhythmic pulse trains. (2 and 3) Responses at later stages of stimulation. Note the appearance of spontaneous spike bursts resembling the evoked ones as a form of 'memory' in the corticothalamic circuit.

sleep. The brain is never 'empty,' and mental activity is present during all stages of normal sleep.

Ponto-Geniculo-Occipital Waves

PGO waves are sharp field potentials that are generally recorded in the visual thalamic lateral geniculate (LG) nucleus and occipital cortex, where they appear in clusters of up to six waves, closely related to gaze direction in dream imagery. Although the term PGO indicates their presence in the visual pathway, these potentials appear in many thalamic nuclei and cortical areas, outside the visual system. This widespread occurrence is due to the generalized thalamic projections of PGO generators, which are cholinergic neurons located in the pedunculopontine tegmental (PPT) nucleus and an adjacent nucleus at the mesopontine junction. Five distinct neuronal types have been recorded within cholinergic nuclei, whose discharges are temporally related to PGO field potentials in the visual thalamic nucleus.

The major input sources of PPT neurons are in adjacent areas of the upper brain stem reticular formation, hypothalamic areas, and cerebral cortex. Impulses in the PGO generators can be triggered by any of these inputs through direct excitation or postinhibitory rebound excitation. Then, PPT neurons can be regarded as the final link in the brain stem–thalamic path that generates PGO waves. Because PGO potentials are thought to represent 'the stuff dreams are made of' and in view of the emotional nature of dreaming mentation in REM sleep, hypothalamic and forebrain structures that store some of the emotionally charged information may be most effective in driving the PGO brain stem neuronal generators.

In naturally sleeping cats – the species of choice for experimental studies because they display sleep patterns similar to those of humans – PGO waves precede other signs of REM sleep by approximately 30–90 s, and they appear during the last period of slow-wave sleep. Thus, there is a transitional period between EEG-synchronized and EEG-activated (REM) sleep that is called the pre-REM period, during which PGO waves appear over the background of a fully synchronized EEG. Thalamic neurons are hyperpolarized during the pre-REM period, when the sleep EEG is still fully synchronized, whereas they are depolarized during REM sleep. These two states (pre-REM and fully developed REM sleep) generate different PGO-related responses of LG neurons to brain stem cholinergic inputs, which influence the signal-to-noise ratio in the visual channel – that is, the ratio between the neuronal activity related to the PGO signal and the background firing of the same neuron. During pre-REM, the activity of thalamic LG cells starts with a short spike burst coinciding with a high-amplitude PGO wave and continues with a train of single spikes. By contrast, during full-blown REM sleep, the rate of LG cells' spontaneous firing is much higher than in pre-REM; LG cells do not fire spike bursts but, rather, single action potentials; and the amplitudes of PGO waves are much lower than during the pre-REM state. The peri-PGO histograms of LG neuronal activities show that the signal-to-noise ratio reaches values of approximately 7 during the pre-REM epoch, whereas the ratio values during REM sleep are approximately 2.

Why all these details? Because PGO waves are commonly regarded as the physiological correlate of dreaming, the greater signal-to-noise ratio in the LG-cortical channel during the pre-REM epoch than during REM sleep suggests that the vivid imagery associated with dreaming sleep may appear before fully developed REM sleep, during a period of apparent slow-wave sleep. Discussing dreaming from experiments in cats is justified in view of the behavioral repertoire typical for dreaming mentation that can be elicited in cats after having prevented muscular atonia by lesions of certain brain stem reticular structures. The idea that PGO waves with greater amplitudes during the pre-REM stage may reflect more vivid imagery during that epoch than even during REM sleep corroborates earlier data showing that after interrupting sleep immediately after the occurrence of the first PGO wave (in the pre-REM stage) and eliminating approximately 30 s of the slow-wave sleep stage that precedes REM sleep, the increased time of the REM sleep rebound was due to phasic events (PGO waves) rather than the loss of REM sleep *per se*. This observation fits in well with data on dream reports from the last epoch of EEG-synchronized sleep, which are indistinguishable from those obtained from REM sleep awakenings.

PGO waves are thought to play a role in development and structural maturation of the brain. PGO waves also exert specific excitatory effects on complex neurons in the visual cortex, and their deprivation may modify the expression of long-term potentiation in immature animals.

See also: Sleep Architecture; Sleep and Sleep States: PET Activation Patterns; Sleep and Sleep States: Hippocampus–Neocortex Dialog; Sleep and Sleep States: Network Reactivation; Sleep and Sleep States: Gene Expression; Sleep Oscillations; Sleep-Dependent Memory Processing.

Further Reading

Achermann P and Borbély A (1997) Low-frequency (<1 Hz) oscillations in the human sleep EEG. *Neuroscience* 81: 213–222.

Contreras D, Destexhe A, Sejnowski TJ, and Steriade M (1996) Control of spatiotemporal coherence of a thalamic oscillation by corticothalamic feedback. *Science* 274: 771–774.

Contreras D and Steriade M (1995) Cellular basis of EEG slow rhythms: A study of dynamic corticothalamic relationships. *Journal of Neuroscience* 15: 604–622.

Gais S, Plihal W, Wagner U, and Born J (2000) Early sleep triggers memory for early visual discrimination skills. *Nature Neuroscience* 3: 1335–1339.

Hobson JA and Pace-Schott EF (2002) The cognitive neuroscience of sleep: Neuronal systems, consciousness and learning. *Nature Reviews Neuroscience* 3: 679–693.

Huber R, Ghilardi MF, Massimini M, and Tononi G (2004) Local sleep and learning. *Nature* 430: 78–81.

Maquet P, Degueldre C, Delfiore G, et al. (1997) Functional neuroanatomy of human slow wave sleep. *Journal of Neuroscience* 17: 2807–2812.

Massimini M, Ferrarelli F, Huber R, Esser SK, Singh H, and Tononi G (2005) Breakdown of cortical effective connectivity during sleep. *Science* 309: 2228–2232.

Massimini M, Huber R, Ferrarelli F, and Tononi G (2004) The sleep slow oscillation as a traveling wave. *Journal of Neuroscience* 24: 6862–6870.

Mölle M, Marshall L, Gais S, and Born J (2002) Grouping of spindle activity during slow oscillations in human non-REM sleep. *Journal of Neuroscience* 22: 10941–10947.

Plihal W and Born J (1997) Effects of early and late nocturnal sleep on declarative and procedural memory. *Journal of Cognitive Neuroscience* 9: 534–547.

Steriade M (2003) *Neuronal Substrates of Sleep and Epilepsy.* Cambridge, UK: Cambridge University Press.

Steriade M and Llinás RR (1988) The functional states of the thalamus and the associated neuronal interplay. *Physiological Reviews* 68: 649–742.

Steriade M and McCarley RW (2005) *Brain Control of Wakefulness and Sleep.* New York: Springer.

Steriade M, Nuñez A, and Amzica F (1993) A novel slow (<1 Hz) oscillation of neocortical neurons *in vivo*: Depolarizing and hyperpolarizing components. *Journal of Neuroscience* 13: 3252–3265.

Steriade M, Paré D, Bouhassira D, Deschênes M, and Oakson G (1989) Phasic activation of lateral geniculate and perigeniculate neurons during sleep with ponto-geniculo-occipital spikes. *Journal of Neuroscience* 9: 2215–2229.

Steriade M and Timofeev I (2003) Neuronal plasticity in thalamocortical networks during sleep and waking oscillations. *Neuron* 37: 563–576.

Steriade M, Timofeev I, and Grenier F (2001) Natural waking and sleep states: A view from inside neocortical neurons. *Journal of Neurophysiology* 85: 1969–1985.

Stickgold R, James L, and Hobson JA (2000) Visual discrimination learning requires sleep after training. *Nature Neuroscience* 3: 1237–1238.

Spiking Neuron Models

W Gerstner, Ecole Polytechnique Fédérale de Lausanne, Lausanne, Switzerland

Introduction: Spikes and the Question of Neural Coding

Neurons communicate with each other by electrical pulses, called action potentials or spikes. Whether the exact timing of action potentials or only the mean firing rate plays a role in neuronal communication is a question of intense debate, often referred to as the problem of neural coding. The question is further complicated by the fact that neuronal firing rates can be defined in at least three different ways: (1) the mean firing rate of a single neuron in a single trial, defined as a temporal average over a sufficiently long time (e.g., number of spikes in a time window of 500 ms, divided by 500 ms); (2) the firing density of a single neuron averaged across several repetitions of the same stimulus, typically defined via the amplitude of a peristimulus-time-histogram as a function of time; and (3) the population rate in a group of neurons with similar properties, defined as an average across the group. From reaction time experiments, it is clear that the first definition of a rate (average across time) cannot be the code used by the neurons. Averaging across several repetitions, as in the second definition, is a useful experimental method but cannot be the strategy of an animal which has to respond to a new stimulus. Finally, while the concept of averaging over groups of equivalent neurons is theoretically appealing, it is hard to see how such groups could be defined in a living brain since the organization into groups might change from one moment to the next, depending on task and stimulus demands.

If rates are such a difficult concept, does that imply that the exact timing of individual spikes matters? Not necessarily. A typical cortical neuron receives input from thousands of other neurons. What matters is probably the number (and spatial distribution across the dendrite) of spike arrivals averaged over an interval of one or a few milliseconds. However, if one spike arrival at an excitatory synapse were removed and replaced by a spike arrival at a different excitatory synapse at a similar dendritic location, the response of the neuron would hardly change. Since the question of coding and of the relevance of exact spike timings for neuronal response is still an open issue, researchers in theoretical neuroscience often use models that take the pulsed (i.e., 'spiking') nature of neuronal signals into account. These are so-called spiking neuron models, as opposed to rate models, in which the activity of neurons is described only in terms of firing rates.

Rate Models in Theoretical Neuroscience

In the field of artificial neural networks, the traditional way of describing neuronal activity has been by means of rate models. In this framework, each unit in a neuronal network is characterized by its rate $r(t)$, which depends nonlinearly on the total stimulation I it received immediately before. In a standard model in discrete time, the rate $r_i(t)$ of a neuron i is given by

$$r_i(t) = g(I_i(t - \mathrm{d}t)) \qquad [1]$$

where $\mathrm{d}t$ is the time step of the simulation and g the nonlinear gain function. Typically, the function g takes a value of zero for a stimulation I below some threshold value and saturates at a maximum value $r^{\max}$ for very strong stimulation. The total stimulation I_i of neuron i has two contributions, that is, the sum over all inputs converging onto neuron i plus potentially some external input I^{ext}:

$$I_i(t) = \sum_k w_{ik} r_k(t) + I^{\text{ext}}(t) \qquad [2]$$

where r_k are the firing rates of other neurons k. In continuous time, eqn [1] is often replaced by a differential equation:

$$\tau \frac{\mathrm{d}r_i}{\mathrm{d}t} = -r_i + g(I_i) \qquad [3]$$

with some time constant τ that describes the response time of the unit to a change in stimulation.

While artificial neural networks using rate models have been successfully used in tasks describing cortex development or memory retrieval, the biological interpretation of the network units is unclear. Each unit i and k in eqn [2] could be interpreted as a single neuron and its rate as a temporally averaged firing rate. In view of the limitations of the firing rate concept discussed above, it must then be concluded that such a single-neuron rate model cannot be used to describe the fast neuronal dynamics during, for example, the rapid reaction of an organism to a new stimulus. Alternatively, each unit could be interpreted as a population of cells and its activity as the population rate. However, in that case the connectivity matrix w_{ij} would refer to the connectivity between populations rather than neurons, and the relevance of model results for electrophysiological measurements is questionable.

Detailed Models of a Spiking Neuron

The classical model of a spiking neuron is the mathematical description of Hodgkin and Huxley of action potential generation in the giant axon of the squid. Generation of spikes in the model arises through the interplay of four nonlinear differential equations. The first equation summarizes the current conservation on a small piece of membrane. A current I^{ext} injected onto the membrane can either charge the capacity C of the membrane or pass through one of the ion channels. With three different ion channel types (one for sodium, one for potassium, and one for all remaining 'leak' components), the change of the voltage is given by

$$C\frac{\mathrm{d}u}{\mathrm{d}t} = I^{\text{ext}} - g_{\text{Na}}m^3h(u - E_{\text{Na}}) - g_{\text{K}}n^4(u - E_{\text{K}}) - g_L(u - E_{\text{L}}) \qquad [4]$$

where g_{Na} and g_{K} are the maximum conductance of the sodium and potassium channel, respectively; E_{Na} and E_{L} are their reversal potentials; and m, h, and n are additional 'gating' variables that describe the state of the channel as a function of time. Each of the three variables m, n, and h follows an equation of the form

$$\frac{\mathrm{d}x}{\mathrm{d}t} = -\frac{x - x_0(u)}{\tau(u)} \qquad [5]$$

with empirical function $x_0(u)$ and $\tau(u)$ derived from the experiments (and different for m, n, and h).

Computer simulations as well as mathematical analysis of the system of four nonlinear differential equations shows that action potentials are generated only if the total stimulation I^{ext} reaches a critical value. To a first degree of approximation, one may therefore conclude that action potential generation is an all-or-none process. However, a closer examination of the behavior shows that there is neither a strict voltage threshold nor a strict current threshold. In particular, for time-dependent inputs (e.g., current steps and ramps or randomly fluctuating current as input), not only the momentary voltage or current amplitude matters, but the stimulation history as well.

Formal Spiking Neuron Models

Although neither the Hodgkin–Huxley model nor real neurons have a strict firing threshold, in practice the process of neuronal action potential generation can often be well approximated as a threshold process. The simplest model in the class of formal spiking neuron models is the leaky integrate-and-fire model. In this model, spikes are triggered whenever the membrane potential u reaches a given threshold θ. Below threshold, the membrane potential is described by its capacity C and input resistance R. Current conservation gives the linear differential equation.

$$C\frac{\mathrm{d}u}{\mathrm{d}t} = -\frac{u}{R} + I^{\text{ext}} \qquad [6]$$

If u reaches the threshold θ, the spike time t^f is noted and the membrane potential reset to a fixed value u_{reset}, before integration of eqn [6] is resumed. The essence of the leaky integrate-and-fire model is a clear separation between a completely linear (passive) subthreshold regime and a strict firing threshold. The leaky integrate-and-fire model is today the standard neuron model in many simulation studies concerning the dynamics of large neuronal networks or the question of neural coding.

Generalizations of the leaky integrate-and-fire model have been proposed in several directions. First, since some neurons exhibit in the subthreshold regime a damped oscillatory response to changes in the input (as opposed to a simple exponential decay), the voltage eqn [6] can be coupled with a second equation. As long as this second equation is linear, the subthreshold behavior of the neuron is still completely linear, that is, doubling the amplitude of an input generates a subthreshold response which is twice as large. Second, refractory effects (i.e., reduced responsiveness of a neuron immediately after firing) have been included. The combination of refractory effects with a linear subthreshold behavior leads to the spike response model with a membrane potential

$$u(t) = \eta(t - \hat{t}) + \int \kappa(t - \hat{t}, s) I^{\text{ext}}(t - s)\mathrm{d}s \qquad [7]$$

where $\hat{t}$ is the firing time of the last spike of the neuron, η describes the form of the action potential and its spike after-potential, and κ the linear response to an input pulse. The next spike occurs if the membrane potential u hits a threshold θ from below, in which case $\hat{t}$ is updated. Hence the main characteristics of the Spike Response Model are identical to those of the leaky integrate-and-fire model, that is, a linear subthreshold regime in combination with a strict firing threshold. However, the spike response model allows refractory effects to be included (since the functions η and κ depend on the time since the last firing) as well as subthreshold oscillations (expressed through an appropriate shape of η and κ).

A third generalization of the standard leaky integrate-and-fire model concerns adaptation. By introduction of a second equation that summarizes processes on a slower timescale, it is possible to describe the slow adaptation of the neuron after a step in the stimulating current.

Fourth, the spike triggered by a strict threshold process at the soma can be combined with one or several additional equations describing the (passive) properties of the dendrite. Finally, the strict threshold can be replaced by a smooth threshold process if eqn [6] is turned into a nonlinear equation:

$$C\frac{du}{dt} = -f(u) + I^{ext} \quad [8]$$

where $f(u)$ describes the nonlinearities of the membrane in the vicinity of the firing threshold. Two standard choices of $f(u)$ are the quadratic integrate-and-fire model $f(u) = a\ (u-u_1)\ (u-u_2)$ and the exponential integrate-and-fire model $f(u) = -(u/R) + b \exp[(u-\theta)/\Delta]$. Both models have free parameters, that is, a, u_1, and u_2 for the quadratic and b, θ, Δ, and R for the exponential integrate-and-fire model, that can be used to adapt the model and put it into a desired firing regime.

Limitations of Formal Spiking Neuron Models

Formal spiking neuron models approximate the electrical properties of neurons by one or a few equations that summarize basic features of normal neuronal behavior with a small number of phenomenological parameters. Formal spiking neurons are therefore not suitable for predicting electrophysiological experiments under nonstandard stimulation conditions. In particular, since all electrical properties of a neuron are summarized in one or two phenomenological equations, these models cannot be used to predict changes of behavior caused by, for example, pharmacological blockage of specific ion channels. Moreover, since the spatial structure of real neurons is not represented in detail, all nonlinear dendritic effects cannot be incorporated into formal spiking neuron models (passive properties, however, can be). Similarly, since the model summarizes neuronal behavior under some reference condition, slow changes in neuronal behavior, caused by slow current ramps or accumulation of intracellular calcium or a simple fatigue of the neuron, for example, cannot be captured.

However, under some stimulation conditions, formal spiking neurons perform surprisingly well. A direct comparison of the spike response model with the Hodgkin–Huxley model during stimulation with random current shows that up to 90% of spike times of the Hodgkin–Huxley model are correctly predicted by the spike response model with a temporal precision of 2 ms. Moreover, a spike response model with a second equation describing adaptation has also been used to predict spike times of layer-V pyramidal neurons in rat cortex under random current injection. The same time-dependent input $I^{ext}(t)$ was given to both a model neuron and a pyramidal neuron. If the fluctuating current had large amplitude, the neuron itself generated spikes reliably with the same timing across several repetitions of the experiments, but less so if the fluctuation amplitude was reduced. Similarly, the model neuron was able to correctly predict the spike times of the pyramidal neuron (up to 70%) if the fluctuation amplitude of the current was high, but much less well if it was low. Thus, under random current injection, formal spiking neurons describe action potential generation in pyramidal neurons to a high degree of accuracy.

Spiking Neurons in Large Networks

A major advantage of formal spiking neurons such as the leaky integrate-and-fire model is their simplicity, which has two important consequences. First, it is possible to simulate neural networks with a large number of neurons at a reasonable numerical cost. Second, network properties such as the mean firing rate of neurons in a network of randomly connected integrate-and-fire units can be studied analytically with tools from mathematical probability theory, statistical physics, and bifurcation theory.

One important insight that has arisen from studies with formal spiking neurons is the importance of the subthreshold regime for cortical activity. In order to have large networks of interacting spiking neurons working in a state in which individual neurons show irregular firing with broad interspike interval distributions, it turns out to be necessary that the total drive from thousands of excitatory inputs is approximately balanced by inhibition. If this is the case, the neuronal membrane potential hovers normally in the subthreshold regime but stays close to the threshold so that neurons are very responsive to small changes in the input.

Furthermore, studies with networks of spiking neurons have been used repeatedly to elucidate the potential of different neural codes. For example, the stability and reproducibility of spatiotemporal spike patterns in networks of integrate-and-fire neurons have been studied in the context of synfire chains, a potential coding mechanism relying on precise spike times. Similarly, it can be understood why and under what conditions a population of spiking neurons responds instantaneously to changes in the input, that is, much faster than the membrane time constant that characterizes the passive response of the membrane. Finally, formal spiking neurons have been used for studying the functional consequences of spike timing-dependent plasticity.

The example of oscillatory activity allows one to see how formal spiking neurons can be used to predict by a purely mathematical argument the firing activity in large networks. For the sake of simplicity, we suppose that the network consists of N neurons with identical properties and that every neuron is connected to all other neurons by synapses of the same strength. Since we are interested in oscillatory activity, we assume that all neurons in the network fire at the same time, except one that lags behind by a small amount. Will this neuron eventually join the group of the others? To answer this question, we calculate the total synaptic input to this specific neuron, generated by the action potentials in the group of synchronous neurons. Knowing the input, we can derive from eqn [6] or eqn [7] the time course of its membrane potential, and from the time course, we can predict its firing time, that is, the moment when the membrane potential hits the threshold. An analogous calculation is repeated to predict the firing time of the group of synchronous neurons and hence the timing difference between the activity of the single neuron and that of the group. The one neuron lagging behind will eventually join the group of synchronous neurons (i.e., the oscillation is stable) if the timing difference is reduced from one firing cycle to the next. This is just a simple example, but similar mathematical arguments can be used to predict the population activity in large networks and answer questions such as: What is the mean firing activity of neurons in the network? Do neurons fire asynchronously, or do the firing times tend to cluster? Does the network activity show spontaneous oscillations? Will the network switch to a different state on a new input? If yes, could this explain short-term memory in neural networks?

To summarize, formal spiking neuron models are a highly simplified and compressed way of describing action potential generation in real neurons. While such an approach has obvious limitations and cannot be used to study detailed properties of isolated neurons (such as active dendrites or effects of pharmacological blockage of specific channels), the models have been useful in the past to elucidate the essence of spike generation in single neurons as well as principles of neuronal coding in large neuronal networks, and they will probably remain important tools for modeling studies in the future.

See also: Action Potential Initiation and Conduction in Axons; Hodgkin–Huxley Models; Population Codes: Theoretic Aspects; Spike-Timing Dependent Plasticity (STDP); Spike-Timing-Dependent Plasticity Models.

Further Reading

Abeles M (1991) *Corticonics*. Cambridge, UK: Cambridge University Press.

Brette R and Gerstner W (2005) Adaptive exponential integrate-and-fire model as an effective description of neuronal activity. *Journal of Neurophysiology* 94: 3637–3642.

Fourcaud-Trocme N, Hansel D, van Vreeswijk C, and Brunel N (2003) How spike generation mechanisms determine the neuronal response to fluctuating input. *Journal of Neuroscience* 23: 11628–11640.

Gerstner W and Kistler WK (2002) *Spiking Neuron Models*. Cambridge, UK: Cambridge University Press.

Izhikevich EM (2004) Which model to use for cortical spiking neurons? *IEEE Transactions on Neural Networks* 15: 1063–1070.

Jolivet R, Rauch A, Lscher H-R, and Gerstner W (2006) Predicting spike timing of neocortical pyramidal neurons by simple threshold models. *Journal of Computational Neuroscience* 21: 35–49.

Koch C and Segev I (2000) The role of single neurons in information processing. *Nature Neuroscience* 3(supplement): 1171–1177.

Rieke F, Warland D, de Ruyter van Steveninck R, and Bialek W (1996) *Spikes Exploring the Neural Code*. Cambridge, MA: MIT Press.

Swim Oscillator Networks

A H Cohen and T Kiemel, University of Maryland, College Park, MD, USA

Introduction

We begin our discussion of modeling swim oscillator networks with a brief review of the uses to which models of such networks are put. After this overview, we examine some types of models in the context of the central pattern generator (CPG) for locomotion of the lamprey. We also mention models of other swim networks.

Models of the lamprey swim network differ in the level or granularity of their description. Biophysical models focus on the specifics at the level of the membrane channel currents and details of the intra- and intersegmental connectivity. Such models have multiple variables per cell or cell type. (Often, one model neuron represents all neurons of a given type in each hemisegment.) Connectionist models have a single variable for each cell type and focus primarily on intra- and intersegmental connectivity. Phase models have a single variable for each segment and focus on intersegmental connectivity.

The choice of level of description for a model depends on both the research question being addressed and the trade-off between detail and simplicity. For example, a biophysical model is required to fully understand the impact of neuromodulators on the CPG. On the other hand, any model type can be used to investigate the production of intersegmental phase lags. Developing a biophysical model can be considered the ultimate goal since it accounts for the CPG's behavior on multiple levels of description. However, using a biophysical model requires estimating many parameters, only some of which can be directly estimated. Connectionist and phase models have fewer parameters, which simplifies both parameter selection and understanding of the resulting model. Given the lack of detailed empirical information, a model will not necessarily reproduce aspects of the CPG's behavior that were not considered when selecting its parameters. For example, all models are tuned to reproduce correct intersegmental phase lags. However, only some models reproduce correct functional intersegmental coupling strength or the details of the functional anatomy of the coordinating system.

The behavior to be captured by the models of swim networks is relatively simple. All swim oscillator networks produce some form of rhythmic output produced by a CPG. The rhythmic output of any swimming network is alternation among the muscles that move the body left/right or up/down, as well as a feature such as a traveling wave to aid in propulsion. In lamprey, the behavioral components of the motor output pattern are clearly defined as alternation between left and right muscles within a single spinal segment and a constant phase delay among the muscles along the side of the body (**Figure 1**). The traveling wave generated by this pattern typically forms a single wavelength along the body, which has been shown to be most efficient for this eel-like body form .

Modeling the Oscillator

We begin with the rhythm generation, or the mechanism for the oscillation between off and on states that accompany the oscillation of the membrane potential seen in the output elements of the CPG, the motor neurons. The oscillatory mechanism is often included with the mechanism for the alternation between the two sides of a single segment, but the two need not be linked. In modeling the oscillator, the first issue is whether the system depends on a single pacemaker or a number of distributed oscillators. The second issue is whether or not the oscillation is a function of membrane properties that generate the periodic changes in the membrane potential or whether it is a function of network connections. Indeed, most often it is a function of both membrane potential mechanisms and network connections, as has been found in the stomatogastric ganglion of Crustacea and the heart ganglia of the leech. In the lamprey, the evidence appears to support this double method as well. There are clearly membrane oscillations that appear in response to NMDA, and there are also network connections that are capable of forming an alternating output in combination with sufficient channel properties that are highly common.

It is also known that the CPG responsible for the oscillation is a distributed system, with each segment, hemisegment, or small group of segments capable of producing a rhythmic discharge of its own motor neurons. The exact minimal unit is still under debate, but there is evidence that it could be a hemisegment. On the other hand, the frequency appears to be a product of the ensemble of oscillators and apparently is not governed by any single oscillator.

Thus, any model of the lamprey swim network must account for rhythm generation in a single segment or hemisegment. There are several models for the network

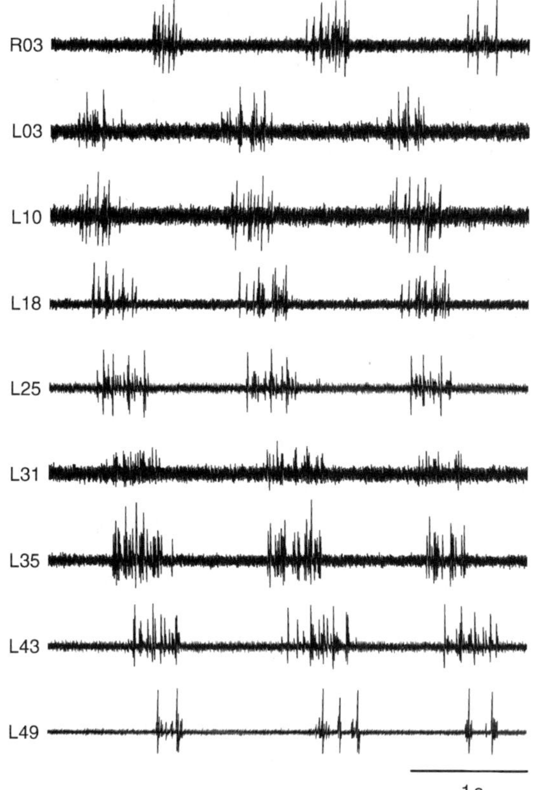

Figure 1 Neural activity recorded from the motor nerves of an isolated 50-segment piece of lamprey spinal cord. Activity from the left and right motor nerves of the same segment exhibits alternation (L03 and R03). Activity from different segments exhibits a rostrocaudal traveling wave. Numbers indicate the segment numbers.

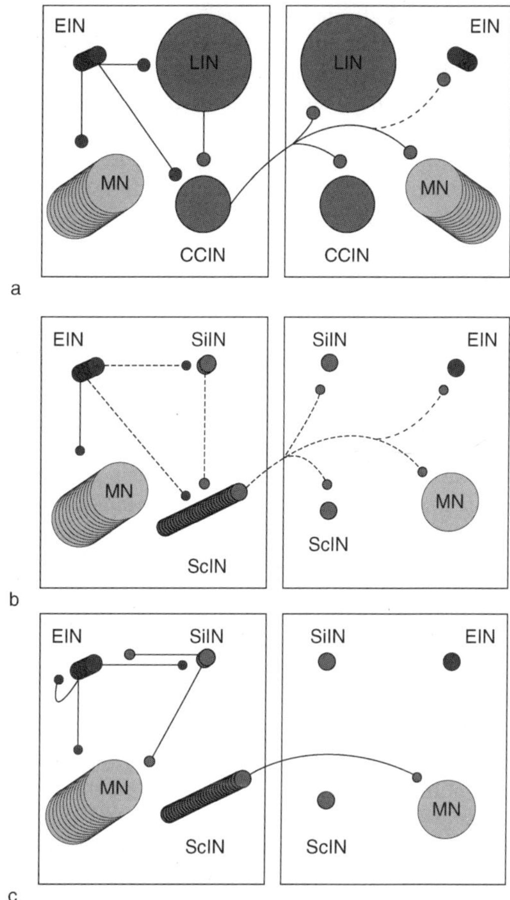

Figure 2 Known (solid lines) and presumed (dashed lines) connections in the lamprey CPG. Cell types are motor neurons (MN), excitatory interneurons (EIN), lateral inhibitory interneurons (LIN), crossed caudal interneurons (CCIN), small ipsilateral inhibitory interneurons (SiIN), and small crossing inhibitory interneurons (ScIN). (a) Connectivity scheme of Buchanan and Grillner based on pairwise recordings from different segments. (b) Segmental network if the LIN and CC interneurons are removed, based on the argument that these neurons provide primarily intersegmental coupling. (c) Evidence of intrasegmental connections. Figure provided by David Parker.

of the segmental unit CPG. The simplest was the original proposed by Buchanan and Grillner based on the experimental evidence of single cell recordings. The current network includes some additional neurons, again based on recordings of single neurons during rhythm generation by the isolated spinal cord, or what has been called 'fictive locomotion.' The basic oscillator model adds channel currents and some modulation. Such a model will almost certainly be missing some important elements of the oscillator, such as neuronal connections and/or channel currents. Nor can it include currents that have not yet been found that are either ligand gated or voltage gated. The current model does include some rather novel currents, such as potassium-dependent sodium channels.

There are many ways to model even a simple system such as the lamprey spinal cord. The issues are the neuronal composition and its connectivity. We present here, for comparison, the model put forth by David Parker, shown in **Figure 2**. The dashed lines represent those connections that are presumed to exist but for which there is no direct evidence. The solid lines represent those for which there is direct evidence. The inference of the connections from the large interneurons, such as the lateral interneurons and crossed caudal interneurons (CCINs), has been based on recordings between segments some distance apart. Although there have been attempts to prove that the large neurons do or do not have connections within their own segment, such evidence is very difficult to obtain directly. It is unclear how the model will be affected by whether or not the inhibitory connections are from the larger CCINs or from the smaller crossed inhibitory interneurons. Unfortunately, answering these questions requires obtaining good recordings of each of the small interneurons in combination with their posited target neurons within a single segment; that task is very difficult. Obtaining the parameter values for the channel currents for each neuron throughout the dynamical changes that are likely to occur within a single cycle is even more difficult. Thus, although the model is a useful way to keep track of the latest view of the oscillator, one must be cautious of strong conclusions based on this or, indeed, any model.

The biophysically based model, in its current configuration, could be used to test the role of a variety of modulatory currents, such as those proposed by Parker and colleagues. This analysis would require that one perform a sensitivity analysis of those currents using perhaps two parameter values simultaneously. Unfortunately, there are far too many parameters in the current model for this kind of analysis to be practical. However, an abstracted form of the model could be developed in which such an analysis could be performed. The results of such a study would suggest which currents and modulators to vary in order to determine more accurately their roles in the development of the rhythm.

The oscillator networks have been modeled in several model systems, including the tadpole of *Xenopus* and the salamander. There are also examples among the invertebrates, including the leech. In some cases, the issues relate to the development of the network, whereas in others they relate to the rhythm generation alone.

In summary, a major difficulty with biophysically detailed models in which the parameters values are not fully known is that there are many 'free' parameters. That is, there are many parameters whose values during the motor behavior are dynamically changing but are known only from static experiments, at best. When one tweaks the parameters to achieve the desired motor output pattern, one can relatively easily change enough parameters to obtain the desired behavioral regime.

We demonstrate this with a discussion of a totally different kind of modeling by Jung and colleagues for the oscillator which used a bifurcation analysis to illustrate the range of potential output patterns that can be assumed by the simple six-neuron network of Williams. The model we consider makes no claims to realism. It has few parameters except the weights of the connections among the classes of the neurons and the descending drive strength that serves as the excitation to the network. In this simple network, we found that a parameter unnecessary for the oscillation was the connectivity of the excitatory neurons. Experimental evidence from the Grillner group has since been presented to counter this possibility, but the results of the model do suggest that one can, with a simple network, produce a relatively large range of behaviors. One must be cautious about any conclusions one draws from any model because the realm of its possible behaviors is manyfold and typically largely unexplored.

Modeling the Traveling Wave Motion

In modeling the traveling wave motion, there are other fundamental issues that must be addressed besides rhythm. The first is the necessity of sensory feedback. Does sensory feedback produce the sequential activation of the segments? In the lamprey CPG and several other CPGs (e.g., leech and *Xenopus*), it has been shown that the traveling wave among the segments appears in the absence of sensory feedback. Sensory feedback may contribute to the traveling wave motion, but it is not necessary for the motion to occur. The next question is whether the delays among the segments are a constant phase of the cycle duration or a constant delay. If they are a constant delay, the mechanism can be relatively easily explained, potentially, as due to conduction delays along the axons connecting the segmental oscillators. However, in most systems the delays are a constant phase angle of the cycle and not a constant delay. Thus, they are due to a computation wherein the delay is changed for each frequency at which the oscillators burst. In the lamprey, for example, this has been shown to be the case. The delays among the segments are a constant phase of the cycle regardless of the frequency even in the complete absence of sensory feedback. That is, in the case of 'fictive swimming,' the delays are roughly appropriate for the frequency seen that is elicited by the addition of excitatory amino acids to the bath holding the isolated spinal cord. The mechanism for the computation of the constant phase delay has been the focus when modeling the intersegmental coordination of the segmental oscillators.

Modeling the traveling wave motion began in 1982 with a paper by Cohen et al. Their model was a phase approximation of a chain of coupled stable limit cycle oscillators. A stable limit cycle oscillator has the property that, following a perturbation, the trajectories of the oscillator's variables return to their original waveforms; the only lasting effect of the perturbation is a phase shift. If stable limit cycle oscillators with similar frequencies are weakly coupled, then it is possible to derive a phase model that approximates the behavior of the system. The state of each oscillator is described by a single variable, its absolute phase, and coupling between oscillators depends only on the relative phases of the oscillators. The behavior of a phase model is determined by the uncoupled frequency of each oscillator and the relative phase coupling functions. There can be a different coupling function for each pair of pre- and postsynaptic oscillators, although typically the coupling function is assumed to depend only on the relative position of the two oscillators in the chain.

Use of a phase approximation simplifies the understanding of intersegmental coordination by dividing the problem into two parts: (1) understanding how the details of the neural dynamics and neural circuitry affect uncoupled oscillator frequencies and the relative phase coupling functions and (2) understanding how the properties of the oscillator frequencies and coupling functions relate to intersegmental coordination. Cohen et al. addressed the second part of the problem. They assumed that coupling functions were sine functions. An important property of a coupling function is its preferred phase, the relative phase that would be produced by unidirectional coupling between two oscillators with equal uncoupled frequencies. The preferred phase of a sine coupling function is either in-phase or anti-phase, depending on the sign of the sine wave's coefficient. Cohen et al. showed that a traveling wave could be produced in two ways: (1) by a gradient of uncoupled oscillator frequencies and nearest-neighbor in-phase coupling and (2) by equal uncoupled oscillator frequencies, nearest-neighbor in-phase coupling, and anti-phase coupling between the first and last oscillator in the chain. These two examples correspond to the two basic mechanisms for producing a traveling wave in a chain of coupled oscillators: a systematic variation in oscillator frequencies (the oscillator frequency mechanism) or non-in-phase coupling functions (the coupling function mechanism). For the lamprey CPG, experimental evidence supports the coupling function mechanism as the source of the traveling wave. For example, when a piece of spinal cord is cut into smaller parts, the relative frequencies of these parts do not show a systematic pattern.

Work by Ermentrout and Kopell has provided a general understanding of the coupling function mechanism for phase models with short-distance coupling. Allowing preferred phases to take on any value, not just in-phase or anti-phase, they showed that the relative strength of ascending and descending coupling plays a critical role in determining intersegmental phase lags. For example, in the case of nearest-neighbor coupling with ascending coupling stronger than descending coupling, phase lags between adjacent oscillators are close to the preferred phase of the ascending coupling, except near the rostral end of the chain. This coupling dominance can be seen in certain swim models, such as the lamprey CPG models of Williams and Ekeberg.

Although the behavior of many swim models can be understood using a phase approximation, there are two important limitations. First, a phase approximation is only guaranteed to be valid in general if coupling is weak. For strong coupling, a phase approximation will be valid only in very restrictive special cases. Second, swim models only exhibit certain properties, such as coupling dominance, if long-distance coupling is absent or very weak. To test whether these two assumptions, weak and predominantly short coupling, hold for the lamprey CPG, we developed a method of estimating functional coupling strength based on recordings from two motor nerves. The method is based on estimating parameters in a model of two coupled phase oscillators and gleans information from cycle-to-cycle variation in cycle periods and intersegmental phase lags. Functional coupling strength is quantified by the measure β, which varies from 0 (no coupling) to 1 (infinitely strong coupling). For a 50-segment piece of spinal cord, functional coupling between the rostral and caudal ends is very strong (**Figure 3**). Also, by inhibiting 20 middle segments, we found that long-distance connections provided substantial coupling. Therefore, as summarized in **Figure 3**, coupling in the lamprey CPG is neither weak nor predominantly short.

The functional coupling strength measure β can be estimated for any model by adding noise to create cycle-to-cycle variations in cycle periods and intersegmental phase lags. We have estimated functional coupling strength for three models: the connectionist model of Williams; the model of Ekeberg, which was

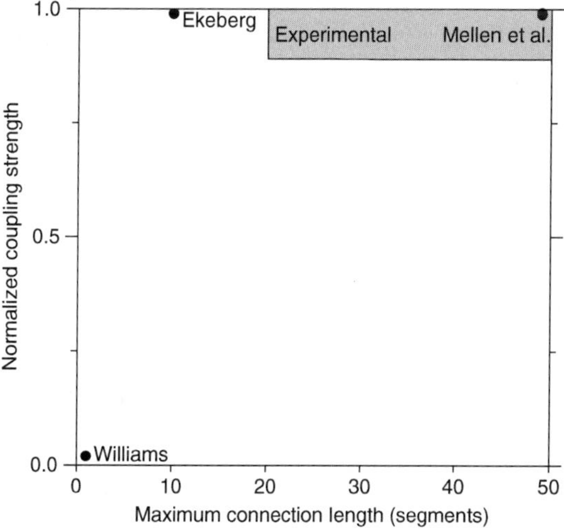

Figure 3 Comparison of experimental estimates of coupling length and function strength to those of various models.

intended as a simplified version of the more-detailed biophysical models of Grillner and colleagues; and the phase model of Mellen et al. **Figure 3** shows β for each model along with its maximum connection length. Note that the Williams model, which has only nearest-neighbor connections, exhibits weak functional coupling, whereas the other two models, which contain longer-distance connections, exhibit strong functional coupling.

The traveling wave of muscle activation along the body is a necessary element of the behavioral motor pattern underlying swimming. A full model for swim behavior should include the known properties of the intersegmental coordinating system fiber anatomy and physiology. Most models have focused on reproducing intersegmental phase lags, not functional intersegmental coupling strength.

Conclusion

It is critically important that models are never mistaken for truth. Regardless of how realistic they appear, they are unlikely to ever include all critical parameters, cells, and connections, at least until new methods for determination of neurons, their channels, and currents as well as their connections can be found. Until then, one can only state that a model contains sufficient anatomical and physiological elements for the generation of the behavioral features of swimming motor output. This holds true for both the rhythmic oscillations and the traveling wave.

One important conclusion from modeling work on the lamprey CPG is that it is advantageous to simultaneously model the system at different levels of description. For systems consisting of coupled oscillators, such as the lamprey and salamander spinal cords and leech nerve cord, phase models can provide insight into how factors such as frequency differences, coupling length, and coupling asymmetry lead to the system's observed behavior. For example, phase models of the lamprey CPG suggest the importance of long connections, but not frequency differences, in setting phase lags. In contrast to phase models, more-detailed models allow us to understand the underlying basis for frequency differences and coupling properties. More-detailed models also potentially allow us to check the validity of a phase model approximation. Thus, the complementary use of detailed models and high-level models often offers the best chance of gaining insight into a complex system's behavior. This should remain true regardless of the details of the underlying physiology of the system. Such systems are notoriously difficult to understand intuitively. Modeling often offers the only sensible approach, as has been shown by a robotic implementation of a salamander by Auke Ijspeert and colleagues in which they demonstrated a potential mechanism for changing gaits in tetrapods.

See also: Central Pattern Generators; Cerebellar Lesions and Effects on Posture, Locomotion and Limb Movement; Computational Approaches to Motor Control; Learning, Action, Inference and Neuromodulation; Pattern Generation; Swimming: Neural Mechanisms.

Further Reading

Buchanan JT (1992) Neural network simulations of coupled locomotor oscillators in the lamprey spinal cord. *Biological Cybernetics* 66(4): 367–374.

Cang J and Friesen WO (2002) Model for intersegmental coordination of leech swimming: Central and sensory mechanisms. *Journal of Neurophysiology* 87(6): 2760–2769.

Cohen AH, Ermentrout GB, Kiemel T, Kopell N, Sigvardt K, and Williams T (1992) Modelling of intersegmental coordination in the lamprey central pattern or for locomotion. *Trends in Neurosciences* 15: 434–438.

Cohen AH, Holmes PJ, and Rand RH (1982) The nature of the coupling between segmental oscillators of the lamprey spinal generator for locomotion: A mathematical model. *Journal of Mathematical Biology* 13: 345–369.

Cohen AH and Wallén P (1980) The neuronal correlate to locomotion in fish: 'Fictive swimming' induced in an *in vitro* preparation of the lamprey spinal cord. *Experimental Brain Research* 41: 11–18.

Ekeberg Ö (1993) A combined neuronal and mechanical model of fish swimming. *Biological Cybernetics* 69: 363–374.

Ijspeert AJ (2001) A connectionist central pattern generator for the aquatic and terrestrial gaits of a simulated salamander. *Biological Cybernetics* 84(5): 331–348.

Jung R, Kiemel T, and Cohen AH (1996) Dynamical behavior of a neural network model of locomotor control in the lamprey. *Journal of Neurophysiology* 75: 1074–1086.

Kiemel T, Gormley KM, Guan L, Williams TL, and Cohen AH (2003) Estimating the strength and direction of functional coupling in the lamprey spinal cord. *Journal of Computational Neuroscience* 13: 233–243.

Kopell N and Ermentrout GB (1990) Phase transitions and other phenomena in chains of coupled oscillators. *SIAM Journal on Applied Mathematics* 50: 1014.

Parker D (2000) Spinal-cord plasticity: Independent and interactive effects of neuromodulator and activity-dependent plasticity. *Molecular Neurobiology* 22(1–3): 55–80.

Roberts A, Tunstall MJ, and Wolf E (1995) Properties of networks controlling locomotion and significance of voltage dependency of NMDA channels: Stimulation study of rhythm generation sustained by positive feedback. *Journal of Neurophysiology* 73(2): 485–495.

Wallén P, Ekeberg Ö, Lansner A, Brodin L, Tråvén H, and Grillner S (1992) A computer-based model for realistic simulations of neural networks: II. The segmental network generating locomotor rhythmicity in the lamprey. *Journal of Neurophysiology* 68: 1939–1950.

Wallén P and Williams TL (1984) Fictive locomotion in the lamprey spinal cord *in vitro* compared with swimming in the intact and spinal animal. *Journal of Physiology* 347: 225–239.

Williams TL (1992) Phase coupling by synaptic spread in chains of coupled neuronal oscillators. *Science* 258(5082): 662–665.

原书词条中英对照表

A

Acetylcholine Neurotransmission in CNS	乙酰胆碱在中枢神经系统中的神经传递
Acetylcholinesterase	乙酰胆碱酯酶
Acetylcholinesterase Inhibitors and Alzheimer's Disease	乙酰胆碱酯酶抑制剂与阿尔茨海默病
Actin Cytoskeleton in Growth Cones, Nerve Terminals, and Dendritic Spines	生长锥、神经末端和树突小棘内的肌动蛋白骨架
Action Potential Initiation and Conduction in Axons	动作电位在轴突上的产生和传导
Active Perception	主动感知
Active Zone	（突触的）活性带
Activity in Visual Development	视觉发育中的活动
Activity-Dependent Metabolism in Glia and Neurons	胶质细胞和神经元的活动依赖性代谢
Activity-Dependent Regulation of Glucose Transporters	葡萄糖转运体的活动依赖性调节
Activity-Dependent Remodeling of Presynaptic Boutons	突触前终扣的活动依赖性重塑
Addiction: Neurobiological Mechanism	成瘾：神经生物学机制
Adenosine	腺苷
Adenosine Receptor Mediated Functions	腺苷受体介导的功能
Adenosine Triphosphate (ATP)	三磷酸腺苷
Adenosine Triphosphate (ATP) as a Neurotransmitter	三磷酸腺苷作为神经递质
Adolescent Brain Development and the Risk of Psychiatric Disorders	青春期大脑发育及精神失常的风险
Adrenal Steroids: Biphasic Effects on Neurons	肾上腺甾类化合物：对神经元的双相影响
Adrenergic Receptors	肾上腺素受体
Adult Cortical Plasticity	成年皮层可塑性
Aggression: Hormonal Basis	侵略性：激素诱因
Aggression: Neurochemical and Molecular Mechanisms	侵略性：神经化学和分子机制
Aging and Memory in Animals	动物的衰老与记忆
Aging and Memory in Humans	人类的衰老与记忆
Aging of the Brain	大脑的衰老
Aging of the Brain and Alzheimer's Disease	大脑的衰老和阿尔茨海默病
Aging: Brain Potential Measures and Reaction Time Studies	衰老：脑电测量和反应时间研究
Aging: Extracellular Space	衰老：细胞外空间

Aging: Invertebrate Models of Normal Brain Aging	衰老：正常脑衰老的无脊椎动物模型
Agnosia	认知不能
Agonistic and Affiliative Signals: Resolutions of Conflict	好斗与亲和信号：冲突的解决
Agraphia	失写症
Alcoholism	酗酒
Alexia	失读症
Allometric Analysis of Brain Size	脑的异速生长分析
Alternative Splicing in the Nervous System	非传统的神经系统剪切
Aluminum	铝
Alzheimer's Disease: An Overview	阿尔茨海默病：概述
Alzheimer's Disease: Molecular Genetics	阿尔茨海默病：分子遗传学
Alzheimer's Disease: MRI Studies	阿尔茨海默病：核磁共振研究
Alzheimer's Disease: Neurodegeneration	阿尔茨海默病：神经退行性变
Alzheimer's Disease: Transgenic Mouse Models	阿尔茨海默病：转基因小鼠模型
Amnesia: Declarative and Nondeclarative Memory	健忘症：陈述性和非陈述性记忆
AMPA Receptor Cell Biology/Trafficking	AMPA 受体细胞生物学/运输
AMPA Receptors: Disease	AMPA 受体：疾病
AMPA Receptors: Molecular Biology and Pharmacology	AMPA 受体：分子生物学及药理学
Amphetamines	苯异丙胺
Amphibian Peptides	两栖动物的多肽
Amygdala: Contributions to Fear	杏仁核：对恐惧情绪的作用
Amygdala: Structure and Circuitry in Primates	杏仁核：灵长类中的结构和环路
Amygdala: Structure and Circuitry in Rodents and Felines	杏仁核：啮齿类和猫科动物中的结构和环路
Amyloid: Vascular and Parenchymal	淀粉体：血管与薄壁组织
Amyotrophic Lateral Sclerosis (ALS)	肌萎缩性脊髓侧索硬化
Amyotrophic Lateral Sclerosis (ALS): Disease Mechanisms	肌萎缩性脊髓侧索硬化：疾病的机制
Angelman Syndrome	安格曼综合征
Angiotensin Actions on and within Brain	血管紧张素在脑中的作用
Angiotensin II	血管紧张素 II
Animal Communication: Honesty and Deception	动物的沟通：诚实与欺骗
Animal Intelligence: The Search for Animal Intelligence	动物的智能：对动物智能的探索
Animal Models of Alzheimer's Disease	阿尔茨海默病的动物模型
Animal Models of Amnesia	健忘症的动物模型
Animal Models of Huntington's Disease	亨廷顿舞蹈病的动物模型
Animal Models of Inherited Retinal Degenerations	遗传性视网膜退行性病变的动物模型
Animal Models of Motor and Sensory Neuron Disease	运动和感觉神经元疾病的动物模型
Animal Models of Parkinson's Disease	帕金森病的动物模型

Animal Models of Stroke 中风的动物模型

Animals and the Biology of Music 动物和音乐的生物基础

Anterior-Posterior Spinal Cord Patterning of the Motor Pool 运动神经元池在前侧-后侧脊髓的模式

Antipsychotic Drugs 安定类药物

Anxiety Disorders 焦虑症

Anxiety: Drug Therapy 焦虑：药物治疗

Apelin 爱帕林肽

Aphasia: Sudden and Progressive 失语症：突发和渐进性

Apoptosis in Nervous System Injury 神经系统损伤中的细胞凋亡

Apoptosis in Neurodegenerative Disease 神经退行性疾病中的细胞凋亡

Appetitive Systems: Amygdala and Striatum 食欲调控系统：杏仁核和纹状体

Apraxia: Disease 失用症：疾病

Apraxia: Sensory System 失用症：感觉系统

Artificial Intelligence 人工智能

Astrocyte: Calcium Signaling 星形胶质细胞：钙信号

Astrocyte: Identification Methods 星形胶质细胞：鉴别手段

Astrocyte: Neurotransmitter and Hormone Receptors 星形胶质细胞：神经递质和激素受体

Astrocyte: Response to Injury 星形胶质细胞：对损伤的反应

Atomic Force Microscopy Methodologies 原子力显微镜方法

Atrial Natriuretic Peptide: Fluid/Mineral Balance 心房钠尿肽：体液/矿物质平衡

Attention and Eye Movements 注意力和眼动

Attention Deficit Hyperactivity Disorder 注意缺陷多动障碍

Attention Deficit Hyperactivity Disorder (ADHD): Mcthylphenidate (Ritalin) and Dopamine 注意缺陷多动障碍：苯哌啶醋酸甲酯(利他林)和多巴胺

Attention: Models 注意力：模型

Attentional Functions in Learning and Memory 学习和记忆中注意力的作用

Attentional Mechanisms in Ventral Pathway 腹侧通路中的注意力机制

Attentional Networks 注意力网络

Attentional Networks in the Parietal Cortex 顶叶皮层中的注意力网络

Attractor Network Models 吸引子网络模型

Audiovocal Communication in Bats 蝙蝠的听觉发声交流

Auditory Cortex Structure and Circuitry 听觉皮层的结构和环路

Auditory Cortex: Models 听觉皮层：模型

Auditory Evoked Potentials 听觉诱发电位

Auditory Localization 听觉的空间定位

Auditory Scene Analysis 听觉场景分析

Auditory System: Central Pathway Plasticity 听觉系统：中枢通路的可塑性

Auditory System: Central Pathways 听觉系统：中枢通路

Auditory System: Efferent Systems to the Auditory Periphery 听觉系统：听觉周边的传入系统

Auditory System: Giant Synaptic Terminals, Endbulbs, and Calyces 听觉系统：巨大突触终端，端球和端萼

Auditory Systems in Insects 昆虫的听觉系统

Auditory/Somatosensory Interactions 听觉/体感相互作用

Autism 自闭症

Autoimmune Autonomic Neuropathy 自身免疫性自主神经疾病

Autonomic and Enteric Nervous System: Apoptosis and Trophic Support During Development 自主和肠神经系统：发育过程中的凋亡和营养支持

Autonomic Disorders 自主神经失调

Autonomic Dysfunction: Drug-Induced 自主神经异常：药物诱发

Autonomic Dysregulation During REM Sleep 快速眼动睡眠中的自主神经失调

Autonomic Failure 自主神经衰竭

Autonomic Nervous System 自主神经系统

Autonomic Nervous System Development 自主神经系统发育

Autonomic Nervous System: Cardiovascular Control 自主神经系统：心血管调控

Autonomic Nervous System: Carotid Body and Chemoception 自主神经系统：颈动脉体和化学感受

Autonomic Nervous System: Central Cardiovascular Control 自主神经系统：心血管的中枢调控

Autonomic Nervous System: Central Control of the Gastrointestinal Tract 自主神经系统：胃肠道的中枢调控

Autonomic Nervous System: Central Respiratory Control 自主神经系统：呼吸的中枢调控

Autonomic Nervous System: Central Thermoregulatory Control 自主神经系统：体温调节的中枢调控

Autonomic Nervous System: Central Urogenital Control 自主神经系统：泌尿生殖的中枢调控

Autonomic Nervous System: Clinical Testing 自主神经系统：临床检查

Autonomic Nervous System: Gastrointestinal Control 自主神经系统：胃肠调控

Autonomic Nervous System: General Overview 自主神经系统：概述

Autonomic Nervous System: Metabolic Function 自主神经系统：代谢功能

Autonomic Nervous System: Neuroanatomy 自主神经系统：神经解剖学

Autonomic Nervous System: Ophthalmic Control 自主神经系统：眼调控

Autonomic Nervous System: Respiratory Control 自主神经系统：呼吸调控

Autonomic Nervous System: Urogenital Control 自主神经系统：泌尿生殖调控

Autonomic Neuroeffector Junction 自主神经神经效应器连接

Autonomic Neuroimmunology 自主神经神经免疫学

Autonomic Neuroplasticity and Aging 自主神经神经可塑性与衰老

Autonomic Neuroplasticity and Regeneration 自主神经神经可塑性与再生

Autonomic Neuroplasticity: Development	自主神经神经可塑性：发育
Autophagy and Neuronal Death	自吞噬与神经元死亡
Aversive Emotions: Genetic Mechanisms of Serotonin	厌恶情绪：5-羟色胺的遗传机制
Aversive Emotions: Molecular Basis of Unconditioned Fear	厌恶情绪：非条件恐惧的分子基础
Awareness: Functional Imaging	意识：功能成像
Axon Guidance by Glia	胶质细胞引导的轴突导向
Axon Guidance: Building Pathways with Molecular Cues in Vertebrate Sensory Systems	轴突导向：脊椎动物感觉系统通过分子线索建立的途径
Axon Guidance: Guidance Cues and Guidepost Cells	轴突导向：引导线索与路标细胞
Axon Guidance: Morphogens as Chemoattractants and Chemorepellants	轴突导向：作为趋化剂和驱化剂的形态发生分子
Axonal and Dendritic Identity and Structure: Control of	轴突及树突的鉴别和结构：控制
Axonal and Dendritic Transport by Dyneins and Kinesins in Neurons	神经元中动力蛋白和驱动蛋白介导的轴突及树突运输
Axonal Injury in Demyelinating Disease and CNS Injury	脱髓鞘病与中枢神经系统损伤中的轴突损伤
Axonal Injury: Neuronal Responses	轴突损伤：神经元反应
Axonal mRNA Transport and Functions	轴突的 mRNA 运输及功能
Axonal Pathfinding	轴突寻路
Axonal Pathfinding: Extracellular Matrix Role	轴突寻路：胞外基质的作用
Axonal Pathfinding: Guidance Activities of Sonic Hedgehog (Shh)	轴突寻路：Shh 的导向活动
Axonal Pathfinding: Netrins	轴突寻路：纺锤蛋白
Axonal Regeneration: Role of Growth and Guidance Cues	轴突再生：生长和导向信号的作用
Axonal Regeneration: Role of the Extracellular Matrix and the Glial Scar	轴突再生：胞外基质和胶质瘢痕的作用
Axonal Transport and ALS	轴突运输与抗淋巴细胞血清
Axonal Transport and Alzheimer's Disease	轴突运输与阿尔茨海默病
Axonal Transport and Huntington's Disease	轴突运输与亨廷顿舞蹈病
Axonal Transport and Neurodegenerative Diseases	轴突运输与神经退行性疾病
Axonal Transport Disorders	轴突运输障碍
Axonal Transport Tracers	轴突运输标记物

B

Babinski's Reflex/Sign	巴宾斯基反射/巴宾斯基征
BAC Transgenesis: Cell-Type Specific Expression in the Nervous System	细菌人工染色体转基因：神经系统中的细胞类型特异性表达
BAC Use in the Study of the CNS	细菌人工染色体技术在中枢神经系统的应用

Balance and Posture Control	平衡和姿势控制
Balance and Posture Control: Human	平衡和姿势控制：人类
Balint Syndrome	巴林特综合征
Barrel Cortex Circuits	桶状皮层环路
Basal Forebrain and Memory	基底前脑和记忆
Basal Ganglia and Oculomotor Control	基底神经节与眼动控制
Basal Ganglia: Acetylcholine Interactions and Behavior	基底神经节：乙酰胆碱的相互作用与行为
Basal Ganglia: Evolution	基底神经节：演化
Basal Ganglia: Functional Models of Normal and Disease States	基底神经节：正常与病理状态的功能模型
Basal Ganglia: Habit	基底神经节：习惯
Basal Ganglia: Internal Organization	基底神经节：内部组织
Basal Ganglia: Motor Functions	基底神经节：运动功能
Basal Ganglia: Physiological Circuits	基底神经节：生理环路
Bayesian Cortical Models	贝叶斯皮层模型
Bayesian Models of Motor Control	运动控制的贝叶斯模型
BDNF in Synaptic Plasticity and Memory	脑源性神经营养因子在突触可塑性与记忆中的作用
Behavioral Hierarchies	行为的等级层次
Bell's Palsy	贝尔麻痹
Bergmann Glial Cells	贝格曼胶质细胞
Bilingualism	双语
Binocular Rivalry	双眼竞争
Biomechanics: Hydroskeletal	生物力学：水骨胳
Bipolar Disorder	双极人格失常
Bird Brain: Evolution	鸟类的大脑：演化
Bird Song Systems: Evolution	鸟鸣系统：演化
Birdsong Learning	鸟鸣学习
Birdsong Learning: Evolutionary, Behavioral, and Hormonal Issues	鸟鸣学习：演化，行为和激素问题
Birdsong: The Neurobiology of Avian Vocal Learning	鸟鸣：禽鸟声音学习的神经生物学
Blindsight: Residual Vision	盲视：残留视觉
Blood Pressure: Baroreceptors	血压：压力感受器
Blood-Brain Barrier and Neurovascular Mechanisms of Neurodegeneration and Injury	血脑屏障与神经退行性变和损伤的神经血管机制
Bone Morphogenetic Protein (BMP) Signaling in the Neuroectoderm	骨形态发生蛋白在神经外胚层的信号传导
Borderline Personality Disorder	边缘型人格异常
Botulinum and Tetanus Toxins	肉毒毒素与破伤风毒素

Brain Adrenergic Neurons	脑肾上腺素能神经元
Brain Asymmetry: Evolution	脑的不对称性：演化
Brain Composition: Age-Related Changes	脑的组成：年龄相关性变化
Brain Connectivity and Brain Size	脑的连接和脑容量
Brain Damage: Functional Reorganization	脑损伤：功能重组
Brain Development: The Generation of Large Brains	脑的发育：大型脑的产生
Brain Evolution: Developmental Constraints and Relative Developmental Growth	脑的演化：发育上的限制和相对发育生长
Brain Evolution: The Radiator Theory	脑的演化：散热器理论
Brain Fossils: Endocasts	脑化石：颅腔模型
Brain Glucose Metabolism: Age, Alzheimer's Disease, and ApoE Allele Effects	脑的葡萄糖代谢：年龄，阿尔茨海默病以及 ApoE 等位基因的影响
Brain Injury: Functional Recovery After	脑损伤后的功能恢复
Brain Injury: Magnetic Resonance Studies of Metabolic Aspects	脑损伤：代谢方面的磁共振研究
Brain Modules: Mosaic Evolution	脑的模块：马赛克演化
Brain Na,K-ATPase	脑的钠-钾 ATP 酶
Brain Scaling Laws	脑尺寸定律
Brain Trauma	脑外伤
Brain Volume: Age-Related Changes	脑容量：年龄相关性变化
Brain–Computer Interface	脑-计算机接口
Brains of Primitive Chordates	原始脊索动物的脑
Brainstem and Cranial Nerves	脑干与颅神经
Brainstem Control of Eye Movements	眼动的脑干控制
Brainstem Respiratory Circuits	脑干呼吸环路
Broca's Area: Evolution	布洛卡区：演化
Brodmann's Areas	布罗德曼氏区

C

CADASIL (Cerebral Autosomal Dominant Arteriopathy with Subcortical Infarcts and Leukoencephalopathy)	常染色体显性遗传脑动脉病合并皮质下梗死和白质脑病
Cadherins and Synapse Organization	钙黏素与突触组织
Cajal's Place in the History of Neuroscience	Cajal 在神经生物学史上的地位
Calcitonin Gene-Related Peptide (CGRP) and Receptors	降钙素基因相关肽及受体
Calcium and Signal Transduction	钙和信号转导
Calcium Channel and Calcium-Activated Potassium Channel Coupling	钙通道及钙激活钾通道偶联

Calcium Channel Subtypes Involved in Neurotransmitter Release	神经递质释放中涉及的钙通道亚型
Calcium Channels	钙通道
Calcium Channels and SNARE Proteins	钙通道和 SNARE 蛋白
Calcium Homeostasis in Glia	神经胶质细胞中的钙稳态调节
Calcium Waves in Glia	神经胶质细胞中的钙波
Calcium Waves: Purinergic Regulation	钙波：嘌呤调控
Calcium-Calmodulin Kinase II (CaMKII) in Learning and Memory	钙-钙调蛋白激酶 II 在学习与记忆中的作用
Canal-Otolith Interactions	耳道-内耳石相互作用
Cardiovascular Function: Central Nervous System Control	心血管功能：中枢神经系统调控
Cataplexy	猝倒症
CCK/Gastrin and Receptors	胆囊收缩素/胃泌素及受体
Cell Adhesion Molecules at Synapses	突触上的细胞黏附分子
Cell Culture: Autonomic and Enteric Neurons	细胞培养：自主和肠神经元
Cell Culture: Primary Neural Cells	细胞培养：原代神经元细胞
Cell Replacement Therapy for Huntington's Disease	亨廷顿舞蹈病的细胞替代疗法
Cell Replacement Therapy: Mechanisms of Functional Recovery	细胞替代疗法：功能恢复的机制
Cell Replacement Therapy: Parkinson's Disease	细胞替代疗法：帕金森病
Cell-Cell Communication Through the Extracellular Space	通过胞外空间的细胞-细胞通信
Cells: 5-Hydroxytryptamine Receptors	细胞：5 -羟色胺受体
Cellular Dynamics Revealed by Digital Holographic Microscopy	数字全息显微镜所揭示的细胞动力学
Central Gustatory System and Ingestive Behavior	中枢味觉系统和摄食行为
Central Pattern Generators	中枢模式发生器
Central Pattern Generators: Sensory Feedback	中枢模式发生器：感觉反馈
Cerebellar Deep Nuclei	小脑深部核团
Cerebellar Lesions and Effects on Posture, Locomotion and Limb Movement	小脑损伤及其对姿势、行进和肢体运动的影响
Cerebellar Microcircuitry	小脑微回路
Cerebellum and Oculomotor Control	小脑和眼动控制
Cerebellum: Clinical Pathology	小脑：临床病理学
Cerebellum: Evolution and Comparative Anatomy	小脑：演化和比较解剖学
Cerebellum: Models	小脑：模型
Cerebral Cortex	大脑皮层
Cerebral Cortex: Inhibitory Cells	大脑皮层：抑制性细胞
Cerebral Cortex: Symmetric vs. Asymmetric Cell Division	大脑皮层：对称与非对称细胞分裂

Cerebral Fissure Patterns	脑裂模式
Cerebrovascular Disease	脑血管病
Cetacean Brains	鲸类动物的脑
Chemical Senses: Overview	化学感受：综述
Chemical Senses: Protozoa	化学感受：原生动物
Chemoaffinity Hypothesis: Development of Topographic Axonal Projections	化学亲和假说：轴突拓扑投射的形成
Cholinergic Neurotransmission in the Autonomic and Somatic Motor Nervous System	自主和躯体运动神经系统中的胆碱能神经传递
Cholinergic Pathways in CNS	中枢神经系统中的胆碱能途径
Cholinergic System	胆碱能系统
Cholinergic System Imaging in the Healthy Aging Process and Alzheimer Disease	正常衰老过程及阿尔茨海默病中的胆碱能系统成像
Chromaffin Cells: Model Cells for Neuronal Cell Biology	嗜铬细胞：神经细胞生物学的模式细胞
Chronic (Repeated) Stress: Consequences, Adaptations	慢性（重复）压力：后果，适应
Cingulate Cortex	扣带皮层
Circadian Function and Therapeutic Potential of Melatonin in Humans	人类褪黑激素的节律功能及治疗潜力
Circadian Gene Expression in the Suprachiasmatic Nucleus	视交叉上核中的节律基因表达
Circadian Genes and the Sleep-Wake Cycle	节律基因与睡-醒周期
Circadian Metabolic Rhythms Regulated by the Suprachiasmatic Nucleus	视交叉上核调节的周期性代谢节律
Circadian Organization	节律组织
Circadian Organization in Non-Mammalian Vertebrates	非哺乳类脊椎动物的节律组织
Circadian Oscillations in the Suprachiasmatic Nucleus	视交叉上核的节律震荡
Circadian Regulation by the Suprachiasmatic Nucleus	视交叉上核的节律调节
Circadian Regulation in Invertebrates	无脊椎动物的节律调节
Circadian Rhythm Models	节律模型
Circadian Rhythms in Sleepiness, Alertness, and Performance	睡眠、清醒和行为中的周期节律
Circadian Rhythms: Influence of Light in Humans	周期节律：人类受光的影响
Circadian Systems: Evolution	周期节律系统：演化
Circumventricular Organs	室周器
Circumventricular Organs in Neuroendocrine Control	室周器在神经内分泌控制中的作用
CIRL/Latrophilins	钙离子非依赖型蛛毒受体/蛛毒素受体
Clathrin and Clathrin-Adaptors	网格蛋白与网格蛋白适配器
Clock Gene Regulation of Endocrine Function	内分泌功能的时钟基因调控

Clock Genes and Metabolic Regulation	时钟基因与代谢调控
Cochlear Development	耳蜗的发育
Cochlear Mechanics	耳蜗的力学特性
Cochlear Prosthesis	耳蜗假体
Cognition in Aging and Age-Related Disease	衰老及年龄相关疾病中的认知
Cognition: An Overview of Neuroimaging Techniques	认知：神经影像技术概论
Cognition: Basal Ganglia Role	认知：基底神经节的作用
Cognition: Cerebellum Role	认知：小脑的作用
Cognition: Neuropharmacology	认知：神经药理学
Cognitive Control and Development	认知控制和发育
Cognitive Deficits in Schizophrenia	精神分裂症中的认知功能缺陷
Cognitive Dysfunction in Psychiatric Disorders	精神疾病中的认知功能障碍
Cognitive Neuroscience: An Overview	认知神经科学：概述
Color Vision	颜色视觉
Coma	昏迷
Coma and Other Pathological Disorders of Consciousness	昏迷及其他意识病理障碍
Command Systems	（神经中枢的）指挥系统
Communication in Frogs and Toads	蛙类及蟾蜍的沟通
Communication in Terrestrial Animals	陆生动物的沟通
Communication in the Honeybee	蜜蜂的沟通
Communication Networks and Eavesdropping in Animals	动物的沟通网络及偷听
Comparative Biology of Invertebrate Neuromuscular Junctions	无脊椎动物神经肌肉接头的比较生物学
Comparative Neurobiology: History	比较神经生物学：历史
Complexins	（突触蛋白）复合体
Computational Approaches to Motor Control	研究运动控制的计算方法
Computational Methods	计算方法
Computational Neuroethology	计算神经行为学
Conditioned Reflex	条件反射
Conditioned Taste Aversion	条件性味觉厌恶
Conditioning: Simple Neural Circuits in the Honeybee	条件化：蜜蜂的简单神经环路
Conditioning: Theories	条件化：理论
Cone Photopigment Evolution	视锥感光色素的演化
Congenital Muscular Dystrophy	先天性肌营养不良
Connectionist Models	联结主义模型
Connectionist Models of Language Processing	语言处理的联结主义模型
Connectivity of Primate Reward Centers	灵长类奖励中心的连接
Consciousness: Neural Basis of Conscious Experience	意识：意识经验的神经基础
Consciousness: Neurophysiology and Visual Awareness in	意识：神经生理学与视觉意识

Consciousness: Philosophy	意识：哲学
Consciousness: Theoretical and Computational Neuroscience	意识：理论与计算神经科学
Consciousness: Theories and Models	意识：理论及模型
Contextual Interactions in Visual Perception	视觉感知中背景的相互作用
Contextual Interactions in Visual Processing	视觉信息处理中背景的相互作用
Cornelia De Lange Syndrome	科妮莉亚德兰格综合征(严重智力迟钝合并多种畸形)
Corpus Callosum: Agenesis	胼胝体：发育不全
Cortical Control of Eye Movements	眼动的皮层控制
Cortical Plasticity and Learning: Mechanisms and Models	皮层可塑性与学习：机制和模型
Cortical Processing of the Reward Value of Food	食物奖励价值的皮层处理
Corticomotoneuronal System	皮层运动神经系统
Corticospinal Development	皮层脊髓的发育
Corticothalamic Connections: Structure and Function	皮层膝体连接：结构和功能
Corticothalamic Connections: Ultrastructure	皮层膝体连接：超结构
Corticotropin-Releasing Hormone and Urocortins: Binding Proteins and Receptors	促肾上腺皮质激素释放与尿皮质素：结合蛋白与受体
Corticotropin-Releasing Hormone: Integration of Adaptive Responses to Stress	促肾上腺皮质激素释放激素：压力适应性反应的整合
Cotransmission	协同传递
Cranial-Cervical Dystonia	颅颈部肌张力障碍
Cross-Modal Interactions Between Vision and Touch	视觉与触觉的跨模态相互作用
Cyclic AMP (cAMP) Role in Learning and Memory	cAMP 在学习与记忆中的作用
Cyclic Nucleotide-Gated and Hyperpolarization-Activated Channels	环核苷酸门控和超极化激活通道
Cysteine-String Proteins (CSPs)	半胱氨酸串蛋白
Cysticercosis: Cerebral	囊虫病：大脑
Cytokine Receptors in Glia	胶质细胞的细胞因子受体
Cytoskeletal Interactions in the Neuron	神经元中的细胞骨架相互作用
Cytoskeleton in Plasticity	细胞骨架在可塑性中的作用

D

d-Serine: From Its Synthesis in Glial Cell to Its Action on Synaptic Transmission and Plasticity	d-丝氨酸：从胶质细胞中的合成到突触传递与可塑性中的作用
Deafness	失聪
Decision-Making and Neuroeconomics	决策与神经经济学
Decision-Making and Vision	决策与视觉

Decision-Making in Financial Markets	金融市场中的决策
Declarative Memory System: Anatomy	陈述性记忆系统：解剖学
Decoding Neuron Transcriptome by SAGE	采用基因表达序列分析解码神经元转录组
Deep Brain Stimulation	脑深部刺激
Deep Brain Stimulation and Movement Disorder Treatment	脑深部刺激与运动障碍治疗
Deep Brain Stimulation and Parkinson's Disease	脑深部刺激与帕金森病
Delayed Reinforcement: Economics	延迟强化：经济学
Delayed Reinforcement: Neuroscience	延迟强化：神经科学
Dementia	痴呆
Dementia and Language	痴呆和语言
Demyelinating Diseases	脱髓鞘病
Demyelination and Demyelinating Antibodies	脱髓鞘与脱髓鞘抗体
Dendrite Development, Synapse Formation and Elimination	树突发育，突触的形成与消除
Dendrites: Localized Translation	树突：局部翻译
Dendritic RNA Transport: Dynamic Spatio-Temporal Control of Neuronal Gene Expression	树突RNA运输：神经元基因表达的动态时空调控
Dendritic Signal Integration	树突信号整合
Dendritic Spine History	树突小棘的历史
Depression and the Brain	抑郁症与脑
Development of Behavior	行为的发育
Development of Drosophila Neuromuscular Junctions	果蝇神经肌肉接头的发育
Developmental Disability and Fragile X Syndrome: Clinical Overview	发育障碍与脆性X染色体综合征：临床概观
Developmental Synaptic Plasticity: LTP, LTD, and Synapse Formation and Elimination	发育突触可塑性：长时程增强、长时程抑制与突触的形成及消除
Diabetes Type 2 and Stress: Impact on Memory and the Hippocampus	2型糖尿病与压力：对记忆和海马区的影响
Diabetic Neuropathy	糖尿病神经病变
Dichotic Listening Studies of Brain Asymmetry	脑不对称性的双耳分听研究
Differentiation: The Cell Cycle Instead	分化：细胞周期
Diffusion Tensor Imaging (DTI)	弥散张量成像
Dopamine	多巴胺
Dopamine-CNS Pathways and Neurophysiology	多巴胺：中枢神经系统途径与神经生理学
Dopamine Control of Arousal	觉醒的多巴胺控制
Dopamine in Perspective	关于多巴胺的正确认识
Dopamine Neurons: Reward and Uncertainty	多巴胺神经元：奖励与不确定性
Dopamine Receptors and Antipsychotic Drugs in Health and Disease	多巴胺受体与健康和病理状态中的抗精神病药物

Dopamine: Cellular Actions	多巴胺：细胞水平的作用
Dopaminergic Agonists and l-DOPA	多巴胺能激动剂与左旋多巴
Dopaminergic Differentiation	多巴胺能分化
Dorsal Root Ganglion Neurons	背根神经节神经元
Double Cortex	双皮层（弥漫性皮层下带异托邦）
Down Syndrome	唐氏综合征
Down Syndrome: A Disorder of Histogenesis	唐氏综合征：组织发生障碍
Dream Function	梦的功能
Dreams and Dreaming: Incorporation of Waking Events	梦与做梦：与清醒状态事件的结合
Dreams and Nightmares in PTSD	创伤后应激障碍中的梦与梦魇
Dreams, Dreaming Theories and Correlates of Nightmares	梦、做梦理论与恶梦的关联
Drosophila Apterous Neurons: From Stem Cell to Unique Neuron	果蝇无翅神经元：从干细胞到独特的神经元
Drug Addiction: Behavioral Neurophysiology	药物成瘾：行为神经生理学
Drug Addiction: Behavioral Pharmacology of Drug Addiction in Rats	药物成瘾：大鼠中药物成瘾性的行为药理学
Drug Addiction: Cellular Mechanisms	药物成瘾：细胞机制
Drug Addiction: Neuroimaging	药物成瘾：神经影像学
Drugs Addiction: Actions	药物成瘾：行为
Dynamin	发动蛋白
Dysautonomia: Familial	自主神经机能异常：家族性
Dyslexia: Neurodevelopmental Basis	诵读困难：神经发育基础
Dystonia: Classification, Genetics and Therapeutics	肌张力障碍：分类、遗传学和疗法
Dystonia: Myoclonus-Dystonia	肌张力障碍：肌阵挛-肌张力障碍
Dystrophin, Associated Proteins, and Muscular Dystrophy	肌营养不良蛋白,相关蛋白与肌肉萎缩症

E

Eating Disorders	饮食障碍症
Echolocation I: Behavior	回声定位 I：行为
Echolocation II: Neurophysiology	回声定位 II：神经生理学
Electrical Perception and Communication	电感知和交流
Electrical Self-Stimulation	自我电刺激
Electrocommunication	电通信
Electroencephalography (EEG)	脑电图
Electrolocation	电定位
Electromyography (EMG) and Nerve Conduction Studies	肌电图与神经传导研究
Electronic Nose	电子鼻

Electrophysiology: EEG and ERP Analysis	电生理学：脑电图与诱发电位分析
Electroretinography	视网膜电流图
Emotion and Vigilance	情绪与警觉
Emotion in Speech	言语中的情绪
Emotion Systems and the Brain	情绪系统和脑
Emotion: Computational Modeling	情绪：计算模型
Emotion: Neuroimaging	情绪：神经影像学
Emotional Control of the Autonomic Nervous System	自主神经系统的情绪控制
Emotional Disorders: Treatment	情绪障碍：治疗
Emotional Hormones and Memory Modulation	情绪激素与记忆调节
Emotional Influences on Memory and Attention	情绪对记忆和注意的影响
Emotional Learning in Humans	人类的情绪学习
Encephalitis	脑炎
Endocannabinoid Role in Synaptic Plasticity and Learning	内源性大麻素在突触可塑性和学习中的作用
Endocrine Function During Sleep and Sleep Deprivation	睡眠及睡眠剥夺时的内分泌功能
Endocrinology of Animal Communication: Behavioral	动物交流的内分泌学：行为方面
Endocytic Traffic in Spines	树突棘的内吞运输
Endocytosis and Presynaptic Scaffolds	内吞作用和突触前支架
Endocytosis: Kiss and Run	内吞作用：一触即跑
Energy Homeostasis: Adiposity Signals	能量稳态：肥胖信号
Energy Homeostasis: Endocannabinoid System	能量稳态：内源性大麻素系统
Energy Homeostasis: Hypothalamic Development	能量稳态：下丘脑发育
Energy Homeostasis: Paraventricular Nucleus (PVN) System	能量稳态：下丘脑室旁核系统
Energy Homeostasis: Thermoregulation	能量稳态：体温调节
Energy Homeostasis: Visceral Control	能量稳态：内脏控制
Engineering Viruses for CNS studies	针对中枢神经系统研究的病毒工程设计
Enteric Nervous System Development	肠神经系统的发育
Enteric Nervous System: Disorders	肠神经系统：紊乱
Enteric Nervous System: Glial Cells and Interstitial Cells of Cajal	肠神经系统：神经胶质细胞与 Cajal 间质细胞
Enteric Nervous System: Neural Circuits and Chemical Coding	肠神经系统：神经环路与化学编码
Enteric Nervous System: Neurotrophic Factors	肠神经系统：神经营养因子
Enteric Nervous System: Physiology	肠神经系统：生理学
Enteric Nervous System: Sensory Pathways	肠神经系统：感觉通路
Entorhinal Cortex	嗅皮层
Entrainment of Circadian Rhythms by Light	光诱导的昼夜节律

Ependymal Cells	室管膜细胞
Eph Receptor Signaling and Spine Morphology	Eph 受体信号与树突小棘形态
Epilepsy	癫痫
Epilepsy: Channelopathies	癫痫：通道病
Epilepsy: Neuronal Death	癫痫：神经元死亡
Episodic Memory	情景记忆
Episodic Memory: Assessment in Animals	情景记忆：动物中的评估
Erectile Dysfunction	勃起功能障碍
Estrus and Menstrual Cycles: Neuroendocrine Control	发情与月经周期：神经内分泌控制
Event-Related Potentials (ERPs)	事件相关电位
Event-Related Potentials (ERPs) and Cognitive Processing	事件相关电位与认知信号处理
Evoked Potentials: Clinical	诱发电位：临床
Evoked Potentials: Recording Methods	诱发电位：记录方法
Evolution of Sensory Receptor Specializations in the Glabrous Skin	光滑皮肤中感觉受体特化的演化
Evolution of the Limbic System	边缘系统的演化
Evolution of Vertebrate Brains	脊椎动物脑的演化
Evolution of Vertebrate Respiratory Control	脊椎动物呼吸控制的演化
Excitotoxicity in Neurodegenerative Disease	神经退行性疾病中的兴奋毒性作用
Executive Function and Higher-Order Cognition: Assessment in Animals	执行功能与高级认知；动物中的评估
Executive Function and Higher-Order Cognition: Computational Models	执行功能与高级认知：计算模型
Executive Function and Higher-Order Cognition: Definition and Neural Substrates	执行功能与高级认知：定义与神经基础
Executive Function and Higher-Order Cognition: EEG Studies	执行功能与高级认知：脑电图研究
Executive Function and Higher-Order Cognition: Neuroimaging	执行功能与高级认知：神经影像学
Executive Functions: Eye Movements and Neuropsychiatric Disorders	执行功能：眼动与神经精神障碍
Exercise in Neurodegenerative Disease and Stroke	锻炼在神经退行性疾病与中风中的作用
Exercise: Optimizing Function and Survival at the Cellular Level	锻炼：在细胞水平优化功能与生存
Exocytosis: Ca^{2+}-Sensitivity	胞吐：钙离子敏感性
Extinction: Anatomy	（条件反射反应的）消失：解剖学
Extracellular Matrix Molecules: Synaptic Plasticity and Learning	胞外基质分子：突触可塑性与学习

Eye and Head Movements	眼与头部运动
Eye Movement Disorders	眼动障碍
Eye Tracking and Mental Illness	眼追踪与精神疾病
Eyeblink Conditioning	眨眼条件反射

F

Facial Expression in Primate Communication	灵长类交流的面部表情
Fatigue	疲劳
Fear Conditioning and Synaptic Plasticity	恐惧条件学习与突触可塑性
Fetal Alcohol Syndrome	胎儿酒精中毒综合征
Finger Movements: Control	手指运动：控制
Flavor Physiology	味觉生理学
Floor Plate Patterning of Ventral Cell Types: Ventral Patterning	腹侧细胞类型的（神经管）底板模式：腹侧模式
Fluid and Electrolyte Homeostasis: Clinical Disease	体液与电解质稳态：临床疾病
Fluorescence Microscopy in the Neurosciences	神经科学中的荧光显微镜
Fluorescent Biomarkers in Neurons	神经元的荧光生物标记
fMRI: BOLD Contrast	功能核磁共振：BOLD 对比度
Folate Deficiency States	叶酸缺乏状态
Food and Water Intake: Regulation	食物和水的摄入：调节
Forebrain Development: Holoprosencephaly (HPE)	前脑发育：前脑无裂畸形
Forebrain Development: Prosomere Model	前脑发育：Prosomere 模型
Forebrain: Early Development	前脑：早期发育
Fovea: Primate	中央凹：灵长类
Fragile X Syndrome	脆性 X 染色体综合征
Fragile X-Associated Tremor Ataxia/Syndrome	脆性 X 染色体相关震颤共济失调/综合征
Free Radicals in Autonomic Functions	自主神经功能中的自由基
Friedreich Ataxia	弗里德希氏共济失调（遗传性共济失调,家族性共济失调）
Frontal Cortex Evolution in Primates	灵长类前额叶的演化
Frontal Eye Fields	额叶眼动区
Frontal Lobe Syndrome	前额叶综合征
Functional Amnesia	功能性失忆
Functional Connectivity	功能连接
Functional Electrical Stimulation	功能电刺激
Functional Imaging of the Motor System	运动系统的功能成像
Functional Neuroimaging Studies of Aging	衰老的功能神经影像学研究

Fusion Pore	融合孔

G

GABA Synthesis and Metabolism	GABA 的合成与代谢
$GABA_A$ Receptor Synaptic Functions	$GABA_A$ 受体的突触功能
$GABA_A$ Receptors and Disease	$GABA_A$ 受体与疾病
$GABA_A$ Receptors: Developmental Roles	$GABA_A$ 受体：发育上的作用
$GABA_A$ Receptors: Molecular Biology, Cell Biology, and Pharmacology	$GABA_A$ 受体：分子生物学,细胞生物学与药理学
$GABA_B$ Receptor Function	$GABA_B$ 受体功能
$GABA_B$ Receptors: Molecular Biology and Pharmacology	$GABA_B$ 受体：分子生物学与药理学
Gain Modulation	增益调节
Galanin and Receptors	甘丙肽和受体
Game Theory and the Economics of Animal Communication	博弈论与动物交流的经济学
Games in Monkeys: Neurophysiology and Motor Decision-Making	猴子的游戏：神经生理学与运动决策
Gamma-Aminobutyric Acid (GABA)	γ 氨基丁酸
Gap Junction Abnormalities and Disorders of the Nervous System	神经系统间隙连接异常和疾病
Gap Junction Communication	间隙连接通信
Gap Junctions and Electrical Synapses	间隙连接与电突触
Gap Junctions and Hemichannels in Glia	神经胶质细胞的间隙连接与半通道
Gap Junctions and Neuronal Oscillations	间隙连接与神经元振荡
Gap Junctions: Metabolic Exchanges	间隙连接：代谢交换
Gastrointestinal Signals: Satiety	胃肠信号：饱腹感
Gastrointestinal Signals: Stimulation	胃肠信号：刺激
Gastrointestinal Tract Role in Neural Control of Metabolism, Food Intake and Body Weight: A Summary	胃肠道在代谢神经控制、食物摄入与体重中的作用：总结
Gene Expression Dysregulation in CNS Pathophysiology	中枢神经系统病理生理学中的基因表达失调
Gene Expression in Normal Aging Brain	正常衰老脑的基因表达
Gene Expression in the Evolution of the Human Brain	人脑演化的基因表达
Gene Expression Regulation: Activity-Dependent	基因表达调节：活动相关性
Gene Expression Regulation: Chromatin Modification in the CNS	基因表达调节：中枢神经系统的染色质修饰
Gene Expression Regulation: Steroid Hormone Effects	基因表达调节：类固醇激素的影响
Gene Therapy and Protection from Stress-Induced Brain Damage	应激所致脑损伤的基因治疗与保护

Gene Therapy: Direct Viral Delivery	基因治疗：直接病毒运输
Gene Therapy: Genetically Modified Cells	基因治疗：基因修饰细胞
Genetic Influence on CNS Gene Expression: Impact on Behavior	遗传对中枢神经系统基因表达的影响：行为方面的影响
Genetic Regulation of Circadian Rhythms in Drosophila	果蝇昼夜节律的遗传调控
Genetics of Circadian Disorders in Humans	人类昼夜节律的遗传学
Genetics of Human Anxiety and Its Disorders	人类焦虑与焦虑症的遗传学
Genomic Disorder and Gene Expression in the Developing CNS	中枢神经系统发育的基因组失调与基因表达
Genomics of Brain Aging: Apolipoprotein E	脑衰老的基因组学：载脂蛋白 E
Genomics of Brain Aging: Nuclear and Mitochondrial Genomes	脑衰老的基因组学：核与线粒体基因组
Genomics of Brain Aging: Twin Studies	脑衰老的基因组学：双胞胎研究
GFL Neurotrophic Factors: Physiology and Pharmacology	GFL 神经营养因子：生理与药理学
Glia and Stroke	胶质细胞与中风
Glia and Synapse Formation: An Overview	胶质细胞与突触形成：概述
Glia Control of Blood Flow	血流的胶质细胞控制
Glial Cells: Astrocytes and Oligodendrocytes during Normal Brain Aging	胶质细胞：正常脑衰老中的星形胶质细胞与少突胶质细胞
Glial Cells: Invertebrate	胶质细胞：无脊椎动物
Glial Cells: Microglia during Normal Brain Aging	胶质细胞：正常脑衰老中的小胶质细胞
Glial Cells: T Cell Interactions	胶质细胞：T 细胞相互作用
Glial Energy Metabolism: A NMR Spectroscopy Perspective	胶质细胞能量代谢：核磁共振光谱方法
Glial Energy Metabolism: Overview	胶质细胞能量代谢：概述
Glial Glutamate and GABA Metabolism	胶质细胞的谷氨酸与 GABA 代谢
Glial Glutamate Transporters	胶质细胞的谷氨酸转运体
Glial Glutamate Transporters: Electrophysiology	胶质细胞的谷氨酸转运体：电生理学
Glial Glycogen Metabolism	胶质细胞的糖原代谢
Glial Growth Factors	胶质细胞生长因子
Glial Influence on Synaptic Transmission	胶质细胞对突触传递的影响
Glial Ion Homeostasis: A Fluorescence Microscopy Approach	胶质细胞离子稳态：荧光显微镜研究
Glial Plasticity and Neuroendocrine Regulation	胶质细胞可塑性与神经内分泌调节
Glial Responses to Injury	胶质细胞对损伤的反应
Glial Responses to Virus Infection	胶质细胞对病毒感染的反应
Glial Steroid Metabolism	胶质细胞类固醇代谢
Glioma	神经胶质瘤
Glutamate	谷氨酸

Glutamate Receptor Clusters: Narp, EphB2 Receptor, Stargazin	谷氨酸受体群：Narp，EphB2 受体，Stargazin
Glutamate Receptor Organization: Ultrastructural Insights	谷氨酸受体组织：超结构研究
Glutamate Regulation of Dendritic Spine Form and Function	树突小棘形成和功能的谷氨酸调控
Glutamatergic and Gabaergic Systems	谷氨酸能与 GABA 能系统
Glycine Receptors: Molecular and Cell Biology	甘氨酸受体：分子与细胞生物学
Glycogen Metabolism in CNS White Matter	中枢神经系统白质的糖原代谢
Glycosylation: General Overview	糖基化：概述
Goal-Directed Behavior Theories	目标导向行为理论
Gonadal Steroid Actions on Brain	性腺激素对脑的作用
Gonadotropin, Neural and Hormonal Control	促性腺激素、神经与激素控制
Gonadotropin-Releasing Hormone: GnRH-1 System	促性腺激素释放激素：GnRH-1 系统
Gravitational Effects on Brain and Behavior	重力对脑和行为的影响
Growth Cones	生长锥
Growth Factors: Neuronal Atrophy	生长因子：神经元萎缩
Growth Hormone	生长激素

H

Hair Cell Differentiation	毛细胞分化
Hair Cell Regeneration	毛细胞再生
Hair Cells: Sensory Transduction	毛细胞：感觉传导
Headache	头痛
Hearing and Echolocation in Dolphins	海豚的听觉及回声定位
Heart Rate Variability: A Neurovisceral Integration Model	心率变异性：脑脊髓交感神经系统整合模型
Hebbian Plasticity	Hebbian 可塑性
Helix-Loop-Helix (bHLH) Proteins: Hes Family	螺旋-环-螺旋蛋白：Hes 家族
Helix-Loop-Helix (bHLH) Proteins: Proneural	螺旋-环-螺旋蛋白：原神经
Hemiplegic Migraine and Channel Disorders	偏瘫偏头痛与通道紊乱
Hemispheric Specialization and Cognition	半球特化及认知
Hepatic Encephalopathy	肝性脑病
Herbal Products and GABA Receptors	草药与 GABA 受体
Hereditary Spastic Paraplegia	遗传性痉挛性截瘫
Heritable Microgyrias	遗传性脑回小畸形
Hibernation	冬眠
Hippocampus	海马区
Hippocampus and Neural Representations	海马区与神经表征
Hippocampus: Computational Models	海马区：计算模型

Hippocampus: Molecular Anatomy	海马区：分子解剖学
Histamine Receptors and their Ligands: Mechanisms and Applications	组胺受体及其配体：机制与应用
History of Neuroscience: Early Neuroscience	神经科学的历史：早期神经科学
Hodgkin-Huxley Models	Hodgkin-Huxley 模型
Holoprosencephaly	前脑无裂畸形
Homeostasis at Multiple Spatial and Temporal Scales	多时空尺度稳态
Homology and Homoplasy	同源和异源同形
Hormonal Signaling to the Brain for the Control of Feeding/Energy Balance	控制进食/能量平衡的脑激素信号
Hormones and Behavior	激素和行为
Hormones and Memory	激素和记忆
Hox Genes Expression	Hox 基因表达
Human Depth Electrodes	人体深部电极
Human Haptics	人的触觉
Human Methods: Psychophysics	人类实验方法：心理物理
Humans	人类
Huntington's Disease	亨廷顿舞蹈病
Huntington's Disease: Neurodegeneration	亨廷顿舞蹈病：神经退行性变
Hyperacuity	（感觉的）超锐度
Hypocretin/Orexin and MCH and Receptors	下丘脑泌素/进食素，黑色素浓集激素及其受体
Hypothalamic Structure-Function Relationships	下丘脑结构与功能的关系
Hypothalamic-Pituitary-Adrenal (HPA) Axis	下丘脑-垂体-肾上腺轴
Hypothalamic-Pituitary-Thyroid Axis: Organization, Neural/Endocrine Control of TRH	下丘脑-垂体-甲状腺轴： 促甲状腺激素释放激素的组织与神经/内分泌控制

I

Ideal Observer Theory	理想观察者理论
Imaging Studies Using Reporter-Gene Transgenic Rats	报告基因转基因大鼠的影像研究
Immune Function During Sleep and Sleep Deprivation	睡眠及睡眠剥夺时的免疫功能
Immune System-Neuroendocrine Interactions	免疫系统-神经内分泌相互作用
Induced Seizures as Therapy in Man	人类（精神失常）的诱发癫痫疗法
Infectious Agents in Neurodegenerative Disease	神经退行性疾病中的传染原
Inflammation in Neurodegenerative Disease and Injury	神经退行性疾病及损伤中的炎症
Information Coding	信息编码
Inherited Macular Degenerations: Animal Models	遗传性黄斑变性：动物模型
Inhibitory Control over Action and Memory	行动和记忆的抑制性控制

Insulin-Like Growth Factor Signaling and Actions in Brain	脑内类胰岛素生长因子信号传递与作用
Intermediate Filaments	中间纤维
Interstitial Axon Branching/Collateral Elimination	间质轴突分支/侧支消减
Intracellular Calcium and Neuronal Death	胞内钙与神经元死亡
Invertebrate Models to Study Learning and Memory: Lymnaea	研究学习与记忆的无脊椎动物模型：椎实螺属
Invertebrate Neurohormone GPCRs	无脊椎动物神经激素 G 蛋白受体
Inwardly Rectifying Potassium Channels	内向整流钾通道
Ion Channel Localization in Axons	离子通道在轴突上的分布
Ion Channel Localization in Cell Bodies and Dendrites	离子通道在胞体及树突上的分布
Ionic Channels in Glia	胶质细胞上的离子通道

J

Joubert Syndrome	朱伯特综合征

K

Kainate Receptor Functions	红藻氨酸受体的功能
Kainate Receptors: Molecular and Cell Biology	红藻氨酸受体：分子和细胞生物学
Kinematics and Dynamics	运动学和动力学
Kinship Signals in Animals	动物的亲缘信号
Kisspeptins and their Receptors	Kisspeptin 与其受体

L

Lamina-Specific Neuronal Connections	层特异性神经元连接
Landau Kleffner Syndrome	Landau-Kleffner 综合征
Language Development	语言的发育
Language Evolution	语言的演化
Language Following Congenital Disorders (not SLI)	先天性疾病对语言的影响
Language in Aged Persons	老年人的语言
Language: Aphasia	语言：失语症
Language: Auditory Processes	语言：听觉过程
Language: Cortical Processes	语言：皮层过程
Language: Learning Impairments	语言：学习损伤
Language: Nonhuman Animals	语言：非人类动物
Large Conductance Calcium-Activated Potassium	高电导钙激活钾通道

Channels	
Large Dense Core Vesicles (LDCVs)	大致密核心囊泡
Latrotoxin	蛛毒素
Learned Flavor Aversions and Preferences	习得的口味厌恶和偏好
Learning and Memory in Invertebrate Models: *Tritonia*	无脊椎动物学习和记忆模型：Tritonia
Learning and Memory in Invertebrates: *Aplysia*	无脊椎动物的学习和记忆：海兔
Learning and Memory in Invertebrates: *C. Elegans*	无脊椎动物的学习和记忆：线虫
Learning and Memory in Invertebrates: *Drosophila*	无脊椎动物的学习和记忆：果蝇
Learning and Memory in Invertebrates: *Hermissenda*	无脊椎动物的学习和记忆：Hermissenda
Learning and Memory in Invertebrates: Honey Bee	无脊椎动物的学习和记忆：蜜蜂
Learning and Memory in Invertebrates: *Limax*	无脊椎动物的学习和记忆：蛞蝓
Learning and Memory in Invertebrates: Mollusks	无脊椎动物的学习和记忆：软体动物
Learning, Action, Inference and Neuromodulation	学习、行动、推理和神经调节
Lexical Impairments Following Brain Injury	脑损伤后词汇能力受损
LIM Kinase and Actin Regulation of Spines	树突小棘的 LIM 激酶和肌动蛋白调控
Lipids and Membranes in Brain Aging	脑衰老过程中的脂和膜
Lipofuscin and Lipofuscinosis	脂褐素及脂褐质
Liprins, ELKS, and RIM-BP Proteins	Liprins、ELKS 和 RIM-BP 蛋白
Lissencephaly	无脑回畸形
Lissencephaly Type I and Periventricular Heterotopia	I 型无脑回畸形与脑室周围异位
Localizing Signal Sources	定位信号源
Long-Term Depression (LTD): Endocannabinoids and Cerebellar LTD	长时程抑制：内源大麻素与小脑 LTD
Long-Term Depression (LTD): Metabotropic Glutamate Receptor (mGluR) and NMDAR-Dependent Forms	长时程抑制：代谢型谷氨酸受体与 NMDA 受体依赖形式
Long-Term Depression: Cerebellum	长时程抑制：小脑
Long-Term Potentiation (LTP)	长时程增强
Long-Term Potentiation (LTP): Mossy Fiber cAMP-Dependent Presynaptic LTP	长时程增强：苔状纤维 cAMP 依赖突触前长时程增强
Long-Term Potentiation (LTP): NMDA Receptor Role	长时程增强：NMDA 受体的作用
Long-Term Potentiation and Long-Term Depression in Experience-Dependent Plasticity	经验依赖可塑性中的长时程增强与长时程抑制
Lysosomal System	溶酶体系统
Lysosome and Endosome Organization and Transport in Neurons	神经元中溶酶体和胞内体的组织和运输

M

Machine Haptics	机器触觉
Macroglial Lineages	大胶质细胞家族
Magnetic Resonance Spectroscopy	磁共振波谱
Magnetic Sense in Animal Navigation	动物的磁感导航
Magnetoencephalography	脑磁图
Magnocellular Neurosecretory System: Organization, Plasticity, Model Peptidergic Neurons	大细胞神经内分泌系统：组织，可塑性，模式肽能神经元
Mammalian Neuropeptide Families	哺乳动物的神经肽家族
Mammalian Sleep and Circadian Rhythms: Flies	哺乳动物睡眠与昼夜节律：蝇类
MAP Kinase Signaling in Learning and Memory	MAP 激酶在学习与记忆中的信号传递
Map Plasticity and Recovery from Stroke	功能图可塑性与中风后恢复
Marsupial Neocortex	有袋动物的新皮层
Mass Spectroscopy of Proteins	蛋白质质谱
Mechanoreceptors	机械力感受器
Mechanosensory Transduction	机械力感觉传导
Medulloblastoma	成神经管细胞瘤
Melanocortins: Brain Effects	黑素皮质素：脑的作用
Melatonin Regulation of Circadian Rhythmicity in Vertebrates	脊椎动物昼夜节律的褪黑素调控
Memory Consolidation: Cerebral Cortex	记忆的巩固：大脑皮层
Memory Consolidation: Systems	记忆的巩固：系统
Memory Disorders	记忆障碍
Memory Representation	记忆的表征
Memory: Computational Models	记忆：计算模型
Memory: Genetic Approaches	记忆：遗传学研究方法
Metabolic Syndrome and Sleep	代谢综合征与睡眠
Metabotropic Glutamate Receptors (mGluRs): Functions	代谢型谷氨酸受体：功能
Metabotropic Glutamate Receptors (mGluRs): Molecular Biology, Pharmacology and Cell Biology	代谢型谷氨酸受体：分子生物学,药理学及细胞生物学
Metal Accumulation during Aging	衰老过程中的金属积累
Metaplasticity	时间累积的突触可塑性
3,4-Methylenedioxymethamphetamine (MDMA, “Ecstasy”)	3,4-二亚甲基双氧苯丙胺(摇头丸)
Microarray Use for the Analysis of the CNS	采用微阵列分析中枢神经系统
Microcephaly Vera	真小脑症
Microglia Identification Methods	小胶质细胞的鉴别方法

Microglia Properties	小胶质细胞的特性
Microglial Response to Injury	小胶质细胞对损伤的反应
Microtubule Associated Proteins in Neurons	神经元中的微管相关蛋白
Microtubules: Organization and Function in Neurons	微管：神经元中的组织和功能
Midbrain Patterning	中脑的模式
Mitochondrial Dysfunction in Nervous System Injury	神经系统损伤中的线粒体功能障碍
Mitochondrial Encephalomyopathies	线粒体脑肌病
Mitochondrial Organization and Transport in Neurons	神经元中的线粒体组织和运输
Molecular Anatomy of the Mammalian Brain	哺乳动物脑的分子解剖学
Monoamine Transporters: Focus on the Regulation of Serotonin Transporter by Cytokines	单胺转运体：聚焦 5-羟色胺转运体的细胞因子调节
Monoamines	单胺
Monoamines: Human Brain Imaging	单胺：人脑成像
Monoamines: Release Studies	单胺：释放研究
Monocarboxylate Transporters	单羧酸转运体
Mood Stabilizers	情绪稳定剂
Morphogens: History	形态发生：历史
Mother-Infant Interaction in the Variable Foraging Demand Model	可变觅食需求模型中的母婴相互作用
Motion Sickness	运动病
Motor Autonomic Transmission	运动自主传输
Motor Control of Feeding and Drinking	摄食和饮水的运动控制
Motor Gait and Falls	运动步态与摔倒
Motor Neuron Specification in Vertebrates	脊椎动物运动神经元的分化
Motor Primitives	原始运动（调节）
Motor Psychophysics	运动心理物理学
Motor Sequences	运动序列
Motor Skill Learning	运动技巧学习
Motor Timing	运动计时
MPTP Parkinsonism Model	MPTP 的帕金森模型
Müller Cells	Müller 细胞
Multimodal Signaling in Animals	动物的多模态信号传递
Multiple Memory Systems	多记忆系统
Multisensory Convergence and Integration	多感觉汇聚与整合
Munc13 and Associated Molecules	Munc13 及其相关分子
Munc18	Munc18 蛋白
Muscarinic Receptors: Autonomic Neurons	毒蕈碱受体：自主神经元
Music	音乐

Musical Illusions	音乐错觉
Myelin: Molecular Architecture of CNS and PNS Myelin Sheath	髓鞘：中枢及外周神经系统髓鞘的分子构建
Myopia	近视
Myosin Transport and Neuronal Function	肌球蛋白运输及神经元功能

N

Napping	午睡
Narcolepsy	阵发性睡眠发作症
Natriuretic Peptides	钠尿肽
Natural Images: Coding Efficiency	自然图像：编码效率
Nausea and Vomiting	恶心和呕吐
Neglect Syndrome and the Spatial Attention Network	忽视综合征与空间注意力网络
Neocortex: Origins	新皮层：起源
Neocortical Organization in Monotremes	单孔目动物的新皮层组织
Neonatal Circuits	新生期回路
Nerve Growth Factor	神经生长因子
Network Control	（呼吸的）神经网络控制
Neural Cell Adhesion Molecules and Synapse Regulation	神经细胞黏附分子与突触调控
Neural Circuitry in the Somatosensory System	体感系统的神经回路
Neural Coding in Primary Motor Cortex	初级运动皮层的神经编码
Neural Coding of Spatial Representations	空间表示的神经编码
Neural Crest	神经嵴
Neural Crest Cell Diversification and Specification: ErbB Role	神经嵴细胞分化与特化：ErbB 的作用
Neural Crest Cell Diversification and Specification: Melanocytes	神经嵴细胞分化与特化：黑色素细胞
Neural Crest Diversification and Specification: Transcriptional Control of Schwann Cell Differentiation	神经嵴分化与特化：施万细胞分化的转录控制
Neural Induction in Chicks	鸡的神经诱导
Neural Integrator Models	神经整合子模型
Neural Oscillators and Dynamical Systems Models	神经振荡与动态系统模型
Neural Patterning: Arealization of the Cortex	神经模式：皮层的区域化
Neural Patterning: Eye Fields	神经模式：眼睛（视网膜）
Neural Patterning: Midbrain-Hindbrain Boundary	神经模式：中脑-后脑边界
Neural Prostheses for Reaching	伸手运动的神经假体
Neural Repair and Regeneration: Inflammatory	神经修复与再生：炎症机制与细胞因子

Mechanisms and Cytokines	
Neural Stem Cells and CNS Diseases	神经干细胞与中枢神经系统疾病
Neural Stem Cells: Adult Neurogenesis	神经干细胞：成年神经发生
Neural Stem Cells: Ocular	神经干细胞：眼
Neural Synchrony and Feature Binding	神经同步化与特征绑定
Neurexins	轴突蛋白
Neuroanatomy Methods in Humans and Animals	人和动物的神经解剖学方法
Neurodegeneration in Psychiatric Illness	精神疾病中的神经退行性疾病
Neuroeconomics: History	神经经济学：历史
Neuroendocrine Aging: Hypothalamic-Pituitary-Gonadal Axis in Women	神经内分泌衰老：女性的下丘脑-垂体-性腺轴
Neuroendocrine Aging: Pituitary Metabolism	神经内分泌衰老：垂体代谢
Neuroendocrine Aging: Pituitary-Adrenal Axis	神经内分泌衰老：垂体-肾上腺轴
Neuroendocrine Aging: Pituitary-Gonadal Axis in Males	神经内分泌衰老：男性的垂体-性腺轴
Neuroendocrine Control of Energy Balance (Central Circuits/Mechanisms)	能量平衡的神经内分泌控制（中央回路/机制）
Neuroendocrine Control: Maternal Behavior	神经内分泌调节作用：母爱行为
Neuroendocrine Peptide Processing	神经内分泌肽加工
Neuroendocrinology	神经内分泌学
Neuroendocrinology of Affective Disorders	情感障碍的神经内分泌学
Neuroendocrinology of Puberty	青春期的神经内分泌学
Neuroendocrinology of Social/Affiliative Behavior	社会/友好行为的神经内分泌学
Neuroethics	神经伦理学
Neuroethological Perspective	神经行为学
Neurofibromatosis Type 1	1型神经纤维瘤病
Neurofibromatosis Type 1: Molecular and Cellular Biology	1型神经纤维瘤病：分子与细胞生物学
Neurofibromatosis Type 2	2型神经纤维瘤病
Neurofibromatosis Type 2: Further Questions and Answers	2型神经纤维瘤病：进一步的问题和解答
Neurofilaments: Organization and Function in Neurons	神经纤维：神经元的组织和功能
Neurogenesis and Neural Precursors, Progenitors, and Stem Cells inthe Adult Brain	成人脑神经发生、神经前体、祖细胞和干细胞
Neurogenesis in the Intact Adult Brain	完整成人大脑的神经发生
Neurohypophyseal System	垂体系统
Neuroimaging	神经影像
Neuroimmune System: Aging	神经免疫系统：衰老
Neuroinformatics	神经信息学
Neuroleptics	抗精神病药
Neuroligins	神经连接蛋白

Neuromodulation	神经调节
Neuromodulation of Calcium Channels	钙通道的神经调节
Neuromodulation of Sodium Channels	钠通道的神经调节
Neuromorphic Systems	神经形态系统
Neuromuscular Connections: Vertebrate Patterns of	神经肌肉连接：脊椎动物模式
Neuromuscular Junction (NMJ): A Target for Natural and Environmental Toxins in Humans	神经肌肉接头：人类中自然和环境毒素的作用位点
Neuromuscular Junction (NMJ): Acetylcholinesterases	神经肌肉接头：乙酰胆碱酯酶
Neuromuscular Junction (NMJ): Activity-Dependent Muscle Fiber Modulation	神经肌肉接头：活性依赖的肌纤维调制
Neuromuscular Junction (NMJ): Aging	神经肌肉接头：衰老
Neuromuscular Junction (NMJ): Inherited and Acquired Disorders	神经肌肉接头：遗传性与获得性疾病
Neuromuscular Junction (NMJ): Mammalian Development	神经肌肉接头：哺乳动物中的发育
Neuromuscular Junction (NMJ): Postsynaptic Basal Lamina	神经肌肉接头：突触后基底膜
Neuromuscular Junction (NMJ): Postsynaptic Events in Neuromuscular Transmission	神经肌肉接头：在神经肌肉突触传递活动中的突触后事件
Neuromuscular Junction (NMJ): Presynaptic Non-Quantal Release of Transmitter	神经肌肉接头：突触前递质的非量子释放
Neuromuscular Junction (NMJ): Presynaptic Schwann Cells and Modulation of Neuromuscular Transmission	神经肌肉接头：突触前施万细胞和神经肌肉接头传递调制
Neuromuscular Junction (NMJ): Presynaptic Short-Term Plasticity of Neuromuscular Transmission	神经肌肉接头：神经肌肉传递中突触前短时程可塑性
Neuromuscular Junction (NMJ): Presynaptic Stretch Effects on Neuromuscular Transmission	神经肌肉接头：突触前牵张对神经肌肉接头传递的效应
Neuromuscular Junction Plasticity in Mammals and Botulinum Toxins	哺乳动物神经肌肉接头可塑性和肉毒毒素
Neuromuscular Junction: Neuronal Regulation of Gene Transcription at the Vertebrate	神经肌肉接头：脊椎动物基因转录的神经调节
Neuromuscular Junction: Synapse Elimination	神经肌肉接头：突触消除
Neuromuscular Transmission Modulation at Invertebrate Neuromuscular Junctions	无脊椎动物神经肌肉接头处神经肌肉接头递质传递的调制效应
Neuron Doctrine: Historical Background	神经元学说：历史背景
Neuron-Glia pH Regulation	神经元-胶质细胞pH调控
Neuronal Angiotensin	神经血管紧张素
Neuronal Motility and Structure: Cdk5 Pathways	神经运动功能和结构：Cdk5基因途径

Neuronal Motility and Structure: MARK and GSK Pathways	神经运动功能和结构：MARK和GSK途径
Neuronal Pacemaking	神经起搏
Neuronal Plasticity after Cortical Damage	皮层损伤后神经元的可塑性
Neuron-Glia Coupling in Glutathione Metabolism	神经元-胶质细胞与谷胱甘肽代谢偶联
Neuropathic Pain	神经病理性疼痛
Neuropathy: Chemically-Induced	神经病变：化学诱导
Neuropathy: Metabolically-Induced	神经病变：代谢诱导
Neuropathy: Peripheral	神经病变：外周
Neuropeptide FF and Receptors	神经肽FF和受体
Neuropeptide Inactivation or Metabolism	神经肽失活或代谢
Neuropeptide Receptors-Drug Development	神经肽受体-药物开发
Neuropeptide Release	神经肽的释放
Neuropeptide S	S神经肽
Neuropeptide Signaling in Invertebrates	无脊椎动物中的神经信号
Neuropeptide Synthesis and Storage	神经肽合成和贮存
Neuropeptide Y (NP Y) and its Receptors	神经肽Y及其受体
Neuropeptides and Coexistence	神经肽与共存
Neuropeptides and Receptors in Glia	神经胶质细胞中的神经肽和受体
Neuropeptides in Autonomic Neurons	自主神经元的神经肽
Neuropeptides Internalization	神经肽内在化
Neuropeptides Phylogeny and Evolution	神经肽系统发育与演化
Neuropeptides: Discovery	神经肽：发现
Neuropeptides: Electrophysiology	神经肽：电生理学
Neuropeptides: Endocrine Cells	神经肽：内分泌细胞
Neuropeptides: Enteric Nervous System	神经肽：肠神经系统
Neuropeptides: Epilepsy	神经肽：癫痫
Neuropeptides: Food Intake	神经肽：食物摄入
Neuropeptides: Mental Disease	神经肽：精神疾病
Neuropeptides: Pain	神经肽：疼痛
Neuropeptides: Sensory Systems	神经肽：感觉系统
Neurophysiology: Past and Present	神经生理学：过去和现在
Neuroplasticity: Computational Approaches	神经可塑性：计算方法
Neuroprotection: Endogenous Mechanisms	神经保护：内生机制
Neuroprotection: Pharmacological Approaches	神经保护作用：药理学方法
Neuroproteomics	神经元蛋白质组学
Neuropsychological Testing	神经心理学测试
Neuropsychology of Primate Reward Processes	灵长类神经心理学奖励过程

Neuropsychology: Theoretical Basis	神经心理学：理论基础
Neurosecretion (Regulated Exocytosis in Neuroendocrine Cells)	神经分泌（调制神经内分泌细胞胞吐作用）
Neurosteroids	神经类固醇
Neurotensin and Receptors	神经降压素和受体
Neurotoxins	神经毒素
Neurotoxins and their Neurotoxicology	神经毒素和神经毒理学
Neurotransmitter and Hormone Receptors on Oligodendrocytes and Schwann Cells	少突胶质细胞和施万细胞的神经递质和激素受体
Neurotransmitter Release from Astrocytes	星形胶质细胞的神经递质的释放
Neurotransmitter Release: Synchronous and Asynchronous	神经递质释放：同步和异步
Neurotransmitters and Growth Factors: Overview	神经递质和生长因子：概述
Neurotrophic Factor Therapy: GDNF and CNTF	神经营养因子治疗：GDNF和CNTF
Neurotrophic Factor Therapy: NGF, BDNF and NT-3	神经营养因子治疗：NGF、BDNF和NT-3
Neurotrophins: Physiology and Pharmacology	神经营养因子：生理学和药理学
Neurulation	神经胚形成
Neutrotransmission and Neuromodulation: Acetylcholine	神经传递和神经调节：乙酰胆碱
Nicotine	尼古丁
Nicotinic Acetylcholine Receptors	烟碱乙酰胆碱受体
Nicotinic Receptors: Autonomic Neurons	烟碱受体：自主神经元
Niemann-Pick Disease	尼曼匹克症
Nightmares	噩梦
Nitric Oxide	一氧化氮
NMDA Receptor Function and Physiological Modulation	NMDA受体的功能和生理上的调节作用
NMDA Receptors and Development	NMDA受体和发育
NMDA Receptors and Disease	NMDA受体与疾病
NMDA Receptors, Cell Biology and Trafficking	NMDA受体、细胞生物学和运输
Nociceptor Responses	伤害性反应
Nogo-A: Its Role in Axon Regeneration	Nogo蛋白A在轴突再生中的作用
Non-Photoreceptor Photoreception	非光感受器介导的光感受
Non-Primate Models of Normal Brain Aging	非灵长类动物的正常脑衰老模型
Noradrenaline	去甲肾上腺素
Norepinephrine: Adrenergic Receptors	去甲肾上腺素：肾上腺素受体
Norepinephrine: CNS Pathways and Neurophysiology	去甲肾上腺素：中枢神经系统通路与神经生理学
Notch Pathway: Lateral Inhibition	Notch通路：侧抑制
Notch Signal Transduction: Molecular and Cellular Mechanisms	Notch信号转导：分子和细胞机制
NSF and SNAPs	可溶性*N*-乙基马来酰亚胺敏感的融合蛋白和

	NSF附着蛋白
Nuclear Movements in Neurons	神经元的核运动
Nucleic Acid Introduction into Primary Neurons and Glia	在初级神经元和神经胶质中转入核酸物质
Numerical Intelligence: Neural Substrates	数值情报：神经基质
Nutrient Sensing: Carbohydrates	营养感应：碳水化合物
Nutrient Sensing: Cellular Metabolism	营养感应：细胞代谢
Nutrition	营养作用
Nystagmus	眼球震颤

O

Obsessive-Compulsive Disorder	强迫症
Octopamine and Other Monoamines in Invertebrates	无脊椎动物的章胺和其他单胺类
Oculomotor Control: Anatomical Pathways	眼动控制：解剖通路
Oculomotor System: Models	动眼系统：模型
Olfaction in Invertebrates: *Drosophila*	无脊椎动物的嗅觉：果蝇
Olfaction in Invertebrates: Honeybee	无脊椎动物的嗅觉：蜜蜂
Olfaction in Invertebrates: *Manduca*	无脊椎动物的嗅觉：烟草天蛾
Olfactory Bulb Anatomy	嗅球解剖学
Olfactory Bulb Mapping	嗅球图谱
Olfactory Bulb Physiology	嗅球生理学
Olfactory Coding	嗅觉编码
Olfactory Cortex Physiology	嗅觉皮层生理学
Olfactory Cortex: Comparative Anatomy	嗅觉皮层：比较解剖学
Olfactory Ensheathing Cells: Regeneration Following Spinal Cord Injury	嗅鞘细胞：脊髓损伤后再生
Olfactory Epithelium	嗅觉上皮
Olfactory Glomeruli: Structure and Circuitry	嗅觉小球：结构和回路
Olfactory Higher Centers Anatomy	嗅觉高级中枢解剖学
Olfactory Insights from Transcriptional Profiling	转录谱对嗅觉的启示
Olfactory Neuron Patterning and Specification	嗅觉神经元的模式和特化
Olfactory Receptor Genes: Human Loss During Evolution	嗅觉受体基因：人类在演化过程中的丢失
Olfactory Receptors	嗅觉受体
Olfactory Receptors: Microarray Analysis	嗅觉受体：微阵列分析
Olfactory System Theory	嗅觉系统理论
Olfactory System: Circuit Dynamics and Neural Coding in the Locust	嗅觉系统：蝗虫的回路动力学和神经编码
Oligodendrocyte and Schwann Cell Identification Methods	少突胶质细胞和施万细胞识别方法

Oligodendrocyte Morphology	少突胶质细胞形态学
Oligodendrocyte Specification	少突胶质细胞详述
Olivocerebellar System	橄榄小脑系统
Operant Conditioning of Reflexes	操作性条件反射
Opioid Peptides and Receptors	阿片肽及其受体
Opsoclonus/Myoclonus and Neuroblastoma	眼阵挛/肌阵挛和神经母细胞瘤
Optic Nerve, Optic Chiasm, and Optic Tracts	视神经，视交叉和视束
Optic Tectum: Development and Plasticity	顶盖：发育和可塑性
Optic Tectum: Sensorimotor Integration	顶盖：感觉运动整合
Optical Imaging of Intrinsic Signals	内源信号光学成像
Optical Monitoring of Exo- and Endocytosis	胞吐和内吞的光学监测
Optokinetic Eye Movements	视动性眼动
Orbitofrontal Cortex: Visual Functions	眶额皮层：视觉功能
Orofacial Motor Control	面部运动调控
Osmoregulation	渗透调节
Otoacoustic Emissions	耳声发射
Oxidative Damage in Neurodegeneration and Injury	神经退行性疾病和损伤中的氧化损伤
Oxytocin (Peripheral/Central Actions and their Regulation)	催产素（外周/中央活动及其调控）

P

P2X Receptors	P2X受体
Pain and Genes	疼痛和基因
Pain and Plasticity	疼痛和可塑性
Pain and the Sympathetic Nervous System	疼痛和交感神经系统
Pain Management	疼痛管理
Pain Pathways: Descending Modulation	疼痛通路：下行调制
Pain: Central	疼痛：中央
Pain: Neuroimaging	疼痛：神经影像
PANDAS (Pediatric Autoimmune Neuropsychiatric Disorders Associated with Streptococcal Infections)	小儿自身免疫性神经精神障碍与链球菌感染
Panic Disorder	惊惶症
Panic Disorder as an Emotional Disorder	惊惶症：一种情绪障碍
Parasitic Diseases: Nervous System Effects	寄生虫病：神经系统的影响
Parasomnias	深眠
Parasympathetic Nervous System	副交感神经系统
Parietal Cortex and Spatial Attention	顶叶皮层和空间注意
Parkinsonian Syndromes	帕金森综合征

Parkinson's Disease: Alpha-Synuclein and Neurodegeneration	帕金森病：α突触核蛋白和神经退行性疾病
Paroxysmal Paralysis	阵发性麻痹
Paroxysmal Sympathetic Storms	阵发性交感神经风暴
Pattern Generation	模式生成
Peptidergic Receptors	肽受体
Perception and Eye Movements	知觉和眼动
Perception of Surfaces and Forms	表面和形状的感知
Perceptual Learning and Sensory Plasticity	知觉学习和感官可塑性
Perceptual Learning: Neural Mechanisms	知觉学习:神经机理
Perfusion MRI	核磁共振灌注成像
Peripheral Circadian Oscillators	周边昼夜振荡器
Peripheral Nerve Regeneration: An Overview	周围神经再生：概述
Perirhinal Cortex	嗅周皮层
Perirhinal Cortex: Neural Representations	嗅周皮层：神经表征
Peroxisomal Disorders and Neurological Disease	过氧化物酶体病和神经疾病
Peroxisomes: Organization and Transport in Neurons	过氧化物酶体：神经元中的组织和运输
Pharmacology of Fear Extinction	消除恐惧的药理学
Pharmacology of Sleep: Adenosine	睡眠的药理学：腺苷
Pheromones and other Chemical Communication in Animals	动物体内的信息素和其他化学通信
Pheromones in Humans and Social Chemosignal	人类信息激素和社会化学信号
Pheromones in Mammals	哺乳动物的信息激素
Phobia and Human Evolution	恐惧症和人类演化
Photolysis of Caged Glutamate for Use in the CNS	笼中谷氨酸的光解在中枢神经系统的应用
Photoperiodic Regulation of Reproductive Cycles	生殖周期的光周期调节
Photoreceptor Adaptation	光感受器适应
Photoreceptor Mosaic	光感受器马赛克
Photoreceptors and Circadian Clocks	光感受器和生物钟
Photoreceptors: Physiology	光感受器：生理学
Phototransduction	光转导
PHR (Pam/Highwire/RPM-1)	Pam/Highwire/PRM-1蛋白
Phrenology	颅相学
Piccolo and Bassoon	（突触相关的）Piccolo与Bassoon分子
Pineal Gland and Melatonin	松果体和褪黑激素
Pituitary Gland (Cell Types, Mediators, Development)	脑垂体（细胞类型，介导子，发育）
Plasticity of Intrinsic Excitability	内在兴奋性的可塑性
Plasticity, and Activity-Dependent Regulation of	可塑性和基因表达的活动依赖性调控

Gene Expression	
Pleasant Touch	愉快的触摸
Population Codes: Theoretic Aspects	群体编码：理论
Population Coding	群体编码
Porphyria: Acute Intermittent	卟啉症：急性间歇
Positron Emission Tomography (PET)	正电子发射断层扫描
Post-Polio Syndrome	后小儿麻痹症
Post-Tetanic Potentiation (PTP)	强直后增强
Posterior Parietal Cortex and Arm Movement	后顶叶皮质和手臂运动
Posterior Parietal Cortex and Tool Usage and Hand Shape	后顶叶皮质和工具的使用和手形
Postsynaptic Density/Architecture at Excitatory Synapses	突触后密度/兴奋性突触结构
Postsynaptic Development: Neuronal Molecular Scaffolds	突触后发育：神经元分子支架
Postsynaptic Specialization Assembly	突触后的特化成分组装
Posttraumatic Stress Disorder as an Emotional Disorder	创伤后应激障碍：作为一种情绪障碍
Posttraumatic Stress Disorder: Neurobiology	创伤后应激障碍：神经生物学
Posttraumatic Stress Disorder: Overview	创伤后应激障碍：概述
Potassium Channel Regulation	钾通道调节
Potassium Homeostasis in Glia	胶质细胞中的钾离子稳态平衡
Prader-Willi Syndrome	Prader-Willi综合征
Prediction Errors in Neural Processing: Imaging in Humans	神经处理中的预测误差：在人类中的成像
Prefrontal Contributions to Reward Encoding	前额叶对奖励编码的贡献
Prefrontal Cortex	前额叶皮层
Prefrontal Cortex: Structure and Anatomy	前额叶皮层：结构和解剖学
Premenstrual Dysphoric Disorder and Postpartum Major Depression: Chronobiology	经前烦躁和产后抑郁症：时间生物学
Premotor Areas: Medial	前运动区：内侧
Premotor Cortex in Primates: Dorsal and Ventral	灵长类的前运动皮层：背侧，腹侧
Prepulse Inhibition of Startle in Humans and Laboratory Models	人类和实验室模型中惊吓的前脉冲抑制
Presynaptic Development and Active Zones	突触前发育和活动区
Presynaptic Development: Functional and Morphological Organization	突触前发育：功能和形态学组织
Presynaptic Endosomes	突触前内体
Presynaptic Events in Neuromuscular Transmission	神经肌肉接头传递活动中的突触前事件
Presynaptic Facilitation	突触前易化
Presynaptic Inhibition	突触前抑制
Presynaptic Receptor Signaling	突触前受体信号
Presynaptic Regulation by Liprins	Liprins蛋白的突触前调节

Presynaptic: Mitochondria and Presynaptic Function	突触前：线粒体和突触前功能
Primate Communication: Evolution	灵长类通信：演化
Primate Interneurons	灵长类的中间神经元
Priming	启动
Prion Diseases	朊病毒疾病
Prion Transport	朊病毒运输
Procedural Learning in Animals	动物的程序学习
Procedural Learning in Humans	人类的程序学习
Procedural Learning: Cerebellum Models	程序学习：小脑模型
Procedural Learning: Classical Conditioning	程序学习：经典条件反射
Procedural Learning: Striatum	程序学习：纹状体
Programmed Cell Death	程序性细胞死亡
Prolactin and its Neuroendocrine Control	催乳素及其神经内分泌控制
Prolactin-Releasing Peptide	催乳素释放肽
Proopiomelanocortin	阿黑皮素原
Proprioception	本体感觉
Prosopagnosia	面容失认症
Proteasome Role in Neurodegeneration	蛋白酶体在神经退行性疾病的作用
Protein Folding and the Role of Chaperone Proteins in Neurodegenerative Disease	蛋白质折叠与神经退行性疾病中分子伴侣蛋白的作用
Psychiatric Disorders Associated with Disturbed Sleep and Circadian Rhythms	与睡眠紊乱和昼夜节律相关的精神疾病
Psychiatric Disorders: Functional Genomics	精神疾病：功能基因组学
Psychiatric Genomics and Expression Profiling	精神病基因组学与表达图谱
Psycholinguistics	心理语言学
Psychopharmacology of Reward and Appetite in Rats	大鼠奖励和食欲的精神药理学
Psychophysics of Attention	注意的心理物理学
Psychotherapeutic Approaches to Psychiatric Disorders	精神疾病的心理治疗途径
Pulsatility in Neuroendocrine Systems	神经内分泌系统的波动性释放
Pulvinar Structure and Circuitry in Primates	灵长类的枕核结构和回路
Purinergic Receptors	嘌呤受体
Purines and Purinoceptors: Molecular Biology Overview	嘌呤和嘌呤受体：分子生物学概述
Pursuit Eye Movements	追踪眼动

R

Rab3	GTP结合蛋白3
Rab3A Interacting Molecules (RIMs)	Rab3a相互作用的分子

Radial Glial Cells: Brain Functions	放射状胶质细胞：脑功能
Reaching and Grasping	伸手和把握
Reading	阅读
Reasoning and Problem Solving: Models	推理和解决问题：模型
Receptor Trafficking	受体运输
Recognition Memory	识别记忆
Red Nucleus	红核
Referentiality and Concepts in Animal Cognition	动物认知中的指涉和概念
Reflex Circuits	反射回路
Regulation of Cell Volume in Neural Cells	神经细胞的细胞体积调控
Reinforcement Models	强化模型
Representation of Color	颜色的表示
Representation of Movement	运动的表示
Representation of Reward	奖励的表示
Respiration	呼吸
Restless Leg Syndrome	不宁腿综合征
Reticular Activating System	网状激活系统
Reticular Formation and the Brain Stem	网状结构和脑干
Reticulospinal System	网状脊髓系统
Retina: An Overview	视网膜：概述
Retinal Amacrine Cells	视网膜无长突细胞
Retinal Bipolar Cells	视网膜双极细胞
Retinal Color Mechanisms	视网膜颜色机制
Retinal Development: An Overview	视网膜发育：概述
Retinal Development: Cell Type Specification	视网膜发育：细胞类型详述
Retinal Ganglion Cells: Anatomy	视网膜视经节细胞：解剖学
Retinal Ganglion Cells: Receptive Fields	视网膜视经节细胞：感受野
Retinal Glia	视网膜神经胶质细胞
Retinal Horizontal Cells	视网膜水平细胞
Retinal Models	视网膜模型
Retinal Pharmacology: Inner Retinal Layers	视网膜药理学：内视网膜层
Retinitis Pigmentosa	视网膜色素变性
Retinoic Acid Signaling and Neural Patterning	视黄酸信号和神经模式
Retinomotor Movements	视网膜运动现象（光感受器与色素上皮运动）
Retrograde Neurotrophic Signaling	逆行神经营养信号
Retrograde Transsynaptic Influences	逆行跨突触的影响
Retronasal Olfaction	鼻后嗅觉
Rett Syndrome	Rett综合征

Reward and Learning	奖励和学习
Reward Decision-Making	奖励决策
Reward Neurophysiology and Orbitofrontal Cortex	奖励的神经生理学和眶额皮层神经
Reward Neurophysiology and Primate Cerebral Cortex	奖励的神经生理学和灵长类大脑皮层
Reward Processing: Human Imaging	奖励加工：人类成像
Reward Systems: Human	奖励系统：人类
Reye Syndrome	瑞氏综合征
Rho GTPases and Spines	Rho GTP酶和树突小棘
Rhodopsin	视紫红质
Ribbon Synapses	带状突触
RNA Binding Protein Methods	RNA结合蛋白方法
RNA Granules: Functions within Presynaptic Terminals and Postsynaptic Spines	RNA的颗粒：在突触前和突触后终端小棘的功能
Rodent Aging	啮齿动物衰老
Rodent Behavior: Approaches	啮齿动物行为：研究方法与思路
Role of NO in Neurodegeneration	一氧化氮在神经退行性疾病中的作用

S

Saccade-Pursuit Interactions	扫视-跟踪的相互作用
Saccades and Visual Search	扫视和视觉搜索
Saccadic Eye Movements	扫视中的眼球运动
Salt Appetite	盐食欲
Schizophrenia: Epidemiology, Clinical Features, Course and Outcome	精神分裂症：流行病学，临床特征，过程和结果
Schizophrenia: Genetics	精神分裂症：遗传学
Schwann Cell Development	施万细胞的发育
Schwann Cell Morphology	施万细胞的形态学
Schwann Cells and Axon Relationship	施万细胞和轴突的联系
Schwann Cells and Plasticity of the Neuromuscular Junction	施万细胞和神经肌肉接头的可塑性
Seasonal Changes in Night-Length and Impact on Human Sleep	夜晚长短的季节性变化及其对人类睡眠的影响
Seasonal Hormonal Changes and Behavior	激素的季节性变化与行为
Seasonal Timing: Neural Mechanisms	季节时序：神经机制
Second Language Acquisition	第二语言的获得
Segawa Dopa Responsive Dystonia	Segawa多巴反应肌张力障碍
Segmentation: Segmental Boundaries, Establishment	分节现象：分割的边界、建立和形态发生

and Morphogenesis (EPH)	
Segmentation: Spinal Cord Segmentation and A-P Somite Patterning	分节现象：脊髓分节和前-后轴体节模式
Seismic and Vibrational Signals in Animals	动物中的地震和振动信号检测
Self-Organizing Maps	自组织功能图
Semantic Memory	语义记忆
Semaphorins	信号素
Sensation from the Face	面部感知
Sensorimotor Control of Manipulation	操作的感觉运动控制
Sensorimotor Integration: Attention and the Premotor Theory	感觉运动整合：注意和前运动理论
Sensorimotor Integration: Barrels, Vibrissae and Topographic Representations	感觉运动整合：桶状、触须和拓扑表征
Sensorimotor Integration: Models	感觉运动整合：模型
Sensorimotor Plasticity and Control of Movement Following Spinal Cord Injury +D18	脊髓损伤后感觉运动的可塑性和运动的控制
Sensory Aging: Chemical Senses	感觉衰老：化学感官
Sensory Aging: Hearing	感觉衰老：听力
Sensory Aging: Vision	感觉衰老：视觉
Sensory Ganglia	感觉神经节
Sensory Re-education	感觉再教育
Sensory System Specializations	感觉系统的特化
Sentence Comprehension	语句理解
Sentence Production	语句生成
Serotonin (5-Hydroxtryptamine; 5-HT): Neurotransmission and Neuromodulation	5-羟色胺：神经传递和神经调控作用
Serotonin (5-Hydroxytryptamine; 5-HT): CNS Pathways and Neurophysiology	5-羟色胺：中枢神经系统的通路和神经生理学
Serotonin (5-Hydroxytryptamine; 5-HT): Receptors	5-羟色胺：受体
Serotonin and the Regulation of Mammalian Circadian Rhythms	5-羟色胺和哺乳动物昼夜节律的调节
Serotonin-Related Psychedelic Drugs	与5-羟色胺相关的迷幻药
Sexual Behavior: Neuroendocrine Control	性行为：神经内分泌的控制
Sexual Differentiation of the Brain	大脑的性分化
Sexual Differentiation of the Central Nervous System	中枢神经系统的性分化
Sexual Selection and the Evolution of Animal Signals	性选择和动物信号的演化
Shape Representation in Inferotemporal Cortex	颞叶下皮层的形状代表特性
Shift Work and Circadian Rhythms	轮班工作及昼夜节律

Short Term and Working Memory	短期和工作记忆
Signal Design Rules in Animal Communication	动物交流中的信号设计规则
Signal Identification: Peripheral and Central Mechanisms	信号识别：周边和中枢系统机制
Signal Production and Amplification in Birds	鸟类的信号产生和放大
Signal Transmission in Natural Environments	自然环境中的信号传递
Single Cell Electroporation	单细胞电穿孔
Single Cell Genomic DNA Analysis	单细胞基因组DNA分析
Single Cell Molecular Analysis Procedures	单细胞分子分析程序
Single Cell Neuronal Circadian Clocks	单细胞神经元生物钟
Single Cell PCR Coupled with Electrophysiology	与电生理学相结合的单细胞PCR技术
Single Photon Emission Computed Tomography (SPECT)	单光子发射计算机断层摄影术
Single Photon Emission Computed Tomography (SPECT): Technique	单光子发射计算机断层摄影术：技术
Single-Nucleotide Polymorphism (SNP) Analysis	单核苷酸多态性分析
siRNA: Utility	小干扰RNA：实用性
Sleep and Circadian Rhythm Disorders in Human Aging and Dementia	与人类衰老和痴呆症相关的睡眠和昼夜节律障碍
Sleep and Sleep States: Cytokines and Neuromodulation	睡眠和睡眠状态：细胞因子与神经调节
Sleep and Sleep States: Gene Expression	睡眠和睡眠状态：基因表达
Sleep and Sleep States: Hippocampus-Neocortex Dialog	睡眠和睡眠状态：海马-新大脑皮质对话
Sleep and Sleep States: Histamine Role	睡眠和睡眠状态：组胺作用
Sleep and Sleep States: Hypothalamic Regulation	睡眠和睡眠状态：下丘脑的调节作用
Sleep and Sleep States: Network Reactivation	睡眠和睡眠状态：网络重新活化
Sleep and Sleep States: PET Activation Patterns	睡眠和睡眠状态：PET活化模式
Sleep and Sleep States: Phylogeny and Ontogeny	睡眠和睡眠状态：系统发生和个体发生
Sleep and Sleep States: Thalamic Regulation	睡眠和睡眠状态：丘脑的调节作用
Sleep and Waking in *Drosophila*	果蝇的睡眠和清醒
Sleep Apnea	睡眠呼吸暂停
Sleep Architecture	睡眠结构
Sleep Deprivation and Brain Function	睡眠剥夺和脑的功能
Sleep Deprivation: Neurobehavioral Changes	睡眠剥夺：神经行为改变
Sleep in Adolescents	青少年睡眠
Sleep in Aging	老年睡眠
Sleep Mentation in REM and NREM: A Neurocognitive Perspective	快速眼动和非快速眼动睡眠中的精神作用：一种神经认知观点
Sleep Oscillations	睡眠振荡
Sleep Oscillations and PGO Waves	睡眠振荡和桥膝枕波
Sleep Research and Sleep Medicine in Historical	睡眠研究及睡眠医学的历史透视

Perspective	
Sleep-Dependent Memory Processing	依赖睡眠的记忆处理
Sleep: Development and Circadian Control	睡眠：发育和昼夜控制
Sleeping Sickness	昏睡病
Sleep-Wake State Regulation by Acetylcholine	乙酰胆碱对睡眠-清醒状态的调控作用
Sleep–Wake State Regulation by Noradrenaline and Serotonin	去甲肾上腺素和血清素对睡眠-清醒状态的调控作用
Slow Axonal Transport	慢速轴突运输
SNAREs	可溶性NSF依附蛋白受体
Social Brain: Evolution	社会脑：演化
Social Cognition	社会认知
Social Communication in Whales and Dolphins	鲸和海豚的社会交往
Social Emotion: Neuroimaging	社会情感：神经影像
Social Interaction	社会交互作用
Social Interaction Effects on Reward and Cognitive Abilities in Monkeys	社会效应对猴子的奖励和认知能力的影响
Social Stress in Adult Primates	成年灵长类动物的社会压力
Sodium Channels	钠通道
Somatosensory Cortex	体感皮层
Somatosensory Cortex: Functional Architecture	体感皮层：功能结构
Somatosensory Pathways (Ascending): Functional Architecture	体感皮层通路（上行）：功能结构
Somatosensory Perception	体感知觉
Somatosensory Plasticity	体感皮层的可塑性
Somatosensory Receptive Fields	体感皮层的感受野
Somatostatin and Receptors	生长激素抑制素及其受体
Sonic Hedgehog and Neural Patterning	音猬因子与神经模式
Sound Localization: Neural Mechanisms	声音定位：神经机制
Sox Gene Expression	Sox基因表达
Spasticity	痉挛
Spatial Cognition	空间认知
Spatial Cognition and Executive Function	空间认知与执行功能
Spatial Cognitive Maps	空间认知图
Spatial Memory: Assessment in Animals	空间记忆：在动物中的评估
Spatial Orientation: Our Whole-Body Motion and Orientation Sense	空间方位：全身运动和方位感
Spatial Transformations for Eye-Hand Coordination	手眼协调的空间变换
Spectrin: Organization and Function in Neurons	血影蛋白：神经元的结构和功能

Speech Perception: Adult	语音感知：成人
Speech Perception: Cortical Processing	语音感知：皮层处理
Speech Perception: Development	语音感知：发育
Speech Perception: Neural Encoding	语音知觉：神经编码
Speech Production: Adult	语音产生：成人
Speech Production: Development	语音产生：发育
Spike-Timing-Dependent Plasticity (STDP)	发放时序依赖型可塑性
Spike-Timing-Dependent Plasticity Models	发放时序依赖型可塑性模型
Spiking Neuron Models	发放神经元模型
Spinal Cord Injuries	脊髓损伤
Spinal Cord Pain Systems	脊髓疼痛系统
Spinal Cord Regeneration after Injury: Bridging by Schwann Cells and Bioimplants	脊髓损伤后的再生：施万细胞和植入性生物材料的搭桥
Spinal Cord Regeneration and Functional Recovery: Strategies	脊髓再生和功能恢复：策略
Spinal Motor Neurons: Properties	脊髓运动神经元：特性
Spine Plasticity	树突小棘可塑性
Spines and Mental Disorders	树突小棘和精神疾病
Spinocerebellar Atrophy	脊髓小脑萎缩
Split-Brain Patients	裂脑患者
Spontaneous Patterned Activity in Developing Neural Circuits	发育中神经回路的自发模式活动
Sporadic Degenerative Ataxias and the Dominantly Inherited Spinocerebellar Ataxias	阵发性退行性共济失调和显性遗传脊髓小脑共济失调
Startle Response	惊吓反应
Statistical Analysis of Visual Perception	视觉感知的统计学分析
Statistical Learning of Language	语言的统计学习
Statistical Tests and Inferences	统计检验和推断
Stem Cells and CNS Repair	干细胞和中枢神经系统的修复
Stereoscopic Vision	立体视觉
Stimulant and Wake-Promoting Substances	兴奋剂和唤醒促进物质
Stomatogastric Ganglion Models	口胃的神经节模型
Strategic Control of Memory	记忆的战略控制
Stress and Cognition	压力和认知
Stress and Neural Involvement in Metabolism	压力和代谢中的神经参与
Stress and Neuronal Plasticity	压力和神经元可塑性
Stress and Parasympathetic Control	压力和副交感神经控制
Stress and Suicide	压力与自杀

Stress and Vulnerability to Brain Damage	压力和易受脑损伤
Stress Response and Self-Esteem	压力反应和自尊
Stress Response: Genetic Consequences	压力反应：遗传后果
Stress Response: Neural and Feedback Regulation of the HPA Axis	压力反应：下丘脑-垂体-肾上腺轴的神经和反馈调节
Stress Response: Sex Differences	压力反应：性别差异
Stress, Cytokines and Depressive Illness	压力，细胞因子和抑郁症
Stress, Dopamine, and Puberty	压力，多巴胺和青春期
Stress, Sex and Adolescent Nicotine Response	压力，性别与青少年尼古丁反应
Stress, the HPA Axis and Depressive Illness	压力，下丘脑-垂体-肾上腺轴和抑郁症
Stress: Definition and History	压力：定义和历史
Stress: Homeostasis, Rheostasis, Allostasis and Allostatic Load	压力：稳态平衡，变阻器式（缓慢连续）调控，非稳态调控和适应负荷
Striatum: Internal Physiology	纹状体：内部生理
Stroke	中风
Stroke: Injury Mechanisms	中风：损伤机理
Stroke: Neonate vs. Adult	中风：新生儿与成人
Substance Abuse and Dependence	药物滥用和依赖性
Substance P/Tachykinins and its/their Receptors	P物质/速激肽及其受体
Suicide	自杀
Superior Colliculus	上丘
Supplementary Eye Fields	补充眼动控制脑区
Swim Oscillator Networks	游泳振荡器网络
Swimming: Neural Mechanisms	游泳：神经机理
Sympathetic Nervous System	交感神经系统
Sympathetic Noradrenergic and Adrenomedullary Hormonal Systems in Stress and Distress	压力与苦恼时的交感神经去甲肾上腺素和肾上腺髓质激素系统
Sympathoadrenal System: Neural Arm of the Stress Response	交感肾上腺髓质系统：压力反应的神经臂
Sympathomimetic Drugs and Adrenergic Receptor Antagonists	模拟交感神经药物和肾上腺素受体拮抗剂
Synapse Formation: Competition and the Role of Activity	突触形成：竞争与活动的作用
Synapsins	突触素
Synapsins and Regulation of the Reserve Pool	突触素及储备池调节
Synaptic Capture and Tagging	突触捕获和标签
Synaptic Depression	突触抑制
Synaptic Mechanisms of Learning	学习的突触机制
Synaptic Plasticity and Place Cell Formation	突触可塑性和位置细胞形成

Synaptic Plasticity: Cerebellum	突触可塑性：小脑
Synaptic Plasticity: Diacylglycerol Signalling role	突触可塑性：二酰基甘油信号作用
Synaptic Plasticity: Learning and Memory in Normal Aging	突触可塑性：正常衰老中的学习和记忆
Synaptic Plasticity: Neuronal Sprouting	突触可塑性：神经突发芽
Synaptic Plasticity: Neuronogenesis and Stem Cells in Normal Brain Aging	突触可塑性：正常脑衰老过程中神经元的形成和干细胞
Synaptic Plasticity: Short-Term Mechanisms	突触可塑性：短时程机制
Synaptic Precursors: Filopodia	突触前体：丝状伪足
Synaptic Transmission: Models	突触传递：模型
Synaptic Vesicle Protein-2 (SV2)	突触囊泡蛋白2（SV2）
Synaptic Vesicles	突触囊泡
Synaptojanin	突触伸蛋白
Synaptosomes	突触体
Synaptotagmins	突触结合蛋白
SynCAMs	同步化钙黏附分子
Synfire Chains	Synfire链
Synucleins	突触核蛋白
Syringomyelia	脊髓空洞症

T

Tactile Coding in Peripheral Neural Populations	外周神经元群的触觉编码
Tactile Texture	触觉纹理
Target Selection for Pursuit and Saccades	追踪和扫视中的目标选择
Task Switching	任务转换
Taste: Vertebrate Central Pathways	味觉：脊椎动物的中枢途径
Taste: Vertebrate Psychophysics	味觉：脊椎动物的精神物理学
Taste: Vertebrate Taste Bud Physiology	味觉：脊椎动物味蕾的生理学
Tay-Sachs Disease	泰萨二氏病
Temperature Sensation	温度感觉
Temporal Processing in the Auditory Pathway	听觉通路中的时域处理
Terminal Differentiation: REST	终端分化：RE-1沉默转录因子
Thalamic Mechanisms in Vision	视觉中丘脑的机制
Thalamus and Oculomotor Control	丘脑和动眼控制
Thalamus: Evolution in Vertebrates	丘脑：脊椎动物的演化
The AIM Model of Dreaming, Sleeping, and Waking Consciousness	做梦、睡觉和清醒的AIM模型

Thermoregulation during Sleep and Sleep Deprivation	睡眠和睡眠剥夺时的温度调节
Thermoregulation: Autonomic, Age-Related Changes	温度调节：自主的、与年龄相关的变化
Thirst	口渴
Thyroid Hormone and Transcriptional Regulation in the CNS	甲状腺激素和中枢神经系统中的转录调控
Tinnitus	耳鸣
TIP39 (Tuberoinfundibular Peptide of 39 Residues)	结状漏斗形肽的39个氨基酸残基
Topographic Maps: Molecular Mechanisms	拓朴图：分子机制
Torsion Dystonia	扭转性肌张力障碍
Tourette Syndrome as a Neurotransmitter Disorder	图雷特综合征：一种神经递质疾病
Tourette's Disorder	图雷特综合征
Trace Monoamines and Receptors in Mammalian CNS	哺乳动物中枢神经系统中的微量单胺及其受体
Transcranial Magnetic Stimulation	经颅磁刺激
Transcription and Reward Systems	转录和奖励系统
Transcription Control and the Circadian Clock	转录控制和生物钟
Transcription Factors in Synaptic Plasticity and Learning and Memory	突触可塑性和学习与记忆中的转录因子
Transcriptional Networks and the Spinal Cord	转录网络和脊髓
Transcriptional Silencing	转录沉默
Transgenic Models of Neurodegenerative Disease	神经退行性疾病的转基因模型
Transient Receptor Potential (TRP) Channels	瞬时受体电位通道
Translational Regulation at the Synapse	突触的翻译调控
Transplantation of Myelin Forming Cells	成髓鞘胶质细胞的移植
Transport Dependent Damage Signaling	转运依赖性损伤信号
Transporter Proteins in Neurons and Glia	神经元和神经胶质细胞的转运体蛋白
Trigeminal Motor System	三叉神经运动系统
Trigeminal Neuralgia	三叉神经痛
Triplicate Repeats: Huntington's disease	三倍重复（基因复制）：亨廷顿舞蹈病
Triune Brain Concept: A Comparative Evolutionary Perspective	三位一体脑概念：比较演化研究
Tuberous Sclerosis	结节状硬化
Tumors of the Brain and the Spinal Cord	脑瘤和脊髓瘤
Two-P-Domain (K2P) Potassium Channels: Leak Conductance Regulators of Excitability	K2P钾通道：兴奋性的泄漏电导调节器
Two-Photon Imaging	双光子成像

U

Ubiquitin-Proteasome System and Plasticity	泛素-蛋白酶体途径和可塑性
Ultrastructural Analysis of Spine Plasticity	突触小棘可塑性的超微结构分析
Ultrastructural Organization of Release Sites in the Calyx of Held	巨型单一突触释放位点的超微结构构筑

V

Variant Creutzfeldt–Jakob Disease	变异克鲁兹弗得-雅柯病
Vascular Issues in Neurodegeneration and Injury	神经退行性病变和损伤中的血管组织
Vasoactive Intestinal Peptide and Pituitary Adenylate Cyclase Activating Peptide Receptors	血管活性肠肽和垂体腺苷酸环化酶激活肽受体
Vasopressin/Oxytocin and Receptors	血管加压素/催产素和受体
Vegetative State	植物状态
VelociGene and VelociMouse: High-Throughput Approaches for Generating Targeted Mutations in Mice on a Genome-Wide Scale	Veloci基因和Veloci小鼠：小鼠在基因组范畴内产生定点基因突变的高通量方法
Vergence Eye Movements	眼动辐合
Vertebrate Eyes: Evolution	脊椎动物的眼球：演化
Vertigo	眩晕
Vesicle Pools	囊泡池
Vesicular Neurotransmitter Transporters	囊泡内神经递质的转运体
Vesicular Sorting to Axons and Dendrites	对轴突和树突的囊泡分选
Vestibular Influences on Cognition	前庭对认知的影响
Vestibular System	前庭系统
Vestibulo-Autonomic Responses	前庭-自主反应
Vestibulo-Ocular Reflex	前庭-眼球反射
Vestibulospinal System and Eye-Head/Neck Movement	前庭脊髓束系统和眼-头/颈运动
Vibrissa Movement, Sensation and Sensorimotor Control	鼻毛运动、感觉和感觉运动的控制
Viral Vectors in the CNS	中枢神经系统的病毒载体
Visceral Pain	内脏痛觉
Viscero-Sensory Functions: Capsaicin	内脏感觉功能：辣椒素
Vision for Action and Perception	行动与知觉中的视觉
Vision: Light and Dark Adaptation	视觉：明适应和暗适应
Vision: Mechanisms of Orientation, Direction and Depth	视觉：方位、方向和深度的机制
Vision: Surface Segmentation	视觉：表面分割

Visual Associative Memory	视觉联想记忆
Visual Attention	视觉注意
Visual Cortex in Humans	人类的视觉皮层
Visual Cortex: Mapping of Functional Architecture Using Optical Imaging	视觉皮层：用光学成像对视皮层功能结构的（空间）绘图
Visual Cortical Models of Orientation Tuning	视觉皮层的方位调谐模型
Visual Deprivation	视觉剥夺
Visual Development	视觉发育
Visual Motion Detection	视觉运动检测
Visual Motion Models	视觉运动模型
Visual Signaling in Animals	动物的视觉信号
Visual System Development: Invertebrates	视觉系统的发育：无脊椎动物
Visual System: Adaptive Regression and Progression in Subterranean Mammals	视觉系统：地下哺乳动物的适应退化及其进展
Visual System: Functional Architecture of Area V2	视系统：V2区的功能结构
Visual System: Invertebrates	视觉系统：无脊椎动物
Visual System: Multiple Visual Areas in Monkeys	视觉系统：猴的多个视觉区域
Visually Guided Behavior	视觉引导行为
Visual-Vestibular Interactions	视觉-前庭的相互作用
Vocal Communication in Birds	鸟类的声音信息通信
Voltage Gated Potassium Channels: Structure and Function of Kv1 to Kv9 Subfamilies	电压门控钾通道：Kv1~Kv9亚家族的结构和功能
Voltage-Gated Calcium Channels	电压门控钙通道
Voltage-Gated Potassium Channels (Kv10–Kv12)	电压门控钾通道(Kv10~Kv12)
Vomeronasal Accessory System	犁鼻器附属系统
Vomeronasal System Evolution	犁鼻器系统的演化
Voxel Based Morphometry	基于立体像素的形态测量学

W

Walking in Invertebrates	无脊椎动物的爬行
Wallerian Degeneration	瓦利伦变性
Wilson's Disease	威尔森病（进行性豆状核变性）
Wnt Pathway and Neural Patterning	Wnt通路和神经模式
Word Learning	词语学习
Word Production	词语产生
Word Recognition	词语识别
Working Memory: Capacity Limitations	工作记忆：容量限制

Writer's Cramp	书写痉挛

Z

Zoster and Postherpetic Neuralgia	带状疱疹后神经痛

（俞洪波 译）

有　奖　征　集　反　馈　意　见

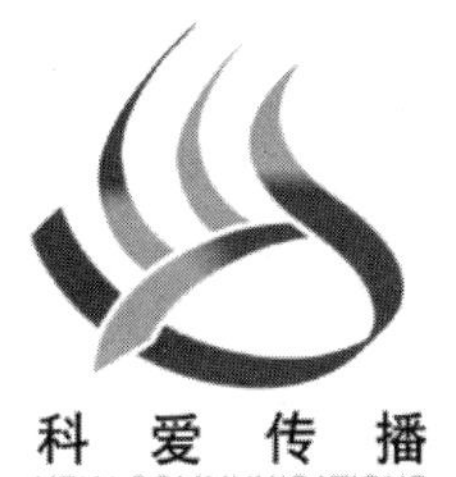

尊敬的读者：

科学出版社科爱森蓝文化传播有限公司（简称“科爱传播”）立足国际合作，致力于为科技专业人士提供优质的信息服务。我们很想通过自己的努力最大限度地满足您的需求，您的哪怕是一点点的建议和意见，都将成为我们改进工作的重要依据。

我们将在每年的 6 月份、12 月份各一次从半年的参与者中抽取幸运者 10 名，幸运者可以从“科爱传播”的出版物中任选价值 1000 元的图书（10 册以内）作为奖品（全部出版物信息可在我们的网站上查到）。

1．您所购买的图书书名：《____》

您于________年___月____日在（通过）________________________购买到此书。

你认为本书的定价：□偏高　□合适　□偏低

你认为本书的内容有约____%对您有用。

2．你认为我们出版物的质量：

内容质量（学术水平、写作水平）：□很好　□较好　□一般　□较差

译介质量（翻译水平、文字水平）：□很好　□较好　□一般　□较差

印制质量（印制、包装）：□很好　□较好　□一般　□较差

3．您所在的专业领域：________________________

4．在你获取专业知识和专业信息的主要渠道中，排在前三位的是：

1．________　2．________　3．________

A.网络　B.期刊　C.图书　D.报纸　E.电视　F.会议　G.内部交流　H.其他：________

5．你还需要哪些类型的图书？

□专著　□教材　□实验手册　□辞典工具书　□文集　□其他：________

□书摘（原版书摘编）　□刊摘（国外学术期刊重要文献摘编）

6．您还希望我们从国外引进哪些专业方向的图书（或期刊）？

7．您建议采用何种引进形式？

□翻译　□影印　□摘编（只从原书中选部分内容引进）

□导读（原文影印加少量中文介绍）　□注解（原文影印加大量中文介绍）

8．您是否愿意与我们合作，参与编写、编译、翻译图书或其他科技信息？

9．请列举您近两年看过的，您认为最有参考价值、对您帮助最大的 1~2 本书：

书名	著作者	出版社	出版日期	定价

10．您还有什么别的意见、建议？（可另附纸）

● 请告诉我们您准确的地址和联系办法：

姓名：__________ 性别：______ 生日：______年__月__日

单位：____________________职务/职称：__________

地址　：______________________________

E-mail：____________________电话：__________

传真：______________ 手机：______________

回邮地址（也可以通过 E-mail 反馈）：

北京东黄城根北街 16 号　科学出版社 科爱传播中心 杨 琴（收）　邮编：100717

联系电话：010-64006871；传真：010-64034056

编辑部电话：010-64034507

投稿及读者反馈：editor@kbooks.cn, keai@mail.sciencep.com

（注：本反馈单复印有效，也可以在线下载：http://www.kbooks.cn）